Textbook of

Laparoscopy for Surgeons and Gynecologists

Video Contents

Textbook of
Laparoscopy for Surgeons and Gynecologists

(Previously known as Textbook of Practical Laparoscopic Surgery)

Fourth Edition

RK Mishra

Director and Chief Surgeon, World Laparoscopy Hospital, Gurugram, Haryana, India
Professor and Chairperson, World Laparoscopy Training Institute, Dubai, UAE
Professor and Chairperson, World Laparoscopy Training Institute, Florida, USA
Professor and Head of Minimal Access Surgery, TGO University
First University Qualified Master Minimal Access Surgeon of India (M.MAS)
Editor-in-Chief, World Journal of Laparoscopic Surgery (WJOLS)
General Secretary, World Association of Laparoscopic Surgeons (WALS)
General Secretary, International College of Robotic Surgeons (ICRS)
Member, European Association for Endoscopic Surgery (EAES)
Member, European Association for Transluminal Surgery (EATS)
Member, Society of American Gastrointestinal and Endoscopic Surgeons (SAGES)
Member, Society of Laparoendoscopic Surgeons (SLS)
Member, Society of Robotic Surgery (SRS)
Member, Clinical Robotic Surgery Association (CRSA)
Fellow, International Medical Sciences Academy (IMSA)
Member, Indian Association of Gastrointestinal Endosurgeons (IAGES)
Member, Association of Surgeons of India (ASI)
Member, Indian Medical Association (IMA)

Foreword

Steven D Wexner

JAYPEE

JAYPEE BROTHERS MEDICAL PUBLISHERS

The Health Sciences Publisher

New Delhi | London

Jaypee Brothers Medical Publishers (P) Ltd

Headquarters
EMCA House
23/23-B, Ansari Road, Daryaganj
New Delhi 110 002, India
Landline: +91-11-23272143, +91-11-23272703
+91-11-23282021, +91-11-23245672
E-mail: jaypee@jaypeebrothers.com

Corporate Office
4838/24, Ansari Road, Daryaganj
New Delhi 110 002, India
Phone: +91-11-43574357
Fax: +91-11-43574314
E-mail: jaypee@jaypeebrothers.com

Overseas Office
J.P. Medical Ltd
83 Victoria Street, London
SW1H 0HW (UK)
Phone: +44 20 3170 8910
E-mail: info@jpmedpub.com

EU GPSR Authorised Representative
Logos Europe, 9 rue Nicolas Poussin
17000, La Rochelle, France
Phone: +33 (0) 6 67 93 73 78
E-mail: contact@logoseurope.eu

Website: www.jaypeebrothers.com
Website: www.jaypeedigital.com

Inquiries for bulk sales may be solicited at: jaypee@jaypeebrothers.com

Textbook of Laparoscopy for Surgeons and Gynecologists

First Edition: 2008

Second Edition: 2009

Third Edition: 2013

Fourth Edition: 2022

Reprint: 2026

ISBN: 978-93-90020-61-4

Printed in India

Dedicated to

My teacher Professor Sir Alfred Cuschieri

Foreword

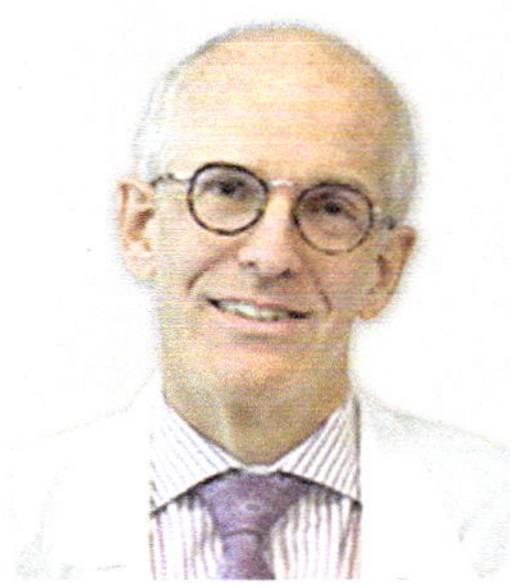

I consider it an honor to be asked by Professor RK Mishra to write the foreword to his *Textbook of Laparoscopy for Surgeons and Gynecologists (Previously known as Textbook of Practical Laparoscopic Surgery)*. Almost 30 years ago, laparoscopy was a revolutionary technology available in a few selected centers and its indications unclear at best. Currently, laparoscopy is the gold standard method of surgery for a wide range of pathology, ranging from cholecystitis and gastroesophageal reflux disease (GERD) to morbid obesity and colon cancer. At present, every gastrointestinal tract surgery is feasible laparoscopically. In most scenarios, the laparoscopic approach has been proven superior with less pain, morbidity, and cost along with shorter hospital stay. Besides, it has gained much popularity for urologic, gynecologic and other intra-abdominal diseases. The demand for education and training in laparoscopic surgery remains high, reflecting its overwhelming surgeon and patient preference. Although many textbooks have been written to help satisfy this void, a few are as easy-to-read and as informative about the gamut of laparoscopic themes. The 50 chapters allow those budding surgeons completely new to laparoscopy to rapidly understand the technical considerations related to these procedures. However, the depth and breadth of the well-illustrated volume also allows the experienced laparoscopic general, urologic, or gynecologic surgeon to become familiar with the new and exciting areas such as robotics and hepatopancreatic operations. The illustrations are all crystal clear, the cutaway enlargements very helpful, and the text explaining them is easy-to-read. The subject matter has been well researched and is written in an authoritative, although not pedantic way as could only be done by a highly experienced laparoscopic surgeon with a wonderful aptitude for sharing his knowledge. Professor RK Mishra has beautifully detailed each area ranging from the history of sterilization techniques to the physics of energy sources to practical methods of port site closure. The constant thread throughout the book is its practical nature this is not a book to be taken from the shelf on rare occasions to use as a reference prior to performing the occasional obscure operation. This book instead one to read cover-to-cover and then to share with one's residents, fellows, theater staff, and associates to ensure that each of them is fluent in the practicalities of laparoscopy. Having written a few books, I know how much work is required to produce such a well-illustrated and superbly written comprehensive textbook. It was immediately apparent to me during my reading that the textbook of practical laparoscopy was a labor of love for Professor RK Mishra and thus will become a cherished and favorite resource for all its readers, including me. I wish to congratulate him on his outstanding achievement and thank him for having allowed me to review it and to write this brief foreword.

Steven D Wexner
MD PhD (Hon) FACS FRCS (England) FRCS (Edinburgh) FRCSI (Hon) Hon FRCS (Glasgow)
Professor
Department of Surgery
Ohio State University, Columbus, OH
Chief of Staff, Cleveland Clinic Florida, Weston, FL, USA
Past President, American College of Surgeons
Past President, Society of American Gastrointestinal Endoscopic Surgeons (2006–2007)
Professor, Department of Surgery, University of Siena, Italy, Jerusalem and Israel
Clinical Professor, Department of Surgery, Division of General Surgery
University of South Florida, College of Medicine, Tampa, FL
Chief of Staff and Chairman, Medical Executive Committee
Cleveland Clinic Hospital, Cleveland, OH
Chairman, Department of Colorectal Surgery, Division of Research and Education
Research Professor of Biomedical Science
Florida Atlantic University
Boca Raton, FL, USA

Preface to the Fourth Edition

Textbook of Laparoscopy for Surgeons and Gynecologists was previously known as the *Textbook of Practical Laparoscopic Surgery*. *Textbook of Practical Laparoscopic Surgery* was well received and has become one of the best-selling books on laparoscopic surgery since its being published in 2007. This book has gained support from surgeons and gynecologists from all over the world for its rich content, concise text, and clinical practicability in operation with helpful tips and notes of laparoscopic surgery. Now this new edition of the book which is in your hand has condensed 50 chapters full of technical detail and clinical skill. To share and exchange information and skills of minimal access surgery is my primary goal in writing this book. The field of laparoscopic and robotic surgery has undergone many changes over the past three decades and minimal access surgery has seen tremendous advances during this period. These innovations in minimal access surgery have contributed to improved diagnosis, faster recovery time, smaller scars, less adhesion formation, fewer complications, lower cost, and, most importantly, better results. I have added in this edition of the book all the latest breakthroughs in 4K video technology, infrared advanced instrumentation, adhesion prevention, the latest technique of tissue extraction, and the latest robotic technology. These new chapters will certainly allow surgeons and gynecologists to routinely perform a number of procedures laparoscopically rather than by laparotomies.

As a professor of minimal access surgery, both in India and in countries around the world, I have realized that not only surgeons and gynecologists in training, but also practicing laparoscopic surgeons would benefit from an instructional book that utilized simplified illustrations to enhance their surgical knowledge. I believe that in combining the knowledge and experience of my 25 years of practice as a laparoscopic surgeon and with simplified, clear drawings and illustrations, this book will be very useful for both young and experienced laparoscopists. All the 50 chapters in this edition have been updated, and many have been rewritten to give readers the most up-to-date information. The book tackles the challenging topic of translating what is taught in the operating room into text and images. Additionally, the book addresses numerous methods to overcome challenges encountered during the laparoscopic procedure. With this book, we have combined all the procedural surgical videos which will give the complete knowledge of operative laparoscopic surgery and I am sure that after reading the book, surgeons and gynecologists will be able to perform all the common minimal access surgeries themselves on their patients.

RK Mishra

Preface to the First Edition

When I was to finish my Master's in Minimal Access Surgery from Ninewells Hospital and Medical School, UK, I was one among the few fortunate students who was called by Chancellor Sir James W Black (Nobel Prize Winner in Medicine 1988) for special meeting. Sir Black advised us to start training of minimal access surgery after completing our degree. He realized the great lack of university trained well-qualified personnel who could propagate art and science of minimal access surgery to the medical fraternity. Sir Black emphasized that training of minimal access surgery is going into the profit-making hands of the industry; and as a qualified minimal access surgeon, this is our duty to disseminate the knowledge of our skill to the entire specialty who wants to use this surgical proficiency. Keeping in mind this instruction of my Chancellor, I started teaching laparoscopy to surgeon gynecologists, urologists and pediatric surgeons all over the world. This book is based on seven years of my teaching experience in minimal access surgery. Within seven years, I have trained more than 1,500 surgeons and gynecologists from every corner of the world.

In recent years progress in medical care has been rapid especially in areas of laparoscopic robotic and natural orifice transluminal endoscopic surgery (NOTES). The major reason of this progress has been the interdisciplinary approach of merging technology with medicine. However, there are limited good books available which are self-sufficient and yet easy to understand. This book has been written to fill this gap. It has grown out of numerous discussions during various educational training programs. The participants have included gynecologists, urologists, and general surgeons from fresh doctors to senior surgeons.

The book is primarily intended for the reader who has some background of conventional operative surgical and gynecological procedures. It is broad in its scope and depth, wherever needed, is provided without being unnecessarily sophisticated. There are plenty of illustrations and diagrams to facilitate faster learning.

The essential section of the book includes the concept of ergonomics, task analysis and practical problems encountered in attempting to venture into laparoscopic operative surgery. An overall view of the latest instruments is presented and detailed explanations in appropriate sections are penned down. The medical terminology is deliberately introductory to facilitate easy understanding. Enough fundamentals are presented within the context of this book to make it reasonably self-sufficient. In fewer than 200 pages, this book guides you through the process of developing a foundation of laparoscopic surgery like developing skill of dissection, suturing, knotting and tissue approximation.

The second section of the book describes comprehensive laparoscopic operative procedure demonstrating a method that is tested, proven, and based upon sound instructional theory. The procedures are written according to systemic task analysis and students are advised to see the DVDs provided with this book. The latter chapters are devoted to special topics of recent advances in minimal access surgery to give the reader a true overall view of the field.

Although I have taken every care to make this book error free, nonetheless mistakes may have been overlooked. I will be grateful for any constructive criticism.

RK Mishra

Acknowledgments

I would like to express my gratitude to all those who gave me the inspiration to write this book. I want to thank my colleagues at surgical skill unit, Ninewells Hospital and Medical School, UK. I express my gratitude to all my fellow doctors and students whose constructive criticism in words of encouragement motivated me to accomplish this work.

I am very grateful to Mr AM Sinha, Department of Biotechnology, All India Institute of Medical Sciences (AIIMS), New Delhi, India whose infectious enthusiasm, innovative ideas, valuable suggestions and proofreading is largely responsible to give the book the present form.

I take this opportunity to thank my junior Dr Rahul Pandey for his hard work and dedication towards this book. His suggestions and ideas were very useful in major chapters of this book. I would like to thank him for efficient proofreading and working out the figures and illustrations in the book.

I would like to thank Shri Jitendar P Vij (Group Chairman), Mr Ankit Vij (Managing Director), Mr MS Mani (Group President), Ms Chetna Malhotra Vohra (Associate Director–Content Strategy), and Ms Pooja Bhandari (Production Head), M/s Jaypee Brothers Medical Publishers (P) Ltd, New Delhi, India. I am really impressed by the efficient publication team, especially Mr Ashwani Kumar (Quality Controller) and Mr Chandra Dutt (DTP Operator). I am grateful to them for their patience and unconditional support.

This work would not have been possible without the unconditional love and support from my family members. I thank my parents Late Dr RP Mishra and Mrs Shanti Mishra. I would like to give my special thanks to my wife Mrs Sadhna Mishra and children Drs Nidhi Mishra, Rishi Mishra, and Ashish Mishra whose patience and love enable to complete this work.

Contents

SECTION 1 ♦ Essentials of Laparoscopy

SECTION 2 ♦ Laparoscopic General Surgical Procedures

SECTION 3 ♦ Laparoscopic Gynecological Procedures

SECTION 4 ♦ Laparoscopic Urology

SECTION 5 ♦ Pediatric Laparoscopy

SECTION 6 ♦ Miscellaneous

SECTION 1

Essentials of Laparoscopy

CHAPTER 1

Chronological Advances in Minimal Access Surgery

INTRODUCTION

Laparoscopy, also known as minimally invasive surgery (MIS) or minimal access surgery, is a revolutionary procedure that has benefitted both the patients and the doctors. The earliest recorded references to endoscopy date to ancient times with Hippocrates. In his description, there is explanation of rectum examination with a speculum. Hippocrates advised injecting a large quantity of air into the intestines through the anus in intestinal obstruction. He advocated the insertion of suppository that was 10 digits long. These descriptions suggest that Hippocrates was well aware of ileus with intestinal obstruction and thought that there were several possible etiologies, including fecal impaction, intussusceptions, and sigmoid volvulus. Moreover, Hippocrates treated these life-threatening conditions with minimally invasive approaches.

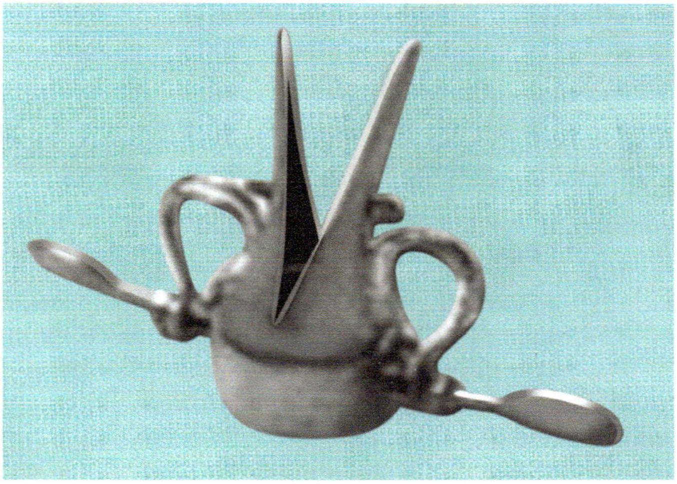

Fig. 1: Lichtleiter endoscope.

1585: Aranzi was the first to use a light source for an endoscopic procedure, focusing sunlight through a flask of water and projecting the light into the nasal cavity.

1706: The term "trocar" was coined in 1706 and is thought to be derived from "trochartor" trois-quarts, a three-faced instrument consisting of a perforator enclosed in a metal cannula.

1806: Philipp Bozzini built an instrument that could be introduced in the human body to visualize the internal organs. He called this instrument "Lichtleiter". Bozzini used an aluminum tube to visualize the genitourinary tract. The tube, illuminated by a wax candle, had fitted mirrors to reflect images **(Fig. 1)**.

1853: Antonin Jean Desormeaux, a French surgeon, first introduced the "Lichtleiter" of Bozzini to a patient. For many surgeons, he is considered as the "Father of Endoscopy".

1867: Desormeaux used an open tube to examine the genitourinary tract, combining alcohol and turpentine with a flame in order to generate a brighter, more condensable beam of light.

1868: Kussmaul performed the first esophagogastroscopy on a professional sword swallower, initiating efforts at instrumentation of the gastrointestinal tract. Mikulicz and Schindler, however, are credited with the advancement of gastroscopy.

1869: Commander Pantaleoni used a modified cystoscope to cauterize a hemorrhagic uterine growth. Pantaleoni thus performed the first diagnostic and therapeutic hysteroscopy.

1901: Dimitri Ott, a Petrograd gynecologist, used head mirrors to reflect light and augment visualization and used access technique in which a speculum was introduced through an incision in the prior vaginal fornix in a pregnant woman.

1901: The first experimental laparoscopy was performed in Berlin in 1901 by the German surgeon, Georg Kelling, who used a cystoscope to peer into the abdomen of a dog after first insufflating it with air. Kelling also used filtered atmospheric air to create a pneumoperitoneum, with the goal of stopping intra-abdominal bleeding (ectopic pregnancy, bleeding ulcers, and pancreatitis), but these studies did not find any response or supporters **(Fig. 2)**.

Kelling proposed a high-pressure insufflation of the abdominal cavity, a technique he called the "luft tamponade" or "air tamponade".

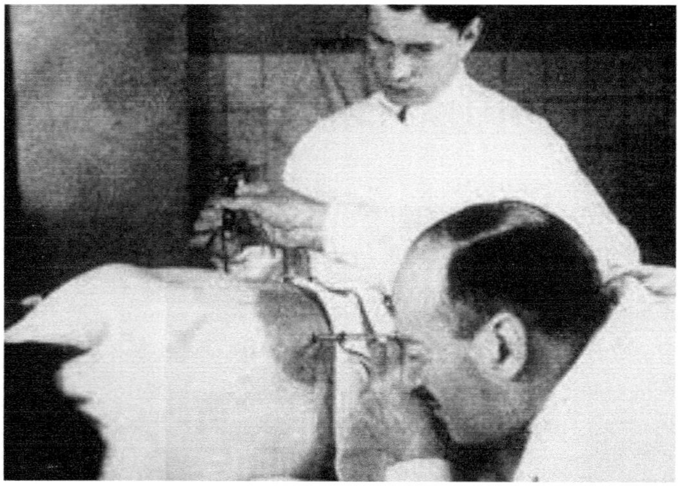

Fig. 2: Kelling performing laparoscopy in dog.

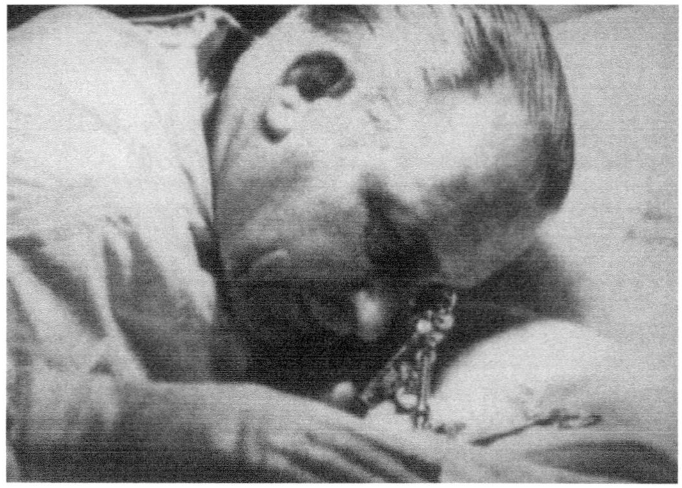

Fig. 3: Heinz Kalk.

1910: HC Jacobaeus of Stockholm published a paper on discussion of the inspection of the peritoneal, pleural, and pericardial cavity.

1911: Bertram M Bernheim of Johns Hopkins Hospital introduced first laparoscopic surgery to the United States. He named it the procedure of minimal access surgery as "organoscopy". The instrument used was a proctoscope of a half inch diameter and ordinary light for illumination was used.

1911: HC Jacobaeus coined the term "laparothorakoskopie" after using this procedure on the thorax and abdomen. He used to introduce the trocar inside the body cavity directly without employing a pneumoperitoneum.

1918: O Goetze developed an automatic pneumoperitoneum needle characterized for its safe introduction to the peritoneal cavity.

The next decade and a half witnessed a decline in technological advancement in endoscopy due to World War I.

1920: Zollikofer of Switzerland discovered the benefit of carbon dioxide (CO_2) gas to use for insufflation rather than filtered atmospheric air or nitrogen.

1929: Kalk, a German physician, introduced the forward oblique (135°) view lens systems. He advocated the use of a separate puncture site for pneumoperitoneum. Goetze of Germany first developed a needle for insufflation.

1929: Heinz Kalk, a German gastroenterologist, developed a 135° lens system and a dual trocar approach. He used laparoscopy as a diagnostic method for liver and gallbladder diseases **(Fig. 3)**.

1934: John C Ruddock, an American surgeon, described laparoscopy as a good diagnostic method, many times, superior than laparotomy. He used the instrument for diagnostic laparoscopy which consisted of built-in forceps with electrocoagulation capacity **(Fig. 4)**.

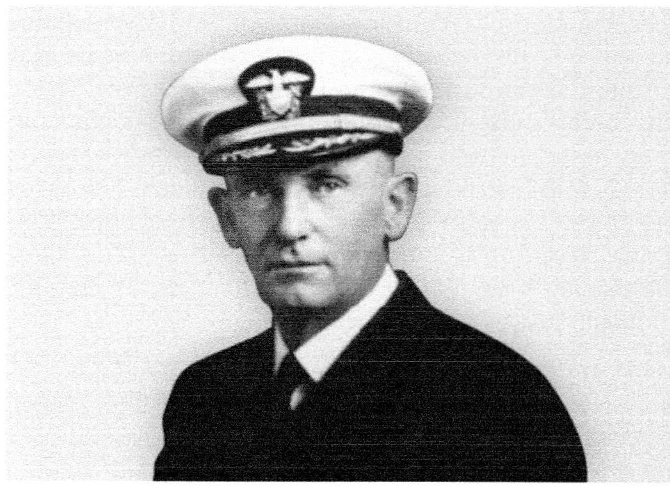

Fig. 4: John C Ruddock.

1936: Boesch of Switzerland is credited with the first laparoscopic tubal sterilization.

1938: Janos Veress of Hungary developed an especially designed spring-loaded needle. Interestingly, he did not promote the use of his Veress needle for laparoscopy purposes. He used Veress needle for the induction of pneumothorax. Veress needle is widely used instrument today to create pneumoperitoneum **(Fig. 5)**.

1939: Richard W Te Linde tried to perform an endoscopic procedure by a culdoscopic approach in the lithotomy position. This method was rapidly abandoned because of the presence of small intestine.

1939: Heinz Kalk published his experience of over 2,000 liver biopsies performed using local anesthesia without mortality.

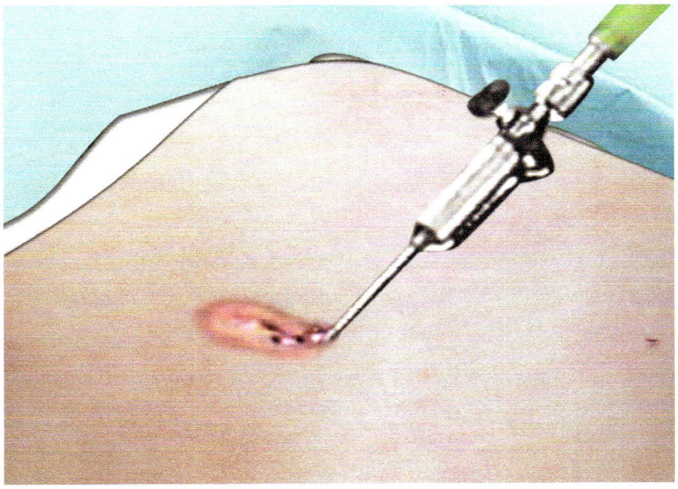

Fig. 5: Veress needle.

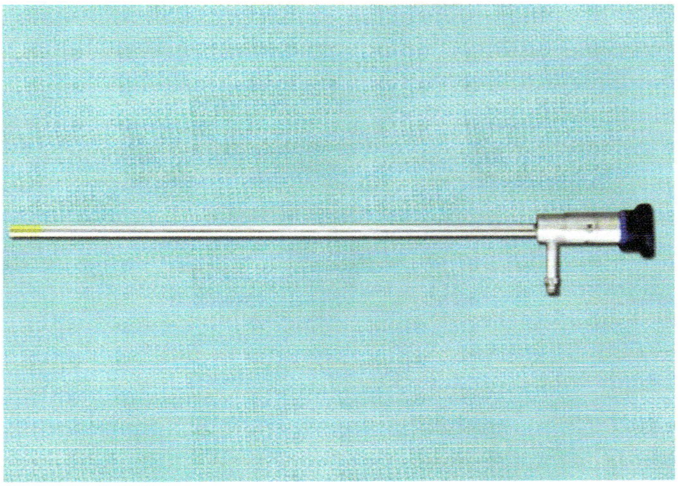

Fig. 6: Laparoscope.

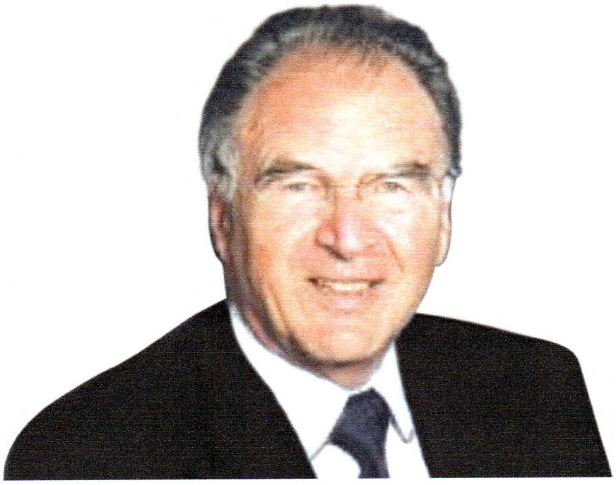

Fig. 7: Kurt Semm.

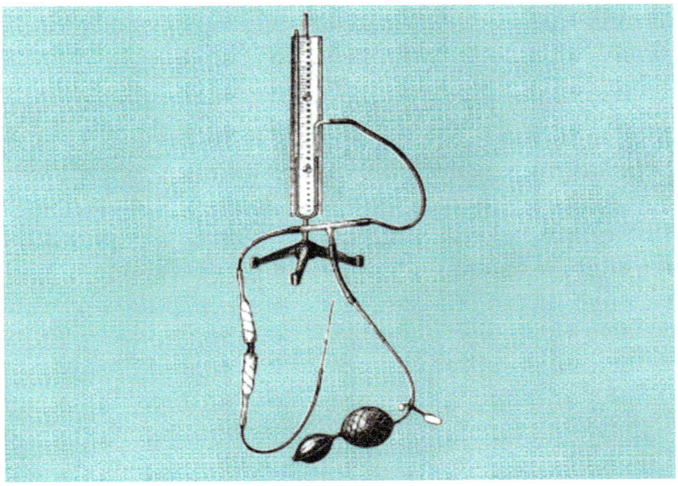

Fig. 8: First insufflator made by Professor Semm.

1944: Raoul Palmer of Paris performed gynecological examinations using laparoscopy **(Fig. 6)** and placing the patients in the Trendelenburg position, so air could fill the pelvis. He also stressed the importance of continuous intra-abdominal pressure monitoring during a laparoscopic procedure.

1953: The rigid rod lens system was discovered by Professor Hopkins. The credit of videoscopic surgery goes to this surgeon who had revolutionized the concept by making this instrument.

1960: Kurt Semm was a German gynecologist, who invented the automatic insufflator **(Fig. 7)**. His experience with this new device was published in 1966. Apart from insufflator, he also perfected many technical refinements including suction irrigator, safer electrocoagulation instruments, intracorporeal and extracorporeal knot tying, and an electrical morcellator for myomas. Though not recognized in his own country, but on the other side of the Atlantic, both American physicians and instrument makers valued the Semm's insufflator for its simple application, clinical value, and safety **(Fig. 8)**.

1960: Patrick Steptoe, a British gynecologist, adapted the techniques of sterilization by two puncture technique.

1972: H Courtenay Clarke showed laparoscopic suturing technique for hemostasis.

1973: Gaylord D Alexander developed techniques of safe local and general anesthesia suitable for laparoscopy.

1977: First laparoscopic-assisted appendicectomy was performed by Dekok. Appendix was exteriorized and ligated outside the abdominal cavity.

1977: Kurt Semm demonstrated endoloop suturing technique in laparoscopic surgery.

1978: Hasson introduced an alternative method of blunt trocar placement. He proposed a blunt minilaparotomy which permits direct visualization of trocar entrance into the peritoneal cavity.

Hasson cannula was a reusable device of similar design to a standard cannula, but attached to an olive-shaped sleeve was developed. This sleeve would slide up and down over the shaft of the cannula and form an airtight seal at the fascial opening. In addition, the sharp trocar was replaced by a blunt obturator. This cannula is held in place by the use of stay sutures passed through the fascial edges and attached to the body of the cannula **(Fig. 9)**.

1980: Patrick Steptoe started to perform laparoscopic procedures first time in UK.

1983: Kurt Semm, a German gynecologist, performed the first laparoscopic appendicectomy. After this surgery, Kurt Semm faced a lot of criticism and censor rather than accolades. The German Board of Surgery condemned him.

1985: The first documented laparoscopic cholecystectomy was performed by Erich Mühe in Germany in 1985. The German surgeon Erich Mühe used his "galloscope", a 3-cm, direct-vision laparoscope of his own design to remove a gallbladder. He presented his work at the 1986, Congress of the German Surgical Society. He, too, suffered skepticism and criticism and was ultimately censored by the courts.

1987: Philippe Mouret has got the credit to perform the first laparoscopic cholecystectomy in Lyons, France using video technique **(Fig. 10)**. Cholecystectomy is the laparoscopic procedure which revolutionized the general surgery. Like Mühe and Semm, Mouret was also strongly criticized. François Dubois, another Frenchman, was the second surgeon to perform videolaparoscopic cholecystectomy in 1988 and was the first to publish his early experience.

1987: Ger reported first laparoscopic repair of inguinal hernia using prototype stapler.

1988: Harry Reich performed laparoscopic lymphadenectomy for treatment of ovarian cancer.

1988: McKernan and Sye performed first cholecystectomy in the USA **(Fig. 11)**.

1989: Harry Reich described first laparoscopic hysterectomy using bipolar desiccation; later, he demonstrated staples and finally sutures for laparoscopic hysterectomy.

1989: Reddick and Olsen reported that common bile duct (CBD) injury after laparoscopic cholecystectomy is five times than with conventional cholecystectomy. As a result of this report, USA government announced that surgeons should perform at least 15 laparoscopic cholecystectomy under supervision before being allowed to do this procedure on their own.

1990: Bailey and Zucker in USA popularized laparoscopic anterior highly selective vagotomy combined with posterior truncal vagotomy. Over the next few years, virtually every abdominal operation was performed and perfected by laparoscopic technique. Laparoscopic splenectomy was performed by Makoto Hashizume, Ed Phillips, Joseph Petelin and John Flowers, and adrenalectomy by Petelin and Gagner.

1994: First robotic arm was designed to hold the telescope with the goal of improving safety and reducing the need of skilled camera operator **(Fig. 12)**.

1996: First live telecast of laparoscopic surgery performed remotely via the internet (robotic telesurgery).

1997: Fully laparoscopic aortofemoral bypass was being performed, led by Dion and Gracia.

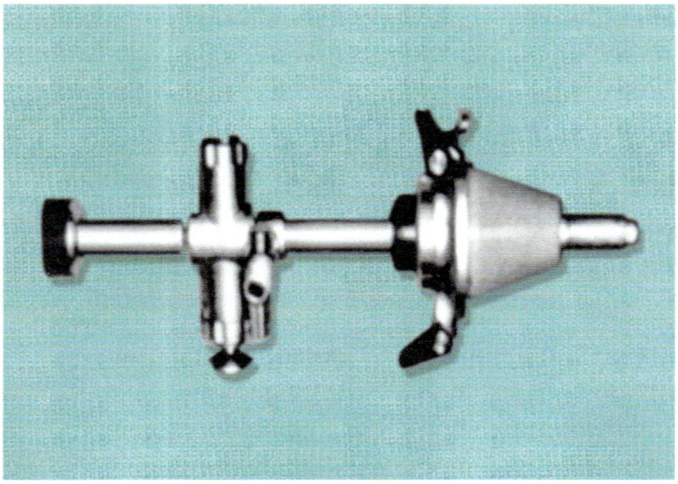

Fig. 9: Hasson cannula.

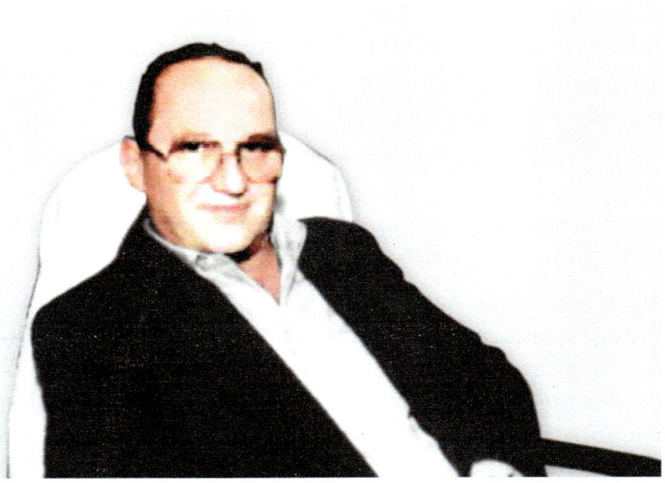

Fig. 10: Philippe Mouret.

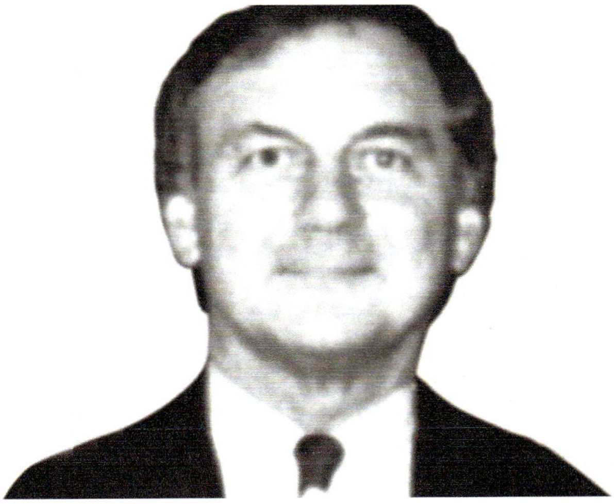

Fig. 11: William Sye.

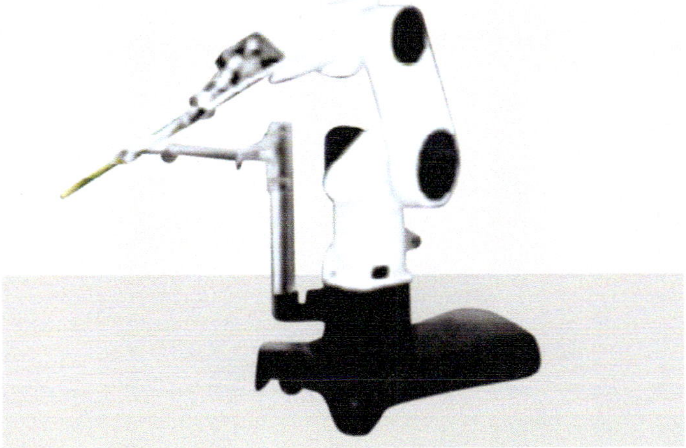

Fig. 12: Robotic arm.

2000: The US Food and Drug Administration (FDA) first time approved the da Vinci Surgical System, making it the first robotic system allowed to be used in American operating rooms.

2001: The Lindbergh operation, named in honor of American aviator Charles Lindbergh, was the first ever transatlantic surgery. Doctors Michel Gagner and Jacques Marescaux removed the gallbladder of a 68-year-old woman in Strasbourg, France from New York. The surgeons used a ZEUS Robotic Surgical System from Computer Motion, Inc., and an ATM fiberoptic connection provided by France Telecom.

2004: Robotic prostatectomy became the first most commonly performed robotic surgery. According to Intuitive Surgical, Inc., the California-based manufacturers of the da Vinci Robot, the number of robotic prostatectomies rose from 36 in 2000 to 8,000 in 2004.

2005: Combining robotically-assisted coronary artery bypass surgery (CABG) with stented angioplasty shows promise for treating extensive coronary artery disease, researchers reported at the American Heart Association Scientific Sessions 2005, Dallas.

The evolution of minimal access therapy aims to minimize the traumatic insult to the patient without compromising the safety and efficacy of the treatment compared with traditional open surgery. If this is achieved, patients recover more quickly, which reduces hospital stay and allows more rapid return to full activity and work within minimum time. This year of 2005 was also known as start of first single-incision laparoscopic surgery (SILS). The evolution of MIS has led to the development of laparoendoscopic single-site surgery (LESS) or SILS. SILS was first performed for the treatment of appendicitis at the Department of Pediatric Surgery, Dokuz Eylul Medical School, Izmir, Turkey.

Recently, SILS and robotic surgery have penetrated all specialties of abdominal surgery. However, evidence-based medicine has failed to show major advantages in SILS and the disadvantage of robotic surgery is the high costs related to purchase and maintenance of technology.

2014: Leonard et al. provided a proof-of-concept Smart Tissue Anastomosis Robot (STAR) which was a vision-guided robotic system for laparoscopic suturing. STARs architecture and interface allowed surgeons to manually select and track incisions and the placement of stitches or automatically performed equally spaced stitches based on the contour of the incision.

2014: The FDA has announced a series of actions aimed at limiting the use of power morcellators in gynecologic surgeries in April 2014. Recommendations are that morcellator should only be used in certain laparoscopic procedures and that they always be used with equipment designed to contain the spread of any minced-up tissue.

2017: Prior to February 2017, laparoscopic cholecystectomy was performed without routine intraoperative imaging of the biliary tree. Beginning February 2017, laparoscopic cholecystectomy was performed with indocyanine green (ICG). 0.5 mL of ICG was given via intravenous infusion 45 minutes prior to surgery. Fluorescence imaging was performed using the PINPOINT endoscopic fluorescence imaging system (Novadaq, Canada). The triangle of Calot was exposed to display the biliary tree. This is followed by dissection of the triangle of Calot to expose the cystic duct and artery. The cystic artery can be independently visualized a few minutes following ICG injection. Hereafter, both structures are safely clipped and divided.

2020: TransEnterix received the FDA clearance to add an artificial intelligence feature to its Senhance Surgical Robotic System **(Fig. 13)**. The new Intelligent Surgical Unit on the

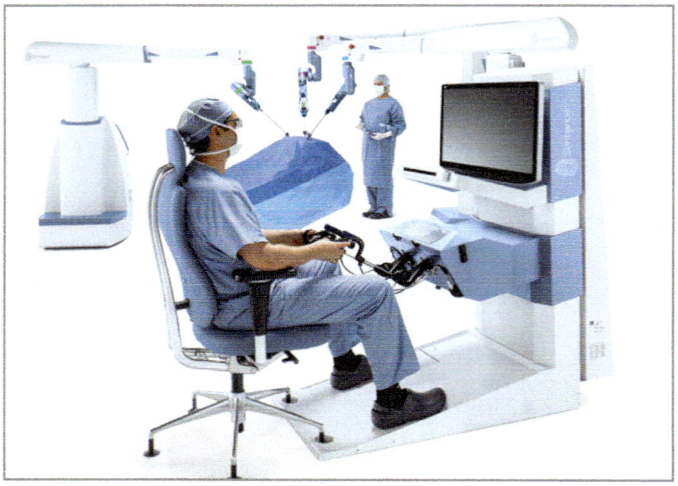

Fig. 13: Senhance Surgical Robotic System.

system enables the camera to automatically move for a surgeon during a procedure, responding to commands, and recognizing certain objects and locations in the surgical field.

BIBLIOGRAPHY

1. Bernheim BM. Organoscopy: cystoscopy of the abdominal cavity. Ann Surg. 1911;53:764-7.
2. Bozzini P. Lichtleiter, eine Erfindung zur Anschau-ung innerer Theile und Krankheiten. J Prakt Arzneikunde. 1806;24:107-13.
3. Desormeaux AJ. The Endoscope, and its Application to the Diagnosis and Treatment of Affections of the Genito-urinary Passages: Lessons Given at Necker Hospital. Chicago: Robert Fergus' Sons Printers; 1867.
4. Fervers C. Die Laparoskopie mit dem Cystoskop. Mediz Klinik. 1933;31:1042-5.
5. Fourestier M, Gladu A, Vulmiere J. Perfection nements al' endoscopie medicale. Realisation bronchoscopique. La Presse Medicale. 1952;60:1292-3.
6. Goetze O. Die Röntgendiagnostik bei gasgefüllten Bauchhöhle. Eine neue Methode. Münch Med Wochenschr. 1918;65:1275-80.
7. Gordon AG, Magos AL. The development of laparoscopic surgery. Baillieres Clin Obstet Gynaecol. 1989;3:429-49.
8. Gow JG, Hopkins HH, Wallace DM. The modern urological endoscope. In: Hopkins HH (Ed). Handbook of Urological Endoscopy. Edinburgh: Churchill Livingstone; 1978.
9. Gunning JE. The history of laparoscopy. J Reprod Med. 1974;12:222-5.
10. Jacobeus HC. Ueberdie Möglichkeitdie Zystoskopiebei Untersuchungseröser Höhlungenanzuwenden. Münch Med Wochenschr. 1910;57:2090-2.
11. Jacobs M, Verdeja JC, Goldstein HS. Minimally invasive colon resection (laparoscopic colectomy). Surg Laparosc Endosc. 1991;1:133-50.
12. Kalk H. Erfahrungenmitder Laparoskopie (Zugleichmit Beschreibunge inesneuen Instrumentes). Zeitschr Klin Med. 1929;111:303-48.
13. Kelling G. Ueber Oesophagoskopie, Gastroskopieund Kölioskopie. Münch Med Wochenschr. 1902;49:21-4.
14. Kurze W. Uebersichtübermeine Erfahrungenmitder Laparo-thoraskopie. Münch Med Wochenschr. 1911;58:2017-9.
15. Lau WY, Leow CK, Li AK. History of endoscopic and laparoscopic surgery. World J Surg. 1997;21:444-53.
16. Mühe B. The first laparoscopic cholecystectomy. Langenbecks Arch Chir. 1986;369:804.
17. Nadeau OE, Kampmeier OF. Endoscopy of the abdomen: abdominoscopy. Surg Gynecol Obstet. 1925;41:259-71.
18. Nitze M. Beobachtungs- und Untersuchungsmethodefür Harnröhre, Harnblase and Rektum. Wiener Mediz Wochenschr. 1879;29:651-2.
19. Orndorff BH. The peritoneoscope in diagnosis of diseases of the abdomen. J Radiol. 1920;1:307-25.
20. Roccavilla A. L'endoscopia delle grandi cavita sierose mediante un nuovo apparecchio ad illuminazione dirtta (laparo-toracoscopia diretta). La Riforma Medica. 1914;30:991-5.
21. Rosin D. History. In: Rosin D (Ed). Minimal Access Medicine and Surgery. Oxford: Radcliffe Medical Press; 1993.
22. Ruddock JC. Peritoneoscopy. Surg Gynecol Obstet. 1937; 65:623-39.
23. Semm K. Endoscopic appendectomy. Endoscopy. 1983;15:59-64.
24. Semm K. Operative Manual for Endoscopic Abdominal Surgery. Chicago: Thieme Medical Publishers; 1987.
25. Semm K. The history of endoscopy. In: Vitale GC, Sanfilippo JS, Perissat J (Eds). Laparoscopic Surgery: An Atlas for General Surgeons. Philadelphia: Lippincott Williams and Wilkins; 1995.
26. Short AR. The uses of coelioscopy. Br Med J. 1925;3:254-5.
27. Steiner OP. Abdominoscopy. Surg Gynecol Obstet. 1924; 38:266-9.
28. Stone WE. Intra-abdominal examination by the aid of the peritoneoscope. J Kan Med Soc. 1924;24:63-6.
29. Veress J. Neues Instrument zur Ausführung von Brust-oder Bauchpunktionen and Pneumothoraxbehandlung. Deutsch Med Wochenschr. 1938;40:1480-1.
30. Vitale GC, Cuschieri A, Perissat J. Guidelines for the future. In: Vitale GC, Sanfilippo JS, Perissat J (Eds). Laparoscopic Surgery: An Atlas for General Surgeons. Philadelphia: Lippincott Williams and Wilkins; 1995.
31. Zollikofer R. Zur Laparoskopie. Schweiz Med Wochenschr. 1924;5:264-5.

CHAPTER 2 Laparoscopic Imaging Systems

INTRODUCTION

It is well-known that laparoscopy is the consequence of advances made in the field of medical engineering. Each surgical specialty has different requirement of instruments. Laparoscopy was initially criticized owing to the cost of specialized instruments and possible complications due to these sharp long instruments. Also, it necessitated difficult hand-eye coordination. Gradually, the technique gained recognition and respect from the medical fraternity since it drastically reduced many of the complications of the open procedure. Minimal access surgery (MAS) has developed rapidly only after grand success of laparoscopic cholecystectomy. Computer-aided designing of laparoscopic instruments is an important branch of medical engineering. It is now possible to control the access through microprocessor controlled laparoscopic instruments. New procedures and instruments are innovated regularly which make it important for the surgeon to be familiar with the developments. Laparoscopy is a technologically-dependent surgery and it is expected that every surgeon should have reasonably good knowledge of these instruments.

LAPAROSCOPIC TROLLEY

The mobile laparoscopic video cart is equipped with locking brakes and has four antistatic rollers. The trolley has a drawer and three shelves **(Fig. 1)**.

The upper shelves have a tilt adjustment and used for supporting the video monitor unit. Included on the trolley is an electrical supply terminal strip, mounted on the rear of the second shelf (from the top). Recently, *ceiling mounted trolleys* are launched by many companies which are ergonomically better and consume less space in operation theater.

IMAGING SYSTEMS

- Light source
- Light cable
- Telescope
- Laparoscopic camera
- Laparoscopic video monitor

The imaging system is a chain of equipment that is link together in place perfectly and functioning well to produce an excellent laparoscopic image. The break in this sequential pass of links of the chain will be rendered our imaging system impotent.

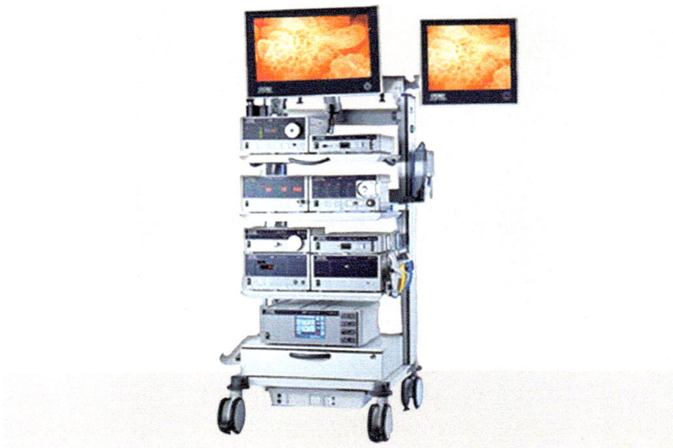

Fig. 1: Laparoscopic trolley.

The classic imaging chain starts with a *light source* and ends in the monitor, requiring seven pieces of equipment, known as the *magnificent seven—light source, fiberoptic light cable, laparoscope, camera head, video signal processor, video cable, and monitor* **(Fig. 2)**. This imaging chain is often supported by a cast of VCRs, photo printers, or digital capture devices. The surgeon and the operating room team must work together to ensure optimal equipment function through careful handling of the equipment in the operating room and during the sterilization process. Yet, when the image is poor, many operating teams become paralyzed, unable to function without the aid of a medical engineer—"understanding can overcome any situation, however, mysterious or insurmountable, it may appear to be". Accordingly, understanding the (imaging) video system will allow the operating surgeon to do the basic troubleshooting for his or her system and not be totally dependent on nursing or technical staff, especially at night when experienced personnel may not be available. The advent of integrated operating suites has not changed the principles of this basic idea.

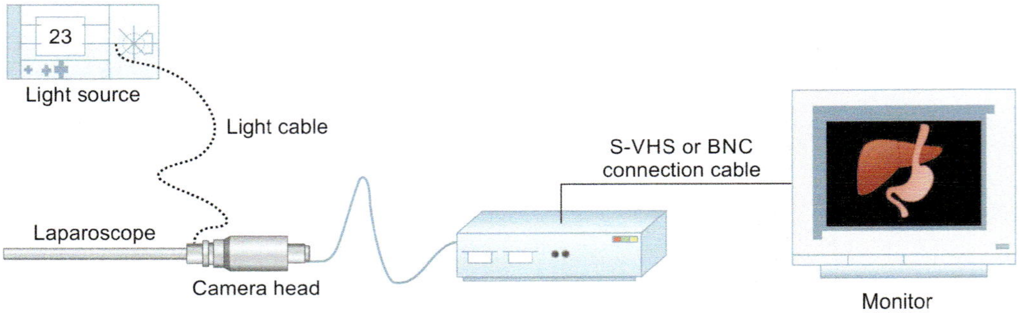

Fig. 2: The magnificent seven of the basic imaging chain.

Light Source

It is clear and easy to say that life, recently, is impossible without light and simply no light, no laparoscopy. The light source is the often-overlooked soldier of the video laparoscopic system.

High-intensity light is created with bulbs of halogen gas, xenon gas, or mercury vapor. The bulbs are available in different wattages "150 W and 300 W" and should be chosen based on the type of procedure being performed. Because light is absorbed by blood, any procedure in which bleeding is encountered may require more light. We use the stronger light sources for all advanced laparoscopy. Availability of light is a challenge in many bariatric procedures where the abdominal cavity is large.

A *good laparoscopic light source* should emit light as much as possible *near the natural sunlight.*

Three types of light source are in use today:

1. Halogen light source
2. Xenon light source
3. Metal halide light source.

The output from the light sources is conducted to the telescope by *light cables* that contain either glass fiber bundles or special fluid.

The halogen light source is used in the medical field since last 20 years, but the spectral temperature of these lights is 3,200 K which makes it too different and too low from natural sunlight. The midday sunlight has approximately 5,600 K color temperature. In practice, the yellow light of the halogen bulb is compensated in the video camera system by white balancing.

A more suitable light source for laparoscopic cameras involves the creation of an electrical arc in a metal halide system or in xenon. This electrical arc is produced in same way as in flash of photographic camera.

Xenon has a more natural color spectrum and a smaller spot size than halogen. The xenon light source emits a spectral temperature of color of approximately 6,000 K on average for a power of 300 W **(Fig. 3)**.

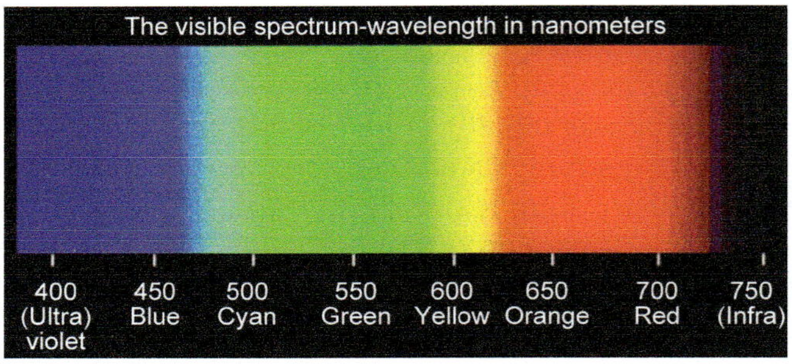

Fig. 3: Spectrum of light.

Arc generated lamps have a spectral temperature that gradually decreases with use and white balance is required before each use. The bulb needs replacing after 250–500 hours of usage, depending on the type of lamp.

One of the main advantages of the laparoscopy is that of obtaining a virtually microsurgical view compared to that obtained by laparotomy. Quality of the image obtained very much depends on the quantity of light available at each step of optical and electronic system.

The interface of the laparoscopic team works with a standard light source.

It is essential for the laparoscopic team, particularly the surgeons, to know about all the switch and function of the light source. All essential details of the equipment and all the action required on the part can be found on the operating manual of the product.

Many light sources record and display the hours of service and alert the biomedical or medical engineer (or the well-informed surgeon) when it is time to make a change. When the lifetime rating of the bulb has been exceeded, the subsequent performance of the light source becomes unpredictable, often slowly dwindling until the surgeon just cannot produce a well-lit scene, despite the fact that a bright light seems to emanate from the laparoscope **(Fig. 4)**.

A typical light source consists of:

- A lamp (bulb)
- A heat filter
- A condensing lens
- Manual or automatic intensity control circuit (shutter).

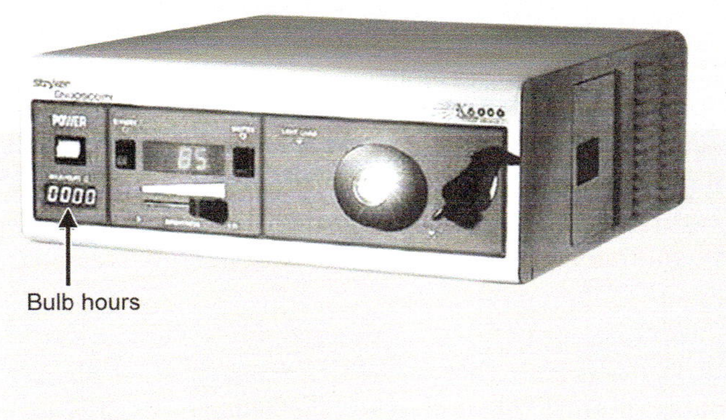

Fig. 4: Xenon light source: Bulb-life display is shown.

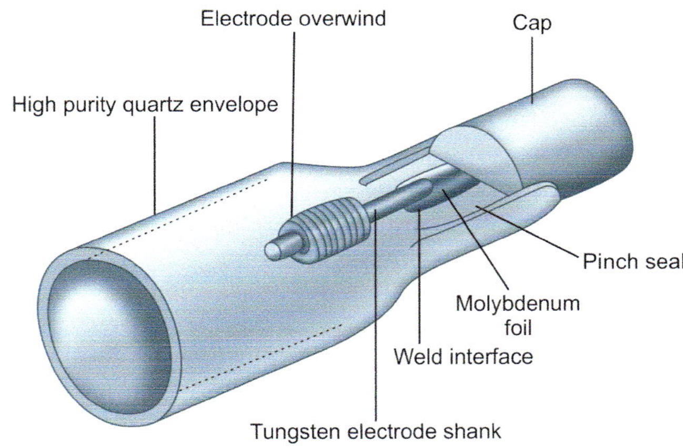

Fig. 5: New generation light source bulb.

Lamp (Bulb)

Lamp or bulb is the most important part of the light source. When the bulb fails, the entire system is out of commission until either the bulb is replaced or a new light is brought to bear.

The quality of light depends on the lamp used. Several modern types of light sources are currently available **(Fig. 5)**. These light sources mainly differ on the type of bulb used.

Three types of lamp are used more recently:
1. Quartz halogen incandescent lamp
2. Xenon lamp
3. Metal halide vapor arc lamp

Halogen bulbs (150 W) or tungsten-halogen bulb: It is an incandescent lamp with a transparent quartz bulb and a compressed gas filling that includes a halogen. Quartz is used instead of glass to permit higher temperatures, higher currents, and therefore greater light output. The lamp gives brilliant light. The halogen combines with the tungsten evaporated from the hot filament to form a compound that is attracted back to the filament, thus extending the filament's life. The halogen gas also prevents the evaporated tungsten from condensing on the bulb and darkening it, an effect that reduces the light output of ordinary incandescent lamps.

First used in the late 1960s in motion-picture production, halogen lamps are now also used in automobile headlights, underwater photography, and residential lighting.

Incandescent (to begin to glow): It is so hot to the point of glowing or emitting intense light rays, as an incandescent light bulb.

Quartz, one of the most common of all rock-forming minerals and one of the most important constituents of the earth's crust. Chemically, it is *silicon dioxide (SiO_2)*. It occurs in crystals of the hexagonal system, commonly having the form of a six-sided prism terminating in a six-sided pyramid; the crystals are often distorted and twins are common. Quartz may be transparent, translucent, or opaque; it may be colorless or colored.

The halogen lamp takes its name from the halogens included in the gas within its tungsten-filament bulb, added to prolong filament life and increase brightness.

Halogen: Any of the elements of the halogen family, consisting of fluorine, chlorine, bromine, iodine, and astatine. They are all monovalent and readily form negative ions.

Halogen bulbs provide highly efficient crisp white light source with excellent color rendering. Electrodes in halogen lamps are made of tungsten filament. This is the only metal with a sufficiently high melting temperature and sufficient vapor pressure at elevated temperatures. They use a halogen gas that allows bulbs to burn (light) more intensely. Halogen bulbs use low voltages and have an average life of 2,000 hours. The color temperature of halogen lamp is around 5,000–5,600 K. These lamps are economical and can be used for laparoscopic surgery if low budget setup is required.

Xenon lamps (300 W):

Xenon (symbol Xe): A colorless, odorless, and highly unreactive gaseous nonmetallic element found in minute quantities in the atmosphere and extracted commercially from liquefied air. Atomic number is 54. The radioactive isotope ^{133}Xe, having a half-life of 5.3 days, is used for diagnostic imaging in assessment of pulmonary function, lung imaging, and cerebral blood flow studies.

Xenon lamps consist of a spherical or ellipsoidal envelope made of quartz glass, which can withstand high thermal loads and high internal pressure. For ultimate image quality, only the highest-grade clear fused silica quartz is used. It is typically doped, although not visible to the human eye, to absorb harmful ultraviolet (UV) radiation generated during operation. The color temperature of xenon lamp is about 6,000–6,400 K. The operating pressures are tens of atmospheres at times, with surface temperatures exceeding 600°C.

The smaller, pointed electrode is called the cathode, which supplies the current to the lamp and facilitates the emission of electrons. To supply a sufficient amount of electrons, the cathode material is doped with thorium. The optimum operating temperature of the cathode tip is approximately 2,000°C. To obtain this precise operating temperature, the cathode tip is pointed and in many cases, it has a groove on the pointed tip to act as a heat choke. This heat choke causes the tip to run at a higher temperature. This configuration of the cathode tip allows for a very high concentration of light from the cathode tip and a very stable arc.

The anode, the larger electrode, receives electrons emitted by the cathode. Once the electrons penetrate the anode face, the resulting energy is converted to heat, most of which radiates away. The large, cylindrical shape of the anode helps to keep the temperature low by radiating the heat from the anode surface.

The advantage of xenon bulb is that it used two electrodes (cathode and anode) and there is no filament as in halogen bulb, so it has somewhat a fixed lifetime with an average of 1,500 hours.

The two most frequently used types of lamps are halogen and xenon. The main difference between them is in the colors obtained. The xenon lamp has a slightly bluish tint. The light emitted by xenon lamp is more natural as compared to halogen lamp. However, most of the cameras at present analyze and compensate these variations by means of automatic "equalization of whites" (2,100–10,000 K), which allows the same image to be obtained with both light sources.

A proper white balancing before start of the operation is essential for obtaining a natural color. The white light is composed of equal proportion of red, blue, and green color. At the time of white balancing, the camera sets its digital coding for these primary colors to equal proportion, assuming that the target is white. If at the time of white balancing, the telescope is not seeing a perfectly white object, the setup of the camera will be incorrect, and the color perception will be poor.

The newer light source of xenon is defined as a cool light, but practically it is not completely heat free and it should be cared for ignition hazard.

Metal halide vapor arc lamp (250 W):
Halide: A halide is a binary compound, of which one part is a halogen atom and the other part is an element or radical that is less electronegative (or more electropositive) than the halogen, to make a fluoride, chloride, bromide, iodide, or astatide compound. Many salts are halides. All group 1 metals form halide compounds which are white solids at room temperature.

A halide ion is a halogen atom bearing a negative charge. The halide ions are fluoride (F^-), chloride (Cl^-), bromide (Br^-), iodide (I^-), and astatide (At^-). Such ions are present in all ionic halide salts.

Metal halides are used in high-intensity discharge lamps called metal halide lamps such as those used in modern street lights. These are more energy efficient than mercury-vapor lamps and have much better color rendition than orange high-pressure sodium lamps. Metal halide lamps are also commonly used in green houses or in rainy climates to supplement natural sunlight.

Examples of halide compounds are: sodium chloride (NaCl), potassium chloride (KCl), potassium iodide (KI), lithium chloride (LiCl), copper (II) chloride ($CuCl_2$), silver chloride (AgCl), and chlorine fluoride (ClF).

Metal halide lamps, a member of the high-intensity discharge (HID) family of lamps, produce high light output for their size, making them a compact, powerful, and efficient light source. By adding rare earth metal salts to the mercury-vapor lamp, it improved luminous efficacy and light color is obtained. Originally created in the late 1960s for industrial use, metal halide lamps are now available in numerous sizes and configurations for commercial and residential applications **(Figs. 6 to 8)**.

Like most HID lamps, metal halide lamps operate under high pressure and temperature and require special fixtures to operate safely.

In metal halide lamp, a mixture of compounds (comprising mostly salts of rare earths and halides as well as the mercury which provides the conduction path) is carefully chosen to produce an output which approximates to "white" light as perceived by the human eye **(Fig. 9)**.

There are two types of metal halide lamp generally used. They are iron iodide lamp and gallium iodide lamp. Iron iodide is a broad emitter and enhances the spectral output of the lamp in the 380 nm. Gallium iodide has the effect of introducing spectral lines at 403 nm and 417 nm of the electromagnetic spectrum **(Fig. 10)**.

The intensity of the light delivered by any lamp also depends on the power supply of the source. However, increasing the power poses a real problem as it generates more heat. At present, the improvements made to the cameras means that it is possible to return to reasonable power levels of 250 W. However, 400 W units are preferable in order to obtain sufficient illumination of the abdomen even when bleeding causes strong light absorption. It is important to remember that a three-chip camera requires more light than single-chip camera, so a 400 W light source is recommended for three-chip camera.

Light-emitting diode light source: Light-emitting diode (LED) technology is rapidly becoming the modern-day benchmark for illumination. New range of LED light source units is available offering high performance, quality, durability, and

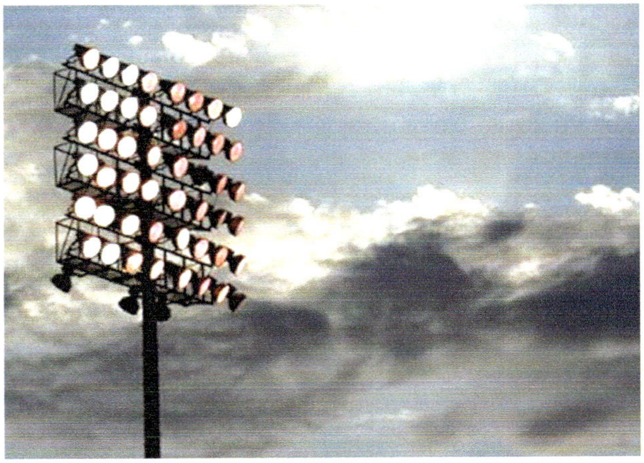

Fig. 6: A metal halide gas discharge lighting system provides illumination for a college baseball game. Note the various colors of the lights as they warm up.

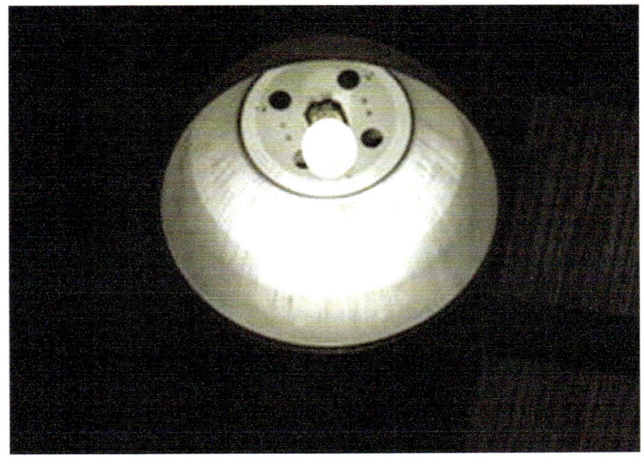

Fig. 7: A low-bay light fixture using a high wattage metal halide lamp of the type used in factories and warehouses.

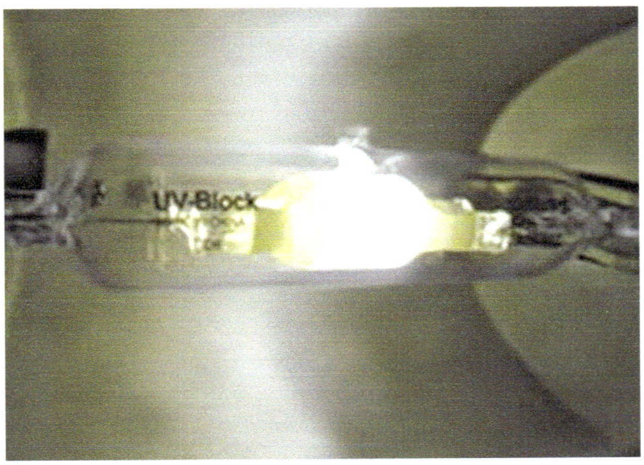

Fig. 8: A linear/tubular metal halide lamp lit up at half power.

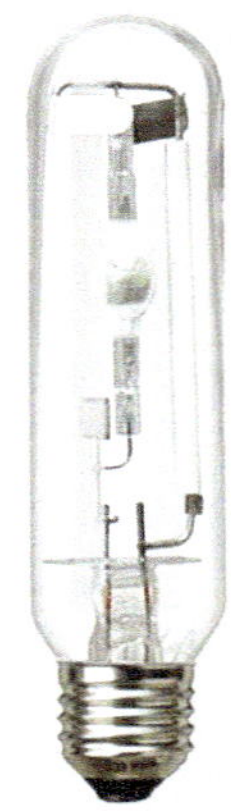

Fig. 9: Metal halide bulb.

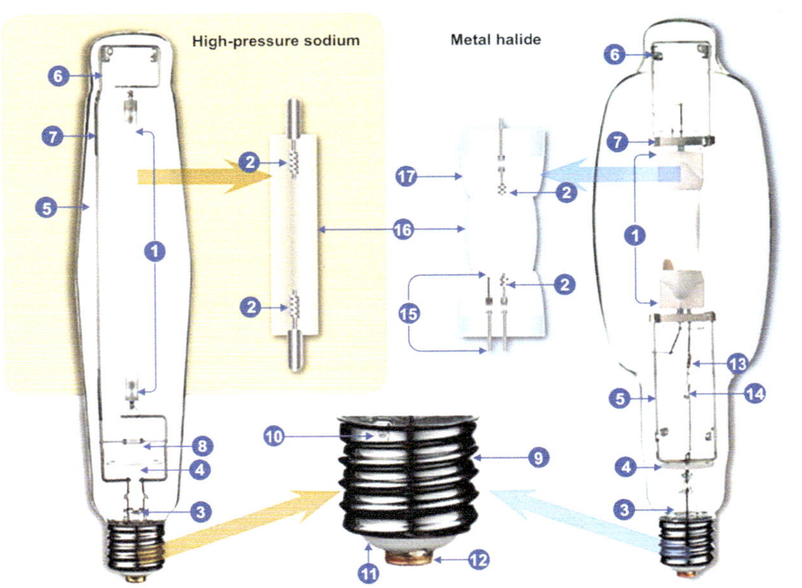

Fig. 10: Internal structure of metal halide tube. (1) ARC tube; (2) Tungsten electrodes; (3) Stem; (4) Ceramic heat shield; (5) Stainless steel frame; (6) Spring supports; (7) Button getter and strip getters; (8) Ceramic spacer; (9) Nickel-plated brass base; (10) EN weld; (11) Ceramic insulator; (12) Deep eyelet; (13) Resistor; (14) Bimetal switch; (15) Starter assembly; (16) HPS ARC tube; (17) End coat.

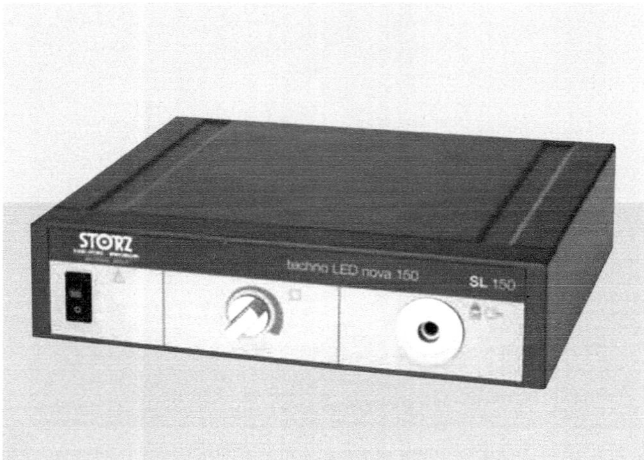

Fig. 11: Light-emitting diode (LED) light source.

economy. The economy is due to the longevity of the lamp units. For example, at an average of 30,000 hours operating life, the LED units offer years of trouble-free performance as well as the inherent cost saving of replacement bulbs. At an average of 30,000 hours, the operating life of LED light sources exceeds the standard life of high-performance light sources. 250 workdays per year at 10 hours each equals an operating life of approximately 10–12 years **(Fig. 11)**. Most incandescent and halogen bulbs are in the Kelvin range (2,700–3,000 K). Fluorescent, metal halide, and LED bulbs can be purchased with color temperature options from 2,700 to 6,500 K.

Why LED Light Source?

Light-emitting diodes offer definite advantages over conventional lamps:

- Purchase costs are quickly justified due to the long life (30,000 hours) and minimal power consumption
- Extremely economical
- Ultra-low maintenance
- Clear return on investment
- High energy efficiency with 90% reduced power consumption over conventional bulb types
- Ready to go, instantly (full light intensity available as soon as the unit is powered on)
- Environmentally friendly.

Heat Filter

For 100% of energy consumed, a normal light source (a light bulb) converts approximately 2% to light and 98% as heat. This heat is mainly due to the infrared spectrum of light and due to obstruction in the pathway of light. If infrared travels through the light cable, the cable will become hot. A heat filter is introduced to filter this infrared in fiberoptic cable. A cool light source lowers this ratio by creating more light, but does not reduce the heat produced to zero. This implies a significant dissipation of heat, which increases as the power rating increases. A *cold light* is light emitted at low temperatures from a source that is not incandescent such as fluorescence or phosphorescence. *Incandescence* is the emission of light (visible electromagnetic radiation) from a hot body as a result of its temperature.

The sources are protected against transmitting too much heat at present. The heat is essentially dissipated in transport, along the cable, in the connection with the endoscope and along the endoscope.

While it is remarkable how little heat is delivered to the tip of the laparoscope, the effects are cumulative. A lighted laparoscope or fiberoptic bundle in direct contact with paper drapes or the patient's skin will cause a burn after 20 or 30 seconds and must be avoided.

Some accidents have been reported due to burning caused by the heat of the optics system. It is therefore important to test the equipment, particularly if assemblies of different brands are used.

Condensing Lens

The purpose of condensing lens is to converge the light emitted by lamp to the area of light cable input. In most of the light source, it is used for increasing the light intensity per square cm of area.

Manual or Automatic Intensity Control Circuit (Shutter)

Manual adjustment allows the light source to be adjusted to a power level defined by the surgeon. In video cameras, close-up viewing is hampered in too much light whereas more distant view is too dark. To address this, the luminosity of most of the current light sources is adjustable.

The advanced light source system is based on the automatic intensity adjustment technology. The video camera transforms the signal into an electronic signal. This electronic signal is coded in order to be transported. The coding dissociates the luminance and chrominance of the image. The luminance is the quantity of light of the signal (black and white) that dictates the quality of the final image. When there is too much light for the image (when the endoscope is near to the tissue), the luminance signal of the oscilloscope increases. On the other hand, when the luminosity is low (distant view or red surroundings), the luminance is low and the electronic signal is much weaker. A good quality luminance signal is calibrated to 1 mV. Overexposed images make the electronic signal pass above 1 mV whereas underexposed images make the signal drop below 1 mV. Light sources equipped with adjustment analyze the luminance. If the signal is significantly higher than 1 mV, they lower the power and bring the signal back within the standards. Conversely, if the signal is too weak, they increase their intensity.

These systems are extremely valuable, permitting work to be performed at different distances from the target in good viewing conditions. However, the cameras currently available are often equipped with a regulation system, which is capable of automatic gain control in poor light condition and the purchase of a light source with adjustment associated with a camera equipped with an adjustment system is a double purchase that is unnecessary.

Troubleshooting of laparoscopic light source: Troubleshooting for inadequate lighting is shown in **Table 1**.

A laparoscopic surgeon should be technically well-acknowledged of the principle of the instrument they are using. The purchase of a costly instrument is not an answer for achieving a good task, ability to handle them is equally important.

Infrared light source: The new infrared LED light source provides real-time endoscopic visibility and near-infrared fluorescence imaging. This enables surgeon to perform minimally invasive surgery (MIS) using standard endoscopic visible light as well as visual assessment of vessels, blood flow, related tissue perfusion, and biliary anatomy near-infrared imaging. In addition, this infrared visualization technology is very useful to transilluminate the ureters with fiberoptic ureteric kit (IRIS U-kits) available **(Fig. 12)**.

TABLE 1: Troubleshooting of light source.

Probable cause	*Remedy*
• Loose connection at source or scope • Light is on "manual-minimum" • Bulb is burned out • Fiberoptics are damaged • Automatic iris adjusting to bright • Reflection from instrument	• Adjust connector • Go to "automatic" • Replace bulb • Replace light cable • Dim room lights • Reposition instruments or switch to "manual"

Light Cable

Minimal access surgery depends on the artificial light available in closed body cavity and before the discovery of light source and light cable; mirrors were used to reflect the light on to the subject where direct light access was not possible.

In 1954, a major breakthrough in technology occurred in the development of fiberoptic cables **(Fig. 13)**. The principle of fiberoptic cable was based on the *total internal reflection of light*. Light can be conducted along a curved glass rod due to multiple total internal reflections. Light would enter at one end of the fiber and emerge at the other end after numerous internal reflections with virtually all of its intensity.

Total Internal Reflection

An effect that combines both refraction and reflection is *total internal reflection* **(Fig. 14)**. Consider light coming from a dense medium like water into a less dense medium like air. When the light coming from the water strikes the surface, part will be reflected and part will be refracted. Measured with respect to the normal line perpendicular to the surface, the reflected light comes off at an angle equal to that at which it is entered while that for the refracted light is larger than the incident angle. In fact, the greater the incident angle, the more the refracted light bends away from the normal. Thus, increasing the angle of incidence from path "1" to "2" will eventually reach a point where the refracted angle is 90°, at which point the light appears to emerge along the surface between the water and air. If the angle of incidence is increased further, the refracted light cannot leave the water. It gets completely reflected. The interesting thing about total internal reflection is that it is really *total*. That is 100% of the light gets reflected back into the more dense medium, as long as the angle at which it is incident to the surface is large enough.

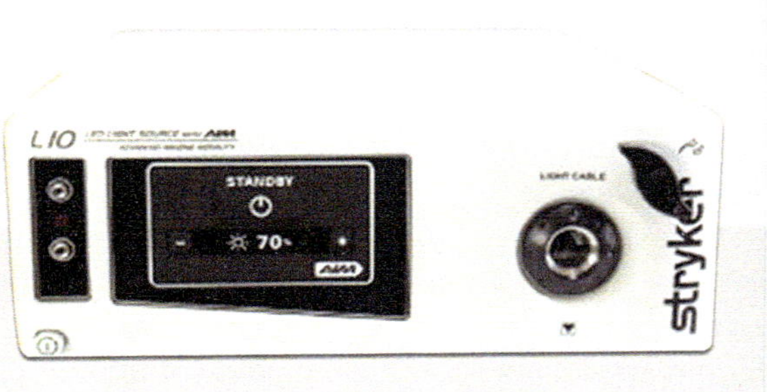

Fig. 12: Light-emitting diode (LED) light source with infrared emission capability.

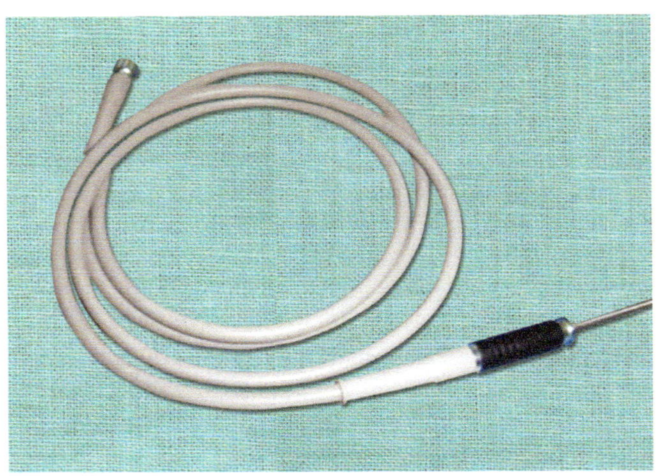

Fig. 13: Fiberoptic light cable.

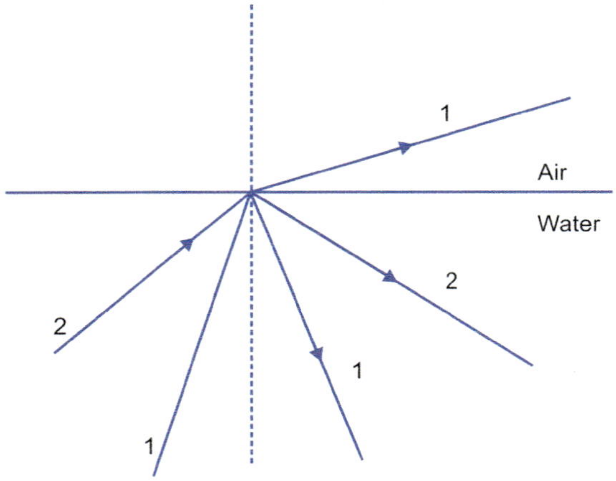

Fig. 14: Refraction of light from water into air.

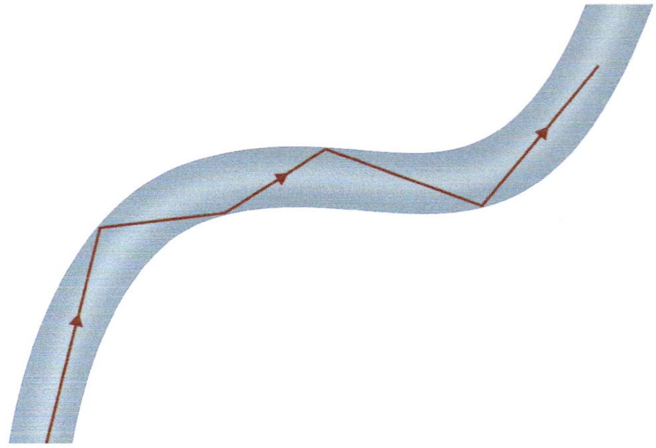

Fig. 15: Fiberoptic cable, total internal reflection.

Fiberoptics uses this property of light to keep light beams focused without significant loss **(Fig. 15)**.

The light enters the glass cable and as long as the bending is not too sudden, it will be totally internally reflected when it hits the sides and thus is guided along the cable. This is used in telephone and TV cables to carry the signals. Light as an information carrier is much faster and more efficient than electrons in an electric current. Also, since light rays do not interact with each other (whereas electrons interact via their electric charge), it is possible to pack a large number of different light signals into the same fiberoptics cable without distortion. You are probably most familiar with fiberoptics cables in novelty items consisting of thin, multicolored strands of glass which carry light beams. Nowadays, there are two types of light cable available:

1. Fiberoptic cable
2. Liquid crystal gel cable

Fiberoptic Cable

Fiberoptic is the science or technology of light transmission through (a bundle of optical fibers) a very fine, flexible glass or plastic fibers.

Fiberoptic cables are made up of a bundle of optical fiber glass threads waged at both ends. The fiber size used is usually 20–150 μ in diameter. A good fiberoptic cable will transmit all the spectrum of light without loss **(Fig. 16)**. They have a very high quality of optical transmission, but are fragile.

The light inside these fibers travels on the principle of total internal reflection without losing much of its intensity. The multimode fiber maintains the intensity of light and the light can be passed in a curved path of light cable **(Fig. 17)**.

As the light cables are used progressively, some optical fibers break **(Fig. 18)**. The loss of optical fibers may be seen when one end of the cable is viewed in daylight. The broken fibers are seen as *black spots*. To avoid the breakage of these fibers, the curvature radius of light cable should be respected and in any circumstances it should not be <15 cm in radius.

If the heat filter or cooling system of light source does not work properly, the fibers of these light cables are burnt (melt) and it will decrease the intensity of light dramatically **(Fig. 19)**. If poor quality fibers are used, it might burn just within a few months of use.

Liquid Crystal Gel Cable

These cables are made up of a sheath that is filled with a clear optical gel (liquid crystal).

Crystal (a clear, transparent mineral or glass resembling ice) is a piece of solid substance, such as quartz, with a regular shape in which plane faces intersect at definite angles, due to the regular internal structure of its atoms, ions, or molecules. Within a crystal, many identical paralleled-piped unit cells, each containing a group of atoms, are packed together to fill all space (see illustration). In scientific nomenclature, the term crystal is usually short for single crystal, a single periodic arrangement of atoms. Most gems are single crystals. However, many materials are polycrystalline, consisting of many small grains, each of which is a single crystal. For example, most metals are polycrystalline **(Fig. 20)**.

Liquid crystal: Substance that flows like a liquid, but maintains some of the ordered structure characteristic of a crystal. Some organic substances do not melt directly when heated, but instead turn from a crystalline solid to a liquid crystalline state. When heated further, a true liquid is formed. Liquid crystals have unique properties. The structures are easily affected by changes in mechanical stress, electromagnetic fields, temperature, and chemical environment.

Liquid crystal gel cables are capable of transmitting up to 30% more light than optic fibers. Due to lighter and better color temperature transmission, this cable is recommended in those circumstances, where documentation (movie, photography, or TV) is performed.

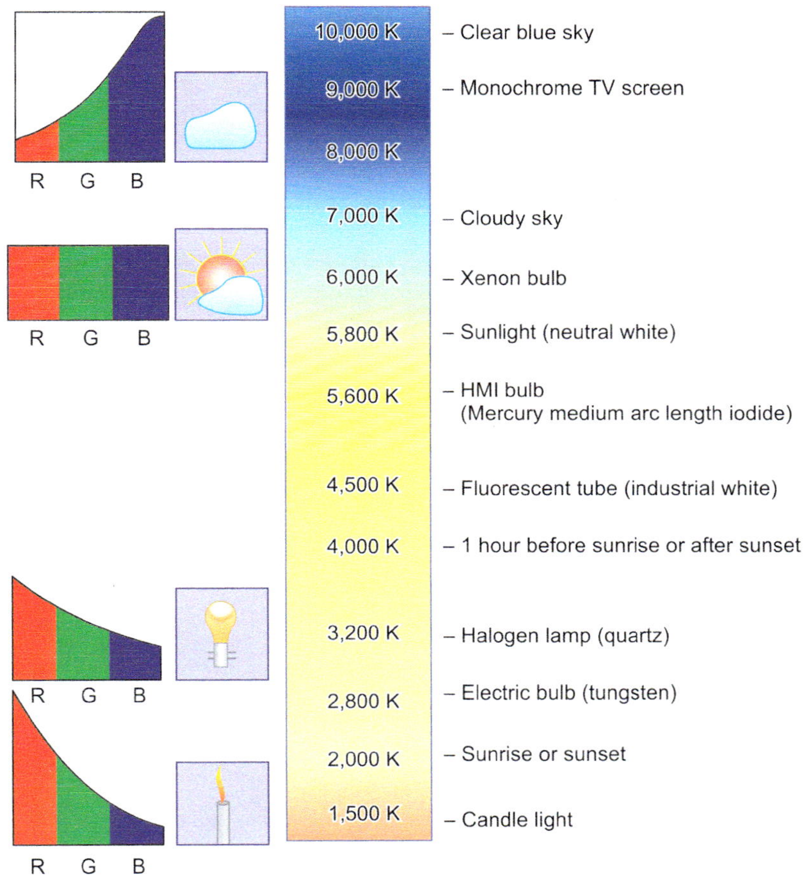

Fig. 16: Spectrum of light.
(HMI: hydrargyrum medium-arc iodide)

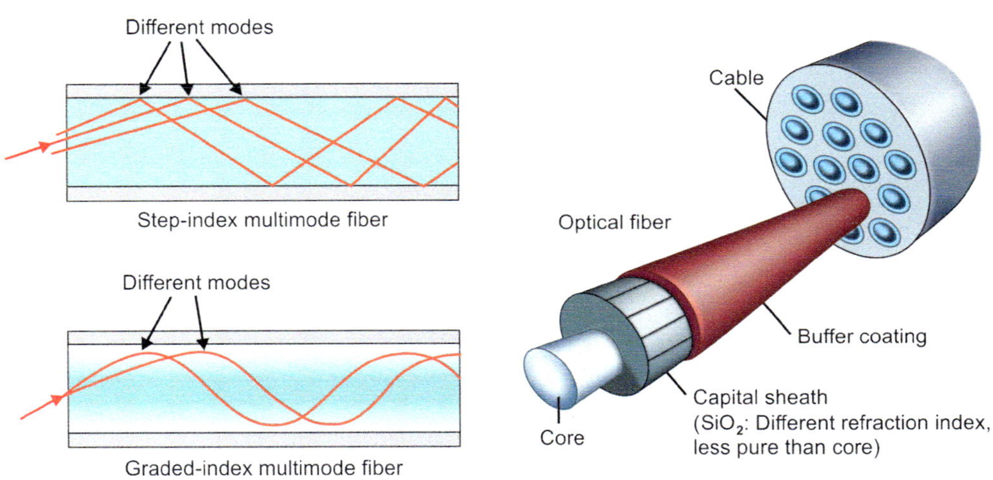

Fig. 17: Multimode fiber.
(SiO_2: silicon dioxide)

The quartz swaging at the ends is extremely fragile, especially when the cable is hot. The slightest shock, on a bench, for example, can cause the quartz end to crack and thus cause a loss in the transmission of the light.

Gel cables transmit more heat than optical fiber cables. These cables are made more rigid by a metal sheath, which makes them more difficult to maintain and to store. In conclusion, even though the choice is a difficult one, we use

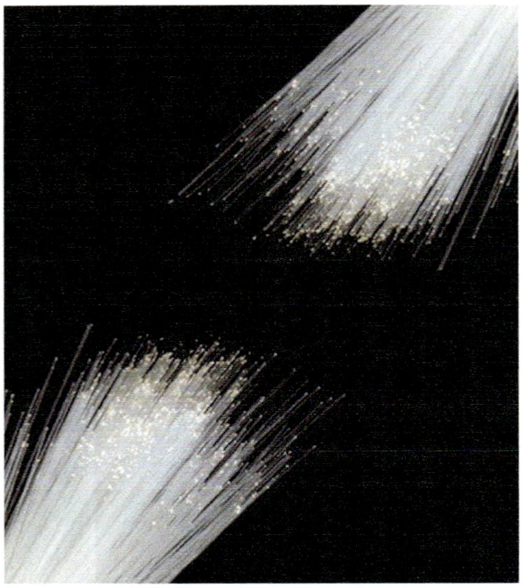

Fig. 18: Broken fibers showing significant loss of light.

optical fiber cables, which are as fragile as the gel cables but their flexibility makes them much easier to maintain.

Attachment of the Light Cable to the Light Source

Conventional attachment has a right angle connection for light source and camera. Recently, new attachment for light cable is available known as display control interface (DCI) **(Fig. 21)**. The benefit of this is that it maintains upright orientation regardless of angle of viewing, using autorotation system. It also provides single-handed control of the entire endoscope camera system.

Maintenance of Light Cable

The following points should be followed for the maintenance of light cable:

- Handle them carefully
- Avoid twisting them

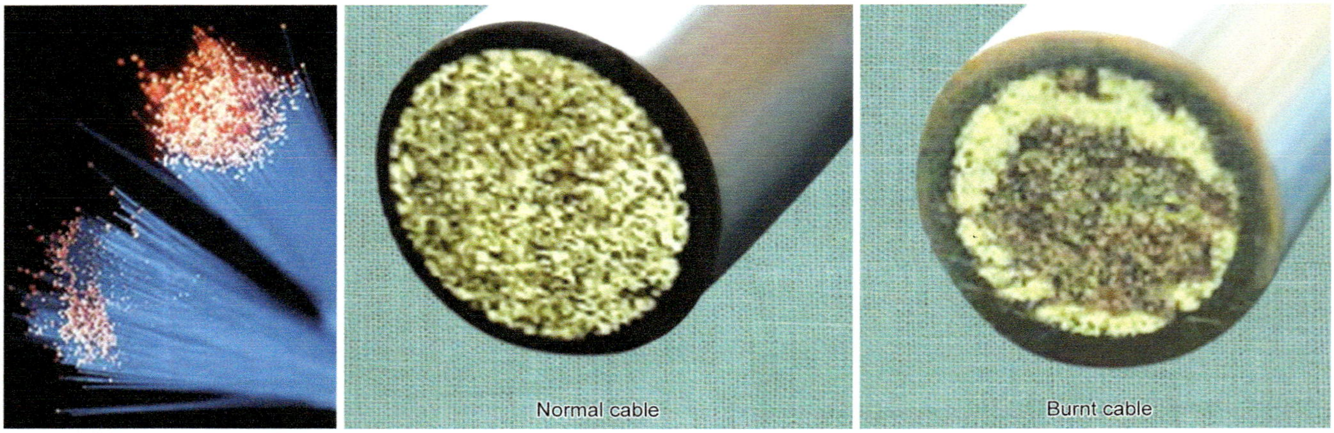

Fig. 19: Burnt fiber causes significant reduction in intensity of light.

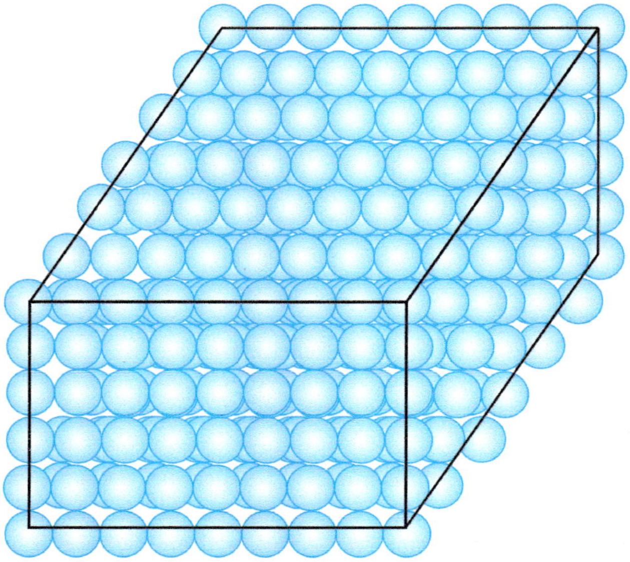

Fig. 20: Structure of a simple crystal.

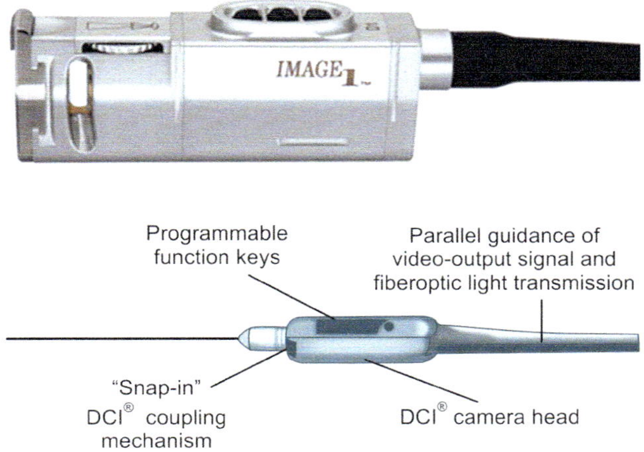

Fig. 21: Display control interface (DCI) attachment of light cable.

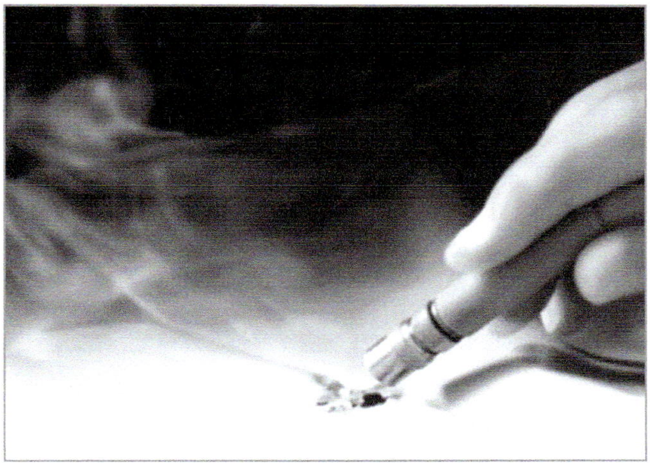

Fig. 22: Negligence with light cable can result in burn.

- After the operation has been completed, the cable should preferably be first disconnected from the endoscope and then disconnected from the light source. In fact, most of the sources currently available have a plug for holding the cable until it cools down.
- The end of the crystal of cable should be periodically cleaned with a cotton swab moistened with alcohol.
- The outer plastic covering of the cable should be cleaned with a mild cleaning agent or disinfectant.
- Distal end of fiberoptic cable should never be placed on or under drapes or next to the patient, when connected to an illuminated light source. The heat generated from the intensity of light may cause burns to the patient or ignite the drapes **(Fig. 22)**.
- The intensity of light source is so high that there is chance of retinal damage if the light will fall directly on eye. Never try to look directly on light source when it is lighted.

Telescope

There are *two types* of telescope: (1) *rigid* and (2) *flexible*.

The *rigid* laparoscopic and thoracoscopic telescopes come in a variety of shapes and sizes and offering several different angles of view. The standard laparoscope consists of a metal shaft between 24 and 33 cm in length.

There are three important structural differences in telescope available in the market:

1. *Number of the rod lens*: From 6 to 18 rod lens system telescopes
2. *Angle of view*: Between 0 and 120° telescopes
3. *Diameter*: 1.5–15 mm of telescopes.

Angle of View

Telescopes offer either a straight-on view with the 0° or can be angled at 25–30° or 45–50°. The 30° telescope provides a total field of view of 152° compared with the 0° telescope, which only provides a field of view of 76° **(Fig. 23)**. The 30° forward oblique angle permits far greater latitude for viewing underlying areas under difficult anatomical conditions **(Fig. 24)**.

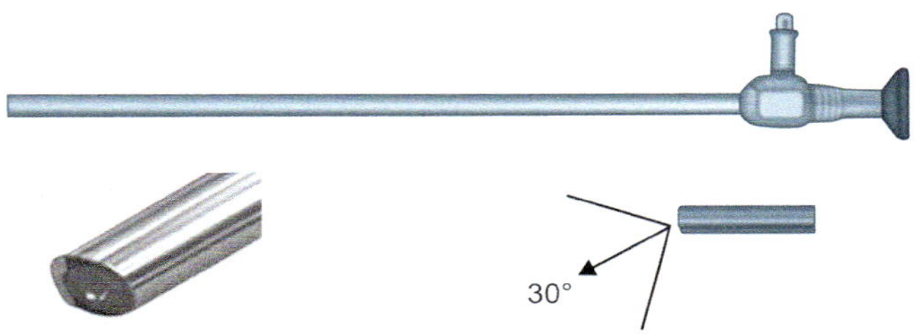

Fig. 23: The 30° telescope provides a total field of view of 152° compared with the 0° telescope, which provides a field of view of only 76°.

Diameter

The most commonly used telescope has a diameter of 10 mm and provides the greatest light and visual acuity. The next most commonly used telescope is the 5 mm laparoscope, which can be placed through one of the working ports for an alternative view. Smaller-diameter laparoscopes, down to a 1.1-mm scope, are available and are used mostly in children. They are not used commonly in adult patients because of an inability to direct enough light into the larger abdominal cavity. Laparoscopes as small as 1 mm have been produced for diagnostic use. The field of view and picture brightness are dramatic improvements over early designs. *Mini* or *micro* 2 mm laparoscopy is reported for diagnostic and even advanced procedures.

One of the problems with working with these smaller laparoscopes (particularly those <3.4 mm) is that they tend to bend easily, leading to potential damage during surgery.

Full screen 5 mm laparoscopes with images comparable to many 10 mm systems are now available.

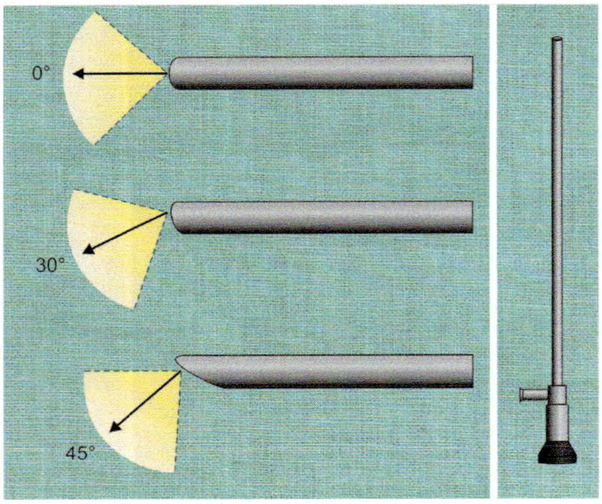

Fig. 24: Angle of laparoscope.

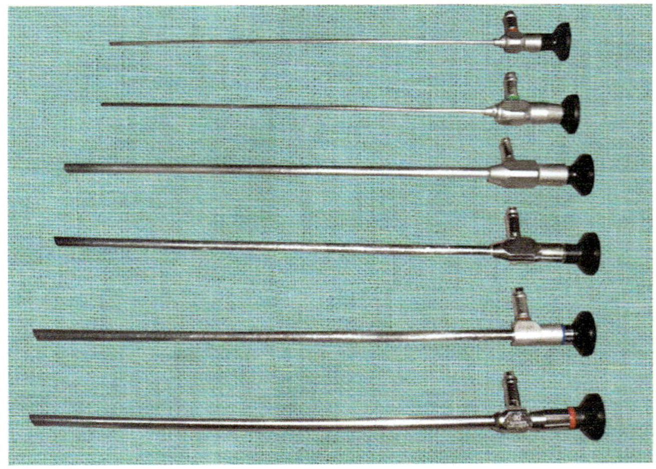

Fig. 25: Different types of laparoscope.

Lens System

There are two lens system designs used with the laparoscopy—(1) the conventional thin lens system and (2) the Hopkins rod-lens system design. The thin lens system, which uses a series of objective lenses to transport the image down the laparoscope, is used less commonly. The Hopkins rod-lens system containing a series of quartz rod lenses that carry the image through the length of the scope to the eyepiece. Rigid rod lens system provides good resolution and better depth perception **(Fig. 25)**. The Hopkins rod-lens system uses more glass than air, so it has improved light transmission **(Fig. 26)**. Normally used telescope is *the Hopkins Forward-Oblique Telescope (30°)*. Its diameter is 10 mm, length is 33 cm, and is autoclavable.

At the distal end, it is a front lens complex [inverting real-image lens system (IRILS)] which creates an inverted and real image of the subject. A number of IRILS transport the image to the eyepiece containing a magnifying lens. In the Hopkins rod-lens system, light is transmitted through glass columns and refracted through intervening air lenses. The camera is attached to the eyepiece of the laparoscope for processing.

Digital laparoscopes, in which the laparoscope and camera head are a single unit with the imaging sensor at the end of the laparoscope, have been available since the early 1990s. This (*chip on stick technology*) has been introduced in which charge-coupled device (CCD) chip will be at the tip inside the abdominal cavity. One of the popular brands of digital laparoscope is Olympus ENDOEYE. The ENDOEYE comes with the fog-free feature, providing clear views throughout the procedure. The advanced multi-CCD chip on the tip technology enables bright, clear images and narrow band imaging (NBI) further enhances visualization of vessels and other tissues on the mucosal surface. The flexible tip can articulate in all directions up to 100° and the focus-free optical design provides greater depth of field, eliminating the need for manual focusing **(Fig. 27)**.

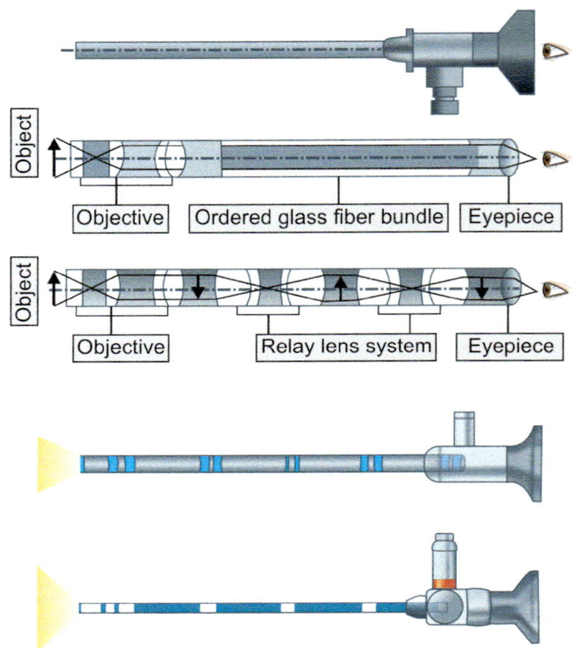

Fig. 26: Inside view of laparoscope.

Telescope Fiber Bundle

The telescope also contains parallel optical fibers bundle that transmits light into the abdomen from the light source via a light cable attached to the side of the telescope. The fiber bundle in the laparoscope and the fiberoptic light cable must be in excellent working order, so as to achieve an optimal well-lighted picture. The fiber bundle located along a tract on the periphery of the telescope and occupies less than half of the circumference of the telescope. It is exit at the inner tip of the telescope that is corresponding to the attachment of the light cable to the side of the telescope.

Three-dimensional Stereoscope

One of the main problems associated with video-assisted MIS is the loss of stereopsis, meaning the perception of depth and three-dimensionality. This occurs when a three-dimensional (3D) image is projected on a two-dimensional (2D) screen and is often the cause of impeded hand-eye coordination and erroneous movements of the tools. Modern laparoscopic stereoscope with dual cameras can provide 3D images in ultra-high definition (UHD) resolution and offer a binocular stereoscopic vision of the operative field comparable to open surgery, making up for the loss of stereovision and representing a definite improvement. There are flexible 3D videoscopes also available which allow the surgeon to reach hidden targets even through tortuous paths and have permitted the emergence of novel techniques that exploit the body's natural openings. In addition, video images can be enhanced with virtual models of structures and tissues, creating an augmented reality environment that has been proven to improve the performance of the surgeon. These new 3D technologies, also used to create completely virtual scenes for surgical preparation and training, are rendered from volumetric data that are obtained from preoperative scans **(Fig. 28)**.

The Olympus VISERA 3D platforms (Olympus, Shinjuku, Tokyo, Japan), for instance, include stereovideoscopes that can bend their tip of 100° in four directions and providing 3D videos in 4K resolution and offering flexibility for applications in laparoscopy and endoscopy. Another example is the 3D-Eye-Flex, developed by Nishiyama et al., an endoscopic video system, that offers a wide angle of view for minimally invasive neurosurgery. This type of technology is already commercially available and has undergone clinical trials, yielding improved performance, shorter learning curve, and greater accuracy and precision **(Fig. 29)**.

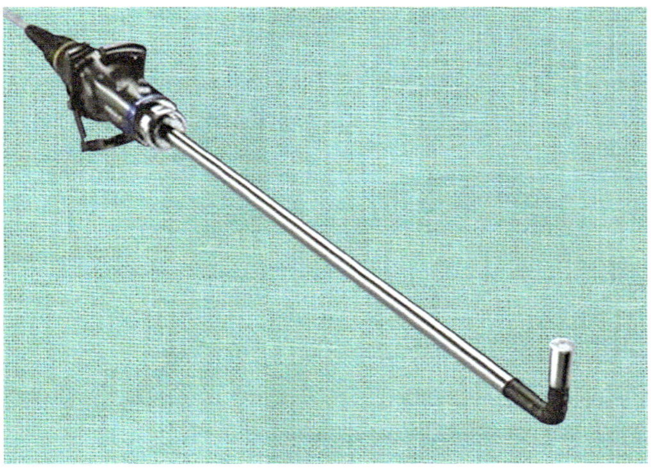

Fig. 27: Chip on stick technology.

Laparoscopic Camera

First medical camera was introduced by Circon Corporation in 1972. Laparoscopic camera is one of the very important instruments and should be of good quality **(Fig. 30)**. Laparoscopic camera available is either of single chip or three chips. We all know that there are three primary colors [red, green, and blue (RGB)]. All the colors are mixture of these three primary colors in different proportion.

The CCD chip or complementary metal oxide semiconductor (CMOS) is an electronic memory that records the intensity of light as a variable charge. Widely used in still cameras, camcorders, and scanners to capture images, CCDs are analog devices. Their charges equate to shades of light for monochrome images or shades of RGB when used with color filters. Three-chip camera uses three CCDs, one for each of the RGB colors **(Figs. 31A and B)**.

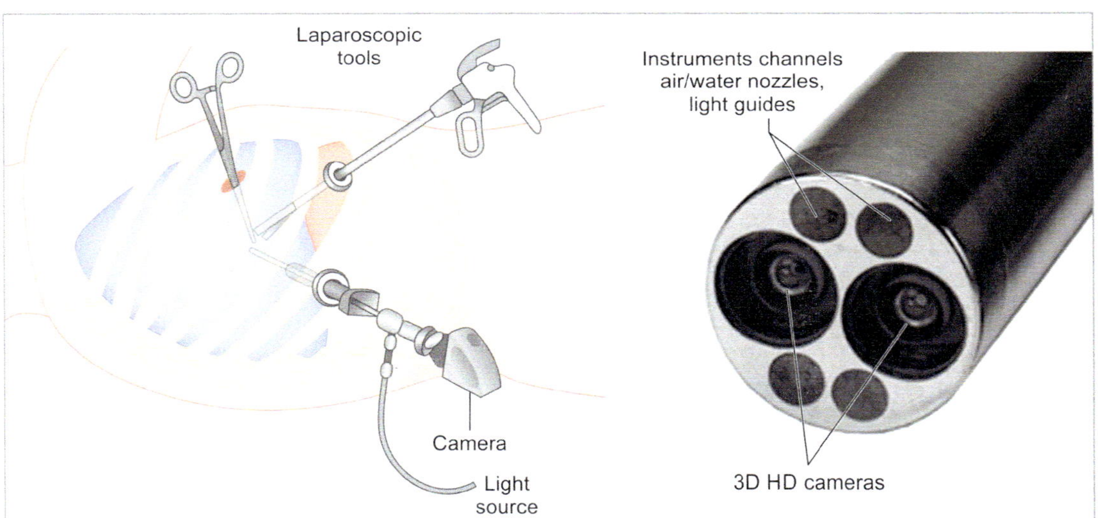

Fig. 28: Stereoscope for three-dimensional (3D) laparoscopic view.

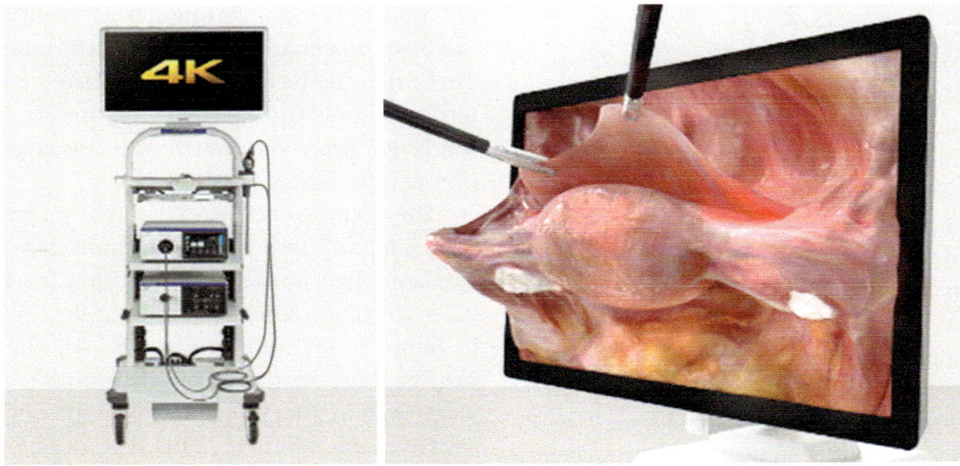

Fig. 29: Olympus VISERA 3D platform.

Why Coupled?

The "coupled" in the name is because the CCD is comprised of an array of imaging pixels and a matching array of storage pixels that are coupled together. After the imaging array is exposed to light, its charges are quickly transferred to the storage array. While the imaging CCDs are being exposed to the next picture, the storage CCDs from the last picture are being read out a row at a time to the analog-to-digital (A/D) converters that transform the charges into binary data (0/1) to be processed **(Fig. 32)**. CCD and CMOS are both image sensors found in digital laparoscopic cameras. They are what is responsible for converting light into electronic signals. The first digital cameras used CCD to turn images from analog light signals into digital pixels. They are made through a special manufacturing process that allows the conversion to take place in the chip without distortion. This creates high quality sensors that produce excellent images. But, because they require special manufacturing, they are more expensive than their newer CMOS counterparts. CMOS chips use transistors at each pixel to move the charge through traditional wires. This offers flexibility because each pixel is treated individually. Traditional manufacturing processes are used to make CMOS. It is the same as creating microchips. Because they are easier to produce, CMOS sensors are cheaper than CCD sensors. Because CMOS technology came after CCD sensors and are cheaper to manufacture, CMOS sensors are the reason that laparoscopic cameras have dropped in price.

The biggest difference is that CCD sensors create high quality images with low noise. CMOS images tend to be higher in noise. CCD sensors are more sensitive to light. CMOS sensors need more light to create a low noise image at proper exposure. This does not mean that CMOS sensors are completely inferior to CCD. CCD has been around for a lot longer in digital cameras and the technology is more advanced. CMOS sensors are catching up and will soon match CCD in terms of resolution and overall quality. They can be manufactured on any standard silicon production line and are much more inexpensive when compared to CCD sensors. Eventually economics will someday make every camera CMOS when the final advances in quality are made. In fact, CMOS sensors are already superior to CCD sensors in terms of power consumption.

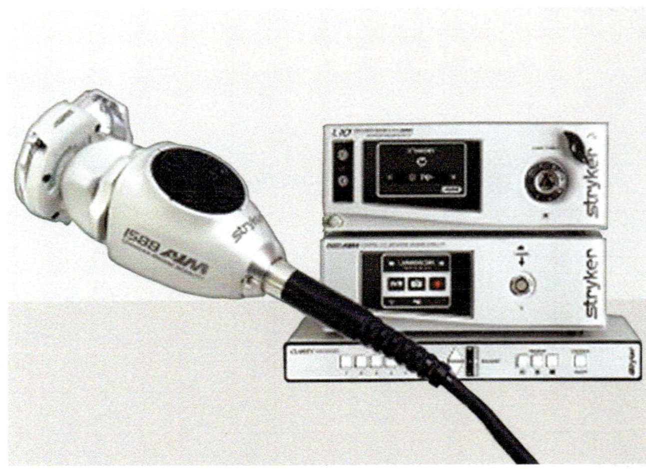

Fig. 30: Laparoscopic camera.

The camera system has two components: (1) *the head* of the camera **(Fig. 33)**, which is attached to the ocular of the telescope and (2) the *controller*, which is usually located on the trolley along with the monitor.

Within the head of camera is an objective zoom lens that focuses the image of the object on the chip and a CCD chip that "sees" an image taken by telescope **(Fig. 34)**. All modern miniature cameras used in minimal access surgery are based on the CCD chip. The CCD then converts optical image into an electrical signal that is sent through the camera cable to camera control unit (CCU). The chip has light-sensitive photoreceptors that generate pixels by transforming the incoming photons into electronic charges. The electronic

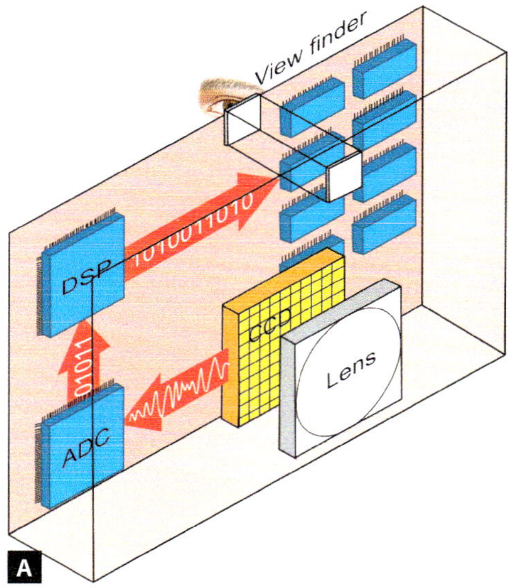

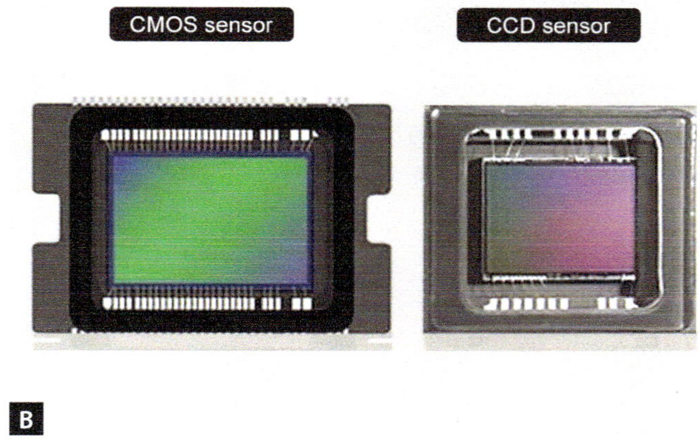

Figs. 31A and B: In a camera, CCD or CMOS takes the place of film. They are exposed to light, recording the intensities, or shades of light as variable charges. In the digital camera above, the variable analog charges in the CCD or CMOS are converted to binary data (0/1) by analog-to-digital converter (ADC) chip.
(CCD: charge-coupled device; CMOS: complementary metal oxide semiconductor; DSP: digital single processing)

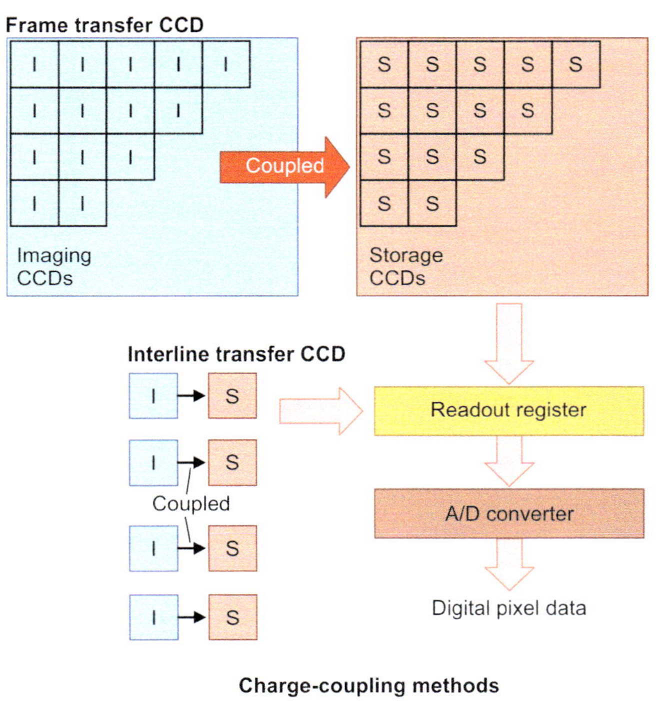

Fig. 32: The storage CCDs are either a separate array (frame transfer) or individual photosites (interline transfer) coupled to each imaging photosite. The charges can be transferred faster with the interline method because each storage component is closer to its imaging counterpart.
(A/D: analog-to-digital; CCDs: charged-coupled devices)

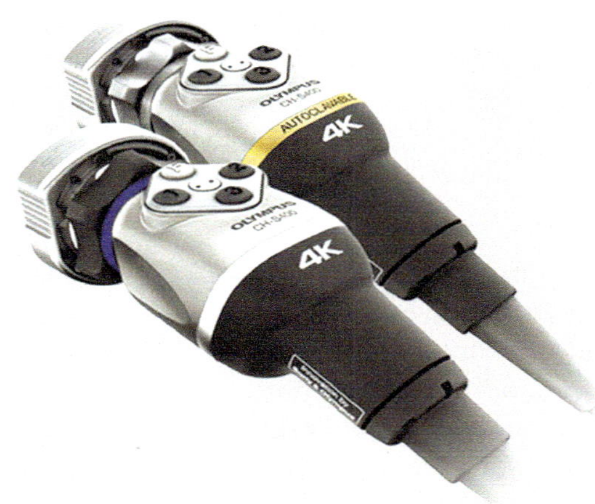

Fig. 33: Head of camera 4K.

charges are then transferred from the pixels into a storage element on the chip. A subsequent scanning at defined time intervals results in a black and white image with gray tones.

Pixel: PIX (picture) + EL (element), picture element is the smallest element of a light-sensitive device, such as cameras that use CCDs. It is the smallest resolved unit of a video image that has specific luminescence and color. Its proportions are determined by the number of lines making up the scanning raster (the pattern of dots that form the image) and the resolution along each line. In the most common form of computer graphics and the CCDs, the thousands of tiny pixels that make up an individual image are projected onto a display screen as illuminated dots that from a distance appear as a continuous image. An electron beam creates the grid of pixels by tracing each horizontal line from left to right, one pixel at a time, from the top line to the bottom line.

The number of pixels determines the resolution. Screen resolution is rated by the number of horizontal and vertical pixels; for example, 1,024 × 768 means 1,024 pixels are displayed in each row and there are 768 rows (lines).

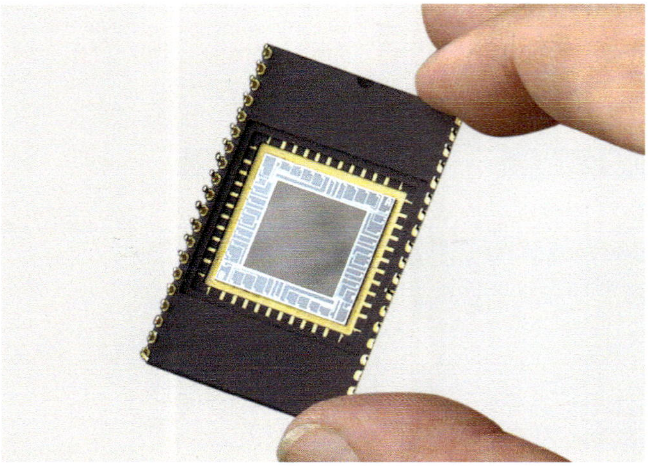

Fig. 34: Charge-coupled device (CCD) camera.

Likewise, bitmapped images are sized in pixels: a 350 × 250 image has 350 pixels across and 250 pixels down. You have probably already noticed the jump from predigital "standard definition" television up to "HD" and "full HD" services that are now available on digital TV, online streaming, and Blu-Ray disks. Compared to earlier standards, this HD footage is detailed, crisp, and it even looks good when viewed on a large TV. But even the best quality, "1,080 pixels" HD footage is only across 1,920 pixels. Recently, 4K or UHD laparoscopic cameras are available. 4K is significantly more detailed, since it has twice as many pixels horizontally and four times as many pixels in total.

Pixels and subpixels: In monochrome systems, the pixel is the smallest addressable unit. With color systems, each pixel contains RGB subpixels and the subpixel is the smallest addressable unit for the screen's electronic circuits. On a display screen, pixels are either phosphorus or liquid crystal elements. For monochrome, the element is either energized fully or not. For grayscale, the pixel is energized with different intensities, creating arrange from light to dark. For color displays, the RGB subpixels are each energized to a particular intensity and the combination of the three color intensities creates the perceived color to the eye. The average chip contains 250,000–380,000 pixels, but 4K video is poised to become the new benchmark for both recording and watching laparoscopic video and it brings a whole host of benefits, right away.

Cameras are classified according to the number of chips. These differ among other things, in the way they relay color information to the monitor. Color separation is used to create a colored video image from the original black and white. In single-chip cameras, color separation is achieved by adding a stripe filter that covers the whole chip. Each stripe accepts one of the complementary colors (magenta, green, cyan, or yellow) and each pixel is assigned to one stripe.

In single-chip camera, these three primary colors are sensed by single chip. In three-chip camera, there are three CCD chips for separate capture and processing of three primary colors (RGB). In three-chip cameras, color separation is achieved with a prism system that overlies the chips. Each chip receives only one of the three primary colors (RGB). This system gives a higher resolution and better image quality because the pixel number is three times greater.

The video information, color, and light are scanned at a rate of 525 lines per frame and 30 frames per second. Picture resolution determines the clarity and detail of the video image. Higher the resolution, the better will be quality of image. The resolution of picture is ascertained by the number of distinct vertical line that can be seen in the picture. The higher the resolution numbers, the sharper and cleaner image will form. The CCU of camera is connected with monitor and monitor converts the electrical image back to the original optical image.

These three-chip camera has unprecedented color reproduction and highest degree of fidelity. Three-chip cameras have high horizontal image resolution of >750 lines.

Chip on Stick Technology

Currently, chip on stick technology has been introduced in which CCD will be at the tip inside the abdominal cavity. It is proved that the resolution of picture will be >250K pixels **(Fig. 27)**.

Focusing of Laparoscopic Camera

Laparoscopic camera needs to be focused before inserting inside the abdominal cavity. At the time of focusing, it should be placed at a distance of approximately 10 cm away from the target for the 10 mm telescope, 5 cm for 5 mm telescope, and 4 cm for 4 mm telescope, with an average distance of approximately 5 mm for all telescopes. This distance is optimum for focusing because at the time of laparoscopic surgery, most of the time we keep the telescope at this distance.

White Balancing of Camera

White balancing should be performed before inserting camera inside the abdominal cavity. White balancing is required to remove added impurities of light which unknowingly we add. During white balancing, digital laparoscopic camera will added counter color to neutralize our added impurity. White balancing is necessary every time before start of surgery because every time there is some added impurities of color due to following variables:

- Difference in voltage
- Differences in color temperature of light sources
- Different cleaning material used to clean the tip of telescope which can stain the tip
- Scratches, wear, and tear of the telescopes eyepiece, object piece, and CCD of camera.

White balancing is done by keeping any white object in front of telescope attached with camera that senses white object as reference. It adjusts its primary color (RGB) to make a pure natural white color.

Laparoscopic Video Monitor

Surgical monitors are slightly different from the TV which we watch at home **(Fig. 35)**. Monitor lasts long so a surgeon gets high-end product with at least 600 lines resolution. The size of the screen varies generally from 8 to 29 inches. The closure the laparoscopic surgeon is to the monitor, the smaller the monitor should be to get better picture. The basic principle of image reproduction is horizontal beam scanning on the face of the picture tube. This plate is coated internally with a fluorescent substance containing phosphorus. This generates electrons when struck by beams from the electron gun. As the beam sweeps horizontally and back, it covers all the picture elements before reaching its original position. This occurs repetitively and rapidly. This method is called horizontal linear scanning. Each picture frame consists of several such lines depending on the type of system used. Distance of monitor from the eye of the surgeon should be five times to the diagonal length of monitor screen. It means that if the monitor is 21 inch it should be kept 105 inch away from the eye of the surgeon. Nowadays, 4K laparoscopic monitor is preferred. It is also known as an ultra-high definition or UHD monitor, is one that supports 4K resolution. This brings up another common question: what is 4K resolution? The answer is simple. Standard HD or 1,080 pixels (as found on Blu-Ray disks and HD televisions) is made up of a picture that is 1,920 pixels in width and 1,080 pixels in height. In total, this results in a picture with more than two million pixels. The width of a picture that has 4K resolution contains almost 4,000 pixels (3,840 pixels to be precise—twice that of 1,080 pixels). With 2,160 pixels along the vertical side, the total number of pixels on a 4K monitor is four times that of a traditional HD monitor.

Endoscopic Vision (Video) Technology Evolution

In the past, endoscopic procedures were done without the aid of monitors. The operator visualized the interiors of the patient directly through the eyepiece of the scope. This method was associated with many difficulties. He was the only person who could observe the procedure leading to poor coordination with other members of the team. As a result, extensive and difficult procedures could not be performed. The magnification was very poor. Surgeons had to face problems with posture leading to discomfort and strain as his eye was always glued to the eyepiece. He had difficulties in orientation due to visualizing with only one eye.

As better methods of communication developed, the introduction of television brought about a significant impact. A good magnification of the image was reproduced. All members of the team could visualize the procedure. Surgeons could operate more comfortably. Complex procedures began to be undertaken and were even recorded.

Soulas in France first used television for endoscopic procedures in 1956. He demonstrated the first televised bronchoscopy. A rigid bronchoscope was attached to a black and white camera that weighed about 100 lbs.

In 1959, a laparoscopic procedure was demonstrated using a closed circuit television program using the "Fourestier method". This method was developed by transmitting an intense beam of light along a quartz rod from the proximal to distal ends of the laparoscope.

The first miniature endoscopic black and white television camera was developed in Australia in 1960 **(Fig. 36)**. It weighed 350 g, was 45 mm wide, and 120 mm long. Because of its small dimensions, it could be attached to the eyepiece.

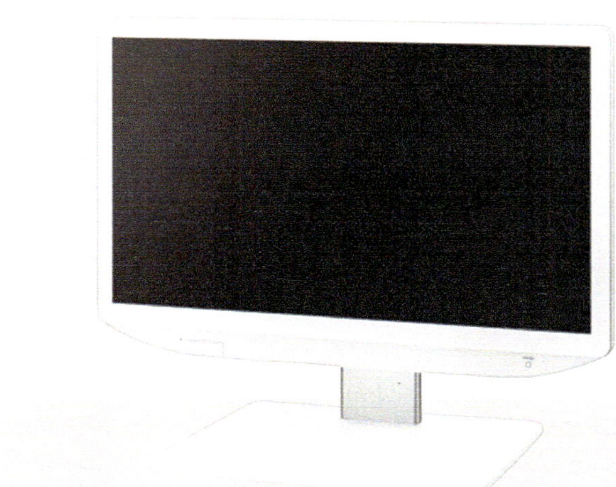

Fig. 35: Laparoscopic 4K monitor.

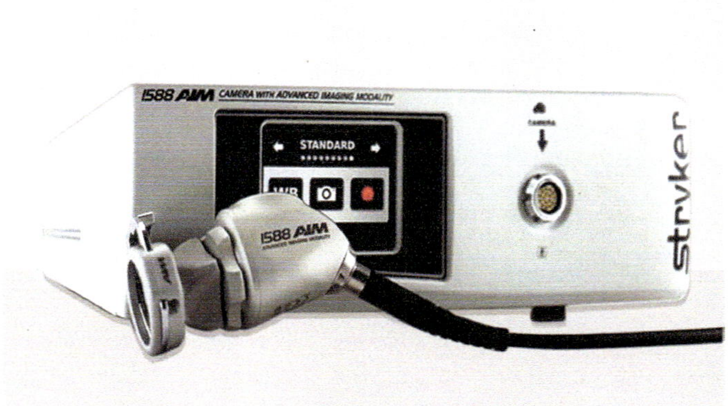

Fig. 36: Endoscopic camera.

TELEVISION SYSTEMS

The existing television systems in use differ according to the country. The USA uses the National Television System Committee (NTSC) system. In European countries, the Phase Alternating Line (PAL) system is in use. There is also a French system called Sequential Color and Memory (SECAM). The broadcasting standards for each are summarized in **Table 2**.

The final image depends upon the number of lines of resolution, scanning lines, pixels, and dot pitch. The number of black and white lines a system can differentiate gives the lines of resolution. These can be horizontal and vertical. Horizontal resolution is the number of vertical lines that can be seen and *vice versa*. Pixels denote the picture elements and they are responsible for picture resolution. The more number of pixels is, the better the resolution. They are represented on the camera chip by an individual photodiode. The restricting factor of information on a scan line is the "dot pitch" that represents phosphorus element size.

The *NTSC system* has certain drawbacks. Not all the lines of resolution are used. The maximum number of lines visible is reduced by 40. Improving the resolution of the camera will not improve monitor resolution. This is due to a fixed vertical resolution. In addition to these problems, if the phase angle is disturbed even a little, it produces unwanted hues.

The *PAL system* is superior in certain aspects. It can overcome this problem by producing alternations over the axis of modulation of the color signed by line. This system also deals with problems of flickering. It involves a process called "interlacing" where odd and even lines in a field are scanned alternatively.

The *SECAM system* is similar to PAL in these aspects, except that the signals are transmitted in sequence.

Formation of the Color Image

Another important aspect one has to keep in mind is the formation of the color image. This is done by superimposing the data for color on the existing black and white picture. The black and white signal is monochromatic signal and combines with the composite color signal. This gives the final color signal.

Luminance (brightness) is delivered by the black and white signal. Chrominance (color) is delivered by the color signal. It is called composite as it contains the three primary color information (RGB). A system that combines luminance and chrominance into one signal is called a compound system.

Color values can be problematic as they can go out of phase. This is due to their high sensitivity. Applying a reference mark for the signal on the scanning line is called as *color burst* and it can prevent this sensitivity. The color on a monitor can be calibrated. This can be done manually by using the standard color bars of NTSC or by using other methods like "blue gun". New monitors do not require this, as calibration can be done automatically.

TABLE 2: Different types of monitor systems.

System	*PAL*	*SECAM*	*NTSC*
Number of lines	625	625	525
Visible lines (maximum)	575	575	486
Field frequency cycles per second (cps)	50	50	60
Frames per second	25	25	30

(NTSC: National Television System Committee; PAL: Phase Alternating Line; SECAM: Sequential Color and Memory)

Monitor Connecting Cables

Images cannot be visualized on the monitor unless they are wired. Monitor cables are of three types. The RGB cable has three wires, one for each primary color. The Y/C cable has two wires, one for the luminance (Y) and one for the chrominance (C) component. The composite cable consists of one pair of wires. An important factor to realize is that no matter what type of cable is used, whether it has better bandwidth or other advantages, the final resolution depends upon the monitor used. For HD and UHD system, we should always use Digital Visual Interface (DVI) or HDMI cable. DVI, which stands for Digital Visual Interface, is the older of the two and arguably on its way out. Functionally, HDMI and DVI cords are basically identical. The DVI video signal is basically the same as HDMI, just without the audio. In laparoscopic surgery, we do not use audio so DVI is used more.

Frames of Reference in Vision

We face many problems with monitors in regard to minimal access surgery. But before dealing with them, a mention of the frames of reference in vision would be apt. NJ Wade's paper on "Frames of Reference in Vision" mentions various frames namely *retinocentric, egocentric, geocentric, and pattern centric.* He applies the set of minimal access surgery and finds a dissociation of pattern centric motion (seen on the monitor) and the area of manipulation. Any visual motor task requires a match between the coordinate systems operating in both vision and motor control. Knowledge of these frames can alter our perspective of the way things happen in minimal access surgery with respect to vision.

Drawbacks with the Monitor

After routine use, we encounter many drawbacks with the monitor. Only a 2D image can be seen on present day monitors. The operative field is represented only by monocular depth cues. Monitor positioning is such that the visual motor axis is disrupted. The monitor distance from the surgeon is also quite far. As a result, the efficiency of the surgeon decreases.

Apart from pictorial depth cues, the picture can be further disturbed by *anticues*. These may originate from the monitor. Glaring effect due to reflection is one of these important anticues.

Imaging Technical Terms

Resolution means the degree of sharpness of a displayed or printed image; simply, the ability of a television or film image to reproduce *fine detail*.

Resolution is defined as (*pixels per inch*) the maximum number of pixels that can be displayed on a screen monitor, expressed as (number of horizontal pixels) × (number of vertical pixels), i.e., 1,024 × 768 pixels. The ratio of horizontal to vertical resolution is usually 4:3, the same as that of conventional television sets.

For *a monitor*, a screen resolution of 1,920 × 1,200 means 1,920 pixels horizontally across each of 1,200 lines, which run vertically from top to bottom.

For *printers and scanners*, resolution is expressed as the number of dots per linear inch [printed *dots per inch (dpi)*]. 300 dpi means 300 × 300 or 90,000 dots per square inch. *Laser printers and plotters* have resolutions from 300 to 1,200 dpi and more whereas most display screens provide <100 dpi **(Figs. 37 and 38)**.

Gain controls the brightness of the image under conditions of low light by recruiting pixels to increase signal strength. Clearly, this step results in some loss of image resolution. This increases light but results in a grainy picture with poorer resolution. It also may create a loss of color accuracy owing to amplification of the noise-to-signal ratio.

The gain should be off at the beginning of a routine procedure (not needed in routine situations). There are two good reasons for this. First, inadequate light at the beginning of the procedure is an indication that a piece of equipment is malfunctioning, a situation that should be rectified before getting too involved with the procedure. Second, the use of "gain" comes at the expense of picture resolution, resulting in a somewhat grainy image on the monitor while turning the brightness knob to maximum produces a very washed-out picture. A good *general rule of thumb* to follow is to look in the right upper quadrant and visualize the space over the liver. The entire dome of the liver and right lateral diaphragm should be well-lit and easily seen. If not, then the lighting system should be evaluated and optimized prior to beginning the dissection **(Figs. 39A and B)**.

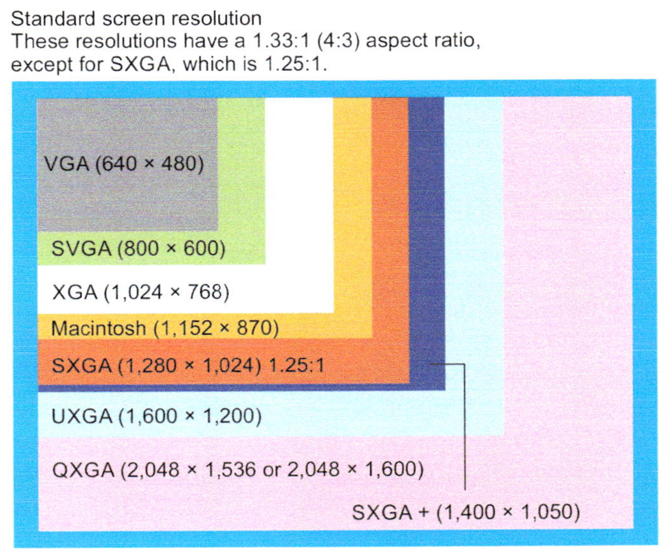

Fig. 37: Standard screen resolution (4:3) aspect ratio, i.e., the height is somewhat approximates to the width.
(QXGA: Quad Extended Graphics Array; SVGA: Super Video Graphics Array; SXGA: Super Extended Graphics Array; UXGA: Ultra Extended Graphics Array; VGA: Video Graphics Array)

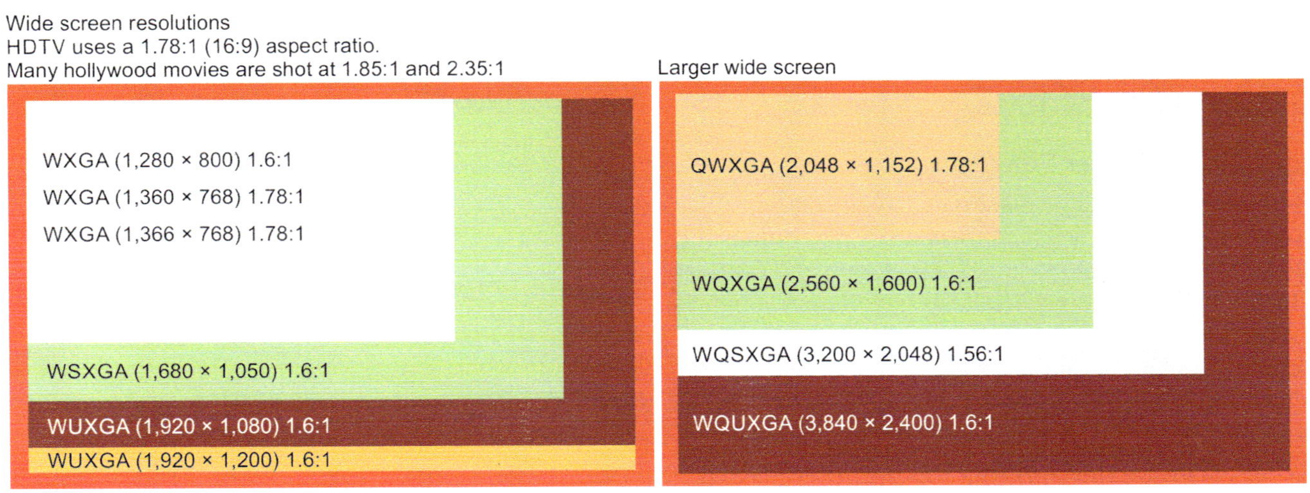

Fig. 38: Wide and larger screen resolution (16:9) aspect ratio, i.e., the width is more than the height.
(QWXGA: Quad Wide Extended Graphics Array; WQSXGA: Wide Quad Super Extended Graphics Array; WQUXGA: Wide Quad Ultra Extended Graphics Array; WSXGA: Wide Super Extended Graphics Array; WUXGA: Wide Ultra Extended Graphics Array; WXGA: Wide Extended Graphics Array)

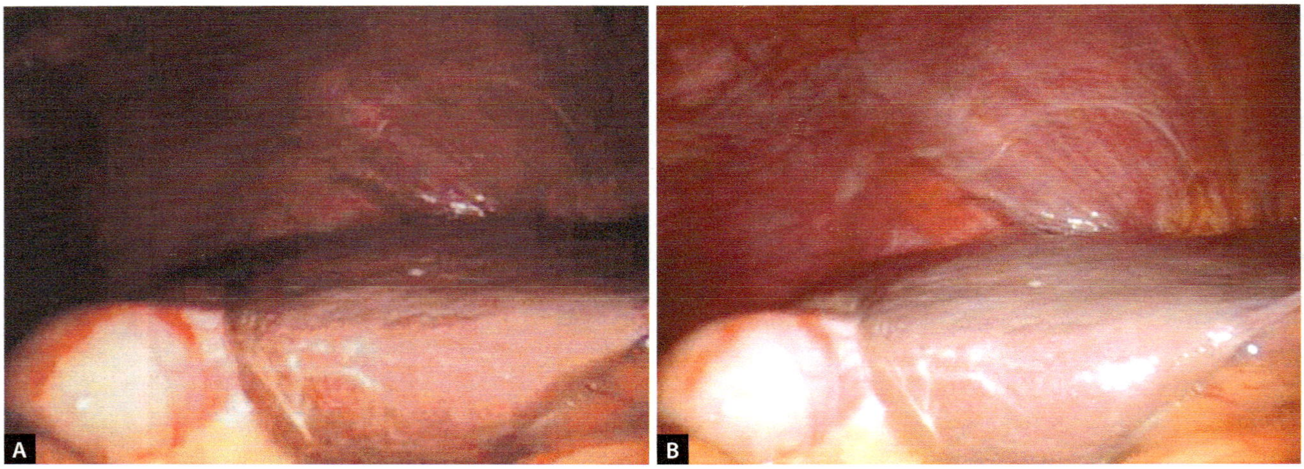

Figs. 39A and B: Gallbladder lighting scene. (A) Poorly lit right upper quadrant. The diaphragm is barely visible; (B) Same patient after faulty light cable is replaced.

Contrast: The extent to which adjacent areas of an optical image, on a monitor screen, differ in brightness. It is the difference in visual properties that makes an object (or its representation in an image) distinguishable from other objects and the background. In visual perception of the real world, contrast is determined by the difference in the color and brightness of the object and other objects within the same field of view. Because the human visual system is more sensitive to contrast than absolute luminescence, we can perceive the world similarly regardless of the huge changes in illumination over the day or from place-to-place **(Fig. 40)**.

Luminescence is a general term applied to all forms of *cool light*, i.e., light emitted by sources other than a hot, incandescent body. It is a process by which an excited material emits light in a process not caused solely by a rise in temperature. The excitation is usually achieved with ultraviolet radiation, X-rays, electrons, alpha particles, electrical fields, or chemical energy. The color or wavelength of the light emitted is determined by the material while the intensity depends on both the material and the input energy. Examples of luminescence include light emissions from neon lamps, luminescent watch dials, television and computer screens, fluorescent lamps, and fireflies.

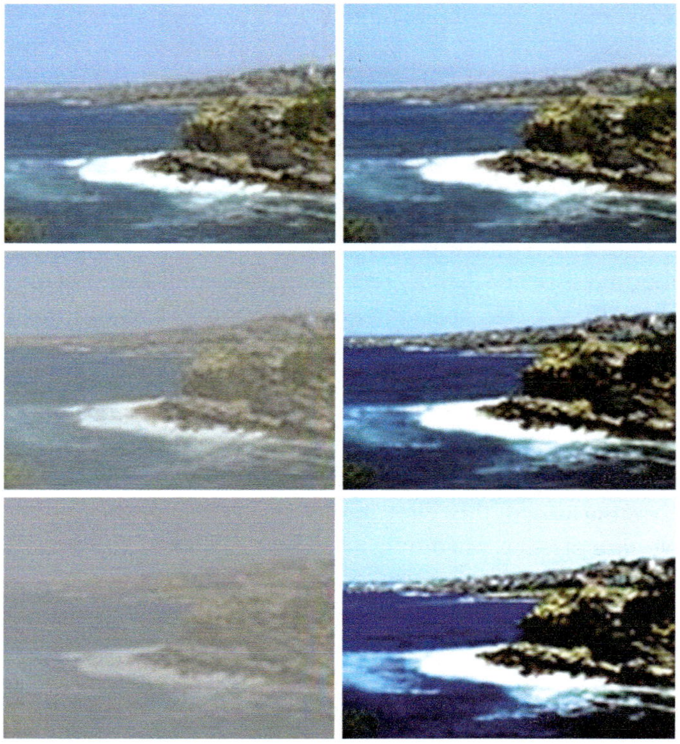

Fig. 40: Changes in the amount of contrast in a photo, left side of the image has low contrast and the right side of the image has higher contrast.

Modulation Transfer Function

The endoscopes transmit resolution and contrast to the monitor. The efficacy by which this occurs determines the more delicate aspects of the image. Resolution and contrast can be measured on an especially designed optical bench and expressed as *modulation transfer function (MTF)*. If there is excessive glare in the picture, then contrast and resolution decrease. Distortions of the image can occur and if these lines seem to curve outward they are called *barrel distortion*. Field curvature occurs when there is improper focus of the center from other parts. *Astigmatism* can occur when some lines of different orientation are present in focus and others are not.

Temporal Aliasing

When a moving object is shown on a monitor, unless the speed with which it is moving is similar to the refresh rate, then jerky movements will occur. This is called temporal aliasing. This can be prevented by the use of filters or by performing slow movements. Fatigue and headache can occur due to disturbance of saccadic eye movements. These are rapid eye movements used to visualize the borders of a field.

Gaze-down Position

When a surgeon has to constantly look in a different direction and operate in another, his efficiency to perform declines. The job becomes even more difficult if the monitor is positioned at a further distance, giving rise to spatial disorientation. A surgeon can perform optimally if he can look and operate in the same direction as in open surgery. This can also be called the gaze-down position.

THREE-DIMENSIONAL VISION

One of the major limitations of minimal access surgery is the loss of depth perception. The surgeon works with an artificial 2D video pictures available on the monitor. There is a need to develop some mechanism to improve depth perception or stereoscopic vision. Stereoscopic vision is needed for precise and fast complex manipulations because perception of space and depth are necessary in surgery.

Stereopsis (Three-dimensional Perception)

Stereopsis refers to perception of 3D shape from any source of depth information. Unlike horses, humans have two eyes located side-by-side in the front of their heads. Due to the close side-by-side positioning, each eye takes a view of the same area from a slightly different angle **(Fig. 41)**.

The two eyes have different views of the visual world and these different views setup disparities that give us information about relative depth of the image that is third dimension of vision. Binocular disparity results when image of an object falls on different areas of the two retinas and binocular vision or stereopsis is impression of depth resulting from differences in the images on these two retinas. We lose stereoscopic vision in laparoscopy because both eyes see same 2D pictures available on the monitor.

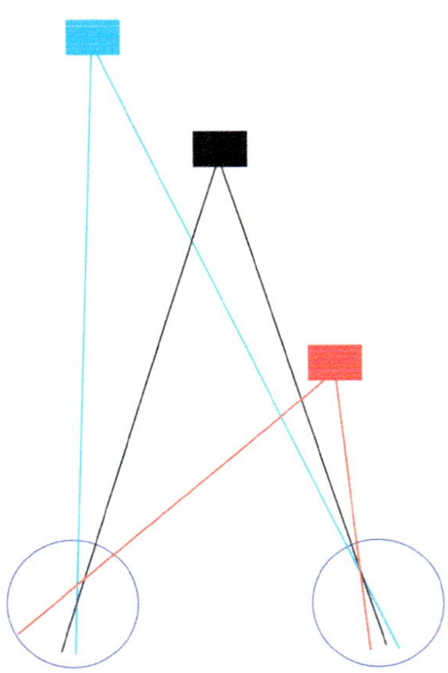

Fig. 41: Difference in angle of light on different retinas.

Stereoscopic vision is simultaneous vision with two eyes (binuclear vision), producing a visual experience of the third-dimension (the depth), i.e., a vivid perception of the relative distances of objects in space. In this experience, the observer seems to see the space between the objects located at different distances from the eyes (the three-dimensions are width, length, and depth).

It is present in normal binocular vision because the two eyes view objects in space from two points, so that the retinal image patterns of the same object points in space are slightly different in the two eyes. The stereoscope, with which different pictures can be presented to each eye, demonstrates the fundamental difference between stereoscopic perception of depth (third-dimension) and the conception of depth and distance from the monocular view.

Humans normally have *binocular vision*, i.e., separate images of the visual field are formed by each eye; the two images fuse to form a single impression. Because each eye forms its own image from a slightly different angle, a stereoscopic effect is obtained and depth, distance, and solidity of an object are appreciated. Stereoscopic color vision is found primarily among the higher primates and it developed fairly late on the evolutionary scale.

Binocular Vision

It refers to vision with two eyes. In binocular vision, the visual axes of the eyes are arranged in such a manner that the images of the object viewed strike the identical portions of the retinas of both eyes. This produces a single stereoscopic image—a view of the world in relief. Binocular vision also makes it possible to determine visually the relative location of objects in space and to judge their distance from each other. When looking with one eye—i.e., with *monocular vision*—the distance of objects can likewise be judged, but not as accurately as with binocular vision.

Physiology of Three-dimensional Vision

Human eye is sensitive to the electromagnetic wavelength between 400 and 700 nm. The "electromagnetic energy" in the range of approximately "400–700 nm", which the human eye can transduce, is called "light". The eyes transduce light energy in the electromagnetic spectrum into nerve impulses.

In 1838, Charles Wheatstone published the first paper on stereopsis entitled "On some remarkable and hitherto unobserved, phenomena of binocular vision". In this, he pointed out that the positional differences in the two eye's images due to their horizontal separation yielded depth information. Prior to this time, the principal problem in the study of binocular vision was "how the world seen as single when we have two different views of it?" People thought that only objects with the same visual directions, falling on corresponding points, would be seen as single, all other points would be double by means of the stereoscope that

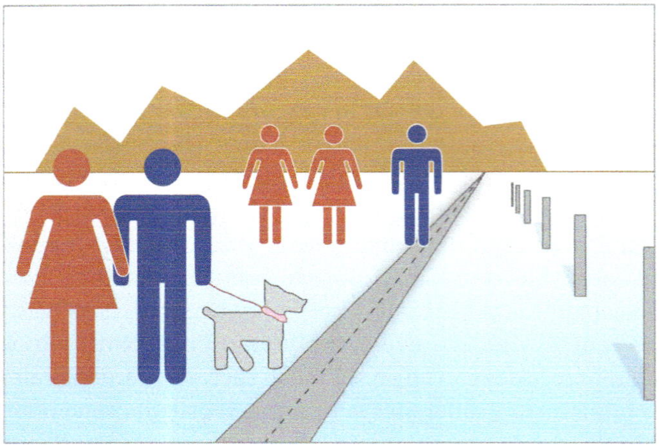

Fig. 42: Different depth cues: The depth cues which are crossed are lost in minimal access surgery.

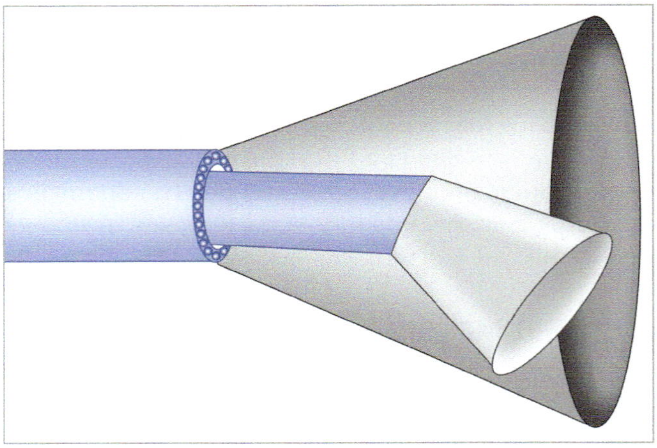

Fig. 43: Shadow telescope by Schurr.

he invented. Wheatstone demonstrated that the stimulation of noncorresponding points yield singleness of vision and results in *the perception of depth.*

Cells in visual cortex are sensitive for binocular vision. Some cells are sensitive for corresponding areas of the left and right retinas and some have sensation for noncorresponding areas of the two retinas. The difference in image on the two retinas of eye is perceived by cortex as *a depth.* Binocular disparity provides the visual system with information concerning the 3D layout of the environment. Recent physiological studies in the primary visual cortex provide a successful account of the mechanisms by which single neurons are able to signal disparity.

Recent studies of visual perception have begun to reveal the connection between neuronal activity in the brain and conscious visual experience. Transcranial magnetic stimulation of the human occipital lobe disrupts the normal perception of objects in ways suggesting that important aspects of visual perception are based on activity in early visual cortical areas. Recordings made with microelectrodes in animals suggest that the perception of the lightness and depth of visual surfaces develops through computations performed across multiple brain areas.

Even though the picture on the monitor is 2D, the operator can assume some depth due to different cues form on ocular vision. This is known as *depth cue* **(Fig. 42)**.

Among the entire depth cue mentioned above, only few monocular are available on the monitor screen. Oculomotor binocular depth cue such as convergence, accommodation, and stereopsis is lost in 2D monitor screen.

Even though the picture is 2D, these depth cues help our brain to interpret a 2D image into virtual 3D feeling. Today, the picture on the screen is 2D but our brain is continuously converting this 2D image in 3D by the help of different monocular depth cues. This conversion of 2D pictures into 3D pictures by brain helps the surgeon to perform a task in laparoscopic surgery.

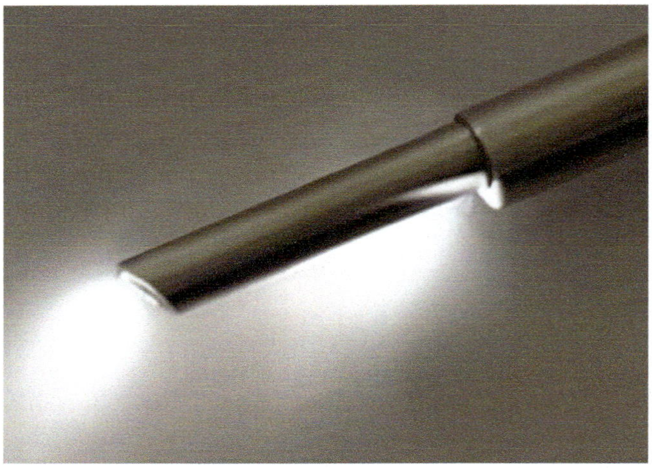

Fig. 44: Shadow telescope of Tübingen University.

A telescope with light delivering through a separate illumination cannula was developed by Schurr in 1996 **(Fig. 43)**.

With slight modification, the section for minimally invasive surgery, University of Tübingen and MGB Endoskopische Geräte GmbH Berlin Company have introduced a new shadow telescope in 1999 **(Fig. 44)**.

Shadow telescope is a rigid 10 mm endoscope with 30° view direction and uses additional illumination fibers ending in an optimized distance behind the front lens. This arrangement of illumination fibers creates a more natural and more plastic appearance, a better balanced contrast, and a well-dosed visible shadow. The shadow gives additional secondary space clues and, therefore, improves orientation and judgment of the 3D properties.

In shadow telescope, angle between the first and second source of illumination is fixed and due to this shadow is also fixed. The second problem with this telescope is that the light which is creating shadow comes from below, but we do not usually experience getting illuminated from the floor. All the light in our day-to-day life is coming from above and most of the time, the shadow we are seeing lies below the object. But in this telescope, the shadow is above the object and so the shadow seems to be unnatural.

INVENTION OF IDEAL SHADOW IN LAPAROSCOPIC SURGERY

The first ideal shadow was introduced in laparoscopic surgery by Dr RK Mishra in the University of Dundee, UK **(Fig. 45)**. This is based on the introduction of one additional light source through a separate port for the generation of natural shadow in minimal access surgery.

Due to the limitations of currently present shadows producing techniques, necessity was felt for development of some newer methods of shadow production. Shadow can play a very powerful role in defining form by giving the object a 3D feel and it is easy to generate. Although shadow is an important depth cue, but too much shadow may cause blurred working field for surgeons and shadow in wrong direction may have adverse effect on the performance of surgeon.

To increase the task performance in minimal access surgery, we recommend certain general rules about shadows. First, light which will cast shadow ideally should come from above. Second, to enhance the task performance with shadow, the contrast of shadow should be mild (22–42%). This useful percentage of contrast can be achieved by equal intensity setting and equal distance of both the light sources from the operating field. Third, too much shadow (>60%) should be avoided because very dark shadow can increase the error rate by interfering with the view of plane of dissection.

THREE-DIMENSIONAL VIDEO SYSTEMS

Three-dimensional Technology Systems

The most commonly used systems depend on rapid time sequential imaging with two cameras and one monitor

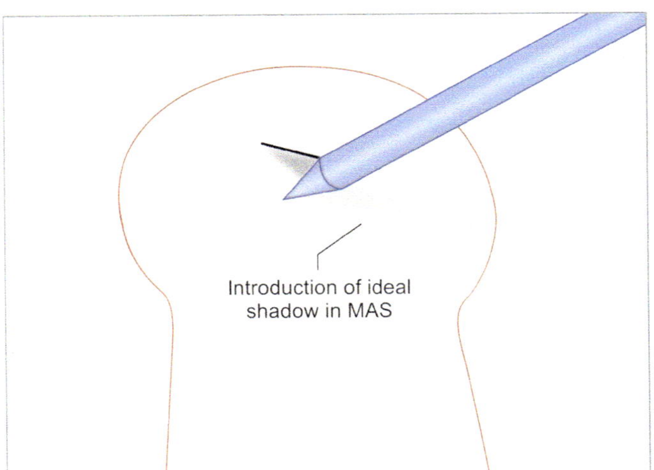

Fig. 45: Shadow in laparoscopy.
(MAS: minimal access surgery)

and are based on the physiological phenomenon of retinal persistence. Both channels alternate (open/close) with sufficient speed (50–60 Hz) to avoid detection of flicker by the human eye. The monitors must therefore have double the frequency (100–120 Hz). Sequential switching between the two eyes is necessary to ensure that the correct image (left and right) falls on the corresponding retina otherwise picture will overlap. This is achieved by wearing special optical glasses that act as alternating shutters to each eye. The current problem with these optical shutters, especially the active battery operated liquid crystal display type shutter is loss of brightness and color degradation. There is no clinically proved evidence that current 3D systems improve performance of laparoscopic surgery.

The current 3D technology is harmful to the surgeon on prolonged use as it gives incorrect depth perception and results in headache and eyestrain.

Another way in which 3D images can be obtained is a mechanism by which the surgeon wears *a polarized glass*. The shutter mechanism is present in the monitor. The final image, however, occurs by the fusion of the two images in the brain. The current 3D systems can only be operated from a very close distance and if placed further will not produce the desired 3D effect.

New Three-dimensional Techniques

With the increasing demands for technological development, many new techniques are currently under trial. These seem to eliminate some of the problems encountered, but only time and repeated use will tell.

Head-mounted display (HMD) is an interesting technique that aims at normalizing the visual-motor axis. It consists of a monitor and the necessary connections mounted to the surgeon's head with the power supply pack attached to the back of the surgeon's shirt. It is not very heavy and also allows the surgeon to view peripherally.

The optical characteristics are:

- Lines of resolution—420 × 320 lines
- Contrast ratio—100:1
- Horizontal field of vision—22°
- Diagonal field—27.5°
- Vertical field—19°.

The surgeon using the display will have to make adjustments to the interpupillary distance, focus, and the distance from his eyes each time. Studies have shown HMD to have certain advantages. It is lightweight, comfortable to position, reduces mental stress, is cheaper than monitor systems, and decreases eyestrain. It allows the surgeon to visualize the operative field directly (the abdomen and ports). The problems, however, are that the picture is granular, definition is not very good, and nausea can occur.

As mentioned before, *the gaze-down position* is said to improve the performance of the surgeon as it brings the alignment between his hands and eyes to normal. This principle has been used in a project called "view-site". This mechanism is used to project the operative field image onto a sterile screen placed on the patient's abdomen close to the original area of surgery. However, it cannot be used for extensive procedures as the image field is small, resolution is not up to the mark, and separation and identification of tissue planes become difficult if bleeding was to occur.

Image display systems are now available which project the image onto a sterile screen overlying the chest of the patient. This aids both cerebral processing of the image and endoscopic manipulations and improves both quality and efficiency of performance **(Fig. 46)**. The limitations of the current "gaze-down" image display systems are diminished resolution and encroachment of the operative field by the sterile screen.

Suspended Image System

An experimental system [*suspended image system (SIS)*] being developed at the University of Dundee and the Central Research Laboratory (EMI) projects the image in air on top of the patient, which means that there is no screen to obstruct the surgeon's movement. This is called the *SIS*. It consists of two components: (1) a high precision retroreflector and (2) a beam splitter. With the help of these, the system can produce images with good resolution and can suspend them on top of the patient in close vicinity to the operative site. The advantages of this method are that there is no distortion, object can be placed anywhere, focal length is not specific, and the image is similar to the original in size. This system is also said to improve the sense of depth, as there are no anticues. Also, the visual-motor axis is correctly aligned for optimal performance.

VISTRAL is a system currently under trial. The advantage of this system is that it does not allow flatness cues to occur in 2D pictures. This improves the sense of depth and it does not require binocular depth cues. It is also said to reduce fatigue and eyestrain. However, this system does not bring about any changes to resolution, brightness, and color.

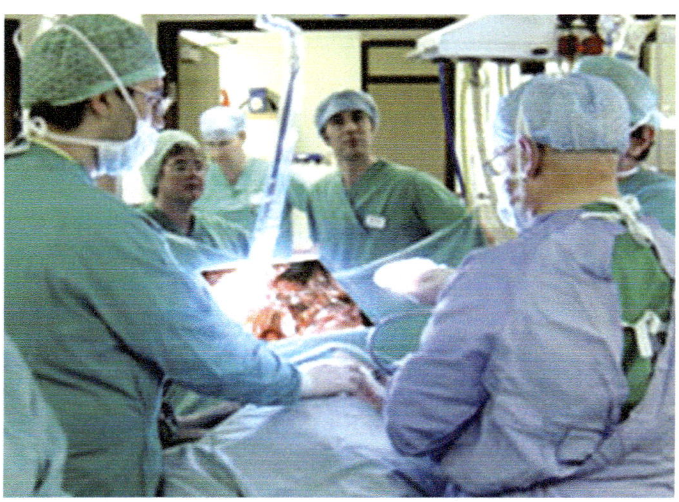

Fig. 46: Projection systems in minimal access surgery.

Augmented reality (AR) is a 3D computer vision technique that is characterized by the real-time fusion of virtual elements on a real space. Currently, AR offers enormous potential in many fields such as education, simulation, architecture, advertising, navigation devices, medicine, and rehabilitation. Minimal access surgery is the branch of medicine where AR has more potential for application. New innovations such as Microsoft HoloLens and the emerging mass market of VR headsets would indicate that these technologies will become familiar to surgeons and inevitability we will find a way to integrate them into our day-to-day practice. The challenge of identifying compelling and valuable experiences for these modalities now begins along with validation of their benefits in all aspects of surgical care. The digital surgical environment is about to drastically change in near future.

Advancement in TV System Technology

High-definition and Ultra-high Definition Television

Another remarkable advancement in technology is the *high-definition television (HDTV) and 4K TV*. It uses component signals, the resolution of the picture is much better, and there are no distortions.

PALplus

The alternatives to HDTV are the PALplus which is an advanced modification of PAL and D2-MAC, HD-MAC which are used for satellite transmissions.

These systems, however, require large amounts of space and can cause problems during transmission. Due to the increased definition, small unwanted movements can be magnified and visual stress can be increased.

Some systems are currently under evaluation and their requirements are given in **Table 3**.

TABLE 3: Different types of TV system.

System	*Japan (NHK/Sony)*	*Europe (EUREKA 95)*	*USA*
Number of lines	1,125	1,250	1,050
Visible lines (92%)	1,035	1,150	966
Pixels per line	1,831	2,035	1,709
Total number of pixels	1,895,085	2,340,250	1,650,894
Field frequency [cycles per second (cps)]	60	50	59
Luminance	20	20	20
Chrominance	7	7	7

BIBLIOGRAPHY

1. Berber E, Pearl JM, Siperstein AE. A simple device for measuring the resolution of videoscopic cameras and laparoscopes in the operating room. Surg Endosc. 2002;16:1111-13.
2. Berci G, Schwaitzberg SD. The importance of understanding the basics of imaging in the era of high-tech endoscopy: Part II. Logic, reality, and utopia. Surg Endosc. 2002;16:1518-22.
3. Bhayani SB, Andriole GL. Three-dimensional (3D) vision: does it improve laparoscopic skills? An assessment of 3D headmounted visualization system. Rev Urol. 2005;7:211-4.
4. Byrn JC, Schluender S, Divino CM, Conrad J, Gurland B, Shlasko E, et al. Three-dimensional imaging improves surgical performance for both novice and experienced operators using the Da Vinci Robot System. Am J Surg. 2007;193:519-22.
5. Chan AC, Chung SC, Yim AP, Lau JY, Ng EK, Li AK. Comparison of two-dimensional vs three-dimensional camera systems in laparoscopic surgery. Surg Endosc. 1997;11:438-40.
6. Ganai S, Seymour NE. VR to OR for camera navigation. In: Westwood JD, Hoffman HM, Robb R, Stredney D (Eds). Medicine Meets Virtual Reality. Amsterdam: IOC Press; 2005. pp. 45-8.
7. Grantcharov TP, Bardram L, Funch-Jensen P, Rosenberg J. Impact of hand dominance, gender, and experience with computer games on performance in virtual reality laparoscopy. Surg Endosc. 2003;17:1082-5.
8. Haluck RS, Gallagher AG, Satava RM, Webster R, Bass TL, Miller CA. Reliability and validity of Endotower, a virtual reality trainer for angled endoscope navigation. Stud Health Technol Inform. 2002;85:179-84.
9. Hanna GB, Cuschieri A. Influence of two-dimensional and three-dimensional imaging on endoscopic bowel suturing. World J Surg. 2000;24:444-9.
10. Hanna GB, Shimi SM, Cuschieri A. Randomized study of the influence of two-dimensional versus three-dimensional imaging on performance of laparoscopic cholecystectomy. Lancet. 1998;351:248-51.
11. Hart SG, Staveland LE. Development of a multi-dimensional workload rating scale: Results of empirical and theoretical research. In: Hancock PA, Meshkati N (Eds). Human Mental Workload. Amsterdam: Elsevier; 1988. pp. 139-83.
12. Herron DM, Lantis JC, Maykel J, Basu C, Schwaitzberg SD. The 3-D monitor and head-mounted display. A quantitative evaluation of advanced laparoscopic viewing technologies. Surg Endosc. 1999;13:751-55.
13. Jones DB, Brewer JD, Soper NJ. The influence of three-dimensional video systems on laparoscopic task performance. Surg Laparosc Endosc. 1996;6:191-7.
14. Korndorffer JR, Hayes DJ, Dunne JB, Sierra R, Touchard CL, Markert RJ, et al. Development and transferability of a cost-effective laparoscopic camera navigation simulator. Surg Endosc. 2005;19:161-7.
15. Korndorffer JR, Stefanidis D, Sierra R, Clayton JL. Validity and reliability of a videotrainer laparoscopic camera navigation simulator. Surg Endosc. 2005;19:S246.
16. McDougall EM, Soble JJ, Wolf JS, Nakada SY, Elashry OM, Clayman RV. Comparison of three-dimensional and two-dimensional laparoscopic video systems. J Endourol. 1996;10:371-4.
17. Mueller MD, Camartin C, Dreher E, Hänggi W. Three-dimensional laparoscopy. Gadget or progress? A randomized trial on the efficacy of three-dimensional laparoscopy. Surg Endosc. 1999;13:469-72.
18. Peitgen K, Walz MV, Walz MV, Holtmann G, Eigler FW. A prospective randomized experimental evaluation of three-dimensional imaging in laparoscopy. Gastrointest Endosc. 1996;44:262-7.
19. Perkins N, Starkes JL, Lee TD, Hutchison C. Learning to use minimal access surgical instruments and two-dimensional remote visual feedback: how difficult is the task for novices? Adv Health Sci Educ Theory Pract. 2002;7:117-31.
20. Schauer PR, Ikramuddin S, Luketich JD. Minilaparoscopy. Semin Laparosc Surg. 1999;6:21-31.
21. Scott DJ, Jones DB. Virtual reality training and teaching tools. In: Soper NJ, Swanstrom LL, Eubanks WS (Eds). Mastery of Endoscopic and Laparoscopic Surgery. Philadelphia: Lippincott Williams and Wilkins; 2005. pp. 146-60.
22. Sun CC, Chiu AW, Chen KK, Chang LS. Assessment of a three-dimensional operating system with skill tests in a pelvic trainer. Urol Int. 2000;64:154-8.
23. Taffinder N, Smith SG, Huber J, Russell RC, Darzi A. The effect of a second-generation 3D endoscope on the laparoscopic precision of novices and experienced surgeons. Surg Endosc. 1999;13:1087-92.
24. Thomsen MN, Lang RD. An experimental comparison of three-dimensional and two-dimensional endoscopic systems in a model. Arthroscopy. 2004;20:419-23.
25. Wickens CD, Hollands J. Engineering Psychology and Human Performance. New Jersey: Prentice Hall; 2000. pp. 11-64.

CHAPTER 3

Laparoscopic Equipment and Instruments

INSUFFLATION SYSTEM

Laproflattor

The electronic carbon dioxide (CO_2) laproflattor is a general-purpose insufflation unit for use in laparoscopic examinations and operations **(Fig. 1)**.

Controlled pressure insufflation of the peritoneal cavity is used to achieve the necessary work space for laparoscopic surgery by distending the anterolateral abdominal wall and depressing the hollow organs and soft tissues. CO_2 is the preferred gas because it does not support combustion. It is very soluble which reduces the risk of gas embolism, and is cheap. Automatic insufflators allow the surgeon to preset the insufflating pressure, and the device supplies gas until the required intra-abdominal pressure (IAP) is reached. The insufflator activates and delivers gas automatically when the IAP falls because of gas escape or leakage from the ports. The required values for pressure and flow can be obtained using jog keys and digital displays. Insufflation pressure can be continuously varied from 0 to 30 mm Hg; total gas flow rate and volumes can be set to any value in the range 0–45 L/min.

Patient safety is ensured by optical and acoustic alarms as well as several mutually independent safety circuits. The detail function and quadromanometric indicators of insufflator is important to understand safety point of view. The important indicators of insufflators are preset pressure, actual pressure, flow rate, and total gas used.

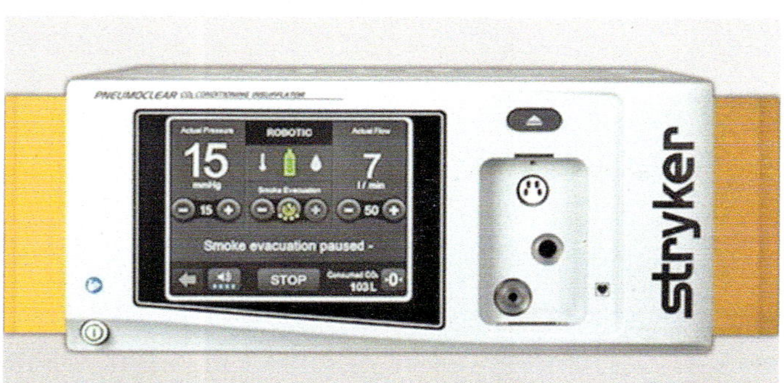

Fig. 1: Insufflator.

Quadromanometric Indicators

Quadromanometric indicators are the four important readings of insufflator. The insufflator is used to monitor:

1. Preset insufflation pressure
2. Actual pressure
3. Gas flow rate
4. Volume of gas consumed

Preset Insufflation Pressure

This is the pressure adjusted by surgeon before starting insufflation. This is the command given by surgeon to insufflator to keep IAP at this level.

The preset pressure ideally should be 12–15 mm Hg. In any circumstance, it should not be more than 18 mm Hg in laparoscopic surgery. However, in extraperitoneal surgery preset pressure can be more than 18 mm Hg. The good quality microprocessor-controlled insufflator always keeps IAP at preset pressure. Whenever IAP decreases due to leak of gas outside, insufflator eject some gas inside to maintain the pressure equal to preset pressure and if IAP increases due to external pressure, insufflator sucks some gas from abdominal cavity to again maintain the pressure to preset pressure.

When surgeon or gynecologist wants to perform diagnostic laparoscopy under local anesthesia, the preset pressure should be set to 8 mm Hg. In some special situation of axilloscopy or arthroscopy, we need to have pressure >19 mm Hg.

Actual Pressure

This is the actual IAP sensed by insufflator. When Veress needle is attached, there is some error in actual pressure reading because of resistance of flow of gas through small caliber of Veress needle. Since continuous flow of insufflating gas through Veress needle usually gives extra 4–8 mm Hg of measured pressure by insufflator, the true IAP can actually be determined by switching the flow from insufflator off for a moment. Many microprocessor-controlled good quality insufflator delivers pulsatile flow of gas when Veress needle is connected, in which the low reading of actual pressure measures the true IAP.

If there is any major gas leak, actual pressure will be less and insufflator will try to maintain the pressure by ejecting gas through its full capacity.

Actual pressure if >20–25 mm Hg has following disadvantage over hemodynamic status of patient:

- Decrease venous return due to vena caval compression leading to:
  - Increased chance of deep vein thrombosis (DVT) of calf
  - Hidden cardiac ischemia can precipitate due to decrease cardiac output
- Decrease tidal volume due to diaphragmatic excursion
- Increase risk of air embolism due to venous intravasation
- Increased risk of surgical emphysema
- Decreased renal perfusion.

Flow Rate

This reflects the rate of flow of CO_2 though the tubing of insufflator. When Veress needle is attached, the flow rate should be adjusted for 1 L/min. Experiment was performed over animal in which direct intravenous (IV) CO_2 was administered and it was found that risk of air embolism is less if rate is within 1 L/min. At the time of access using Veress needle technique, sometime Veress needle may be inadvertently enter inside a vessel but if the flow rate is 1 L/min there is less chance of serious complication. When initial pneumoperitoneum is achieved and cannula is inside abdominal cavity, the insufflators flow rate may be set at maximum, to compensate loss of CO_2 due to use of suction irrigation instrument. This should be remembered that if insufflator is set to its maximum flow rate then also it will allow flow only if the actual pressure is less than preset pressure otherwise it will not pump any gas. Some surgeon keeps initial flow rate with Veress needle to 1 L/min and as soon as they confirm that gas is going satisfactorily inside the abdominal cavity (percussion examination and seeing obliteration of liver dullness) then they increases flow rate. No matter how much flow rate you set for Veress needle, the eye of normal caliber Veress needle can give way CO_2 flow at maximum 2.5 L/min. When the flow of CO_2 is >7 L/min inside the abdominal cavity through cannula, there is always a risk of hypothermia to patient. To avoid hypothermia in all modern microprocessor-controlled laproflattor, there is electronic heating system which maintains the temperature of CO_2.

Total Gas Used

This is the fourth indicator of insufflator. Normal size human abdominal cavity needs 1.5 L CO_2 to achieve intra-abdominal actual pressure of 12 mm Hg. In some big size abdominal cavity and in multipara patients, sometime we need 3 L of CO_2 (rarely 5–6 L) to get desired pressure of 12 mm Hg. Whenever there is less or more amount of gas is used to inflate a normal abdominal cavity, surgeon should suspect some errors in pneumoperitoneum technique. These errors may be leak or may be preperitoneal space creation or extravasations of gas. The detail principles and techniques of safe access are discussed in Chapter 6: Abdominal Access Techniques.

SUCTION/IRRIGATION SYSTEM

It is used for flushing the abdominal cavity and cleaning during endoscopic operative intrusions **(Fig. 2)**.

It has been designed for use with the 26173 AR suction/ instillation tube. Its electrically driven pressure/suction pump is protected against entry of bodily secretions. The suction irrigation machine is used frequently at the time of laparoscopy to make the field of vision clear. Most of the surgeons use normal saline or Ringer's lactate for irrigation purposes. Sometime heparinized saline is used to dissolve blood clot to facilitate proper suction in case of excessive intra-abdominal bleeding.

Irrigation and Suction Tubes

A suction-irrigation probe can be a versatile instrument. Laparoscopic suction and irrigation tube is one of the very important instruments which surgeon should practice frequently **(Fig. 3)**. Vision is one of the limitations of laparoscopic surgery. The blood is the darkest color inside abdominal cavity and excess of blood inside absorbs most of the light. Whenever there is bleeding, one should first try to suck it out. Controlled suction and irrigation enhance the observation and improve operative technique. Suction and

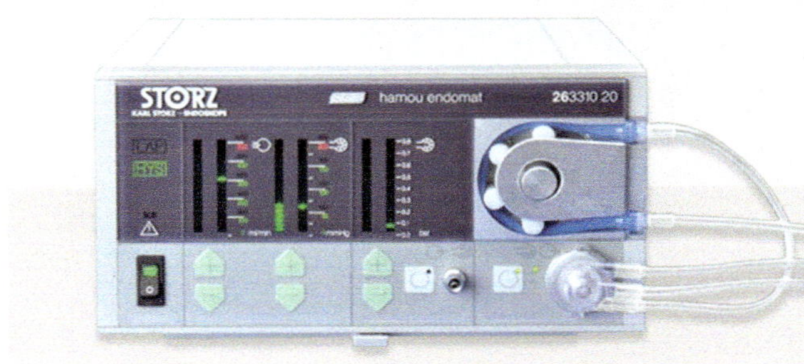

Fig. 2: Laparoscopic suction irrigation machine.

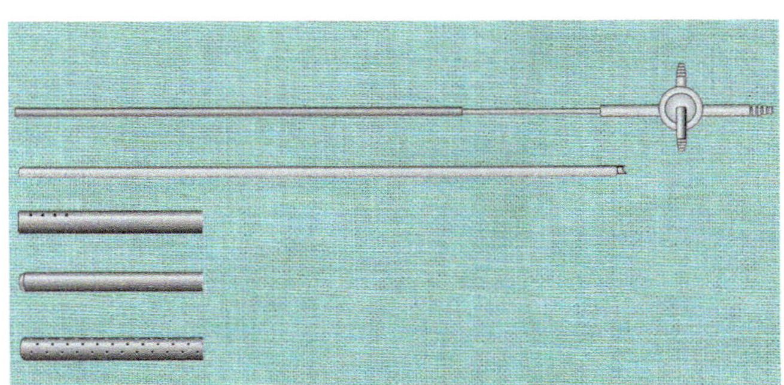

Fig. 3: Laparoscopic irrigation and suction tubes.

irrigation tube also can be used for blunt dissection. At the time of using suction and irrigation, the tip of the suction irrigation cannula should be dipped inside blood, otherwise the gas will be sucked and surgeon will lose his vision due to loss of pneumoperitoneum. 10-mm suction tube should be used if there is >1,500 mL of hemoperitoneum or if there is blood clots inside the abdominal cavity. Sometime small spilled stones can also be sucked with the help of laparoscopic irrigation suction tube at the time of laparoscopic cholecystectomy. It is very useful instrument for doing peritoneal toilet in case of appendicular or duodenal perforation.

ENERGY SOURCE SYSTEM

Electrosurgery is the use of radiofrequency alternating current to cut and coagulate tissues. It has proven a major advance in surgery by minimizing blood lose, reducing operative time, and providing a clear and clean surgical field without the need to tie off all blood vessels.

In laparoscopy, cutting and the establishment of hemostasis forms the core of laparoscopic surgery. For a laparoscopic hernia repair, both monopolar and bipolar modes are required.

Coagulating and Dissecting Electrodes

Spatula and hook are the main electrodes used for monopolar cutting and coagulation **(Fig. 4)**.

Spatula is either "W" shaped or blunt. Hooks are also of various shapes, e.g., "L" shaped, "J" shaped or "U" shaped **(Fig. 5)**.

Hooks are simple instrument whose distal tip can vary slightly. They must be insulated along the entire length because they are used with the monopolar current. The hook with ceramic cone protecting the distal end is available which protects efficiently against current diffusion **(Fig. 6)**.

Some ball-shaped, barrel-shaped or straight coagulation electrodes are also available to achieve proper hemostasis. These blunt electrodes are particularly useful when there is generalized oozing of blood and surgeon cannot see specific bleeder point, e.g., bleeding from the gallbladder bed at the time of laparoscopic cholecystectomy. These blunt electrosurgical instruments are also used for fulguration at the time of ablation of endometriosis.

Bipolar Forceps

Bipolar forceps are one of the very important electrosurgical instruments in minimal access surgery **(Fig. 7)**.

It is safer than monopolar instruments because electron travels only through the tissue held between the jaw and patient's body is not a part of circuit. Both the jaws of bipolar are insulated and the patient return plate is not necessary to be attached **(Fig. 8)**.

The detailed principle of electrosurgery is discussed later in laparoscopic dissection techniques.

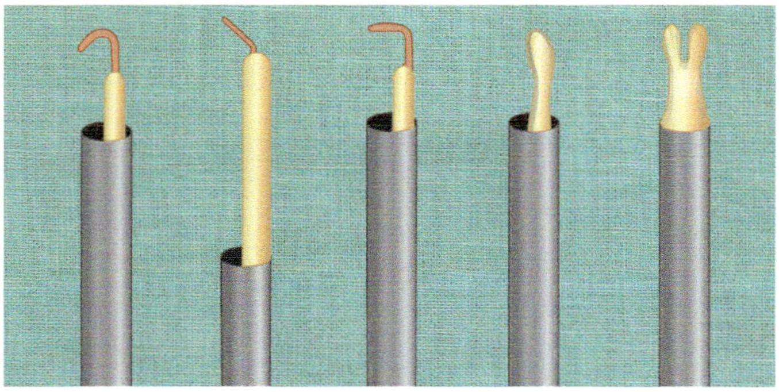

Fig. 4: Spatula.

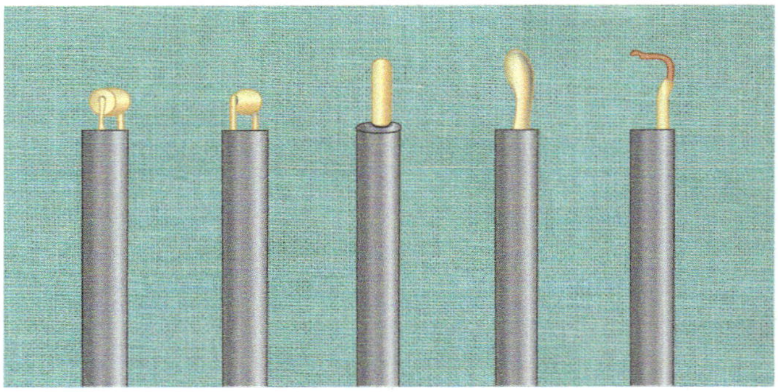

Fig. 5: Various types of hooks.

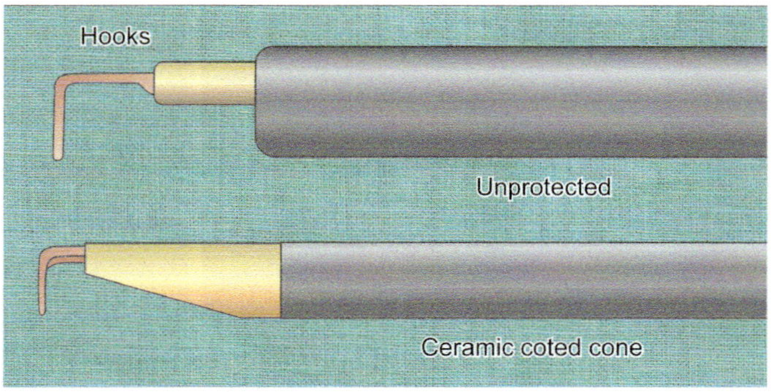

Fig. 6: Ceramic coating of hook.

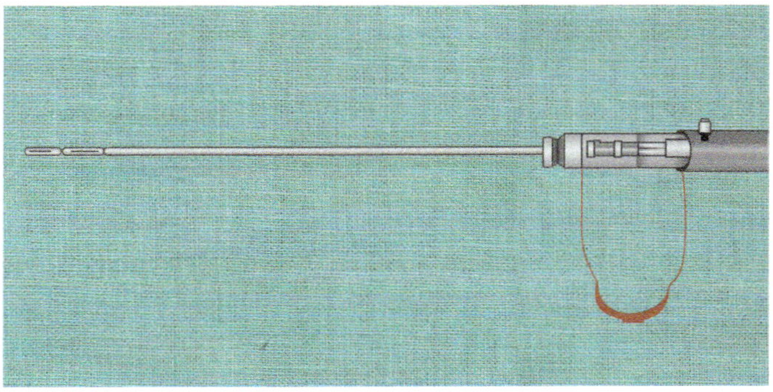

Fig. 7: Bipolar forceps.

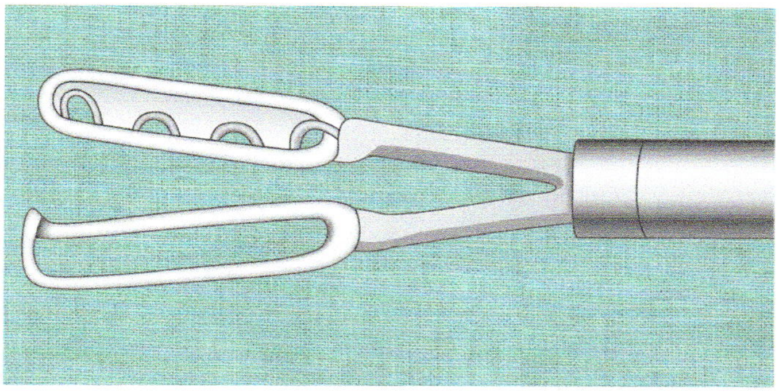

Fig. 8: Jaw of bipolar forceps.

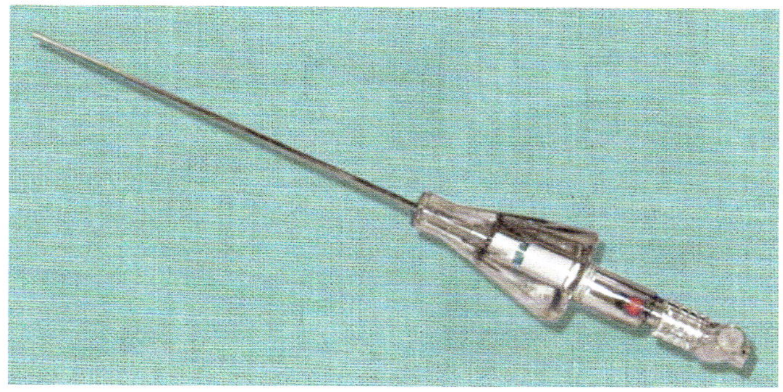

Fig. 9: Veress needle.

LAPAROSCOPIC WORKING INSTRUMENT

Disposable or Reusable Instrument

Several factors should be considered at the time of choosing laparoscopic instrument, including cost, availability, and reliability. Reusable instruments are expensive initially but in long run they are cost-effective. The cost of disposable instruments is less compared to reusable but patient cost is increased. In developing countries, disposable instruments are very rarely used because labor cost is low compare to the cost of disposable instrument. In Europe and the United States of America, surgeons often choose to use disposable instrument in order to save high labor cost. The main advantage of disposable instrument is high performance due to its sharpness and reduced chance of disease transmission due to certified high-end factory sterilization. However, once discarded, environment concerns are raised about disposal and biodegradability of disposable instruments. Ideally, disposable instrument should not be used repeatedly because handling, sorting, storing, and sterilization make these instruments questionable. The disposable instruments are not sterilized properly by dipping in glutaraldehyde because they are not dismountable. Insulation of disposable instrument also can be torn easily which can lead to electrosurgical injuries.

Insufflation Cannulas

Veress Needle

Veress needle was invented by a chest physician for aspiration of pleural effusion keeping in mind that its spring mechanism and blunt tip will prevent the injury of lung tissue **(Fig. 9)**.

Veress needle consists of an outer cannula with a beveled needle point for cutting through tissues. Inside the cannula is an inner stylet, which is loaded with a spring that "springs forward" in response to the sudden decrease in pressure encountered upon crossing the abdominal wall and entering the peritoneal cavity. The lateral hole on this stylet enables CO_2 gas to be delivered intra-abdominally.

Veress needle is used for creating initial pneumoperitoneum so that the trocar can enter safely and the distance of abdominal wall from the abdominal viscera should increase. Veress needle technique is the most widely practiced way of access. Before using Veress needle every time, it should be checked for its potency and spring action. Veress needle is available in three length 80 mm, 100 mm, and 120 mm. In obese patient 120 mm and in very thin patient with scaphoid abdomen 80 mm Veress needle should be used. Veress needle should be held like a dart at the time of insertion.

Hasson Cannula

In an effort to decrease the incidence of injuries associated with the blind access of the peritoneal cavity with the Veress needle and the initial trocar, Hassan proposed a blunt (open) minilaparotomy access. He develops a reusable device of similar design to a standard cannula but attached an olive-shaped cone (sleeve) **(Fig. 10)**.

This cone would slide up and down the shaft of the cannula and would form an airtight seal at the fascial opening. In addition, the sharp trocar was replaced by a blunt obturator. This cannula is held in place by the use of stay sutures passed through the fascial edges and attached to the body of the cannula **(Fig. 11)**.

The reason the olive sleeve is designed to slide up and down the shaft of the cannula is to allow for variations in abdominal wall thickness. The tension provided by the fascial sutures when attached to the device serves to create a seal to prevent gas leakage. To adjust the length of the cannula within the abdominal wall, the fascial sutures require detachment from the device, adjustment of the olive sleeve and reattachment of the sutures.

Several disposable open-access devices have been released. They are similar to the reusable system originally described by Hasson except that the stay sutures are attached directly to the olive, allowing manipulation of the cannula depth without detaching the stay sutures. The basic method of peritoneal access, however, has remained the same.

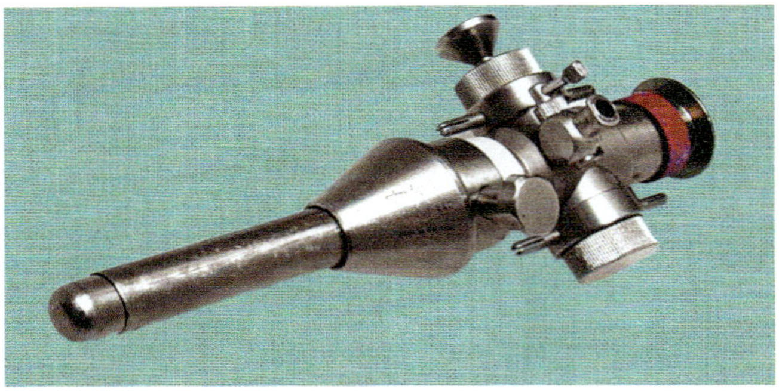

Fig. 10: Hasson trocar and cannula.

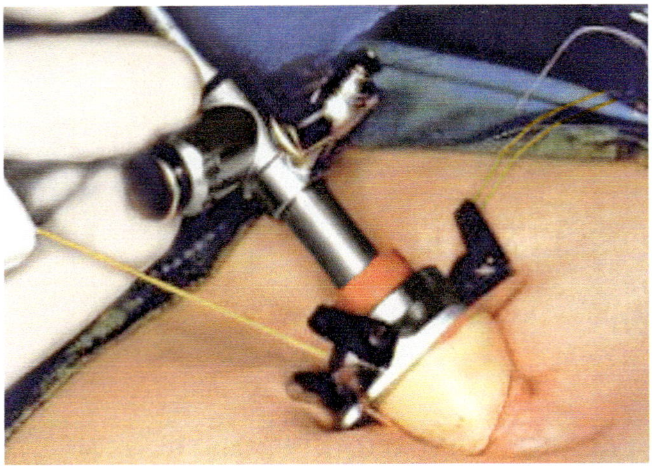

Fig. 11: Hasson cannula in proper position.

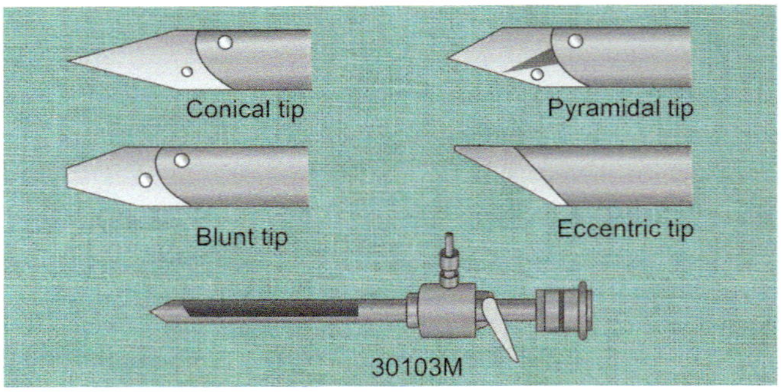

Fig. 12: Tip of the trocar.

PORT ACCESS INSTRUMENT

Trocar and Cannula

The word "trocar" is usually used to refer to the entire assembly but actual trocar is a stylet which is introduced through the cannula. The trocars are available with different types of tips. The cutting tips of these trocars are either in the shape of a three-edged pyramid or a flat two-edged blade.

Conical-tipped trocars are supposed to be less traumatic to the tissue. The tip can be penetrated through the parietal wall without cutting and decreased risk of herniation or hemorrhage is reported.

Cannulas are in general made from plastic or metal. Plastic devices whether they are transparent or opaque, need to be designed in such a way as to minimize the reflection of light from the telescope. Reusable and disposable trocars are constructed by a combination of metal and plastic. The tip of disposable trocar has a two-edged blade. These are very effective at penetrating the abdominal wall by cutting the tissue as they pass through. Most of the disposable plastic trocars have spring-loaded mechanism that withdraws the sharp tip immediately after it passes through the abdominal wall to reduce the incidence of injury of viscera. Trocar and cannula are of different sizes and diameter depending upon the instrument for which it is used. The diameter of cannula ranges from 3 to 30 mm; the most common size is 5 mm and 10 mm. The metal trocar has different types of tips, i.e., pyramidal tip, eccentric tip, conical tip or blunt tip depending on the surgeon's experience **(Fig. 12)**.

All the cannulas have valve mechanism at the top **(Figs. 13A and B)**.

Valves of cannula provide internal air seals, which allow instruments to move in and out within cannula without the loss of pneumoperitoneum. These valves can be oblique, transverse, or in piston configuration.

These valves can be manually or automatically retractable during instrument passage. Trumpet type valves are also present which provide excellent seals, but they are not as practical as some of the other systems. They require both hands during instrument insertion, which may explain why they are less often used in advanced laparoscopic cases. The flexible valves limit the leakage of CO_2 during work whatever the diameter of the instrument used.

It should be remembered that sharp trocars although looking dangerous are actually better than blunt one because they need less force to introduce inside the abdominal cavity and chances of inadvertent forceful entry of full length of trocar are less. There is always a difference in the marked exterior diameter of the cannula and the interior usable diameter. The end of the cannula is either straight or oblique. An oblique tip is felt to facilitate the easy passage of the trocar through the abdominal wall.

Trocar and cannula should be held in proper way in hand so that head of the trocar should rest on the thenar eminence, the middle finger should rest over the gas inlet and index finger is pointed toward the sharp end of the trocar.

Visiport

The Visiport is a kind of optical trocars which is a disposable and expendable visual entry tool which includes a cannula and hollow trocar with cutting blade at tip **(Fig. 14)**. It is applied after insufflation of CO_2 in the abdomen. This technique of inserting Visiport is palmed via surgeon's hand and maintained perpendicular to distend patient's CO_2 to abdomen. When accurate anatomical status of trocar tip

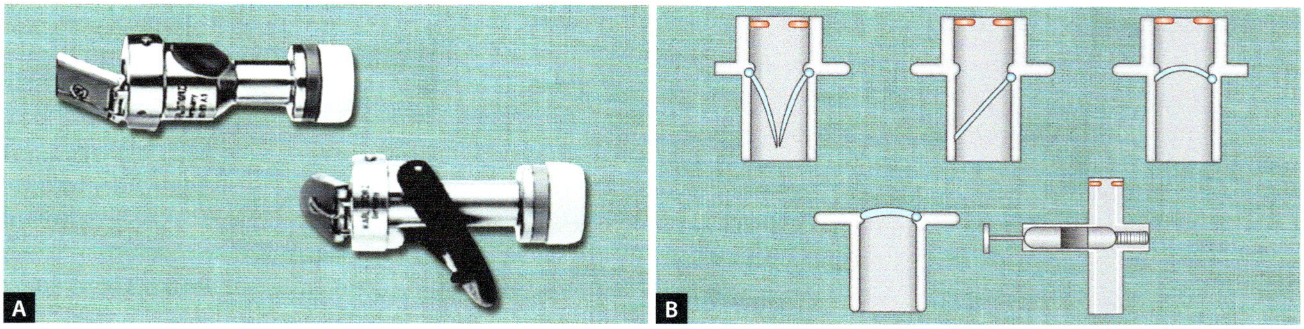

Figs. 13A and B: (A) Different valve mechanism of cannula; (B) Different valve mechanism of cannula (internal view).

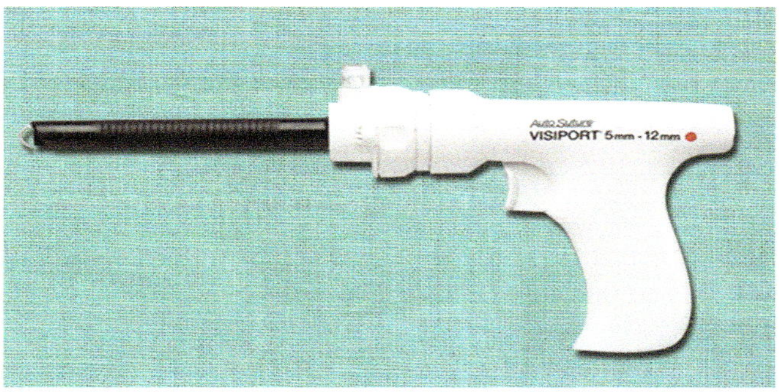

Fig. 14: Visiport.

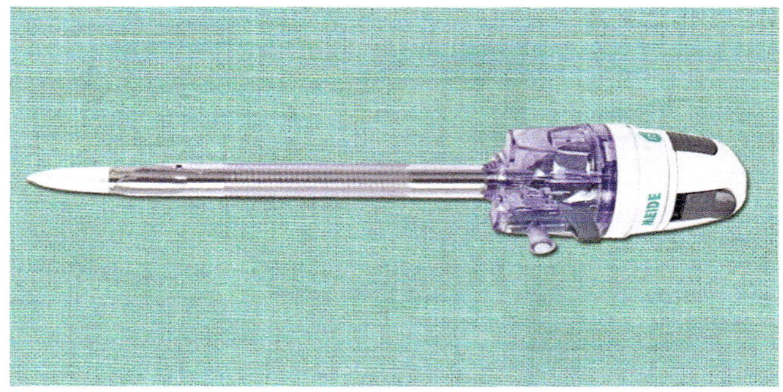

Fig. 15: Bladeless optical trocar.

is checked by visualization of layers of abdominal wall on monitor, downward axial pressure is used and activated to trigger cutting blade. Downward pressure causes trocar to advance optical bladed tip and its situation is checked again and again seeing on the monitor. These sequences are repeated till the peritoneal cavity is arrived. This is not fired till the accurate anatomical status of trocar tip is known. However, none of the laparoscopic entry methods have distinct superiority over other. On the other words, Visiport technique is also associated with abundant complication. Visiport optical trocar technique is faster for initial trocar placement than Hasson technique. However, it is associated with complications compared to open Hasson technique. Therefore, there is benefit with respect to speed for initial trocar placement and harm based on complications of sharp cutting blade in Visiport trocar system.

Bladeless Optical Trocar

There are many single-use bladeless optical trocar systems available which provide a versatile, operationally flexible, and unique mode of entry into the abdominal cavity for any laparoscopic procedure **(Fig. 15)**. The distinctively engineered visual tip greatly reduces wound defect size as well as insertion force into the abdominal cavity. Injuries due to blind entry and a sharp blade are virtually eliminated with the use of bladeless optical tip trocar system. The optical tip provides direct visualization of the various tissue layers when accompanied by a laparoscope during insertion. Because the bladeless tip separates and dissects without cutting, trauma to the abdominal wall and vessels are minimized.

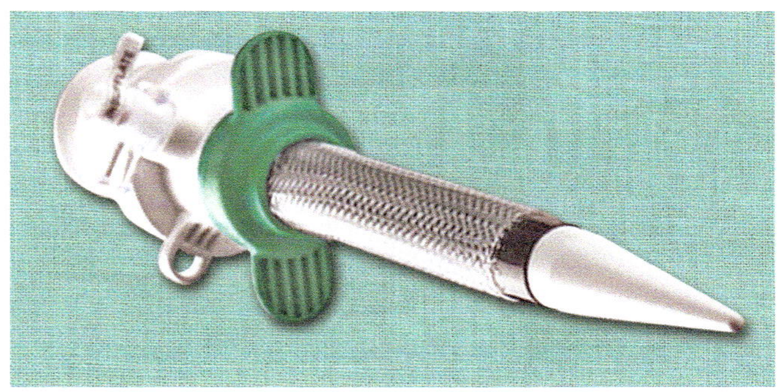

Fig. 16: Step radially expanding trocar.

Step Trocar

Step radially expanding technology allows the VersaStep bladeless trocars to yield smaller fascial defects for an equivalent cannula size compared to conventional bladed trocars. The VersaStep bladeless trocars use Step radial dilation technology. The VersaStep system can be found in a 70 mm, 110 mm or 150 mm working length and can be 5 mm, 11 mm, 12 mm or 15 mm in diameter. The trocars are designed to keep fascial issues from being a threat. It can keep gas completely airtight within the abdominal cavity and can help allow instruments from 4.5 mm, 12 mm or 15 mm to be exchanged as needed. In this technology initially less diameter trocar is introduced which is stretchable. Over this stretchable cannula again desired diameter of trocar is pushed to radially dilate the abdominal port wound. This results in less chance of hernia. This trocar system is strictly disposable and cannot be used second time as outer sheath breaks after single use **(Fig. 16)**.

LAPAROSCOPIC HAND INSTRUMENTS

Laparoscopic hand instruments vary in diameter from 1.8 to 12 mm but majority of instruments are designed to pass through 5–10 mm of cannula. The hand instruments used in laparoscopic surgery are of different length (varies company-to-company and length of laparoscopic instrument varies from 18 to 45 cm) but they are ergonomically convenient to work if they have same length of approximately 36 cm in adult and 28 cm in pediatric practice. Shorter instruments 18–25 cm are adapted for cervical and pediatric surgery. Certain procedures for adult can also be performed with shorter instruments where the space is constricted. 45-cm instruments are used in obese or very tall patients. For better ergonomics, half of the instruments should be inside the abdomen and half outside. If half of the instrument is in and half out, it behaves like class 1 lever and it stabilizes the port nicely so the surgery will be convenient.

Most of the laparoscopic procedures require a mixture of sharp and blunt dissection techniques, often using the same instrument in a number of different ways. Many laparoscopic instruments are available in both reusable and disposable version **(Figs. 17A to C)**.

Most reusable instruments are partially dismountable so that it can be cleaned and washed properly. Some manufacturers have produced modular system where part of the instrument can be changed to suit the surgeon's favorite attachment like handle or working tip.

Most laparoscopic instruments such as graspers and scissors have basic opening and closing function **(Figs. 18A and B)**. Many instrument manufacturers during past few years are able to rotate at 360° angle which increases the degree of freedom of these instruments **(Fig. 19)**.

Certain types of instrument offer angulations at their tip in addition to usual 4° of freedom. These instruments are

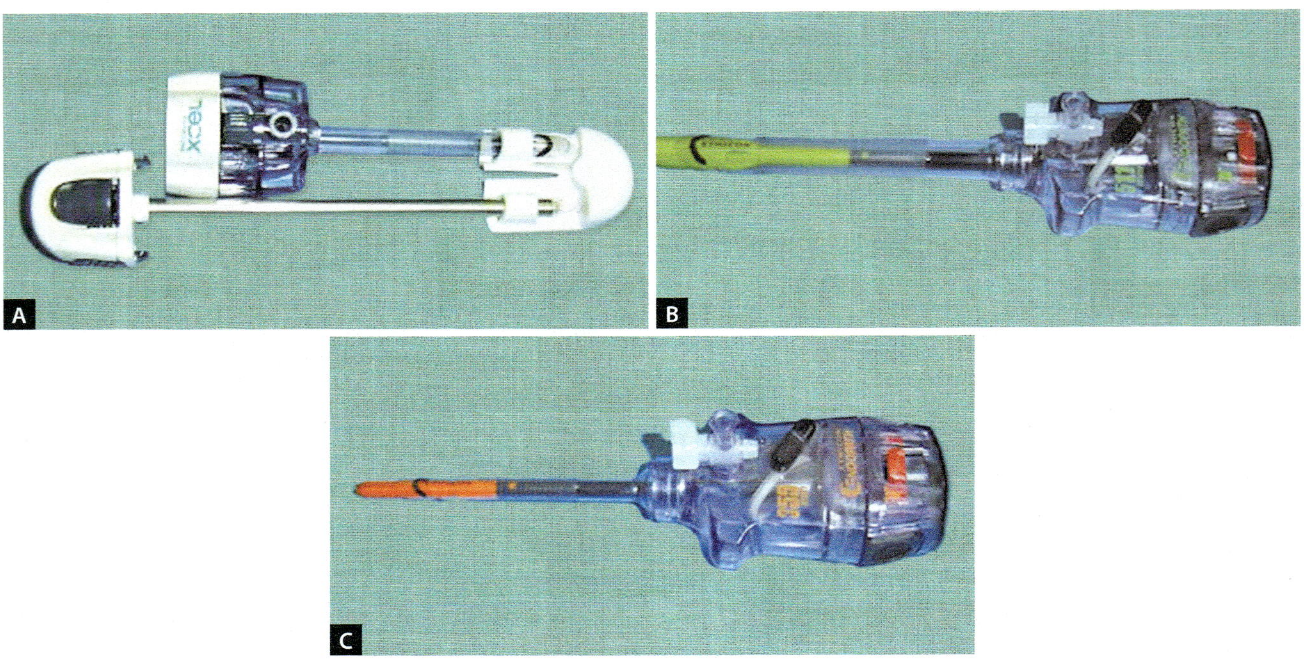

Figs. 17A to C: (A) Disposable trocar and cannula; (B and C) Disposable trocar and cannula (another view).

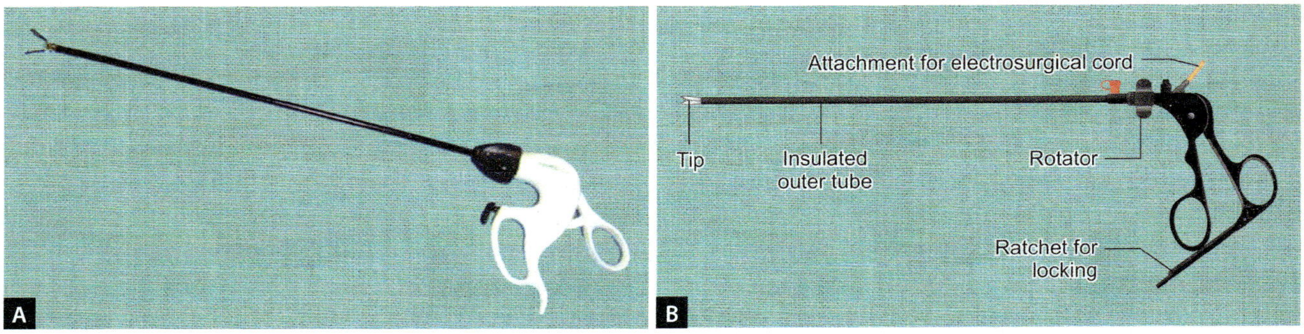

Figs. 18A and B: (A) Disposable grasper; (B) Reusable graspers.

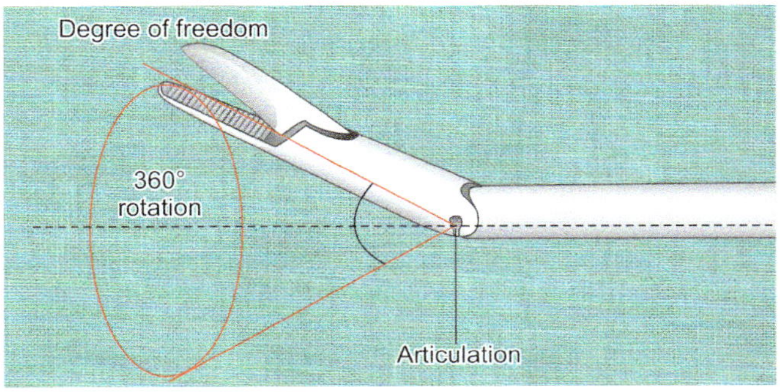

Fig. 19: Articulation of hand instrument.

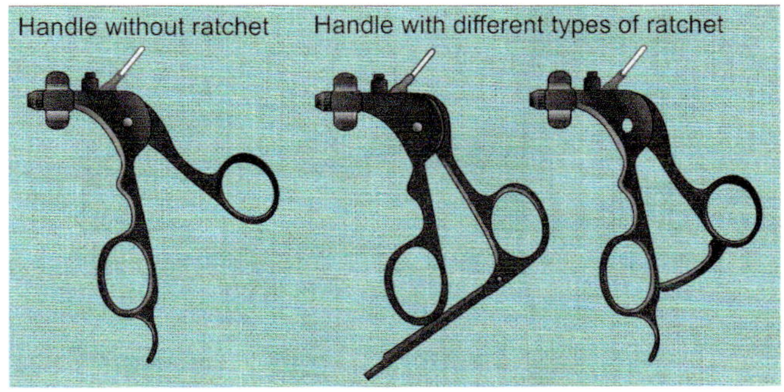

Fig. 20: Different types of handle of hand instrument.

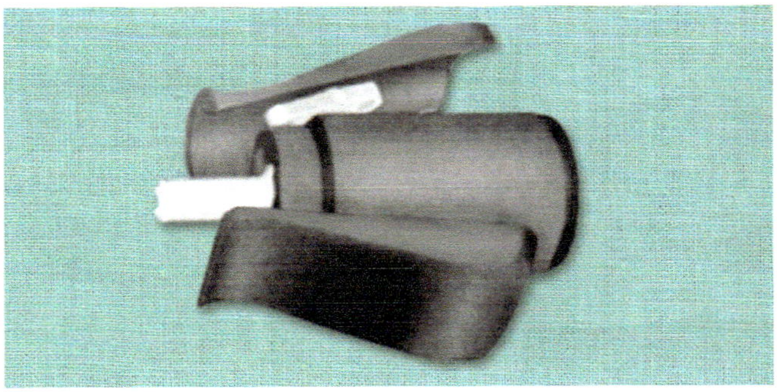

Fig. 21: Cuschieri ball handle.

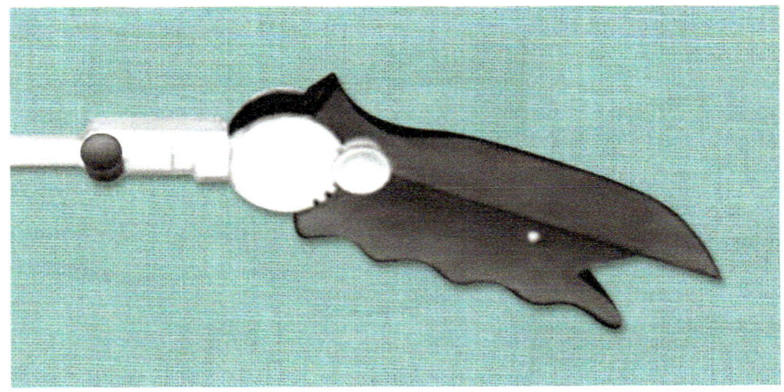

Fig. 22: Cuschieri pencil handle.

used to avoid obstacles and for the lateral grasping when the instrument is placed outside of the visual field. This feature is available for both reusable as well as disposable instrument. The complex mechanism of such instrument makes their sterilization very difficult.

A variety of instruments, especially retractors have been developed with multiple articulations along the shaft. When these are fixed with the tightened cable, the instrument assumes a rigid shape which could not have been introduced through the cannula.

Most of the hand instruments haves three detachable parts:

1. Handle
2. Insulated outer tube
3. Insert which makes the tip of the instrument.

Different Handles of Hand Instrument

Certain instrument handles are designed to allow locking of the jaw **(Fig. 20)**.

This can be very useful when the tissue needs to be grasped firmly for long period of time preventing the surgeon's hand from getting fatigue. The locking mechanism is usually incorporated into the handle so that surgeon can easily lock or release the jaws. These systems usually have a ratchet so that the jaws can be closed in different position and to different pressure. Most of the laparoscopic instrument handles have attachments for unipolar electrosurgical lead and many have rotator mechanism to rotate the tip of the instrument.

Some multifunctional laparoscopic handles have attachment for suction and irrigation and sometime hand switch for cutting and coagulation switch of electrosurgery. Cuschieri ball handle, invented by Professor Sir Alfred Cuschieri, lies comfortably in surgeon's palm **(Fig. 21)**.

This design reduces the fatigue of surgeon and eases rotation of the instrument by allowing rotation within the palm rather than using wrist rotation. Squeezing the front of the handle between the thumb and the first finger increases the jaw closing force; squeezing the rear of the handle between the thenar eminence of the thumb and last finger opens the jaws.

Cuschieri pencil handle also has great ergonomic value especially when used with needle holder **(Fig. 22)**.

This multifunctional laparoscopic handle allows the angle between the handle and the instrument to be altered to suit the surgeon's wrist angle. The conveniently placed lever of this pencil handle when pressed can change the angle. Just like ball handle, pressure at the front increases the jaw closing force while pressure at the rear opens the jaw **(Fig. 23)**.

OUTER SHEATH OF HAND INSTRUMENT

The insulation covering of outer sheath of hand instrument should be of good quality in hand instrument to prevent accidental electric burn to bowel or other viscera **(Fig. 24)**.

Insulation covering may be of silicon or plastic. At the time of cleaning the hand instrument, utmost care should

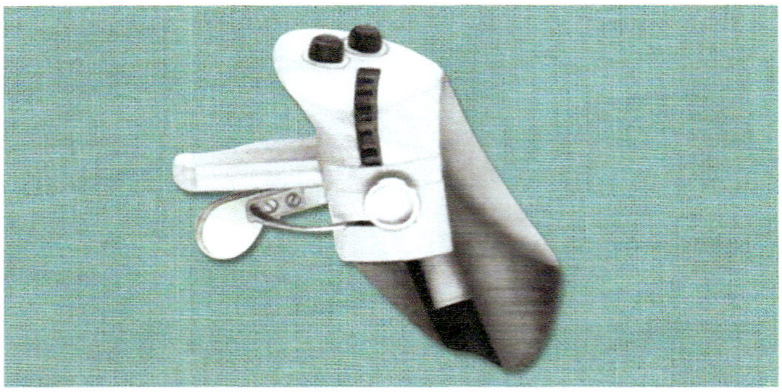

Fig. 23: Multifunctional laparoscopic handle.

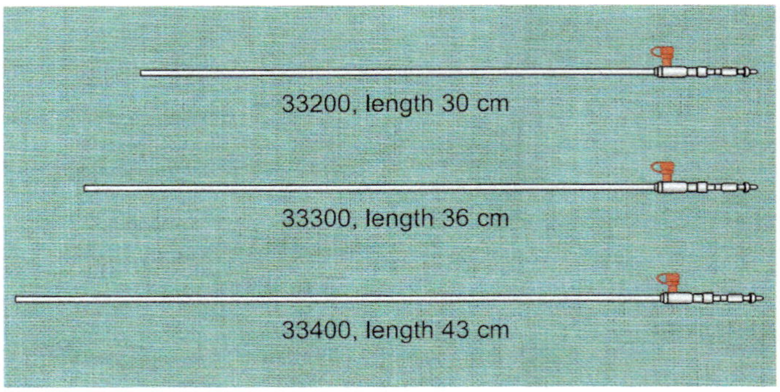

Fig. 24: Outer sheath of hand instrument.

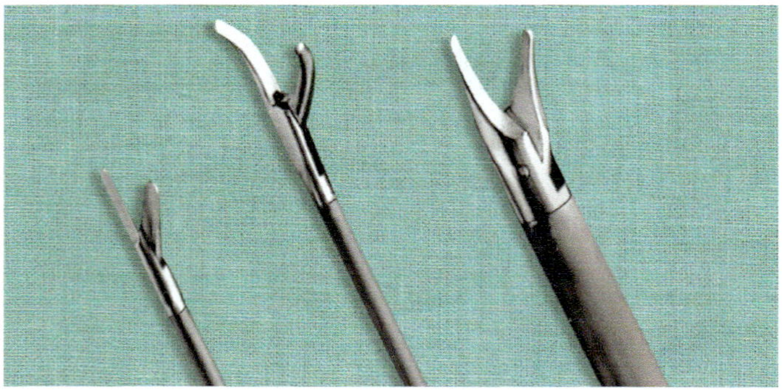

Fig. 25: Insert of hand instrument.

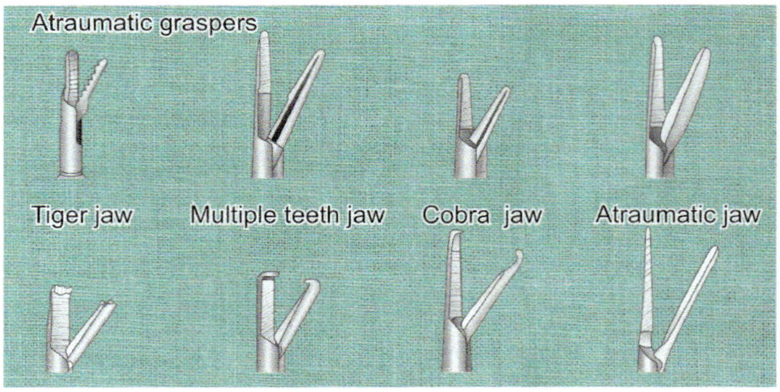

Fig. 26: Different jaw of graspers.

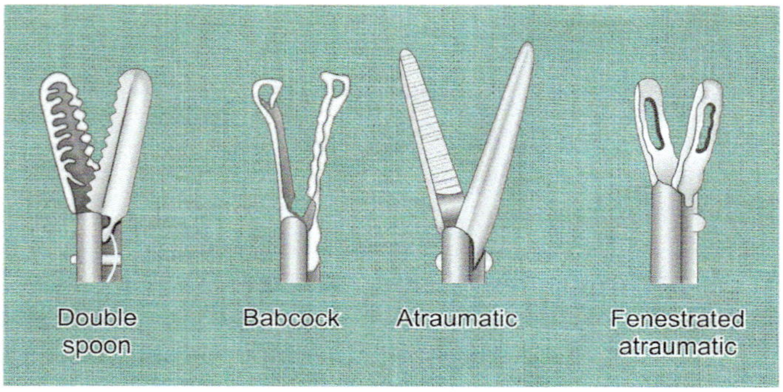

Fig. 27: Double-action jaw graspers.

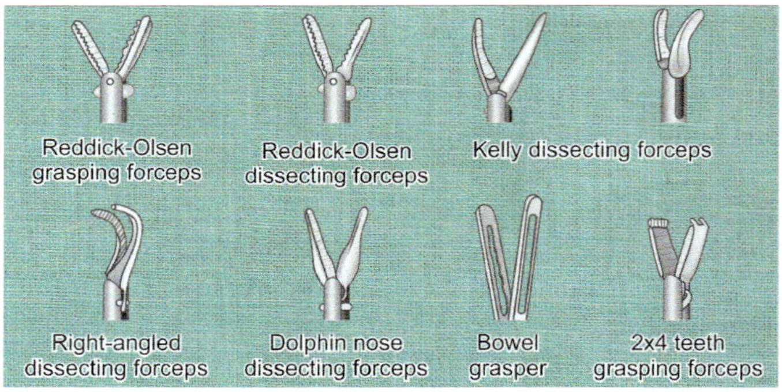

Fig. 28: Serrated jaw graspers.

be taken so that insulation should not be scratched with any sharp contact. A pin hole breach in insulation is not easily seen by naked eye but may be dangerous at the time of electrosurgery.

Insert of Hand Instrument

Insert of hand instrument varies only at tip **(Fig. 25)**.

It may be graspers scissors, or forceps. This grasper may have single-action jaw or double-action jaw. Single-action jaw opens less than double-action jaw but close with greater force. Thus, most of the needle holders are single-action jaw. The necessary wider opening in double-action jaw is present in grasper and dissecting forceps. Single-action graspers and dissectors are used where more force is required **(Fig. 26)**.

Single-action Jaw Graspers

These graspers are good when you do not have control over depth and surgeon wants to work in single plane in controlled manner particularly during adhesiolysis.

Double-action Jaw Graspers

These are shown in **Figures 27 and 28**.

INSTRUMENTS FOR SHARP DISSECTION

- Scissors
- Electrosurgery hook
- High-frequency (HF) electrosurgery spatula (Berci)
- HF electrosurgery knife
- Knife.

Scissors

Jean-Claude Margueron of Emar in 14th century BC invented scissors. Scissors are one of the oldest surgical instruments used by surgeons. Scissors are used to perform many tasks in open surgical procedure but its use in minimal access surgery is restricted. In minimal access surgery, scissors require greater skill because in inexperienced hand it may cause unnecessary bleeding and damage to important structures.

Mechanism of Cutting

The scissors have three parts:
1. Blade
2. Fulcrum
3. Handle

The cutting force of the scissors works on the law of lever. The force applied on the blade can be calculated by length of the handle and force applied on the grip of handle. A pair of scissors is an example of first-class levers connected together at the joint known as fulcrum.

There are three types of lever. Scissors works on the principle of class 1 lever **(Fig. 29)**. In class 1 lever, the pivot (fulcrum) is between the effort and the load. The more length of the handle or the fulcrum of the scissors, the less force of cutting will be required. The laparoscopic scissors do not apply the exact law of lever because of the cylinder action of the long shaft, but the design of handle helps in the amplification of force by lever action.

Scissors function by the combination of:
- Gripping
- Squeezing
- Tearing

When the blades of scissors close, its sharp edges grind against each other and any tissue which comes between the blades of scissors will get cut. The scissors-tissue interaction can be described in five stages:

Engagement

In the process of engagement, the two blades of the scissors engage a piece of tissue to cut. The amount of tissue engaged should not be more than the space between the jaw of blades otherwise the chance of slipping of tissue is more. After engagement, the force applied on the handle of the scissors initiates cutting.

Elastic Deformation

This stage starts just after the engagement of tissue between the blades of the scissors. In this process, the tissues between the two blades of scissors start deforming. This stage is called elastic deformation, because if the force on the handle of scissors is removed then the tissue deformity will return to its normal state.

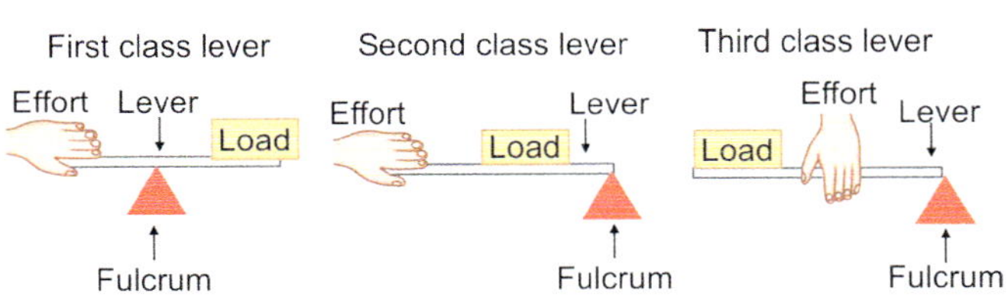

Fig. 29: Types of lever.

Plastic Deformation

Further force on the handle of scissors will cause the tissue between the blades to go into a plastic deformed state, which is irreversible. After undergoing this state of tissue deformation, even if further process of cutting is stopped the impression on the tissue remains.

Fracture

Further increased force on the fulcrum of scissors will result in the fracture of intercellular plane of the tissue. This stage of cutting is peculiar to scissors because unlike the scalpel, the site of tissue fracture is intercellular.

Separation

After the fracture, the tissue separates along line of the blade of scissors, and then this whole process of cutting will continue on the engaged tissue.

Histology of the Tissue After Cutting

Histological examination of the tissue after cutting with scissors shows that there is separation of tissue through intracellular plane. Microscopic examination shows serrated cut margin along the line of tissue separation.

TYPES OF LAPAROSCOPIC SCISSORS

There are different kinds of laparoscopic scissors based on the shape and indications for using them. All these are available in reusable and disposable type **(Fig. 30)**.

Straight Scissors

The blade of this scissors is straight and it is widely used as an instrument for mechanical dissection in laparoscopic surgery.

Straight scissors can give controlled depth of cutting because it has only one moving jaw **(Fig. 31)**. At the time of cutting, the fixed jaw should be down and moving jaw should be up.

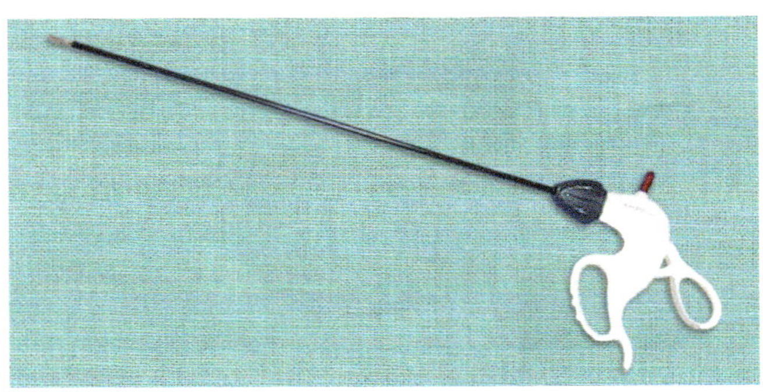

Fig. 30: Disposable scissors.

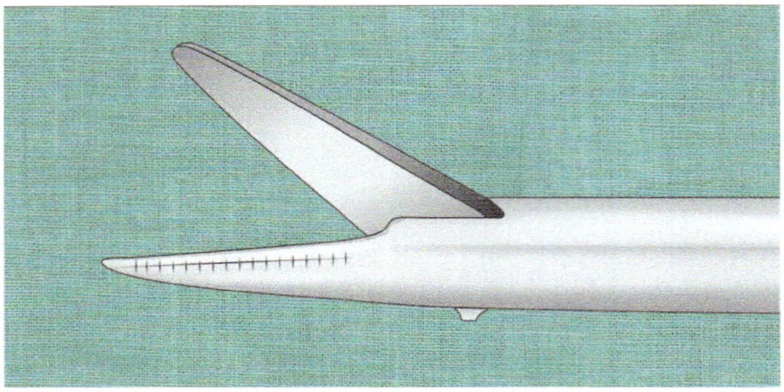

Fig. 31: Straight scissor.

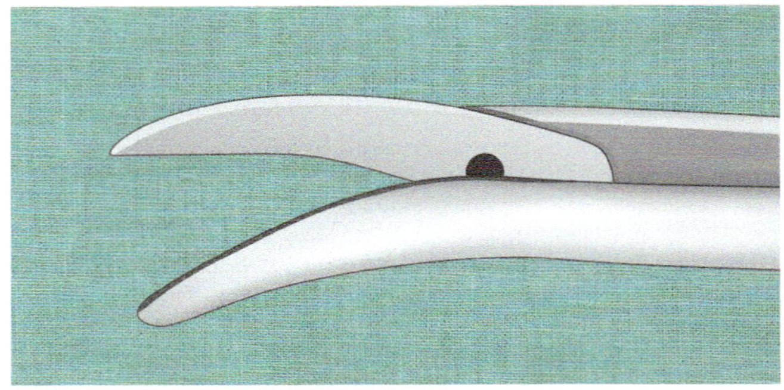

Fig. 32: Curved scissor.

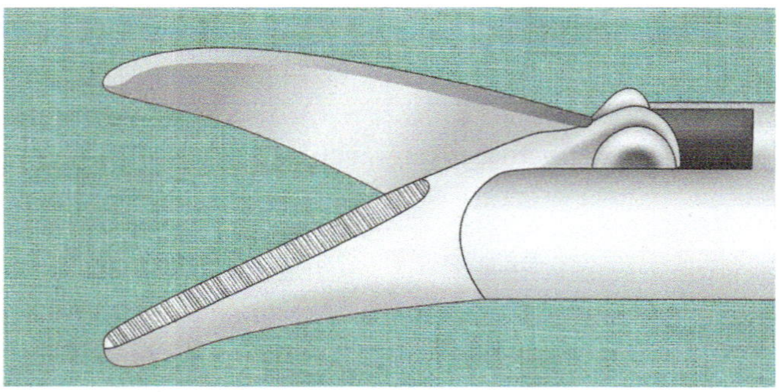

Fig. 33: Serrated scissor.

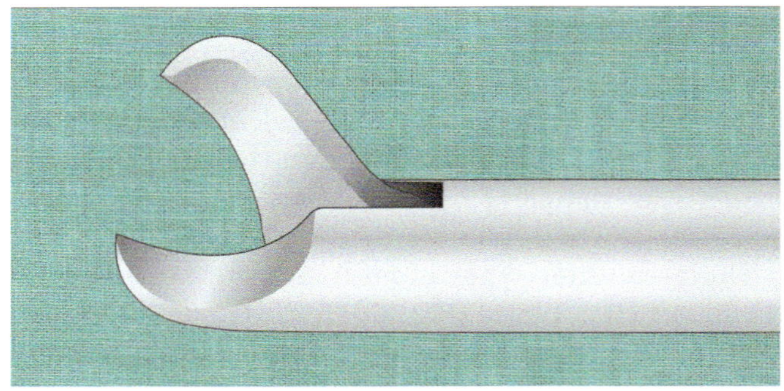

Fig. 34: Hook scissor.

Curved Scissors

The blade of this scissors is slightly curved and this is the most widely used scissors in laparoscopic surgery **(Fig. 32)**.

These scissors are mounted on a curved handle which is either fixed or retractable. The types with a fixed curvature proximal to the scissor blades require introduction through flexible valveless ports. The surgeon prefers this scissor because the curvature of the blade of the scissors abolishes the angle of laparoscopic instruments manipulation and better view through telescope is achieved.

Serrated Scissors

The main advantage of this scissors is that the serrated edges prevent the tissue to slip out of the blades. It is a useful instrument in cutting a slippery tissue or ligature. Serrated scissors may be straight or curved **(Fig. 33)**.

Hook Scissors

The sharp edge of both blades is in the shape of a flattened C. The blades can be partially closed, trapping tissue in the hollow of the blades without dividing it and allowing it to be slightly retracted. This allows the surgeon to double check before he closes the blades completely.

The main advantage of this scissors is that it encircles the structure before cutting: tissue is held between its jaws and there is no chance of slipping. The hook scissors are especially useful for cutting secured duct or artery in laparoscopic surgery. The cutting of nerve bundle in neurectomy becomes very easy with the help of this scissors. Hook scissors are also helpful in partial cutting of cystic duct for intraoperative cholangiography. All the other scissors cut from proximal to distal whereas the hook scissors cut distal to proximal **(Fig. 34)**.

Micro-tip Scissors

These very fine scissors are either straight or angled, and are used to partially transect the cystic duct. The main advantage of this scissor is to cut the ducts partially for facilitating cannulation. It may be used for cutting the cystic duct for performing intraoperative cholangiogram. Exploration of small ducts such as common bile duct (CBD) is very helpful with microscissors due to its fine small blades. Fine microscissors are also available in its curved form **(Fig. 35)**.

The use of scissors endoscopically requires little modification of open techniques.

The basic instrument is a miniaturized, long handled version of conventional scissors and can be single or double action. There are some special types of scissors used in endoscopic surgery.

Insulated Scissors

These allow the use of electrocautery through the scissors. However, when using nondisposable instruments, electrocoagulation using the open blades leads to blunting of the edges. Electrocoagulation using the scissors is thus limited, and when carried out is applied only with the blades

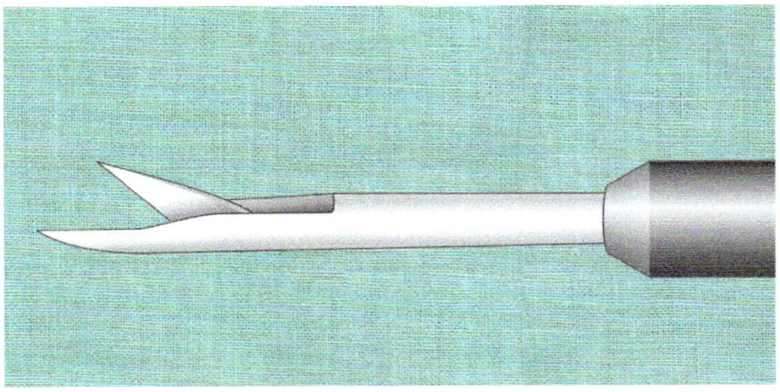

Fig. 35: Micro-tip scissor.

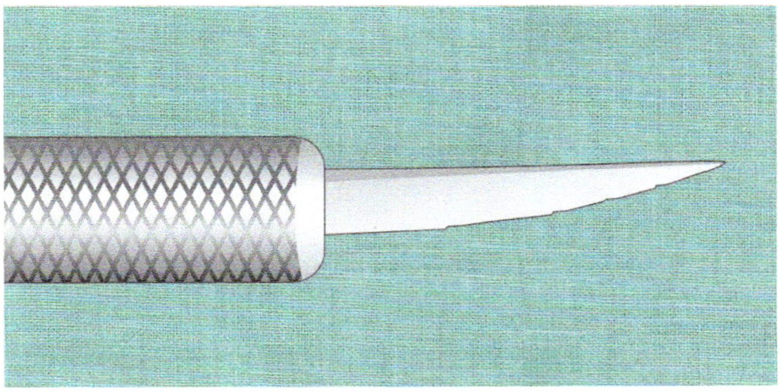

Fig. 36: Endoknife.

closed. Scissor dissection is usually carried out with a grasper in the other hand. If this instrument is insulated, then any vessels encountered can be easily coagulated by the grasper. A further disadvantage associated with electrocoagulation with the scissors results from the long noninsulated segment required to accommodate the blades and hinge mechanism. For safe practice, this requires to be kept in view, and this limits the magnification available to the surgeon.

Scissors have the following advantages:
- Inexpensive
- Safe in safe hand
- Operator determined precise action
- Closed blades can work for blunt dissection and electrocautery
- Piercing tissue with closed blades and then opening helps in obtaining a good plane of dissection.

Scissors have the following disadvantages:
- Nonhemostatic
- Accidental chances of cutting small ducts and vessels
- If overlooked, due to its pointed end, there is chance of injury to viscera
- If used for electric coagulation, its blades get blunt easily.

ENDOKNIFE (SCALPEL)

The knife is not used frequently in endoscopic surgery due to the problems associated with the safety of a blade, which cannot be closed or deactivated. However, it does have some important uses.

In our practice, a disposable blade (Beaver) is mounted on a metal rod, which has a socket at the distal end into which it can be screwed **(Fig. 36)**.

The most common use of the knife is for opening the hepatic duct or CBD during exploration for stones. A small, clean cut, linear stab wound is created in the anterior wall. Great care is required during incision and removal of the knife. However, a sharp curved scissors is better and safer than the endoknife for the choledochotomy.

Biopsy Forceps

Punch, cutting and dissecting biopsy forceps are used to take biopsies at the time of laparoscopic surgery **(Fig. 37)**.

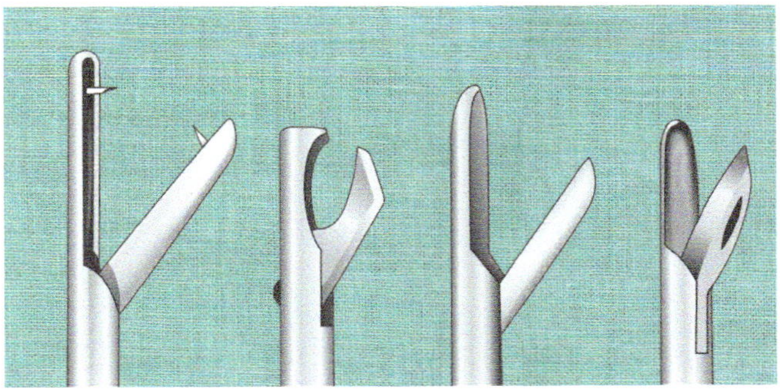

Fig. 37: Biopsy forceps.

The toothed punch biopsy forceps have special teeth which prevent accidental drop of tissue inside the abdominal cavity.

Aspiration Needle

These long needles are used in laparoscopy to aspirate fluid from distended ovarian cysts, gallbladder, or any localized pocket of pus in liver **(Fig. 38)**.

It may be used for drilling of polycystic ovary. Aspiration needle should be inserted inside the abdominal cavity with extreme precaution because if the pathway of entry or exit is ignored it can cause perforation of viscera.

Fan Retractor

These retractors are used to retract liver, stomach, spleen or bowel whenever they interfere in vision or they come in way of other working instrument **(Fig. 39)**.

There are many newer varieties of retractors available which are less traumatic. Cuschieri liver retractor is one of them which is very useful in fundoplication **(Fig. 40)**.

This liver retractor has a distal end which can be rotated by moving handle. Retractor is introduced in abdominal cavity when it is straight. Once it is inside the abdomen, the distal end can take various shapes just like serpent. This retractor can also be used for simple, atraumatic manipulation of bowel.

Nathanson Liver Retractor

Nathanson liver retractor is used to fully support and retracts the liver during laparoscopic upper gastrointestinal (GI)

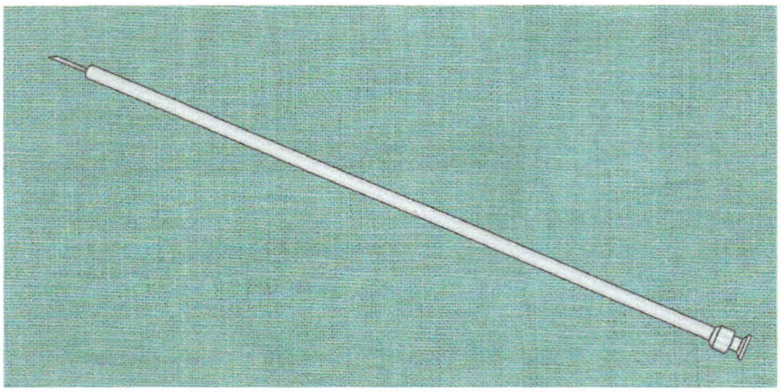

Fig. 38: Aspiration needle.

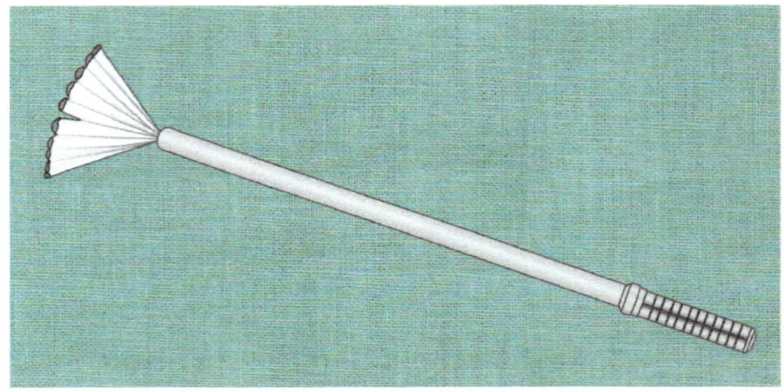

Fig. 39: Fan retractor.

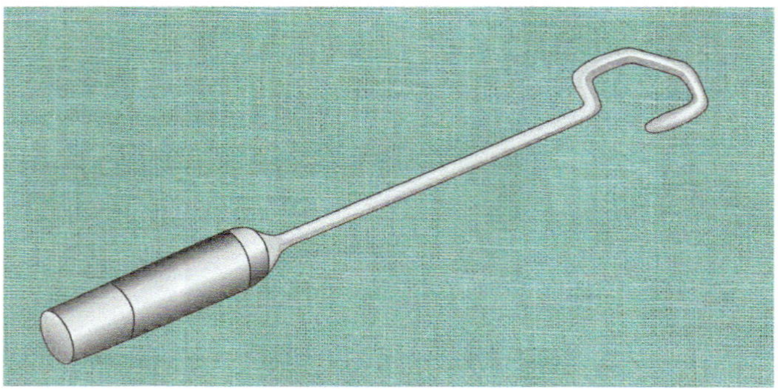

Fig. 40: Cuschieri liver retractor.

surgery, enabling a better view of the operating field. Complex laparoscopic upper GI procedures necessitate the use of the Nathanson retractor for retraction of the left lobe of liver. This retractor is usually inserted in the epigastric region by blunt force, first introducing 5-mm epigastric port, following removal of a 5-mm port. This liver retractor is self-supported by clamping to the operating table **(Fig. 41)**.

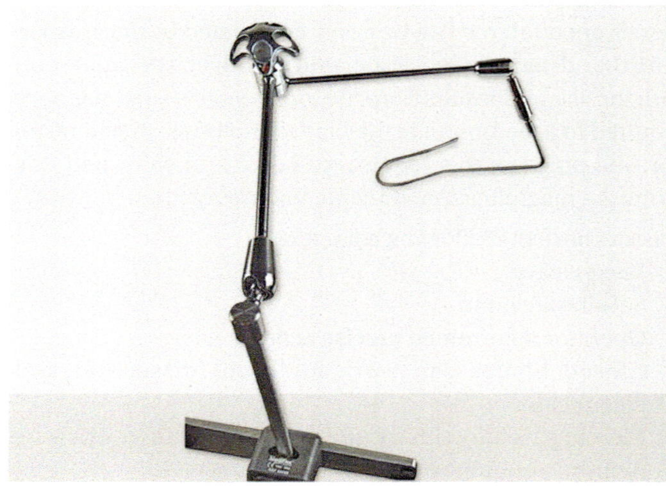

Fig. 41: Nathanson liver retractor.

NEEDLE HOLDERS

Needle holders should grasp the needle rock solid hard to prevent rotation **(Figs. 42 and 43)**.

Hence, until now, reusable needle holders are not available.

Needle holders have different types of jaws **(Fig. 44)**.

Flat grasping surface makes it possible to turn needle in all direction as in conventional surgery. Dome-shaped indentation at the tip automatically orients the needle in a particular direction although this function is not always useful, it can sometime make it easier to grasp the needle. Laparoscopic knotting and suturing should be learnt on a good quality endotrainer. The art and science of laparoscopic suturing and knotting is explained later in tissue approximation technique. Surgeons should slowly learn these techniques. They will develop their confidence once capable of suturing inside abdominal cavity and as a result conversion rate will also decrease.

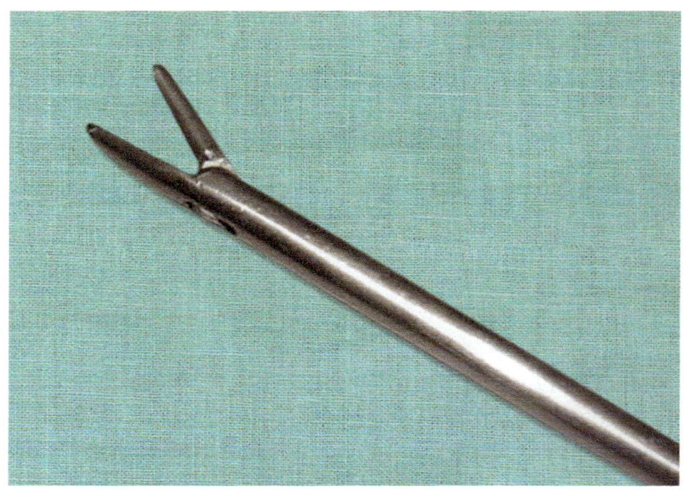

Fig. 42: Jaw of needle holder.

Many automatic laparoscopic suturing devices are invented for intracorporeal suturing but none of them are substitutes of manual laparoscopic suturing because these devices can work only under appropriate tissue plane suitable for their application **(Figs. 45A to C)**.

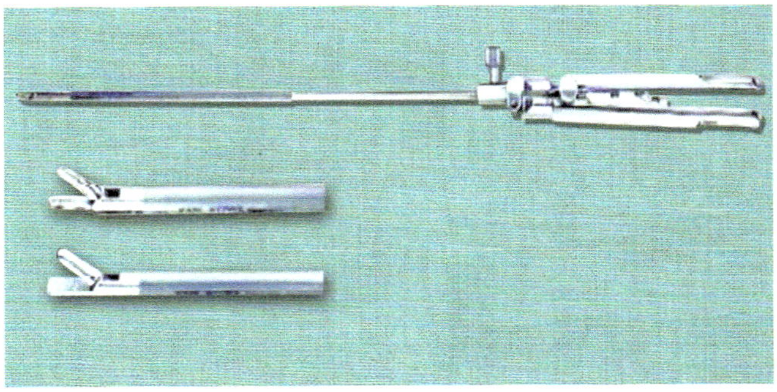

Fig. 43: Laparoscopic straight handle needle holder.

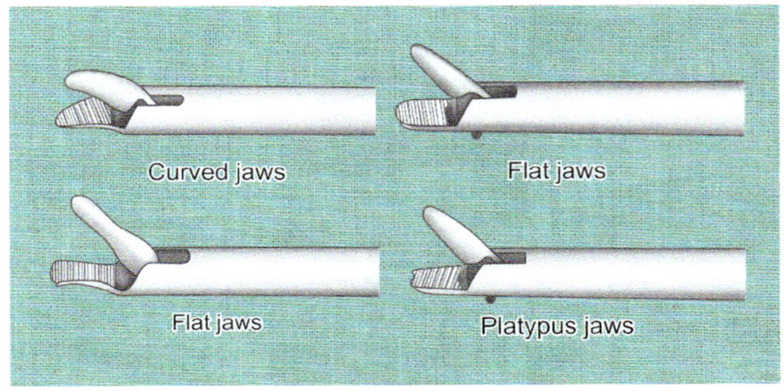

Fig. 44: Different types of jaws of needle holder.

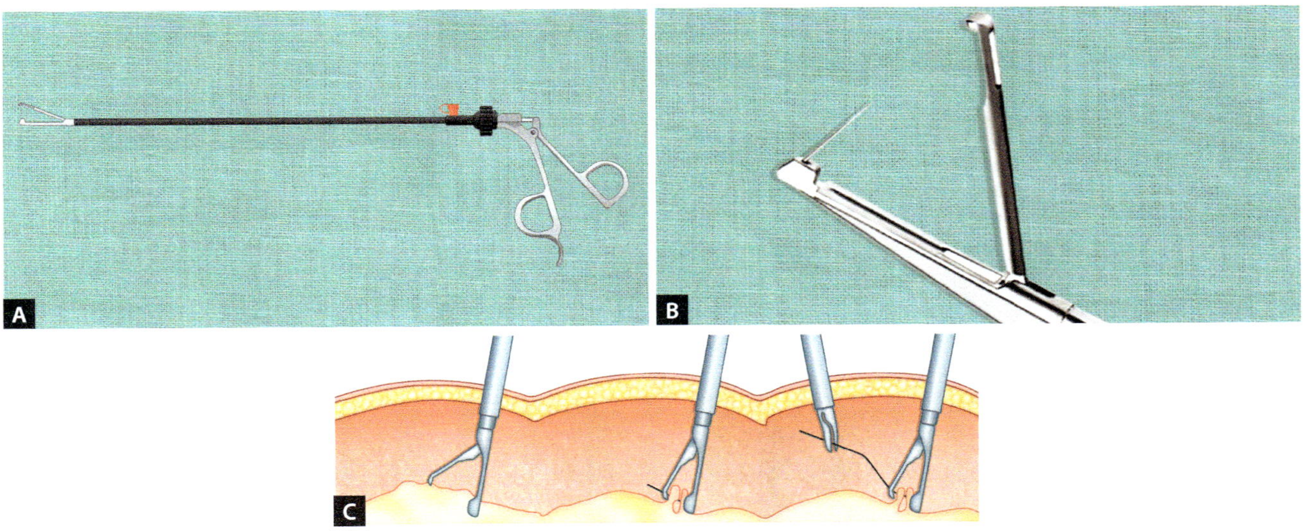

Figs. 45A to C: (A) Laparoscopic autosuturing instrument; (B) Autosuturing device; (C) Autosuturing device (mechanism).

ROBOTIZED LAPAROSCOPIC NEEDLE HOLDERS

JAIMY™ Advance, the first motorized laparoscopic 5 mm needle holder, is first of its kind robotized needle holder. This easy to use, reusable and unique but expensive robotic needle facilitates advanced laparoscopic suturing. It is developed to fit all hand sizes and simple one-handed operation. With bidirectional flexion and unlimited rotation of its end-effector, this needle holder can access difficult to reach areas in the abdominal cavity. It overcomes the ergonomic restrictions of conventional laparoscopy without increasing incision size, hence making complex procedures easier. Reusable, space saving and easy to use, motorized needle holder takes minimally invasive surgery a step further. Although it must be practiced using by the surgeon and if surgeon is good in laparoscopic suturing by conventional needle holder, this device is not required **(Fig. 46)**.

KNOT PUSHER

Although pretied loops are available in the market but surgeon should learn how to tie these extracorporeal knots.

Pretied loop can be used for any free structure like appendix but for continuous structure like cystic duct, surgeon has to perform extracorporeal knotting intraoperatively **(Fig. 47)**.

For extracorporeal knotting, knot pushers are used. These knot pushers are of either closed jaw or of open jaw type **(Fig. 48)**.

LAPAROSCOPIC CLIP APPLICATOR

Disposable preloaded clip applicators are available in 5 mm and 10 mm diameter **(Figs. 49 and 50)**.

These are expensive, but nice to use because the loading time of clip can be minimized. Disposable clip applier comes with 20 preloaded clips **(Fig. 51)**.

In case of emergency, when bleeding has to be stopped immediately one after another, clip can be applied rapidly with the help of these clip applicators.

Titanium is most widely used metal in minimal access surgery for tissue approximation. It rarely reacts with human body and this is why it is popular. It is easy to apply and can be left inside abdominal cavity. After few weeks, it is covered

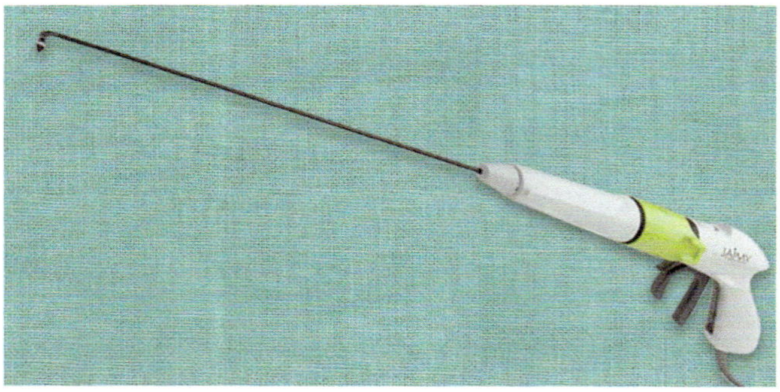

Fig. 46: Robotized laparoscopic needle holder.

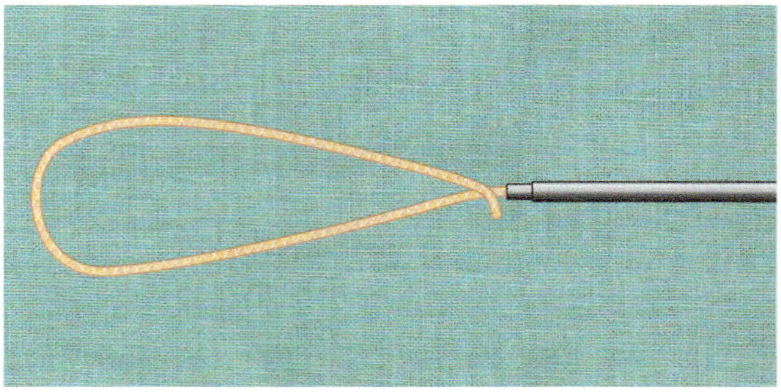

Fig. 47: Pretied loop.

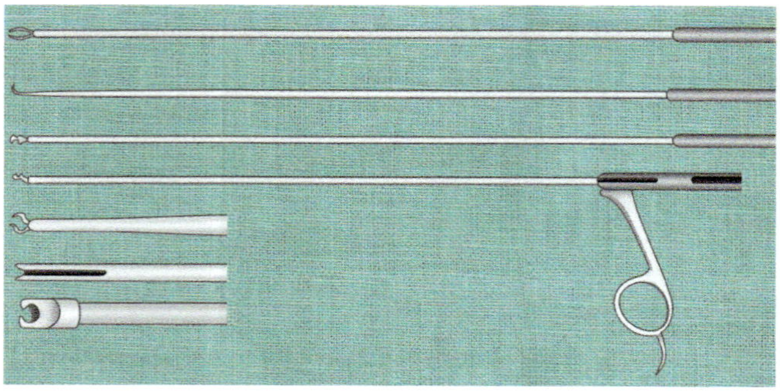

Fig. 48: Laparoscopic knot pusher.

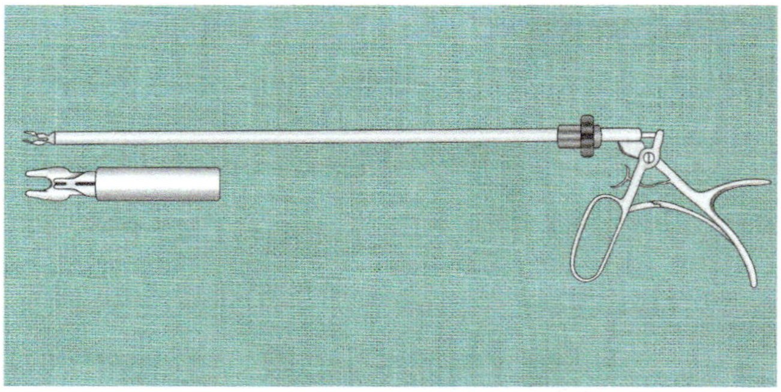

Fig. 49: Laparoscopic clip applicator.

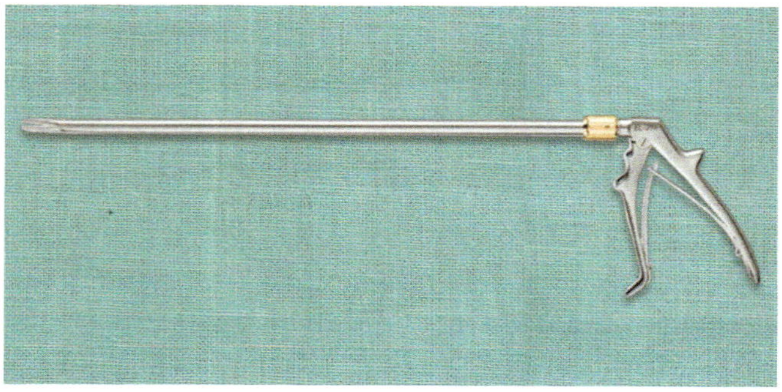

Fig. 50: Laparoscopic reusable clip applicator.

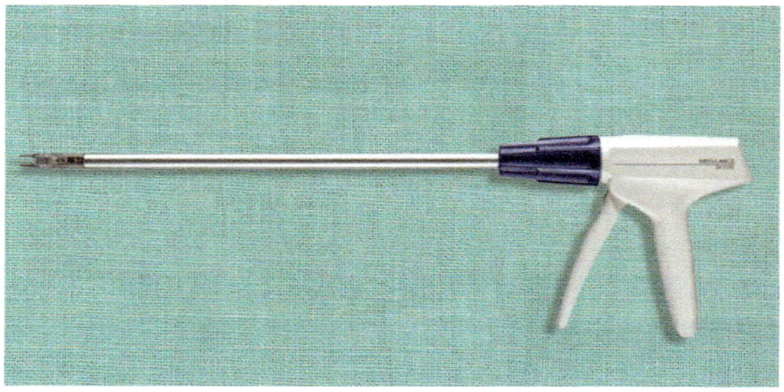

Fig. 51: Laparoscopic disposable clip applicator.

by fibrous tissue. Titanium clip is used by 99% of surgeons for clipping cystic duct and cystic artery at the time of laparoscopic cholecystectomy. Recently, silicon clips have been launched. Absorbable clips (Absolok, Ethicon) are preferred to clip cystic ducts nowadays. It adds to safety by working at the tip and it does not have chance to form cystic duct clip stone. The absorbable soft clips can also be used in running stitches at the beginning and at the termination of knotting.

Medium large size clip is of 9 mm and used most frequently for cystic duct and cystic artery **(Fig. 52)**.

The medium size clip is 7 mm in length and can be used to clip cystic artery or thin cystic duct. The large size clip is 11 mm in length and it is used to control thick wide cystic ducts or large mesenteric vessels. The jaw of clip applicator should be at right angle to the structure and before clipping surgeon should take care that both the jaws are seen. If one of the jaws is hidden, there is always a possibility that some tissue will get entrapped between the jaw of clip and clip will be loose. At the time of securing any duct or artery with titanium clip,

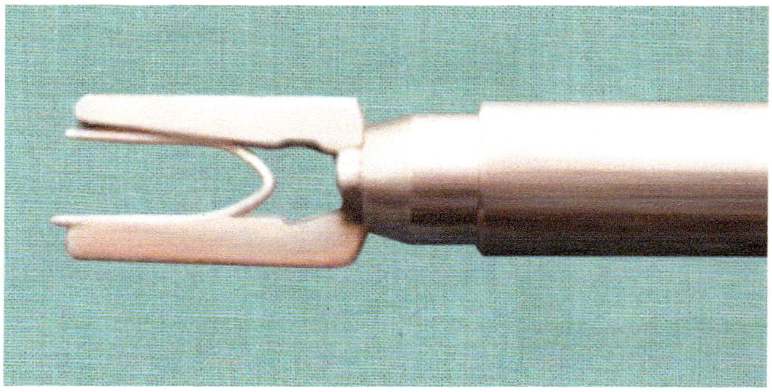

Fig. 52: Clip loaded over laparoscopic clip applicator.

three clips are generally applied. Two clips are left toward the structure which is secured and one clip is toward the tissue which surgeon wants to remove to prevent spillage of fluid **(Fig. 53)**.

The distance between first and second clip should be 3 mm and distance between second and third clip should be 6 mm so that after cutting in between second and third clip there will be 3 mm stump both the sides. The clip should not be applied very near to each other, because clips are held in position by dumbbell formation and if they are very near to each other, they will nullify the dumbbell formation of each other and both the clips will be loose.

Cystic Duct Clip Stone

Recently, many cases have been reported of cystic duct clip stone and this is the reason why in many institutions clipping of cystic duct is replaced by extracorporeal knotting.

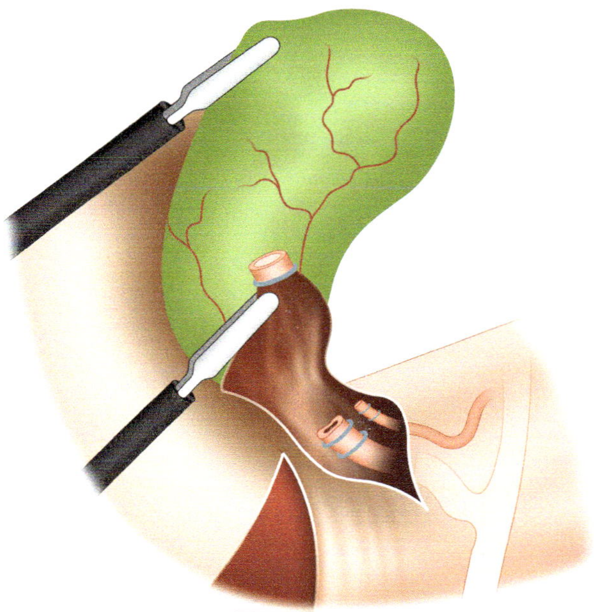

Fig. 53: Clip on cystic duct and artery.

If titanium clip is applied on the cystic duct, sometime it may crush one of the walls of cystic duct and it may get internalized inside the lumen of cystic duct. Inside the lumen of cystic duct, it acts as a nidus for the deposition of bile pigment and the formation of stone. The cross-section of these stones, the clip inside is seen glistening such as pupil of a cat and so it is also known as "cat eye stone". These stones can slip inside the CBD and may cause CBD obstruction.

Although the reported case of CBD obstruction is very less, the surgeon should try to ligate cystic duct to avoid this complication.

Falope Ring Applicator

Falope Ring® applicator is used for application of silastic ring to perform tube ligation. These may be fitted with one or two silastic rings **(Figs. 54A to C)**.

Myoma Fixation Screw

When performing a laparoscopic myomectomy, it is difficult to stabilize a smooth, hard fibroid. This is used to fix the subserous or intramural myoma at the time of laparoscopic myomectomy. Myoma screw can also be used to fix and retract big size uterus at the time of laparoscopic hysterectomy **(Fig. 55)**.

Uterine Manipulator

Uterine manipulator is one of the very essential instruments for mobilization of the uterus, identification of the vaginal fornices and sealing of the vagina during hysterectomy **(Fig. 56)**. There are different types of uterine manipulator. Their most obvious function is to suitably mobilize the uterus. By anteverting or retroverting the uterus, gynecologists get a good exposure of both the anterior wall and vesicouterine fold, the posterior wall and uterosacral ligaments. Lateral movements allow the exposure of the infundibulopelvic ligaments, utero-ovarian ligaments, and the anterior and posterior leaves of the broad ligament. These movements are

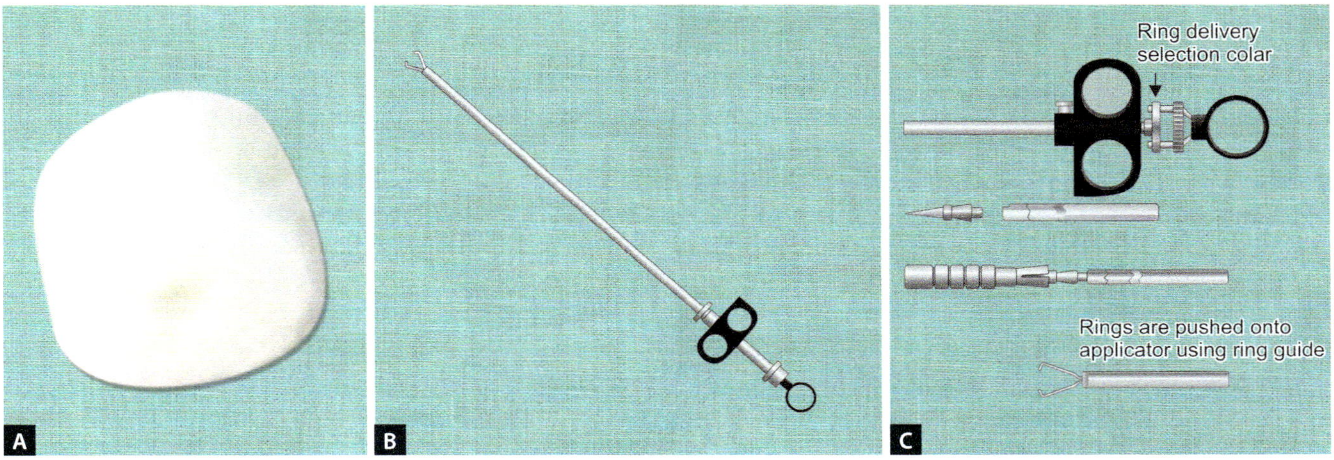

Figs. 54A to C: (A) Falope ring; (B) Falope ring applicator; (C) Handle of Falope ring applicator (mechanism).

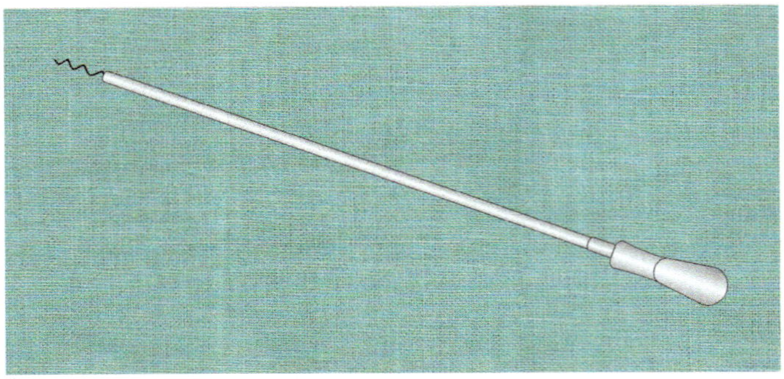

Fig. 55: Myoma screw.

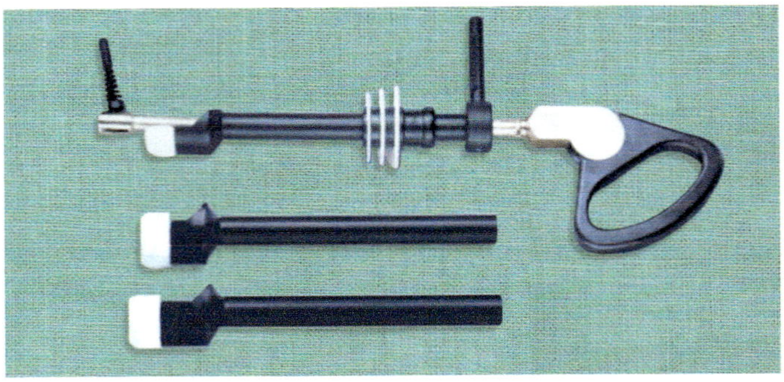

Fig. 56: Clermont-Ferrand uterine manipulator.

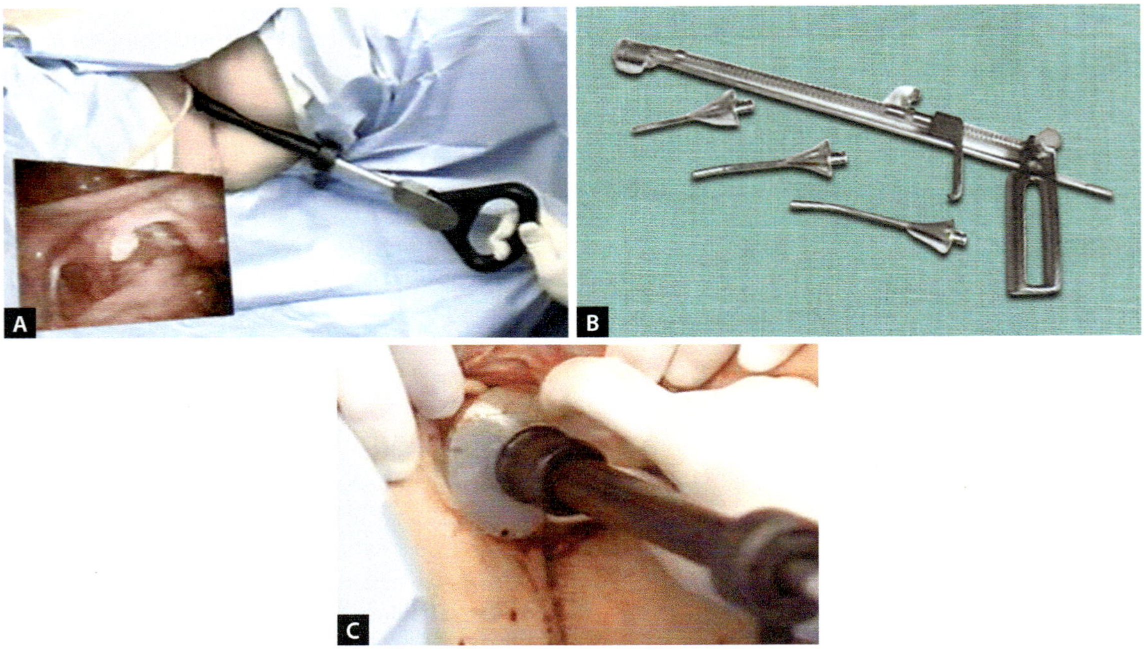

Figs. 57A to C: (A) Lateral traction over uterus by uterine manipulator; (B) Different attachments of uterine manipulator; (C) Sealing of vagina with cuff of uterine manipulator for total laparoscopic hysterectomy (TLH).

important in cases of large uterus. The elevation movement is important in cases of rectovaginal endometriosis in which the uterus needs to be moved upward into the abdomen, providing the best exposure of the uterosacral ligaments and the cul-de-sac. The ideal uterine manipulator should be inexpensive, convenient and quick to use, safe especially by avoiding the need for dilatation and a tenaculum, and have the ability to inject solutions into the uterine cavity and most importantly offer the optimal range of motion of the uterus while avoiding the need for an assistant.

Uterine manipulator is used in most of the advanced gynecological procedures. Most uterine manipulators are essentially rigid instruments that are attached or fixed to the uterus, protrude from the vagina, and require the use of a tenaculum to grasp the cervix, which occasionally may bleed.

The Clermont-Ferrand uterine manipulator provides a good 140° movement of the uterus in the anterior and posterior directions **(Figs. 57A to C)**. In addition, it has the ability to flex the uterus on itself. Its graduated snap-in mechanism, which has five different positions, gives stability to the uterus at various angles, and the snap-in release button allows unrestricted movement. The manipulator rod, when pushed forward, helps to delineate the vaginal fornices with the help of an anatomical blade attached anteriorly. It has a series of silicon seal to maintain the pneumoperitoneum after the colpotomy incision. It is a reusable instrument. Though versatile, this instrument has its drawbacks; it requires cervical dilatation up to Hegar number 9 before its insertion in the cervix, so may not be useful in cases of cervical stenosis. It is pretty complex to assemble and requires a fair amount of training to use this device properly. Clermont-Ferrand uterine manipulator seems to be a good choice for operative laparoscopies involving hysterectomy, endometriosis in the posterior cul-de-sac, and sling surgeries **(Fig. 56)**.

The RUMI manipulator with the Koh colpotomizer from CooperSurgical is a versatile uterine manipulator. Not only does it have extremely good uterine manipulation in the anterior, posterior, and lateral planes, it also helps with the very easy delineation of the vaginal fornices. The Koh-cup distances the ureter form the uterine vessels and facilitates its easy coagulation. This device helps to complete laparoscopic dissection of the cervix and vagina much more easily, resulting in greater efficacy and less blood loss while eliminating the difficulties pertaining to vaginal access. This enhanced uterine mobility also speeds uterovesical peritoneal dissection and inferior displacement of the bladder. Furthermore, the RUMI manipulator allows for significant lateral uterine displacement, improving visualization and ease of dissection of the uterine vasculature and broad ligament. Only drawback of this uterine manipulator is that it is partially disposable **(Fig. 58)**.

The Mangeshikar uterine manipulator is a reusable, completely detachable, low-cost uterine manipulator **(Fig. 59)**. Though specifically designed for total laparoscopic hysterectomy, it can be used in almost all gynecological laparoscopic surgeries. By appropriately mobilizing the handle, the uterus along with the adnexa can be manipulated from side to side and can be rotated along its long axis, thus enabling anteversion and retroversion as well as dextro- and levorotation. Sliding in the vaginal delineator helps identify the vaginal fornices and choosing the right-sized delineator drum helps maintain the pneumoperitoneum.

Thus, the Mangeshikar uterine manipulator offers advantages in its ability to perform a completely laparoscopic hysterectomy and other gynecological surgery by maintaining the loss of pneumoperitoneum. The significant uterine mobility that this system provides facilitates dissection of the ascending uterine arteries in a manner that reduces the risks of ureteric injury. Mangeshikar uterine manipulator is fully autoclavable and reusable system.

Tissue Morcellator

The morcellator is used to grasp the tissue to be removed and cuts it into small bits, which are forced into the hollow part of the instrument **(Fig. 60)**.

It can be designed to remove a myoma or an ovary. It can be introduced through a 10-mm port or through the colpotomy wound **(Fig. 61)**.

Tissue Morcellator and Its Complications

The Food and Drug Administration (FDA) currently estimates that a hidden uterine sarcoma may be present in approximately 1 in 225 to 1 in 580 women undergoing surgery for uterine fibroids based on recent publications. The FDA also estimates that a leiomyosarcoma may be present in approximately 1 in 495 to 1 in 1,100 women undergoing surgery for uterine fibroids based on recent studies. Prior to 2014, the clinical community estimated uterine sarcomas to be present much less frequently, in as few as 1 in 10,000

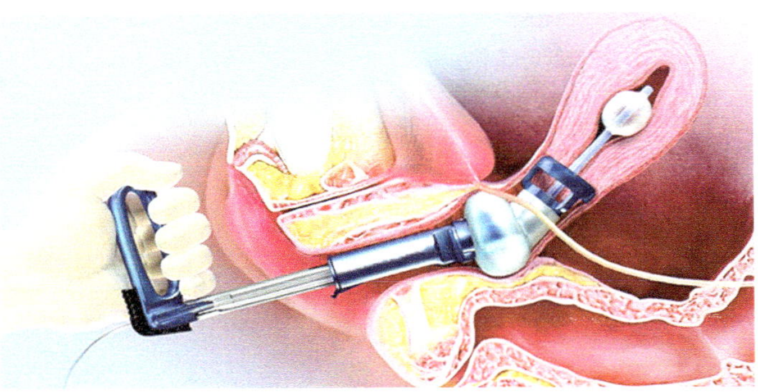

Fig. 58: RUMI uterine manipulator.

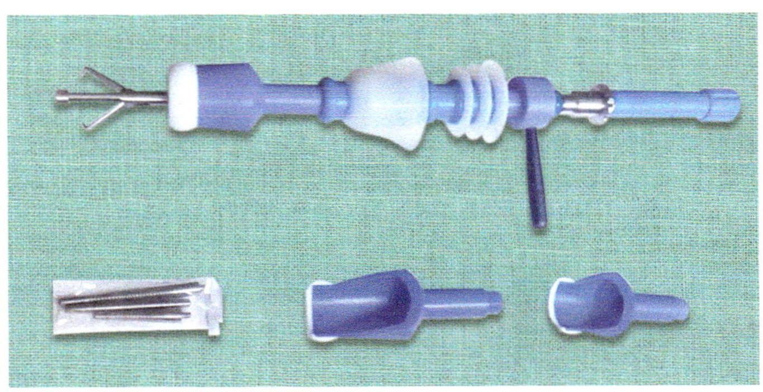

Fig. 59: Mangeshikar uterine manipulator.

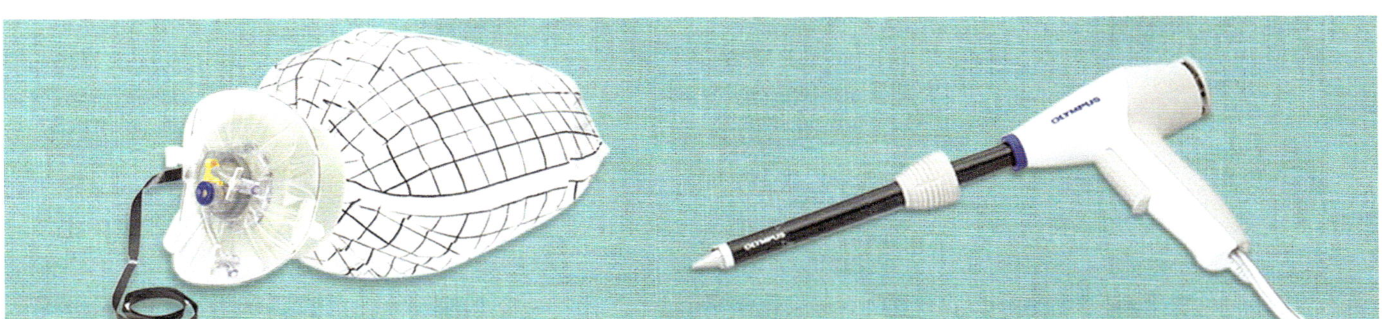

Fig. 60: Tissue morcellator.

women undergoing surgery for uterine fibroids. Several studies show that using a laparoscopic power morcellator during gynecological laparoscopic surgery in women with hidden uterine sarcomas is associated with lowering their chances of long-term survival without cancer. While these studies have limitations, women who have had fibroid surgery with a laparoscopic power morcellator later found to have a hidden uterine sarcoma, have lower disease-free survival, when compared to women who were treated with manual morcellation or without morcellation.

Uterine sarcomas and uterine fibroids may have similar signs and symptoms. At this time, there is no reliable method for predicting or testing whether a woman with fibroids may have a uterine sarcoma. The FDA recommends gynecologist share this information with patients and warns against using laparoscopic power morcellators in gynecologic surgeries to treat patients with suspected or confirmed cancer, and in women over age 50 having a myomectomy or hysterectomy for uterine fibroids.

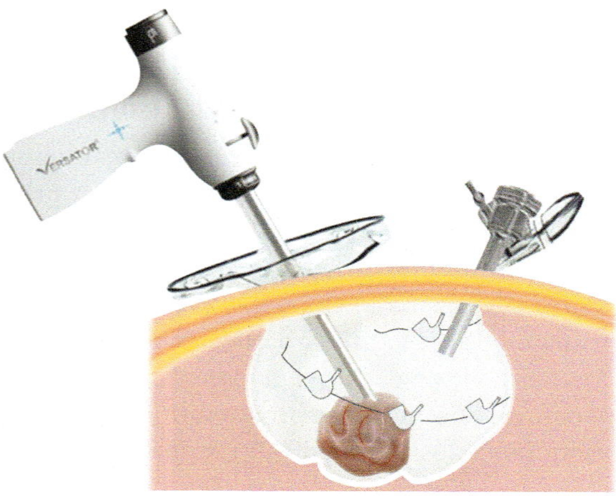

Fig. 61: Morcellation of myoma in myomectomy.

Morcellator Use with Tissue Containment System

The FDA recommends that gynecologist use tissue containment systems when using laparoscopic power morcellators, and that they ensure the laparoscopic power morcellator and tissue containment system are compatible. Legally marketed laparoscopic power morcellation containment systems are intended to isolate and contain tissue that is considered benign. Based on testing and clinical data, use of a containment system confines morcellated tissue within the containment system.

Due to this increased risk, we continue to recommend use of laparoscopic power morcellation only in appropriate women undergoing myomectomy or hysterectomy. In addition, it is good that when morcellation is appropriate, only contained morcellation be performed. MorSafe® is an innovative single-use disposable device intended to be used as a receptacle for benign tissue mass during gynecological procedures such as laparoscopic myomectomy or laparoscopic hysterectomy. MorSafe® is to be used in conjunction with the morcellator to safely contain and remove the shredded benign tissue mass. The device has unique features to allow for quick deployment, insufflation, morcellation, and spill-proof withdrawal of the bag **(Fig. 62)**.

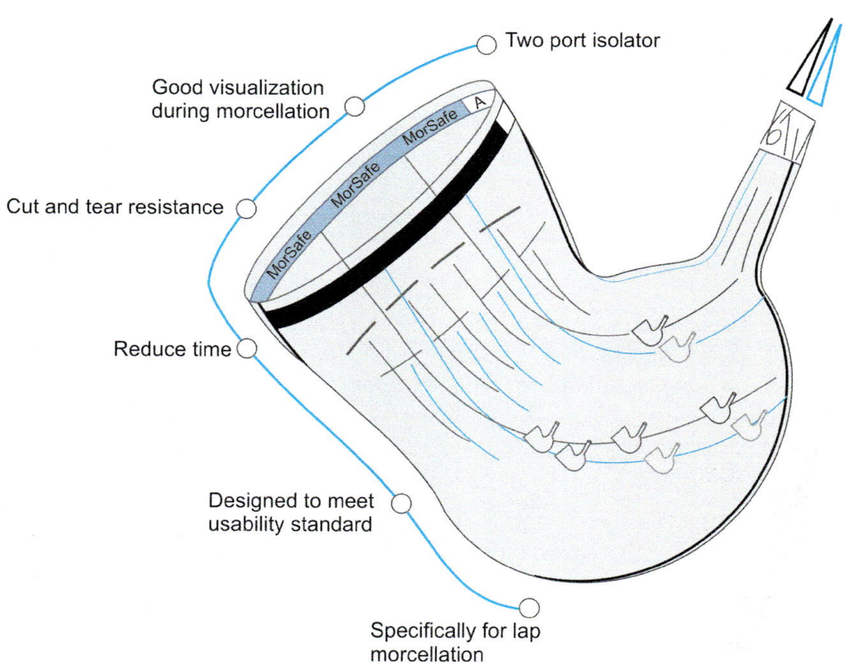

Fig. 62: MorSafe® tissue containment system.

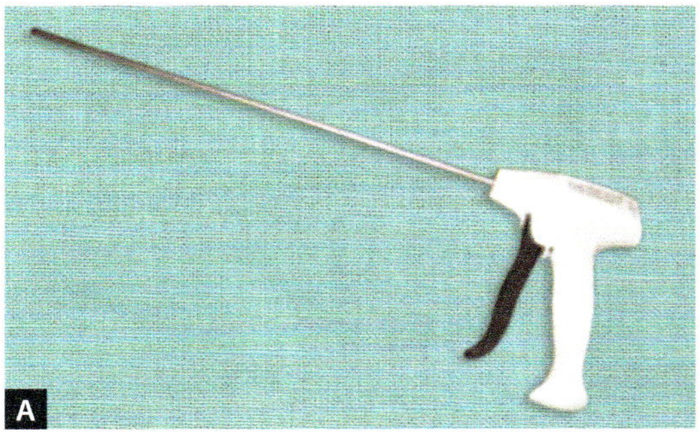

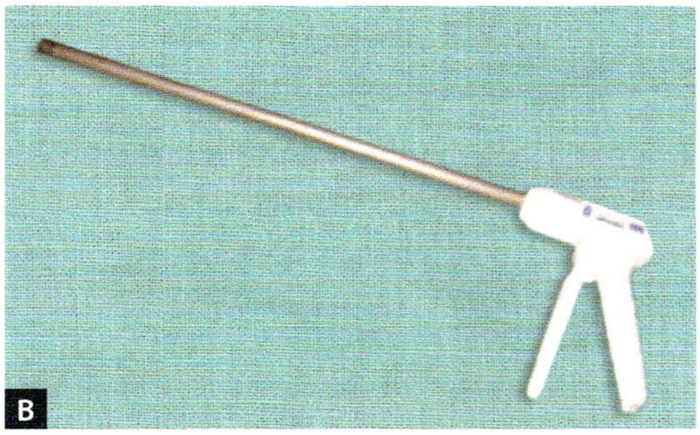

Figs. 63A and B: Endoanchor and tacker.

TABLE 1: Different types of implant for fixing mesh.

Feature	*ESS endoanchor*	*Protack*	*Tacker*
Number of implants	20	30	20
Geometry of implant	Anchor	Helical Fastener	Helical Fastener
Implant material	Nitinol	Titanium	Titanium
Implant length	5.9 mm	3.8 mm	3.6 mm
Implant width	6.7 mm	4 mm	3.4 mm
Port size required	5 mm	5 mm	5 mm
Shaft length	360 mm	356 mm	356 mm
Trigger fire orientation	Release to deploy	Depress to deploy	Depress to deploy

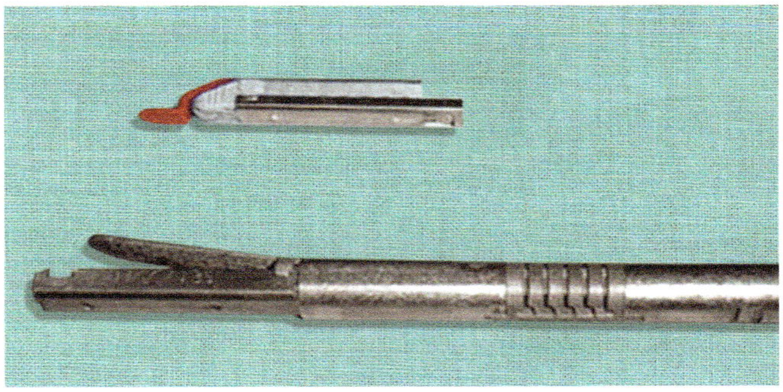

Fig. 64: Jaw of stapler.

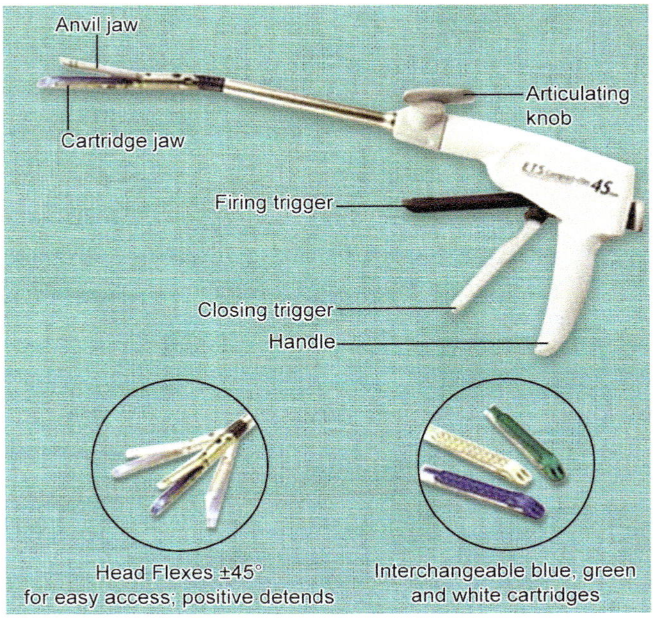

Fig. 65: Endopath ETS Compact-FLEX45 articulating endoscopic linear cutters.

MorSafe®, with its unique two-port design, offers the surgeon superior visibility during the surgery compared to a single-port approach. Designed to fit and take the shape of the abdomen, it has been constructed utilizing a special tear-resistant material to prevent leakage. It also contains a special ring in the bag opening to allow the surgeon ultimate control of the bag opening and easy access to the interior of the bag during surgery.

Hernia Stapler, Endoanchor and Tacker

For fixing mesh in hernia surgery, many preloaded devices are available **(Figs. 63A and B)**.

Currently, three popular brands of implants to fix the mesh are available. These are tacker, protack or anchor. The comparative chart of these implants is shown in **Table 1**.

There are many varieties of laparoscopic stapler **(Fig. 64)**.

The LONG45A Endocutter manufactured by Ethicon has a shaft that is 10 cm and it allows easier access during laparoscopic weight loss surgery, such as gastric bypass, where longer instruments are needed for morbidly obese patients. The ETS 45 and ETS-FLEX45 endoscopic linear cutters provide a 45-mm staple and cut line **(Fig. 65)**.

The 34-cm shaft length makes the device suitable for many minimally invasive surgical procedures. The cutters are intended for transaction, resection, and/or creation of anastomosis in minimally access surgical procedures.

Laparoscopic surgical instruments are extremely variable and increasing number of instruments is being designed for specific application. Instruments are getting complex with greater functionality and freedom of movement. Such instruments reflect the trend toward the automation of procedure. In the future, such developments ultimately will lead to full robotization.

Laparoscopic Linear Stapler

Laparoscopic linear stapler is very useful device for tissue approximation. Staples are made available in various sizes and heights so that the surgeon can choose the one that provides appropriate homeostasis/tissue apposition without significant ischemia or tissue destruction. Dimensions of commonly available staple cartridges that are used to accommodate different tissue thicknesses for appropriate tissue management are shown in **Figure 66**.

If the closed staple height is too high, then it may inadequately oppose the tissues and result in leakage, bleeding, and/or dehiscence. Conversely, if the staple height selected is too low, then ischemia, serosal shearing, or "cheese wiring" may result, potentially leading to leakage or frank necrosis. There are at least three staple heights for most linear staplers. Most modern laparoscopic staplers bend each staple into a B-shape staple form, which helps to secure the tissue in place. However, malformed staples can occur because staple leg bending depends on several tissue/stapler characteristics including tissue thickness, tissue viscosity, staple height, and other staple properties (thickness, bending characteristics, type of metal, etc.). Staples are designed to form consistently, and staples that are not forming as intended should be investigated.

Color	*Rows*	*Tissue type*	*Open staple height*	*Closed staple height*
Gray	6	Mesentery	2.0 mm	0.75 mm
White	6	Vascular	2.5 mm	1.0 mm
Blue	6	Standard	3.5 mm	1.5 mm
Gold	6	Standard/thick	3.8 mm	1.8 mm
Green	6	Thick	4.1 mm	2.0 mm

Fig. 66: Color of staple cartridge used for different tissue thicknesses.

Echelon Flex Endopath Staplers

The Echelon flex endopath staplers designed to deliver reliable performance across a wide range of tissue types and thicknesses on a one-handed, easy to use platform. Enhanced system-wide compression aids in proper staple formation, which is necessary to achieve a leak resistant and hemostatic staple line. Compression before firing gently exudes fluid from targeted tissue before firing **(Figs. 67 and 68)**.

Tri-Staple

Endo GIA™ articulating endoscopic linear stapler with Tri-Staple™ is Covidien product and it is designed to work in harmony with the natural properties of tissue to optimize performance before, during, and after stapling **(Figs. 69 and 70)**. With its stepped cartridge face, Tri-Staple™ technology delivers optimum tissue compression, optimizing interaction between the tissue and staple. It has the following advantages.

- Generates less stress on tissue during compression and clamping
- Allows greater perfusion into the staple line
- Provides superior performance in variable thicknesses.

Tri-Staple™ technology improves staple line strength, leak resistance, and hemostasis when compared to the universal reloads. No single stapler can address the wide range of tissue management issues surgeons face on a daily basis. The current review focused on bariatric, thoracic, and colorectal studies. It was shown that different types

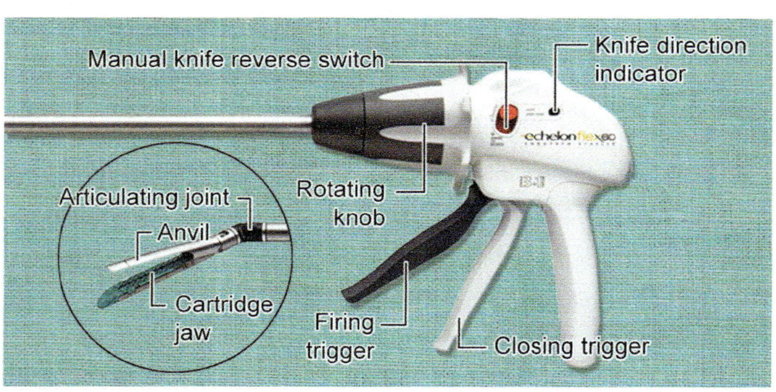

Fig. 67: Endopath articulating endoscopic linear cutter.

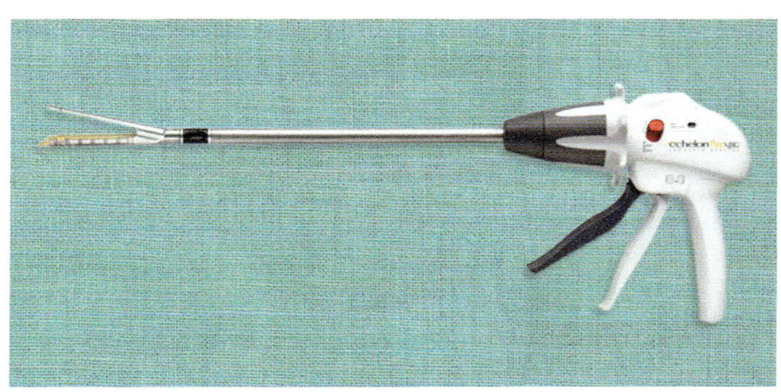

Fig. 68: Endopath articulating endoscopic linear stapler.

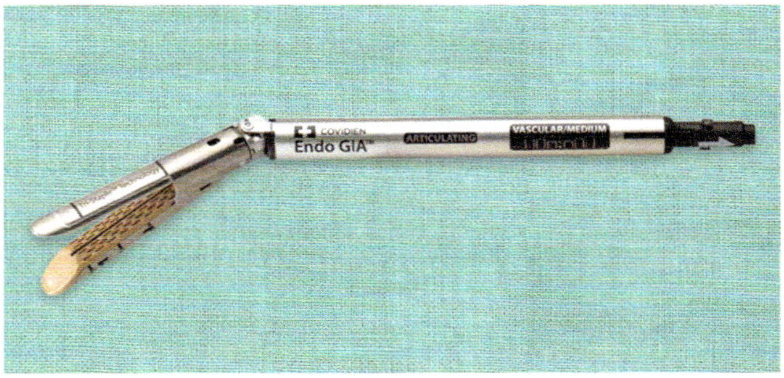

Fig. 69: Covidien Endo GIA® articulating endoscopic linear stapler cartridge.

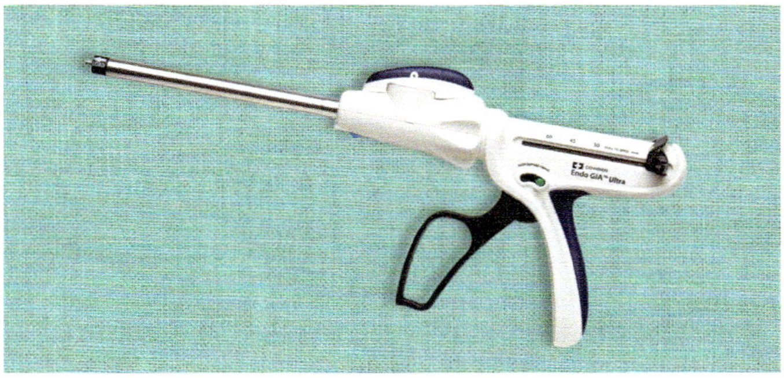

Fig. 70: Covidien Endo GIA® articulating endoscopic linear stapler gun.

of tissues have different thicknesses and biomechanical properties that may require the use of staples of different heights or the use of a different types of stapler (linear vs. curved vs. circular) to construct a stable anastomosis. Each tissue type has its own challenges, and the pathology of the tissue must also be taken into account.

BIBLIOGRAPHY

1. Bhayani SB, Andriole GL. Three-dimensional (3D) vision: does it improve laparoscopic skills? An assessment of 3D head-mounted visualization system. Rev Urol. 2005;7:211-4.
2. Byrn JC, Schluender S, Divino CM, Conrad J, Gurland B, Shlasko E, et al. Three-dimensional imaging improves surgical performance for both novice and experienced operators using the Da Vinci Robot System. Am J Surg. 2007;193:519-22.
3. Chan AC, Chung SC, Yim AP, Lau JY, Ng EK, Li AK. Comparison of two-dimensional vs three-dimensional camera systems in laparoscopic surgery. Surg Endosc. 1997;11:438-40.
4. Ericsson KA. Deliberate practice and the acquisition and maintenance of expert performance in medicine and related domains. Acad Med. 2004;79:S70-81.
5. Everbusch A, Grantcharov TP. Learning curves and impact of psychomotor training on performance in simulated colonoscopy: a randomized trial using a virtual reality endoscopy trainer. Surg Endosc. 2004;18:1514-8.
6. Fraser SA, Freldman LS, Stanbridge D, Fried GM. Characterizing the learning curve for a basic laparoscopic drill. Surg Endosc. 2005;19:1572-8.
7. Ganai S, Seymour NE. VR to OR for camera navigation. In: Westwood JD, Haluck RS, Hoffman HM, Mogel GT, Phillips R, Robb RA, Vosburgh KG (Eds). Medicine Meets Virtual Reality, Vol. 111. Amsterdam: IOC Press; 2005. pp. 45-8.
8. Grantcharov TP, Bardram L, Funch-Jensen P, Rosenberg J. Impact of hand dominance, gender, and experience with computer games on performance in virtual reality laparoscopy. Surg Endosc. 2003;17:1082-5.
9. Grantcharov TP, Bardram L, Funch-Jensen P, Rosenberg J. Learning curves and impact of previous operative experience on performance on virtual reality simulator to test laparoscopic surgical skills. Am J Surg. 2003;185:146-9.
10. Haluck RS, Gallagher AG, Satava RM, Webster R, Bass TL, Miller CA. Reliability and validity of Endotower, a virtual reality trainer for angled endoscope navigation. Stud Health Technol Inform. 2002;85:179-84.
11. Haluck RS, Webster RW, Snyder AJ, Melkonian MG, Mohler BJ, Dise ML, et al. A virtual reality surgical trainer for navigation in laparoscopic surgery. Stud Health Technol Inform. 2001;81:171-6.
12. Hanna GB, Cuschieri A. Influence of two-dimensional and three-dimensional imaging on endoscopic bowel suturing. World J Surg. 2000;24:444-9.
13. Hanna GB, Shimi SM, Cuschieri A. Randomized study of the influence of two-dimensional vs three-dimensional imaging on performance of laparoscopic cholecystectomy. Lancet. 1998;351:248-51.
14. Hart SG, Staveland LE. Development of a multi-dimensional workload rating scale: results of empirical and theoretical research. In: Hancock PA, Meshkati N (Eds). Human Mental Workload. Amsterdam: Elsevier; 1988. pp. 139-83.
15. Jones DB, Brewer JD, Soper NJ. The influence of three-dimensional video systems on laparoscopic task performance. Surg Laparosc Endosc. 1996;6:191-7.
16. Korndorffer JR Jr, Hayes DJ, Dunne JB, Sierra R, Touchard CL, Markert RJ, et al. Development and transferability of a cost-effective laparoscopic camera navigation simulator. Surg Endosc. 2005;19:161-7.
17. Korndorffer JR Jr, Stefanidis D, Sierra R, Clayton JL. Validity and reliability of a videotrainer laparoscopic camera navigation simulator. Surg Endosc. 2005;19:S246.
18. Maithel S, Sierra R, Korndorffer J, Neumann P, Dawson S, Callery M, et al. Construct and face validity of MIST-VR, Endotower, and CELTS: are we ready for skills assessment using simulators? Surg Endosc. 2006;20:104-12.
19. McDougall EM, Soble JJ, Wolf JS Jr, Nakada SY, Elashry OM, Clayman RV. Comparison of three-dimensional and two-dimensional laparoscopic video systems. J Endourol. 1996;10:371-4.
20. O'Donnell RD, Eggemeier FT. Workload assessment methodology. In: Boff KR, Kaufman L, Thomas JP (Eds). Handbook of Perception and Human Performance, Cognitive Processes and Performance. New York: John Wiley; 1986. pp. 42-9.
21. Peitgen K, Walz MV, Walz MV, Holtmann G, Eigler FW. A prospective randomized experimental evaluation of three-dimensional imaging in laparoscopy. Gastrointest Endosc. 1996;44:262-7.
22. Perkins N, Starkes JL, Lee TD, Hutchison C. Learning to use minimal access surgical instruments and two-dimensional remote visual feedback: how difficult is the task for novices? Adv Health Sci Educ Theory Pract. 2002;7:117-31.
23. Peters JH, Fried GM, Swanstrom LL, Soper NJ, Sillin LF, Schirmer B, et al. Development and validation of a comprehensive program of education and assessment of the basic fundamentals of laparoscopic surgery. Surgery. 2004;135:21-7.
24. Powers TW, Bentrem DJ, Nagle AP, Toyama MT, Murphy SA, Murayama KM. Hand dominance and performance in a laparoscopic skills curriculum. Surg Endosc. 2005;19:673-7.

25. Reed JF 3rd. Analysis of two-treatment, two-period crossover trials in emergency medicine. Ann Emerg Med. 2004;43:54-8.
26. Risucci D, Geiss A, Gellman L, Pinard B, Rosser J. Surgeon-specific factors in the acquisition of laparoscopic surgical skills. Am J Surg. 2001;181:289-93.
27. Scott DJ, Jones DB. Virtual reality training and teaching tools. In: Soper NJ, Swanstrom LL, Eubanks WS (Eds). Mastery of Endoscopic and Laparoscopic Surgery. Philadelphia: Lippincott Williams and Wilkins; 2005. pp. 146-60.
28. Stefanidis D, Korndorffer JR Jr, Sierra R, Touchard C, Dunne JB, Scott DJ. Skill retention following proficiency-based laparoscopic simulator training. Surgery. 2005;138:165-70.
29. Stefanidis D, Korndorffer JR, Scott DJ. Robotic laparoscopic fundoplication. Curr Treat Options Gastroenterol. 2005;8: 71-83.
30. Sun CC, Chiu AW, Chen KK, Chang LS. Assessment of a three-dimensional operating system with skill tests in a pelvic trainer. Urol Int. 2000;64:154-8.
31. Taffinder N, Smith SG, Huber J, Russell RC, Darzi A. The effect of a second-generation 3D endoscope on the laparoscopic precision of novices and experienced surgeons. Surg Endosc. 1999;13:1087-92.
32. Thomsen MN, Lang RD. An experimental comparison of three-dimensional and two-dimensional endoscopic systems in a model. Arthroscopy. 2004;20:419-23.
33. Torkington J, Smith SG, Rees B, Darzi A. The role of the basic surgical skills course in the acquisition and retention of laparoscopic skills. Surg Endosc. 2001;15:1071-5.
34. Votanopoulos K, Brunicardi FC, Thornby J, Bellows CF. Impact of three-dimensional vision in laparoscopic training. World J Surg. 2008;32:110-8.
35. Wickens CD, Hollands JG. Engineering Psychology and Human Performance. Upper Saddle River, NJ: Prentice Hall; 2000. p. 1164.
36. Windsor JA, Zoha F. The laparoscopic performance of novice surgical trainees: testing for acquisition, loss, and reacquisition of psychomotor skills. Surg Endosc. 2005;19:1058-63.

CHAPTER 4

Sterilization of Laparoscopic Instruments

Sterilization is the process by which surgical items are rendered free of viable microorganisms, including spores. The purpose of effective laparoscopic instrument sterilization is to provide the surgeon with a sterile product.

HISTORY

According to ancient writings, most primitive people regarded disease as the work of evil spirits or as coming from supernatural powers. Hippocrates (460–370 BC) began the shift of the healing process from mystical rites to a practical approach. Marcus Terentius Varro (117–26 BC) proposed a germ theory by stating, "Small creatures, invisible to the eye, fill the atmosphere, and breathed through the nose cause dangerous diseases." Seventeenth century advancements in anatomy, physiology, and medical instrumentation included the development of the microscope in 1683 by Antonie van Leeuwenhoek which allowed bacteria to be studied. Research into surgery and anatomy continued during the eighteenth century. In the 1850s, Pasteur proved that fermentation, putrefaction, infection, and souring are caused by the growth of microbes. Lord Joseph Lister was the one who successfully identified the implications for surgical infections. Lister believed that infection could be prevented if he could prevent the airborne microbes from entering the wound. Further advances in aseptic techniques from 1881 to 1882 were possible when a German bacteriologist, Robert Koch, introduced methods of steam sterilization and developed the first nonpressure flowing steam sterilizer.

LEGISLATION IN STERILIZATION

The sterilization of laparoscopic instruments must comply with safety standards. These vary depending upon legislation of the individual countries.

In Germany, legislation requires steam autoclaving at 134°C for 5 minutes. However, in France, sterilization is practiced at this temperature for 18 minutes. In the United States of America, Food and Drug Administration (FDA) has established different sterilization criteria regarding sterilization of reusable instruments. General requirement for characterization of sterilizing agent and the development, validation and routine control of a sterilization process for laparoscopic instrument is provided by the manufacturer and sterilization should be performed strictly according to the manufacturer's guidelines.

Cleaning

All used instruments, regardless of size, should be completely immersed in distilled water before leaving the operating room. The first step of the high-level disinfection process is thorough cleaning **(Fig. 1)**. Cleaning removes debris, mucus, blood, and tissue (bioburden) which would interfere with the action of the disinfectant. Current recommendations specify disassembly of most laparoscopic equipment prior to sterilization. If the surgical assistants are unfamiliar with the proper assembly of laparoscopic instruments, it may cause patient injury from equipment malfunction. Because of the intricate internal parts of laparoscopic instruments, questions have been raised about the efficacy of cleaning and sterilization techniques.

In the instruments which cannot be dismantled, there is separate channel to irrigate water under pressure to clean it properly. At least 300 mL of water should be flushed through these instruments to clean it properly.

Approximately 99.8% of the bioburden can be removed by meticulous cleaning. Cleaning may be accomplished via manual or mechanical washing or enzyme detergent application **(Figs. 2 and 3)**.

Ultrasonic Technology for Cleaning

- Energy from high-frequency sound waves
- Vigorous microscopic implosions of tiny vapor bubbles
- Millions of scrubbing bubbles do the job of cleaning
- Ultrasonic cleaners facilitate removal of organic material, decreasing the risk of contaminants.

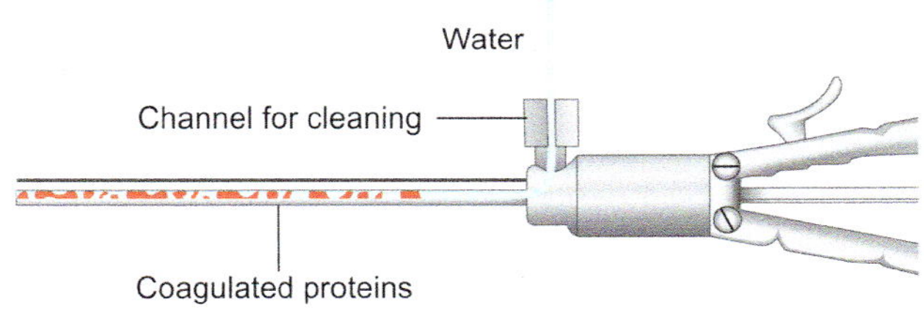

Fig. 1: Incomplete cleaning can result in accumulation of coagulated protein inside channel of the instrument.

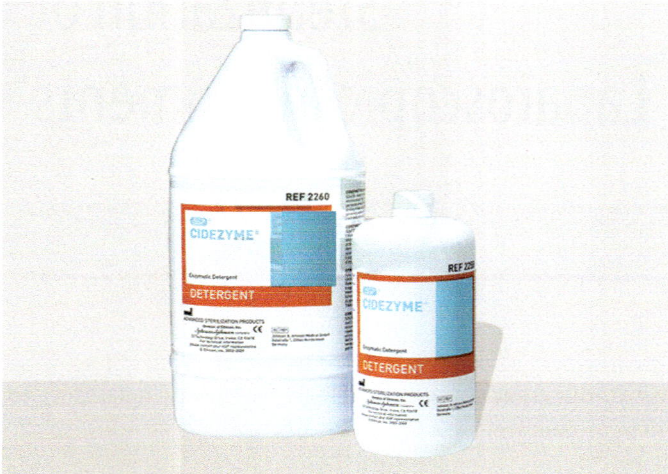

Fig. 2: Enzyme-based laparoscopic instrument cleaner.

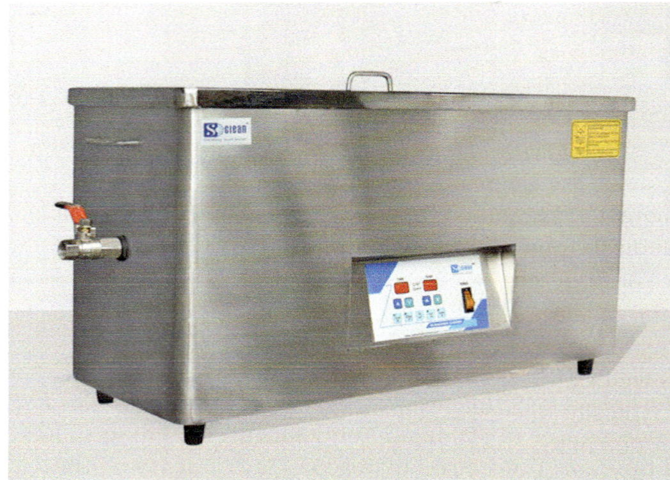

Fig. 3: Ultrasonic laparoscopic instrument cleaner.

The cleaning agent selected should be:

- Able to remove organic and inorganic soil
- Able to prevent waterborne deposits
- Low foaming
- Able to be rinsed completely
- Compatible with the materials being cleaned.

Enzymatic Laparoscopic Instrument Cleaner

The enzyme-based laparoscopic instrument cleaner has been shown in **Figure 2**.

Enzyme-based cleaner has an enzymatic detergent solution. The solution gets into hard-to-reach parts of your equipment for thorough cleaning. The enzymatic cleaning detergent has the following advantages.

- Increased activity on proteins (like blood, feces, and mucous) with protease enzyme
- Advanced formulation quickly and thoroughly penetrates organic matter
- The safe, biodegradable base is easy on you and the environment.

Following cleaning, items to be disinfected must be rinsed thoroughly to remove any residual detergent. After cleaning, instruments are subjected to sterilization.

Sterilization

The two methods of sterilization most commonly used for laparoscopic instruments are:

1. Steam sterilization
2. Chemical sterilization

Autoclaving by means of steam was the oldest, safest and most cost-effective method of sterilization. When steam is placed under pressure and the temperature is raised, the moist heat produces changes within the cell protein, thereby rendering it harmless over a prescribed period of time. The relationship between temperature, pressure and time of exposure is the critical factor in the destruction of microbes. Although steam sterilization in effective an inexpensive it is not suitable for all laparoscopic instruments.

The growth and expansion of minimal access surgical procedures require specialized surgical instrumentation. Most of the laparoscopic instrument can be safely autoclaved but some of the laparoscopic instruments cannot withstand the prolonged heat and moisture of the steam sterilization process. Laparoscopic cameras, laparoscopes, light cables, and flexible endoscopes are damaged by heat. Therefore, alternative methods of sterilization were needed to effectively sterilize moisture-stable, moisture-sensitive, and heat-sensitive items that require rapid, frequent processing in the clinical setting.

One of the most common types of alternative of steam sterilization is chemical sterilization. Many chemicals are proven to have sterilizing property. Laparoscopic camera [charge-coupled device (CCD)] is damaged by chemical sterilization with repeated exposure. In these expensive devices, a sterile plastic sleeve or sterile thick cloth sleeve should be used to avoid contamination.

Ethylene Oxide

One of the most common types of chemical sterilization uses ethylene oxide (EtO) gas, which is in use since the 1950s. EtO is colorless at ordinary temperatures, has an odor similar to that of ether and is extremely toxic and flammable. Mixture of EtO with an inert gas such as carbon dioxide or a chlorofluorocarbon (CFC) was used to make it noninflammable. The most common combination was 12% EtO and 88% freon. A newer formulation uses EtO plus a hydrochlorofluorocarbon (HCFC).

Ethylene oxide sterilization depends on four parameters:

1. Time
2. Temperature

3. Gas concentration
4. Relative humidity

All EtO sterilizers operate at low temperature, typically between 49 and 60°C (130–140°F) and relative humidity of 40–60%. The humidity must be not <30% in order to hydrate the items during the sterilization process. These characteristics make EtO sterilization suitable for complex medical equipment.

Both temperature and humidity have a profound influence on the destruction of microorganisms because they affect penetration of the gas through bacterial cell walls, as well as through the wrapping and packaging materials. It typically takes between 3 and 6 hours for the sterilization portion of the cycle to be completed.

Additionally, items sterilized by EtO must be aerated to make them safe for personnel handling and patient use. The main disadvantages associated with EtO are the lengthy cycle time, the cost, and its potential hazards to patients and staff; the main advantage is that it can sterilize heat- or moisture-sensitive medical equipment without deleterious effects on the material used in the laparoscopic devices. Therefore, the EtO sterilization and aeration processes can take up to 20 hours and should be used only when time is not a factor.

Hydrogen Peroxide Gas Plasma

Hydrogen peroxide is an oxidizing agent that affects sterilization by oxidation of key cellular components. Gas plasmas have been referred to as the fourth state of matter (i.e., liquids, solids, gases, and gas plasmas). The cloud of plasma is composed of ions, electrons, and neutral atomic particles that produce a visible glow. Hydrogen peroxide is bactericidal, virucidal, sporicidal, and fungicidal, even at low concentration and temperature. Gas plasmas are generated in an enclosed chamber under deep vacuum using radio-frequency or microwave energy to excite the gas molecules and produce charged particles, many of which are in the form of free radicals. A free radical is an atom with an unpaired electron and is a highly reactive species. The mechanism of action of this device is the production of free radicals within a plasma field that are capable of interacting with essential cell components (e.g., enzymes, nucleic acids) and thereby disrupt the metabolism of microorganisms. The type of seed gas used, and the depth of the vacuum are two important variables that can determine the effectiveness of this process.

A solution of hydrogen peroxide and water (59% nominal peroxide by weight) is vaporized and allowed to surround and interact with the devices to be sterilized. Applying a strong electrical field then creates plasma. The plasma breaks down the peroxide into a "cloud" of highly energized species that recombine, turning the hydrogen peroxide into water and oxygen. No aeration time is required and the instruments may either be used immediately or placed on a shelf for later use. A load of surgical instruments may be sterilized in <1 hour **(Fig. 4)**.

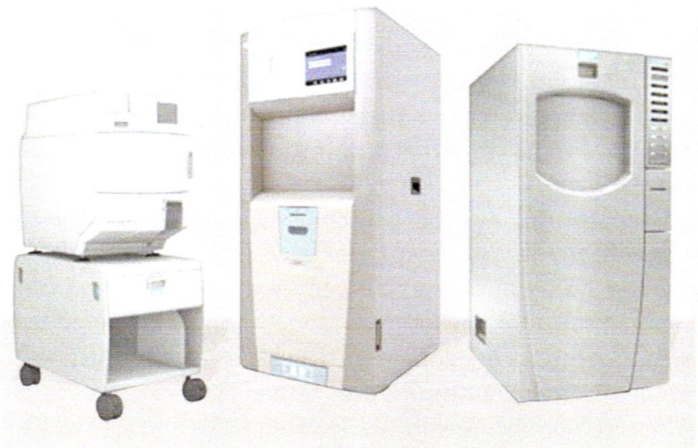

Fig. 4: Hydrogen peroxide gas plasma.

A newer version of the unit improves sterilizer efficacy by using two cycles with a hydrogen peroxide diffusion stage and a plasma stage per sterilization cycle. This revision, which is achieved by a software modification, reduces total processing time from 60 to 30 minutes. Laparoscopic instruments that cannot tolerate high temperatures and humidity of autoclaving, such as some hand instruments, electrical devices, and corrosion-susceptible metal alloys, can be sterilized by hydrogen peroxide gas plasma very efficiently. This method has been compatible with most (>95%) laparoscopic instruments.

Peracetic Acid

Liquid peroxyacetic acid, or peracetic acid, is a biocidal oxidizer that maintains its efficacy in the presence of high levels of organic debris. Peracetic acid is acetic acid plus an extra oxygen atom and reacts with most cellular components to cause cell death. The peracetic acid solution is heated to 50–56°C (122–131°F) during the 20–30 minutes cycle. Peracetic acid must be used in combination with anticorrosive additives.

Parameters for peracetic acid sterilizers include:

- Relatively short cycle times
- Availability of the items for immediate use
- Sterilant can be discharged into the drainage system since it is not hazardous
- No aeration time is required for the sterilized items
- Items must be rinsed with copious amounts of sterile water after the sterilization process.

Items processed by this method should be used immediately after processing, since the containers are wet and are not protected from the environment. This system must also be monitored for sterility with live spores.

Glutaraldehyde

An activated 2% aqueous glutaraldehyde solution is recognized as an effective liquid chemical sterilant. Glutaraldehyde is most frequently used as a high-level disinfectant for lensed instruments because it is non-corrosive and has minimal harmful effect on the instrument **(Fig. 5)**.

Sterilization can be achieved with an activated 2% glutaraldehyde solution after the item is completely immersed for 10 hours at 25°C in especially designed tray. Before immersion, the item must be thoroughly cleaned and dried. During immersion, all surfaces of the item must be in contact with the solution. After immersion, the item must be rinsed thoroughly with sterile water prior to use **(Fig. 6)**.

Cidex should be used maximum 15 times or 21 days after activation, whichever may be earlier. Once activated, the solution should be discarded after 21 days, so it is important to write the date of activation and date of expiry in the space provided on the Cidex tray **(Fig. 7)**. If the instrument is not cleaned properly, the activated glutaraldehyde becomes dirty just after few use and turns into blackish solution. In this case, it should be rejected before specified period of time. It is important that surgeon should read carefully the literature provided by the manufacturer.

Ortho-phthalaldehyde

For laparoscopic instruments, 0.55% ortho-phthalaldehyde (OPA) is good option, it is nonglutaraldehyde solution for disinfection of delicate instruments. In fact, OPA solution is one of the gentlest reprocessing options available, which means it can substantially reduce instrument damage and repair costs. OPA solution offers excellent materials compatibility and can therefore be used to disinfect a wide range of medical instruments made of aluminum, brass, copper, stainless steel, plastics, elastomers. It is good not only because of its speed and efficiency but also because of its environmental safety. It comes with the trade name of Cidex OPA **(Fig. 8)**.

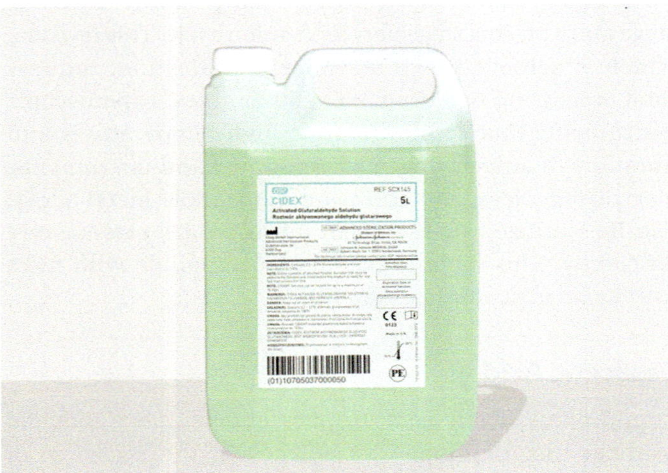

Fig. 5: Cidex (2% glutaraldehyde).

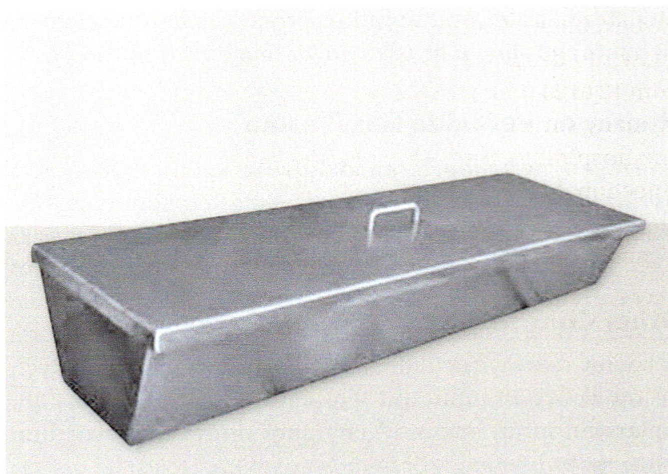

Fig. 6: Cidex tray used for laparoscopic instrument sterilization.

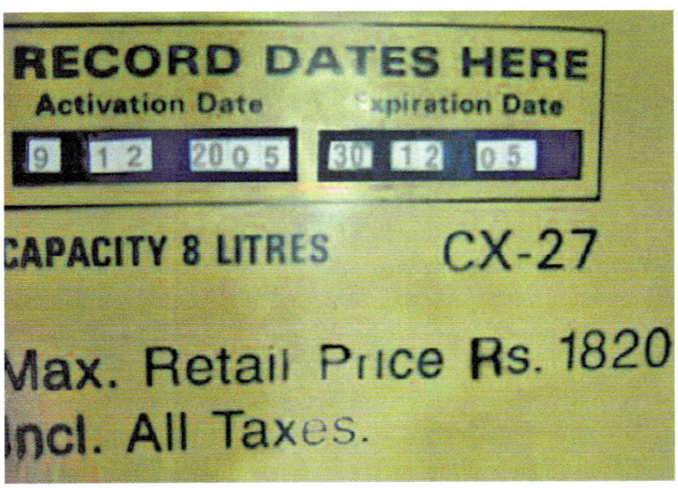

Fig. 7: Labeling of Cidex tray (activation date and expiration date).

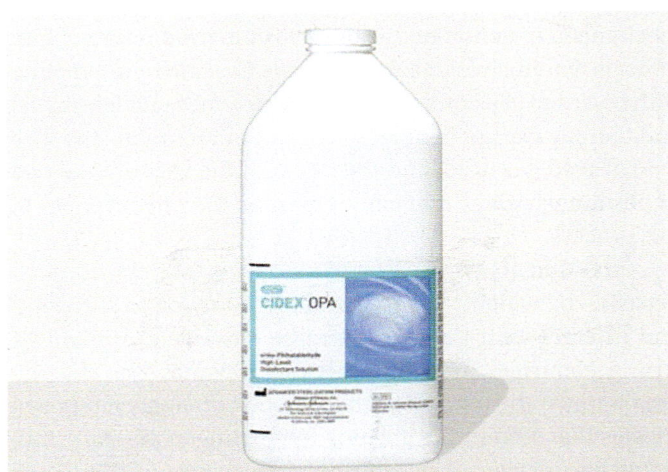

Fig. 8: Cidex® ortho-phthalaldehyde (OPA) high-level disinfectant.

It has following advantages:
- No activation or mixing required
- It can be used in both automated and manual reprocessing
- Two years shelf-life and 75 days open-bottle shelf-life
- Rapid 5 minutes immersion time at a minimum of 25°C in an automatic endoscope reprocessor
- Efficient 12 minutes soak time at room temperature (20°C) for manual reprocessing
- Effective against glutaraldehyde-resistant *Mycobacterium.*

Formaldehyde

Bactericidal properties and use of formaldehyde include: 37% aqueous solution (formalin) or 8% formaldehyde in 70% isopropyl alcohol kills microorganisms by coagulating intracellular protein. Solution is effective at room temperature.

Specially designed airtight formalin chambers are available **(Fig. 9)**. Eight to ten formalin tablets wrapped with moist gauze piece should be placed in the chamber and the door should be closed. The vapor of formalin acts for 1 week, after 1 week, tablets should be changed. Although known to destroy spores, it is rarely used because it takes from 12 to 24 hours to be effective. Formalin chamber is used by many surgeons to carry their sterilized instrument from one hospital to another. Pungent odor of formalin is quite objectionable and irritating to the eyes and nasal passages. The vapors can be toxic and ongoing controversy exists regarding its carcinogenic effects.

Other Chemical Disinfectant

Recently, nonaldehyde instrument disinfectant is available for rapid decontamination of noninvasive and heat labile laparoscopic instruments. It contains halogenated tertiary amines, polyhexamethylene biguanide hydrochloride, ethyl alcohol B, dodecylamine, and sulfamic acid. Contact time for bactericidal, fungicidal, and virucidal protection is 10 minutes. For sporicidal protection, contact time is 30 minutes.

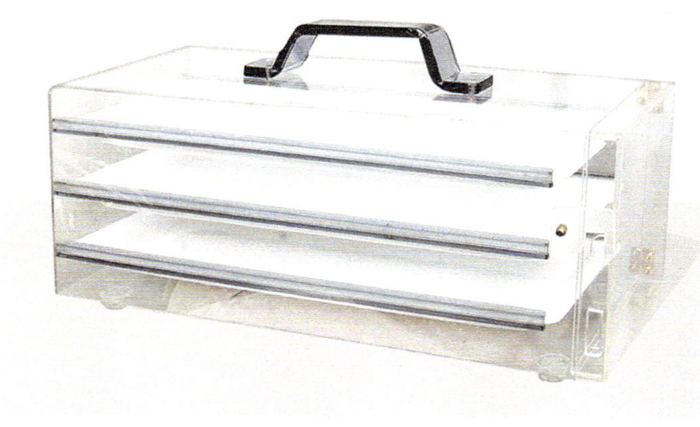

Fig. 9: Formalin chamber.

CONCLUSION

Most of the laparoscopic instrument can be easily sterilized if the person knows how to dissemble, clean and use specific chemical for sterilization. Manufacturer's instruction is important to follow if desired effect has to be achieved. Expensive instruments should be handled carefully and all the insulated instruments should be checked thoroughly for any breach in insulation before sterilization. Apart from newer generation chemical disinfectant, low-temperature steam with formaldehyde has been widely used in healthcare facilities in Northern Europe for the sterilization of reusable medical devices that cannot withstand steam sterilization.

Other key considerations in the sterilization process which should be taken care are:
- Packaging of the items after sterilization
- Monitoring the sterilization process
- Shelf life of the sterilized items
- Cost implications

BIBLIOGRAPHY

1. Barthram C, McClymont W. The use of a checklist for anaesthetic machines. Anaesthesia. 1992;47:1066-9.
2. Berge JA, Gramstad L, Grimnes S. An evaluation of a time-saving anaesthetic machine checkout procedure. Eur J Anaesthesiol. 1994;11:493-8.
3. Berge JA, Gramstad L, Jensen O. A training simulator for detecting equipment failure in the anaesthetic machine. Eur J Anaesthesiol. 1993;10:19-24.
4. Blike G, Biddle C. Preanesthesia detection of equipment faults by anesthesia providers at an academic hospital: comparison of standard practice and a new electronic checklist. AANA J. 2000;68:497-505.
5. Burner ST, Waldo DR, McKusich DR. National health expenditures projections through 2030. Health Care Financ Rev. 1992;14(1):1-29.
6. Calland JF, Guerlain S, Adams RB, Tribble CG, Foley E, Chekan EG. A systems approach to surgical safety. Surg Endosc. 2002; 16:1005-15.
7. Civil Aviation Authority (CAA) (2000). Guidance on the design, presentation and use of electronic checklists. CAP 708. Safety Regulation Group. [online] Available from http://www.caa.co.uk/docs/33/CAP708.PDF [Last accessed May, 2020].
8. Civil Aviation Authority (CAA) (2006). Guidance on the design presentation and use of emergency and abnormal checklists. CAP 676. Safety Regulation Group. [online] Available from http://www.caa.co.uk/docs/33/CAP676.PDF [Last accessed May, 2020].
9. Dankelman J, Grimbergen CA. Systems approach to reduce errors in surgery. Surg Endosc. 2005;19:1017-21.
10. DeFontes J, Surbida S. Preoperative safety briefing project. Perm J. 2004;8:21-7.
11. Degani A, Wiener EL. Cockpit checklists: concepts, design, and use. Hum Factors. 1993;35(2):28-43.
12. Degani A, Wiener EL. Human Factors of Flight-Deck Checklists: The Normal Checklist. NASA Contractor Report 177549; 1990.

13. Diamond T, Mole DJ. Anatomical orientation and cross-checking: the key to safer laparoscopic cholecystectomy. Br J Surg. 2005;92:663-4.
14. Eiseman B, Borlase BC. Measurement of cost effectiveness. In: Eiseman B, Stahlgren L (Eds). Cost Effective Surgical Practice. Philadelphia: WB Saunders; 1978. pp. 1-5.
15. Ginzberg E. High-tech medicine and rising health care costs. JAMA. 1990;263(13):1820-2.
16. Gwinnutt CL, Driscoll PA. Advanced trauma life support. Eur J Anaesthesiol. 1996;13:95-101.
17. Hart EM, Owen H. Errors and omissions in anesthesia: a pilot study using a pilot's checklist. Anesth Analg. 2005;101:246-50, table of contents.
18. Helmreich RL. On error management: lessons from aviation. BMJ. 2000;320:781-5.
19. Jordan AM. Hospital charges for laparoscopic and open cholecystectomy. JAMA. 1991;266(24):3425.
20. Kendell J, Barthram C. Revised checklist for anaesthetic machines. Anaesthesia. 1998;53:887-90.
21. Kohn LT, Corrigan JM, Donaldson MS. To Err Is Human: Building a Safer Health System. Institute of Medicine, Washington DC: National Academies Press; 1999. pp. 1-14.
22. Kwaan MR, Studdert DM, Zinner MJ, Gawande AA. Incidence, patterns, and prevention of wrong-site surgery. Arch Surg. 2006;141:353-7; discussion 357-8.
23. Leape L. The preventability of medical injury. In: Bogner MS (Ed). Human Error in Medicine. Hillsdale, NJ: Lawrence Erlbaum Associates; 1994.
24. Leonard M, Graham S, Bonacum D. The human factor: the critical importance of effective teamwork and communication in providing safe care. Qual Saf Health Care. 2004;13(Suppl 1): i85-i90.
25. Lingard L, Espin S, Rubin B, Whyte S, Colmenares M, Baker GR, et al. Getting teams to talk: development and pilot implementation of a checklist to promote interprofessional communication in the OR. Qual Saf Health Care. 2005;14(5):340-6.
26. Makary MA, Holzmueller CG, Thompson D, Rowen L, Heitmiller ES, Maley WR, et al. Operating room briefings: working on the same page. Jt Comm J Qual Patient Saf. 2006;32(6):351-5.
27. Makary MA, Mukherjee A, Sexton JB, Syin D, Goodrich E, Hartmann E, et al. Operating room briefings and wrong-site surgery. J Am Coll Surg. 2007;204:236-43.
28. Manley R, Cuddeford JD. An assessment of the effectiveness of the revised FDA checklist. AANA J. 1996;64:277-82.
29. March MG, Crowley JJ. An evaluation of anesthesiologists' present checkout methods and the validity of the FDA checklist. Anesthesiology. 1991;75:724-9.
30. McIntyre RC, Foster MA, Weil KC, Cohen MM. A comparison of outcome and cost of open vs. laparoscopic cholecystectomy. J Laparoendosc Surg. 1992;2:143-8; discussion 149.
31. Meijer DW. Safety of the laparoscopy setup. Minim Invasive Ther Allied Technol. 2003;12:125-8.
32. Michaels RK, Makary MA, Dahab Y, Frassica FJ, Heitmiller E, Rowen LC, et al. Achieving the National Quality Forum's "Never Events": prevention of wrong site, wrong procedure, and wrong patient operations. Ann Surg. 2007;245:526-32.
33. Palmer E, Degani A. Electronic checklists: evaluation of two levels of automation. Proceedings of the Sixth International Aviation Psychology Symposium. Columbus, OH: The Ohio State University; 1994.
34. Peters JH, Ellison L, Innes JT, Liss JL, Nichols KE, Lomano JM, et al. Safety and efficacy of laparoscopic cholecystectomy. A prospective analysis of 100 initial patients. Ann Surg. 1991;213:3-12.
35. Punt MM, Stefels CN, Grimbergen CA, Dankelman J. Evaluation of voice control, touch panel control, and assistant control during steering of an endoscope. Minim Invasive Ther Allied Technol. 2005;14:181-7.
36. Reason J. Human Error. New York: Cambridge University Press; 1990.
37. Reason J. Human error: models and management. BMJ. 2000;320:768-70.
38. Reichert M. Laparoscopic instruments: patient care, cost issues. AORN J. 1993;57(3):637-55.
39. Rouse SH, Rouse WB. Computer-based manuals for procedural information. IEEE Trans Syst Man Cybern. 1980;10(8):506-10.
40. Saufl NM. Universal protocol for preventing wrong site, wrong procedure, wrong person surgery. J Perianesth Nurs. 2004;19:348-51.
41. Schieber GJ, Poullier JP, Greenwald LM. U.S. health expenditure performance: an international comparison and data update. Health Care Financ Rev. 1992;13(4):1-87.
42. Stufflebeam DL (2000). Guidelines for developing evaluation checklists: the checklists development checklist (CDC). [online] Available from http://www.wmich.edu/evalctr/checklists/guidelines_cdc.pdf [Last accessed May, 2020].
43. Technology Assessment Committee of the American Society for Gastrointestinal Endoscopy Position statement report on transmission of microorganisms. Gastrointestinal Endosc. 1993;36(6):885-8.
44. Undre S, Healey AN, Darzi A, Vincent CA. Observational assessment of surgical teamwork: a feasibility study. World J Surg. 2006;30:1774-83.
45. Universal protocol for preventing wrong site, wrong procedure, wrong person surgery. [online] Available from http://www.jointcommission.org/PatientSafety/UniversalProtocol/ [Last accessed May, 2020].
46. Verdaasdonk EG, Stassen LP, van der Elst M, Karsten TM, Dankelman J. Problems with technical equipment during laparoscopic surgery: an observational study. Surg Endosc. 2007;21:275-9.
47. Verdaasdonk EG, Stassen LP, Widhiasmara PP, Dankelman J. Requirements for the design and implementation of checklists for surgical processes. Surg Endosc. 2009;23:715-26.
48. Vincent C, Moorthy K, Sarker SK, Chang A, Darzi AW. Systems approaches to surgical quality and safety: from concept to measurement. Ann Surg. 2004;239:475-82.
49. Wagner C, de Bruijne M. Onbedoelde schade in Nederlandse ziekenhuizen. Amsterdam/Utrecht: EMGO en NIVEL, Nederlands Instituut voor Onderzoek van de Gezondheidszorg; 2007. p. 20.

CHAPTER 5

Anesthesia in Laparoscopic Surgery

INTRODUCTION

The anesthetic problems during minimal access surgery are related to the cardiopulmonary effects of pneumoperitoneum, carbon dioxide (CO_2) absorption, extraperitoneal gas insufflation, venous embolism, and inadvertent injuries to intra-abdominal organs. Optimal anesthetic care of patients undergoing laparoscopic surgery is very much important. Good anesthetic techniques facilitate risk-free surgery and allow early detection and reduction of complications.

In young patients, fit for diagnostic laparoscopy, general anesthesia is the preferred method and does not impose any increased risk. Adequate anesthesia and analgesia are essential and endotracheal intubation and controlled ventilation should be considered. The pneumoperitoneum can be created safely under local anesthesia provided that the patient is adequately sedated throughout the procedure. For successful laparoscopy under local anesthesia, intravenous (IV) medication for sedation should be given.

EVALUATION AND PREPARATION OF PATIENT FOR LAPAROSCOPIC SURGERY

A thorough preanesthetic assessment is mandatory and all comorbidities should be optimized in case the procedure needs to be converted to an open one. Premedication should include a short-acting anxiolytic, an H_2-receptor antagonist, and an analgesic for preemptive analgesia.

Many of the patients scheduled to undergo laparoscopic surgery are young women undergoing gynecological laparoscopy. Young women undergoing gynecological procedures under general anesthesia are at high risk of postoperative nausea and vomiting. Laparoscopy itself is also associated with postoperative nausea and vomiting, probably due to stretching of the abdominal cavity or residual irritant effects of retained CO_2. Anesthesiologists should plan their anesthetic to prevent and treat postoperative nausea and vomiting in these patients.

A second group of patients that cause concern are those with significant cardiac disease. Most of these patients tolerate abdominal insufflation at low pressures currently used (<18 mm Hg) surprisingly well. If the operation is to be of short duration, few patients with cardiac disease, other than those with severe congestive heart failure, require invasive monitoring. However, insufflation can be associated with a moderately reduced cardiac index, increased cardiac filling pressures, systemic blood pressure, and systemic vascular resistance. In addition, hypercarbia from insufflated CO_2 may be detrimental to patients with cardiac disease by stimulating the sympathetic nervous system and vasopressin release. Therefore, for extensive laparoscopic procedures, direct arterial and pulmonary artery catheterization and/or transesophageal echocardiography may be necessary for monitoring.

A third group of patients of concern are those with severe emphysema, asthma, cystic fibrosis, or other pulmonary disease. Often, these are patients who would benefit from a laparoscopic operation as opposed to an open procedure because of improved postoperative pulmonary function following procedures performed laparoscopically. However, some of these patients may not be able to be adequately ventilated to eliminate the CO_2 absorbed during laparoscopy. It is important for patients with severe lung disease to be in optimum medical condition prior to having surgery.

The anesthesiologist must be certain that the patient does not have an upper respiratory tract infection or other conditions that may impair pulmonary function at the time of surgery. Prior preparation with a course of bronchodilators, steroids, and/or antibiotics may be necessary. In these patients, an intra-arterial catheter for arterial blood sampling for gas analysis as well as direct arterial pressure monitoring is essential, since the end-tidal carbon dioxide ($EtCO_2$) tension often does not accurately reflect the arterial CO_2 tension and may be significantly lower.

Laparoscopic procedures offer numerous advantages in obese patients including less postoperative pain, pneumonia and wound site infection, better respiratory functions and cosmetic appearance, shorter duration of recovery and discharge, and lower total cost. Full understanding of pathophysiological changes is necessary for an optimal anesthetic care. These patients are at risk of other comorbidities such as hypertension, diabetes mellitus, cardiac problems, and respiratory problems and should be thoroughly examined and managed before planning for surgery. Thromboprophylaxis is essential in the morbidly obese patients scheduled for bariatric surgery. Low-molecular-weight heparin, enoxaparin 0.6 mL subcutaneous (SC), dalteparin 5,000 IU SC, or fondaparinux 2.5 mg SC is given 12 hours before surgery. Mechanical thromboprophylaxis with sequential compression devices is mandatory.

A laparoscopic surgeon should develop communication and understanding with his anesthetist. Adequate preoperative assessment of the patient and the disease minimizes the risk of general anesthesia. Necessary measures should be undertaken to correct any metabolic or hematological abnormalities such as hypokalemia, hyponatremia, hyperglycemia, azotemia, anemia, and coagulation defects. All the required preanesthetic laboratory data should be available including blood grouping and testing for the hepatitis B antigen and human immunodeficiency virus (HIV). Patients should have an electrocardiogram and chest X-ray.

PHYSIOLOGICAL CHANGES DURING LAPAROSCOPY

The introduction of gas into the peritoneal cavity under pressure may cause pain, respiratory distress, and possibly cardiac embarrassment. Further, Trendelenburg position is necessary for access but extreme Trendelenburg position enhances respiratory and cardiac embarrassment.

Pneumoperitoneum at the time of laparoscopic surgery causes upward displacement of the diaphragm, resulting in the reduction in lung volumes including functional residual capacity (FRC). Pulmonary compliance is reduced and airway resistance is increased due to high intra-abdominal pressure (IAP). The anesthetist often uses high airway pressure to overcome the IAP for a given tidal volume, which increases the risk of hemodynamic changes and barotraumas.

The impaired diaphragmatic mobility gives rise to uneven distribution of ventilation to the nondependent part of the lung, resulting in ventilation-perfusion (V/Q) mismatch with hypercarbia and hypoxemia. The ventilatory impairment is even more severe if there is associated airway and alveolar collapse. Increased IAP also predisposes to regurgitation of gastric contents and pulmonary aspiration.

Insufflation of CO_2 is usually accompanied by hypercapnia. The reason initially proposed to explain this hypercapnia was that CO_2 was reabsorbed from the peritoneal cavity. This explanation was all the more plausible in that it was based on the capacity of CO_2 to diffuse and the exchange capacities of the peritoneal serosa. Recent studies reveal a two-phase phenomenon, with absorption proportional to intraperitoneal pressure for low insufflation pressures, then a drop in the rate of this reabsorption probably due to the peritoneal circulation being crushed under the effect of the pressure. The variations in arterial partial pressure of carbon dioxide ($PaCO_2$) observed during the second phase with high IAPs which act against reabsorption essentially depend on a change in the V/Q ratio with an increase in the dead space.

The hypercapnia mechanism is different with extraperitoneal insufflation. In this case, the pressure effect limiting reabsorption from the peritoneum no longer applies. The increase in pressure increases the diffusion space by dilacerations of the tissues and thus the CO_2 reabsorption surface. Reabsorption is thus directly proportional to the pressure and volume of CO_2 insufflated in extraperitoneal insufflation. Severe hypercapnia is thus possible, if not to say frequent, in these situations. On the other hand, provided the hypercapnia is controlled, the circulatory effect of extraperitoneal insufflation is lower than those of intraperitoneal insufflation.

The increase in intrathoracic pressures induced by the increase in IAP can be limiting factors for laparoscopic surgery in certain patients. Insufflation of the pneumoperitoneum in laparoscopic surgery is accompanied by a decrease of some 30% in pulmonary compliance. The resistance of the air passages increases in the same proportions. The resulting increase in pressure in the air passages can have adverse consequences for patients with bubbles of emphysema. These patients and all those who suffer from dystrophy of the pulmonary parenchyma will find it difficult to cope with the often considerable hyperventilation required by hypercapnia, with volumes per minute sometimes reaching two or three times than normal.

Venous gas embolism is a fatal complication of pneumoperitoneum. Veress needle or the trocar may directly puncture the arteries or blood flow across an opening in an injured vessel, may sometimes draw gas into the vessel and leads to gas embolism.

A slow infusion of air <1 L/min is absorbed across the pulmonary capillary-alveolar membranes without causing any damage. At higher infusion rates, the gas bubbles lodging in the peripheral pulmonary arterioles provoke neutrophil clumping, activation of the coagulation cascade, and platelet aggregation. This may lead to pulmonary vasoconstriction, bronchospasm, pulmonary edema, and pulmonary hemorrhage. Gas bubbles attached to fibrin deposits and platelet aggregates mechanically obstruct the pulmonary vasculature and increases the pulmonary vascular resistance.

The increased right heart afterload leads to acute right heart failure with arrhythmia, ischemia, hypotension, and elevated central venous pressure. Sometimes, paradoxical embolism is seen through a patent foramen ovale.

Elevated IAP produces physiological changes in the hemodynamic by its effects on systemic vascular resistance, venous return, and myocardial performance. Systemic venous return increases when IAP is elevated. Effects on venous return and cardiac output depend on the magnitude of the IAP. Venous return initially increases with IAP below 10 mm Hg. This paradox is due to reduction in the blood volume sequestrated in the splanchnic vasculature which increases cardiac output and arterial pressure. When IAP exceeds 20 mm Hg, the inferior vena cava is compressed. Venous return from the lower half of the body is impeded resulting in a fall in cardiac output.

A number of animal studies have been devoted to variations in cardiac output induced by the increase in intraperitoneal pressure. The results are consistent with a fall in cardiac output proportional to the intraperitoneal pressure. In low abdominal pressure (5 mm Hg), cardiac output remains unchanged. The drop in right transmural auricular pressure indicates a reduction in the venous return which is demonstrated by a reduction in flow, through the vena cava, the degree of which is proportional to the intra-abdominal pressure.

The cardiac output is governed by the myocardial function, the postloading, and by the venous return, the latter in turn depending on venous resistance and mean systemic pressure. With an IAP of 5 mm Hg, the venous return improves. Under these conditions, the intraperitoneal pressure remains lower than the pressure in the vena cava which results in a flushing effect, with no obstructive phenomena in the lower vena cava. When the intraperitoneal pressure rises above the intravascular pressure, a subdiaphragmatic narrowing of the lower vena cava slows the flow of blood. The abdominal blood volume is reduced due to the pressure and a reflux into the venous system of the lower limb occurs.

The increase in vascular resistance can be explained by the splanchnic vascular compression, but the persistence of high resistance after exsufflation, means a humoral factor could be suggested. During the increase in intraperitoneal pressure, a considerable rise in antidiuretic hormone is found and its vasopressive effects are well-known. This secretion would seem to be dependent on the drop in cardiac flow rate. A simultaneous rise in the level of plasma norepinephrine, whose vasoconstrictor effects are equivalent to those of vasopressin, has also been reported. The increase in vascular resistance is correlated with a rise in arterial pressure in so far as inotropism is sufficient.

The circulation of kidney becomes much compromised with increased IAP. Renal blood flow and glomerular filtration rate decrease because of increase in renal vascular resistance, reduction in glomerular filtration gradient, and decrease in cardiac output. The increase in systemic vascular resistance impairs left ventricular function and cardiac output. Arterial pressure, however, remains relatively unchanged, which conceals the fall in cardiac output. High intrathoracic pressure during intermittent positive pressure ventilation adds in impairment of venous return and cardiac output, particularly if positive end-expiratory pressure (PEEP) is also applied. The elevation in IAP produces lactic acidosis, probably by severely lowering cardiac output and by impairing hepatic clearance of blood lactate.

Stretching of the peritoneum sometimes leads to stimulation of vagus nerve and can provoke arrhythmias such as atrioventricular dissociation, nodal rhythm, sinus bradycardia, and asystole. This shock is more commonly seen with rapid stretching of the peritoneum at the beginning of peritoneal insufflation.

Faulty pneumoperitoneum may give rise to subcutaneous emphysema, pneumomediastinum, pneumopericardium, and pneumothorax. However, gas can also dissect through existing defects in the diaphragm or along surgically traumatized tissue planes in the retroperitoneum, the diaphragm, or the falciform ligament. Gas can leak into the subcutaneous tissues connected with poor positioning of a trocar sleeve (2.7% of cases of severe hypercapnia in a series of cholecystectomies published by Wieden); CO_2 is seen to spread outside the abdominal cavity during laparoscopic-assisted hysterectomy, with or without lymphadenectomy and during bladder neck suspensions. In laparoscopic gynecological surgery, because this effusion originates in the pelvis, it mostly affects the sides and loins and generally remains hidden by the drapes until the end of the operation. Only the very abundant, rare forms can be diagnosed by the anesthetist during the operation, when they shift toward to the upper part of the thorax. In this case, the capnographic signs (slow and regular increase in CO_2 expired) will provide an alert during the anesthesia.

Major factors that alter physiology during laparoscopic surgeries are:

- Pneumoperitoneum
- Carbon dioxide
- Positioning

Effects of reverse Trendelenburg position during laparoscopy are:

- Decreased preload
- Decreased mean arterial pressure
- Blood pooling to lower extremities leading to increased risk of venous thromboembolism
- Improved pulmonary functions

Effects of Trendelenburg position during laparoscopy are:

- *Respiratory*:
  - Decreased vital capacity
  - Decreased FRC
  - Abdominal contents restrict movement of diaphragm
  - Decreased compliance
  - Increased V/Q abnormalities
- *Circulatory*: The changes seen in healthy patients are minimal and consist of increased venous return and

cardiac output. The changes are more severe in patients with cardiovascular comorbidities and can be seen as increased central venous pressure and pulmonary artery occlusion pressure with decrease in cardiac output. There may be increase venous return and myocardial oxygen (O_2) demand leading to acute heart failure.

Pneumoperitoneum may lead to vagally-mediated reflexes such as bronchospasm, bradycardia, and sinus arrest. This is seen especially in young women when CO_2 insufflation is done rapidly. Similarly, cardiovascular collapse and gas emboli may also be seen.

Carbon dioxide stimulates sympathoadrenal system and may lead to increase cardiac output, heart rate, blood pressure, and force myocardial contraction. It increases cerebral blood flow and intracranial pressure. In neuroendocrine system, it increases epinephrine, norepinephrine, renin, cortisol, aldosterone, and antidiuretic hormone. It causes direct vasodilation of the splanchnic capillary beds whereas causes oliguria and decrease in glomerular filtration rate.

GENERAL ANESTHESIA

General anesthesia with tracheal intubation and controlled ventilation is recommended. This provides optimal control of CO_2, facilitates surgical access, and protects against aspiration of gastric contents.

Traditional volume controlled ventilation ensures an adequate tidal volume, but there is an increased risk of high inflation pressures and barotrauma, especially in bariatric surgery for the morbidly obese. Use of pressure controlled ventilation minimizes peak pressure and improves oxygenation in such situations.

Anesthesia for laparoscopy can be achieved with a variety of agents and techniques. General anesthesia using balanced anesthesia technique including IV induction agents such as thiopentone, propofol, etomidate, and inhalational agents like isoflurane, desflurane, and sevoflurane can be used **(Fig. 1)**. An ideal general anesthesia machine should have:

- Spontaneous breathing with computerized ventilation
- Manual ventilation
- Volume controlled ventilation
- Pressure controlled ventilation
- Computerized pressure support

Muscle relaxation can be done with atracurium, cisatracurium, vecuronium, and rocuronium. Pain can be controlled with opioids such as fentanyl and remifentanil along with nonopioid adjuvants such as paracetamol and dexmedetomidine.

Few anesthetist advocates use of laryngeal mask airways (LMAs), which avoid the postintubations or throat and laryngeal sequelae, but this is associated with a risk of inhalation of gastric content and gastric distension. However, the ProSeal LMA has been found to be as effective as a tracheal tube for pulmonary ventilation in laparoscopic surgery.

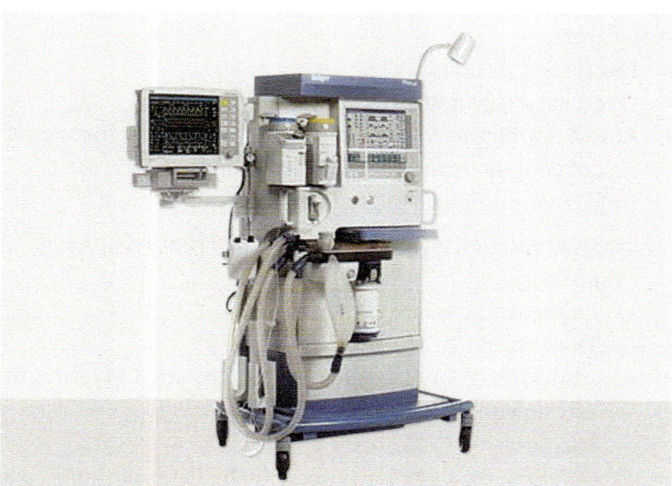

Fig. 1: Ideal anesthesia machine.

REGIONAL ANESTHESIA

Spinal anesthesia is reported enthusiastically for diagnostic laparoscopy without significant complications. Regional anesthesia may be useful for pelvic procedures but if high block is used it interferes with the respiratory status of patient. Bilateral lower intercostal nerve block has also been used, but it is time-consuming and it can cause pneumothorax.

Table 1 shows the comparison of general and regional anesthesia for laparoscopy.

TABLE 1: Comparison of general and regional anesthesia for laparoscopy.

	Advantages	*Disadvantages*
Regional anesthesia	• Avoids use of different drugs • Awake and spontaneously breathing patient • Faster recovery and ambulation • Less postoperative pain • No airway manipulation • Decreased PONV	• Significant hypotension • Shoulder discomfort due to diaphragmatic irritation • Patient anxiety • Risk of postoperative urinary retention • Risk of hypoventilation and desaturation, if supplemented with sedation • High level of block is required
General anesthesia	• Respiratory changes are well tolerated • Risk of aspiration minimal to nil	• Delayed recovery (especialy in old, obese, and compromised patients) • More postoperative pain • Increased PONV

(PONV: postoperative nausea and vomiting)

LOCAL ANESTHESIA

Many surgeons have done sufficient number of laparoscopic procedures under local anesthesia with IV sedation and results are encouraging with minimal morbidity and negligible mortality. Laparoscopy under local anesthesia should be performed with an anesthetist being present to monitor the patient's cardiac and respiratory functions. IV sedation should be administered with IV diazepam and pethidine. Preferred local anesthetic agent is 1% lignocaine without adrenaline or lidocaine without epinephrine. The anesthetic agent should be administered at the sites of insertion of the needle and all trocars.

If local anesthesia is used, anesthetist should perform valuable service by providing "vocal local technique". Anesthetist should talk constantly to the patient that everything is going well. One of the most difficult situations of local anesthesia is that the patient, rather than the surgeon, becomes the center of attraction for all noises and comments made in the room during surgery.

It is important to understand that under local anesthesia, adequate sedation and analgesia are administered to keep the patient somnolent but responsive. Continuous monitoring of all the vitals is essential throughout the procedure. Secondly, it is essential that a pneumoperitoneum of approximately 1.5–3 L be present under pressure.

ANESTHETIST'S ROLE IN LAPAROSCOPY

The role of anesthetist in laparoscopic surgery is vital. The laparoscopic surgery should never be performed if anesthetist has no experience in minimal access surgical anesthesia. It is up to anesthetist to identify whether he is capable of performing realistically without compromising the safety of the patients. It is only on these clearly established bases that safe laparoscopy can be contemplated.

Pregnant Women

Pregnant women undergoing laparoscopic surgery present several challenges to the anesthesiologist. The effect of carboperitoneum and increased IAP on the uteroplacental blood flow and its overall effect on the well-being of the fetus are the main concerns. In addition, space constraint, trocar insertion, and surgical manipulation are compounding factors. The gravid uterus pressing on the diaphragm leads to further decrease in FRC, increase in V/Q mismatch, and an increase in the arterioalveolar gradient. Special considerations in such patients include placing the patient in left lateral decubitus position, using open Hasson technique for gaining access to the abdominal cavity, maintaining the IAP as low as possible and continuously monitoring the maternal $EtCO_2$.

Fast-track Laparoscopic Bariatric Surgery

Target control infusions of remifentanil and propofol, maintenance with bispectral index (BIS)-titrated desflurane, multimodal analgesia, and antiemetic prophylaxis result in a successful and safe "short-stay" bariatric surgery program.

Pheochromocytoma

Low IAP (<10 mm Hg) along with slow insufflation of CO_2 and gradual positioning of the patient has been found to produce minimal changes in catecholamine levels and hemodynamics and is therefore recommended.

Pediatric

The physiological effects of laparoscopy in children are similar to adults, but the effects of the pneumoperitoneum and the extremes of patient position (Trendelenburg or reverse Trendelenburg) are more profound in neonates and infants. To minimize the negative physiological effects of pneumoperitoneum, it is recommended to have a slower rate of gas insufflation (1 L/min) and a lower IAP (6–8 cmH_2O in infants and up to 12 cmH_2O in older children). Induction of anesthesia can be performed safely using either IV or inhalational techniques. Children are generally more prone to intraoperative hypothermia than adults. In laparoscopic surgeries, the core temperature can drop further if the insufflation gas is cold. Temperature monitoring must be done routinely and patient warming measures such as fluid warming system and cutaneous warming measures should be used to prevent hypothermia.

Thoracoscopy

Initially these procedures were conducted with local anesthetic injected at the point of entry or under intercostal block. This often resulted in hypoxia and hypercarbia due to the pneumothorax. Thoracoscopic surgery is now traditionally done under general anesthesia and one-lung ventilation.

PATIENT SELECTION

- Patients with cardiac pathology must be subjected to a thorough preoperative assessment taking the particular hemodynamic conditions imposed by laparoscopic surgery into account.
- Patients presenting with decompensated congestive cardiomyopathy are at highest risk of laparoscopic surgery because the hemodynamic repercussions would be too difficult to manage, even with the help of invasive monitoring techniques.
- The increase in systemic vascular resistance and the O_2 requirements of the myocardium could be the risk factor in cardiac patients. For these patients, the postoperative benefits of laparoscopic surgery must be weighed against

the intraoperative risks. Preoperative investigation in these patients enables this risk to be evaluated more closely. The cardiac reserve must be assessed carefully; in particular, myocardial contractility and the ejection fraction should be estimated.

- The drop in venous return during peritoneal insufflation is one of the important factors which are responsible for drop in cardiac output during laparoscopic surgery. This drop in venous return is more important when the hypovolemia develops due to excessive bleeding, indicating that hypovolemia is a contraindication, at least for as long as their circulating volume has not been restored to normal. This point is particularly important for ruptured ectopic pregnancy or during laparoscopic surgical exploration of abdominal injuries.

MONITORING

Careful monitoring of a patient undergoing laparoscopic surgical procedure is very important. The American Society of Anesthesiologists (ASA) standard monitoring is mandatory for all patients. A multiparameter monitor **(Fig. 2)** is essential. Peak and plateau airway pressure can be measured from the anesthesia machine. An intra-arterial blood pressure (IBP), cardiac filling pressures, and frequent blood gas monitoring are indicated in high-risk patients undergoing major surgery.

- Electrocardiogram (ECG)
- Rate of respiration
- Pulse oximetry
- Noninvasive blood pressure (NIBP)
- Temperature
- End-tidal carbon dioxide
- Intraperitoneal pressure

Routine Monitoring

The stethoscope remains an important instrument enabling anesthetist to auscultate both the lungs after any change in position and after insufflation of the pneumoperitoneum because it pushes back the tracheal carina, can displace intubation to the right. The use of a stethoscope in the precordial position is a good practice in order to detect gas embolism, but requires permanent auscultation.

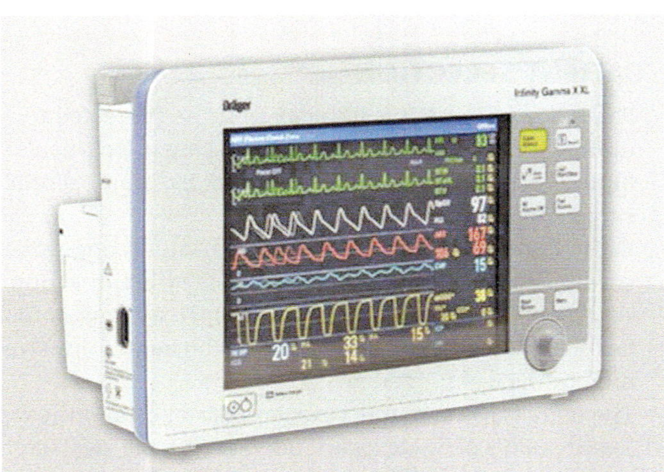

Fig. 2: Multiparameter monitor.

Electrocardioscopic monitoring during laparoscopy enables arrhythmia, which may occur due to hypercapnia, to be rapidly detected. At the time of laparoscopic surgery, sudden appearance of a microvoltage can be the sign of subcutaneous emphysema or pneumomediastinum.

Oximetry monitoring [peripheral oxygen saturation (SpO_2)] is essential part of any surgery, but it is especially important in laparoscopic surgery because the dim lighting in the laparoscopic surgery theater and the wearing of protective glasses, if a laser is being used, make it difficult to recognize cyanosis. In any case, the latter is a late clinical sign of hypoxia. Variations in saturation are not specific during laparoscopic surgery. Desaturation is a late sign of complications such as gas embolism, pneumothorax, selective intubation, or a shunt effect due to excessively high intraperitoneal pressure.

During laparoscopic surgery, control of intraperitoneal pressure is an integral part of the anesthesia monitoring. The insufflator must be microprocessor controlled; it must be reliable and subjected to regular checks. Excessive intraperitoneal pressure must trigger an alert and an immediate halt in insufflation. As the majority of older insufflators do not have safety valve for a reduction in intraperitoneal pressure, this must be carried out by manual exsufflation via opening the valve of cannula.

Monitoring of the neuromuscular block is also important. Proper relaxation is good for laparoscopic surgery. Stable and deep myoresolution improves the laparoscopic surgeon's view and limits the peritoneal insufflation pressures. In addition, the wide range of operating times and the rapidity with which an operation is terminated means it is essential to know exactly what the neuromuscular block situation is at any point in time. When equipment for reading the muscular activity in the thumb is not available, the simplest stimulation is a train-of-four on a temporal branch of the facial nerve and observation of the contraction of the orbicular eye muscle.

Intraperitoneal insufflation of dry and unheated gas, possibly accompanied by irrigation with cold liquids, results in heat loss during laparoscopic surgery which is at least equal to that with laparotomy. Temperature monitoring associated with measures to combat heat loss is also essential when procedures take several hours. It is important to remember that excessive leakage of gas through the cannula causes rapid hypothermia to the patient.

Cardiovascular Monitoring

Measurement via the bloodstream enables arterial pressure to be monitored in real time. In addition, the appearance of cyclic variations in time with ventilation is an excellent indication of drops in preloading which prompt the intraperitoneal insufflation pressure to be limited, to increase filling, or even to accentuate the Trendelenburg position when possible. Installation of an arterial entry point also helps with blood gas measurements.

Measurement of central venous pressure is traditionally used to supervise the filling pressures in the right heart. This becomes difficult during laparoscopic surgery because of the changes in position which require continual changes at cell level and particularly because of the increase in intrathoracic pressure transmitted from the peritoneal area via the diaphragm. It is important to perform simultaneous measurement of intrathoracic pressure which is obtained by esophageal pressure and to deduct this from the measured central venous pressure.

Catheterization of the right heart using a Swan-Ganz probe has been used for monitoring during laparoscopic surgery **(Fig. 3)**. As for central venous pressure, the values measured need to be corrected according to the intrathoracic pressure. An increase in pulmonary arterial pressure is an early sign of gas embolism. Aspiration of the gas bubbles by the proximal orifice placed in the right atrium theoretically helps to minimize the consequences of air embolism. The use of a Swan-Ganz probe during laparoscopy for patients with coronary disease helps adapt the anesthesia protocol and therapy, for simple measurement of arterial pressure is insufficient in 80% of these cases. Nevertheless in the course of general anesthesia with controlled ventilation when arterial oxygen saturation (SaO_2), hemoglobin, and O_2 consumption are stable, a change in venous oxygen saturation (SvO_2) is often the sign of a change in cardiac flow rate.

Because right heart catheterization is an invasive procedure, several studies have reported the use of cardiac flow rate monitoring by electrical bioimpedance during laparoscopic surgery. The principle is founded on continuous measurement of the blood flow rate in the thorax by analysis of the variations in conductivity relative to an electrical field. Transthoracic electrical bioimpedance brings a certain number of advantages:

- Low risk (noninvasive monitoring)
- Easy and simple to use
- Continuous measurement in real time
- Not limited in time
- Inexpensive
- Reliability seems to be satisfactory as compared to other methods.

It is important that the skin be carefully prepared and the electrodes are of good quality and correctly positioned.

However, its use in standard monitoring is still limited due in large part to the frequent difficulties encountered in interpreting the variations.

Some studies have been made of hemodynamic monitoring during laparoscopic surgery using trans-esophageal ultrasound cardiography. Whereas the advantages of this technique for monitoring and diagnosis are considerable, the cost remains an important barrier. Interpretation can also be difficult because of the variations in the viewing axis of the heart according to peritoneal pressure and the variable patient's position.

Measurement of the cardiac flow rate by pulsed Doppler velocimetry can be carried out by either the transesophageal or the suprasternum route at the time of laparoscopic surgery. The basic principle is the same as with any Doppler device with a piezoelectric transducer transmitter and a transducer

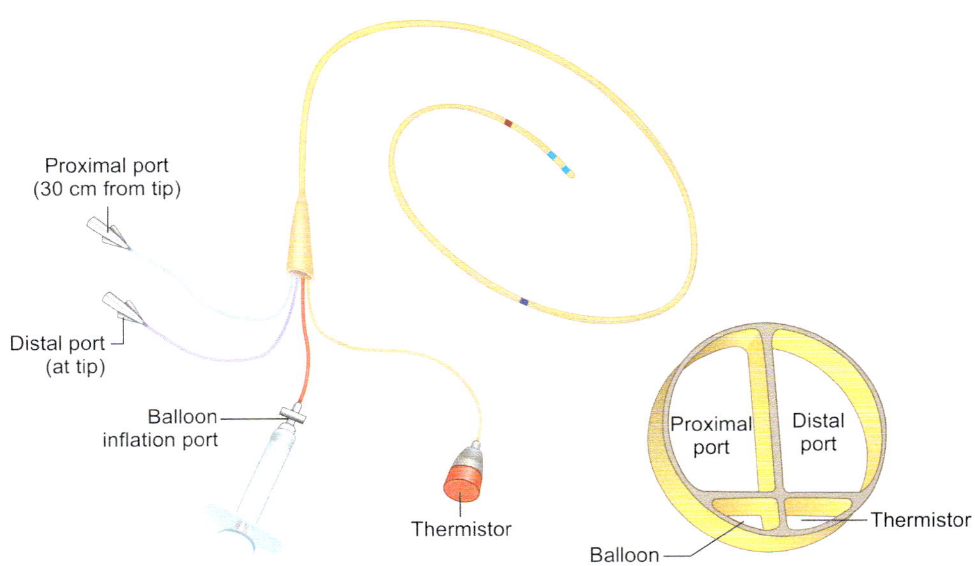

Fig. 3: Swan-Ganz catheter.

receiver which receives the return echoes modified by the Doppler effect when they bounce off mobile structures such as wall of the heart, vessels, or red blood cells. Based on the effective diameter of the aorta which can either be calculated from the cardiac flow rate measured by another method or estimated from the patient's biometric factors, the ejection volume can be deduced and thus the continuous cardiac flow rate.

Respiratory Monitoring

Quantitative waveform capnography is the continuous, noninvasive measurement and graphical display of end-tidal carbon dioxide [$EtCO_2$, also called end-tidal carbon dioxide pressure ($PetCO_2$)]. Capnography uses a sample chamber/sensor placed for optimum evaluation of expired CO_2 **(Fig. 4)**. The inhaled and exhaled CO_2 is graphically displayed on a capnograph as a waveform on the monitor along with its corresponding numerical measurement.

As an assessment tool during laparoscopic surgery, capnography can help the anesthetist determine a number of things. It is a direct measurement of ventilation in the lungs, CO_2 absorption causing hypercarbia, and it also indirectly measures metabolism and circulation. For example, an increase in CO_2 absorption during laparoscopy will increase the $EtCO_2$ and a decrease in perfusion will lower the delivery of CO_2 to the lungs. This will cause a decrease in the $EtCO_2$ and this will be observable on the waveform as well as with the numerical measurement. Capnography is a continuous and noninvasive method for CO_2 measurement and it has become the standard of care for basic respiratory monitoring for intubated patients during laparoscopic surgery. The $PetCO_2$ provides evidence of production of CO_2 by the cellular metabolism, absorbed through the peritoneal cavity and pulmonary exchanges **(Figs. 5A and B)**. A rapid increase in $PetCO_2$ is a serious complication. Thus, continuous and careful monitoring of $EtCO_2$ by capnography is a useful and effective noninvasive monitoring technique in anesthesia for laparoscopy. The $EtCO_2$ immediately reflects changes in circulatory status and ventilation as well as detects complications related to CO_2 pneumoperitoneum (hypercarbia, subcutaneous emphysema, gas embolism, pneumothorax, etc.). Thus, $EtCO_2$ monitoring is mandatory and essential monitoring during laparoscopic surgery for the safe conduct of general anesthesia.

- A rapid rise of a few millimeters of mercury returning a few minutes later to the base figures may be the sign of minimal CO_2 gas embolism.
- A more gradual and persistent rise is often the sign of extraperitoneal diffusion of CO_2 (preperitoneal, subcutaneous, retroperitoneal, mediastinal, etc.). This increase in expired CO_2 continues after exsufflation of the pneumoperitoneum, indeed often several hours after the laparoscopic procedure, justifying a follow-up of hypercapnia in the recovery room.
- The CO_2 is transported by the circulatory system from the peripheral areas toward the lungs. Any disturbance in the circulation will reduce the CO_2 expired. A rapid drop in $PetCO_2$ may be the sign of a drop in cardiac flow rate or a decreased venous return, but also pulmonary arterial obliteration. This is what happens in massive gas embolism which shows up as a drop in $PetCO_2$ proportional in size and duration to the volume of the CO_2 embolus.

Classically, the $PetCO_2$ values are 2–6 mm Hg lower than $PaCO_2$. During anesthesia with artificial ventilation, the V/Q ratio often >1, so a $PaCO_2$-$PetCO_2$ gradient of 10–15 mm Hg must be expected. However, during laparoscopic surgery, the change in the arterial CO_2-$EtCO_2$ gradient is very variable.

Changes in position such as the Trendelenburg or the lateral reclined position can modify the value of the $PetCO_2$. Furthermore, it is shown that in cases of cardiovascular

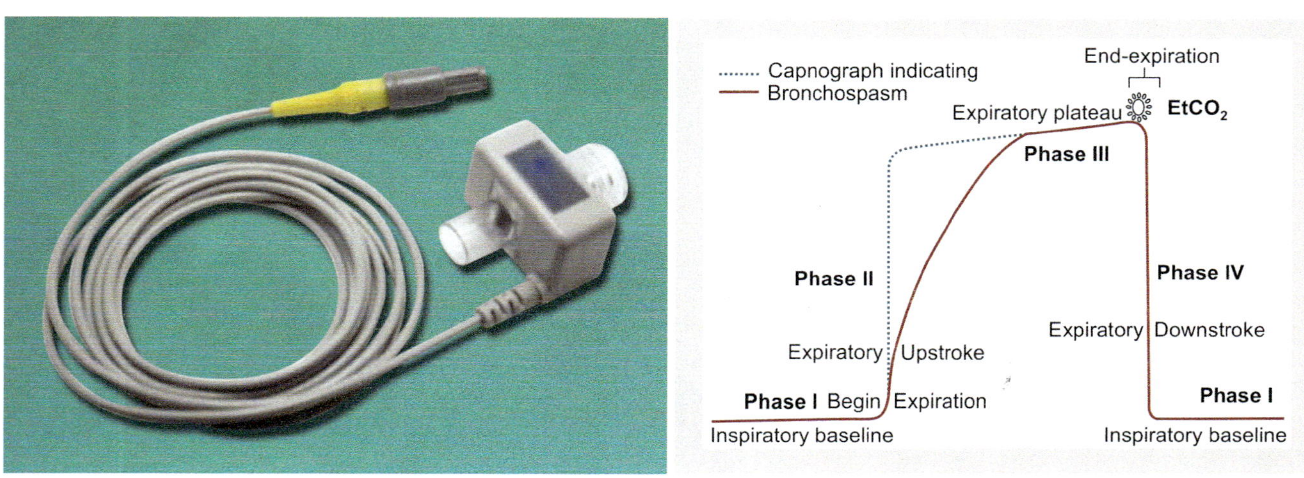

Fig. 4: Capnograph.
($EtCO_2$: end-tidal carbon dioxide)

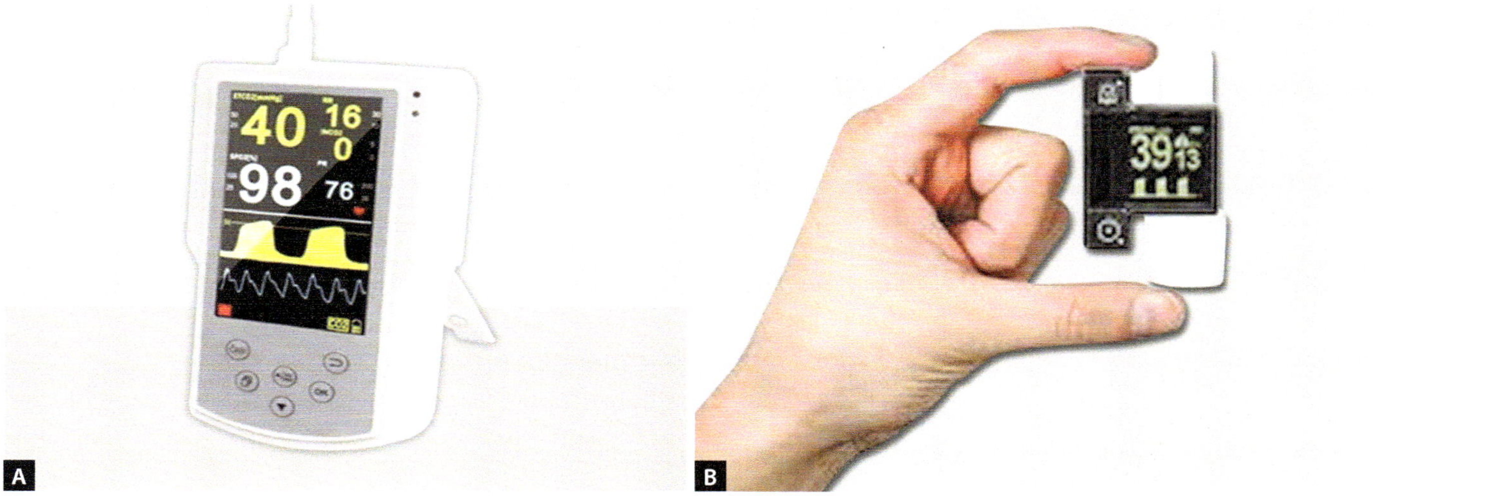

Figs. 5A and B: Portable carbon dioxide (CO_2) monitor.

disease, the correlation between $PetCO_2$ and $PaCO_2$ was less good when compared with patients with no such pathology and the same is true with obese patients. A recent study confirms that in patients with respiratory impairment, the increase in $PaCO_2$ is underestimated by $PetCO_2$. So, for these patients with respiratory or heart pathology, it is particularly useful to duplicate the $PetCO_2$ measurement by arterial gasometry at the beginning of the operation and every time there is an important variation in $PetCO_2$.

In view of this uncertainty, transcutaneous CO_2 monitoring would give a better idea of $PaCO_2$, but this also raises a certain number of technical problems (heating of electrodes, difficulties with measurements in adults, etc.).

Anesthetist should keep following points in mind at the time of laparoscopic surgery:

- The patient voids urine just prior to entering the operating room.
- No shaving is necessary.
- All patients undergoing laparoscopy should have an empty bowel. In the unlikely event of bowel damage, there is much less risk of contamination if the bowel is empty.
- The position of leg is important considering different laparoscopic procedures. Pressure stocking prevents deep vein thrombosis (DVT).
- Good muscle relaxation reduces the IAP required for adequate working room in abdominal cavity.
- The inflation of stomach should be avoided during artificial ventilation using mask as this increases the risk of gastric injury during trocar insertion or instrumentation.
- The distended stomach also hampers the visibility of Calot's triangle at the time of laparoscopic cholecystectomy or laparoscopic bile duct surgery.
- Tracheal intubation and intermittent positive pressure ventilation should be routinely used. This ensures airway protection and controls pulmonary ventilation to avoid hypocarbia.
- The ventilatory pattern should be adjusted according to respiratory and hemodynamic performance of the individual patient.
- Ventilation with large tidal volumes (12–15 mL/kg) prevents alveolar atelectasis and hypoxemia and allows adequate alveolar ventilation and CO_2 elimination.
- Halothane increases the incidence of arrhythmia during laparoscopic surgery, especially in the presence of hypercarbia.
- Isoflurane is the preferred volatile anesthetic agent in minimal access surgery as it has less arrhythmogenic and myocardial depressant effects.
- Patients should receive adequate airway humidification and protection against unintentional hypothermia because generally the duration of operation is more in laparoscopic surgery.
- Excessive IV sedation should be avoided because it diminishes airway reflexes against pulmonary aspiration in the event of regurgitation.
- Monitoring of $PetCO_2$ is mandatory during laparoscopic surgery. The continuous monitoring of $PetCO_2$ allows adjustment of the minute ventilation to maintain normal concentration of CO_2 and O_2.
- Airway pressure monitor is mandatory for anesthetized patients receiving intermittent positive pressure ventilation.

INTRAOPERATIVE COMPLICATIONS

If anesthetic consideration is not taken properly, arrhythmias have been associated with laparoscopy. The most common are junctional rhythms, bigeminy, and asystole. Bradycardia has been reported due to rapid insufflation, especially in older patients. The increasing pressure on the peritoneum increases vagal tone and bradycardia may develop. This bradycardia may be increased secondary to absorption of CO_2. Atropine has proven effective in restoring vagal tone.

The development of a CO_2 gas embolus is a rarely encountered emergency. It develops due to intravasations of CO_2 used in laparoscopic surgery. Some apparent signs of air embolism include a sudden drop in $EtCO_2$, a drop in blood pressure, and development of an arrhythmia. A classic "waterwheel" or "millwheel" murmur will be heard in cardiac auscultatory area. Should such an event be suspected, further insufflation should be immediately stopped and abdomen should be deflated. The patient should be turned toward left and head-down to deviate the bubbles of CO_2 away from heart. The patient should be hyperventilated with 100% O_2. If a central line is present, aspiration of the embolus should be attempted.

Pulmonary edema can result from aggressive fluid replacement or irrigating fluid absorption. Fluid management is even more difficult in gynecological procedure where hysteroscopy is combined. Pulmonary edema is prevented by monitoring fluid input and output. Intraoperative diuretics should be administered if a large discrepancy between fluid input and output is found. If a patient develops respiratory distress, pulmonary edema should always be considered. Rales couple with classic chest radiographic findings that will confirm the diagnosis.

ADJUNCTS DURING LAPAROSCOPIC SURGERY

Patients with compromised cardiovascular status, obese, old age, and respiratory diseases may have an exaggerated response to pneumoperitoneum. An anesthesiologist aims at controlling and modifying these hemodynamic changes. Various pharmacological agents such as opioids, dexmedetomidine, clonidine, beta-blockers, nitroglycerin (NTG), pregabalin, gabapentin, and magnesium sulfate ($MgSO_4$) have been tried with varying success to provide hemodynamic stability during pneumoperitoneum.

Dexmedetomidine

Dexmedetomidine, an alpha-2 agonist, acts by inhibiting the release of catecholamines and vasopressin. It is known to provide excellent sedation and analgesia with minimal respiratory depression. Dexmedetomidine was found to reduce the requirements of other anesthetic agents and opioids, with minimal side effects, when used at a loading dose of 0.5–1 μg/kg over 10–15 minutes followed by a continuous infusion of 0.2–0.5 μg/kg/h.

Clonidine

Clonidine, an alpha-2 agonist similar to dexmedetomidine, is a potent antihypertensive drug that suppresses renin-angiotensin-aldosterone system (RAAS). Clonidine administered in a dose of 4.5 μg/kg was found to decrease mean arterial pressure (MAP) and heart rate (HR) significantly during and after pneumoperitoneum.

Beta-blockers

Beta-blockers as esmolol, an ultra-short-acting cardio-selective beta-1 receptor antagonist, has been routinely used in a loading dose of 1 mg/kg over 5 minutes followed by 0.5 mg/kg/h in attenuation of stress response to laparoscopy.

Magnesium Sulfate

Administration of $MgSO_4$ was found to attenuate the increase in arterial pressure during CO_2 pneumoperitoneum.

Pregabalin

Pregabalin, an antiepileptic drug, is effective in controlling neuropathic component of acute nociceptive pain of surgery by inhibiting voltage-gated calcium channels. The hemodynamic stability provided by oral premedication might enable laparoscopic surgery in obese, hypertensive, and cardiac compromised patients with no risk of postoperative respiratory depression.

POSTOPERATIVE CONSIDERATIONS

At the end of the procedure, antagonism of the residual muscle relaxation should be reversed by appropriate dose of reversal agents. When patient is awake, he or she should be extubated and transferred to the recovery room in a semirecumbent position. Before extubation, the patient's stomach may be emptied with an orogastric tube. During the next 5 hours in the postoperative period, analgesia should be achieved. Patients spend a minimum of an hour in the recovery room. Vital signs and O_2 saturation are monitored and supplemental O_2 is administered by mask or nasal prongs.

Nausea is frequent after general anesthesia and laparoscopic surgeries. IV droperidol, ondansetron, or dexamethasone can be given for prevention of postoperative nausea and vomiting (PONV).

Multimodal analgesia with nonsteroidal anti-inflammatory drugs (NSAIDs), short-acting opioids, dexmedetomidine, and local infiltration of local anesthetics provide superior pain relief with reduced PONV and early discharge. Following laparoscopic cholecystectomy surgeries, ropivacaine nebulization of intraperitoneal cavity, with or without fentanyl, provides highly effective postoperative analgesia, with decreased incidence of shoulder pain. Furthermore, addition of fentanyl to ropivacaine prolongs the duration of analgesia. Another approach is ultrasound-guided peripheral nerve blocks such as transverse abdominis plane (TAP) block and posterior quadratus lumborum block (QLB).

The urine output should be at rate of 100 mL/h and that should continue for 18 hours postoperatively. The nursing management included O_2 therapy, early mobilization, incentive spirometry, and chest physiotherapy. These should repeat at 2 hours interval. She or he should be transferred to the surgical ward and may be discharged home next day if everything is alright. On the morning of the first postoperative day, the patient should be mobile, pain free, and should start soft diet.

All procedures under anesthesia carry small but inherent risks and patient should understand these before agreeing to undergo the procedure. However, the risks of anesthesia for elective surgery under modern conditions are very small indeed.

BIBLIOGRAPHY

1. Andrei VE, Schein M, Margolis M, Rucinski JC, Wise L. Liver enzymes are commonly elevated following laparoscopic cholecystectomy: is elevated intra-abdominal pressure the cause? Dig Surg. 1998;15:256-9.
2. Andrei VE, Schein M, Wise L. Small bowel ischemia following laparoscopic cholecystectomy. Dig Surg. 1999;16:522-4.
3. Bandyopadhyay D, Kapadia CR. Large bowel ischemia following laparoscopic inguinal hernioplasty. Surg Endosc. 2003;17:520-1.
4. Ben-Haim M, Rosenthal RJ. Causes of arterial hypertension and splanchnic ischemia during acute elevations in intra-abdominal pressure with CO_2 pneumoperitoneum: a complex central nervous system mediated response. Int J Colorectal Dis. 1999;14:227-36.
5. Boussuges A, Blanc P, Molenat F, Bergmann E, Sainty JM. Haemoconcentration in neurological decompression illness. Int J Sports Med. 1996;17:351-5.
6. Brunner F, Frick P, Bühlmann A. Post-decompression shock due to extravasation of plasma. Lancet. 1964;1:1071-3.
7. Case EH, Stiles JA. The effects of various surgical positions on vital capacity. Anesthesiology. 1946;7:29-31.
8. Collins VJ. Principles of Anesthesiology, 2nd edition. Philadelphia: Lea and Febiger; 1976.
9. Cunningham AJ, Turner J, Rosenbaum S, Rafferty T. Transoesophageal echocardiographic assessment of haemodynamic function during laparoscopic cholecystectomy. Br J Anaesth. 1993;70:621-5.
10. Diakun TA. Carbon dioxide embolism: Successful resuscitation with cardiopulmonary bypass. Anesthesiology. 1991;74:1151-3.
11. Donald JS, Gamble CJ, Shaw R. The cardiac output in man. Am J Physiol. 1934;109:666.
12. Dorsay DA, Green FL, Baysinger CL. Hemodynamic changes during laparoscopic cholecystectomy monitored with transesophageal echocardiography. Surg Endosc. 1995;9:128-34.
13. Dorsay DA, Greene FL, Baysinger CL. Hemodynamic changes during laparoscopic cholecystectomy monitored with transesophegeal echocardiography. Surg Endosc. 1995;9:128-34.
14. Feig BW, Berger DH, Dougherty TB, Dupuis JF, His B, Hickey RC, et al. Pharmacologic intervention can reestablish baseline hemodynamic parameters during laparoscopy. Surgery. 1994;116:733-71.
15. Gannedahl P, Odeberg S, Brodin LA, Sollevi A. Effects of posture and pneumoperitoneum during anaesthesia on the indices of left ventricular filling. Acta Anaesthesiol Scand. 1996;40:160-6.
16. Girardis M, Broi UD, Antonutto G, Pasetto A. The effect of laparoscopic cholecystectomy on cardiovascular function and pulmonary gas exchange. Anesth Analg. 1996;83:134-40.
17. Glantzounis GK, Tselepis AD, Tambaki AP, Trikalinos TA, Manataki AD, Galaris DA, et al. Laparoscopic surgery-induced changes in oxidative stress markers in human plasma. Surg Endosc. 2001;15:1315-9.
18. Hachenberg T, Ebel C, Czorny M, Thomas H, Wendt M. Intrathoracic and pulmonary blood volume during CO_2 pneumoperitoneum in humans. Acta Anaesthesiol Scand. 1998;42:794-8.
19. Hasson HM, Galanopoulos C, Langerman A. Ischemic necrosis of small bowel following laparoscopic surgery. JSLS. 2004;8:159-63.
20. Henderson Y, Haggard HW. The circulation in man in head down position and a method for measuring the venous return to the heart. J Pharm Exp Therap. 1918;11:189-201.
21. Hirvonen EA, Nuutinen LS, Kauko M. Hemodynamic changes due to Trendelenburg positioning and pneumoperitoneum during laparoscopic hysterectomy. Acta Anaesthesiol Scand. 1995;39:949-55.
22. Ho HS, Saunders CJ, Gunther RA, Wolfe BM. Effector of hemodynamics during laparoscopy: CO_2 absorption or intra-abdominal pressure? J Surg Res. 1995;59:497-503.
23. Ido K, Suzuki T, Taniguchi Y, Kawamoto C, Isoda N, Nagamine N, et al. Femoral vein stasis during laparoscopic cholecystectomy: effects of graded elastic compression leg bandages in preventing thrombus formation. Gastrointest Endosc. 1995;42:151-5.
24. Irwin MG, Ng JKF. Transoesophageal acoustic quantification for evaluation of cardiac function during laparoscopic surgery. Anaesthesia. 2001;56:623-9.
25. Ishizaki Y, Bandai Y, Shimomura K, Abe H, Ohtomo Y, Idezuki Y. Safe intra-abdominal pressure of carbon dioxide pneumoperitoneum during laparoscopic surgery. Surgery. 1993;114:549-54.
26. Joris JL, Hamoir EE, Hartstein GM, Meurisse MR, Hubert BM, Charlier CJ, et al. Hemodynamic changes and catecholamine release during laparoscopic adrenalectomy for pheochromocytoma. Anesth Analg. 1999;88:16-21.
27. Joris JL, Noirot DP, Legrand MJ, Jacquet NJ, Lamy ML. Hemodynamic changes during laparoscopic cholecystectomy. Anesth Analg. 1993;76:1067-71.
28. Koivusalo AM, Kellokumpu I, Scheinin M, Tikkanen I, Makisalo H, Lindgren L. A comparison of gasless mechanical and conventional carbon dioxide pneumoperitoneum methods for laparoscopic cholecystectomy. Anesth Analg. 1998;86:153-8.
29. Kubal K, Komatsu T, Sanchala V. Trendelenburg position used during venous cannulation increases myocardial oxygen demands. Anesth Analg. 1984;63:239.
30. Makinen MT. Comparison of body temperature changes during laparoscopic and open cholecystectomy. Acta Anaesthesiol Scand. 1997;41:736-40.
31. Mariano ER, Furukawa L, Woo RK, Albanese CT, Brock-Utne JG. Anesthetic concerns for robot-assisted laparoscopy in an infant. Anesth Analg. 2004;99:1665-7.
32. Matzen S, Perko G, Groth S, Friedman DB, Secher NH. Blood volume distribution during head-up tilt induced central hypovolaemia in man. Clin Physiol. 1991;11:411-22.
33. McDougall EM, Monk TG, Wolf JS, Hicks M, Clayman RV, Gardner S, et al. The effect of prolonged pneumoperitoneum on renal function in an animal model. J Am Coll Surg. 1996;182:317-28.
34. Miller R. Miller's Anesthesia, 6th edition. Philadelphia: Elsevier; 2005.
35. Myre K, Rostrup M, Buanes T, Stokland O. Plasma catecholamines and haemodynamic changes during pneumoperitoneum. Acta Anaesthesiol Scand. 1998;42:343-7.
36. Nguyen NT, Perez RV, Fleming N, Rivers R, Wolfe BM. Effect of prolonged pneumoperitoneum on intraoperative urine output during laparoscopic gastric bypass. J Am Coll Surg. 2002;195:476-83.

37. O'Leary E, Hubbart K, Tormey W, Cunningham AJ. Laparoscopic cholecystectomy: haemodynamic and neuroendocrine responses after pneumoperitoneum and changes in position. Br J Anaesth. 1996;76:640-4.
38. Odeberg S, Ljungqvist O, Svenberg T, Gannedahl P, Bäckdahl M, von Rosen A, et al. Haemodynamic effects of pneumoperitoneum and the influence of posture during anesthesia for laparoscopic surgery. Acta Anaesthesiol Scand. 1994;38:276-83.
39. Oliver SB, Cucchiara RF, Warner MA, Muir JJ. Unexpected focal neurologic deficit on emergence from anesthesia: a report of three cases. Anesthesiology. 1987;67:823-6.
40. Razvi HA, Fields D, Vargas JC, Vaughan ED, Vukasin A, Sosa RE. Oliguria during laparoscopic surgery: evidence for direct renal parenchymal compression as an etiologic factor. J Endourol. 1996;10:1-4.
41. Root B, Levy MN, Pollack S, Lubert M, Pathak K. Gas embolism death after laparoscopy delayed by "trapping" in portal circulation. Anesth Analg. 1978;57:232-7.
42. Schwenk W, Bohm B, Fugener A, Muller JM. Intermittent pneumatic sequential compression (ISC) of the lower extremities prevents venous stasis during laparoscopic cholecystectomy: a prospective randomized study. Surg Endosc. 1998;12:7-11.
43. Shuto K, Kitano S, Yoshida T, Bandoh T, Mitarai Y, Kobayashi M. Hemodynamic and arterial blood gas changes during carbon dioxide and helium pneumoperitoneum in pigs. Surg Endosc. 1995;9:1173-8.
44. Sprung J, Whalley DG, Falcone T, Warner DO, Hubmayr RD, Hammel J. The impact of morbid obesity, pneumoperitoneum and posture on respiratory system mechanics and oxygenation during laparoscopy. Anesth Analg. 2002;94:1345-50.
45. Stewart BT, Stitz RW, Tuch MM, Lumley JW. Hypothermia in open and laparoscopic colorectal surgery. Dis Colon Rectum. 1999;42:1292-5.
46. Taura P, Lopez A, Lacy AM, Anglada T, Beltran J, Fernandez-Cruz L, et al. Prolonged pneumoperitoneum at 15 mm Hg causes lactic acidosis. Surg Endosc. 1998;12:198-201.
47. Walder AD, Aitkenhead AR. Role of vasopressin in the haemodynamic response to laparoscopic cholecystectomy. Br J Anaesth. 1997;78:264-6.
48. Wilcox S, Vandam LD. Alas, poor Trendelenburg and his position! A critique of its uses and effectiveness. Anesth Analg. 1998;67:574-8.
49. Winter R, Munro M. Lingual and buccal nerve neuropathy in a patient in the prone position: a case report. Anesthesiology. 1989;71:452-4.

CHAPTER 6

Abdominal Access Techniques

INTRODUCTION

Minimal access surgery (MAS) a new surgical and interventional approach, was called by different name and one of the popular is minimally invasive surgery. However, unique complications are associated with gaining access to the abdomen for laparoscopic surgery. The technique of first entry inside the human body with telescope and instruments is called access technique. The hallmark of the new approaches is the reduction in the trauma of access. The technique for access to the peritoneal cavity, choice of access technique, placement locations, and port placement is very important in MAS. Technique of access is different for different minimal access surgical procedures. Thoracoscopy, retroperitoneoscopy, axilloscopy, and arthroscopy all have different ways of access. In this chapter, we will discuss various abdominal access techniques.

It is important to know that approximately 20% of laparoscopic complications are caused at the time of initial access. Developing access skill is one of the important achievements for the surgeon practicing MAS. First entry or access in laparoscopy is of two types: (1) closed access and (2) open access.

ANATOMY OF ANTERIOR ABDOMINAL WALL

Knowledge of the surgical anatomy of the abdominal wall is essential for the safe access in laparoscopic surgery. Laparoscopic instruments traverse the skin, subcutaneous fat, variable myofascial layers, preperitoneal fat, and parietal peritoneum. There are three large, flat muscles (external oblique, internal oblique, and transversus abdominis) and one long vertically oriented segmental muscle (rectus abdominis) on each side. The layers of the abdominal wall in the midline include skin, subcutaneous fat, and a fascial layer (linea alba) that is a coalescence of the anterior and posterior rectus sheath. Four major arteries on each side are also present which form an anastomotic arcade that supplies the abdominal wall. The superior and inferior epigastric artery and the branches provide the major blood supply to the rectus abdominis muscle and other medial structures **(Fig. 1)**.

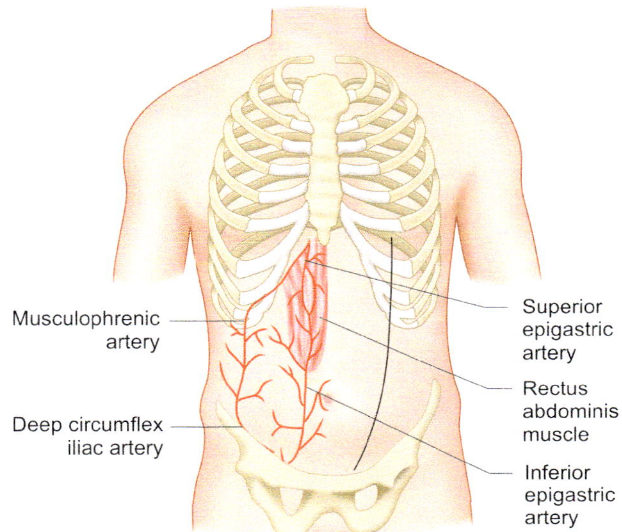

Fig. 1: Anterior abdominal wall anatomy.

Among all these arteries, the most important for laparoscopic surgeon is the inferior epigastric artery and vein. The inferior epigastric vessel landmark is less variable compared to superior epigastric. Bleeding from inferior epigastric is a big problem because it is larger in diameter than superior epigastric.

Umbilicus is the site of choice for access in majority of laparoscopic procedure. The umbilicus is a fusion of fascial layers and is devoid of subcutaneous fat. The median umbilical ligament which is obliterated urachus and paired medial umbilical ligaments, i.e., obliterated umbilical arteries are peritoneal folds that join at the inferior crease of the umbilicus, forming a tough layer. This umbilical tube scar remains after the umbilical cord obliterates which makes an attractive site of primary access of Veress needle and trocar. At the level of umbilicus, skin fascia and peritoneum are fused together, with the minimum fat. The midline of abdominal wall is free of muscle fibers, nerves and vessels except at its inferior edge where pyramidalis muscle is sometimes found. Therefore, Veress needle or trocar insertion in these locations rarely cause much bleeding. If a defect in the umbilical fascia suggests an umbilical hernia or if any midline incision scar of previous laparoscopy is found or if any anomalies of the urachus may also exist umbilicus should not be used for primary access. If an umbilical hernia or urachal anomaly is suspected, alternative access sites may need to be considered.

The colon is attached to the lateral abdominal wall along both gutters and puncture laterally for secondary trocars should be under video control to avoid visceral injury. When left subcostal site is chosen for access it should be 2 cm below the costal margin in midclavicular line called Palmer's point. The costal margin provides good resistance as the needle is introduced. When puncture site lateral to the midline is used, it is prudent to choose location lateral to the linea semilunaris to avoid injury of superior and inferior epigastric vessels. In obese patients, the linea semilunaris may not be visible. In these, location of inferior artery can be localized by careful transillumination.

Access to preperitoneal space is gained by penetrating almost all the layers of abdominal wall except peritoneum. The open technique of access is preferable in this situation. After incising the fascia with the scalpel, fingered dissection is advisable to avoid puncture of peritoneum.

CLOSED ACCESS TECHNIQUE

To start any laparoscopic procedure the peritoneal cavity needs to be accessed, first to establish pneumoperitoneum and subsequently to place a port for the laparoscope and add the placement of additional ports for various laparoscopic instruments. In closed access technique, pneumoperitoneum is created by Veress needle (named for Janos Veress) **(Fig. 2)**. The Veress needle was originally developed by Janos Veress to give patients with tuberculosis iatrogenic pneumothorax without damaging the underlying lung parenchyma **(Fig. 3)**. It has a small-bore (1.8–2.2 mm) needle with a spring-loaded protective obturator with a side hole that recoils to cover the end of the needle, allowing entry into a body cavity without traumatizing the underlying organs **(Fig. 4)**. Maximum flow of gas through the eye of Veress needle is 2.5 L/min only but for safety it should be kept at 1 L/min to prevent accidental gas embolism **(Fig. 5)**. This is a blind technique and most practiced way of access by surgeons and gynecologists worldwide. When choosing site of closed access, previous surgical incisions, or any anatomical abnormality, should be noted. Sites that have not been previously instrumented are preferred for initial access. Closed technique of access merely by Veress needle insertion and creation of pneumoperitoneum is an easy way of access but it is not possible in some of the minimal access surgical procedures such as axilloscopy, retroperitoneoscopy, and totally extraperitoneal approach of hernia repair. In general, closed technique by Veress needle is possible only if there is a preformed cavity like abdomen.

Creation of pneumoperitoneum is one of the most important steps in laparoscopy. The aim is to build up a good protective cushion of gas to ensure the safe entry of trocar and cannula.

Veress Needle Insertion

The standard method of insufflations of the abdominal cavity is via a Veress needle inserted through a small skin incision over inferior crease of umbilicus. Disposable and reusable metal Veress needles are available commercially in different lengths (8–20 cm), i.e., long for obese patients, short for thin or pediatric patients.

Before using Veress needle, it should be checked for its patency and spring action. Spring action of Veress needle can be checked by pulling the head out. The disposable

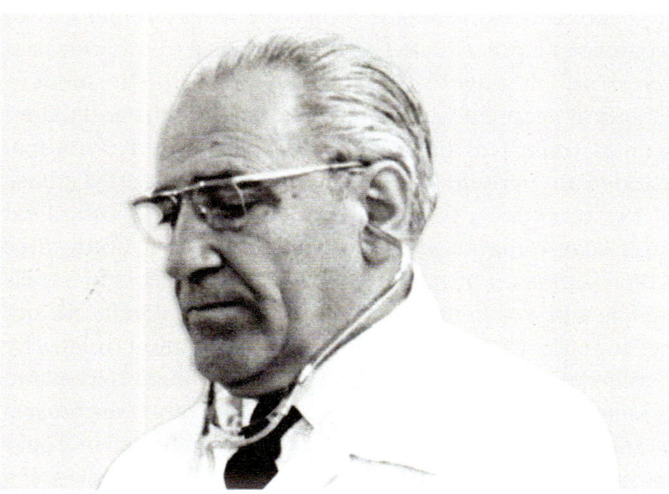

Fig. 2: Veress needle inventor—Janos Veress.

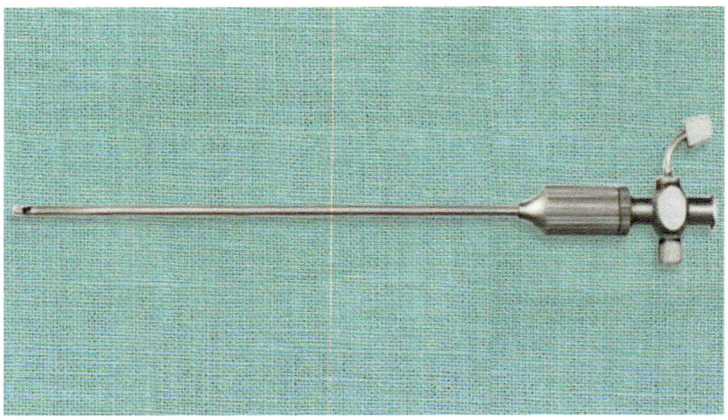

Fig. 3: Veress needle.

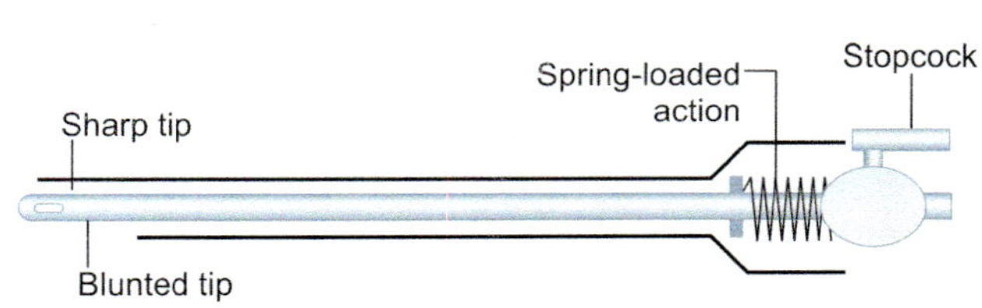

Fig. 4: Parts of Veress needle.

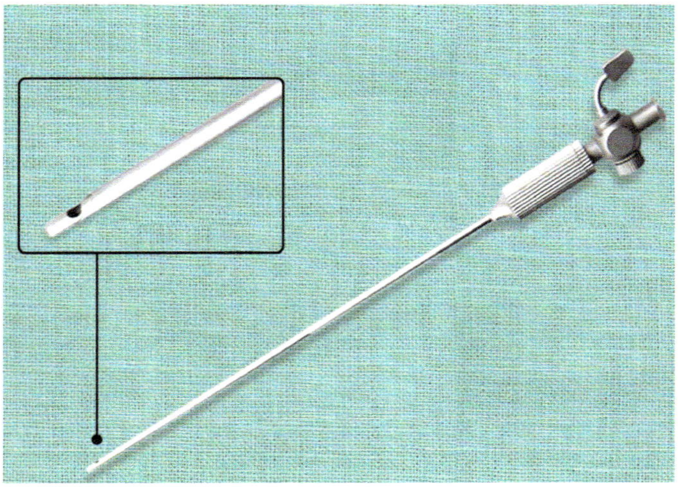

Fig. 5: Eye of Veress needle.

Veress needle spring action can be checked by pressing the sharp end against any sterilized draping.

Insufflation via the Veress needle creates a cushion of gas over the bowel for insertion of the first trocar. Insufflation then retracts the anterior abdominal wall, exposing the operative field.

Preparation of Patient

The patient should be nil orally since the morning of surgery. In some of the procedure such as laparoscopic hysterectomy or colorectal surgery where distended bowel may interfere, it is good to prepare bowel prior to the night of surgery by giving some mild purgative (polyethylene glycol). Bowel preparation can minimize the need of accessory port to retract the bowel.

Before coming to operation theater, patient should always void urine. The full urinary bladder may get perforation at the time of insertion of Veress needle or trocar. If the laparoscopic procedure is of short duration and is going to be performed of upper abdomen, then Foley catheterization is not necessary. If gynecological operative surgery or any major general surgical lower abdominal procedure has to be performed (such as hernia or adhesiolysis), it is wise to insert Foley catheter.

If surgeon is going to perform any upper abdominal procedures such as cholecystectomy, fundoplication, duodenal perforation, hiatus hernia, etc., it is good practice to have nasogastric tube in place. A distended stomach will not allow proper visualization of Calot's triangle and then surgeon has to apply more traction over fundus or Hartmann's pouch, and this may cause tenting of common bile duct (CBD) followed by accidental injury. In gynecological or lower abdominal minor laparoscopic procedure, it is not necessary to put nasogastric tube.

In MAS, shaving of skin is not must and if necessary, it should be done on operation table itself by surgeon.

Operating Room Setup

An organized well-equipped operation theater is essential for successful laparoscopy. The entire surgical team should be familiar with the instruments and their function. Each instrument should be inspected periodically for loose or broken tips even if the same instrument was used during a previous procedure. It is necessary to confirm proper sterilization of instruments because the surgeon ultimately is responsible for the proper functioning of all instrument and equipment.

The entire instrument should be placed according to wish of the surgeon so that it should be ergonomically perfect for that surgery. The coaxial alignment should be maintained. Coaxial alignment means the eye of the surgeon, target of dissection, and monitor should be placed in same axis.

Patient Position

Initially at the time of pneumoperitoneum by Veress needle, patient should be placed supine with 15° head down. The benefit of this Trendelenburg's position is that bowel will be pulled up and there will be more room in pelvic cavity for safe entry of Veress needle. It is important to remember that patient should be placed in head-down position only if surgeon is planning to insert Veress needle pointing toward pelvis cavity. If surgeon is planning to insert Veress needle perpendicular to abdominal wall as in case of very obese patient, previous midline incision or diagnostic laparoscopy in local anesthesia, the patient should be placed in supine position otherwise all the bowel will come just below the umbilicus and there is increased risk of bowel injury.

In gynecological laparoscopic procedures or if laparoscopy is planned to be performed together with hysteroscopy, patient should be positioned in lithotomy position and one assistant should be positioned between the leg of patient **(Fig. 6)**. Patient's leg should be comfortably supported by padded obstetric leg holders or Allen stirrups which minimize the risk of venous thrombosis. In these procedures, surgeon needs to use uterine manipulator for proper visualization of female reproductive organs. The assistant seating between the legs of patient will keep on watching the hand movement of surgeon on monitor and he should give traction with the handle of uterine monitor in appropriate direction. If thoracoscopy or retroperitoneoscopy is planned, then patient is placed in lateral position **(Fig. 7)**.

Position of Surgical Team

The laparoscopic surgeon is very much dependent and helpless with eye fixed on monitor. At the time of laparoscopic surgery, surgeon is largely depending on his correct standing position. If the surgery is of upper abdomen, French surgeons like to stand between the legs of patient, popularly known as

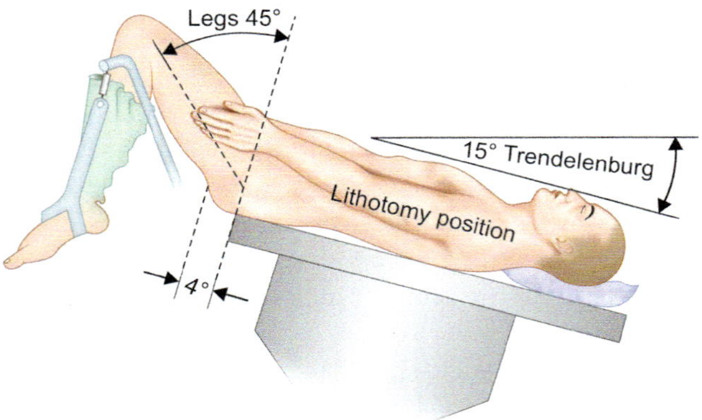

Fig. 6: Patient position in gynecological laparoscopy.

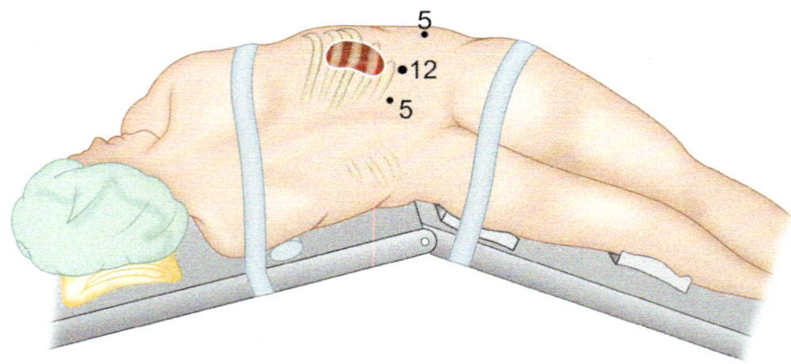

Fig. 7: Patient position in retroperitoneoscopy.

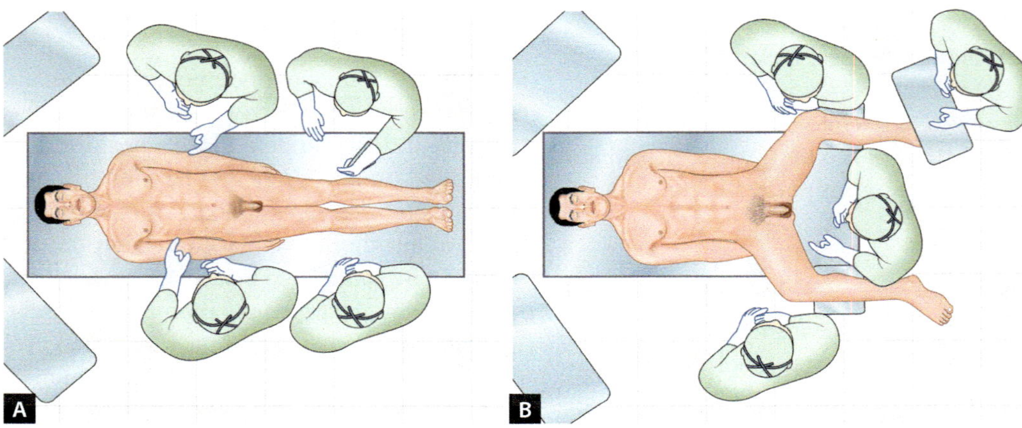

Figs. 8A and B: American versus French position.

"French position" **(Figs. 8A and B)**. The American surgeons like to operate from left in cases of upper abdominal surgery such as cholecystectomy called as "American position".

It is not always wise to remain standing in any one fixed position and surgeon can walk to the other side of operation table to achieve proper ergonomics. In most of the cases at the time of initial access, right-handed surgeon should stand on left side of the patient so that he can hold the Veress needle with right dominant hand. If surgeon is left-handed, he should stand right to the patient at the time of access and insert the Veress needle or trocar with left hand. This helps in inserting Veress needle and trocar toward pelvis by dominant hand. Once the initial Veress needle and first optical trocar has been introduced surgeon should stand opposite to the organ which he wants to operate on. Once all the ports are in position, the surgeon should come opposite to the side of pathology to start surgery and he should achieve coaxial alignment means eye of the surgeon, target of dissection, and center of monitor should be in one linear axis. In cholecystectomy, appendectomy, right-sided hernia or right ovarian cyst, surgeon should stand left to the patient. In left-sided pathology such as left ovarian cyst and left-sided hernia, it is ergonomically better for surgeon to stand right to the patient **(Fig. 9)**.

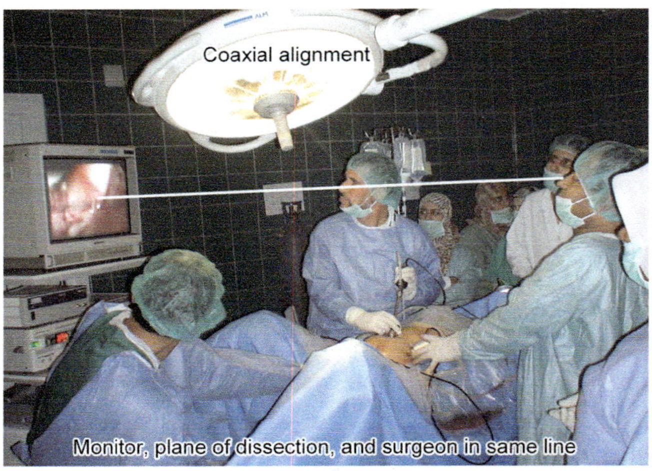

Fig. 9: Surgeons stands left to the patient in most of the right-sided pathology.

In most of the upper abdominal surgery, camera assistant should stand left to the surgeon and in lower abdominal surgery, he or she should stand right to the surgeon. Camera assistant while holding telescope can pass his or her hand between body and arm of surgeon so that sometime surgeon can help him to focus his camera correctly. Camera assistant can be placed opposite to the surgeon to stand but in this case, it is better to have two monitors on both the side of patient, one for surgeon and one for camera stand and other members of surgical team. The surgeon should work in the most comfortable and less tiring position possible with shoulder relaxed, arms alongside of the body, elbows at 90° angle and forearm horizontal.

Preparation for Access

Before starting access, abdomen should be examined for any palpable lump. It is wise to tell the patient to void urine before coming to operating room but if the bladder is found full at the time of palpation. Foley catheter and nasogastric tube should be applied once patient is anesthetized. Remember that full bladder or distended stomach may be injured very easily by Veress needle or trocar.

Once the patient is cleaned painted and draped, all the connection should be attached, followed by focusing and white balancing of camera. At the time of focusing, the distance between the gauge piece and tip of the telescope should be 6–8 cm.

Choice of Gas for Pneumoperitoneum

At first, pneumoperitoneum was created by filtered room air. Carbon dioxide (CO_2) and nitrous oxide (N_2O) are now preferred gas because of increased risk of air embolism with room air. CO_2 is used for insufflation as it is 200 times more diffusible than oxygen and 20 times more absorbable than room air. It is rapidly cleared from the body by the lungs and will not support combustion. N_2O is only 68% as rapidly absorbed in blood as CO_2. N_2O has one advantage over CO_2 that it has mild analgesic effect, and hence no pain if diagnostic laparoscopy is performed under local anesthesia. CO_2 has the advantage of being noncombustible and allows the concomitant use of electrocoagulation and laser irradiation. For short operative procedures such as sterilization or drilling, under local anesthetic N_2O may also be used. During prolonged laparoscopic procedure, N_2O should not be a preferred gas for pneumoperitoneum because it supports combustion better than air. CO_2 when comes in contact with peritoneal fluid converts into carbonic acid. Carbonic acid irritates diaphragm causing shoulder tip pain and discomfort in abdomen. Carbonic acid has one advantage also that it alters pH of peritoneal fluid (acidotic changes) and it is mild antiseptic, so the chances of infection may be slightly less compared to any other gas. Helium gas being inert in nature is also tried in many centers, but it does not have any added benefit over CO_2. Helium may be a suitable alternative to CO_2 for creating pneumoperitoneum in patients with severe cardiorespiratory disease. Some of the study suggest that pneumoperitoneum with helium will not be associated with profound circulatory depression or oxygen transport abnormalities. In addition, the use of helium is not associated with acid-base disturbances, although central venous filling pressures are similarly increased as with the use of CO_2 pneumoperitoneum. However, helium is expensive gas and because of its low water solubility helium has a lower safety margin than CO_2 in the event of gas embolism.

Introduction of Veress Needle

To access the abdomen with a closed approach using a Veress needle:

- Apply two Allis forceps to evert the inferior crease of umbilicus **(Fig. 10)**.
- Give a 2-mm smiling incision in the skin and the subcutaneous tissue over inferior crease of umbilicus **(Fig. 11)**.
- Hold shaft of the Veress needle as a dart **(Fig. 12)**.
- Guard the length of Veress needle needed to reach the peritoneal cavity **(Fig. 13)**.
- Place the needle through the incision to the level of the fascia **(Fig. 14)**.

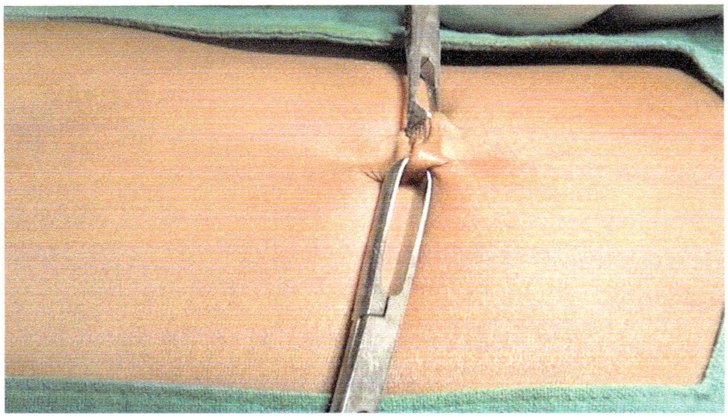

Fig. 10: Two Allis forceps is applied over crease of umbilicus.

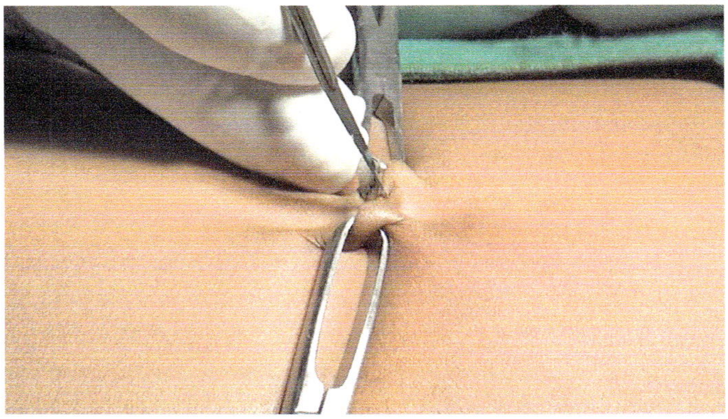

Fig. 11: 2-mm stab wound over inferior crease of umbilicus.

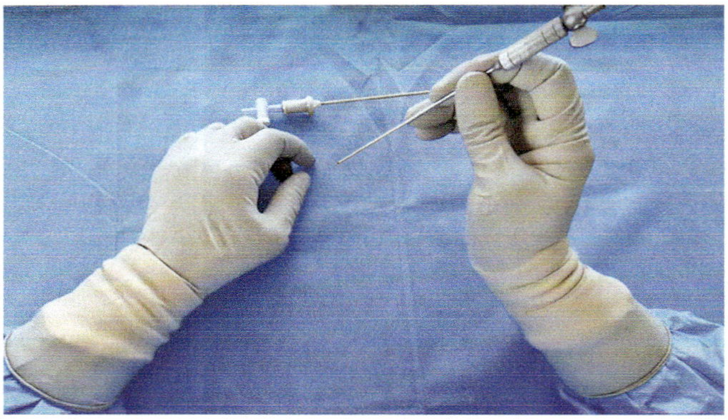

Fig. 12: Veress needle should be held like a dart.

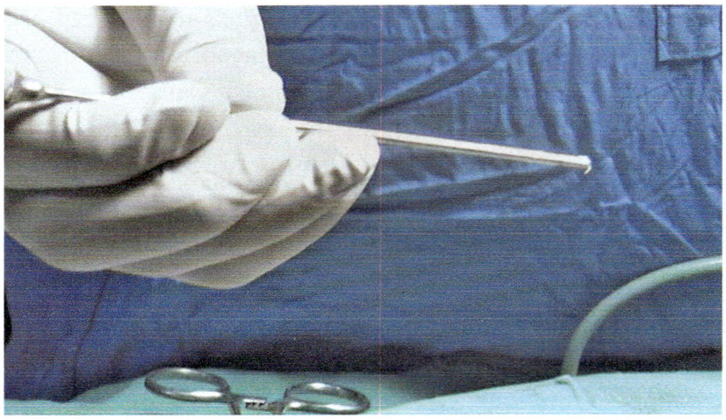

Fig. 13: Guard the required length of Veress needle.

- Grasp and elevate the abdominal wall with your left hand. It is important to note that grasping only the skin while not including the fascia may increase the rate of failed entry **(Fig. 14)**.
- Hold the Veress needle just over the previously incised site and insert it through the incision at a 45° angle toward anus but keep perpendicular to the abdominal wall. This can be only achieved by lifting the abdominal wall adequately by left hand **(Fig. 14)**.
- While inserting the Veress needle feel for two "pops". The first occurs when the needle passes through the abdominal fascia and the second as it passes through the parietal peritoneum. More lateral access sites may have additional "pops" if more than one layer of fascia is traversed.
- As soon as the needle enters the peritoneal space, the displaced hub of the needle will "click" as the protective sheath recoils to cover the end of the needle. After entering in abdominal cavity, the intra-abdominal needle will also move more freely than a needle within the abdominal wall.

Veress needle should be held like a dart **(Fig. 12)**. At the time of insertion, there should be 45° of elevation angle. Elevation angle is angle between instrument and body of patient. To get an elevation angle of 45° the distal end of the Veress needle should be pointed toward anus **(Fig. 14)**. To prevent creation of preperitoneal slip of tip of Veress needle, it is necessary that Veress needle should be perpendicular to the abdominal wall. However, there is a fear of injury of great vessels or bowel if Veress needle is inserted perpendicular to the abdominal wall. To avoid both the difficulty (creation of preperitoneal space and injury to bowel or great vessels), the lower abdominal wall should be lifted in such a way that it should lie at 90° angle in relation to the Veress needle but in relation to the body of patient Veress needle will be at an angle of 45° pointed toward anus. Lifting of abdominal wall should be adequate so that the distance of abdominal wall from viscera should increase. If less than required dose of muscle relaxant is given in muscular patient, lifting of abdominal wall may be difficult. In multipara patient, lifting lower abdominal wall is very easy.

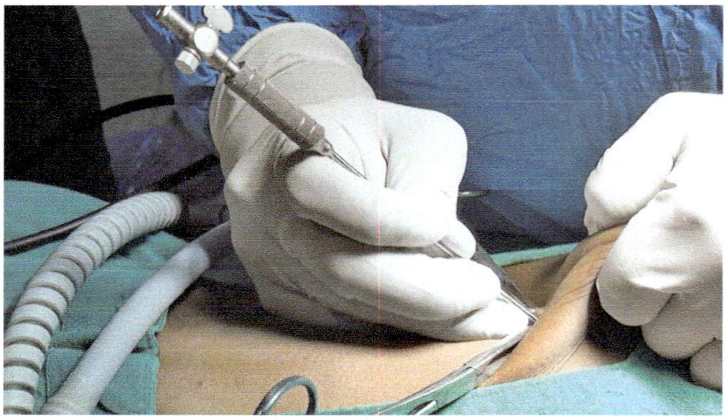

Fig. 14: Veress needle should be pointed toward anus but perpendicular to abdominal wall.

Several tests are available for confirming Veress needle placement. These include one of the following:

Needle Movement Test

Once the Veress needle is inside the abdominal cavity, the tip of Veress needle should be free and if surgeon will gently move the tip of needle there should not be feel of any resistance. It is very important to remember that Veress needle should not be moved inside the abdominal cavity much, otherwise there is a risk of laceration of bowel to be punctured.

Irrigation Test

A 10-mL syringe should be taken in one hand and surgeon should try to inject at least 5 mL of normal saline through Veress needle. If tip of Veress needle is inside the abdominal cavity, there will be free flow of saline otherwise some resistance is felt in injecting saline **(Fig. 15)**.

Aspiration Test

After injecting saline, surgeon should try to aspirate that saline back through Veress needle **(Fig. 16)**. If the tip of Veress

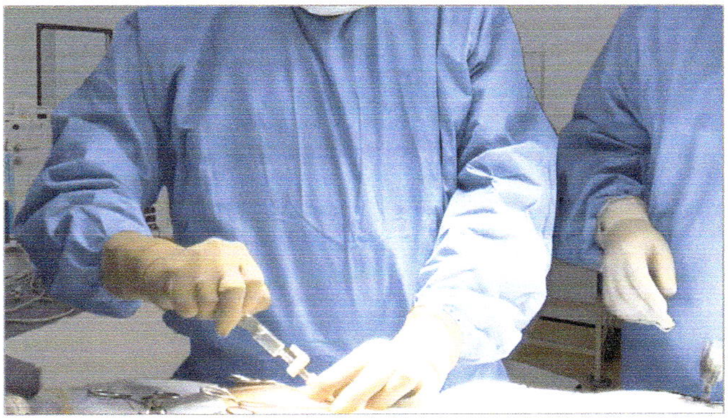

Fig. 15: Irrigation test.

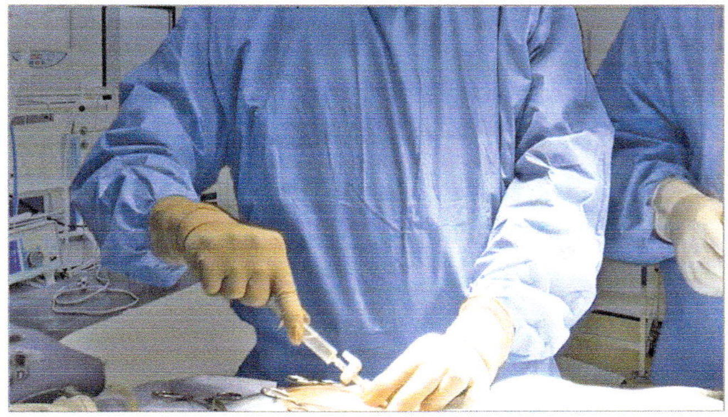

Fig. 16: Aspiration test.

needle is in abdominal cavity, the irrigated water cannot be sucked. But if it is in preperitoneal space or in muscle fiber or above; the rectus the injected water can be aspirated back. In aspiration test, if more irrigated fluid is coming, then surgeon should suspect ascites, some cysts or perforation of urinary bladder. If fecal matter is seen then perforation of bowel may be the reason and if blood is coming then the vessel injury is the cause. If any fresh blood or fecal fluid is aspirated in the syringe, surgeon should not remove the Veress needle and urgent laparotomy is required. Leaving Veress needle in position is helpful in two ways. First, it is easy to find the punctured area after laparotomy and secondly, the further bleeding will be less.

Hanging Drop Test

Few drops of saline should be poured over the Veress needle and abdominal wall should be lifted slightly, if tip of the Veress needle is inside the abdominal cavity the hanging drop should be sucked inside because inside the abdomen, there is negative pressure. If tip of the Veress needle is anywhere else, the hanging drop test will be negative **(Figs. 17A and B)**. Once it is confirmed that Veress needle is inside the abdominal cavity, the tubing of insufflator is attached and flow is started.

Measurement of Intra-abdominal Pressure

Measure intra-abdominal pressure by attaching the Veress needle to the laparoscopic insufflator. An intra-abdominal position of the needle is suggested for intra-abdominal pressure ≤10 mm Hg. In one large observational study, confirmation of low intraperitoneal pressure was the most reliable method to confirm Veress needle placement.

Once an intra-abdominal position of the needle is verified, initiate gas insufflation (typically CO_2). A properly placed Veress needle will allow free flow of gas. Tympany should be appreciated with percussion of the abdomen in the right upper quadrant.

For many years, surgeons have been using towel clip to elevate the abdominal wall. This towel clip technique of lifting abdominal wall was advocated by Johns Hopkins University but after some time it was realized that towel clip technique increases the distance of skin from rest of the abdominal wall more than distance of abdominal wall from viscera. Abdominal wall should be held full thickness with the help of thenar, hypothenar and all the four fingers **(Fig. 14)**. It is lifted in such a way that angle between Veress needles to abdominal wall should be 90° and angle between Veress needle and patient should be 45°. At the time of entry of Veress needle, surgeon can hear and feel two click sounds. The first click sound is due to rectus sheath and second click sound is due to puncture of peritoneum. Anterior and posterior rectus forms one sheath at the level of umbilicus, so there will be only one click for rectus.

If any other area of abdominal wall is selected for access surgeon will get three click sounds. Once these two click sound is felt, surgeon should stop pushing Veress needle further inside and he should use various indicators to know how far he has accessed. Once the desire length of Veress needle is introduced in abdomen, the tubing of insufflator should be attached to Veress needle **(Fig. 15)**. It is important to keep nice hold on Veress needle throughout while gas is flowing; otherwise Veress needle can slip out and may create preperitoneal insufflation **(Fig. 16)**.

Insufflation of Gas Test, Quadromanometric Test

Tubing of the insufflator should be tightly attached with the help of Luer lock of Veress needle **(Figs. 18 and 19)**. For safe access, surgeon should always see carefully all the four indicators of insufflator at the time of creation of pneumoperitoneum. If the gas is flowing inside the abdominal cavity, there should be proportionate rise in actual pressure with total gas used. Suppose only with the entry of 200–300 mL of gas, if actual pressure is equal to preset pressure of 12 mm Hg, that means gas is not going in free abdominal cavity, it may be in preperitoneal space or inside omentum or may be in bowel. If gas is flown >5 L without any distention of abdomen that may be due to leakage or gas may be going inside the vessel.

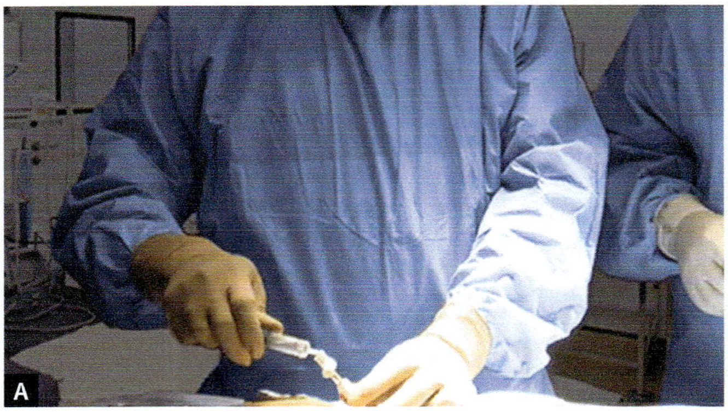

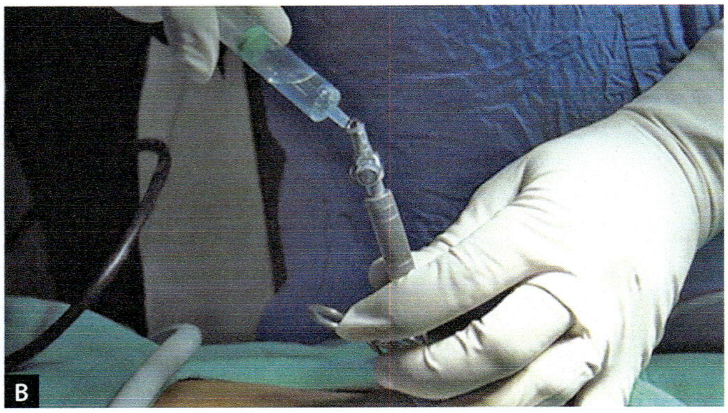

Figs. 17A and B: Hanging drop test.

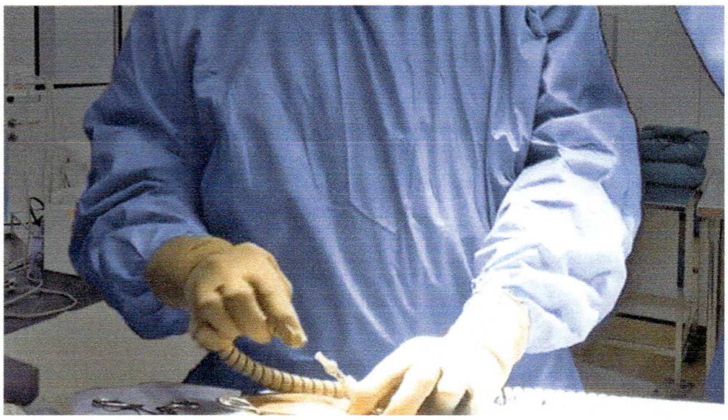

Fig. 18: Attaching gas tubing with careful hold of Veress needle and counter twist over Luer lock of insufflator tubing.

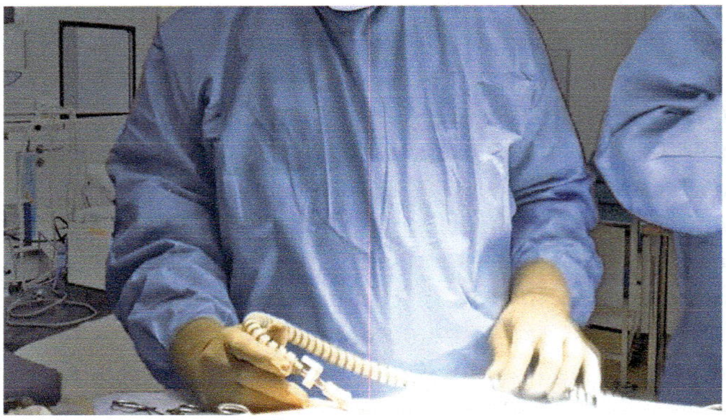

Fig. 19: Beginning of insufflation with careful hold over Veress needle.

Quadromanometric Indicators of Insufflator (Figs. 20A and B)

Quadromanometric indicators are the four important readings of insufflator the insufflator is used to monitor:

1. Preset insufflation pressure
2. Actual pressure
3. Gas flow rate
4. Volume of gas consumed.

Preset pressure: This is the pressure adjusted by surgeon before starting insufflation. This is the command given by surgeon to insufflator to keep intra-abdominal pressure at this level.

The preset pressure ideally should be 12 mm Hg. In any circumstance, it should not be >18 mm Hg. Good quality insufflator always keeps intra-abdominal pressure at preset pressure. Whenever intra-abdominal pressure decreases due to leak of gas outside, insufflator eject some gas inside to maintain the pressure, equal to preset pressure. If intra-abdominal pressure increases due to external pressure; insufflator sucks some gas from abdominal cavity, to maintain the pressure to preset pressure. When surgeon or gynecologist wants to perform diagnostic laparoscopy under local anesthesia, the preset pressure should be set to 8 mm Hg. In some special situation of axilloscopy or arthroscopy, we need to have pressure >19 mm Hg.

Actual pressure: This is the actual intra-abdominal pressure sensed by insufflator. When Veress needle is attached, there is some errors in actual pressure reading because of resistance of flow of gas through small caliber of Veress needle. Since continuous flow of insufflating gas through Veress needle usually gives extra 4–8 mm Hg of measured pressure by insufflator, the true intra-abdominal pressure can be determined by switching the flow from insufflator off for a moment. Many microprocessors controlled good quality insufflator deliver pulsatile flow of gas when Veress needle is connected, in which the low reading of actual pressure measures the true intra-abdominal pressure. If there is any major gas leak, actual pressure will be less, and insufflator will try to maintain the pressure by ejecting gas through its full capacity.

Actual pressures of >20–25 mm Hg has following disadvantage over hemodynamic status of patient.

- Decrease venous return due to vena caval compression leading to:
  - Increased chance of deep vein thrombosis (DVT) of calf
  - Hidden cardiac ischemia can precipitate due to decrease cardiac output
- Decrease tidal volume due to diaphragmatic excursion
- Increase risk of air embolism due to venous intravasation
- Increased risk of surgical emphysema.

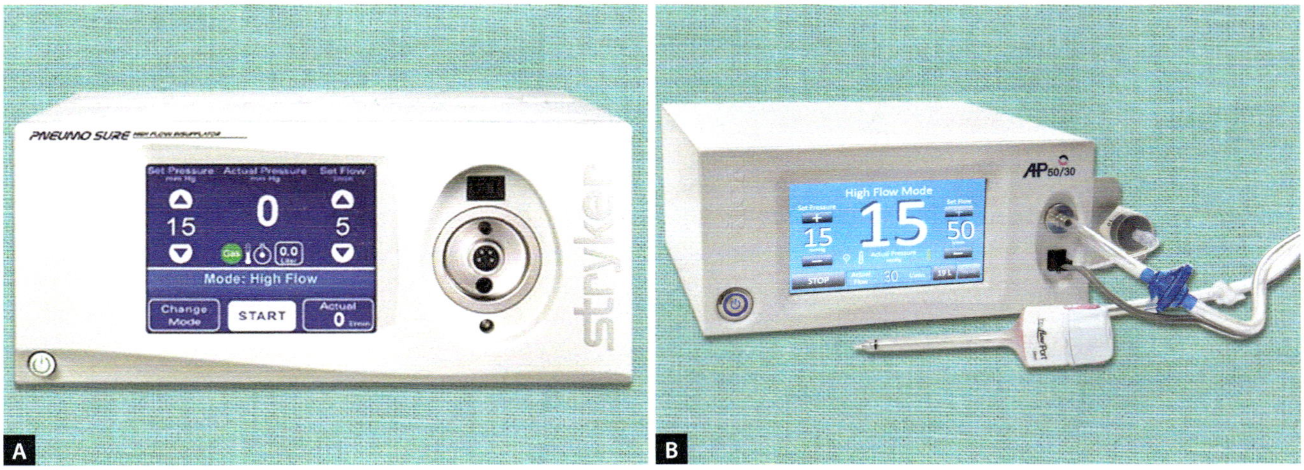

Figs. 20A and B: Quadromanometric indicators.

Flow rate: This reflects the rate of flow of CO_2 through the tubing of insufflator. When Veress needle is attached, the flow rate should be adjusted to 1 L/min. Studies were performed over animal in which direct intravenous (IV) CO_2 were administered, and it was found that risk of air embolism is less if rate is within 1 L/min. At the time of access using Veress needle technique, sometime Veress needle may inadvertently enter inside a vessel but if the flow rate is 1 L/min there is a less chance of serious complication. When initial pneumoperitoneum is achieved and cannula is inside abdominal cavity, the insufflators flow rate may be set at maximum, to compensate loss of CO_2 due to use of suction irrigation instrument. This should be remembered that if insufflator is set to its maximum flow rate then also it will allow flow only if the actual pressure is less than preset pressure otherwise it will not pump any gas. Most of the surgeons keep initial flow rate with Veress needle to 1 L/min and as soon as they confirm that gas is going satisfactorily inside the abdominal cavity by percussion examination and seeing obliteration of liver dullness **(Fig. 21)**, then they increase flow rate to 3 L/min. No matter how much flow rate you set for Veress needle, the eye of normal caliber Veress needle can give away CO_2 flow at maximum 2.5 L/min. Once cannula is in place flow rate can be increase but when the flow of CO_2 is >10 L/min inside the abdominal cavity through cannula and there is leak, there is always a risk of hypothermia and dryness of intestine. To avoid this hypothermia in all modern microprocessor controlled Laproflattor, there is an electronic heating system which maintains the temperature of CO_2.

Total gas used: As soon as 100–200 mL of gas is inside the abdominal cavity, surgeon should do percussion of the right hypochondrium and liver dullness should obliterate with tympanic sound **(Fig. 21)**. This is the fourth indicator of insufflator. Normal size human abdominal cavity needs 1.5-L CO_2 to achieve intra-abdominal actual pressure of 12 mm Hg. In some big size abdominal cavity and in multipara patients, sometimes we need 3 L of CO_2 (rarely 5–6 L) to get desired pressure of 12 mm Hg. Whenever there is less or more amount of gas used to inflate a normal abdominal cavity, surgeon should suspect some errors in pneumoperitoneum technique. These errors may be leakage or may be preperitoneal space creation or extravasation of gas.

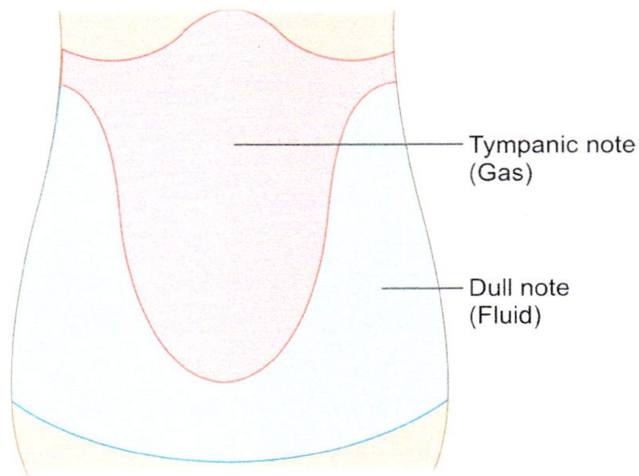

Fig. 21: Tapping over right hypochondrium will demonstrate obliteration of liver dullness.

PRIMARY TROCAR INSERTION

Technical errors in the insertion of trocars after creation of pneumoperitoneum are the most common causes of injury, resulting from inadequate stabilization of the abdominal wall, excessive resistance to trocar insertion, and excessive, misdirected or uncontrolled force applied by the surgeon along the axis of the trocar. It is important to stabilize the abdominal wall by full insufflation, complete muscle relaxation, to increase the distance between the anterior abdominal wall and the retroperitoneal vessels and the abdominal organs. It is important to ensure that the skin incision is of enough length and that the reusable trocar tip is sharp so that no resistance is offered.

Trocar and cannula design currently available have several basic features in common. They come in a variety of sizes and the central trocar may have a pyramidal, conical or rounded tip **(Figs. 22 and 23)**. They have a valve system and a gas input with a tap. These cannulas have flap, bicuspid or magnetic valves and care should be taken when passing telescope through the port that lens of telescope should not hit the valve otherwise it can be damaged. Some disposable cannula has a safety system with a cylinder jumps forward after penetration of abdominal wall and forms a shield over the sharp trocar tip. This is not fool proof due to shield lag. In the most recent disposable cannula, the trocar itself is spring loaded. Few optical trocars are also available which has been discussed in Chapter 3: Laparoscopic Equipment and Instrument.

The first trocar and cannula inserted is usually 11 mm in diameter. This will accommodate a 10-mm telescope and leave enough space in the cannula for rapid gas insufflation, if required.

Steps of Primary Trocar Insertion

Patient Position

As for Veress needle insertion, patient should be placed supine with 10–20° head down. The cephalocaudal relationship between the aortic bifurcation and the umbilicus has been studied radiologically. The umbilicus is often located directly above or cephalad to the aortic bifurcation and is consistently located cephalad to where the left common iliac vein crosses the midline. The aortic bifurcation is located more caudal to the umbilicus in the Trendelenburg's position than in the supine position.

Site

The same site of Veress needle entry should be used for primary trocar insertion. Inferior or superior crease of umbilicus can be used in average built patient and transumbilical incision can be used in obese patient. Before introduction of trocar, surgeon should confirm pneumoperitoneum. After adequate distention of abdominal cavity, the actual pressure should be equal to the preset pressure and gas flow should be stopped.

Before introduction of trocar, the initial 2-mm stab puncture wound of skin for Veress needle should be extended to 11 mm **(Fig. 24)**. It should be remembered that most common cause of forceful entry inside the abdominal cavity with primary trocar is small skin incision. To avoid inadvertent injury of bowel due to forceful uncontrolled entry, the incision of skin should not be <11 mm in size. The skin incision for trocar should be smiling in shape (U-shaped) along the crease of umbilicus to get a better cosmetic value. After giving 11-mm incision with 11 number blades, surgeon should spread fatty tissues with Kelly clamp or mosquito forceps **(Fig. 25)**. This will also dilate the obliterated vitellointestinal duct which was demonstrated first time by Scandinavian surgeons so it is called Scandinavian technique.

Introduction of Primary Trocar

Surgeon should hold the trocar in proper way. Head of trocar should rest on thenar eminence, middle finger should encircle air inlet and index finger should point toward sharp end **(Fig. 26)**.

After holding the trocar properly in hand, full thickness of abdominal wall should be lifted by fingers thenar and hypothenar muscles. After creation of pneumoperitoneum, lifting of abdominal wall is difficult because it slips. To overcome this, it should be grasped to counter the pressure exerted by the tip of trocar.

Angle of Insertion

Initially, angle of insertion for primary trocar should be perpendicular to abdominal wall but once surgeon feels

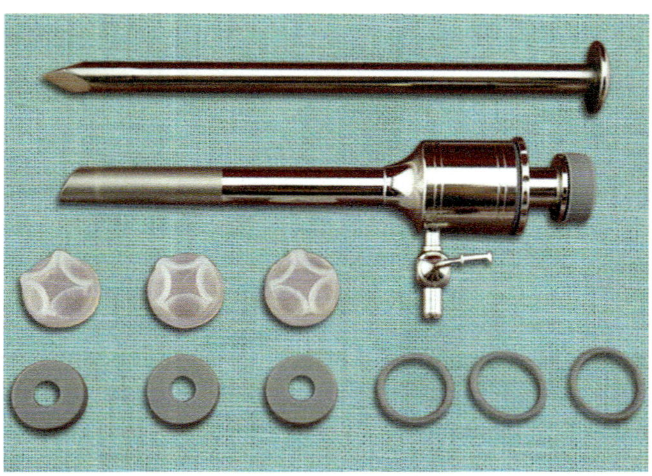

Fig. 22: Reusable trocar and cannula.

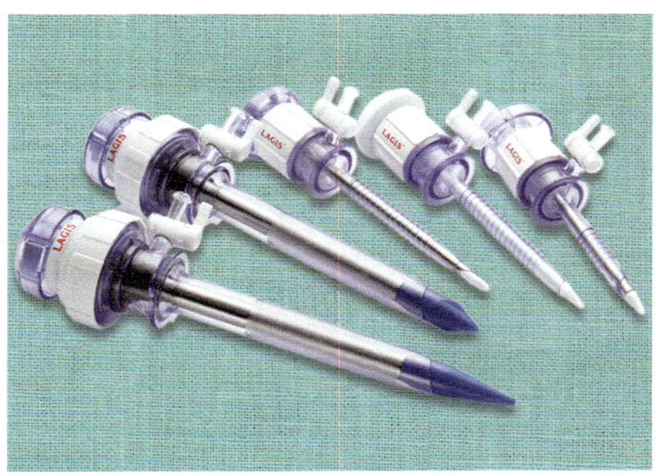

Fig. 23: Disposable trocar and cannula.

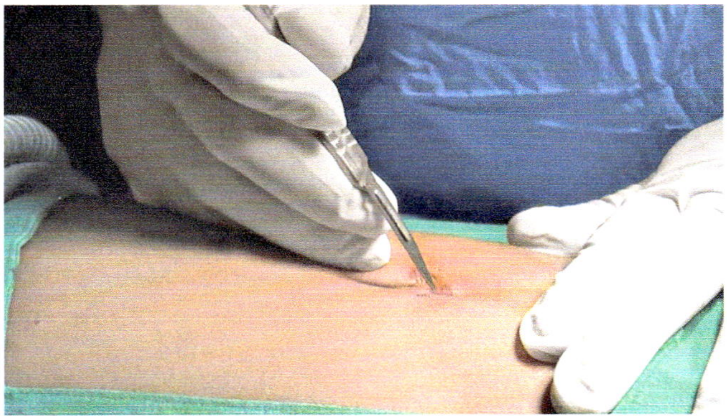

Fig. 24: 2-mm stab wound should be extended to 11 mm.

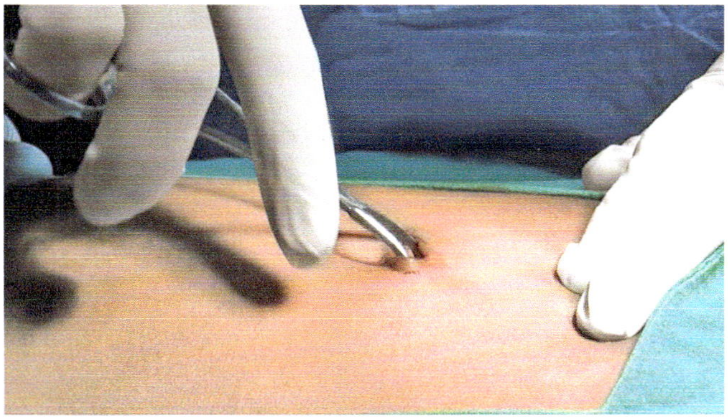

Fig. 25: Mosquito forceps tip introduced through stab wound.

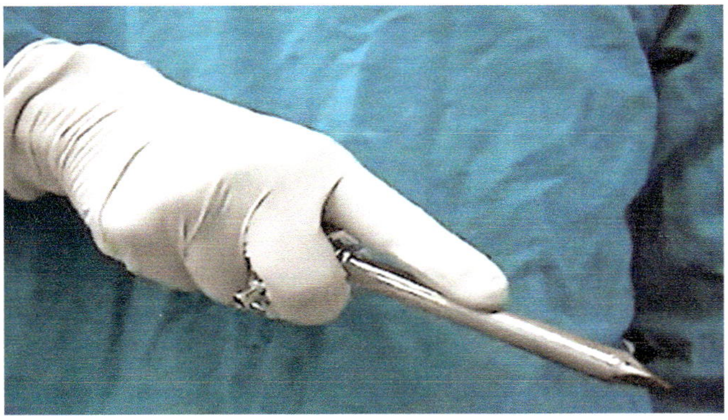

Fig. 26: The trocar and cannula should be held like a pistol.

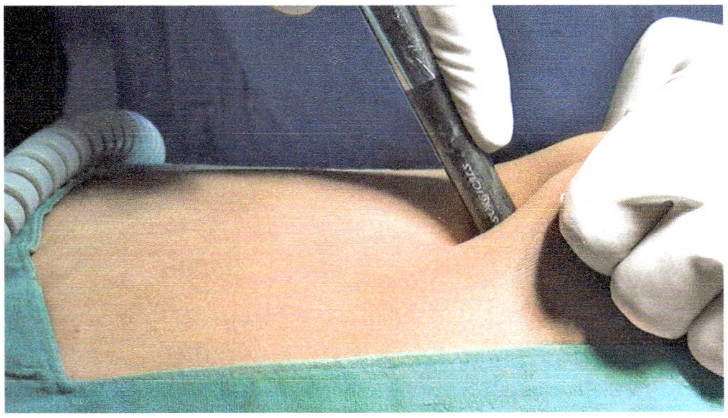

Fig. 27: Insertion of trocar by screwing fashion.

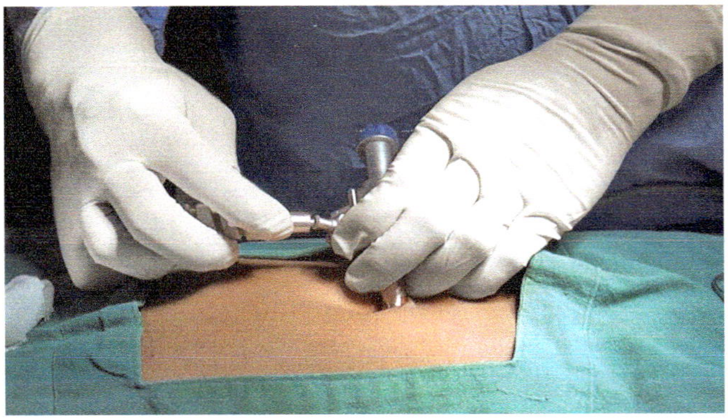

Fig. 28: Insufflator tubing in reattached once optical port is introduced.

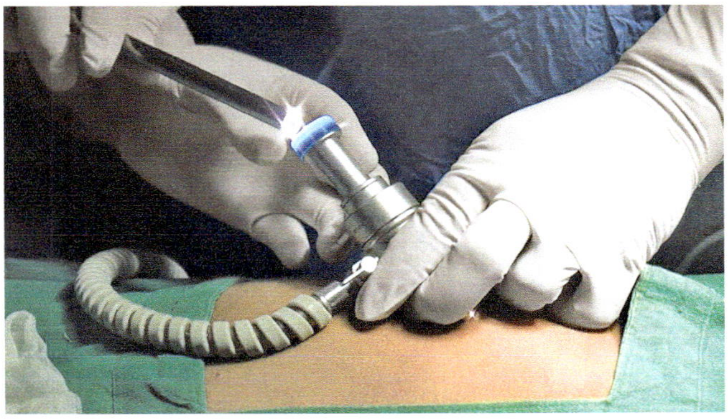

Fig. 29: Introduction of telescope.

giving way sensation, the trocar should be tilted to 60–70° angle. Insertion of trocar should be in screwing fashion in case of pyramidal trocar. In disposable bladed trocar, screwing the trocar should not be done **(Fig. 27)**.

Confirmation of Entry of Primary Trocar

- Audible click if disposable trocar or safety trocar is used.
- Whooshing sound if reusable trocar is used (gas passes from the small hole at the tip of pyramidal shaped trocar to the head of trocar).
- Loss of resistance felt both in disposable as well as reusable trocar.

Once the trocar entry in abdominal cavity is confirmed, cannula is stabilized with left hand and trocar is removed by right hand. After removing trocar, cannula is pushed slightly further inside the abdominal cavity to prevent coming cannula in preperitoneal space with movement of abdominal wall with respiration. Once cannula is in place tubing of insufflator is attached again and flow is restarted to refill the CO_2 at preset pressure **(Fig. 28)**. Telescope is introduced slowly keeping the oblique cut edge down in case of 30° telescope **(Fig. 29)**. At the time of introduction of telescope, it is wise to keep valve of cannula open to prevent scratch over tip of telescope.

Once the telescope is inside, the elevation angle of the telescope should be 90° with panoramic vision. The site just below the entry of primary port is examined for any vessel or bowel injury **(Fig. 30)**. Sometime, there may be few drops of blood found just below the site of entry but these few drops of blood are trickled blood through umbilical wound. If surgeon has any doubt about perforation of bowel or injury to vessel, he should evaluate this area again after putting other ports.

Working Ports

To select the site for secondary port, transillumination with illuminated telescope tip should be done first to locate avascular area to avoid injury of subcutaneous vessels. With the help of mosquito forceps, any remaining skin fiber is breached, and the subcutaneous fat should be cleared. Initially, the direction of entry of trocar is perpendicular but as soon as the tip of trocar is seen, the direction of trocar should be changed toward the free space to prevent any injury of underlying viscera **(Fig. 31)**.

Subsequent Ports

Subsequent ports are inserted under direct vision at locations appropriate for the procedure and to the anatomy of the individual. If the port is on the opposite side of the patient, it can be introduced same way but if surgeon is not able to bend enough to opposite side, his right index finger can be placed over the head of the trocar and left hand should guard the shaft of cannula. Alternatively, trocars of opposite side can be introduced by the assistant **(Fig. 32)**. With slow rotatory movement of right hand, first the tip of trocar should be perpendicular to the skin but as soon as tip of trocar is seen direction of trocar should change toward the anterior abdominal wall. Alternatively, surgeon can go to another side of the patient and he can introduce the trocar in conventional way.

In same manner, all the working port should be introduced, and instruments are inserted to start the surgery **(Fig. 33)**. It should be remembered that distance between two ports should never be <5 cm. The "Baseball diamond concept" discussed in Chapter 7: Principle of Laparoscopic Port Position is the most appropriate method to decide the site of introduction of working port. The positioning of operative ports is an important factor in determining the ease with which a procedure is carried out. It is a skill which must be learnt.

Slipping of Port

Sometimes, the port wound becomes bigger than the diameter of cannula and it tends to slip out frequently.

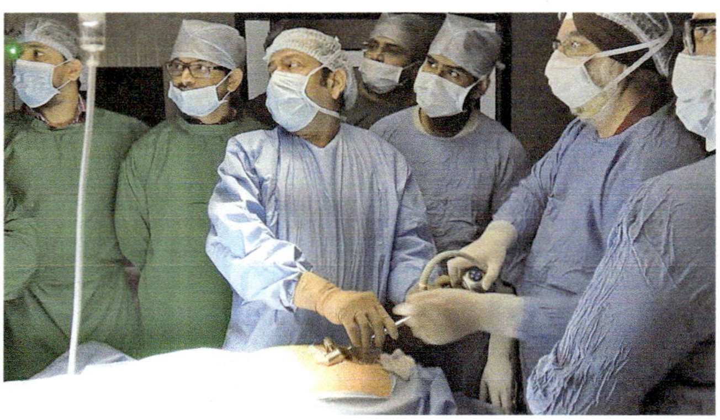

Fig. 30: Initial diagnosis of injury after access.

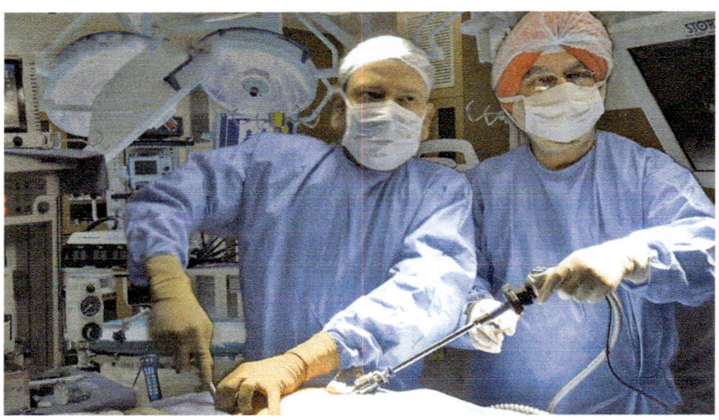

Fig. 31: Introduction of secondary port.

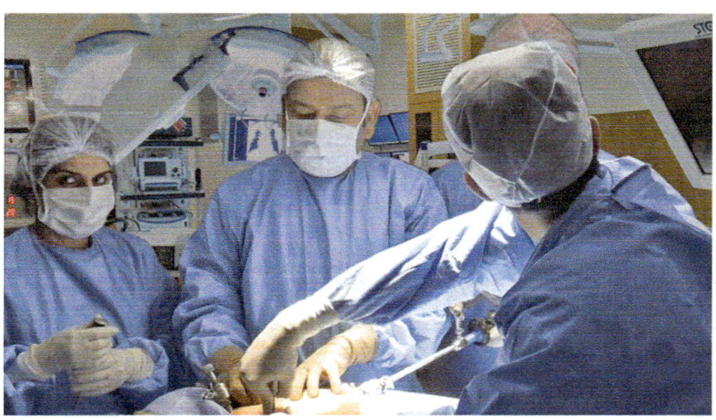

Fig. 32: Introduction of secondary trocar.

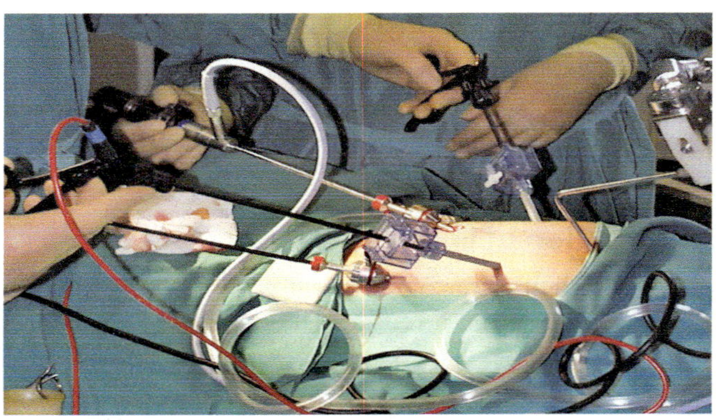

Fig. 33: All the ports and instruments should be positioned properly without entangling each other.

In these situations, a simple stitch over skin and fixing of the cannula with the help of sterile adhesive tape helps. In pediatric laparoscopic surgery, stabilizing the port is necessary. Reusable metal cannula has trumpet or flap valves. The flap valves can be manually opened when introducing or removing an instrument. This avoids damaging delicate instruments such as tip of telescope or blunting sharp instruments such as aspiration needle and scissors. A reducer tube is used with large cannula to maintain the gas seal and this automatically opens the valve. Several cannulas modeled on the Hasson cannula is available for use during open laparoscopic procedures. Different sized converters (gaskets) are available for disposable cannula to maintain the gas seal.

OPEN ACCESS

Open access technique was developed by Hasson in 1974 **(Figs. 34 to 40)**. The choice of site may be based on the surgeon's preference or the presence of a previous regional incision that may have adhesions. Hasson trocar is used in open technique which is available both in disposable and reusable model **(Figs. 34 and 35)**. Open access technique is like minilaparotomy and the cannula is introduced inside. Hasson's technique involves direct open visualization of the tissues at every layer until the peritoneum is opened, followed by placement of anchoring sutures in the fascia to secure a conical collar. The trocar is then placed through the collar to establish pneumoperitoneum and access. Disadvantages include persistent uncontrolled CO_2 leakage in many cases, increased incision size, and increased time for placement. This technique generally adds to the length of the procedure, taking longer to perform at the beginning and the end of the procedure compared with a closed Veress needle technique. Even though the Hasson technique is most commonly used in the periumbilical region, this method can be used anywhere on the abdominal wall and is particularly useful when there is a concern for abdominal wall adhesions in a patient with a prior laparotomy.

In this, there is a direct entry by open technique, without creating pneumoperitoneum and insufflator is connected once blunt trocar is inside the abdominal cavity under direct vision. There are various ways of open access such as Hasson's technique, Scandinavian technique, and Fielding technique.

Some surgeons and gynecologists practice blind trocar insertion without pneumoperitoneum. The incidence of injury due to this type of access is much higher. This type of direct trocar entry is practiced by gynecologists for sterilization. Sterilization may be performed because in multipara patients the lower abdominal wall is lax; making the fascia thinner and easy elevation by hand is possible. Bleeding due to accidental damage to a major vessel during this initial stage is one of the most dangerous complications of laparoscopic surgery.

The Hasson trocar system was initially developed for laparoscopy in patients who have had a previous laparotomy. After seeing benefit of open access technique, many surgeons started using open access technique routinely in all their patients. An access wound was made using traditional open techniques and the Hasson trocar and cannula was designed to both fix the port and seal this larger wound round the port. It requires the use of sutures to prevent slippage of port. This involved making a small entry wound directly through the scar tissue of the umbilicus and then dilating this up by passage of a blunt, preferable conically tipped trocar and cannula **(Figs. 39 and 40)**.

Steps of Open Access Technique

A transverse incision is made in the subumbilical region and the upper skin flap is retracted with an Allis forceps. The lower flap is retracted using a small right-angled retractor. Subcutaneous tissue is dissected till the linea alba and the

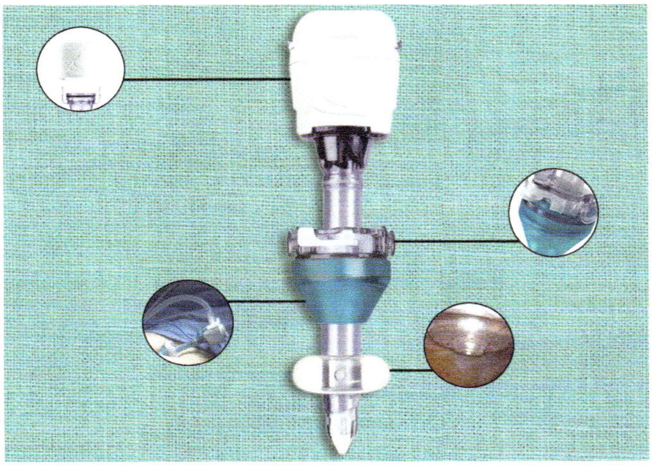

Fig. 34: Disposable Hasson trocar.

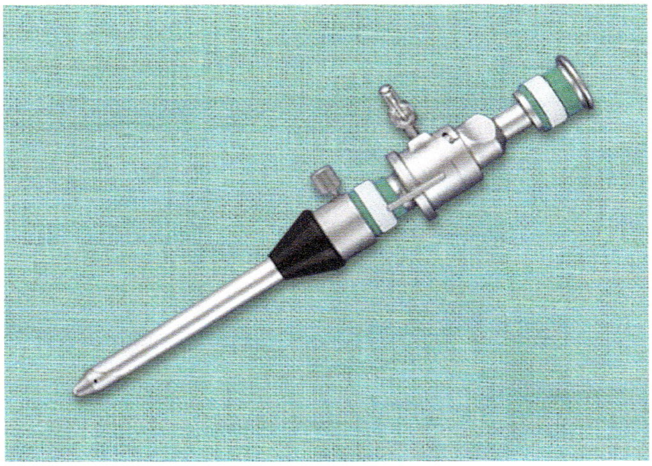

Fig. 35: Reusable Hasson trocar.

rectus sheath is visualized. Stay sutures are taken on either side of the midline.

- Make a transverse or longitudinal incision in the skin just below the umbilicus **(Fig. 36)**.
- Stay suture is given both the end of transverse incision.
- Both the stays are pulled up to make a bridge-like elevation of rectus.
- Rectus sheath is incised in the midline along the line of linea alba pointing upward. Incision should not penetrate the peritoneum; otherwise any adhesion with the peritoneum may be punctured **(Figs. 38A and B)**.
- Incise the fascia until a small amount of preperitoneal fat is identified. Place stay sutures in the fascial edges.
- The stay sutures aid with retraction of the abdominal wall and can be used to secure the port to the fascia, preventing its displacement during the surgery.
- A hemostat is stabbed into the peritoneum while holding the stays up **(Fig. 37)**.
- The give-way of the peritoneum can be felt as peritoneum is perforated and then the hemostat is opened to widen the opening.
- Open the peritoneum bluntly, sweep the underside of the abdominal wall with the index finger to clear omentum or bowel, and confirm the absence of adhesions in the region of the incision **(Figs. 36 to 38)**.
- Surgeon should insert his finger to feel all around inside the abdominal cavity to feel any possible adhesion.
- Small tiny adhesion felt can be broken with gentle sweeping movement of finger.
- Blunt trocar-cannula should be inserted for the first port after visualizing the intraperitoneal viscera **(Fig. 39)**.
- Care is taken not to make a big incision; cannula dilates the smaller incision to give an airtight fit.
- If incision is big, rectus string should be tightened to hold the port in proper position **(Fig. 40)**.
- Attach the gas (typically CO_2) to the port and insufflate the abdomen. Fast insufflation should be avoided to prevent vasovagal shock.

Advantages of Open Technique

- Definite, small risk of injury with blind Veress needle technique irrespective of experience.
- Particularly useful in previous abdominal surgery or underlying adhesions.
- The incidence of injury to adhesion although not eliminated is significantly reduced by entry into the peritoneal cavity under direct vision.
- There is a decreased risk of injury to the retroperitoneal vessels. The trocar is blunt, and the angle of entry allows

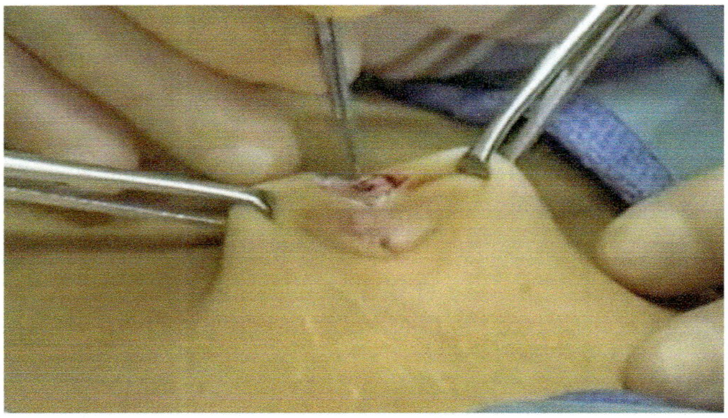

Fig. 36: Skin incision for open technique.

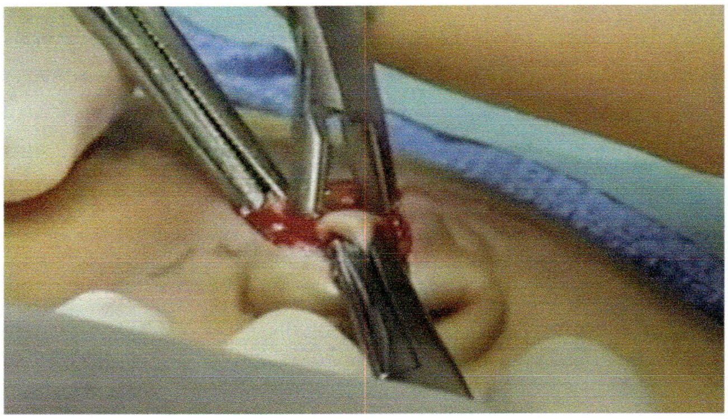

Fig. 37: Hemostat is stabbed into the peritoneum.

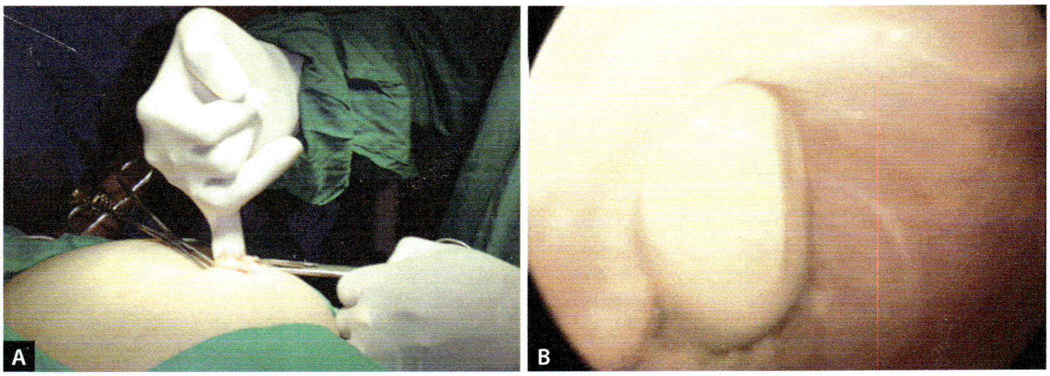

Figs. 38A and B: Finger insertion after open access will confirm adhesion.

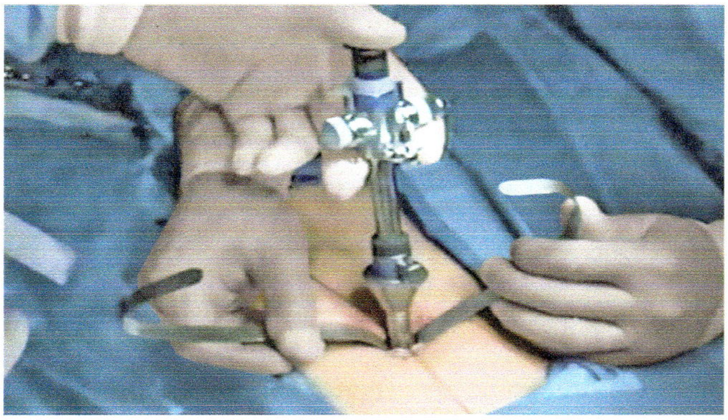

Fig. 39: Introduction of Hasson trocar.

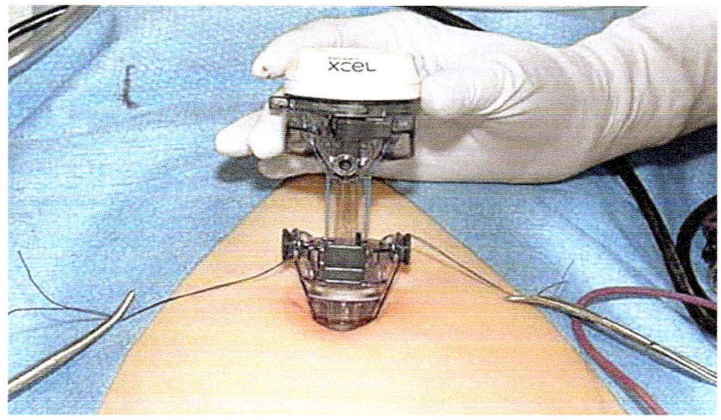

Fig. 40: Fixation of Hasson trocar.

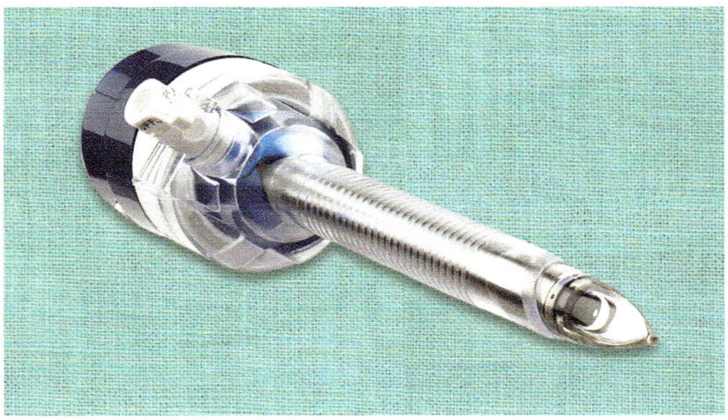

Fig. 41: Optical trocar.

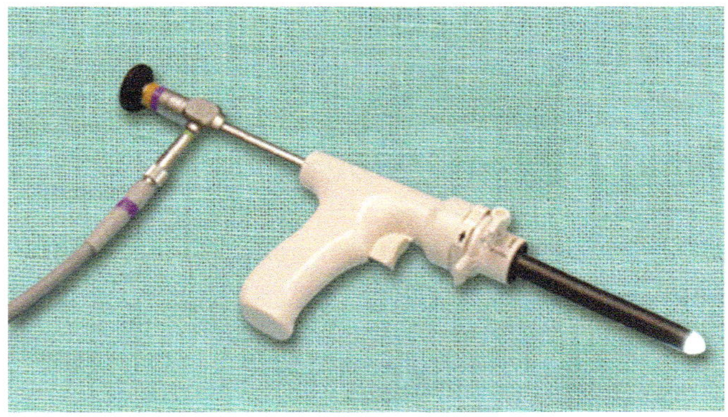

Fig. 42: Visiport.

the surgeon to maneuver the cannula at an angle, which avoids viscera, while still assuring peritoneal placement.

- The risk of extraperitoneal insufflation is eliminated. Placement under direct vision ensures that insufflation of gas is actually into the peritoneal cavity.
- The likelihood of hernia formation is decreased because the fascia is closed as part of the technique.
- Increasing number of surgeons performing laparoscopy without experience and in these group open technique may be easy.
- Useful in muscular man and children with strong abdominal wall.
- Useful for gynecologists or surgeon lacking enough upper arm strength to elevate the abdominal wall of patient.
- An open technique, which involves creating a minilaparotomy into which a special cannula is inserted, may be adopted. This procedure has its own complications and requires skilled execution.

Visual Entry Technique

The visual entry technique accesses the abdominal cavity with a specialized optical port that has a transparent tip, allowing each layer of the abdominal wall to be seen with a 0° laparoscope as it is being traversed **(Fig. 41)**. Commercially available optical trocar/ports include Optiview, Kii optical access system, and Visiport **(Fig. 42)**. The way each of these devices affects tissue dissection as the tip advances differs in minor ways. These devices are typically used for primary port placement after Veress needle abdominal insufflation or secondary port placement after pneumoperitoneum has already been established.

Open Fielding Technique

This technique developed by Fielding in 1992 involves a small incision over the everted umbilicus at a point where the skin and peritoneum are adjacent. Fielding technique is useful in patients with abdominal incisions from previous surgery provided there is no midline incision, portal hypertension and recanalized umbilical vein, and umbilical abnormalities, such as urachal cyst, sinus or umbilical hernia. Thorough skin preparation of the umbilicus is carried out and the everted umbilicus is incised from the apex in a caudal direction. Two small retractors are inserted to expose the cylindrical umbilical tube running from the undersurface of the umbilical skin down to the linea alba.

This tube is then cut from its apex downward toward its junction with the linea alba. Further, blunt dissection through this plane permits direct entry into the peritoneum. Once the peritoneal cavity is breached, the primary port can be inserted directly, and insufflation started. A blunt internal trocar facilitates insertion of this port and an external grip that can be attached to the port assist to secure it in position. Suture is usually not required to prevent gas leakage because the umbilicus has been everted so the angle of insertion of the laparoscopic port becomes oblique and the incision required is relatively small. However, one may be needed to stabilize the port.

Scarred Abdomen

Additional precautions are necessary during the access procedure in patients with abdominal scars. It may be inadvisable to insert the Veress needle below the umbilicus in a patient with a scar in this area (or an umbilical hernia). Insufflation through unscarred such as subcostal region, or if this is scarred, the iliac fossa is better. A general guideline is to choose the quadrant of the abdomen opposite to that of the scar.

Contraindications of Umbilical Entry

- Previous midline incision
- Portal hypertension with recanalized umbilical artery with advanced cirrhosis of the liver
- Umbilical abnormalities viz. urachal cyst, sinus, hernia.

PNEUMOPERITONEUM IN SPECIAL CONDITIONS

Palmer's Technique

This access was advocated by Palmer in the 1940s because visceral parietal adhesions are rarely encountered in this area **(Fig. 43)**. A small incision is made to allow the insertion of the Veress needle through left subcostal margin **(Fig. 44)**. In addition, some authors feel that because the abdominal wall in the area is supported by the rigid thoracic wall, insertion of the needle is more controlled than in the periumbilical area. Palmer's technique is particular useful in cases where umbilical entry is contraindicated, it is preferred to use left upper quadrate for entry of Veress needle. The Veress needle is introduced through left hypochondria, i.e., Palmer's point 2 cm below the left subcostal margin in midclavicular line **(Fig. 45)**. Special care should be taken that there should not be hepatosplenomegaly. After access though Palmer's point, umbilicus site is rechecked for any adhesion or other abnormalities. If necessary, umbilicus port may be introduced under vision.

Mishra's Technique

This access technique we have developed where little modification of Palmer's technique is done. We give incision 2 cm above the costal margin in midclavicular line called Mishra's point **(Fig. 46)**. To introduce Veress needle at Mishra's point abdominal wall is stretched down and brought below the costal margin. Advantage of this technique is there is no incidence of hernia because after surgery incision retract back to 2 cm above the costal margin **(Fig. 47)**. During insertion of Veress needle or trocar through the palmer's point, the tip of the trocar should be pointed toward the stomach to prevent injury of splenic flexor of colon. It is very important that nasogastric tube should be in place and stomach should be deflated **(Fig. 48)**.

Obese Patients

In obese patient, incision site should be transumbilical (base of umbilicus) for the insertion of Veress needle, because it is the thinnest abdominal wall and even in obese patient, the amount of fat in transumbilical region is less compared to other areas of the abdominal wall. Direction of Veress needle entry in obese patient should be perpendicular to abdominal wall and patient should be in supine position not in Trendelenburg's position **(Fig. 49)**. Once the Veress needle is inside pneumoperitoneum should be created up to 18 mm Hg. Once the actual pressure is equal to preset pressure and at least 1.5–3 L of gas is introduced, Veress needle is removed. After removing Veress needle, the initial incision is enlarged up to 11 mm. After enlarging the initial incision, fat should be cleared up to anterior rectus sheath with the help of hemostat and little finger. In obese patients, it is difficult to lift the abdominal wall alone, assistant's hand should be asked for help to have a better grip **(Fig. 50)**. If bariatric surgery or fundoplication is planned, then Veress needle

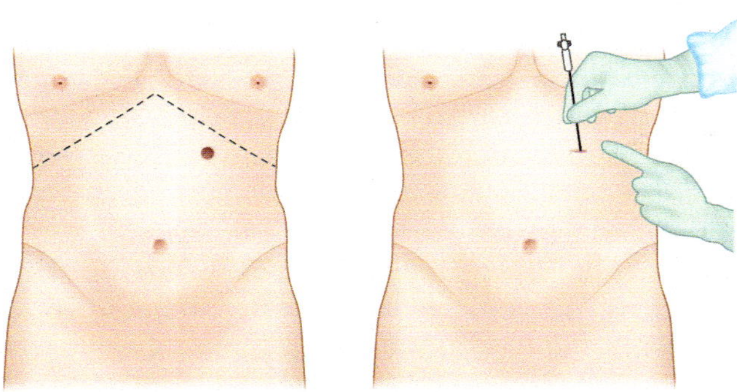

Fig. 43: Palmer's point of access.

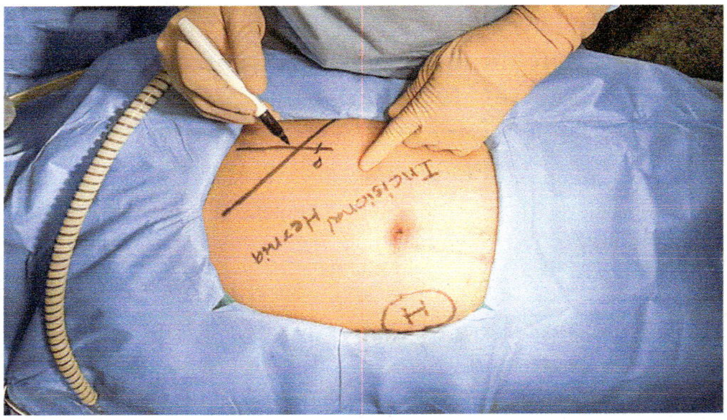

Fig. 44: Palmer's point 2 cm below the costal margin.

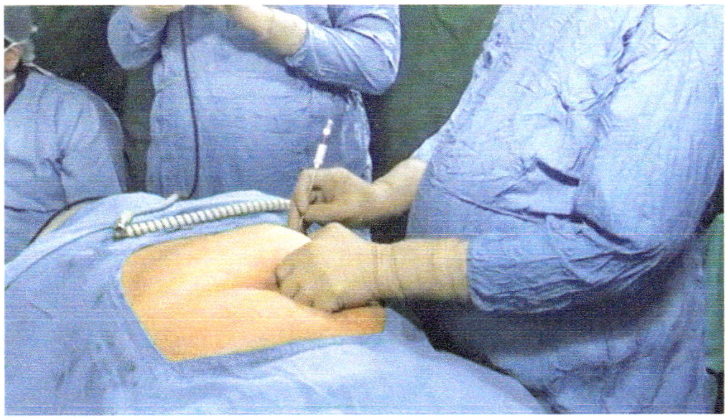

Fig. 45: Veress needle insertion through Palmer's point.

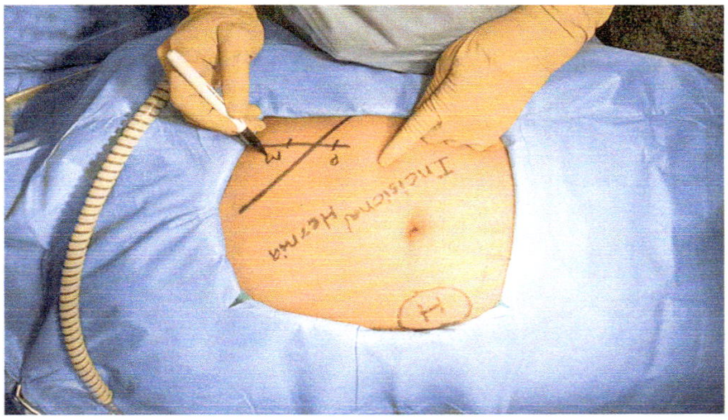

Fig. 46: Mishra's point 2 cm above the costal margin.

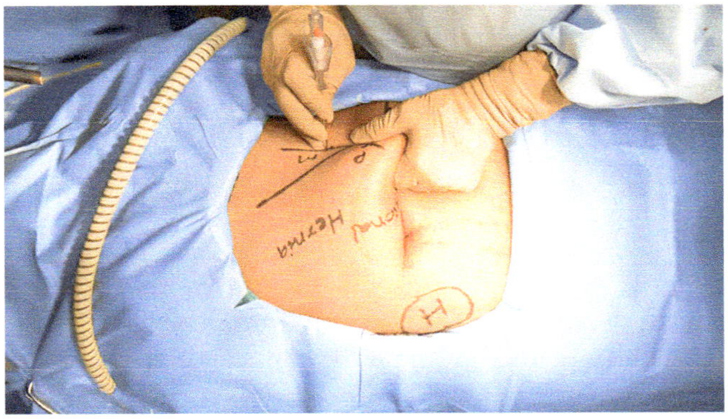

Fig. 47: Veress needle insertion through Mishra's point.

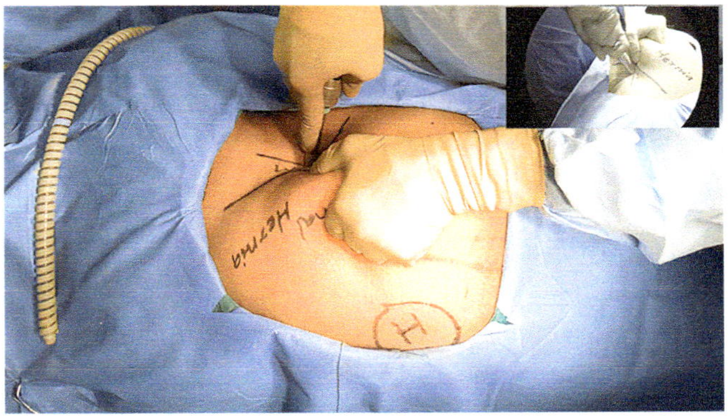

Fig. 48: Trocar insertion through Mishra's point.

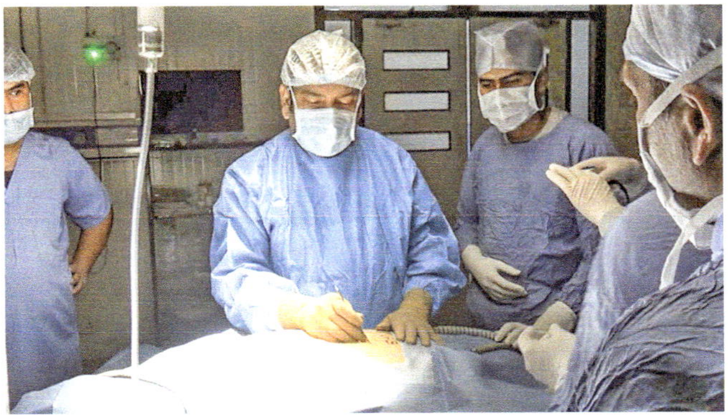

Fig. 49: Patient should be in supine position not in Trendelenburg's position.

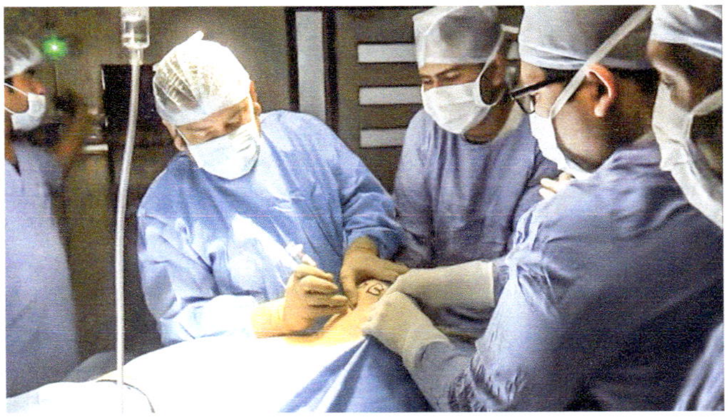

Fig. 50: Veress needle introduction in obese patient.

and primary trocar need to be introduced supraumbilical so that the telescope can show the diaphragm and posterior mediastinum during esophageal mobilization.

ENTRY IN CASES OF MORBID OBESITY

Abdominal access can be challenging in the patient with a thick abdominal wall; however, all types of entry access can be safely performed by experienced surgeons. In morbid obese patient, the umbilicus is well below the aortic bifurcation in supine position. When using the Veress needle technique in obese patients, the left upper quadrant is preferred by many surgeons for initial placement (Palmer's point). If supraumbilical access is used to perform bariatric surgery assistant's help should be taken to lift the abdominal wall **(Fig. 50)**. Longer port 20 cm in length is required in case of obese patient **(Fig. 51)**. The irrigation test, aspiration test, the saline drop test, and an opening pressure of <10 mm Hg should all be used to confirm proper placement of the needle. When using the Hasson technique for patients with a large amount of subcutaneous fat, the incision should be made large enough to identify the abdominal wall fascia and peritoneum.

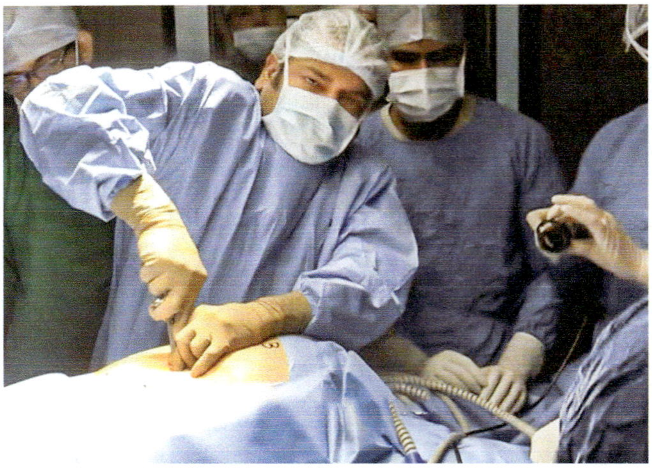

Fig. 51: Optical trocar entry in obese patients.

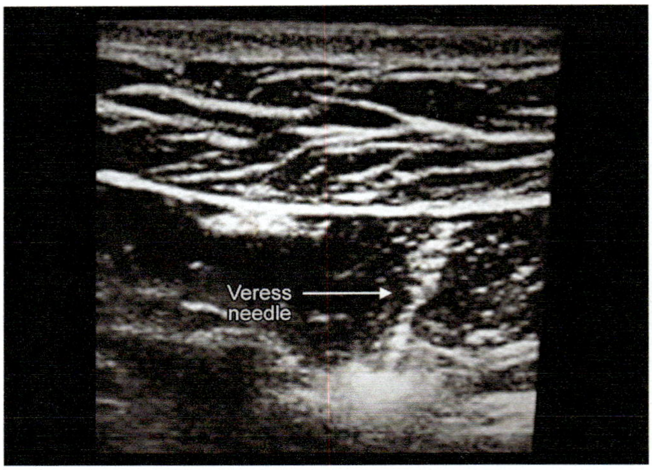

Fig. 52: Ultrasound-guided entry.

The area beneath the Veress needle insertion site inside the abdomen should be inspected for injuries during the initial laparoscopic evaluation of the abdomen.

Ultrasound Visceral Slide

There is a simple preoperative test that can help to identify a safe region for Veress needle insertion in the scarred abdomen. The preoperative detection of anterior abdominal wall adhesions by ultrasonic scanning is a simple and reliable technique of ultrasonic detection and mapping of abdominal wall adhesions. In patients with portal hypertension, a major risk factor upon entry into the abdomen is injury to large, engorged paraumbilical vessels in the anterior abdominal wall **(Fig. 52)**. Major blood loss often results from just entering the abdomen. Use of ultrasound-guided access into the peritoneum for laparoscopic surgery is also a safe and effective approach in a patient presenting with portal hypertension. This technique demonstrates an effective tool in the surgical armamentarium for entering the abdomen in patients with caput medusae. Once the Veress needle has been inserted, there should still be concern about the risk of causing damage with the trocar. The following techniques have been described for this situation.

Sounding Test

A fine spinal needle, attached to a saline-filled syringe, is passed into the inflated abdomen. As the needle is slowly advanced, while aspirating, a stream of bubbles is seen in the saline until the needle tip contacts tissue. The needle is then withdrawn toward the surface and the process repeated several times, in different directions, thereby "mapping" the gas filled cavity and any solid structures.

Complications of Access Technique

The rate of serious complications associated with a laparoscopic approach is overall low. Half of the complications occur at the time of abdominal access for camera or port placement. Complications can also arise from abdominal insufflation, tissue dissection, and hemostasis. Conversion to an open procedure may be needed to manage complications that have been identified intraoperatively, while others may be recognized in postoperative period. Severe complications such as vascular injury and bowel perforation can be catastrophic and are the main cause of procedure-specific morbidity and mortality related to laparoscopic surgery. Improper trocar insertion causes most of the operative complications of laparoscopic surgery. Examples are injury to the bowel, major vessels, bladder, inferior epigastric vessels, and subcutaneous emphysema. Other complications include thermal injury to the bowel, abdominal wall contusions, trocar site herniation with possible bowel obstruction, and trocar site tumor implants. However, the overall incidence of complications is relatively low (about 2%). There have been a few case reports of vulvar edema and surgical emphysema after laparoscopic surgery. The mechanism is unclear, but the condition is self-limited and resolves with conservative management. Patients with an abdominal wall hematoma from laparoscopic access who are hemodynamically stable and with no signs of hematoma expansion can be managed conservatively.

Access Injuries

The incidence of abdominal access injury was 5–30/10,000 procedures. Bowel and retroperitoneal vascular injuries comprised 76% of all injuries, and almost 50% of small and large bowel injuries were unrecognized for at least 24 hours. The overall reported rate of vascular injury arterial or venous injury ranges from 0.1 to 6.4/1,000 laparoscopies. Most injuries involve minor vessels; however, underreporting is common. Bladed disposable trocars with sharp blades are more likely to injure vessels compared with smooth, pyramidal tip trocars that push the vessel out of the way.

The types and proportion of organ injury during abdominal access were as follows:

- Small bowel (25%)
- Iliac artery (19%)
- Colon (12%)
- Iliac or another retroperitoneal vein (9%)
- Secondary branches of a mesenteric vessel (7%)
- Aorta (6%)
- Inferior vena cava (4%)
- Abdominal wall vessels (4%)
- Bladder (3%)
- Liver (2%)
- Other (<2%)

Port-site metastasis refers to cancer growth at a port incision site after laparoscopic tumor resection. Port-site metastasis occurs after 1–2% of laparoscopic procedures performed in the presence of intraperitoneal malignancy, which is equivalent to the rate of wound metastasis after laparotomy performed under similar conditions. Mechanism of metastasis includes hematogenous spread or direct contamination by tumor cells, secondary effects from pneumoperitoneum-related immune suppression, and surgical technique. Although it is not clear whether port-site metastases can be prevented, suggested measures to minimize the risk of port-site metastases include the use of wound protectors and specimen extraction bags, instillation of agents to prevent tumor growth, and port-site excision.

Access Injury Risk Factors

It is shown that patients who have had prior open surgery for intra-abdominal or pelvic disease have a higher risk of complications related to adhesions compared with patients who do not have this history. Other conditions that increase the risk of complications include extensive bowel distention, very large abdominal or pelvic mass-like large fibroid or abdominal cyst, and diaphragmatic hernia. In addition, patients with poor cardiopulmonary reserve due to severe chronic obstructive pulmonary disease (COPD) and cardiac disease may not be candidates for abdominal insufflation given the physiologic changes related to pneumoperitoneum. For patients with risk factors for complications, the laparoscopic approach and approach to abdominal access need to be carefully planned; an open approach may be preferred. If possible, these patients can be a candidate of gasless laparoscopic surgery. The frequency of complications during access technique may be related to surgeon experience and the number of the specific procedures performed for some, but not all, types of minimal access surgical procedures.

Mild-to-Moderate Hypotension

In cases of moderate hypotension, the surgeon should consider discontinuing gas insufflation immediately and reducing intra-abdominal pressure to 8.0 mm Hg. 360° scan of the abdominal cavity should be performed immediately to rule out retroperitoneal bleeding. If bleeding or expanding hematoma is seen, one should proceed immediately to long midline laparotomy and compression of the bleeding vessel. Blood should be aspirated; bleeder is exposed, and bleeding should be controlled with vascular clamps. When necessary, operator should obtain assistance of a vascular surgeon.

Withdrawal of Instruments and Ports

Once the surgery is finished, all the instrument should be removed carefully under vision. All the accessory port should be removed, and the gas is removed by releasing the valve of 10 mm cannulas. The primary port should be taken out in the end **(Fig. 53)**.

If last port is suddenly withdrawn sudden suction effect of cannula can pull the omentum or bowel inside the port wound, the chances of port-site hernia and adhesion are much higher in this case. It is a good practice to insert some blunt instrument or telescope inside the abdomen while removing the last cannula out over that instrument, to prevent inadvertent entrapment of omentum or bowel **(Figs. 54A and B)**.

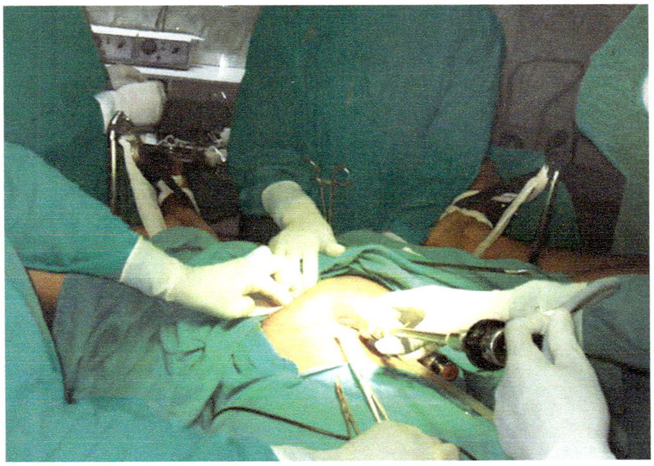

Fig. 53: The tip of telescope should be introduced in and cannula is pulled over telescope to prevent suction of omentum or bowel.

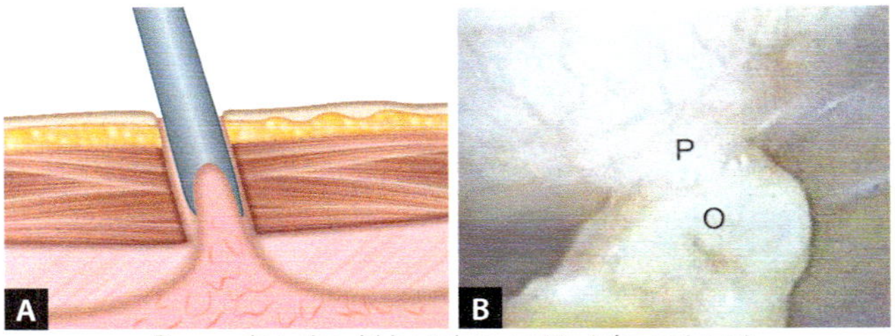

Precaution should be taken not to take out port suddenly, without removing complete gas

Figs. 54A and B: Adhesion may form if cannula is pulled rapidly at the end of surgery (P: peritoneum; O: omentum).

PORT CLOSURE TECHNIQUES

The access technique will result in breach in continuity of abdominal wall which need to be repaired at the end of surgery. All the 10 mm or >10 mm port should be repaired properly to prevent any future possibility of hernia. The rectus sheath is only necessary to suture with Vicryl. Only one stitch is required in middle which will convert 10 mm wound into 5 mm. The 5 mm port wounds are not necessary to repair **(Figs. 55A to D)**.

Various types of port closure instruments are available. The suture passer is a convenient instrument for port closure, it is used to pass the thread on the side of cannula and then it is tied externally **(Figs. 56A and B)**. For port closure, specially designed port closure instruments are also available commercially, such as port closure needle and aneurism needle. After closing the rectus sheath, the skin can be closed by intradermal, skin stapler or by any of the surgical skin glues available.

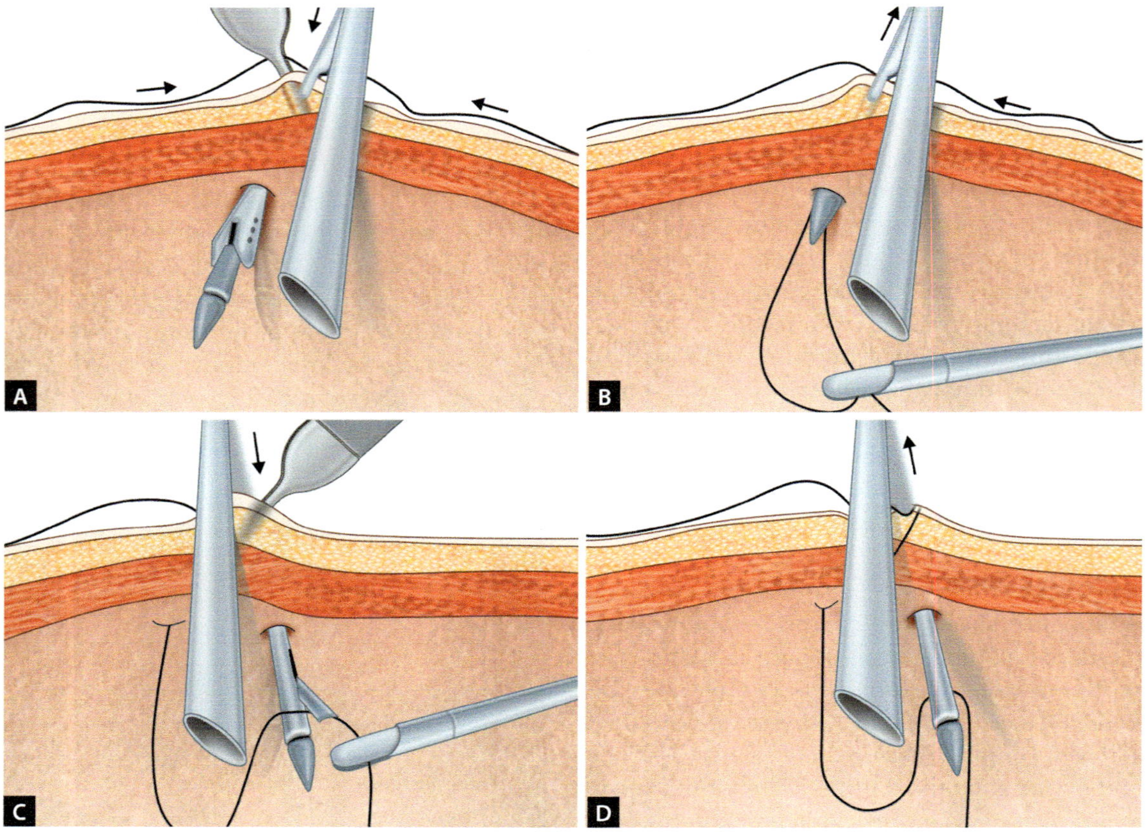

Figs. 55A to D: Port closure with the help of suture passer.

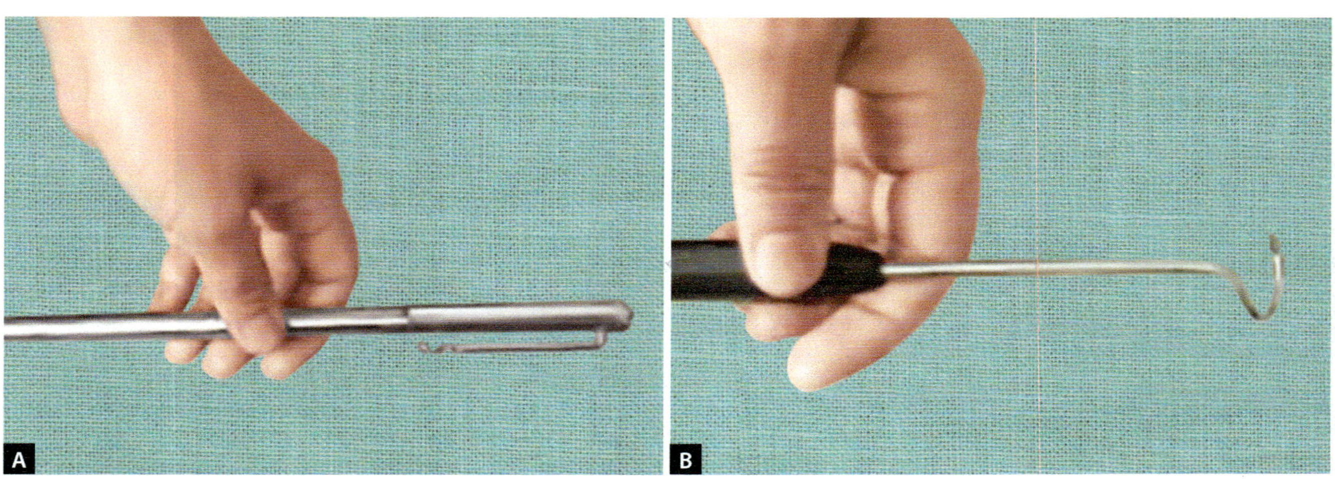

Figs. 56A and B: Port closure needle and aneurysm needle.

Gasless Laparoscopic Surgery

Conventional laparoscopic surgery requires pneumoperitoneum to elevate the abdominal wall for proper exposure. A continuous insufflation of a noncombustible gas in a sealed environment is essential part of MAS. Many undesirable physiological side effects have been observed with CO_2 pneumoperitoneum. Furthermore, it has been necessary to retrain surgeons to use specialized instruments in order to operate on video images. Abdominal lifting mechanical devices can provide working space without pneumoperitoneum. With gasless technique, conventional instruments can be used, direct visualization of abdominal viscera is possible, and digital examination of abdominal contents can be performed without the fear of losing exposure. Since these procedures are being performed in an isobaric abdominal cavity, the risk of body fluid contamination to operating team is diminished when compared to open or traditional laparoscopic surgery. Gasless laparoscopic surgery is primarily advocated for the patients who are at high risk of pneumoperitoneum. A variety of abdominal lift devices have been developed recently to provide good working space. Although gasless laparoscopic surgery is good for patient with high risk of pneumoperitoneum, due to intraoperative problems and complications and because of suboptimal exposure, gasless laparoscopic surgery is still not considered as the prime modality for every patient. All the gasless systems can be used on their own or with low pressure insufflation (4–6 mm Hg).

Three Basic Types

1. Rubber tube sling abdominal wall lifts
2. Planar intraperitoneal abdominal wall retraction lift devices
3. Subcutaneous abdominal wall lift devices.

None of these techniques gives as good a laparoscopic exposure as the pressurized pneumoperitoneum because they produce a tent-like elevation of the abdominal wall rather than an elevated expansion and they do not depress the hollow organs and omentum. Exposure is improved when low pressure insufflation is added.

Several devices for gasless laparoscopy have been developed recently. The Laparolift (Origin Medsystems) is commercially available device routinely used by many surgeons and gynecologist worldwide **(Figs. 57 to 59)**.

It consists of an adjustable arm that is attached to the side of the operating table and sterilely draped **(Figs. 60A and B)**. The surgeon can raise and lower it electronically. The arm is connected to the Laparofan, a disposable sterile device with two metal blades (available in 10 cm and 15 cm lengths) that are inserted through the umbilical incision in an overlapped position. After entering the peritoneal space, the Laparofan paddles are spread. Using the dovetail connector, the Laparofan retractor is attached to the Laparolift arm and raised, creating a working cavity for laparoscopic surgery. It is intended to be used as a substitute for, or in conjunction

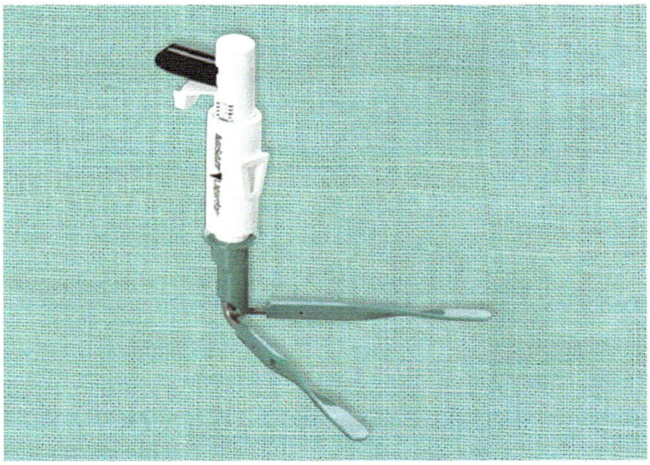

Fig. 58: Laparofan attached with laparolift after introduction inside abdominal cavity.

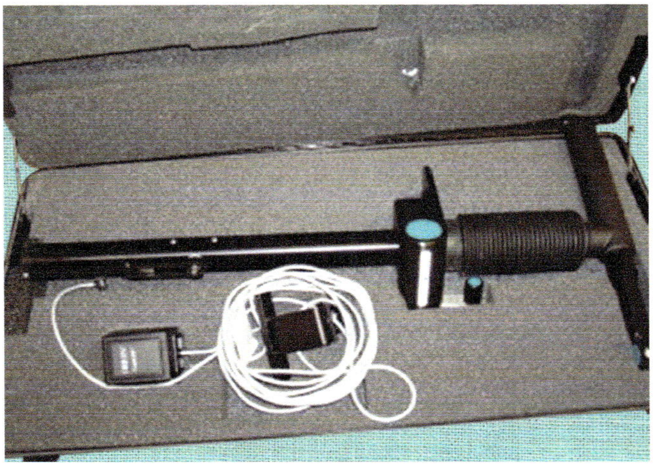

Fig. 57: Laparolift.

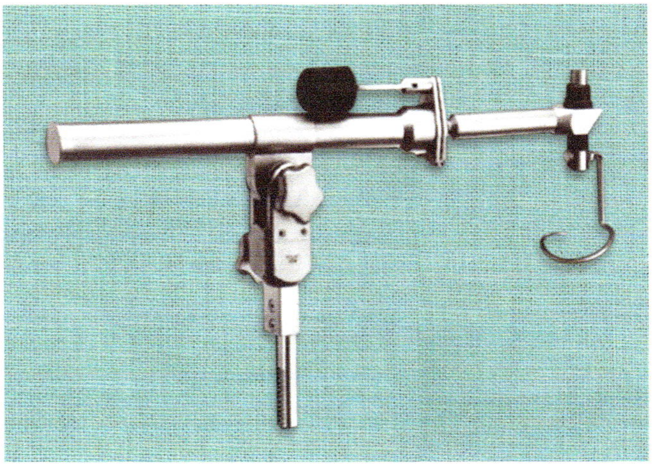

Fig. 59: Abdolift (another variety of abdominal lifting device).

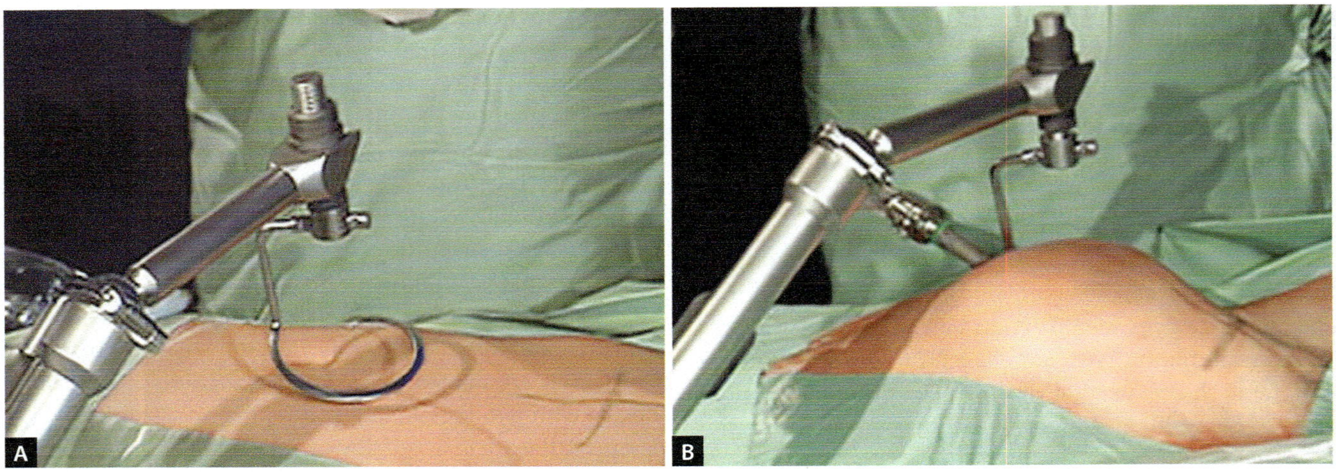

Figs. 60A and B: Abdolift lifting the abdominal cavity.

BOX 1: Problems due to pneumoperitoneum.

- Hypothermia
- Cardiac arrhythmia
- Cardiovascular collapse
- Pulmonary insufficiency
- Gas embolism
- Venous thrombosis
- Cerebral edema/ischemia
- Ocular hypertension
- Extraperitoneal insufflation (subcutaneous emphysema, pneumomediastinum)

with, pneumoperitoneum for abdominal wall retraction. The blades are then splayed out and locked into a V by tabs on the plastic handle, which is fixed to the end of the adjustable arm. The maximum lifting force of 13.6 kg is equivalent to a pneumoperitoneum pressure of 15 mm Hg. The laparoscope is inserted through the same incision, cephalad to the Laparofan.

The physiologic changes associated with CO_2 pneumoperitoneum are well tolerated in healthy patients but may result in life-threatening cardiac arrhythmia, myocardial infarction, cardiac failure, or pulmonary insufficiency in compromised patients who cannot compensate for these alterations in hemodynamic **(Box 1)**. A gasless laparoscopic approach could provide an added margin of safety for these patients. Patients undergoing laparoscopic surgery for malignancy or laparoscopically assisted vaginal hysterectomy may also benefit from gasless laparoscopy. Another potential advantage of gasless laparoscopy is the ability to use continuous suction and conventional laparotomy instruments **(Figs. 61 and 62)**.

Disadvantages of Gasless Laparoscopic Surgery

- Marked guttering effect of lateral abdominal wall results after lifting anterior abdominal wall.
- Anterior abdominal adhesion can make insertion of these mechanical devise difficult and visualization almost impossible.
- It is a space occupying as instrument takes all the ergonomically good space of port position.
- It only elevates anterior abdominal wall whereas gas creates workable space in whole abdominal cavity.
- Sometime causes pressure necrosis of superior or inferior epigastric vessels.
- Bigger incision is required in the umbilicus.
- Difficult to perform in presence of ileus.
- Difficult peritoneal toileting at remote places.

Studies to date have demonstrated that surgical procedures with gasless laparoscopy are technically more difficult than those performed with adequate pneumoperitoneum owing to impaired visualization from bowel in the pelvis. As with any new laparoscopic device, the initial enthusiasm over gasless laparoscopy has been tempered by actual clinical experience. However, because gasless laparoscopy still promises significant advantages over CO_2 pneumoperitoneum in high-risk patient, it is anticipated that interest in this technique will continue with improvements that will eliminate the current limitations to its use.

OPEN VERSUS CLOSED ACCESS TECHNIQUE

Knowledge of proper access techniques is crucial to avoid these complications. However, no significant differences in overall complication rates have been found for closed compared with open techniques for primary abdominal insufflation, when performed by experienced surgeons. Proper selection of patients, knowledge of laparoscopic surgical anatomy, and attention to proper abdominal access techniques are necessary to avoid complications. Risk factors for complications include prior laparoscopy, abdominal adhesions, excessive bowel distention, very large abdominal or pelvic masses, and diaphragmatic hernia. Patients with poor cardiopulmonary reserve may not tolerate pneumoperitoneum. For patients with risk factors for laparoscopic complications, an open surgical access should be preferred.

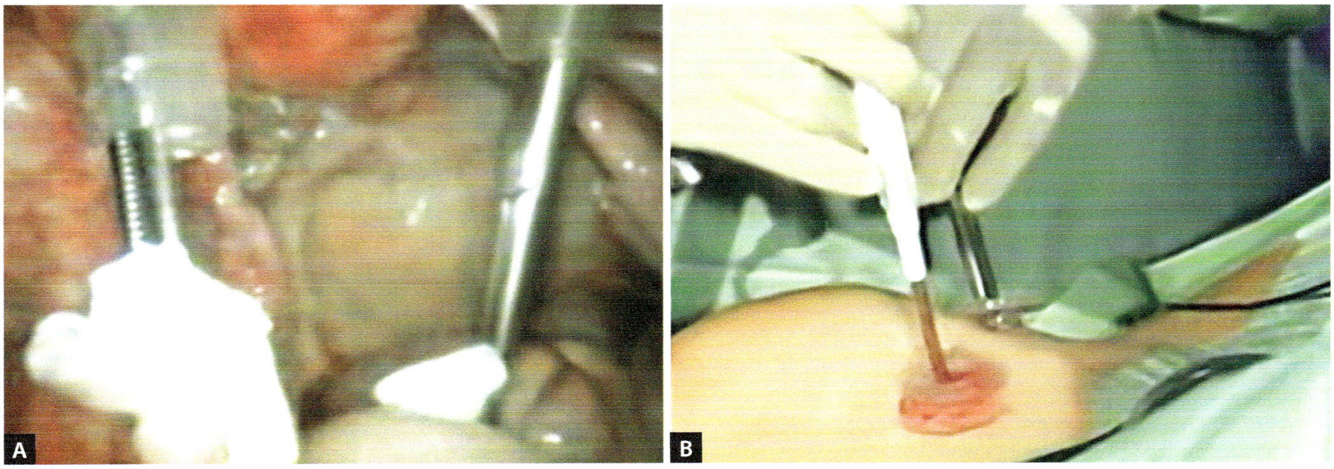

Figs. 61A and B: Use of open surgical instrument in gasless laparoscopic surgery.

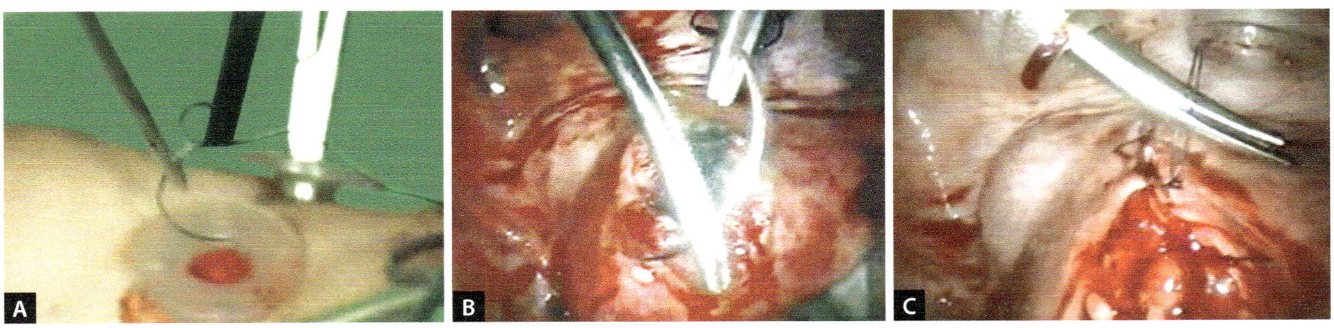

Figs. 62A to C: Use of open needle holder and suturing technique in gasless laparoscopic.

BIBLIOGRAPHY

1. Bemelman WA, Dunker MS, Busch OR, Den Boer KT, De Wit LT, Gouma DJ. Efficacy of establishment of pneumoperitoneum with the Veress needle, Hasson trocar, and modified blunt trocar (TrocDoc): a randomized study. J Laparoendosc Adv Surg Tech A. 2000;10:325-30.
2. Bernik TR, Trocciola SM, Mayer DA, Patane J, Czura CJ, Wallack MK. Balloon blunt-tip trocar for laparoscopic cholecystectomy: improvement over the traditional Hasson and Veress needle methods. J Laparoendosc Adv Surg Tech A. 2001;11:73-8.
3. Bhoyrul S, Payne J, Steffes B, Swansrtom L, Way LW. A randomized prospective study of radially expanding trocars in laparoscopic surgery. J Gastrointestinal Surg. 2000;4:392-7.
4. Bhoyrul S, Vierra MA, Nezhat CR, Krummel TM, Way LW. Trocar injuries in laparoscopic surgery. J Am Coll Surg. 2001;192(6):677-83.
5. Bonjer HJ, Hazebroek EJ, Kazemier G, Giuffrida MC, Meijer WS, Lange JF. Open vs closed establishment of pneumoperitoneum in laparoscopic surgery. Br J Surg. 1997;84:599-602.
6. Champault G, Cazacu F, Taffinder N. Serious trocar accidents in laparoscopic surgery: a French survey of 103,852 operations. Surg Laparosc Endosc. 1996;6:367-70.
7. Cogliandolo A, Manganaro T, Saitta FP, Micali B. Blind vs open approach to laparoscopic cholecystectomy. Surg Laparosc Endosc. 1998;8:353-5.
8. Eden CG, King D, Kooiman GG, Adams TH, Sullivan ME, Vass JA. Transperitoneal or extraperitoneal laparoscopic radical prostatectomy: does the approach matter? J Urol. 2004; 172:2218-23.
9. Endogru T, Teber D, Frede T, Marrero R, Hammady A, Seemann O, et al. Comparison of transperitoneal and extraperitoneal laparoscopic radical prostatectomy using match-pair analysis. Eur Urol. 2004;46:312-20.
10. Gill IS, Clayman RV, Albala DM, Aso Y, Chiu AW, Das S, et al. Retroperitoneal and pelvic extraperitoneal laparoscopy: an international perspective. Urology. 1998;52:566-71.
11. Guillonneau B, Vallancien G. Laparoscopic radical prostatectomy: the Montsouris experience. J Urol. 2000;163:418-22.
12. Gutt CN, Oniu T, Schemmer P, Kraus T, Buchler MW. Circulatory and respiratory complications of carbon dioxide insufflation. Dig Surg. 2004;21:95-105.
13. Guven S, Guven ES, Ayhan A. Vulvar edema as a rare complication of laparoscopy. J Am Assoc Gynecol Laparosc. 2004;11:429-32.
14. Hanney RM, Carmalt HL, Merret N, Tait N. Use of the Hasson cannula producing major vascular injury at laparoscopy. Surg Endosc. 1999;13:1238-40.
15. Hashizume M, Sugimachi K. Needle and trocar injury during laparoscopic surgery in Japan. Surg Endosc. 1997;11:1198-201.
16. Hasson HM. Open laparoscopy as a method of access in laparoscopic surgery. Gynaecol Endosc. 1999;8:353-62.
17. Hoznek A, Antiphon P, Borkowski T, Gettman MT, Katz R, Salomon L, et al. Assessment of surgical technique and perioperative morbidity associated with extraperitoneal versus transperitoneal laparoscopic radical prostatectomy. Urology. 2003;61:617-22.
18. Khoury N. A comparative study of laparoscopic extraperitoneal and transabdominal preperitoneal hernioplasty. J Laparoendosc Surg. 1995;5:349-55.
19. Liao CH, Chueh SC, Lai MK, Hsiao PJ, Chen J. Laparoscopic adrenalectomy for potentially malignant adrenal tumors greater than 5 centimeters. J Clin Endocrinol Metab. 2006;91:3080-3.

20. Magrina JF. Complications of laparoscopic surgery. Clin Obstet Gynecol. 2002;45:469-80.
21. Marcovici I, Shadigian E. Operative laparoscopy and vulvar hematoma: an unusual association. JSLS. 2001;5:87-8.
22. McCormack K, Wake BL, Fraser C, Vale L, Perez J, Grant A. Transabdominal pre-peritoneal (TAPP) versus totally extraperitoneal (TEP) laparoscopic techniques for inguinal hernia repair: a systematic review. Hernia. 2005;9:109-14.
23. Merlin TL, Hiller JE, Maddern GJ, Jamieson GG, Brown AR, Kolbe A. Systematic review of the safety and effectiveness of methods used to establish pneumoperitoneum in laparoscopic surgery. Br J Surg. 2003;90:668-79.
24. Neudecker J, Sauerland S, Neugebauer E, Bergamaschi R, Bonjer J, Cuschieri A, et al. The European Association for Endoscopic Surgery clinical practice guideline on the pneumoperitoneum for laparoscopic surgery. Surg Endosc. 2002;16:1121-43.
25. Ost MC, Tan BJ, Lee BR. Urological laparoscopy: basic physiological considerations and immunological consequences. J Urol. 2005;174:1183-8.
26. Pados G, Vavilis D, Pantazis K, Agorastos T, Bontis JN. Unilateral vulvar edema after operative laparoscopy: a case report and literature review. Fertil Steril. 2005;83:471-3.
27. Peitgen K, Nimtz K, Hellinger A, Walz MK. Offener zugang oder Veress-nadel bei laparoskopischen eingriffen? Ergebnisse einer prospektiv randomisierten studie. Chirurg. 1997;68:910-3.
28. Porpiglia F, Terrone C, Tarabuzzi R, Billia M, Grande S, Musso F, et al. Transperitoneal versus extraperitoneal laparoscopic radical prostatectomy: experience of a single center. Urology. 2006;68:376-80.
29. Raboy A, Ferzli G, Albert P. Initial experience with extraperitoneal endoscopic radical retropubic prostatectomy. Urology. 1997; 50:849-53.
30. Remzi M, Klingler HC, Tinzl MV, Fong YK, Lodde M, Kiss B, et al. Morbidity of laparoscopic extraperitoneal versus transperitoneal radical prostatectomy versus open retropubic radical prostatectomy. Eur Urol. 2005;48:83-9; discussion 89..
31. Rodriguez AR, Kapoor R, Pow-Sang JM. Laparoscopic extraperitoneal radical prostatectomy in complex surgical cases. J Urol. 2007;177:1765-70.
32. Rozet F, Galiano M, Cathelineau X, Barret E, Cathala N, Vallancien G. Extraperitoneal laparoscopic radical prostatectomy: a prospective evaluation of 600 cases. J Urol. 2005;174:908-11.
33. Ruiz L, Salomon L, Hoznek A, Vordos D, Yiou R, de la Taille A, et al. Comparison of early oncologic results of laparoscopic radical prostatectomy by extraperitoneal versus transperitoneal approach. Eur Urol. 2004;46:50-6.
34. Semm K, Semm I. Safe insertion of trocars and the Veress needle using standard equipment and the 11 security steps. Gynaecol Endosc. 1999;8:339-47.
35. Stolzenburg JU, Do M, Rabenalt R, Pfeiffer H, Horn L, Truss MC, et al. Endoscopic extraperitoneal radical prostatectomy: initial experience after 70 procedures. J Urol. 2003;169:2066-71.
36. Tamme C, Scheidbach H, Hampe C, Schneider C, Köckerling F. Totally extraperitoneal endoscopic inguinal hernia repair (TEP). Surg Endosc. 2003;17:190-5.

CHAPTER 7

Principles of Laparoscopic Port Position

INTRODUCTION

The relative position of the instrument ports is very important in the performance of surgical procedures endoscopically. The angle the instruments make with the operative site and to each other should mimic as far as possible to the natural relationship of the hands and eyes during conventional surgery. It is proved that the most common cause of stressful minimal access surgery is wrong port position. The umbilicus commonly is selected as the site for primary trocar insertion because it offers the shortest distance between the skin and the anterior peritoneum and is cosmetically appealing.

There are different sites of primary optical port in laparoscopic surgery:

- Supraumbilical
- *Umbilical*:
  - Superior crease of umbilicus **(Fig. 1)**
  - Inferior crease of umbilicus **(Fig. 2)**
  - Transumbilical **(Fig. 3)**
- Infraumbilical **(Fig. 4)**
- Palmer's point **(Fig. 5)**.

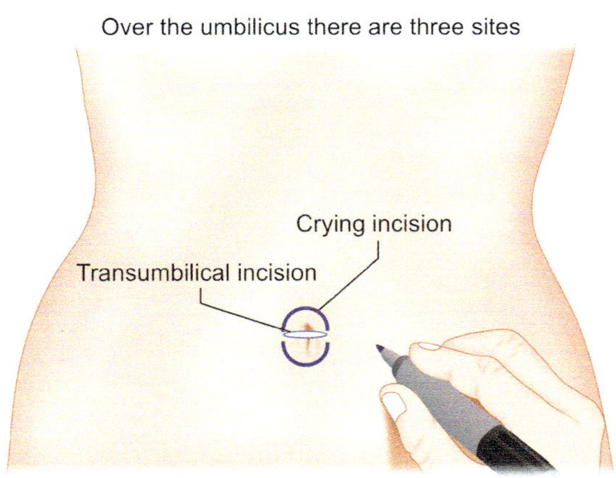

Fig. 1: Superior crease of umbilicus.

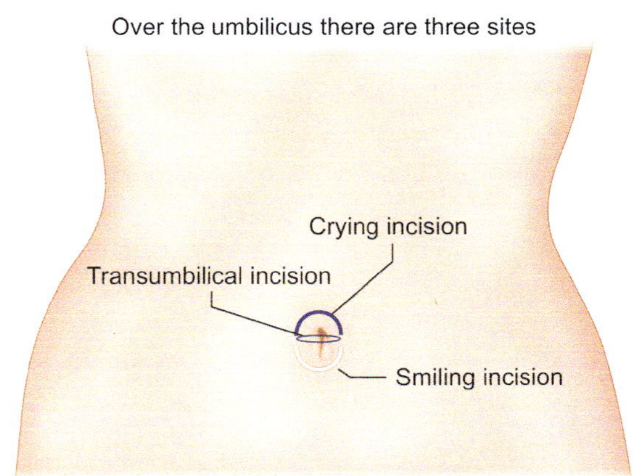

Fig. 2: Inferior crease of umbilicus.

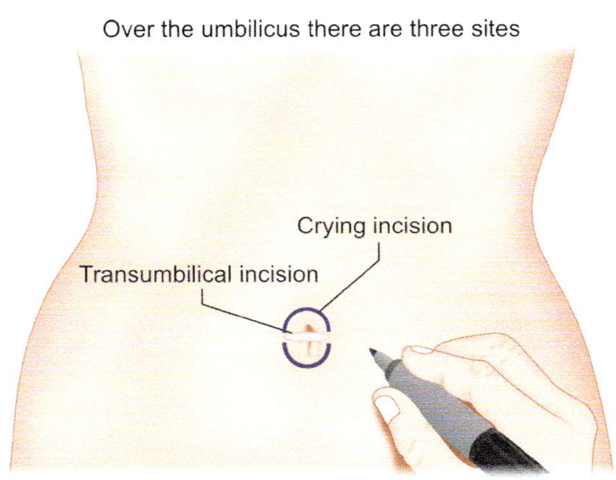

Fig. 3: Transumbilical port.

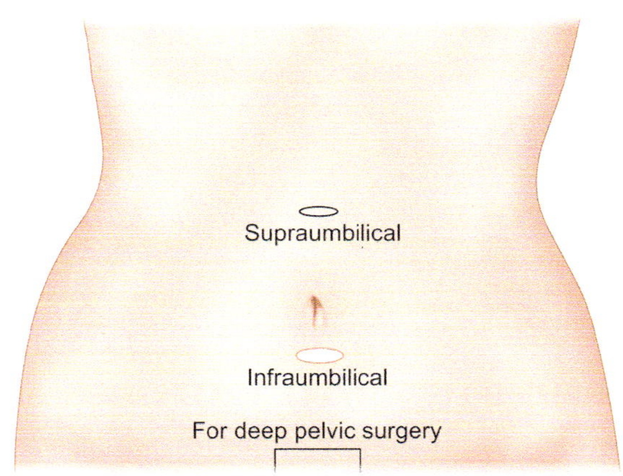

Fig. 4: Infraumbilical port.

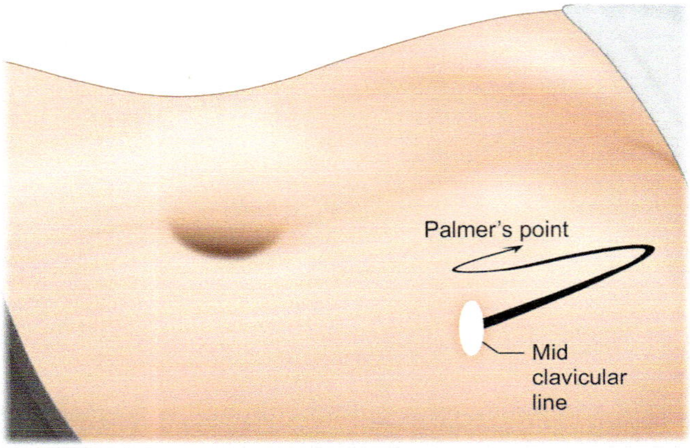

Fig. 5: Palmer's point.

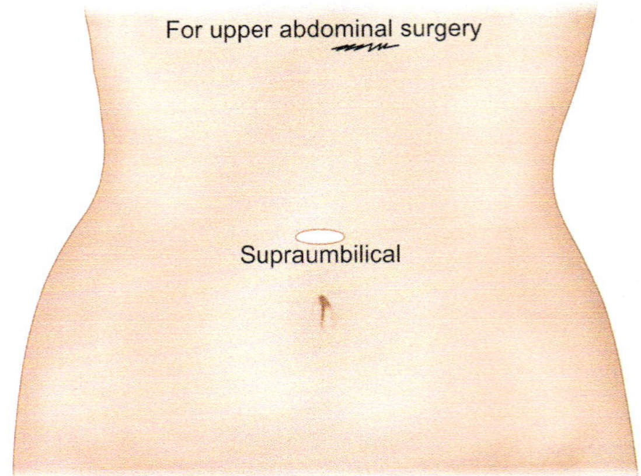

Fig. 6: Supraumbilical port.

SUPRAUMBILICAL PORT POSITION

Despite its common use and its relation to vital abdominal structures, there are often in gynecology when an umbilical port is not ergonomically optimum. Supraumbilical primary trocar is highly advantageous for upper abdominal surgery such as fundoplication, Heller myotomy, hiatus hernia, and most of the bariatric surgery **(Fig. 6)**. It is also an optimum port position for most of the gynecological surgery. Advances in laparoscopy have demonstrated that supraumbilical primary ports can be desirable in complex cases with large masses. It helps to increase the distance from enlarged pelvic pathology and thereby improve exposure and surgical efficiency. Supraumbilical port use has been reported in the literature to enable minimally invasive surgical management of large fibroid uteri at the time of myomectomy or hysterectomy and of large ovarian cyst. This port position is also useful in pregnant patients with gravid uterus. In these instances, creating distance between the primary trocar and the uterus is especially important to avoid any penetrating injury to the gravid uterus from trocar insertion. Supraumbilical port use is also reported in the literature by gynecologic oncologists for laparoscopic excision of large ovarian cancers. The supraumbilical primary port is also frequently used in robotic surgery when increased interport distances are desirable to eliminate robotic arm collisions. Reports in the literature describe the common locations of the supraumbilical port site that are 5 cm above the umbilicus and at least 6–10 cm above a second-trimester gravid uterus or very large uterus and ovarian cyst. In obese patient where umbilicus is displaced down, xiphisternum should be used to plan supraumbilical port. For upper abdominal surgery and most of the bariatric surgery, supraumbilical port incisions should be given 18 cm below the xiphisternum.

INFRAUMBILICAL PORT POSITION

This port position is less commonly used in laparoscopic surgery. Infraumbilical port is used 3–5 cm below the umbilicus. Infraumbilical port should not be confused with the port of inferior crease of umbilicus. This port position is used in following surgery:

- Single puncture sterilization
- For upper abdominal surgery (cholecystectomy or duodenal perforation) in very small height patient.

PRIMARY PORT POSITION

The central location and ability of the umbilicus to camouflage scars make it an attractive primary port site for laparoscopic surgery. There are many drawbacks with umbilicus as well. Umbilicus is a naturally weak area due to absence of all the layers. Weakness is also due to its location at the midpoint of the abdomen's greatest diameter.

It is easy to believe that there is a difference between the umbilicus and other trocar sites in both susceptibility to infection and postoperative incisional herniation.

The study showed that the increased infection rate at the umbilicus seems to be related to retrieval of infected organs through the umbilicus and not to the umbilicus itself. When umbilicus was used to retrieve gallbladder after cholecystectomy, the rate of infection was high due to port contamination with infected gallbladder. Excluding cholecystectomy, the umbilical infection rate was 2% similar to that of any alternative site. The postoperative ventral hernia rate was at 0.8%, the same at the umbilicus as elsewhere if the port >10 mm size is not repaired. It is now proved that the wound infection at the umbilicus is similar to that at other sites; postoperative ventral hernia at the umbilicus is similar to that at other sites and most of the infection after laparoscopic cholecystectomy is due to the contamination of wound due to infected gallbladder.

There are three sites over umbilicus for optical port:

1. Superior crease of umbilicus
2. Transumbilical
3. Inferior crease of umbilicus.

As it is discussed in previous chapter, inferior crease of umbilicus is most attractive site for primary entry due to presence of obliterated umbilical tube. Surgeon can access abdominal cavity through inferior crease of umbilicus by smiling incision. Detail steps of first entry are discussed in Chapter 6: Abdominal Access Techniques. In this chapter, we will discuss basic principle of secondary port position using baseball diamond concept.

CONTRALATERAL PORT POSITION IN LAPAROSCOPIC SURGERY

In contralateral port position, telescope is placed in between the two-working ports. In contralateral port position, manipulation angle (angle between two working instrument) should be 60° and azimuth angle (angle between telescope and one working instrument) is generally 30° either side.

SECONDARY PORT POSITION

The obligatory passage of the laparoscopic instruments through the abdominal wall generates a fixed point after which all movements are reversed. For instance, when the hand moves to the left, the end of the instruments moves right and when the hand moves downward, the end of the instrument moves upward. For some surgeon's, the fulcrum effect is not a problem, but for others it is an insurmountable obstacle to the performance of advanced laparoscopy.

Because the handling of laparoscopic instruments is through the fixed point at abdominal wall, the force feedback felt by the surgeon will depend on the length of the instrument inferior to this fixed point.

BASEBALL DIAMOND CONCEPT OF PORT POSITION

A satisfactory relationship includes **(Figs. 7A and B)**:

- An angle of 60° between the two instrument tips
- Tangential approach to the site
- Appropriate working distance.

First Decide the Target

Target may be in suprapubic region for laparoscopically-assisted vaginal hysterectomy (LAVH), right iliac fossa for appendicectomy, right upper quadrant for laparoscopic cholecystectomy, or left upper quadrant for fundoplication **(Fig. 8)**.

Draw the Line of Optimum Area

For optimum task performance, half to two-thirds instrument should be inside the abdomen. The size of adult laparoscopic instrument is 36 cm and pediatrics instrument is 28 cm **(Figs. 9 and 10)**.

Telescope and Instruments

- Telescope should be in the middle of working instrument **(Fig. 11)**
- Manipulation angle of instruments should be 60° **(Fig. 12)**.

Rule of Diamond for Laparoscopically-assisted Vaginal Hysterectomy

These factors combined with the specific anatomy will determine individual port sites. For standard operations such as cholecystectomy, standard port sites related to surface marking may suffice, but as more advanced or varied situations are tackled we recommend that you master the skill of individual port placement using the internal view. In general, the optic and the two main operating ports usually lie at the points of a flattened triangle, the optic being centrally and more distally placed. Try to keep ports at least 5 cm apart **(Figs. 13 and 14)**.

Manipulation angle 60° is essential for optimum task performance in laparoscopic surgery **(Figs. 12 and 15)**.

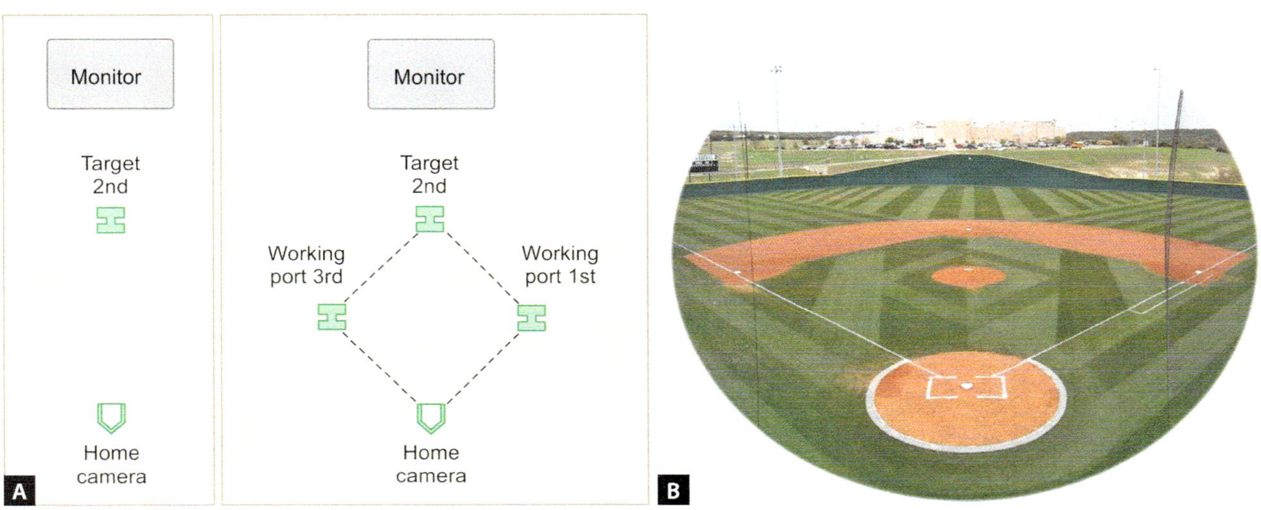

Figs. 7A and B: (A) Baseball diamond concept of port position; (B) Ports simulate field of a baseball.

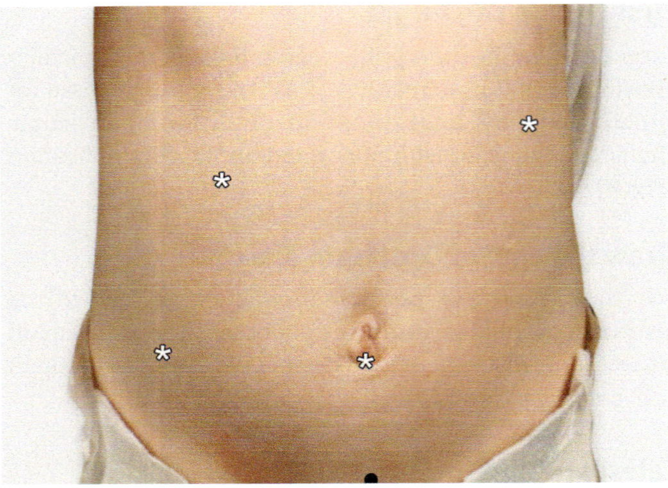

Fig. 8: First decide the target.

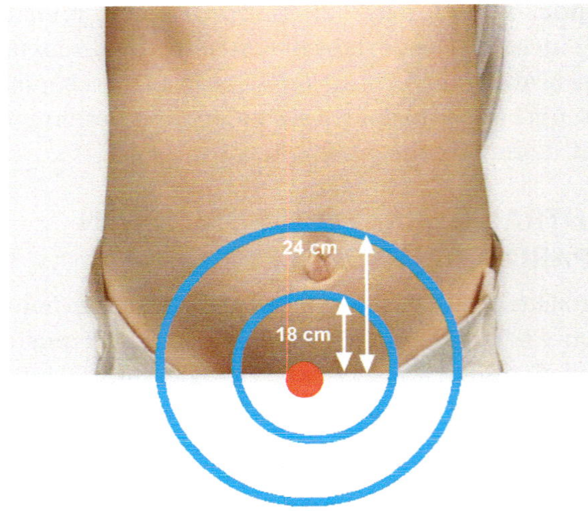

Fig. 9: Draw two arcs on the abdominal wall at 18 cm and 24 cm from that point and note area in between.

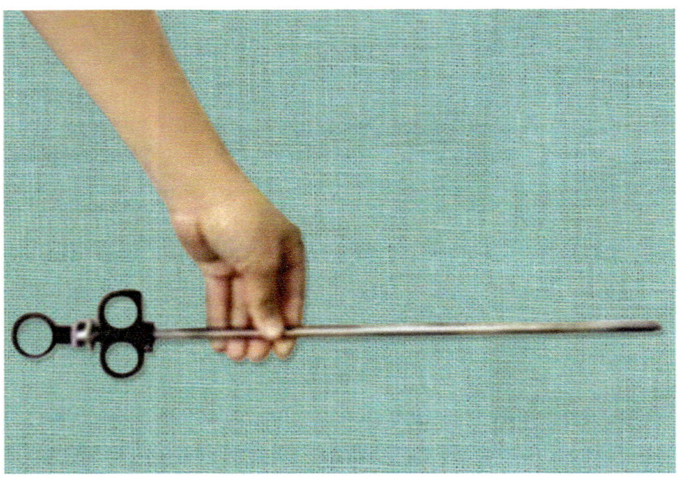

Fig. 10: Measure the length of instrument.

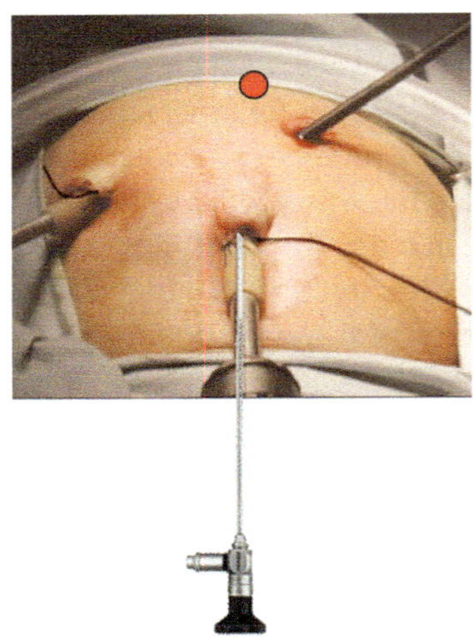

Fig. 11: Telescope should be in the center of working instrument.

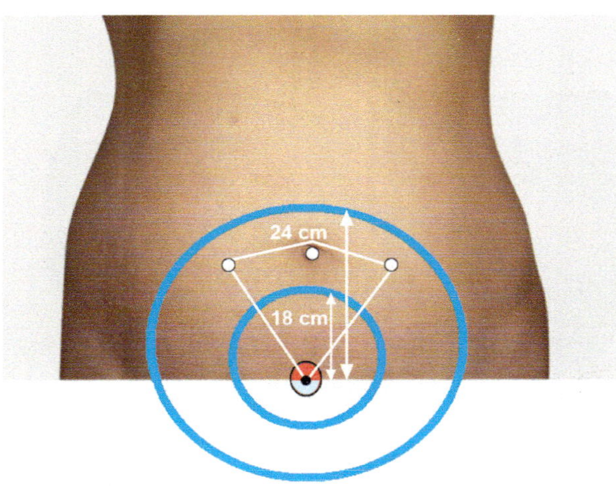

Fig. 12: Manipulation angle 60° is angle between tips of instrument.

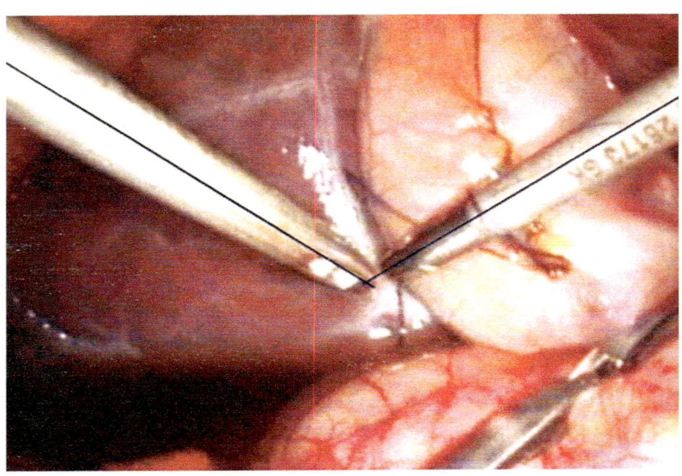

Fig. 13: 18 cm and 24 cm arc should be drawn.

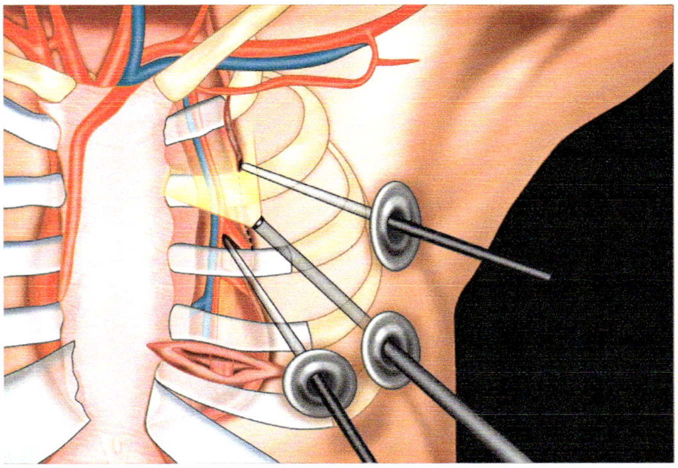

Fig. 14: Port position in thoracoscopic surgery.

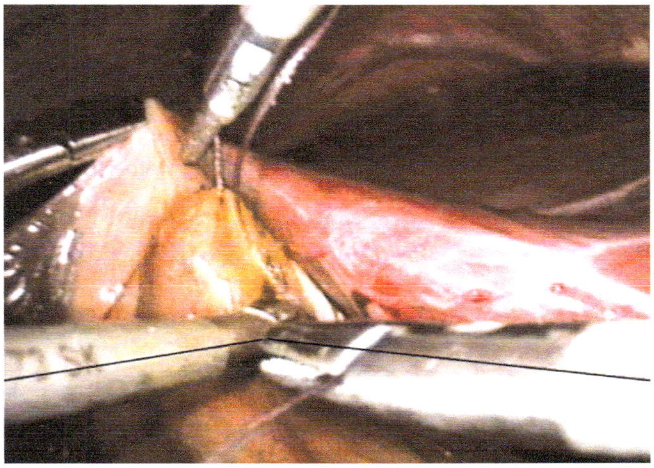

Fig. 15: Manipulation angle of 60° is ideal.

PORT POSITION IN VARIOUS SURGERIES

Port position in various surgeries is described in **Figures 16 to 29**.

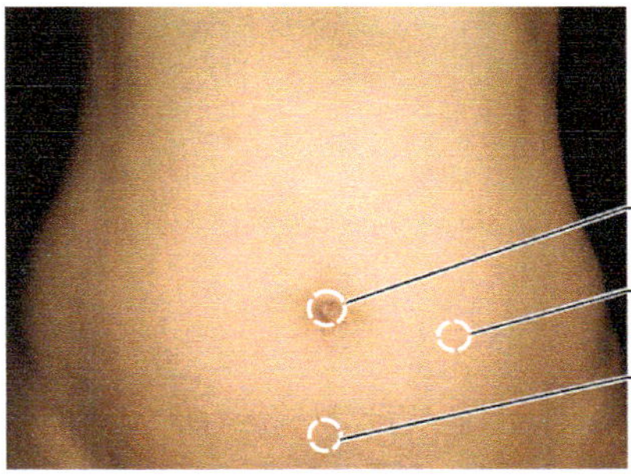

Fig. 16: Port position for diagnostic laparoscopy.

DRAWBACKS OF INCORRECT PORT POSITION

Swording

Swording occurs when the telescope or the shaft of the assistant's instrument obstruct the operator's instruments. If this occurs, you may need to consider:

- Repositioning retracting instruments
- Rotation of an angled telescope allowing alteration of the position of the end of the telescope
- Withdrawal of the telescope
- Transposition of the operator's instruments
- Additional port placement
- Changing the instruments to a different port.

IPSILATERAL PORT POSITION IN LAPAROSCOPIC SURGERY (FIG. 30)

In ipsilateral port position, telescope is placed on one side and two-working ports are placed on another side. In ipsilateral port position, manipulation angle (angle between two working instrument) should be 30° and azimuth angle (angle between telescope and one working instrument) is generally 30° for first working instrument and 60° for second working instrument. Main advantage of ipsilateral port position is that surgeon does not have any physical contact with camera holder. Another advantage of ipsilateral port position is that surgeon does not has to abduct his or her arm because manipulation angle is only 30°, so arm will be on the side of body without any abduction. Laparoscopic ipsilateral port position is particularly useful in gynecological laparoscopy **(Fig. 31)**. However, ipsilateral port position has little difficult port position for suturing and knotting. Due to ergonomic physical comfort and ability to move freely without touching the camera person, ipsilateral port position is very popular among female gynecologists.

Important points to be remember during placing the port in laparoscopic surgery:

- Laparoscopic instrument should behave like type I lever
- Telescope should be in the middle of working instrument approximately 24 cm from the target of dissection
- Manipulation angle should be 60° for contralateral and 30° for ipsilateral port position
- Elevation angle (angle between instrument and body of the patient) should be ideally 30°
- Distance between telescope and instrument should not be <5 cm
- Distance between two working instruments should not be >15 cm
- Azimuth angle should be minimum 15° and maximum 45°. Ideally, it should be 30° either side for contralateral port position and 30° and 60° on same side in ipsilateral port position
- Shadow of the telescope should be below the object, so light cable should be up as much as possible.

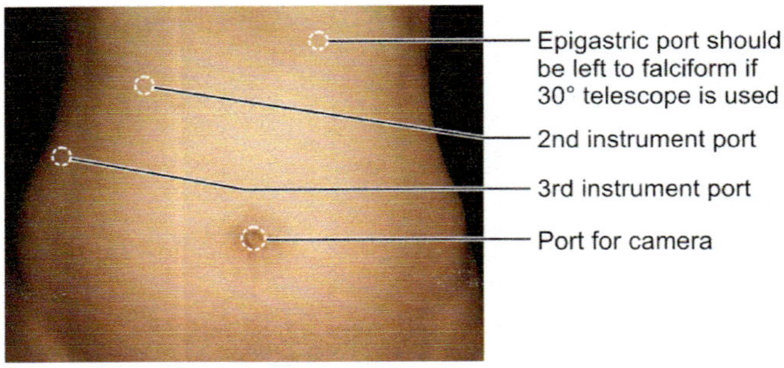

Fig. 17: Port position for cholecystectomy.

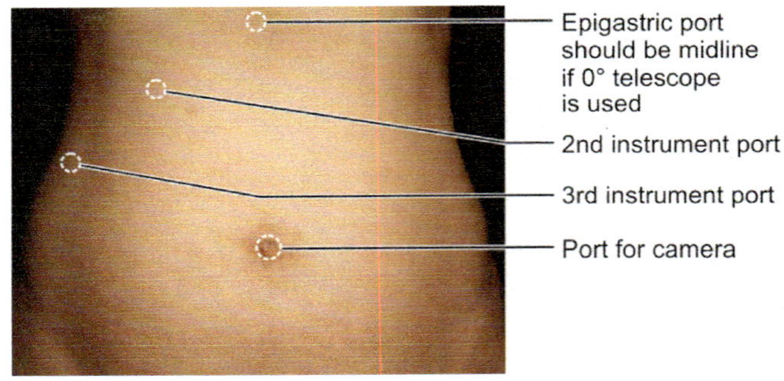

Fig. 18: Alternative port position for cholecystectomy.

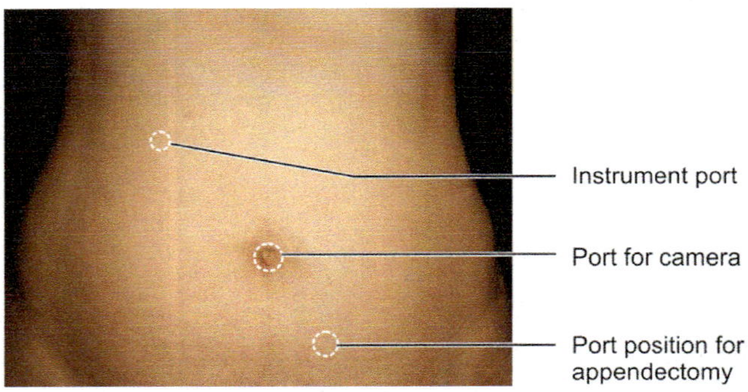

Fig. 19: Port position for appendectomy.

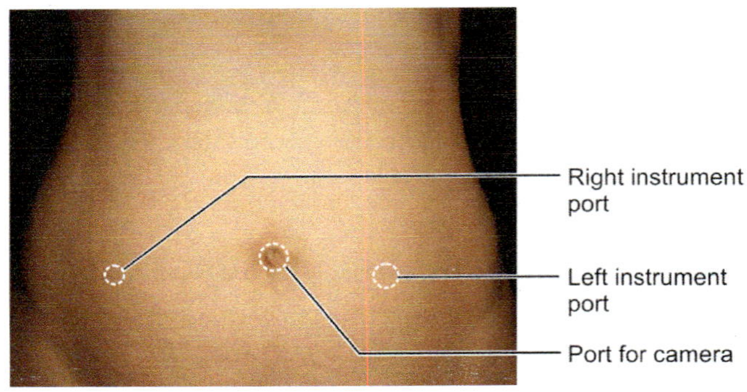

Fig. 20: Port position for bilateral hernia, laparoscopically-assisted vaginal hysterectomy (LAVH), and most of the gynecological procedures.

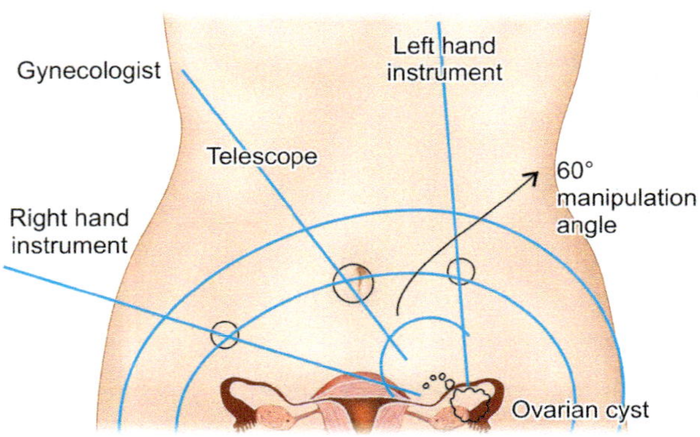

Fig. 21: Port position for left-sided laparoscopic ovarian cystectomy.

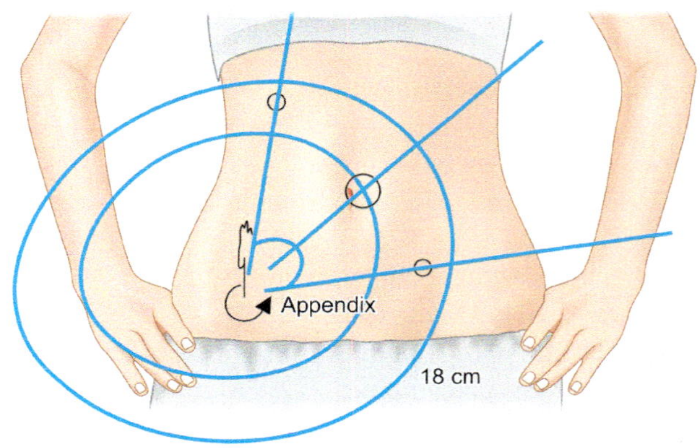

Fig. 22: Contralateral port position for laparoscopic appendectomy.

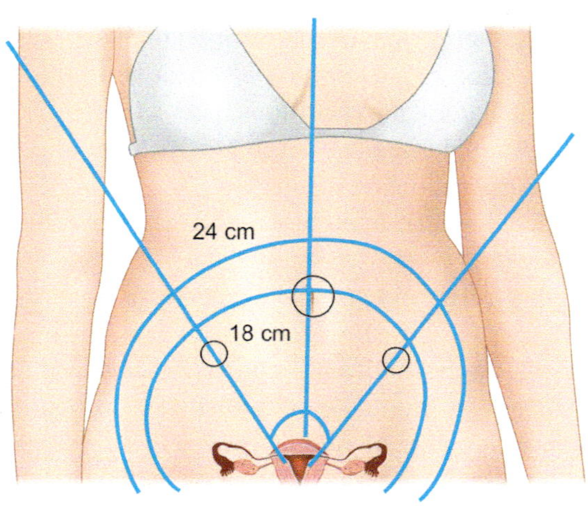

Fig. 23: Contralateral port position for small uterus laparoscopic hysterectomy.

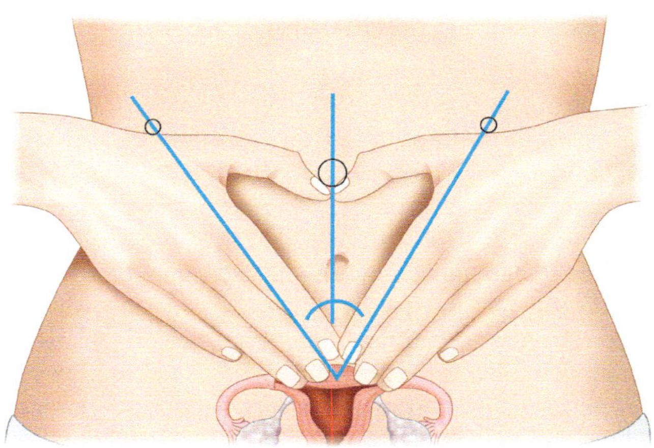

Fig. 24: Contralateral port position for large uterus laparoscopic hysterectomy.

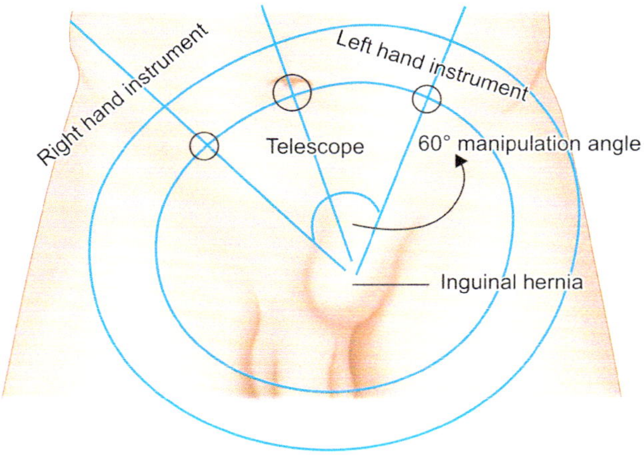

Fig. 25: Contralateral port position for left-sided laparoscopic inguinal hernia.

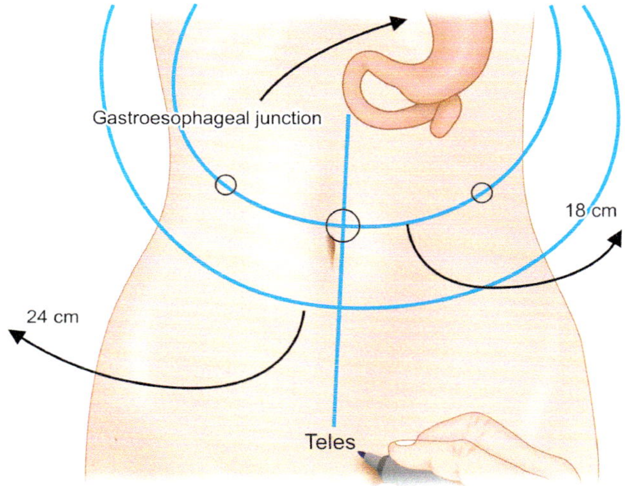

Fig. 26: Contralateral port position for laparoscopic fundoplication.

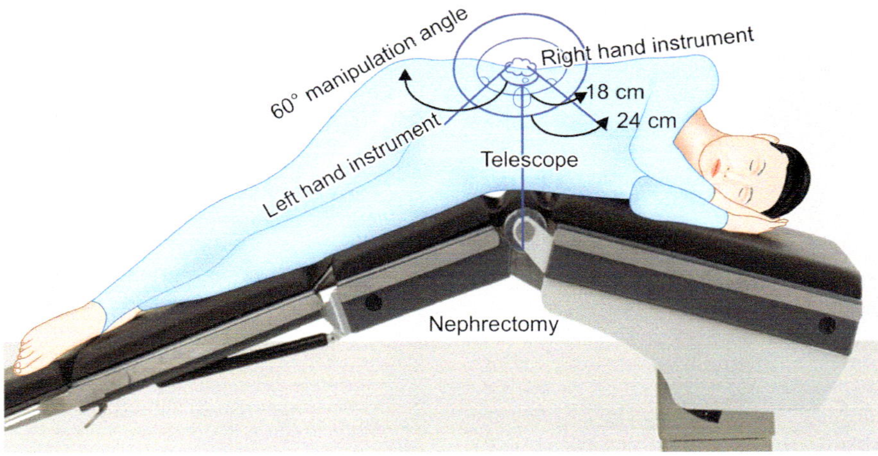

Fig. 27: Contralateral port position for laparoscopic nephrectomy.

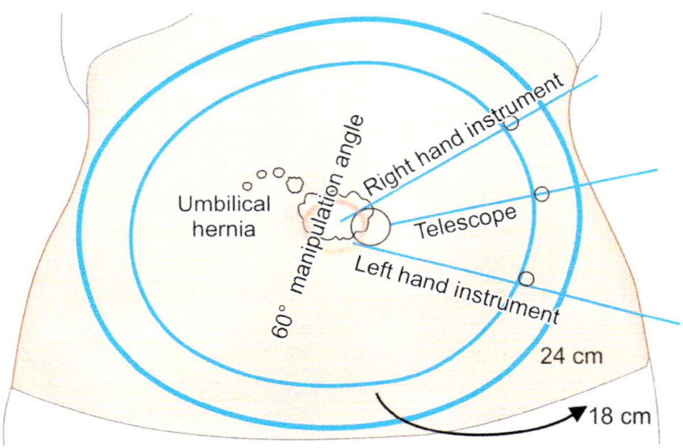

Fig. 28: Contralateral port position for laparoscopic umbilical hernia.

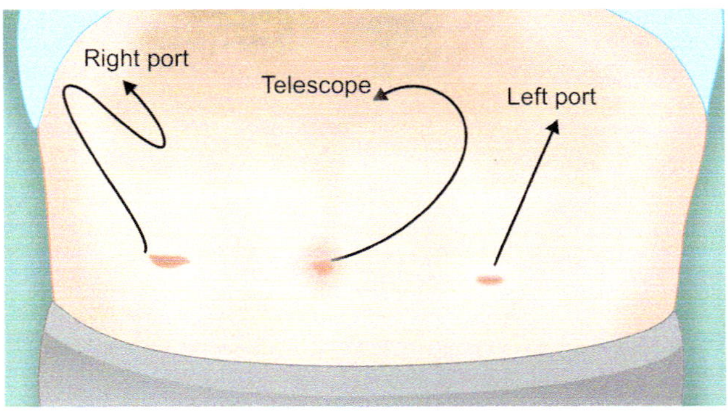

Fig. 29: Contralateral port position for laparoscopic bilateral inguinal hernia.

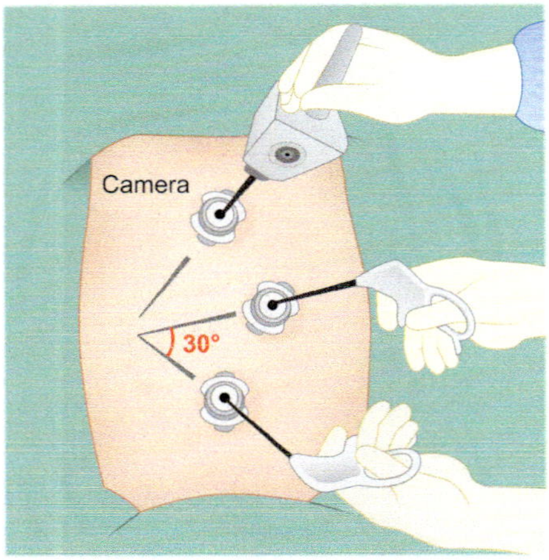

Fig. 30: Ipsilateral port position for laparoscopic appendectomy.

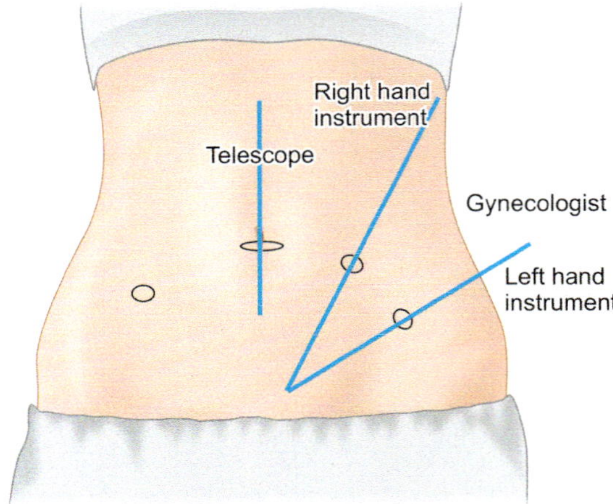

Fig. 31: Ipsilateral port position for laparoscopic gynecological surgery.

BIBLIOGRAPHY

1. Abu-Rafea B, Vilos GA, Vilos AG, Ahmad R, Hollett-Caines J, Al-Omran M. High-pressure laparoscopic entry does not adversely affect cardiopulmonary function in healthy women. J Minim Invasive Gynecol. 2005;12(6):475-9.
2. Abu-Rafea B, Vilos GA, Vilos AG, Hollett-Caines J, Al-Omran M. Effect of body habitus and parity on insufflated CO_2 volume at various intra-abdominal pressures during laparoscopic access in women. J Minim Invasive Gynecol. 2006;13(3):205-10.
3. Agresta F, De Simone P, Ciardo LF, Bedin N. Direct trocar insertion vs. Veress needle in nonobese patients undergoing laparoscopic procedures: a randomized prospective single-center study. Surg Endosc. 2004;18(12):1778-81.
4. Ahmad G, Duffy JMN, Watson AJS. Laparoscopic entry techniques and complications. Int J Gynecol Obstet. 2007; 99(1):52-5.
5. Angelini L, Lirici MM, Papaspyropoulos V, Sossi FL. Combination of subcutaneous abdominal wall retraction and optical trocar to minimize pneumoperitoneum-related effects and needle and trocar injuries in laparoscopic surgery. Surg Endosc. 1997;11(10):1006-9.
6. Baggish MS. Analysis of 31 cases of major-vessel injury associated with gynecologic laparoscopy operations. J Gynecol Surg. 2003;19(2):63-73.
7. Bateman BG, Kolp LA, Hoeger K. Complications of laparoscopy—operative and diagnostic. Fertil Steril. 1996; 66(1):30-5.
8. Bemelman WA, Dunker MS, Busch OR, Den Boer KT, de Wit LT, Gouma DJ. Efficacy of establishment of pneumoperitoneum with the Veress needle, Hasson trocar, and modified blunt trocar (TrocDoc): a randomized study. J Laparoendosc Adv Surg Tech A. 2000;10(6):325-30.
9. Bhoyrul S, Payne J, Steffes B, Swanstrom L, Way LW. A randomized prospective study of radially expanding trocars in laparoscopic surgery. J Gastrointest Surg. 2000;4(4):392-7.
10. Bhoyrul S, Vierra MA, Nezhat CR, Krummel TM, Way LW. Trocar injuries in laparoscopic surgery. J Am Coll Surg. 2001;192(6): 677-83.
11. Bishoff JT, Allaf ME, Kirkels W, Moore RG, Kavoussi LR, Schroder F. Laparoscopic bowel injury: incidence and clinical presentation. J Urol. 1999;161(3):887-90.
12. Bonjer HJ, Hazebroek EJ, Kazemier G, Giuffrida MC, Meijer WS, Lange JF. Open versus closed establishment of pneumoperitoneum in laparoscopic surgery. Br J Surg. 1997;84(5):599-602.
13. Briel JW, Plaisier PW, Meijer WS, Lange JF. Is it necessary to lift the abdominal wall when preparing a pneumoperitoneum? A randomized study. Surg Endosc. 2000;14(9):862-4.
14. Brosens I, Gordon A, Campo R, Gordts S. Bowel injury in gynecologic laparoscopy. J Am Assoc Gynecol Laparosc. 2003;10(1):9-13.
15. Byron JW, Markenson G, Miyazawa K. A randomized comparison of Veress needle and direct trocar insertion for laparoscopy. Surg Gynecol Obstet. 1993;177(3):259-62.
16. Catarci M, Carlini M, Gentileschi P, Santoro E. Major and minor injuries during the creation of pneumoperitoneum. A multicenter study on 12,919 cases. Surg Endosc. 2001; 15(6):566-9.
17. Champault G, Cazacu F. Laparoscopic surgery: injuries caused by trocars. (French Survey 1994) in reference to 103,852 interventions. J Chir (Paris). 1995;132(3):109-13.
18. Chandler JG, Corson SL, Way LW. Three spectra of laparoscopic entry access injuries. J Am Coll Surg. 2001;192(4):478-90.
19. Chapron C, Cravello L, Chopin N, Kreiker G, Blanc B, Dubuisson JB. Complications during set-up procedures for laparoscopy in gynecology: open laparoscopy does not reduce the risk of major complications. Acta Obstet Gynecol Scand. 2003;82(12):1125-9.
20. Chapron C, Fauconnier A, Goffinet F, Bréart G, Dubuisson JB. Laparoscopic surgery is not inherently dangerous for patients presenting with benign gynaecologic pathology. Results of a meta-analysis. Hum Reprod. 2002;17(5):1334-42.
21. Chapron C, Pierre F, Harchaoui Y, Lacroix S, Béguin S, Querleu D, et al. Gastrointestinal injuries during gynaecological laparoscopy. Hum Reprod. 1999;14(2):333-7.
22. Chapron C, Pierre F, Querleu D, Dubuisson JB. Major vascular complications from gynecologic laparoscopy. Gynecol Obstet Fertil. 2000;28(12):880-7.
23. Chapron C, Pierre F, Querleu D, Dubuisson JB. Complications of gynaecological laparoscopy. Gynecol Obstet Fertil. 2001;29(9):605-12.
24. Chapron C, Querleu D, Bruhat MA, Madelenat P, Fernandez H, Pierre F, et al. Surgical complications of diagnostic and operative gynaecological laparoscopy: a series of 29,966 cases. Hum Reprod. 1998;13(4):867-72.
25. Chapron C, Querleu D, Mage G, Madelenat P, Dubuisson JB, Audebert A, et al. Complications of gynecologic laparoscopy. Multicentric study of 7,604 laparoscopies. J Gynecol Obstet Biol Reprod (Paris). 1992;21(2):207-13.
26. Chapron CM, Pierre F, Lacroix S, Querleu D, Lansac J, Dubuisson JB. Major vascular injuries during gynecologic laparoscopy. J Am Coll Surg. 1997;185(5):461-5.
27. Chin K, Newton J. Survey of training in minimal access surgery in the West Midlands region of the UK. Gynaecol Endosc. 1996;5(6):329-3.

28. Corson SL, Chandler JG, Way LW. Survey of laparoscopic entry injuries provoking litigation. J Am Assoc Gynecol Laparosc. 2001;8(3):341-7.
29. Cravello L, Banet J, Agostini A, Bretelle F, Roger V, Blanc B. Open laparoscopy: analysis of complications due to first trocar insertion. Gynecol Obstet Fertil. 2002;30(4):286-90.
30. de Azevedo OC, Azevedo JL, Sorbello AA, Miguel GP, Wilson JL, de Godoy AC. Evaluation of tests performed to confirm the position of the Veress needle for creation of pneumoperitoneum in selected patients: a prospective clinical trial. Acta Cir Bras. 2006;21(6):385-91.
31. Driscoll V. Case in focus: Bowel injury during laparoscopic sterilization—Vanessa Palmer v Cardiff & Vale NHS Trust. AvMA Med Legal J. 2004;10(3):109-11.
32. El-Banna M, Abdel-Atty M, El-Meteini M, Aly S. Management of laparoscopic-related bowel injuries. Surg Endosc. 2000;14(9):779-82.
33. Ellis H. Medicolegal consequences of postoperative intra-abdominal adhesions. J R Soc Med. 2001;94(7):331-2.
34. Epstein J, Arora A, Ellis H. Surface anatomy of the inferior epigastric artery in relation to laparoscopic injury. Clin Anat. 2004;17(5):400-8.
35. Ferriman A. Laparoscopic surgery: two-thirds of injuries initially missed. West J Med. 2000;173(6):372.
36. Fuller J, Ashar BS, Carey-Corrado J. Trocar-associated injuries and fatalities: an analysis of 1399 reports to the FDA. J Minim Invasive Gynecol. 2005;12(4):302-7.
37. Galen DI, Jacobson A, Weckstein LN, Kaplan RA, DeNevi KL. Reduction of cannula-related laparoscopic complications using a radially expanding access device. J Am Assoc Gynecol Laparosc. 1999;6(1):79-84.
38. Garry R. A consensus document concerning laparoscopic entry techniques: Middlesbrough, March 19-20 1999. Gynaecol Endosc. 1999;4(8):403-6.
39. Geers J, Holden C. Major vascular injury as a complication of laparoscopic surgery: a report of three cases and review of the literature. Am Surg. 1996;62(5):377-9.
40. Gett RM, Joseph MG. A safe technique for the insertion of the Hasson cannula. Aust N Z J Surg. 2004;74(9):797-8.
41. Gordts S, Watrelot A, Campo R, Brosens I. Risk and outcome of bowel injury during transvaginal pelvic endoscopy. Fertil Steril. 2001;76(6):1238-41.
42. Gunenc MZ, Yesildaglar N, Bingol B, Onalan G, Tabak S, Gokmen B. The safety and efficacy of direct trocar insertion with elevation of the rectus sheath instead of the skin for pneumoperitoneum. Surg Laparosc Endosc Percutan Tech. 2005;15(2):80-1.
43. Hanney RM, Alle KM, Cregan PC. Major vascular injury and laparoscopy. Aust N Z J Surg. 1995;65(7):533-5.
44. Harkki-Siren P, Kurki T. A nationwide analysis of laparoscopic complications. Obstet Gynecol. 1997;89(1):108-12.
45. Harkki-Siren P, Sjoberg J, Kurki T. Major complications of laparoscopy: a follow-up Finnish study. Obstet Gynecol. 1999;94(1):94-8.
46. Hart R, Doherty DA, Karthigasu K, Garry R. The value of virtual reality-simulator training in the development of laparoscopic surgical skills. J Minim Invasive Gynecol. 2006;13(2):126-33.
47. Hasson HM. Open laparoscopy as a method of access in laparoscopic surgery. Gynaecol Endosc. 1999;8(6):353-62.
48. Hasson HM, Rotman C, Rana N, Kumari NA. Open laparoscopy: 29-year experience. Obstet Gynecol. 2000;96(5 Pt 1):763-6.
49. Hender K. What is the Safety of Open (Hasson) Technique versus Closed (Blind Veress Needle) Technique for Laparoscopy? Centre for Clinical Effectiveness—Evidence Report. Clayton, Victoria: Centre for Clinical Effectiveness; 2001.
50. Hill DJ, Maher PJ. Direct cannula entry for laparoscopy. J Am Assoc Gynecol Laparosc. 1996;4(1):77-9.
51. Hurd WW, Amesse LS, Gruber JS, Horowitz GM, Cha GM, Hurteau JA. Visualization of the epigastric vessels and bladder before laparoscopic trocar placement. Fertil Steril. 2003;80(1):209-12.
52. Hurd WW, Bude RO, DeLancey JO, Newman JS. The location of abdominal wall blood vessels in relationship to abdominal landmarks apparent at laparoscopy. Am J Obstet Gynecol. 1994;171(3):642-6.
53. Jacobson MT, Osias J, Bizhang R, Tsang M, Lata S, Helmy M, et al. The direct trocar technique: an alternative approach to abdominal entry for laparoscopy. JSLS. 2002;6(2):169-74.
54. Jansen FW, Kapiteyn K, Trimbos-Kemper T, Hermans J, Trimbos JB. Complications of laparoscopy: a prospective multicentre observational study. Br J Obstet Gynaecol. 1997;104(5):595-600.
55. Jansen FW, Kolkman W, Bakkum EA, de Kroon CD, Trimbos-Kemper TC, Trimbos JB. Complications of laparoscopy: an inquiry about closed-versus open-entry technique. Am J Obstet Gynecol. 2004;190(3):634-8.
56. Jansen FW, Wind J, Cremeres JEL, Bemelman WA. 146: Entry-related Complications in Laparoscopy and Their Medical Liability Insurance. J Minim Invasive Gynecol. 2007; 14(6 Suppl):S54-5.
57. Kaali SG, Barad DH. Incidence of bowel injury due to dense adhesions at the sight of direct trocar insertion. J Reprod Med. 1992;37(7):617-8.
58. Kaloo P, Cooper M, Molloy D. A survey of entry techniques and complications of members of the Australian Gynaecological Endoscopy Society. Aust N Z J Obstet Gynaecol. 2002; 42(3):264-6.
59. Kaloo P, Cooper M, Reid G. A prospective multicentre study of laparoscopic complications related to the direct-entry technique. Gynaecol Endosc. 2002;11(2):67-70.
60. Kolkman W, Wolterbeek R, Jansen FW. Gynecological laparoscopy in residency training program: Dutch perspectives. Surg Endosc. 2005;19(11):1498-502.
61. Lalchandani S, Philips K. Laparoscopic entry technique—a survey of practices of consultant gynaecologists. Gynecol Surg. 2005;2(4):245-9.
62. Larobina M, Nottle P. Complete evidence regarding major vascular injuries during laparoscopic access. Surg Laparosc Endosc Percutan Tech. 2005;15(3):119-23.
63. Leng J, Lang J, Huang R, Liu Z, Sun D. Complications in laparoscopic gynecologic surgery. Chin Med Sci J. 2000;15(4):222-6.
64. Leonard F, Lecuru F, Rizk E, Chasset S, Robin F, Taurelle R. Perioperative morbidity of gynecological laparoscopy. A prospective monocenter observational study. Acta Obstet Gynecol Scand. 2000;79(2):129-34.
65. Lingam K, Cole RA. Laparoscopic entry port visited: a survey of practices of consultant gynaecologists in Scotland. Gynaecol Endosc. 2001;10(5):335-42.
66. Mac CC, Lecuru F, Rizk E, Robin F, Boucaya V, Taurelle R. Morbidity in laparoscopic gynecological surgery: results of a prospective single-center study. Surg Endosc. 1999;13(1):57-61.
67. Marret H, Golfier F, Cassignol A, Raudrant D. Methods for laparoscopy: open laparoscopy or closed laparoscopy? Attitude of the French Central University Hospital. Gynecol Obstet Fertil. 2001;29(10):673-9.
68. Marret H, Harchaoui Y, Chapron C, Lansac J, Pierre F. Trocar injuries during laparoscopic gynaecological surgery. Report from the French Society of Gynaecological Laparoscopy. Gynaecol Endosc. 1998;7(5):235-41.
69. Mayol J, Garcia-Aguilar J, Ortiz-Oshiro E, Diego Carmona JA, Fernandez-Represa JA. Risks of the minimal access approach for laparoscopic surgery: multivariate analysis of morbidity related to umbilical trocar insertion. World J Surg. 1997;21(5):529-33.
70. McKernan JB, Champion JK. Access techniques: Veress needle—initial blind trocar insertion versus open laparoscopy with the Hasson trocar. Endosc Surg Allied Technol. 1995;3(1):35-8.

71. Merlin TL, Hiller JE, Maddern GJ, Jamieson GG, Brown AR, Kolbe A. Systematic review of the safety and effectiveness of methods used to establish pneumoperitoneum in laparoscopic surgery. Br J Surg. 2003;90(6):668-79.
72. Merlin T, Jamieson G, Brown A, Maddern G, Hiller J, Kolbe A. A Systematic Review of the Methods Used to Establish Laparoscopic Pneumoperitoneum. New York: Centre for Reviews and Dissemination; 2001.
73. Moberg AC, Montgomery A. Primary access-related complications with laparoscopy: comparison of blind and open techniques. Surg Endosc. 2005;19(9):1196-9.
74. Molloy D, Kaloo PD, Cooper M, Nguyen TV. Laparoscopic entry: a literature review and analysis of techniques and complications of primary port entry. Aust N Z J Obstet Gynaecol. 2002;42(3):246-54.
75. Munro MG. Laparoscopic access: complications, technologies, and techniques. Curr Opin Obstet Gynecol. 2002;14(4):365-74.
76. Narendran M, Baggish MS. Mean distance between primary trocar insertion site and major retroperitoneal vessels during routine laparoscopy. J Gynecol Surg. 2002;18(4):121-7.
77. Nezhat C, Childers J, Nezhat F, Nezhat CH, Seidman DS. Major retroperitoneal vascular injury during laparoscopic surgery. Hum Reprod. 1997;12(3):480-3.
78. Nezhat CH, Nezhat F, Brill AI, Nezhat C. Normal variations of abdominal and pelvic anatomy evaluated at laparoscopy. Obstet Gynecol. 1999;94(2):238-42.
79. Nezhat FR, Silfen SL, Evans D, Nezhat C. Comparison of direct insertion of disposable and standard reusable laparoscopic trocars and previous pneumoperitoneum with Veress needle. Obstet Gynecol. 1991;78(1):148-50.
80. Nordestgaard AG, Bodily KC, Osborne RW, Buttorff JD. Major vascular injuries during laparoscopic procedures. Am J Surg. 1995;169(5):543-5.
81. Pasic RP, Kantardzic M, Templeman C, Levine RL. Insufflation techniques in gynecologic laparoscopy. Surg Laparosc Endosc Percutan Tech. 2006;16(1):18-23.
82. Philips PA, Amaral JF. Abdominal access complications in laparoscopic surgery. J Am Coll Surg. 2001;192(4):525-36.
83. Rahman MM, Mamun AA. Direct trocar insertion: alternative abdominal entry technique for laparoscopic surgery. Mymensingh Med J. 2003;12(1):45-7.
84. Reich H, Rasmussen C, Vidali A. Peritoneal hyperdistention for trocar insertion. Gynaecol Endosc. 1999;8(6):375-7.
85. Reich H, Ribeiro SC, Rasmussen C, Rosenberg J, Vidali A. High-pressure trocar insertion technique. JSLS. 1999;3(1):45-8.
86. Rein H. Complications and litigation in gynecologic endoscopy. Curr Opin Obstet Gynecol. 2001;13(4):425-9.
87. Rosen DM, Lam AM, Chapman M, Carlton M, Cario GM. Methods of creating pneumoperitoneum: a review of techniques and complications. Obstet Gynecol Surv. 1998;53(3):167-74.
88. Roviaro GC, Varoli F, Saguatti L, Vergani C, Maciocco M, Scarduelli A. Major vascular injuries in laparoscopic surgery. Surg Endosc. 2002;16(8):1192-6.
89. Roy GM, Bazzurini L, Solima E, Luciano AA. Safe technique for laparoscopic entry into the abdominal cavity. J Am Assoc Gynecol Laparosc. 2001;8(4):519-28.
90. Royal Australian and New Zealand College of Obstetricians and Gynaecologists (RANZCOG) (2006). Use of the Veress needle to obtain pneumoperitoneum prior to laparoscopy. Consensus statement of the Royal Australian and New Zealand College of Obstetricians and Gynaecologists (RANZCOG) and the Australian Gynaecological Endoscopy and Surgery Society (AGES). [online] Available from https://ranzcog.edu.au/RANZCOG_SITE/media/RANZCOG-MEDIA/Women%27s%20Health/Statement%20and%20guidelines/Clinical%20-%20Gynaecology/Use-of-the-Veress-Needle-(C-Gyn-7)-review-July-2017.pdf?ext=.pdf [Last accessed June, 2020].
91. Saber AA, Meslemani AM, Davis R, Pimentel R. Safety zones for anterior abdominal wall entry during laparoscopy: a CT scan mapping of epigastric vessels. Ann Surg. 2004;239(2):182-5.
92. Saville LE, Woods MS. Laparoscopy and major retroperitoneal vascular injuries (MRVI). Surg Endosc. 1995;9(10):1096-100.
93. Schafer M, Lauper M, Krahenbuhl L. Trocar and Veress needle injuries during laparoscopy. Surg Endosc. 2001;15(3):275-80.
94. Schrenk P, Woisetschlager R, Rieger R, Wayand W. Mechanism, management, and prevention of laparoscopic bowel injuries. Gastrointest Endosc. 1996;43(6):572-4.
95. Soderstrom RM. Bowel injury litigation after laparoscopy. J Am Assoc Gynecol Laparosc. 1993;1(1):74-7.
96. Soderstrom RM. Injuries to major blood vessels during endoscopy. J Am Assoc Gynecol Laparosc. 1997;4(3): 395-8.
97. Sokol AI, Chuang K, Milad MP. Risk factors for conversion to laparotomy during gynecologic laparoscopy. J Am Assoc Gynecol Laparosc. 2003;10(4):469-73.
98. Sriprasad S, Yu DF, Muir GH, Poulsen J, Sidhu PS. Positional anatomy of vessels that may be damaged at laparoscopy: new access criteria based on CT and ultrasonography to avoid vascular injury. J Endourol. 2006;20(7):498-503.
99. Sutton CJ. Medico-legal implications of keyhole surgery. Med Leg J. 1996;64(Pt 3):101-13.
100. Sutton CJG, Philips K. Preventing Gynaecological Laparoscopic Injury. Guideline No. 48. Surg Endosc. 2007;21(8):2094-9.
101. Teoh B, Sen R, Abbott J. An evaluation of four tests used to ascertain Veress needle placement at closed laparoscopy. J Minim Invasive Gynecol. 2005;12(2):153-8.
102. Ternamian AM. Laparoscopy without trocars. Surg Endosc. 1997;11(8):815-8.
103. Ternamian AM, Deitel M. Endoscopic threaded imaging port (EndoTIP) for laparoscopy: experience with different body weights. Obes Surg. 1999;9(1):44-7.
104. Tsaltas J, Pearce S, Lawrence A, Meads A, Mezzatesta J, Nicolson S. Safer laparoscopic trocar entry: It's all about pressure. Aust N Z J Obstet Gynaecol. 2004;44(4):349-50.
105. Vilos AG, Vilos GA, Abu-Rafea B, Hollett-Caines J, Al-Omran M. Effect of body habitus and parity on the initial Veress intraperitoneal CO_2 insufflation pressure during laparoscopic access in women. J Minim Invasive Gynecol. 2006;13(2):108-13.
106. Vilos GA. Litigation of laparoscopic major vessel injuries in Canada. J Am Assoc Gynecol Laparosc. 2000;7(4):503-9.
107. Vilos GA. Laparoscopic bowel injuries: forty litigated gynaecological cases in Canada. J Obstet Gynaecol Can. 2002;24(3):224-30.
108. Vilos GA, Ternamian A, Dempster J, Laberge PY. Laparoscopic entry: a review of techniques, technologies, and complications. Society of Obstetricians and Gynaecologists of Canada Clinical Practice Guideline. J Obstet Gynaecol Can. 2007;29(5):433-47.
109. Wang PH, Lee WL, Yuan CC, Chao HT, Liu WM, Yu KJ, et al. Major complications of operative and diagnostic laparoscopy for gynecologic disease. J Am Assoc Gynecol Laparosc. 2001; 8(1):68-73.
110. Wind J, Cremers JE, Berge Henegouwen MI, Gouma DJ, Jansen FW, Bemelman WA. Medical liability insurance claims on entry-related complications in laparoscopy. Surg Endosc. 2007;21(11):2094-9.
111. Woolcot R. The efficacy and safety of different techniques for trocar insertion in laparoscopic surgery. Minim Invasive Ther Allied Technol. 2001;10(1):11-4.
112. Yim SF, Yuen PM. Randomized double-masked comparison of radially expanding access device and conventional cutting tip trocar in laparoscopy. Obstet Gynecol. 2001;97(3):435-8.

CHAPTER 8

Laparoscopic Dissection Techniques

INTRODUCTION

Dissection is defined as the separation of tissues with hemostasis. It consists of a sensory visual and tactile component, an access component involving tissue manipulation, and instrument maneuverability. These are combined to achieve exposure, i.e., developing a suitable space for seeing and handling target structures.

Precision and meticulous hemostasis is essential requirement in minimal access surgery (MAS). Endoscopic dissection, in contrast to dissection in conventional surgery, possesses several limitations. Three-dimensional direct visions are replaced by two-dimensional indirect visions in laparoscopic surgery. Illumination and the video image quality are still limited despite recent advances in video systems such as digitization and three-chip endocamera. Movement of the functional tip of laparoscopic instruments is restricted along with the kinematics response. The loss of tactile sensation in endoscopic surgery is yet another limiting factor.

Endoscopic dissection and manipulation of tissue within a confined space require a two-handed approach, assisting and dissecting both task are performed by surgeon himself. A passive assisting instrument (usually a grasper) provides countertraction and exposure for the active dissecting instrument. The active instrument may be nonenergized (e.g., scissors and scalpel) or energized with electricity (diathermy), ultrasound, or light energy.

TYPES OF LAPAROSCOPIC DISSECTION

A variety of mechanisms have been used to divide tissue and enable hemostasis. They all involve some form of physical energy being applied to the appropriate tissue. The amount of energy required for dissection depends on the type and constituency of the tissue. The properties of tissues may vary in different directions and for different disease states. This in totality influences the choice of the modality for dissection.

The ideal dissection technique requires a modality that can accomplish meticulous hemostasis and will be tissue selective without causing inadvertent tissue damage. It must be safe for both patient and surgical team when in regular use and when inactive in storage. In this respect, built-in safety measures are mandatory. An ideal dissecting modality should be efficient in both power delivery and in space requirement. The modality must be cost-effective also. The initial expenditure needed to acquire and setup the necessary equipment must be taken into account along with subsequent operational and maintenance costs.

In reality, there is no single "ideal" dissecting modality for entire minimal access surgical procedures. In actual practice, a combination of energy forms is applied with selection of the most appropriate one at each particular phase or type of the operation.

The available modalities for dissection in MAS include:

- Blunt dissection
- Sharp scalpel and scissors dissection
- High-frequency radiowave electrosurgery
- Radiofrequency ablation
- Ultrasonic dissection
- High-velocity and high-pressure water-jet dissection
- Laser surgery

Blunt Dissection

Instrument Used

- Closed scissors tips used as blunt dissector
- Scissor points used to separate by spreading the jaw
- Grasper—straight and curved
- Inactive suction cannula
- Heel of inactive electrosurgery (hook or spatula)
- Pledget

Methods

- Distraction
- Separation
- Teasing
- Wiping

Pledget Dissection

Endoscopic pledget dissection was first introduced in the University of Dundee in 1987. A special endoscopic pledget or peanut swab 5.0 mm ratcheted holder, manufactured by Storz (with strong jaws and inward facing tongs at the end of the jaws for security), is used in a manner similar to that employed in open surgery. The holder grasping, the pledget, is introduced inside a reducer tube through an 11.0-mm cannula. The blunt dissection is safe and is used to open planes and expose structures especially when the anatomy is obscured by adhesions. The movement consists of forward and backward wipes accompanied by clockwise/counterclockwise rotation of the pledget swab. It is also useful for controlled small bleeder by compressions before this is secured by clipping or electrocoagulation. The pledget swab is particularly useful for blunt dissection in Calot's triangle during cholecystectomy. It is economical, simple to use, and maintains a dry operative field while performing dissection. This type of dissecting modality is also utilized in hemostatically separating gallbladder from its bed, bladder from the uterus, or the rectum from the sacral attachment **(Fig. 1)**.

Removal of pledget must be carried out under vision to ensure that the swab is inside the reducer tube before withdrawal of the instrument, otherwise there is a real risk of losing the small pledget swab in the peritoneal cavity.

The pledget is an invaluable tool for the rapid dissection of loose areolar planes when it is wiped or pushed against the line of cleavage to separate the tissues.

Pledget is useful in maneuvers to control minor hemorrhage. The pledget can be placed over the bleeding point to apply pressure. When used on an oozing operative field, it adsorbs some of the blood and may clarify the anatomical position.

It is important to follow routine practice to minimize loss of the peanut swab inside the abdomen:

- Always use a reducer tube to insert and remove the swab.
- Employ a safe system (ratchet and elastic band) to maintain the grip of instrument used for insertion.
- Keep the pledget in view from insertion to retraction into the introducer tube. Be sure it is retrieved into the introducer, not the cannular end.

Tissue Stripping and Tissue Distraction

These are other safe and effective forms of blunt dissection. The latter is applied for seromyotomy. Insignificant hemostatic capability is the main disadvantage of blunt dissection **(Fig. 2)**.

Sharp Dissection

Sharp scalpel is used mainly for division by cutting. Although inexpensive, its use is restricted in laparoscopic surgery. The lack of hemostasis, the potential of injury from the tip when inserting through the port, and the kinematics problems restrict its use to common bile duct division.

Scissors Dissection

It is one of the most frequent methods in laparoscopic surgery. It offers the benefits of being cheap, safe, and precise operator determined action. However, being nonhemostasis renders it far from ideal as a dissecting modality **(Fig. 3)**.

Electrosurgical Dissection

Electrosurgery is the most convenient way of dissection in MAS combined with most risky method of dissection. Most of the complication in laparoscopic surgery is due to use of energized instrument (1%) **(Fig. 4)**.

Before understanding the principle of electrosurgery, following definitions should be known:

- *Current*: Flow of electrons
- *Circuit*: Pathway for flow of electrons
- *Voltage*: Force that causes electron to flow
- *Resistance*: Obstacle to the flow of electron.

There are two basic principles of electricity:

1. Electrical current ultimately flows to ground
2. It always follows the path of least resistance.

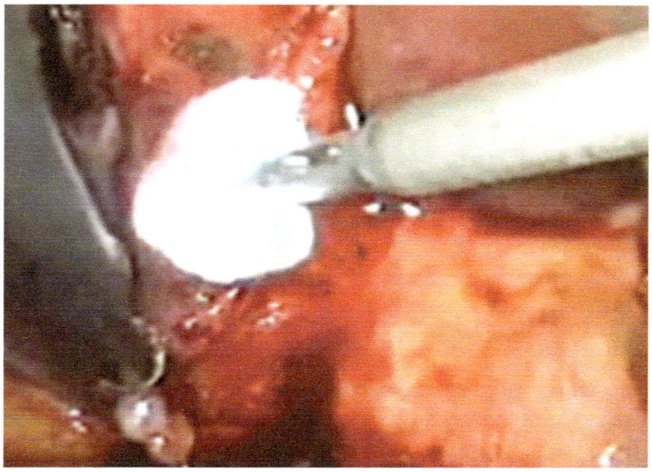

Fig. 1: Pledget dissection.

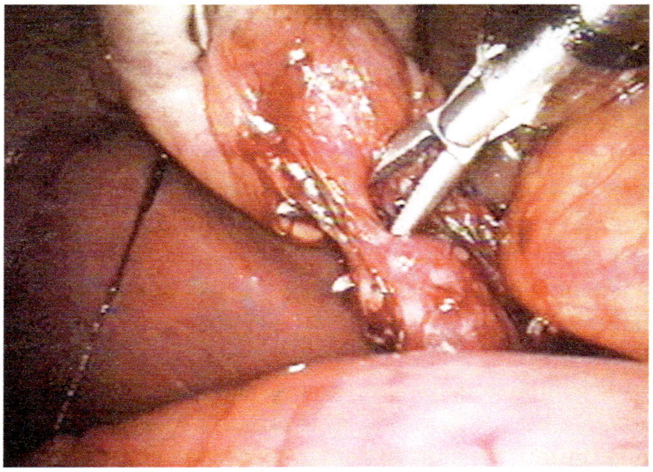

Fig. 2: Tissue stripping and dissection.

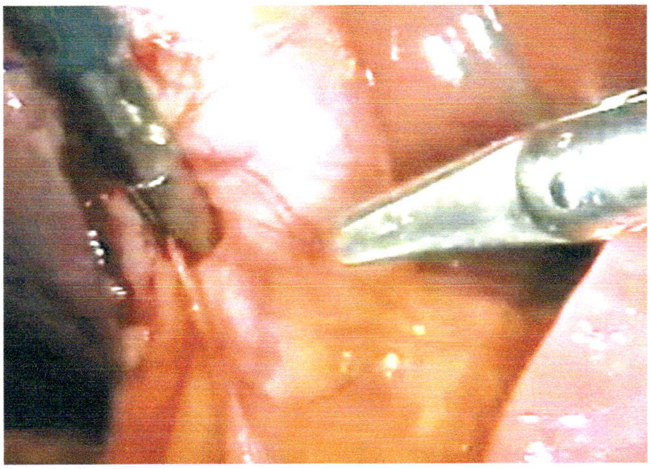

Fig. 3: Scissor dissection.

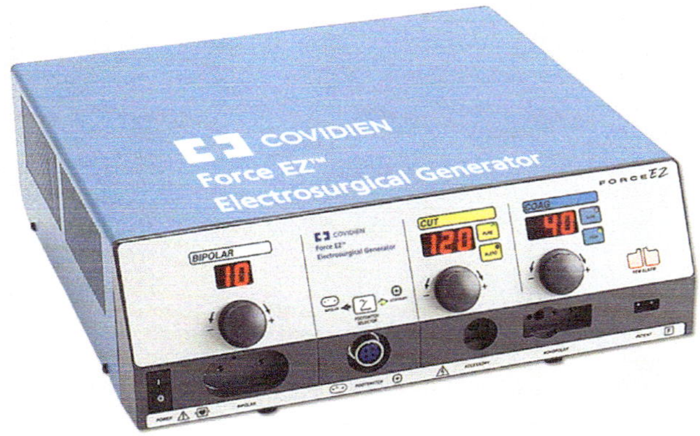

Fig. 4: High-frequency electrosurgical generator.

High-frequency Electrosurgical Dissection

Our household appliances have the 50–60 Hz frequency. This frequency is beneficial because if faulty instrument has current and inadvertently someone touches, then he will be thrown away and the person getting shock will be safe. If the frequency is >100 kHz, muscle and nerve stimulation ceases whereas all other property of electric current is still there. High-frequency electrosurgery is the application of high-frequency currents (in the frequency range of 300 kHz up to several MHz) to coagulate, fulgurate, spray coagulates, or ablates tissue. Knowledge of how this and other physical modes interact with biological materials is becoming increasingly important to the surgeon for safe and consistent surgery **(Fig. 5)**.

- Standard electrical current alternates at a frequency of 50 cycles per second (Hz)
- Nerve and muscle stimulation ceases at 100,000 cycles per second (100 kHz)
- Electrosurgery can be performed safely at frequencies above 100 kHz.

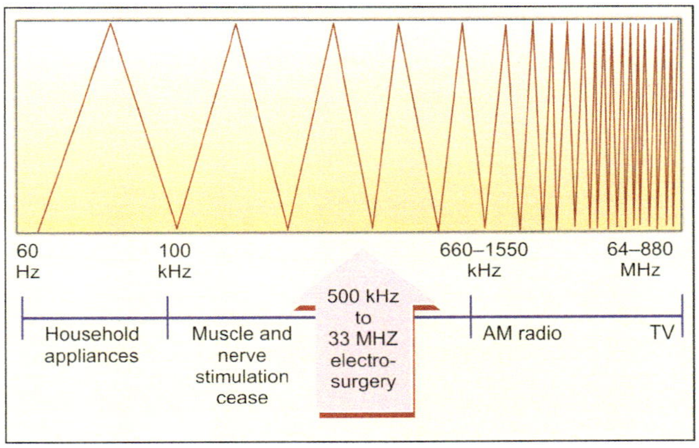

Fig. 5: Frequency range of electrosurgery.

High-frequency Monopolar Electrosurgery

The monopolar circuit is composed of the generator, active electrode, patient, and patient return electrode. The patient's tissue provides the resistance, producing heat **(Fig. 6)**.

Monopolar diathermy is used in endoscopic surgery for coagulation and for dissection (cutting). During monopolar diathermy, current is conducted from the instrument through the tissues to a skin pad (neutral electrode) connected back to the generator. Heating occurs at site of small cross-section and low electrical conductivity. A high current density occurs in the tissue in immediate contact with the instrument and heat is generated.

Burn = Intensity of current × Time/area

Burn is directly proportional to the intensity of current. Intensity of current can be adjusted by the knob provided in the generator's control panel. If the intensity setting is more, the burn will be more. Intensity actually denotes ampere or number of electrons that flows through the pathway.

Burn is also directly proportional to time. Time is paddle application time. Surgeon should always keep in mind that continuous activation of paddle can result in many complications. Intermittent activation is always better than continuous activation **(Figs. 7 and 8)**.

Burn is inversely proportional to area. One of the major problem in electrosurgery is patient will get burn at the site where area is narrowest. This may cause remote injury with the use of monopolar diathermy. The surgeon should hold the tissue with the point of instrument to catch the minimum amount of tissue at one time. If a bunch of tissue is caught, there is always fear of remote injury.

Patient return electrodes: Silicon and metal patient return plates are available. The silicon is better because it does not have any sharp edge and the resistance is less **(Fig. 9)**. Patient return electrode is required only in unipolar electrosurgery because the patient's body is a part of circuit and the patient return plate will take the current back to the generator. If the patient return plate is not attached properly

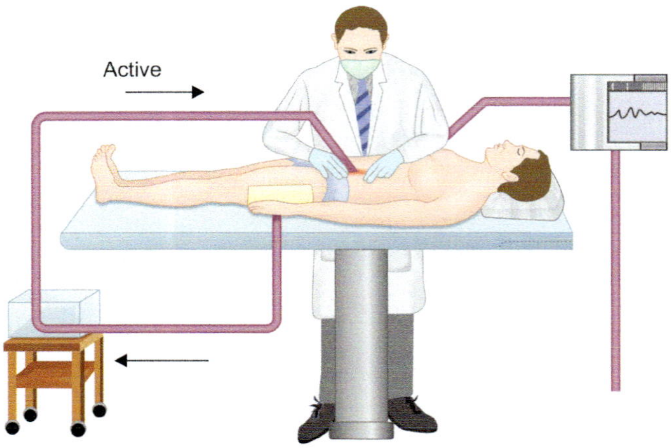

Fig. 6: Circuit of monopolar current.

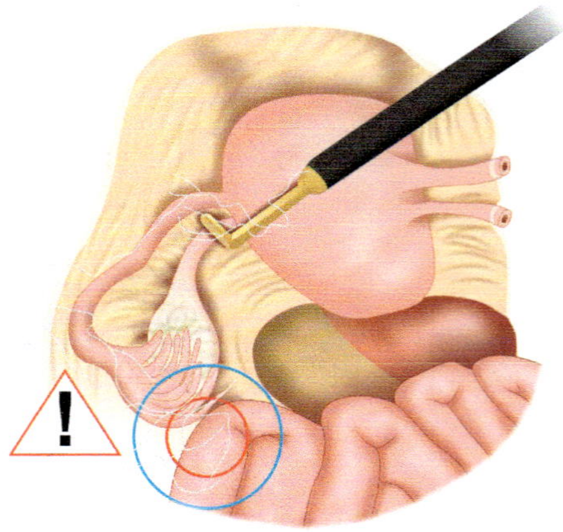

Fig. 7: Remote injury.

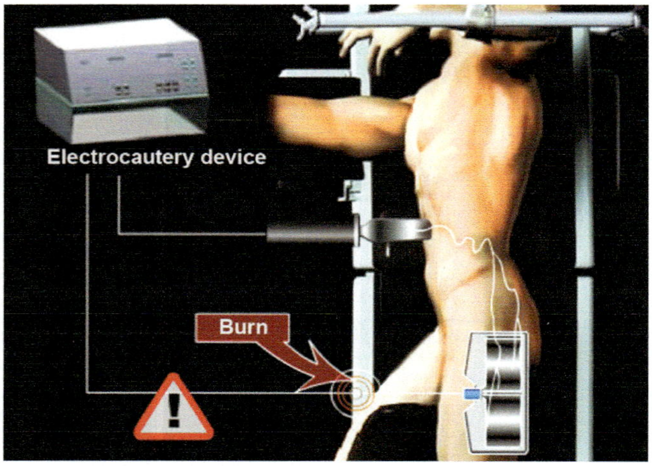

Fig. 8: Remote injury with electrocautery device.

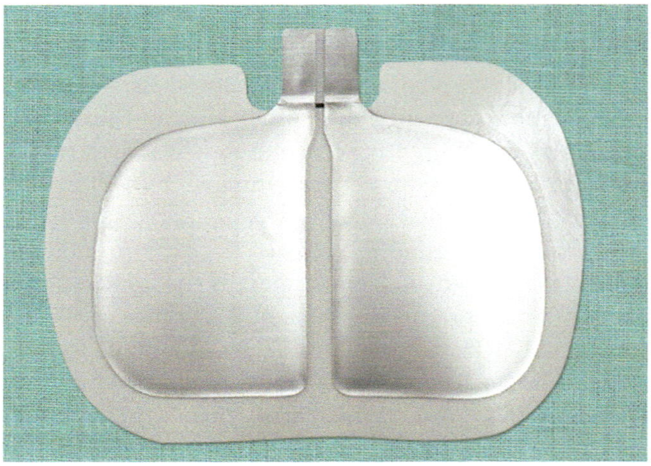

Fig. 9: High-quality patient return plate.

to the body of the patient or the size of the patient return plate is very small, patient can get electric burn at the point of attachment of this patient return plate. Ideally, the size of patient return plate should not be $<100\ cm^2$.

At the time of location of patient return plate attachment, surgeon should keep in mind the following points **(Fig. 10)**:

- *Choose*: Well-vascularized muscle mass to have more area of contact.
- *Avoid*:
  - Vascular insufficiency should be avoided because of high resistance
  - Irregular body contours can prevent plate to be in firm contact
  - Bony prominences will not allow the surrounding skin to be in contact.
- *Consider*:
  - Plate should be nearer to incision site
  - Plate should be placed according to patient's position, so it should not be displaced
  - Plate should be away from other equipment such as cardiac monitor.

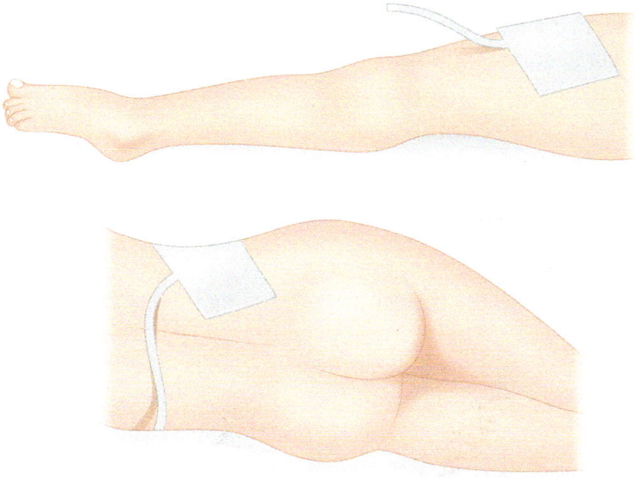

Fig. 10: Patient return plate.

The effect of high-frequency current on the tissues depends on:

- Temperature generated
- Shape and dimensions of the contact point (broader damage with broader contact)

- Time of activation (short bursts reduce depth and charring)
- Distance from the electrode **(Fig. 11)**
- Conductivity of the tissue (bleeding results in a change in conductivity)
- Power output from the generator (voltage)
- Amplitude and current wave form time curve of the signal (cutting or coagulating settings).

Bipolar Diathermy

A bipolar system is inherently safer as the interaction is restricted to the immediate vicinity of contact and the current does not pass through the patient, but instead returns to the generator via the receiving pole after passage through the grasped tissue **(Fig. 12)**.

Bipolar Electrosurgery

- Active output and patient return functions both are at the site of surgery
- Current path is confined to tissue grasped between forceps **(Fig. 13)**
- Return electrode should not be applied for bipolar procedures.

Tripolar Electrosurgery

Bipolar probes are now available for coagulation as well as for cutting. The cutting system is not strictly bipolar and is hence referred to as tripolar **(Fig. 14)**.

It has four functions in one and the same instrument namely:

1. Dissecting
2. Grasping
3. Bipolar coagulation
4. Bipolar cut

Use of the Diathermy Hook

These are generally L-shaped or open C-shaped, blunt ended rods mounted on an insulated handle. The active, noninsulated part is limited in size. The hook is a delicate

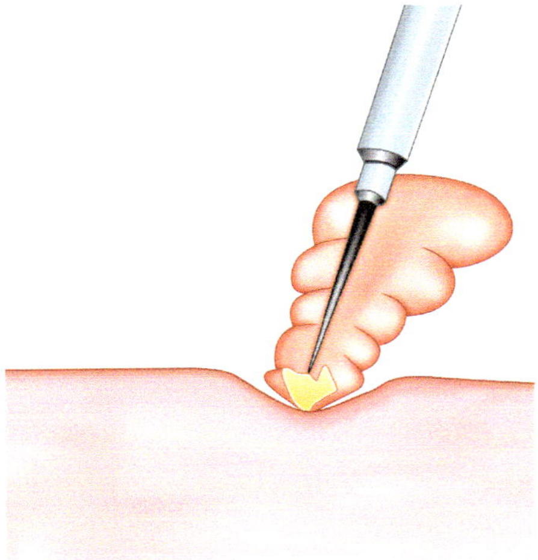

Fig. 11: Effect of cutting current.

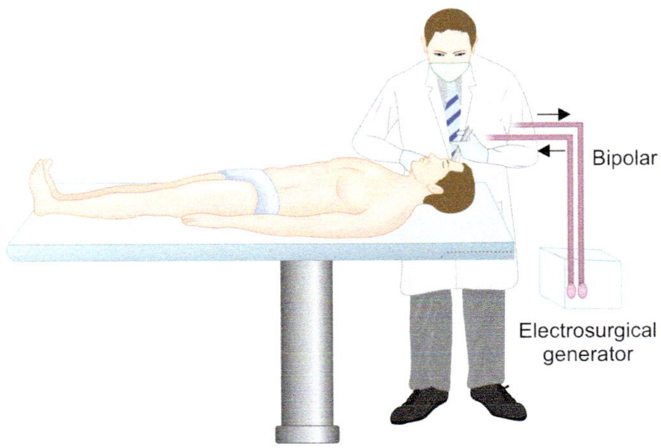

Fig. 12: Circuit of bipolar current.

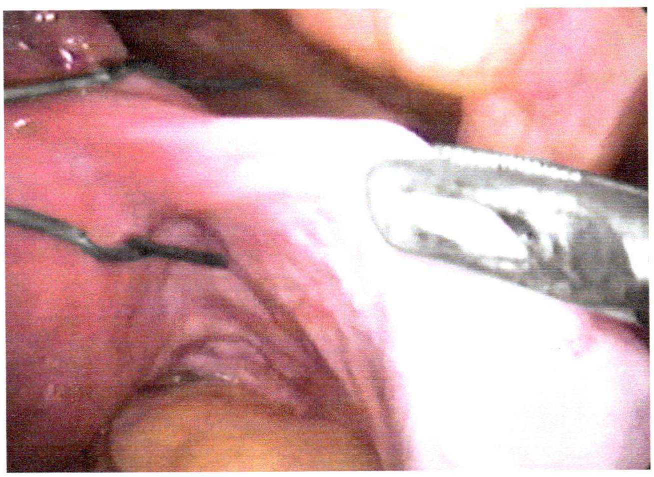

Fig. 13: Bipolar forceps used in laparoscopically-assisted vaginal hysterectomy (LAVH).

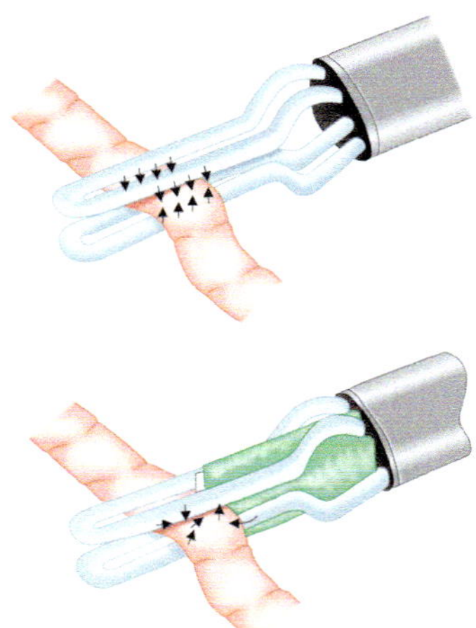

Fig. 14: Tripolar device.

instrument and should be protected during insertion by manual opening of the cannula valve or use of a reducing tube. As electrosurgery generates smoke (which is harmful), many handles of electrosurgical hooks have a suction attachment at the other end of the handle.

Electrosurgical Hooks (Fig. 15)

Electrosurgical instruments such as the hook are useful as blunt dissectors prior to activation. They are used to isolate the tissue to be divided by the current. The tip is passed into or under a layer of the tissue being dissected, which is then hooked and tented up (to increase its impedance and thus limit the spread of current when applied). Small portions of tissue are tackled, so that an assessment of the tissue caught on the hook can be made before coagulation or cutting current is applied to the instrument. The hook can be used to clear unwanted tissue beside linear structures by passing the hook into the tissues parallel to the structure and then rotating it to hook up strands of unwanted tissue. The tissue to be divided is held away from underlying tissue to prevent inadvertent damage. Short bursts of coagulating current can be followed by the use of cutting current, if the tissue has not already separated. The use of the hook can be summarized as "hook, look, and cook".

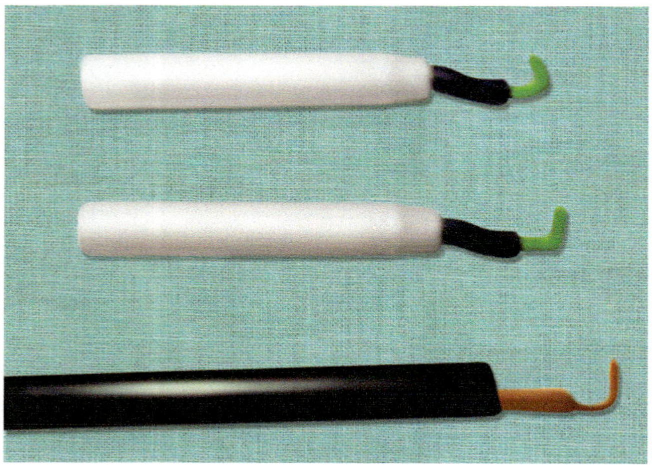

Fig. 15: Different types of hook.

The hook or the spatula may be used to mark out and coagulate a line for division. The heel of the hook is used with the high-frequency current set to soft coagulation. Short bursts are applied and the hook moved along to create a "dotted" line of coagulated tissue. When deeper penetration is desired, the hook is appropriate instrument. This type of contact is best reserved for situation where no significant damage can be caused by current penetration **(Fig. 16)**.

Monopolar electrosurgery has become the most widely used cutting and coagulating technique in MAS. It has proven to be versatile, cost-effective, and demonstrated superior efficacy for coagulation. By varying the voltage, current, or waveform, tissue can be cut cleanly (pure cut); coagulated to achieve hemostasis (coag mode) or a "blend cut" that combines these two functions can also be produced. Finally, a dispersed coagulation mode known as fulguration allows coagulation of diffuse bleeding **(Fig. 17)**.

Cutting current is low-voltage high-frequency current. Due to high frequency, the ions inside the cell get turbulence and cells brust (explode or evaporize). Cutting current can be obtained by pressing the yellow paddle of electrosurgical generator. To cut any structure, it is important that surgeon should apply the sharp tip of electrosurgical instrument and the tissue should not be held firmly. At the time of cutting, it is wise that tissue should be under tension. Ideally, direct touch with the tissue should be avoided in case of cutting current. It should be spark wave from some distance **(Fig. 18)**.

Electrosurgical coagulation is achieved by high-voltage low-frequency current. This low frequency is not sufficient to cause the explosion of cell, but heat inside the cell is increased.

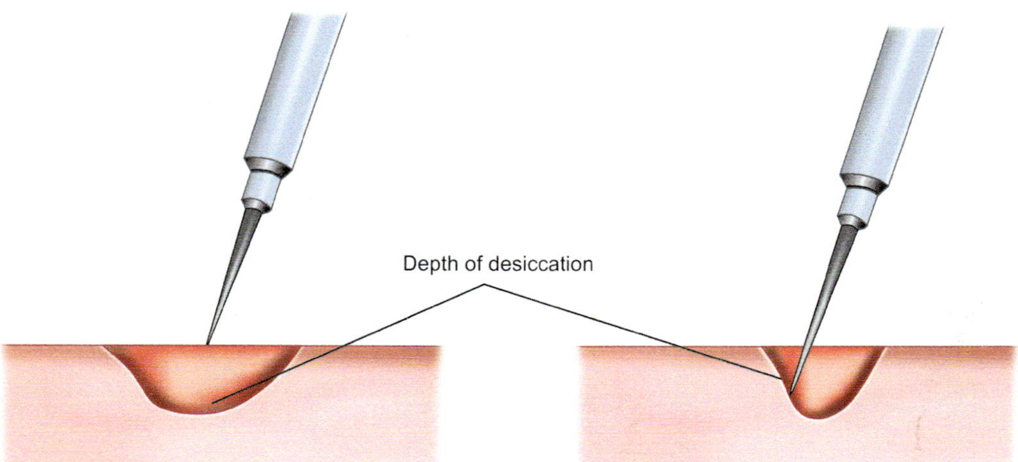

Fig. 16: Depth of desiccation is proportional to paddle application time.

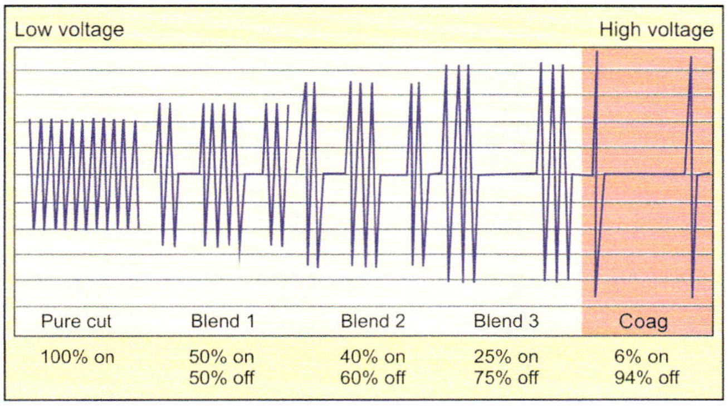

Fig. 17: Different types of electrosurgery.

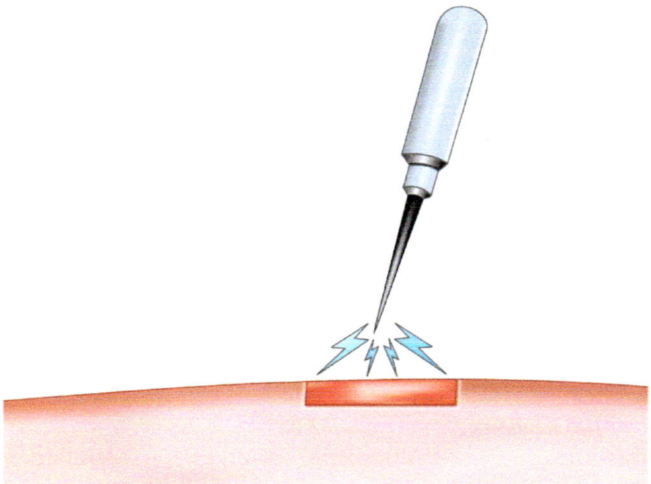

Fig. 18: Fulguration.

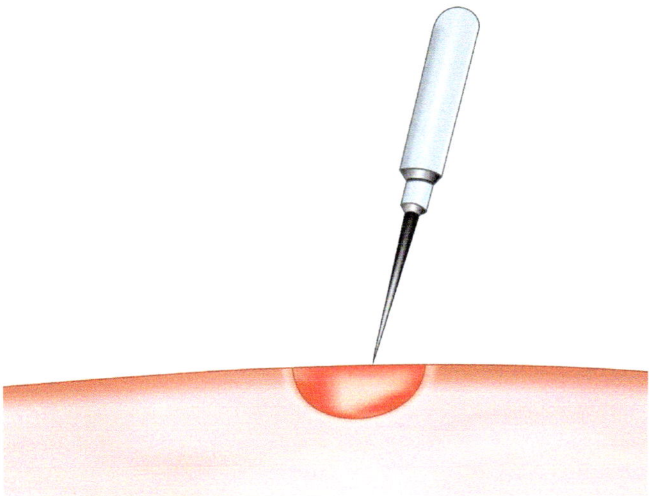

Fig. 19: Desiccation with more collateral damage.

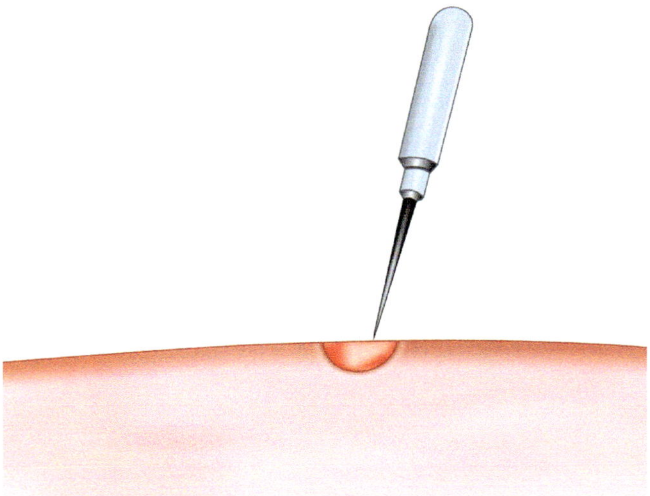

Fig. 20: Desiccation with less collateral damage.

Due to increased intracellular temperature, the protein inside the cell coagulates and shrinks. Shrinkage of protein will cause constriction in the lumen of bleeding vessels and the vessels are sealed. Permanency of coagulated tissue and its sealing effect depends upon melted collagen. At the time of electrosurgical monopolar coagulation, the temperature of tissue causes the collagen to melt. These melted collagens solidify again once the active instrument is off from the tissue. It is important to remember that if the tissue is burnt more than required, the melted collagen burns, turns into charcoal, and the sealing strength of the lumen of any vessel will decrease. Surgeons and gynecologists should always try to avoid overcooking of the tissue.

Electrosurgical coagulation is of two types:

1. *Fulguration*: Fulguration is coagulation current from some distance **(Fig. 18)**. It is also known as spray mode. At the time of fulguration, lateral spread of energy is more than depth. We want to use fulguration everywhere, where superficial burn is required and deeper injury may cause damage of underlying structure. The example of good use fulguration is ablation in cases of endometriosis and fulguration of gallbladder bed at the time of cholecystectomy, if there is generalized oozing from liver. Direct touch with tissue should be avoided to achieve maximum effect. Fulguration is coagulation current from some distance.
2. *Desiccation*: Electrosurgical desiccation occurs when the electrode is in direct contact with the tissue. Most of the time with the unipolar or bipolar electrosurgery, we do desiccation only. The tissue damage in depth and width is same in desiccation. The extent of collateral damage in desiccation is more compared to cutting current. The extent of collateral damage of desiccation can be minimized by minimizing the paddle application time **(Figs. 19 and 20)**.

However, monopolar laparoscopic electrosurgery can compromise patient safety under certain circumstances. Thermal injury to nontargeted internal organs may occur firstly, as a result of imprecise mechanical operation of a laparoscopic instrument and secondly, through diversion of electrical current to other paths. These stray current may be released either through insulation failure, direct coupling, or capacitive coupling. Other problems encountered include effect on pacemakers, return electrode burns, toxic smoke, charring of instruments, and minimal control of energy delivery **(Fig. 21)**.

Bipolar electrodes design although virtually eliminating complication from insulation failure, capacitive coupling, and direct coupling **(Figs. 22 to 24)**.

The primary electrothermal tissue effect is limited to desiccation, not cutting. It requires slightly more time than monopolar coagulation because of lower power settings and bipolar generator output characteristics. It is not an effective method of making a "pure cut".

- Hemostasis over a large area is not possible
- Grasping dense tissue between both the active and return electrodes is difficult.

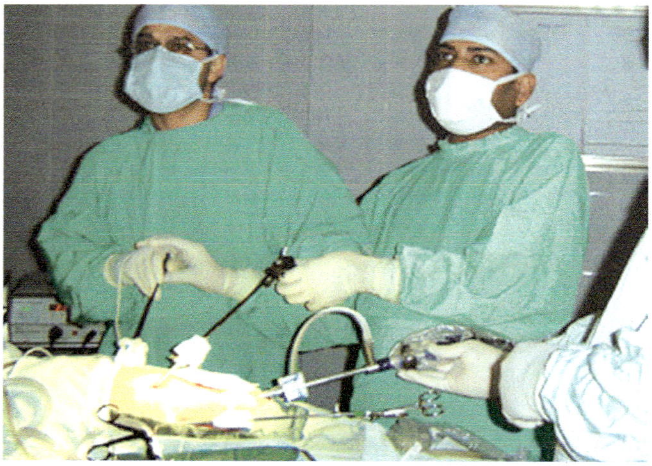

Fig. 21: Overshooting should be avoided.

Safety during Electrosurgery

Laparoscopic dissection requires more extensive dissection and thus meticulous hemostasis becomes particularly important. Any loss of view will result in loss of control and hence decreased safety. Hemorrhage, even to a minor extent, tends to obscure their operative field and is to be avoided. This means that vessels of a size that in open surgery could be divided without particular attention need to be secured prior to division when working endoscopically. Dissection must be more meticulous to proceed smoothly to avoid any unacknowledged injury.

The magnification produced by the endoscope may initially confuse the surgeon as to the extent of electrical injury. However, an inexperienced endoscopic surgeon is well-advised to convert if he have any doubt about his ability to control the situation expeditiously.

Safety Considerations in Minimal Access Surgery

The potential for accidental damage with electrosurgery must always be borne in mind at the time of MAS. Following are the most commonly encountered problems specific to the MAS:

- Overshooting
- Overcooking
- Direct coupling
- Capacitive coupling
- Insulation failure

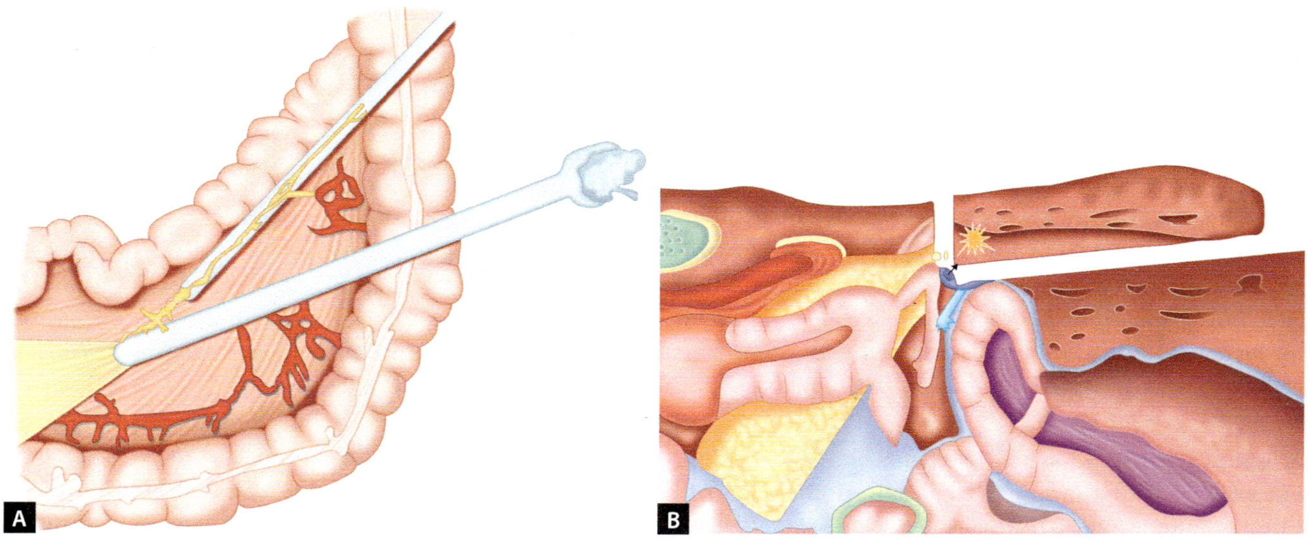

Figs. 22A and B: Direct coupling.

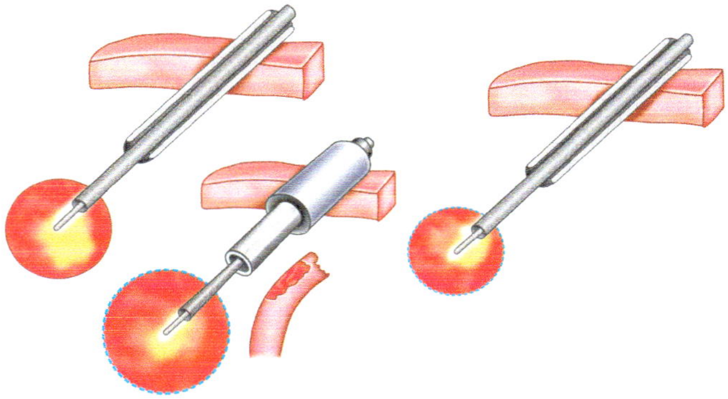

Fig. 23: Capacitive coupling.

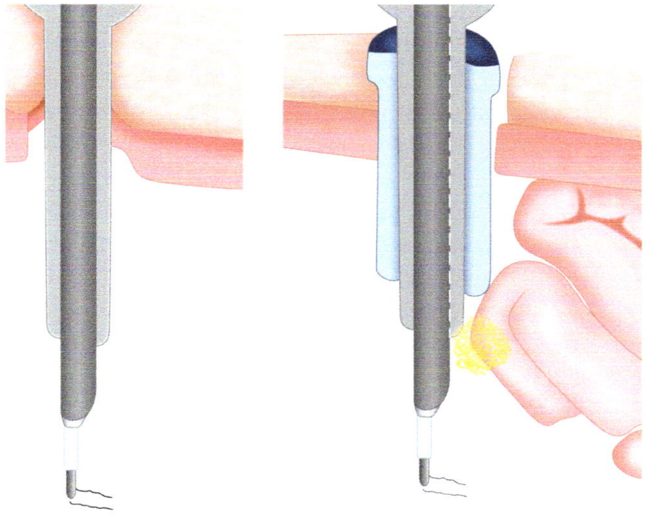

Fig. 24: Burn due to capacitive coupling.

Overshooting: Overshooting means the tip of energized instrument going beyond the field of vision during electrosurgery. Overshooting is one of the common mistakes done by beginners. Surgeon should be careful that if they are cutting any structure they should apply less force, otherwise their instrument will overshoot once the structure is cut and the energized instrument can heat any nearby viscera leading to perforation.

During initial learning phase of laparoscopy, the trainer surgeon should keep hold on the hand of trainee at the time of electrosurgery to prevent any inadvertent injury by overshooting. At the time of laparoscopic cholecystectomy, if hook overshoots, it may hit diaphragm or duodenum. If overshooting is not under the control of surgeon, he should try to keep the tip of hook toward the anterior abdominal wall, so that only peritoneum will be injured.

Overcooking: Proper hemostasis requires optimum application of energy over the tissue. Due to visual limitations and fear of impending bleeding, laparoscopic surgeons have a tendency of overcooking. It is important to remember that instead of more secure coagulation overcooking can create rebleeding. To understand the effect of overcooking, it is important to know physiology of tissue sealing.

Coagulation current is high-voltage low-frequency current. At this current, the ions inside the cell will move but it cannot explode. Due to increase in intracellular heat, the protein inside the cell will be denatured, coagulated, and shrink. Due to shrinkage of tissue, the lumen of small bleeder obliterates and bleeding stops. At the same time due to heat, the collagen of tissue melts and once the paddle of electrosurgical generator is off, the melted collagen will cool down and solidify.

Overcooking results in charring of melted collagen and the sealing strength of tissue is decreased. It could be understood just by the example of sealing of polythene over a flame of candle. If you want to seal the polythene bag but applying more temperature on polythene by putting it over direct flame, instead of getting sealed, the polythene will start burning. One should know the sealing temperature of polythene so that required temperature is applied, the polythene will melt and once cooled will solidify. Similarly, the burnt collagen does not have any tissue sealing property and bleeding may start again if it is overcooked.

Most common causes of overcooking or charring of tissue are:

- High power setting of electrosurgical generator
- Prolonged activation of foot paddle
- Keeping the jaw closed permanently in contact of tissue
- Poorly engineered electrosurgical generator.

Direct coupling: If the active electrode touches a noninsulated metal instrument within the abdomen, it will convey energy to the second instrument, which may in turn, if the current density is high enough, transfer it to surrounding tissues and cause a thermal burn. For example, the active electrode could come in contact or in close proximity (<2 mm) to a laparoscope, creating an arc of current between the two. The laparoscope could then brush against surrounding tissue, causing a severe burn to the bowel and other structures. The burns may not be in the visual field of the surgeon and therefore will not be recognized and dealt with in a timely fashion.

To prevent direct coupling, the active electrode should not be in close proximity to or touching another metal instrument before the generator is activated. Bowel is particularly susceptible to this kind of collateral damage from sparks and stray currents. Recognition of this complication may be delayed until the postoperative period with serious consequences. Check that the electrode is touching the target tissue, and only that tissue, before you activate the generator. Note that when target tissue is coagulated (desiccated), the impedance increases and the current may arc to adjacent tissue, following the path of least resistance.

We should be careful that all metal instruments such as laparoscopes pass through conductive metal trocars. This way, if the active electrode touches the instrument, the current will simply flow from the instrument to the metal trocar. As long as the trocar is in contact with a relatively large portion of the abdominal wall, the current will not concentrate. Instead, it will dissipate harmlessly from the trocar through the abdomen and back through adjacent tissue to the return electrode. If the trocar is completely or partially constructed of plastic, however, the energy may not be able to dissipate back through the body. The metal within the trocar will build up a charge, which could eventually arc to adjacent tissue and back to the return electrode, but at a harmful level of current. In doing so, it may travel through the bowel, skin, or even the operator's hands, causing burns **(Fig. 23)**.

To avoid direct coupling, surgeon should not activate the generator while the active electrode is touching or in close proximity to another metal object.

Capacitive coupling: This now never arise but occurred in the early days of laparoscopic surgery with the use of plastic fixation screws to fix metal ports to the abdominal wall, so as to prevent them from being accidentally pulled out or pushed when instruments were withdrawn during the course of an operation.

The physics underlying this injury is fairly straightforward. Whenever current is applied through an insulated instrument inserted through a metal trocar (port), some radiofrequency electric charge is transferred to the metal cannula by every activation (even if the insulation of the instrument is perfect). This effect is known as capacitance coupling.

There is absolutely no problem if the metal cannula is in contact with the full thickness of the abdominal wall, as the charge accumulated by the cannula is immediately discharged over a wide contact area (low power density like the neutral return electrode plate) and hence no damage is done.

However, if the cannula is isolated from the abdominal wall, by a plastic screw (acting as an insulator), the cannula cannot discharge and thus accumulates a substantial charge with repeated activation of the electrosurgical instrument. Thus, in essence, it becomes an electric accumulator. Should at any stage, the tip of the cannula inside the abdomen touches tissue or bowel, the accumulated charge will discharge immediately through a single point of contact, i.e., with a high power density sufficient to cause an electrical burn. Since this occurs away from the site of action of the operation, it is usually overlooked. Capacitive coupling is not a problem if plastic fixation screws are not used.

The phenomenon of "capacitance" is the ability of two conductors to transmit electrical flow even if they are separated by an intact layer of insulation. Capacitive coupling can occur even in the best-case scenario, i.e., when the insulation around the active electrode is intact and the tip of the electrode is not touching anything metal. If the active, insulated electrode is wrapped around a towel clamp, or placed inside a metal trocar sleeve, or comes in close contact with any conductive substance for an extended period of time, the current in the active electrode may induce a current in the second conductor.

As long as the induced current can dissipate easily, through a large surface of tissue, it would not present a problem. The danger occurs if the second conductor contains some insulating material, as in the case of a metal cannula held in place by a plastic anchor. The plastic anchor will prevent the energy from dissipating and increase the likelihood of a thermal burn. Burns from capacitance current may occur when the surface area is <3 cm^2 or the current density is approximately 7 W/cm^2.

As with direct coupling, the best way to prevent this phenomenon is to use the active electrode monitoring system that prevents current from capacitive coupling from building to dangerous levels. Also, you should avoid all plastic-metal hybrid instruments, including cannulas, trocars, and clamps, when doing electrosurgery.

Insulation failure: During a laparoendoscopic procedure, only about 10% of an insulated instrument is visible on the video monitor at any one time, which means about 90% of that electrode remains outside the surgeon's field of view, where it can cause the most damage. Whenever a defective instrument is introduced into the patient, electric current can escape to contiguous tissue or organs, but the surgeon is not aware that a thermal burn at a peripheral site has occurred. It is estimated that 67% of such injuries are not recognized at the time of surgery. Sadly, manifestations of these unsuspected injuries do not appear until several days after the actual surgery and so, when the impaired patient presents, his or her clinical symptoms are already severe. Diagnosis is difficult and often delayed and the damage can be irreversible. Complications include perforated bowel diaphragm, urinary bladder, permanent disfigurement, fecal peritonitis cases, etc. **(Fig. 25)**.

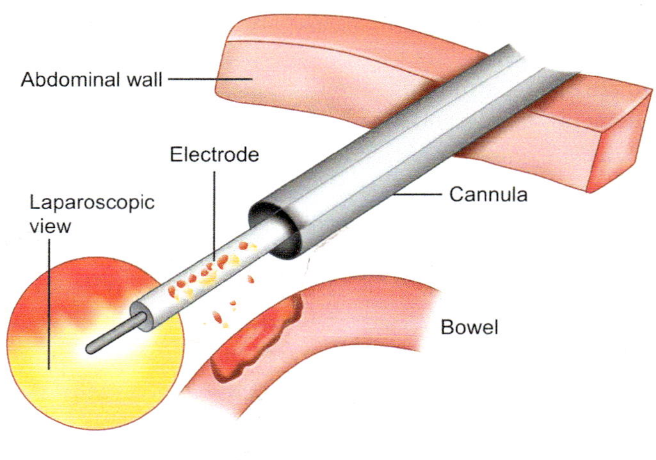

Fig. 25: Insulation failure.

Continued regular use of cleaning and sterilization can cause the layer of insulation covering the shaft of the active electrode to break down. Tiny, visually undetectable tears are actually more dangerous than large cracks, since the current escaping from these miniscule breaks is more concentrated and therefore capable of causing sparks (averaging 700°C). These sparks can cause severe burns and even ignite fires, especially in oxygen-rich environments. In fact, all insulated electrodes should be considered suspicious, unless adequate safety measures are introduced.

Unfortunately, many surgeons unknowingly contribute to the problem. Routine use of the high-voltage "coagulation" current may actually compromise insulation integrity. The higher the voltage, the greater the risk that the current will break through weak insulation.

Surgeon should always use the lowest voltage. All electrosurgery systems will allow to use a "coagulation" or "cutting" waveform of current.

In most cases, we should try to use the cutting current for both cutting and coagulation. The coagulation mode is necessary only when you need to fulgurate or stop diffuse bleeding on highly vascularized tissue. Using the lowest voltage, it may reduce the wear on the insulation and minimize the chance that the current can escape through hairline cracks.

The surgeon should test for insulation defects in the operating room, after the set has been opened. This step can significantly reduce the number of accidental electrosurgical burns because it will prevent a surgeon from inserting a potentially lethal instrument into the patient's abdomen. Insulation that degraded during that final sterilization cycle cannot be detected until this point in time, so it is critical that inspection in the operating room itself be made an integral part of hospital protocol. It is advisable to keep a supply of single-use electrodes available to replace any found to be faulty during the preoperative scan. One can also devise a vigorous and ongoing inspection plan with a qualified technician to ensure that all reusable electrosurgical tools are scanned and reinsulated as needed.

If the instruments are rescanned in the operating room following surgery, the surgeon can be secure in the knowledge that no stray electrical current escaped into adjacent, but unseen sites and so if any postoperative clinical complications were to arise, he or she could more easily isolate the cause. Conversely, if the postoperative scan revealed that insulation was damaged during the procedure, he or she may elect to take aggressive steps to investigate further. For documentation purposes, the results of both scans can be recorded in the patient record.

We should always keep in mind that using the cutting current minimizes, but does not eliminate the risk of insulation failure. To really be sure that the insulation is not compromised, it is recommended to use an electrosurgical unit that employs active electrode monitoring (AEM) technology. This technology is called "ElectroShield" (Electroscope, Inc., Boulder, Colorado) and it virtually eliminates these types of electrical burns.

The traditional system for inspection in the sterile processing department is hardly foolproof and its weaknesses must be addressed. Because the margin for error is so great, risk managers and physicians alike are insisting on alternatives that will ensure patient safety and reduce liability exposure. AEM protects against thermal burns in two ways. First, it encases the insulated electrode in a protective metal shield that is connected to the generator; the entire probe is also covered with an extra layer of insulation. The extra conductive and insulating layers ensure that stray current is contained and flows right back to the generator. Second, the system monitors the electrical circuit so if stray energy reaches dangerous levels, the unit shuts off automatically and sounds an alarm before a burn can occur. Electroscope's AEM system operates on a principle similar to ground fault interrupter (GFI) outlets in our home. It protects against insulation breaks by grounding electricity in unpredictable elements, eliminating stray burns to the patient. This is presently considered the standard of care in endoscopic electrosurgery.

Surgical Smoke

Dissection with electrocautery produces a great deal of smoke. Carbon monoxide at levels as high as 1,900 ppm, many times higher than the Environmental Protection Agency Standard of 35 ppm for a 1-hour exposure, are produced by electrocautery in the hypoxic environment of the carbon dioxide-filled abdomen. Fortunately, carbon monoxide is a very insoluble molecule and does not cross the peritoneum. Carbon monoxide absorption is therefore not a problem for patients undergoing laparoscopy. However, contamination by carbon monoxide and other toxic or infectious byproducts of electrocautery may affect the operating room personnel if the smoke is vented into the room.

When an electrosurgical probe heats tissue and vaporizes cellular fluid, one byproduct is surgical smoke. We know that these fumes, which can contain viral deoxyribonucleic acid (DNA), bacteria, carcinogens, and irritants, are malodorous and can cause upper respiratory irritation. We do not yet know whether they are capable of causing cancer or spreading infectious disease. Surgical smoke can also obscure the operative site and causes the surgeon to inadvertently touch the electrode to nontargeted tissue.

Surgical masks do not adequately filter surgical smoke, the particles are too small. A much better solution is a smoke evacuation system, a high-flow suction, and filtering device that remove the particles from the air. Two kinds are available commercially. One uses a handheld nozzle, which is intended to be positioned at the surgical site.

To avoid complication of laparoscopic electrosurgery, following important points are:

- Inspect insulation carefully
- Use lowest possible power setting
- Use a low voltage waveform (cut)
- Use brief intermittent activation versus prolonged activation
- Do not activate in open circuit
- Do not activate in close proximity or direct contact with another instrument
- Use bipolar electrosurgery when appropriate
- Select an all metal cannula system as the safest choice. Do not use hybrid cannula systems that mix metal with plastic
- Utilize available technology, such as a tissue response generator to reduce capacitive coupling or an active electrode monitoring system, to eliminate concerns about insulation failure and capacitive coupling.

Argon Beamer Coagulator

The argon beamer is used in conjunction with monopolar electrosurgery to produce fulguration or superficial coagulation **(Fig. 26)**. Less smoke is produced because there is lesser depth of tissue damage. The system emits a high-energy jet of argon plasma possessing thermal and kinetic energy that can be used to coagulate a tissue surface including small vessels and lymphatics. Since its introduction, plasma jet has been used safely in both open and endoscopic cases in orthopedics, oncology, gastroenterology, liver surgery, plastic surgery of the abdomen and face, and in thoracic surgery.

Neutral argon plasma can be utilized as a multi-functional device that has vaporization, coagulation, and superficial cutting capacities with minimal thermal spread and acceptable outcomes. The use of neutral argon plasma appears to be efficacious and safe for laparoscopic surgery

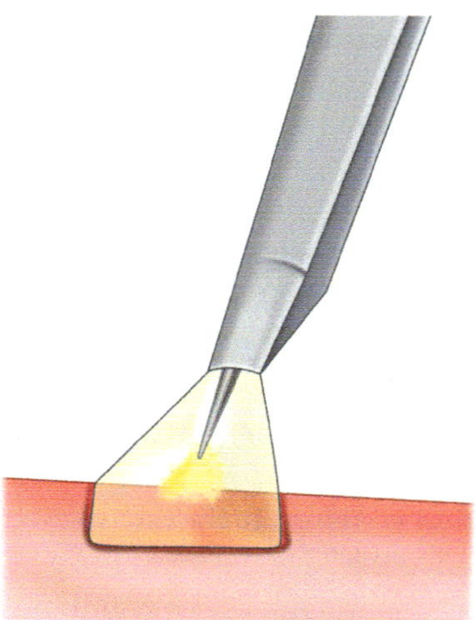

Fig. 26: Argon electrosurgery.

such as endometriosis, presacral neurectomy, liver resection, myoma bed bleeding control, etc.

Despite these advantages, the argon beamer suffers from a very significant drawback in laparoscopic surgery, namely increased intra-abdominal pressure to potentially dangerous levels due to high-flow infusion of argon gas.

Ultrasonic Dissection

Ultrasonic dissectors are of two types: (1) low-power systems which cleave water containing tissues by cavitations leaving organized structures with low water content intact, e.g., blood vessels, bile ducts, etc., and (2) high-power systems which cleave loose areolar tissues by frictional heating and thus cut and coagulate the edges at the same time. Thus, low-power systems are used for liver surgery (CUSA, Selector) and do not coagulate vessels. High-power systems (Autosonix, Ultracision) are used extensively especially in fundoplication and laparoscopic colon surgery. It is important to remember that high-power ultrasonic dissection systems may cause collateral damage by excessive heating and this is well-documented in clinical practice.

Ultrasonic surgical dissection allows coagulation and cutting with less instrument traffic (reduction in operating time), less smoke, and no electrical current.

- Mechanical energy at 55,500 vibrations/s
- Disrupts hydrogen bonds and forms a coagulum
- Temperature by harmonic scalpel (80–100°C)
- Temperature through electrocoagulation (200–300°C)
- Less collateral damage, less tissue necrosis.

The ultrasonic shears (harmonic scalpel) is ideal for dividing and simultaneously sealing small and medium vessels by tamponade and heat. However, larger vessels, >2 mm in diameter, need additional measures (clips, tie, or staple) to control bleeding. Other disadvantages of the harmonic scalpel include lack of tissue selectivity and relatively expensive. Ultrasonic dissecting applicators are also designed in hook, spatula, or ball coagulator shapes **(Figs. 27A and B)**.

The cavitational ultrasonic aspirator has the advantage of removing debris and is tissue selective, e.g., divides liver but spares bile ducts and vessels. It affords safe rapid dissection with reduction in tissue damage and blood loss compared to the harmonic scalpel. The problems associated with its use are evacuation of the pneumoperitoneum together with vibration and irrigation which cloud the telescope lens necessitating frequent cleaning **(Fig. 28A)**.

It is not correct that ultrasonic generators are without any risk. If bowel or blood vessels touch directly to the vibrating jaw, it can be punctured.

High-velocity Water-jet Dissection

High-velocity high-pressure water-jet dissection involves the use of relatively simple devices to produce clean cutting of

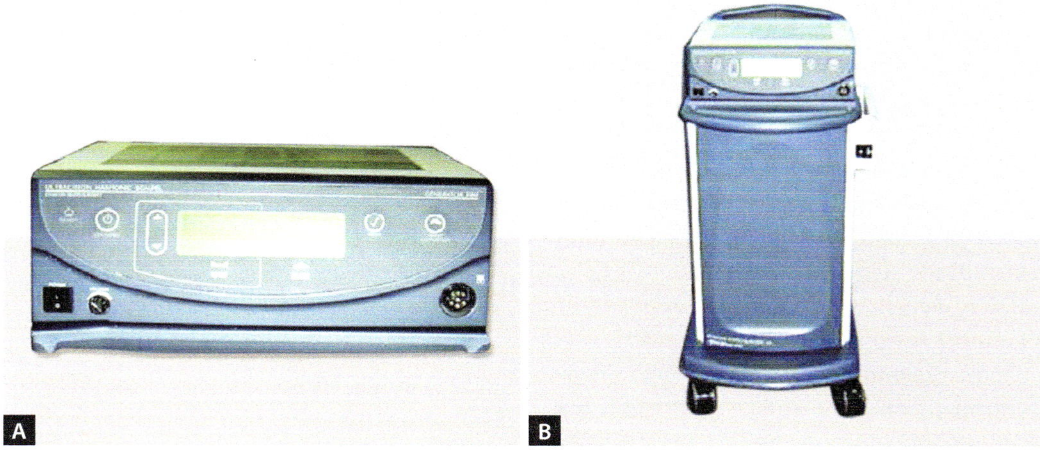

Figs. 27A and B: Ultrasonic generator.

reproducible depth. Other advantages are the cleansing of the operating field by the turbulent flow zone and the small amount of water required to complete dissection.

Specific problems were identified with the use of this modality. The "hailstorm" effect results in excessive misting which obscures vision. This has been solved to some extent by incorporating a hood over the nozzle. The nonhemostatic nature of this modality, difficulty in gauging distance, and poor control of the depth of the cut are additional drawbacks. The spraying of tissue fragments renders it also oncologically unsound. The present use of water-jet dissection is limited to dissection of solid organs.

Hydrodissection

Hydrodissection uses the force of pulsatile irrigation with crystalloid solutions to separate tissue planes **(Fig. 28B)**. The operating field at the same time is kept clear. Like water-jet dissection, no hemostasis is achievable. The use of this dissecting modality is restricted to pelvic lymphadenectomy and pleurectomy in thoracoscopic surgery. Today, the hydrodissection technique is frequently used with success in cataract, urologic, and plastic surgery. Hydrodissection is also used in laparoscopic surgery as an adjunct to electrocauterization to facilitate the dissection of fascial planes. The mechanical benefits of hydrodissection infiltrates the serosal layers with saline, it both creates and reveals the correct plane between adherent tissues and subsequently makes separation easier.

Hydrodissection is a safe technique that can be applied as an adjunct to electrocauterization, which facilitates dissection in the correct plane during many laparoscopic surgeries such as cholecystectomy, hernia, colectomy, and endometriosis surgery. Although hydrodissection does not have additional benefits in terms of dissection time, postoperative outcome, or overall survival, it can be useful for inexperienced surgeons, especially for those in the learning phase. Hydro-Surg™ Plus Irrigator is designed to provide controlled powered irrigation to, and aspiration of fluids/smoke from, the operative site during laparoscopic surgical procedures (e.g., laparoscopic cholecystectomy and laparoscopic gynecological procedures). It may also be used for resection of filmy adhesions by hydrodissection and peritoneal lavage. Appropriate fluids include those which have a specific gravity of approximately 1 (e.g., saline). Additional specialty probe tips are available from Davol including insulated and nonconductive tips for use with electrosurgery. Suction/irrigation probe tips, when included, have a nonreflective surface to help avoid laser beam reflection. With proper adapter, a laser fiber and laser fiber sheath can be passed through the probe handle and tip.

Laser Dissection

The laser devices release photons which induce molecular vibration and create heat when they interact with the tissue and create heat. LASER is an acronym for "light amplification by stimulated emission of radiation" **(Fig. 28C)**. Each lasing substance has a unique atomic and molecular structure and so the waveform and frequency. Laser light is monochromatic and cannot be separated into colors when passed through prism. The amount of power delivered by laser is measured in Watts. The basic components in a laser unit are a pumping system, lasing medium, optical cavity, and operating system. The operating system controls delivery of laser into tissue when activated by surgeon. The surgeon controls power control knob. There are many modes of power delivery such as continuous, pulse, superpulse, and ultrapulse modes.

The primary difference from other source of energy is that generally tissue is not directly touched by surgical instrument. Thus, the depth of incision is not controlled by pressure exerted on the tissue but by the power density delivered by surgeon. The unique property of laser is determined by its wavelength and tissue absorption. By changing the power setting, desired tissue effect such as ablation, fulguration, coagulation, or vaporization can be achieved. These days laser is not used frequently in general laparoscopic surgery as they offer no advantages over more user friendly and safer forms of energized dissection and coagulation systems.

The previous generation of lasers (with gas vapor chambers) was large, very expensive, and required special power supply (three-phase electricity) and maintenance. In addition, they lacked portability. The current generation of solid-state lasers diode array has overcome all these disadvantages and may well be used for certain applications of laparoscopic general surgery in the future. Currently, laser ablation is used largely in gynecological laparoscopic surgery, e.g., ablation of endometriosis and much less commonly for the photoablation of secondary tumors of the liver. The most effective use of carbon dioxide (CO_2) laser beam is laser knife that gives high precision for dissection over sensitive areas such as bladder, ureter, and major blood vessels.

The degree and extent of thermal damage produced by laser depends on the structure, water content, pigmentation, optical and thermal properties, and perfusion of the tissue. The properties of a particular laser beam are also other determinants of heat damage. Therefore, each of the various types of laser available have a specific clinical application.

In gynecology, the argon laser coagulator is the ideal method of treating small red endometriotic deposits. Tissue absorption of light is low and hemoglobin absorption is high at its operating wavelengths of 488 nm and 514 nm, i.e., selective absorption.

The CO_2 laser is best suited for extremely superficial ablation. It is relatively inexpensive (compared to other lasers) and has the ability to vaporize a very thin surface of tissue. On the other hand, photocoagulation of vascular lesions is ineffective using CO_2 laser. This type of laser also has the potential for injuring structures in the abdomen distant from the site under laparoscopic view.

The contact neodymium-doped yttrium aluminum garnet (Nd:YAG) laser virtually eliminates the free beam effect and is therefore suitable for laparoscopic application. The thermal injury from contact laser is superficial. No additional protection is needed for the endocamera since they are already fitted with infrared filters. However, Nd:YAG laser dissection was found to be significantly slower and produced more blood loss than monopolar electrosurgery in laparoscopic cholecystectomy.

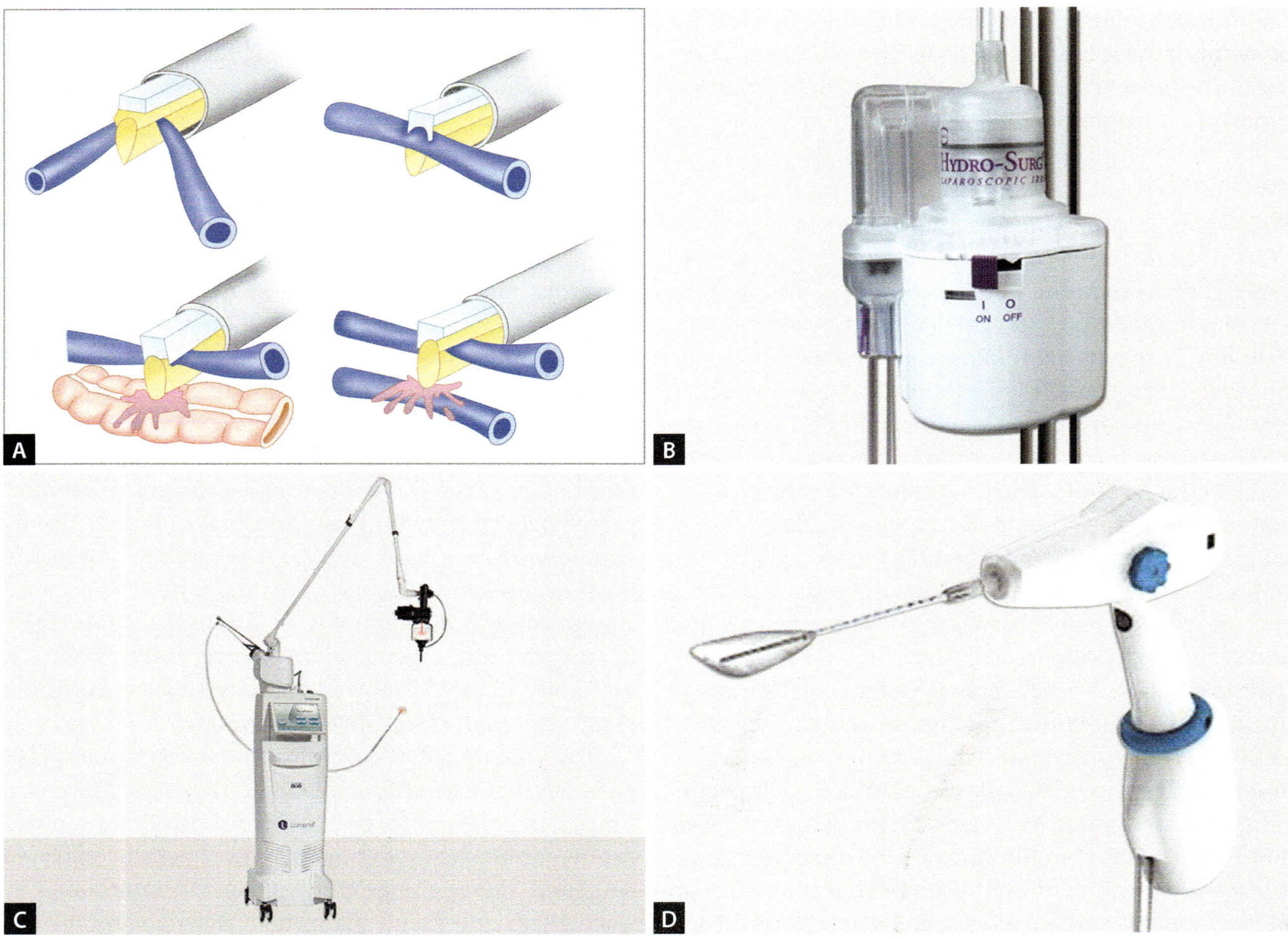

Figs. 28A to D: (A) Harmonic scalpel; (B) Hydro-Surg™ Plus Irrigator; (C) Laser generator; (D) Cryotherapy device.

All lasers including potassium-titanyl-phosphate (KTP) and the more recently developed solid state have several major drawbacks in common. They are expensive, inefficient, produce toxic smoke, nontunable, require specialized theater, and achieve variable penetration. Safety issues such as heat cumulative effect, burns due to accidental exposure, and retinal damage also contribute toward preventing widespread use of laser.

It is now obvious that from the range of available dissecting modalities in laparoscopic surgery, none has proven to be ideal. Utility of a particular modality is dictated by how close it meets the requirements to achieve safe, effective, and hemostatic tissue division under the specific circumstances. The surgeon must be able to use the appropriate combination of modalities in order to exploit the benefit each has to offer during dissection.

When properly used, laser, microelectrode, ultrasonic dissector, tissue response generator, and mechanical instruments are equally effective in any surgery. The choice of instrument should be on the instrument with surgeon that is more comfortable and he has the skill and experience for that particular instrument.

Cryotherapy and Radiofrequency Ablation

Both are used in the laparoscopic ablation of secondary tumor deposits in the liver, usually when the lesions are inoperable for whatever reason, laparoscopic cryotherapy with implantable probe destroys tumors by rapid freezing to -40°C or lower.

The lesion revascularizes for a short period (12–14 hours) on thawing but because the vasculature and the tumor parenchyma are damaged beyond repair, hemorrhagic infraction ensues. With radiofrequency thermal ablation, a radiofrequency current is transmitted through the probe implanted in the tumor. The radiofrequency current causes molecular and ionic agitation which heats the tissues (much like the microwave) and hence the tumor is heated to destruction. Both modalities are operated with laparoscopic contact ultrasonographic scanning.

Cryotherapy device is also used to ablate the endometrial lining of a woman's uterus and reduce heavy menstrual bleeding **(Fig. 28D)**. The cryotherapy device has a slim probe that inserts through the cervix and then into the uterus. Once inserted, a freezing agent is released and the endometrial lining of the uterus is destroyed. The device is intended to be used in premenopausal women with heavy menstrual bleeding due to benign (noncancerous) causes who do not want to become pregnant in the future. Use of cryotherapy destroys the endometrial lining of the uterus to reduce menstrual bleeding. In the pivotal clinical study, 76% of women observed a reduction in menstrual blood loss from an excessive level to normal or less than normal levels.

Tissue Response Electrosurgical Generator

The tissue response generator has unique vessel sealing ability. These vessel sealing produces significantly reduced thermal spread compared to existing bipolar instruments. These generators precisely confine its effects to the target tissue or vessel with virtually no charring and with minimal thermal spread to adjacent tissue **(Figs. 29 and 30)**. These generator uses seal mechanism by sensing body's collagen to actually change the nature of the vessel walls by obliterating the lumen. The collagen and elastin within the tissue melt and reform to create the seal zone. These electrosurgical generator works by fusing the collagen in vessel walls to create a permanent seal. The jaw of electrosurgical forceps using this technology leaves no foreign material behind to potentially interfere with future diagnosis. The system uses the body's own collagen to reform the tissue, creating a permanent seal which resists dislodgment.

Tissue response generator has following advantages:
- It can be used with confidence on vessels up to 7 mm
- It seals all the tissue bundles without dissection and isolation

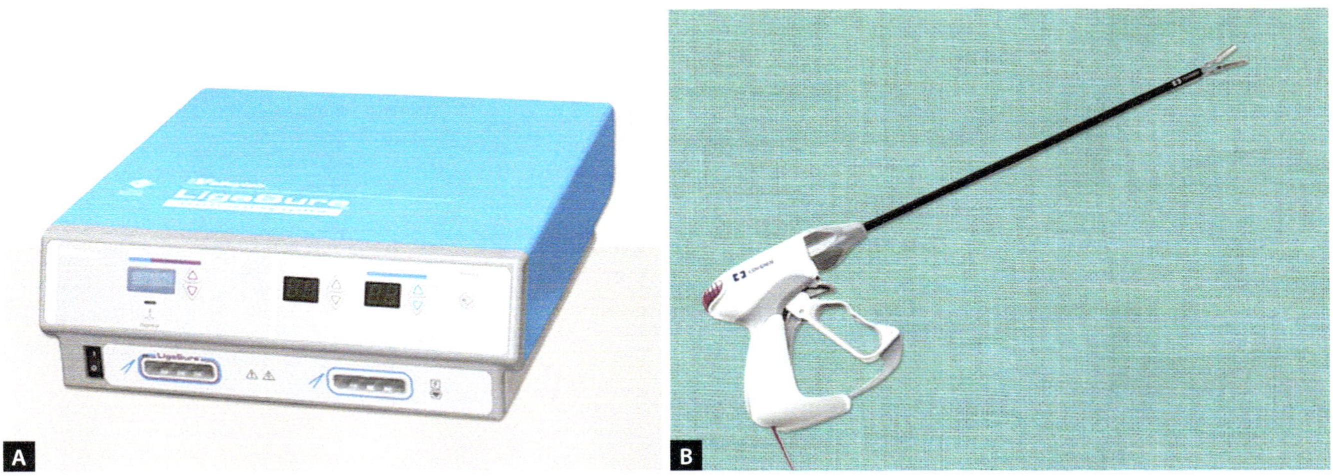

Figs. 29A and B: Tissue response generator (LigaSure™).

- It causes minimal thermal spread
- It has good effect to the target tissue
- The unique energy output results in virtually no sticking

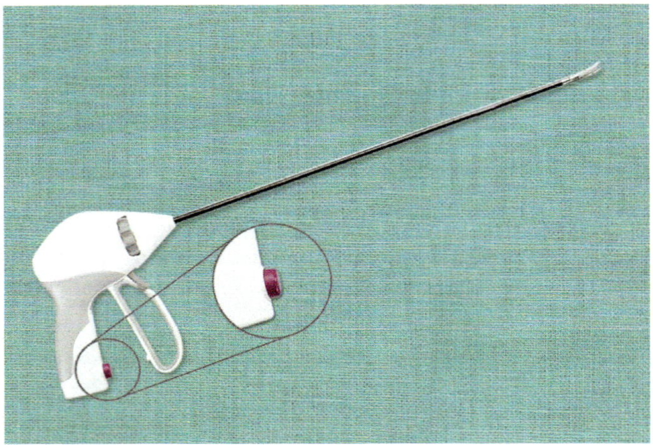

Fig. 30: LigaSure™.

- Reduced sticking and charring
- Minimized need for multiple applications
- No dislodged clips
- No foreign material is left behind.

In 1916, the physicist Lord Rayleigh discovered the effect of cavitation while investigating damage to a ship's propeller. He concluded that the collapse of the bubbles created a small jet stream of water, which was responsible for the structural damage. Using a similar principle, high speed mechanical waves can be used in nonelastic media, such as water, to create a cavitation effect. If this phenomenon is applied to water-rich tissues, such as liver, the final effect is the destruction of all the cells, preserving structures rich in collagen (low in water), such as blood vessels, nerves. The Cavitron Ultrasonic Surgical Aspirator (CUSA) device generates ultrasonic waves in the range of 23 kHz to produce tissue cavitation **(Figs. 31A and B)**. This mechanical energy is delivered through a hollow 3 mm tip that vibrates

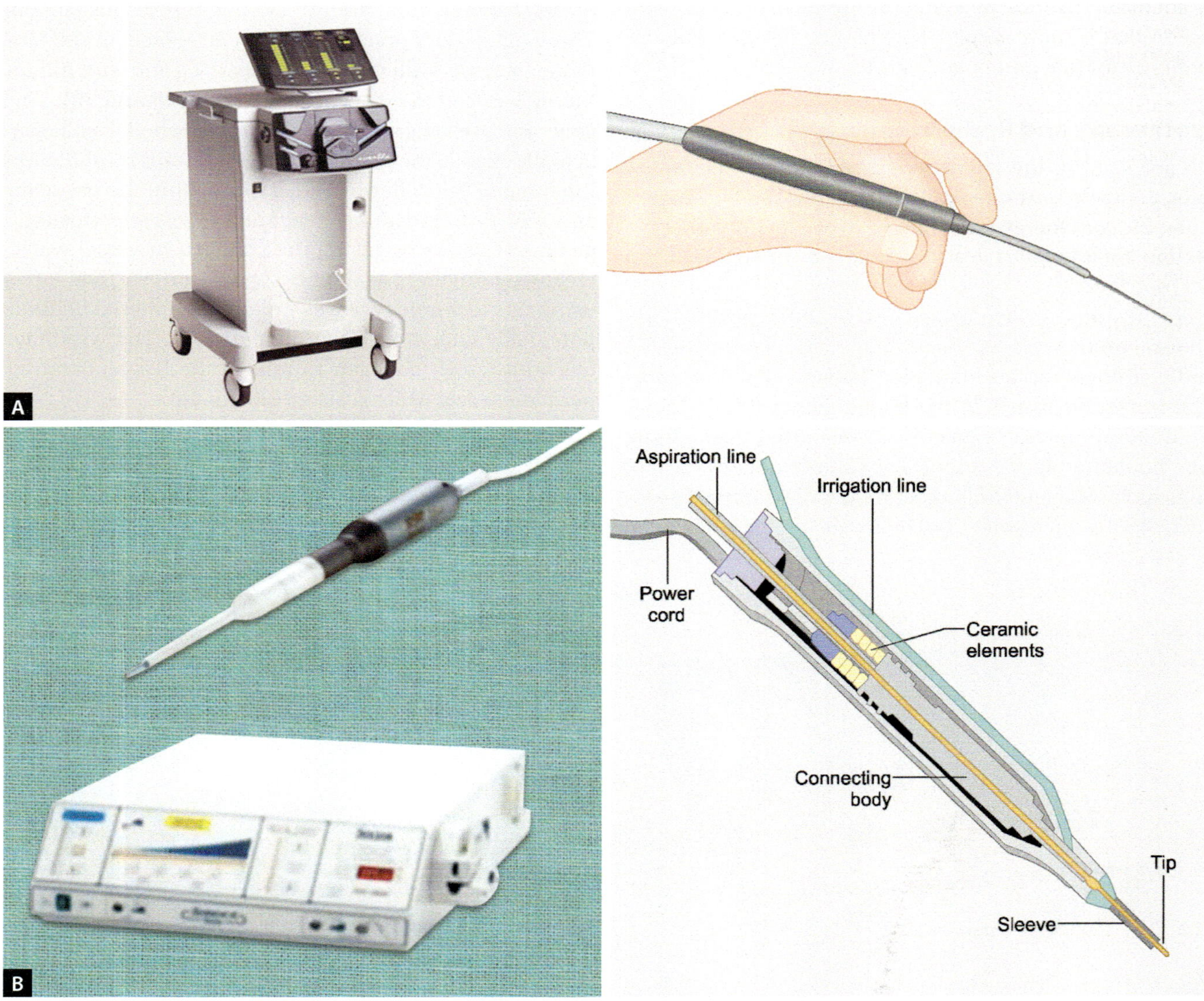

Figs. 31A and B: Cavitron Ultrasonic Surgical Aspirator (CUSA).

at 23,000 cycles per second. The entire device is embedded with an irrigator and aspirator in order to dispose off the tissue debris.

BIBLIOGRAPHY

1. Bagdasarian RW, Bolton JS, Bowen JC, Fuhrman GM, Richardson WS. Steep learning curve of laparoscopic splenectomy. J Laparoendosc Adv Surg Tech A. 2000;10:319-23.
2. Basdanis G, Papadopoulos VN, Michalopoulos A, Apostolidis S, Harlaftis N. Randomized clinical trial of stapled hemorrhoidectomy vs. open with LigaSure for prolapsed piles. Surg Endosc. 2005;19:235-9.
3. Berman RS, Yahanda AM, Mansfield PF, Hemmila MR, Sweeney JF, Porter GA, et al. Laparoscopic splenectomy in patients with hematologic malignancies. Am J Surg. 1999;178:530-6.
4. Brunt LM, Langer JC, Quasebarth MA. Comparative analysis of laparoscopic versus open splenectomy. Am J Surg. 1996;172: 596-601.
5. Carbonell AM, Joels CS, Kercher KW, Matthews BD, Sing RF, Heniford BT. A comparison of laparoscopic bipolar vessel sealing devices in the hemostasis of small-, medium-, and large-sized arteries. J Laparoendosc Adv Surg Tech A. 2003;13:377-80.
6. Crawford ED, Kennedy JS, Sieve V. Use of the Ligasure Vessel Sealing System in urologic cancer surgery. Grand Round Urol. 1999;1:10-7.
7. Delaitre B, Champault G, Barrat C, Gossot D, Bresler L, Meyer C, et al. Laparoscopic splenectomy for hematologic disease. Study of 275 cases. French Society of Laparoscopic Surgery. Ann Chir. 2000;125:522-9.
8. Dexter SPL, Martin IG, Alao D, Norfolk DR, McMahon MJ. Laparoscopic splenectomy: the suspended pedicle technique. Surg Endosc. 1996;10:393-6.
9. Diaz J, Eisenstat M, Chung R. A case-controlled study of laparoscopic splenectomy. Am J Surg. 1997;173:148-50.
10. Dubay DA, Franz MG. Acute wound healing: the biology of acute wound failure. Surg Clin North Am. 2003;83:463-81.
11. Franciosi C, Caprotti R, Romano F, Porta GC, Real G, Colombo G, et al. Laparoscopic versus open splenectomy: a comparative study. Surg Laparosc Endosc Percutan Tech. 2000;5:291-5.
12. Glasgow RE, Yee LF, Mulvihill SJ. Laparoscopic splenectomy. The emerging standard. Surg Endosc. 1997;11:108-12.
13. Goldstein SL, Harold KL, Lentzner A, Matthews BD, Kercher KW, Sing RF, et al. Comparison of thermal spread after ureteral ligation with the Laparosonic ultrasonic shears and the LigaSure system. J Laparoendosc Adv Surg Tech A. 2002;12:61-3.
14. Harrell AG, Kercher KW, Heniford BT. Energy sources in laparoscopy. Semin Laparosc Surg. 2004;11:201-9.
15. Heniford BT, Matthews BD, Sing RF, Backus C, Pratt B, Greene FL. Initial results with an electrothermal bipolar vessel sealer. Surg Endosc. 2001;15:799-801.
16. Horgan PG. A novel technique for parenchymal division during hepatectomy. Am J Surg. 2001;181:236-7.
17. Howard TJ, Mimms S. Use of a new sealing device to simplify jejunal resection during pancreaticoduodenectomy. Am J Surg. 2005;190:504-6.
18. Katkhouda N, Hurwitz MB, Rivera RT, Chandra M, Waldrep DJ, Gugheneim J, et al. Laparoscopic splenectomy: outcome and efficacy in 103 consecutive patients. Ann Surg. 1998;228:568-78.
19. Katkhouda N, Mavor E. Laparoscopic splenectomy. Surg Clin North Am. 2000;80:1285-97.
20. Katkhouda N, Waldrep DJ, Feinstein D, Soliman H, Stain SC, Ortega AE, et al. Unsolved issues in laparoscopic splenectomy. Am J Surg. 1996;172:585-90.
21. Kennedy JS, Buysse SP, Lowes KR, Ryan TP. Recent innovation in bipolar electrosurgery. Minim Invasive Ther Allied Technol. 1999;8:95-9.
22. Kennedy JS, Shanahan PL, Buysse SP, Ryan TP, Pearce JA, Thomsen S. Large vessel ligation using bipolar energy: a chronic animal study and histologic evaluation. 7th International meeting of the Society for Minimally Invasive Therapy; 1999.
23. Kennedy JS, Shanahan PL, Taylor KD, Chandler JG. High-burst strength feedback controlled bipolar vessel sealing. Surg Endosc. 1998;12:876-8.
24. Klingler PJ, Tsiotos GG, Glaser KS, Hinder RA. Laparoscopic splenectomy: evolution and current status. Surg Laparosc Endosc. 1999;9:1-8.
25. Lawes DA, Palazzo FF, Francis DL, Clifton MA. One year follow-up of a randomized trial comparing LigaSure with open haemorrhoidectomy. Colorectal Dis. 2004;6:233-5.
26. Meijer DW, Gossot D, Jakimowicz JJ, De Wit LT, Bannemberg JJ, Gouma DJ. Splenectomy revised: manually assisted splenectomy with the dexterity device: a feasibility study in 22 patients. J Laparoendosc Adv Surg Tech A. 1999;9:507-10.
27. Meyer G, Wichmann MW, Rau HG, Hiller E, Schildberg FW. Laparoscopic splenectomy for idiopathic thrombocytopenic purpura. A 1-year follow-up study. Surg Endosc. 1998;12: 1348-52.
28. Muller JM, Desambre R, Junghans T, Bohm B. Extended left emicolectomy using Ligasure Vessel Sealing System. Munich: 116th Surgical Congress; 1999.
29. Park A, Birgisson G, Mastrangelo MJ, Marcaccio M, Witzke D. Laparoscopic splenectomy: outcomes and lessons learned from over 200 cases. Surgery. 2000;128:660-7.
30. Park A, Marcaccio M, Sternbach M, Witzke D, Fitzgerald P. Laparoscopic versus open splenectomy. Arch Surg. 1999; 134:1263-9.
31. Poulin EC, Mamazza J, Schlachta CM. Splenic artery embolization before laparoscopic splenectomy. An update. Surg Endosc. 1998;2:870-5.
32. Romano F, Franciosi C, Caprotti R, Uggeri F, Uggeri F. Hepatic surgery using the LigaSure vessel sealing system. World J Surg. 2005;29:110-2.
33. Santini M, Vicidomini G, Baldi A, Gallo G, Laperuta P, Busiello L, et al. Use of an electrothermal bipolar tissue sealing system in lung surgery. Eur J Cardiothorac Surg. 2006;29:226-30.
34. Schulze S, Krisitiansen VB, Fischer HB, Rosenberg J. Sealing of cystic duct with bipolar electrocoagulation. Surg Endosc. 2002;16:342-4.
35. Shields CE, Schechter DA, Tezlaf P, Baily AL, Dycus S, Cosgriff N. Method for creating ideal tissue fusion in soft-tissue structures using radiofrequency energy (RF). Surg Technol Int. 2004;13:49-55.
36. Shigemura N, Akashi A, Nakagiri T, Ohta M, Matsuda H. A new tissue sealing technique using the LigaSure system for nonanatomical pulmonary resection: preliminary results of sutureless and stapleless thoracoscopic surgery. Ann Thorac Surg. 2004;77:1415-8.
37. Shimomatsuya T, Horiuchi T. Laparoscopic splenectomy for treatment of patients with idiopathic thrombocytopenic purpura. Comparison with open splenectomy. Surg Endosc. 1999;13: 563-6.
38. Steed DL. Wound-healing trajectories. Surg Clin North Am. 2003;83:547-55.
39. Stumpf M, Klinge U, Wilms A, Zabrocki R, Rosch R, Junge K, et al. Changes of the extracellular matrix as a risk factor for anastomotic leakage after large bowel surgery. Surgery. 2005; 137:229-34.

40. Takada M, Ichihara T, Kuroda Y. Comparative study of electrothermal bipolar vessel sealer and ultrasonic coagulating shears in laparoscopic colectomy. Surg Endosc. 2005;19:226-8.
41. Targarona EM, Balague C, Marin J, Neto RB, Martinez C, Garriga J, et al. Energy sources for laparoscopic colectomy: a prospective randomized comparison of conventional electrosurgery, bipolar computer-controlled electrosurgery and ultrasonic dissection. Operative outcome and costs analysis. Surg Innov. 2005;12:339-44.
42. Targarona EM, Espert JJ, Balague C, Piulachs J, Artigas V, Trias M. Splenomegaly should not be considered a contra-indication for laparoscopic splenectomy. Ann Surg. 1998;228: 35-9.
43. Trias M, Targarona EM, Espert JJ, Balague C. Laparoscopic surgery for splenic disorders. Lessons learned from a series of 64 cases. Surg Endosc. 1998;12:66-72.
44. Walsh RM, Heniford BT, Brody F, Ponsky J. The ascendance of laparoscopic splenectomy. Am Surg. 2001;67:48-53.
45. Watson DI, Coventry BJ, Chin T, Gill PG, Malycha P. Laparoscopic versus open splenectomy for immune thrombocytopenic purpura. Surgery. 1997;121:18-22.
46. Witte MB, Barbul A. Repair of full-thickness bowel injury. Crit Care Med. 2003;31:S538-46.
47. Yang HR, Wang YC, Chung PK, Jeng LB, Chen RJ. Laparoscopic appendectomy using the LigaSure vessel sealing system. J Laparoendosc Adv Surg Tech A. 2005;15:353-56.

CHAPTER 9

Laparoscopic Tissue Approximation Techniques

INTRODUCTION

Knots are used since the time of primitive man for trapping animals and making weapons. Today's laparoscopic knots are basically a modification of knots used by Seamen, Fishermen, Weavers, or Hangmen. In much of the literature on laparoscopic surgery, the learning curve for performing the technique is described as steep. In fact, laparoscopy is more than a new technique; it is a completely different way of operating as far as tissue approximation is concerned. The visualization is different, the instruments are different, and the tactile aspects are very different. Laparoscopic suturing and knotting is a skill that requires a great deal of practice: "As a young surgeon in training, you sit up all night, night after night, and tying knots over and over and over again until you become perfect".

There are many ways of laparoscopic tissue approximation, but most commonly used one are:

- Laparoscopic extracorporeal and intracorporeal knots
- Surgical glues which act as a tissue adhesive
- Laparoscopic clips
- Laparoscopic staplers
- Laser welding.

LAPAROSCOPIC SUTURING AND KNOTTING

It is important to remember that knot is either exactly right or is hopelessly wrong and never nearly right.

There are three steps of knot tying:

1. Configuration (tying)
2. Shaping (drawing)
3. Securing (locking or snuggling).

Choice of Suture Material

Ideal Suture Characteristics

The choice of suture material influences wound healing. Ideal suture characteristics include:

- Good knot security
- Adequate tensile strength
- Flexibility and ease of handling
- Inertness and nonallergenic nature
- Resistance to infection
- Smooth passage through tissue
- Absorbability, when desirable.

Surgeons should choose sutures that they are comfortable with and that are suited to the intended application. This choice should be based on the duration of tensile strength. For internal sutures, least number of knots should be used to ensure knot security and avoid an excessive knot burden and consequent foreign body reaction.

Types of Sutures

Sutures traditionally have been classified into natural (i.e., naturally occurring) and synthetic (man-made). The use of natural sutures is declining for a number of reasons such as tissue reaction, infection, and weak knots. Examples of natural sutures include catgut and silk. Suture material is also classified into absorbable and nonabsorbable.

Absorbable Sutures

The natural absorbable (catgut) tend to have unpredictable rates of absorption and tissue reaction. For the most part, these sutures have short half-lives, so they are not good for wound closure where strength is desirable. Their use is being discontinued.

The synthetic absorbable are broken down by hydrolyzation. They generally have a longer half-life, less tissue reaction, and a more consistent breakdown rate. The synthetic absorbable, polyglycolic acid (Dexon®) or polyglactin 910 (Vicryl®), has decreased tissue reaction compared to the natural absorbable. Knot security is fair and can be used for extracorporeal knotting.

Polyglactin 910 (Vicryl®) keeps 75% of its tensile strength for about 2 weeks and 50% by 3 weeks. The coated sutures decrease the drag through tissue, so it is easier to use, but there are variable rates of absorption. Polyglactin 910 is a good suture material for intracorporeal suturing.

Poliglecaprone 25 (Monocryl®) is a monofilament product that has easy passage through tissue, good handling, and is inert. It keeps tensile strength for only a week, but stays in the wound for almost 4 months. It is good for anastomosis, gynecologic work, and small vessel ligation and epithelial approximation. This material can be used for both extra- and intracorporeal suturing.

The delayed absorbable monofilament sutures such as polydioxanone (PDS®) and polyglyconate (Maxon®), used for abdominal wound closure, have good tensile strength and low tissue reaction, but the knots are not as strong. PDS is considered as ideal material for extracorporeal knotting by many surgeons and gynecologists.

Polydioxanone is also good for contaminated fields because it has a low affinity for bacteria. It is good for general use, tissue approximation, biliary work, anastomosis, fascial closures, heart surgery, and orthopedics.

Panacryl® is a braided synthetic absorbable suture. It has good tensile strength, low tissue reaction, and fairly good knot security. It maintains 60% of its tensile strength at 6 months. It may be a good substitute for a nonabsorbable suture because it has complete absorption in 2.5 years. It is good for fascial closures, closing tissues under tension, and it might have a role in the compromised patient where you presume that there is going to be inadequate or delayed wound healing.

Nonabsorbable Sutures

The natural nonabsorbables, cotton and silk, should be relegated to the past. Even though they have good knot security and are easy to tie, they provoke a lot of tissue reaction. Synthetic nonabsorbable sutures in common use include nylon, polyester, and stainless steel. The role of this material in laparoscopic surgery is very limited and can be used if the other materials are not available.

Suture Size

The narrower the suture, the lower is its tensile strength. Narrower sutures cause less scarring. In addition, a narrower suture will harbor fewer bacteria.

Surgeons should use the smallest suture that they are comfortable with and that will give optimal security of wound closure with minimal wound tension.

Usually, 2/0 or 3/0 is used in most of the minimal access surgical procedure with the exception of the fallopian tube, where 6/0 may be preferred.

Knots

The knot is the most important part of the suture closure *in vivo*; the knot is the determining factor in suture strength in 95% of sutures tested. Complex knots have twice the security of simple knots.

However, increasing complexity of the knot simply leads to the suture strength being the weak link. The size of the knot is also important. If you use the same suture and increase from three to five throws, the foreign body volume is increased by 50%.

LAPAROSCOPIC NEEDLE

In general surgery, needles are either straight or curved. With increasing proficiency, curved needle can also be used but in laparoscopic surgery most intuitive needle is Endoski needle. Endoski needle has advantage of both straight and curved needle **(Fig. 1A)**.

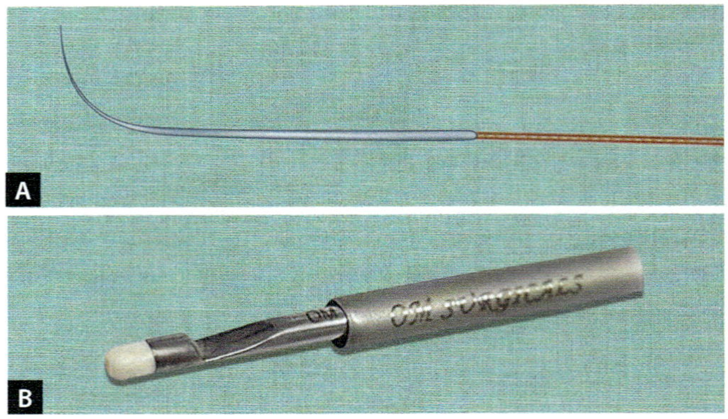

Figs. 1A and B: (A) Endoski needle; (B) Bhandarkar Knot Pusher.

Endoski Needle

The distal end is tapered half circle and proximal shaft of the needle is straight. The shaft of the needle is 1.5 times the length of curved portion of Endoski needle.

In our day-to-day practice, we can convert half-circled needle into Endoski-shaped needle by making proximal half of the needle straight.

LAPAROSCOPIC SUTURE MATERIAL

Although it is a personal preference and varies surgeon to surgeon but considering handicap of laparoscopic setting following is recommended:

- For extracorporeal suturing of small tubular structure such as cystic duct and small blood vessels—dry chromic catgut
- For extracorporeal suturing of thick tubular structure such as appendix and large blood vessels—PDS
- For intracorporeal continuous or interrupted suturing— Vicryl®
- For intracorporeal interrupted suturing in the repair of hernia, fundoplication, and rectopexy—dacron (polyester) or silk.

Types of Laparoscopic Surgical Knots

- *Extracorporeal (tied outside the body and then slipped inside using a push rod)*:
  - Roeder's knot
  - Meltzer's knot
  - Tayside knot
- *Intracorporeal (tied with the help of needle holder within the body cavity)*:
  - Square knot
  - Surgeon's knot
  - Tumble square knot
  - Dundee jamming knot
  - Aberdeen termination.

A long length of ligature is required (90 cm) for extracorporeal suturing. It must be long enough to have the knot pusher threaded onto it, to be passed into the abdomen, round the structure to be ligated and to be brought out again, and still have sufficient length for the surgeon to tie his/her knot effectively. The type of extracorporeal knot chosen to complete the loop depends on the clinical situation and the material used.

Roeder's Knot (Figs. 2A to L)

Roeder's knot is one of the most used extracorporeal knot. Bhandarkar Knot Pusher is ideal to tie extracorporeal all the knots including Roeder's knot **(Fig. 1B)**. The index finger of the assistant may be used to make extracorporeal knot. The left hand should be used to hold the short limb and the right hand should be used to hold the long limb of thread. The short limb of the thread is crossed over the long limb. The intersection point of thread should be pinched by left hand index finger and thumb. At the time of making intersection, surgeon should keep sufficient length of short limb to make it comfortably. It is important to remember that left hand is used only to hold the intersection point while the right hand will make the necessary hitches and loops.

Properly configured Roeder's knot loop diameter should be approximately 4 cm. Large size loop is difficult to manipulate inside the abdominal cavity and very short loop

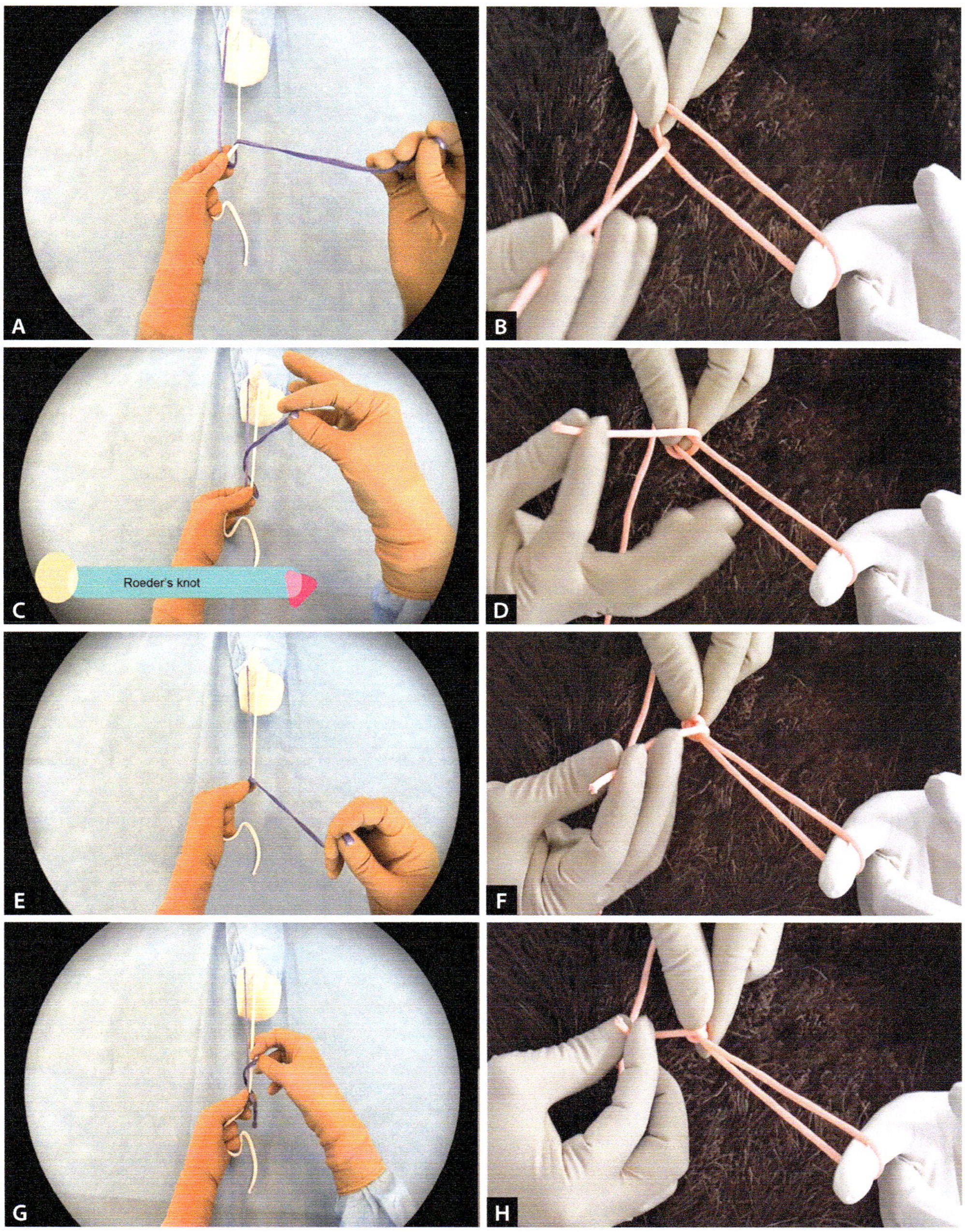

Figs. 2A to H

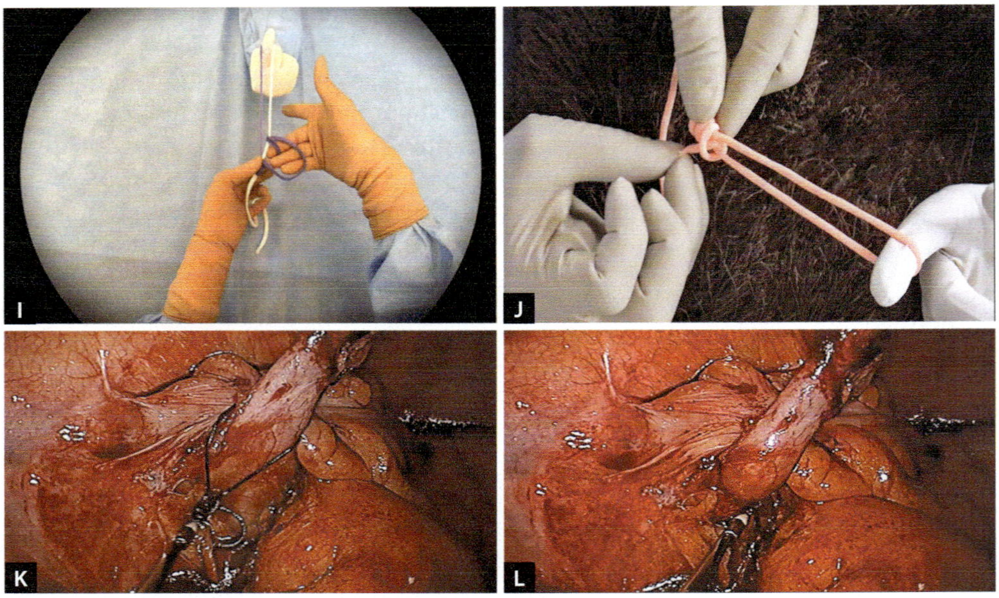

Figs. 2I to L

Figs. 2A to L: (A and B) First hitch; (C and D) First wind; (E and F) Second wind; (G and H) Third wind; (I and J) The last lock (half knot); and (K and L) Roeder's knot applied on the appendix.

is difficult to reach up to the base of the structure which is to be tied.

Roeder's knot can be remembered as 1:3:1.

- One hitch
- Three winds
- One locking hitch.

The steps below describe how to tie Roeder's knot:

- The length of suture used in the extracorporeal knot for free structure is 90 cm.
- Take the Bhandarkar Knot Pusher in left hand and pass 2 cm suture through the eye in the tail end of the Bhandarkar Knot Pusher by right hand.
- The knot pusher is now reversely feed in the 3 mm reducer. Reverse feeding is important.
- Once the reducer is feeded, the thread is pulled out from the eye of the tail of knot pusher. The job of the eye in the tail is just to pass the suture safely from the reducer.
- Now the other end of the suture is passed through the eye of the head end using right hand.
- Ask the assistant for a finger and the extracorporeal slip knot is tied.
- The configuration of Roeder's knot is 1-3-1 in which the first 1 stands for the single hitch, 3 stand for three winds, and 1 stands for single lock at the end.
- After making the knot, make the diameter of loop 6 cm by sliding the loop by right hand finger and thumb.
- After that, hide the knot and its loop under the reducer.
- Now the knot pusher and the reducer are introduced through the 5-mm or 10-mm port. If it is introduced through the 10-mm port, additional 5 mm reducer should be introduced over 3 mm reducer to prevent the leakage of the gas.
- An atraumatic grasper should also be introduced from the contralateral port.
- The loop of the knot should go near the free structure.
- The atraumatic grasper should have introduced in the loop and after that it should hold the tip of the free structure over which you want to tie.
- Now the knot pusher should go to feed the loop behind the structure. The same way like our hands goes behind when we put garland on someone's neck.
- The knot now can be slide to the desire place where you want to tie the knot by stabilizing the knot pusher with left hand and pulling the suture with right hand.
- It should be done in such a fashion that structure should not know that it is getting tied. Any traction of pulling and pushing should never be exerted over the tubular structure which you are ligating.
- After tightening the knot consecutively three times, the knot pusher and 3 mm reducer are pulled and hook scissors are introduced from the same port and the suture is cut leaving 1 cm tail.
- The extracorporeal Roeder's knot is very strong knot and one knot is sufficient to tie any tubular structure like appendix, fallopian tube, a piece of omentum, small pedunculated myoma, or paraovarian simple cyst.

Meltzer's Slip Knot (Figs. 3A to U)

This modification of the Roeder's knot was described in 1991 by Meltzer for use with PDS and has now superseded the use of Roeder's knot. It has components:

- Two hitches
- Three winds
- Two half locking hitches.

  Meltzer's knot can be remembered as 2:3:2.

Tying a Meltzer's knot: Following are the steps to tie extracorporeal Meltzer's knot:

- The length of suture used in the extracorporeal knot for free structure should be 90 cm or 120 cm.
- Take the Bhandarkar Knot Pusher in left hand and pass 2 cm suture through the eye in the tail end of the Bhandarkar Knot Pusher by right hand.
- The knot pusher is now reversely feed in the 3 mm reducer. Reverse feeding is important.

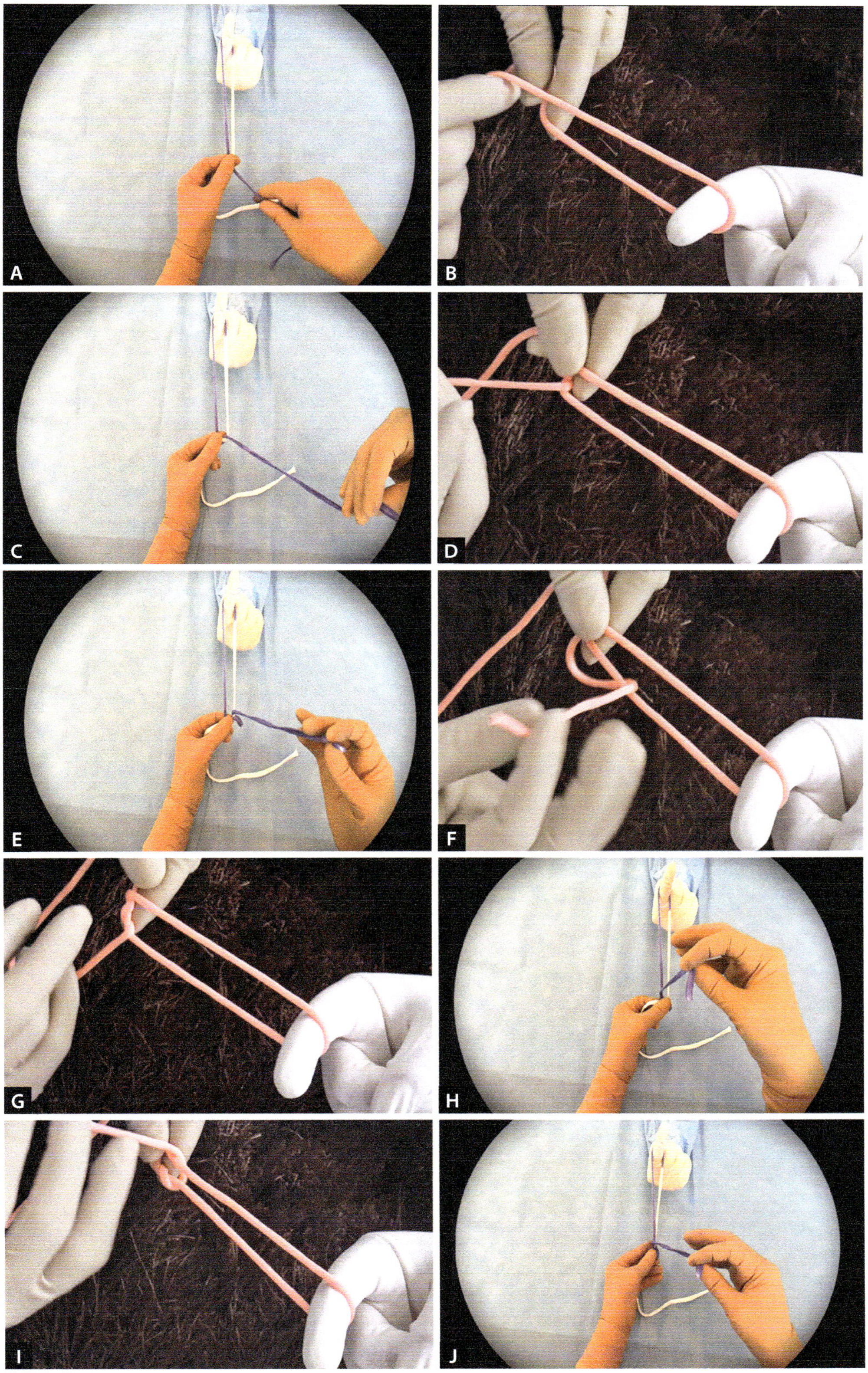

Figs. 3A to J

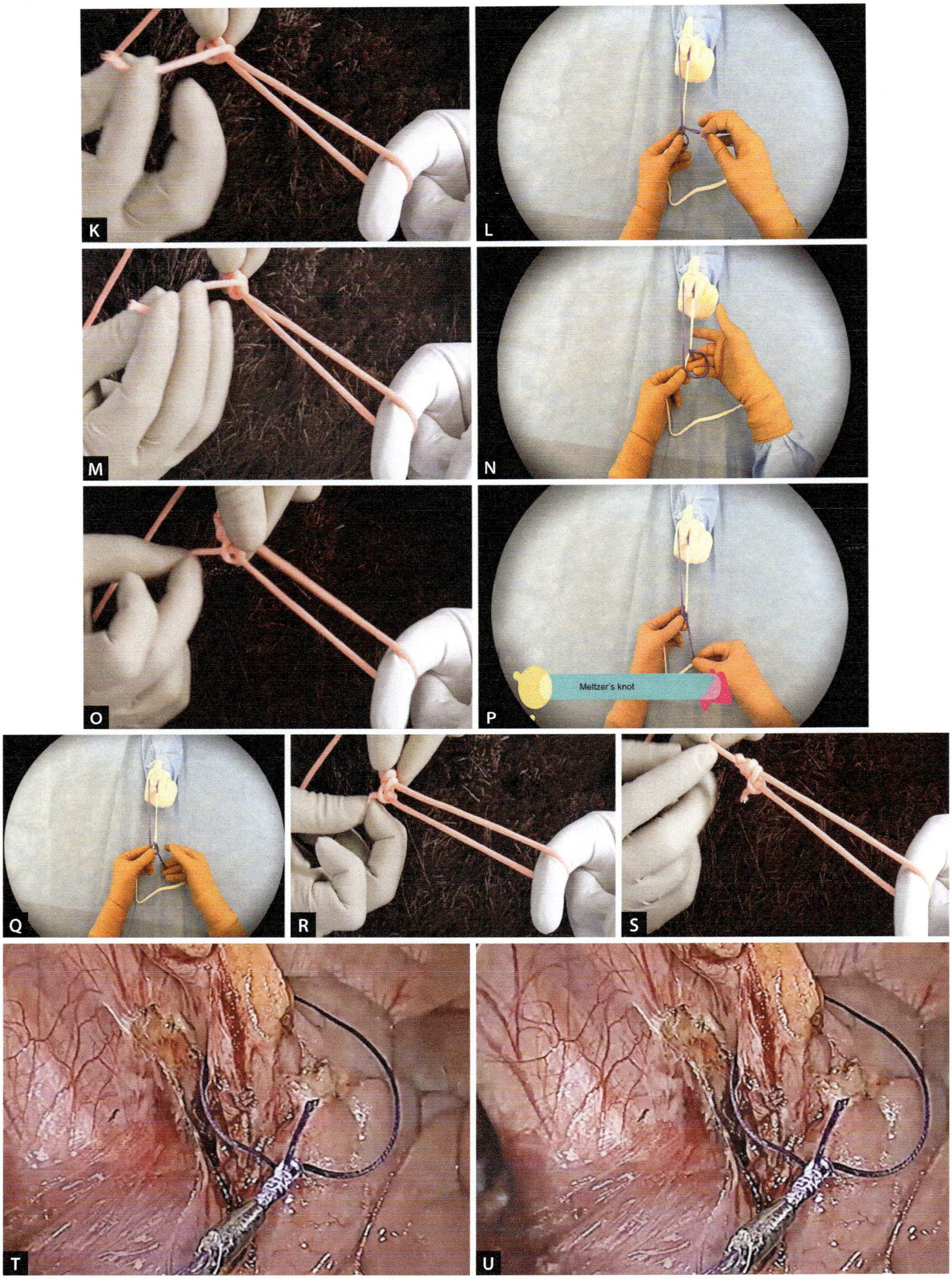

Figs. 3K to U

Figs. 3A to U: (A and B) Shorter thread (suture) over the longer thread; (C and D) First hitch; (E and F) Second hitch; (G) Both the hitch; (H and I) First wind; (J and K) Second wind; (L and M) Third wind; (N and O) First lock (first half knot); (P and Q) Second lock (second half knot); (R) Completion of Meltzer's knot; (S) Complete Meltzer's knot ready to slide; and (T and U) Meltzer's knot tied to the appendix.

- Once the reducer is feeded, the thread is pulled out from the eye of the tail of knot pusher. The job of the eye in the tail is just to pass the suture safely from the reducer.
- Now the other end of the suture is passed through the eye of the head end using right hand.
- Ask the assistant for a finger and the extracorporeal slip knot is tied. You always start tying the knot putting the shorter end of the suture over the longer.
- There are three types of extracorporeal knot: (1) Roeder's knot, (2) Meltzer's knot, and (3) Mishra's knot. Meltzer's knot is ideal for monofilament suture materials.
- The configuration of Meltzer's knot is 2:3:2 in which the 2 stand for two hitches.
- The 3 stand for three consecutive winds.
- The last 2 stand for two locks (half knot). This knot is secure up to 12 mm tubular structure.
- Make the diameter of loop 6 cm by sliding the loop by right hand finger and thumb.
- After that, hide the knot and its loop under the reducer.
- Now the knot pusher and the reducer are introduced through the 5-mm or 10-mm port. If it is introduced through the 10-mm port, additional 5 mm reducer should be introduced over 3 mm reducer to prevent the leakage of the gas.
- An atraumatic grasper should also be introduced from the contralateral port.
- The loop of the knot should go near the free structure.
- The atraumatic grasper should have introduced in the loop and after that it should hold the tip of the free structure over which you want to tie.
- Now the knot pusher should go to feed the loop behind the structure. The same way like our hands goes behind when we put garland on someone's neck.
- The knot now can be slide to the desire place where you want to tie the knot by stabilizing the knot pusher with left hand and pulling the suture with right hand.
- It should be done in such a fashion that structure should not know that it is getting tied. Any traction of pulling and pushing should never be exerted over the tubular structure which you are ligating.
- After tightening the knot consecutively three times, the knot pusher and 3 mm reducer are pulled and hook scissors are introduced from the same port and the suture is cut leaving 1 cm tail.
- The extracorporeal Meltzer's knot is extraordinarily strong knot and one knot is sufficient to tie any tubular structures such as appendix, fallopian tube, a piece of omentum, small pedunculated myoma, or paraovarian simple cyst.

Applications: The Meltzer's knot is now used by most of the surgeons instead of the Roeder's knot to tie the medial end of the cystic duct during cholecystectomy and to fix the cystic duct drainage cannula after transcystic clearance of ductal stones, as catgut is no longer available **(Figs. 4A to C)**. PDS is the suture material of choice for Meltzer's knot.

Tayside Knot (Figs. 5A to O)

The Tayside knot is safe for use with any braided material. It supplies a degree of resistance to reverse slippage equivalent to a surgeon's knot.

- *Step 1*: A single hitch is taken first just as Roeder's knot.
- *Step 2*: Four and half rounds are taken approximately 1 cm below the first hitch over long limb of thread.
- *Step 3*: A locking hitch is made by passing tail through the second and third loop.
- *Step 4*: Finally the first hitch is brought closer to the locking hitch by spreading the first loop.
- *Step 5*: The knot is stacked properly and the extra tail (if any) is cut. Once the knot is configured properly, it should be checked by sliding over the long thread.

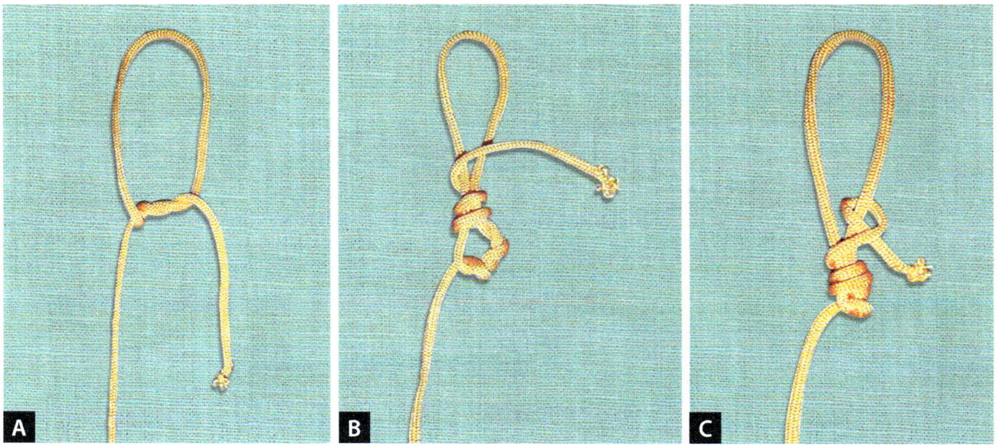

Figs. 4A to C: Steps of Meltzer's slip knot.

Applications: The Tayside knot is suitable for use with all braided sutures (2/0 or stronger) as well as Dacron. It is used with Dacron for ligation of vessels such as the azygous vein, splenic artery/vein, or the inferior mesenteric artery/vein.

Using a Pretied Loop (Fig. 6)

- The loop is drawn up into the metal sleeve.
- The tube is then introduced through an abdominal port.
- Once inside the abdomen, the loop is advanced using the push rod.
- A grasping forceps are placed through the loop and used to grasp the tissue to be ligated.
- The loop is delivered over the tissue and the knot and push rod is positioned at the base of the tissue.
- The loop is then tightened around the tissue by tensioning the long end and applying pressure to the knot via the push rod causing it to slide.
- The knot is locked firmly in place.
- The graspers are removed and replaced by suture scissors to divide the long end prior to removal.

Pretied loops are available commercially. They are packaged with the following items, assembled ready for use:

- A push rod
- A pretied loop
- A metal or silicon introducer tube.

The pretied loop has one long tail of suture material, which is threaded through the plastic push rod and encapsulated by the end. The region at the end of the push rod is designed to be broken, so the thread may be pulled

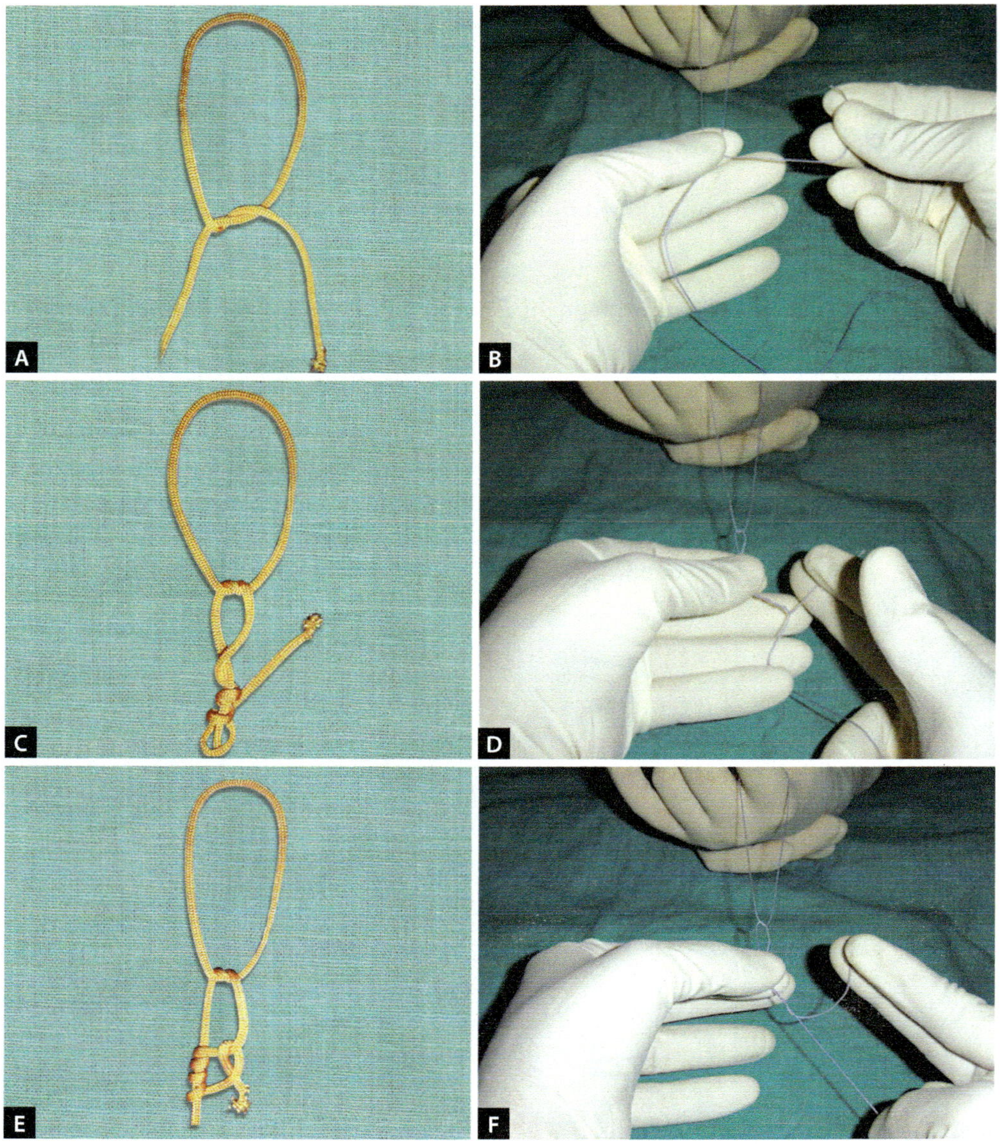

Figs. 5A to F

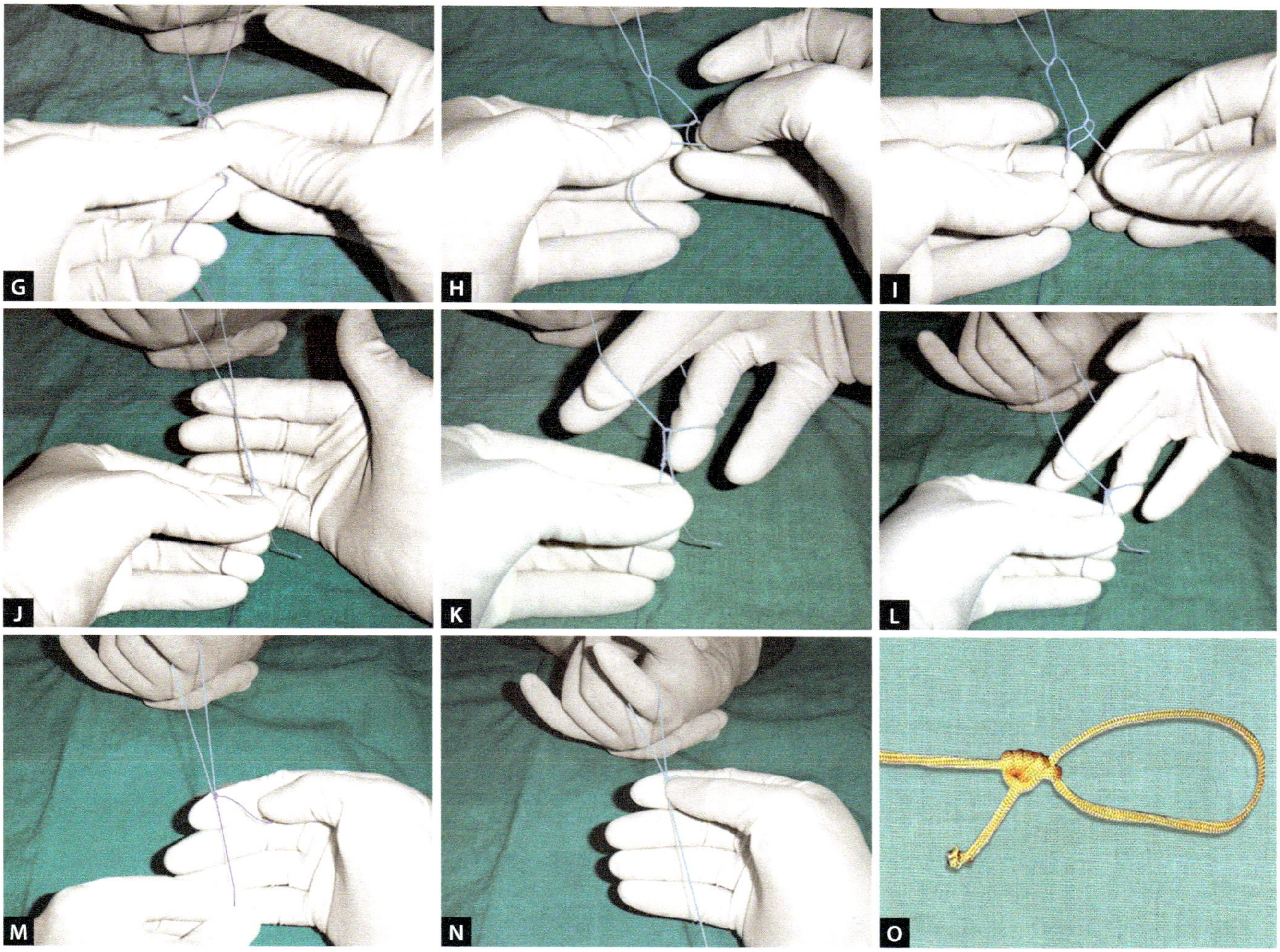

Figs. 5G to O

Figs. 5A to O: Various steps of Tayside knot.

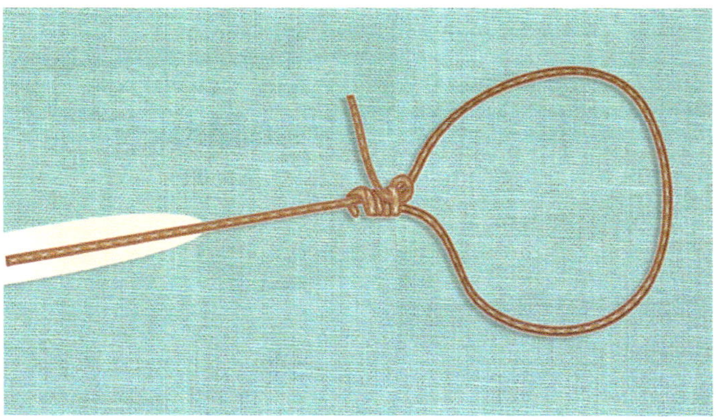

Fig. 6: Roeder's loop.

through the remainder of the rod. The push rod is passed through the metal introducer tube.

Clinical uses: Preformed loops are used to ligate tissue, e.g., the base of the appendix, lung bullae, and a hole in the gallbladder during cholecystectomy. If multiple loops are required, the push rod and introducer can be reloaded with a length of ligature and additional loops fashioned by a surgeon with knowledge of external slip knots.

A preformed loop can also be used to secure a divided vessel after it has been isolated by a grasper. A slight modification of this technique allows it to be used to secure smaller identified vessels. One end is clipped and the other is controlled by a grasper, which has already been passed through a loop. The vessel is divided and the loop slides into place and tightened before the grasper releases the vessel.

Endoloops are also useful for sealing a perforated organ if this is to be removed, e.g., perforation of the gallbladder during laparoscopic cholecystectomy where closure is necessary to prevent escape of gallstones into the peritoneal cavity.

On no account endoloops can be used to close a perforation in any organ that is not going to be resected and removed, as the tissue included in the closed endoloop will slough off a few days later, because of ischemia, resulting in peritonitis.

INSTRUMENTATION

Needle

Endoski Needle

Although conventional open surgical needles (half circle) can be used endoscopically, the Endoski needle developed in Dundee is designed specifically for endoscopic use and is a hybrid of the straight and half circle needle. It carries an atraumatic suture and has a straight shaft and a terminal tapering curve (that corresponds to one-fourth of a circle), giving it the shape of a miniature ski. The shaft is a modified rectangle, which becomes more and more rounded toward the tip so that the curved portion of the needle is round bodied. This combination allows for an easier grip of the shaft by the jaws of the needle holder and smooth passage of the curved portion of the needle through the tissues.

Needle Holders

The most commonly used is 5 mm Cuschieri needle holders. These have single action tapered jaws. The handles are spring loaded and the most recent versions have diamond coating for gripping the suture material without damage. A relaxed "open hand" grip is strongly recommended for these instruments. Please note that there are a wide variety of needle holders (or drivers). In practice, it is vital for each surgeon to become accustomed to a particular type and use that pair all the time. This is crucial for efficient and safe suturing.

Needle Control

Introduction into the Body Cavity

We recommend the use of the introducer tube to protect all ligatures and sutures from the cannula valve mechanisms.

The suture material on the Endoski needle is trimmed to a suitable length. For a continuous suture, this will be approximately 15–20 cm **(Fig. 10)**.

The suture length must never exceed 20 cm as this will result in very difficult intracorporeal suturing since the length is magnified (2.5 times) by the imaging system.

The needle holder is first passed through an introducer tube. The tail of the suture is held next to the tip of the needle and the suture is picked up by the needle holder at its midpoint. It is then withdrawn into the introducer tube until neither the needle nor the tail is visible. The introducer tube can then be passed through a port and the needle is extruded from the tube. The suture is watched into the abdomen and placed on a convenient surface, e.g., the flat, smooth anterior surface of the stomach.

To Insert the Needle

- Pass the needle holder through the reducing tube.
- Pick up the suture material with the needle holder at a point midway from the tip of the needle and the tail of the thread.
- Withdraw the suture and needle inside the tube so that it is completely out of sight.
- Insert the tube through an appropriate port.
- Extrude the needle and suture from the tube by advancing the needle holder and position on a safe surface, e.g., the anterior surface of the stomach.

Manipulation

- A trailing needle is a safe needle.
- A held needle should always be in view.
- Tips of the two needle holders must always be in view.
- Two needle holders must never cross each other by moving parallel to each other from one side to the other.

The ability to maneuver the needle into the desired position in the needle holder jaw is one of the first skills you must acquire. It is well-worth practicing the techniques for this as it will make all subsequent tasks much easier. This task causes much frustration until it can be achieved at will.

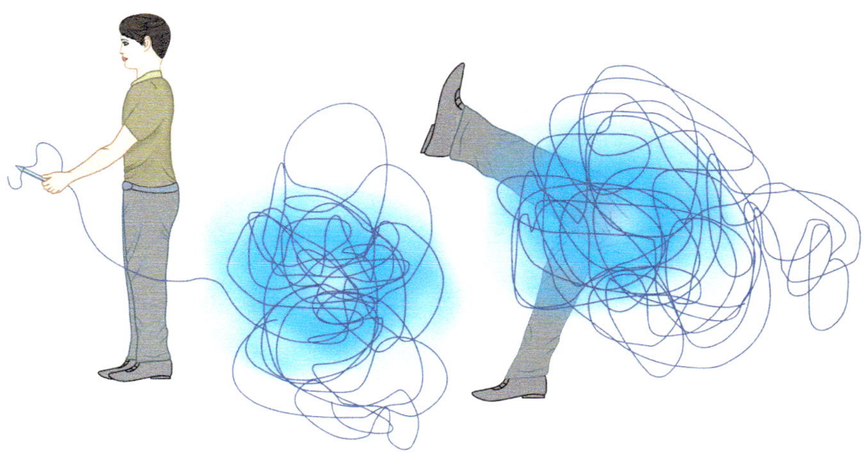

Fig. 10: The length of suture should not be more than 20 cm.

The first step is to arrange the needle to the required orientation on the tissues (preferably on a serosal surface and not fatty tissue). Recommended techniques to get the needle in the right attitude on the tissues include the "nudge", the "push", and the "twist" techniques. This maneuver should be better demonstrated for learning.

Position

The needle must next be positioned correctly in the jaws of the needle holder. Ideally the needle is grasped in the right orientation by the tips of the jaws. It is a mistake to grasp the needle by the back of the jaws as this impairs precision needle driving through the tissues and also reduces the grasping force so that needle swivel is more likely.

For a right-handed surgeon in a straightforward situation, the needle is held in the right hand (RH) needle holder with the tip pointing to the left. The tip of the needle points upward and the shaft of the needle should make an obtuse angle with the shaft of the holder.

The key elements in achieving this are:
- The needle position on the tissues
- The angle of approach of the holder
- The pickup actions.

Adjustments to the angle can be made using:
- Other needle holder
- Surrounding tissue
- Tensioned suture material.

Passage through the Tissues

Position the needle appropriately in the needle holder and identify the position of the first entry point. Place the tip of the needle at this position so that the sharp tip enters the tissue at right angles.

When approximately half of the curve of the needle has entered the tissue (corresponding to 2.0 mm), the wrist is supinated and lifted slightly to passage the curved section of the needle through the tissue. When the point of the needle is seen to emerge at the exit point, the grasp is maintained and the needle end (not tip) is grasped by the other (assisting) needle holder before it is released by the dominant needle holder. For the second bite (in other tissue edge), the dominant needle holder can retrieve the needle directly from the assisting needle holder provided the needle is in a favorable position for direct transfer. Otherwise, it is more ergonomic to drop the needle and pick it up by the dominant holder. Once the two edges have been passaged, the needle is dropped and the suture is pulled to the desired point by an instrument-to-instrument technique through the tissues. A trailing needle does less harm than one that is held rigid in the holder. A grasped needle must always be in view.

Tensioning

A continuous suture is initially tensioned by pulling through the suture material. Further tightening can be achieved by use of the dominant needle holder although one must be careful not to fray or damage the suture. The open jaws of needle holder are placed on the side of the suture as it exits from the tissues. They can then be used to apply counterpressure on the tissues as the suture is pulled tight by the assisting needle driver. Tension in a suture line is then maintained by occasional locking sutures and the appropriate use of an assistant. In clinical practice, tension on the suture line is kept by the assistant using a special suture holder that does not damage the suture which has rounded jaws.

Microsurgical Tying

This is a precise choreographed set of actions. Each maneuver is designed to help make the whole process smooth and reproducible with economy of movement and structured choreography, so that suturing is efficient with minimum of wasted time. Note the following important points:
- The passive and active role of the holders
- The formation of the initial "C"
- Its relation to the tail of the suture
- The conscious assessment of position
- The use of the natural bias of the thread
- Appropriate rotations of the needle active and passive needle holder that must be manipulated in consort
- Note the importance of keeping the ends of the two needle holders in the operative field
- Note the importance of two-handedness for efficient suturing.

Steps of Surgeon's Knot (Figs. 11A to H)

- A "C" loop is made.
- The instrument of the side of "C" should be kept above the "C" and two winds are taken with the help of right instrument.
- Winds are slipped in the line of left instrument.
- Knot is tightened with the help of both the instruments.
- First knot of surgeon's knot is complete.
- A reverse "C" is made and single wind is taken over the right instrument with the help of left instrument.
- Again "C" loop is made and single winds are taken to complete surgeon's knot.
- Surgeon's knot contains double wrap on the first throw, followed by two opposing, alternating single throws.

Tumble Square Knot (Figs. 12A to G)

This is a simple square knot which can be changed to slipping configuration by tightening of a same side of thread.
- A square knot is tied.
- Same side of thread should be straightened with the help of two Maryland or needle holders.

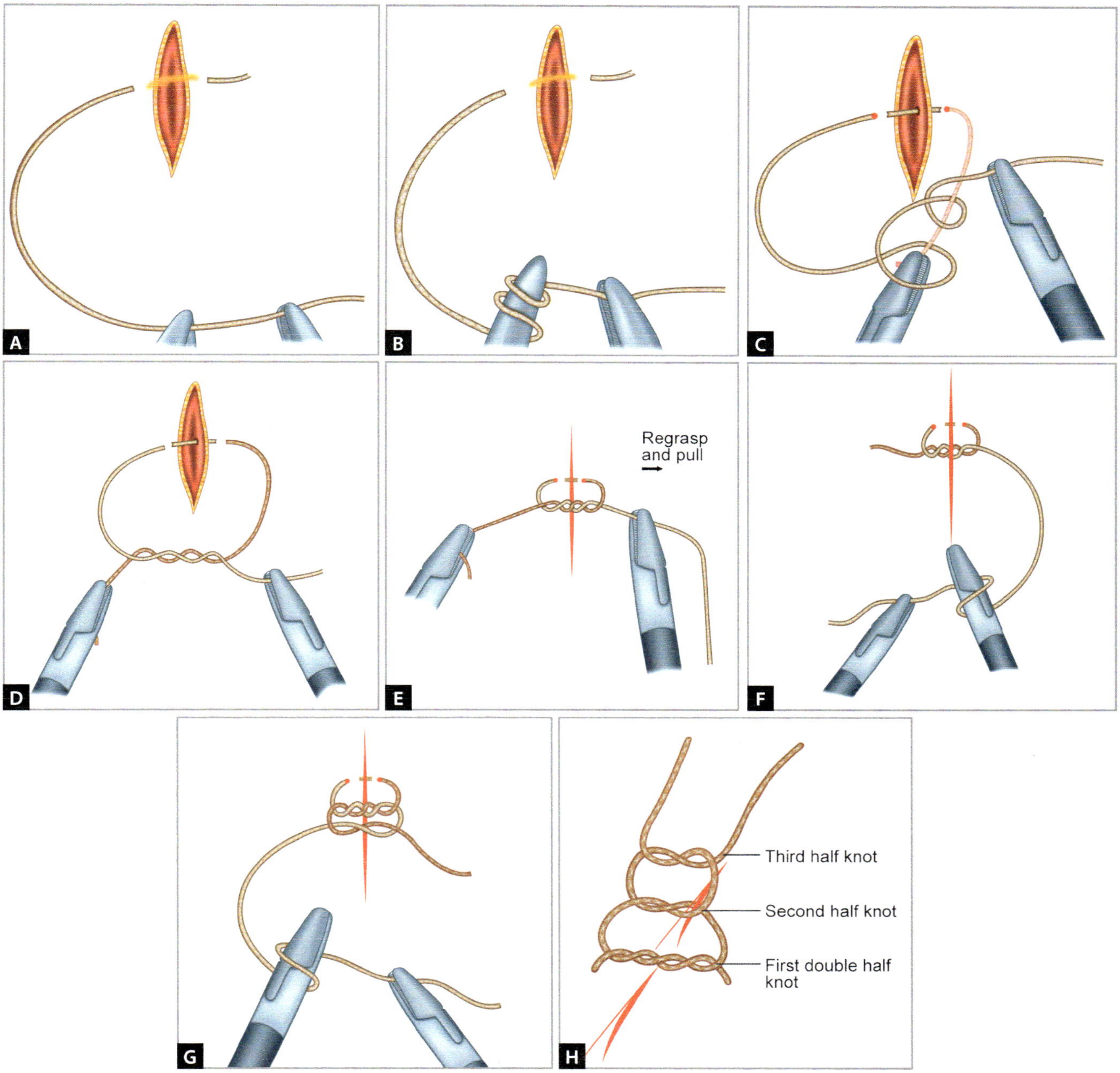

Figs. 11A to H: Various steps of surgeon's knot.

- After straightening of same side of thread, it is ready to slide.
- Closed jaw of Maryland forceps will slide the knot.
- After tightening, the knot is locked again by pulling both the thread.
- One more knot is tied to prevent slipping of Tumble square knot.

CONTINUOUS SUTURING

It is common practice to start a continuous suture with a Dundee Jamming slip knot. An equally acceptable alternative is an internal tied knot if the surgeon is proficient.

A continuous suture can be finished in a number of ways. We recommend the Aberdeen termination, an internal tie to a convenient tail or a slipping loop tied to itself.

Dundee Jamming Slip Knot

This is a recommended way of starting a continuous suture. This knot has an external component but is completed, once inside the body cavity, after the first bite of tissue has been taken.

The external component has following steps:

- A simple slipping loop
- Passage of the tail through the first loop

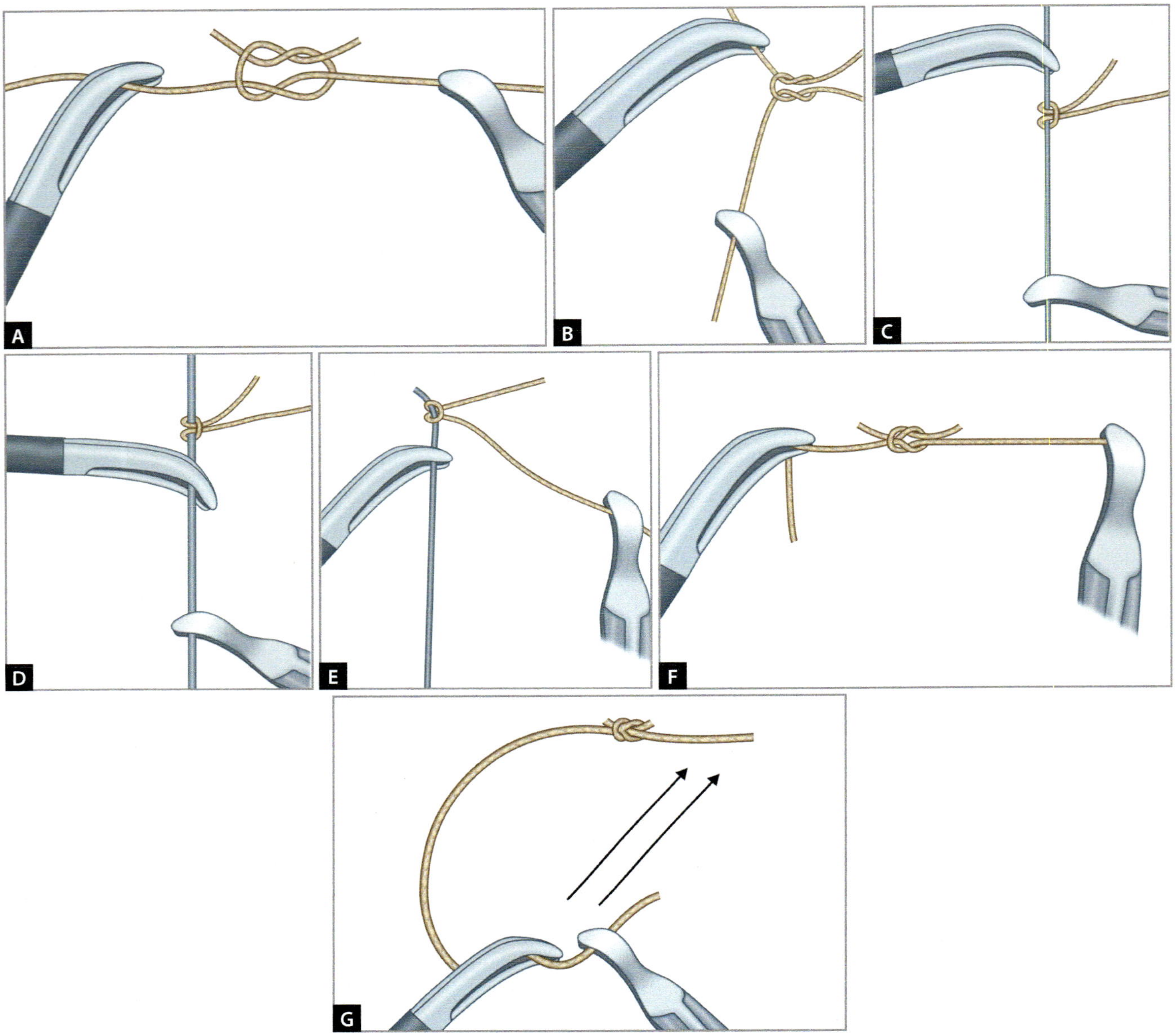

Figs. 12A to G: Various steps of Tumble square knot.

- Creating a second loop
- Tensioning of the second loop.

The second loop should slip only from the tail, the knot should not be tightened at this stage, and the length of both the loop and of the tail should be at least 1 cm.

Once inside, the knot is locked by passage of the standing part of the suture through the loop, which is then slipped to lock the knot.

Starting a Continuous Suture

- Tie the external component of the Dundee Jamming slip knot at the end of an atraumatic suture or start with an intracorporeal surgeon's knot.
- Pass an atraumatic grasper through an introducer tube.
- Pick up the suture at a point midway from the tail of the suture to the needle tip.
- Draw suture and needle completely inside the introducer tube, being careful not to slip the Dundee Jamming slip knot.
- Pass the introducer through the 11 mm cannula.
- Extrude the suture and deposit it on a safe surface (e.g., the anterior surface of the stomach).
- Pick up the needle and take the first bite of the tissue or tissues to be sutured.
- Pull the thread through until the Dundee Jamming slip knot just impinges on the tissue.
- Pass the needle holder carefully through the loop of the Dundee Jamming slip knot and pick up the thread attached to the needle at a point near to its exit from the tissues.
- Pull the needle holder and thread with the trailing needle back through the loop.

- Next take hold of the tail of the loop and the standing part of the thread and pull first on the tail and then on the standing part, locking the knot.
- Trim the tail. You are now ready to start your continuous suture.

Applications

It is used in any continuous suture, e.g., closure of viscerotomies following stapled anastomosis, sutured anastomosis such as cholecystojejunostomy, gastrojejunostomy, etc. It can also be used as an interrupted suture, when additional one or two hitches are advised for security (in our practice, an internally tied knot would be used in preference for an interrupted suture).

Aberdeen Termination

This is an adaptation of a termination commonly used in abdominal closure following open surgery. The continuous suture is finished by the formation of three interlocking loops. In order to simplify the maintenance of tension in the suture line, the penultimate stitch can be locked. A further bite is then taken and the suture pulled through, though not completely. A small loop of suture is left, enough that the needle holder can be passed through it to pick up the standing part of the suture. A loop of this is then drawn through the first loop, which is tightened down onto the tissues. The needle holder is then passed through the new loop to repeat the maneuver three times.

It is important that each loop can be tightened as you proceed. To do this, tension must be applied to the leg of the loop, which exits, from the tissues or the preceding loop. The standing part and needle are delivered completely through the last loop. The standing part is held up and the suture is tensioned with counterpressure from the jaws of the needle holder placed on either side of the suture. The suture is cutoff leaving a reasonable length (approximately 1 cm).

EXTRACORPOREAL MISHRA'S KNOT

Mishra's knot is very string extracorporeal knot which can ligate any tubular structure up to 18 mm. Bhandarkar Knot Pusher is ideal to tie extracorporeal Mishra's knot. The index finger of the assistant is used to make extracorporeal Mishra's knot. The left hand should be used to hold the short limb and the right hand should be used to hold the long limb of thread. The short limb of the thread is crossed over the long limb. The intersection point of thread should be pinched by left hand index finger and thumb. At the time of making intersection, surgeon should keep sufficient length of short limb to make it comfortably. It is important to remember that left hand is used only to hold the intersection point while the right hand will make the necessary hitches and loops. All the movement of right hand is from below up.

Properly configured Mishra's knot loop diameter should be approximately 6 cm. Large size loop is difficult to manipulate inside the abdominal cavity and very short loop is difficult to reach up to the base of the structure which is to be tied.

Mishra's knot can be remembered as 1:1:1:1:1:1:1.

- One hitch
- One wind
- One lock
- Second wind
- Second lock
- Third wind
- Third lock.

The steps below describe how to tie Mishra's knot **(Figs. 13A to R)**:

- The length of suture used in the extracorporeal Mishra's knot is 90 cm.
- Take the Bhandarkar Knot Pusher in left hand and pass 2 cm suture through the eye in the tail end of the Bhandarkar Knot Pusher by right hand.
- The knot pusher is now reversely feed in the 3 mm reducer. Reverse feeding is important.
- Once the reducer is feeded, the thread is pulled out from the eye of the tail of knot pusher. The job of the eye in the tail is just to pass the suture safely from the reducer.
- Now the other end of the suture is passed through the eye of the head end using right hand.
- Ask the assistant for a finger and the extracorporeal slip knot is tied. You always start tying the knot putting the shorter end of the suture over the longer.
- There are three types of popular extracorporeal knot: (1) Roeder's knot, (2) Meltzer's knot, and (3) Mishra's knot. All the knots have different configuration.
- The configuration of Mishra's knot is 1:1:1:1:1:1:1. The first three 1 stands for one hitch, one wind, and one lock.
- The fourth and fifth 1 stand for second wind and second lock.
- The sixth and seventh 1 stand for third wind and the final lock. It is the most secure knot among the three for the structure up to 18 mm tubular structure.
- Make the diameter of loop 6 cm by sliding the loop by right hand finger and thumb.
- After that, hide the knot and its loop under the reducer.
- Now the knot pusher and the reducer are introduced through the 5-mm or 10-mm port. If it is introduced through the 10-mm port, additional 5 mm reducer should be introduced over 3 mm reducer to prevent the leakage of the gas.
- An atraumatic grasper should also be introduced from the contralateral port.
- The loop of the knot should go near the free structure.
- The atraumatic grasper should have introduced in the loop and after that it should hold the tip of the free structure over which you want to tie.

- Now the knot pusher should go to feed the loop behind the structure. The same way like our hands goes behind when we put garland on someone's neck.
- The knot now can be slide to the desire place where you want to tie the knot by stabilizing the knot pusher with left hand and pulling the suture with right hand.

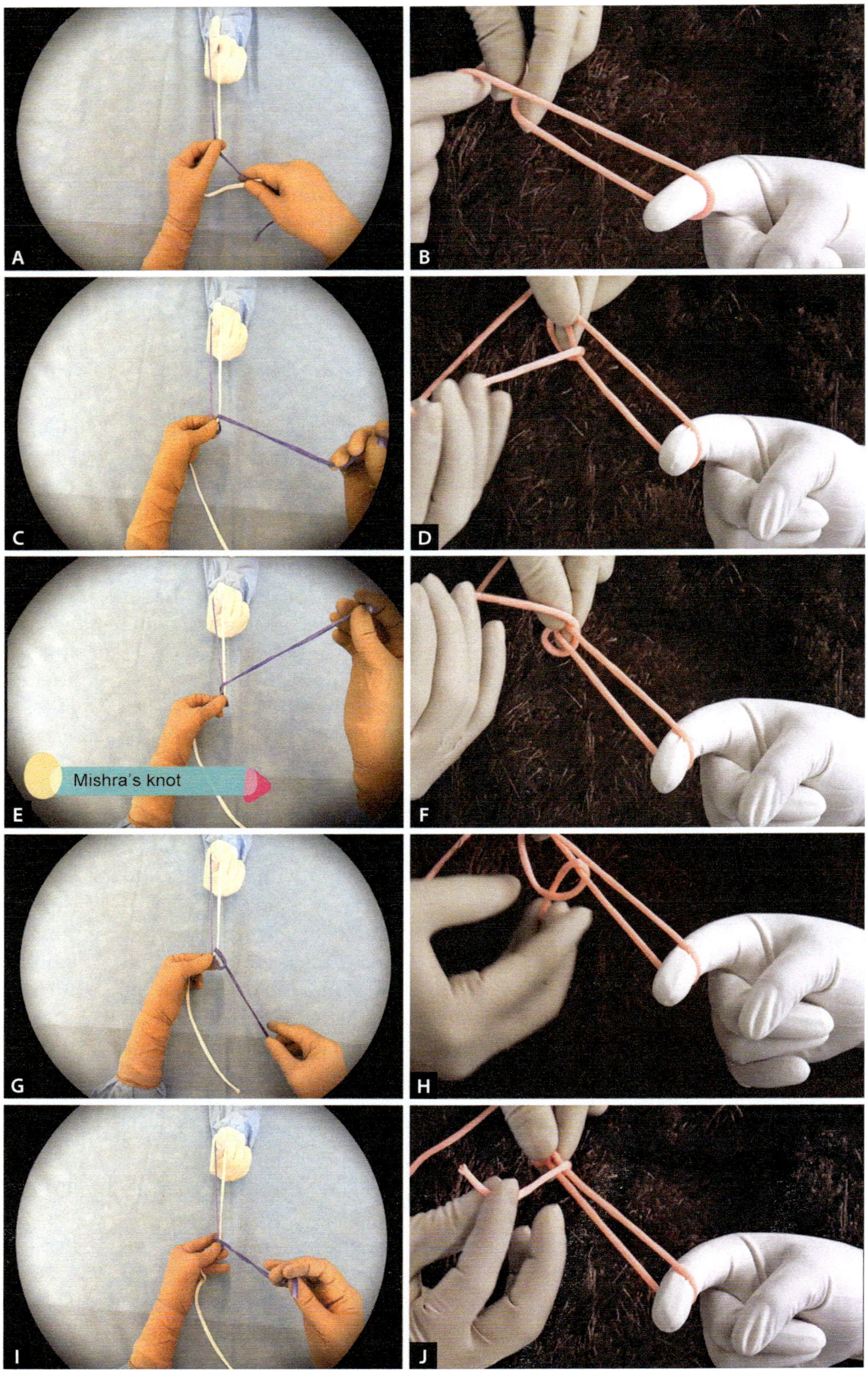

Figs. 13A to J

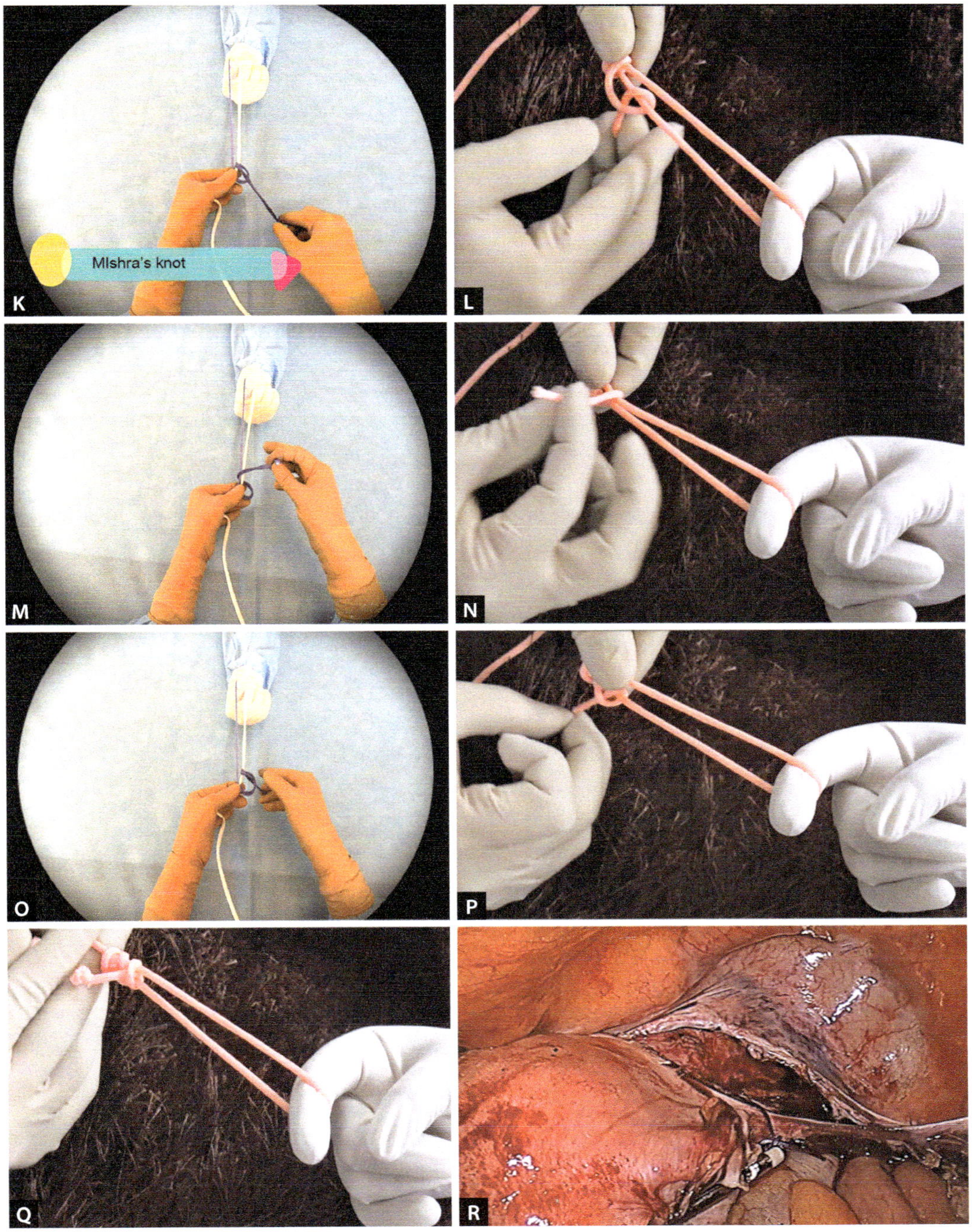

Figs. 13K to R

Figs. 13A to R: (A and B) Shorter left limb is over longer right limb; (C and D) First hitch of Mishra's knot; (E and F) First wind of Mishra's knot; (G and H) First lock half knot of Mishra's knot; (I and J) Second wind of Mishra's knot; (K and L) Second lock half knot of Mishra's knot; (M and N) Third wind of Mishra's knot; (O and P) Third lock half knot of Mishra's knot; (Q) Complete Mishra's knot; and (R) Mishra's knot applied in the uterine artery.

- It should be done in such a fashion that structure should not know that it is getting tied. Any traction of pulling and pushing should never be exerted over the tubular structure which you are ligating.
- After tightening the knot consecutively three times, the knot pusher and 3 mm reducer are pulled and hook scissors are introduced from the same port and the suture is cut leaving 1 cm tail.
- The extracorporeal knot is very strong knot and one knot is sufficient to tie any tubular structures such as appendix, fallopian tube, a piece of omentum, small pedunculated myoma, or paraovarian simple cyst. This knot can also be used to do in mass ligation of cholecystectomy or partial cholecystectomy, ligation of uterine artery, splenic vessels, and renal vessels.

EXTRACORPOREAL WESTON KNOT

Weston knot is an extracorporeal knot which was first started by arthroscopic surgeons but now it is more used by gynecologist. This knot has advantage that there is no need of knot pusher. Another advantage of this knot is that many knots can be applied by only one 9 cm suture. This knot is used to close vaginal vault with needle or to do muffing of gastric band or can also be used for crural approximation in fundoplication.

- Taking suture 790 cm or preferably 150 cm with Endoski needle which is proximal two-thirds straight and distal one-third curved.
- Insert Maryland in the reducer.
- Hold the suture with Maryland at the tail end and pull it out through the reducer and then hold it near the needle and hide it in the reducer.
- Insert the Maryland with the reducer into the abdomen.
- Drop the needle over the tissue in such a way that the tip should be in the left and the tail in the right side.
- Align the needle by the following three techniques:
  1. Pressing the needle by the upper jaw of the needle holder at the junction of one-third and two-thirds.
  2. Holding the needle by the left hand at the curvature and pulling the suture up near the needle by the right hand.
  3. Hang the needle by the left hand like a pendulum and go with the open jaw of the needle holder keeping the moving jaw to the left and dragging it to the right.
- Stabilize the tissue by the left hand and take a bite by keeping the needle at 90° angle to the tissue and rotating the tip of the needle to bring it to the other side.
- Bring the tip of the needle one-third out and catch it with the left instrument, keeping the convex end toward the tissue.
- Guard the tissue by the needle holder, keeping the concave part of the instrument toward the tissue and pulling the needle by the left hand instrument.
- Feed the suture four times.
- Hold the suture by the needle holder as soon as the needle is out.
- The configuration of Weston knot is 1-1-1.
- Weston knot is a self-locking sliding knot, which has one hitch, one reverse hitch, and one final wrap and lock. The steps of Weston knot are **(Figs. 14A to O)**:

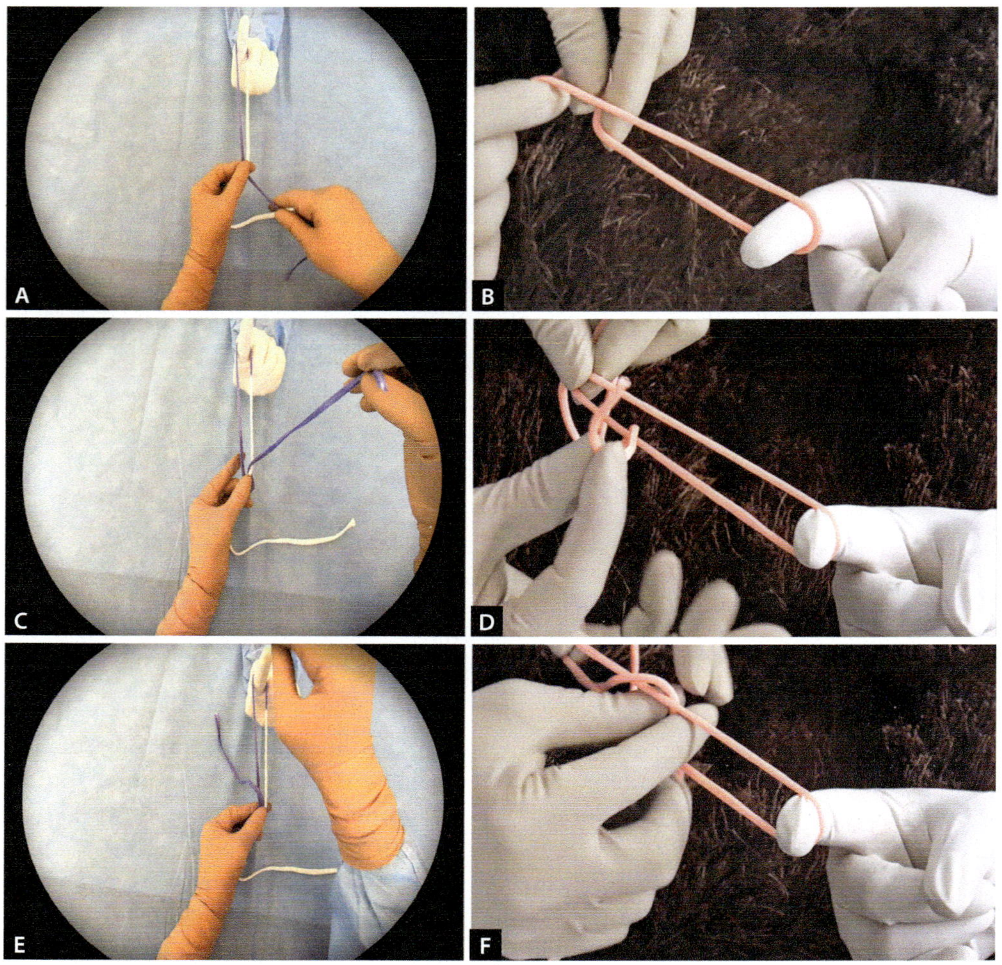

Figs. 14A to F

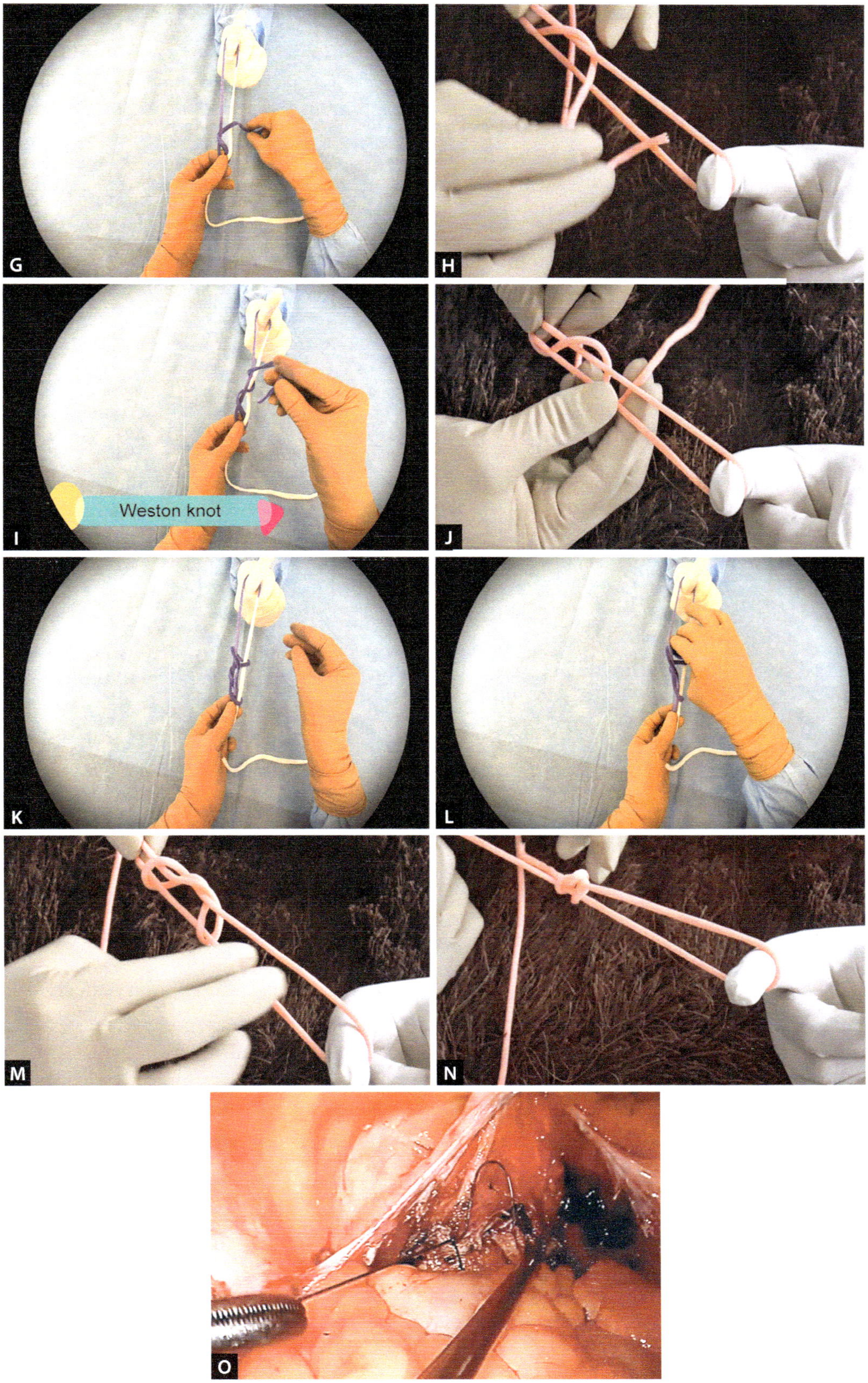

Figs. 14G to O

Figs. 14A to O: (A and B) Shorter thread (suture) over the longer one; (C and D) First hitch; (E and F) Thread placed toward the left side; (G and H) The thread passed between the two limbs to make a reverse hitch; (I and J) Encircling of both the limbs from below upward; (K and L) Encircling both the limbs and locking it in the first hitch; (M) Stacking the Weston knot; (N) Completed Weston knot; and (O) Weston knot applied in the vault closure.

- *Step 1*: The index finger of the assistant may be used to make Weston knot. The left hand should be used to hold the short limb and the right hand should be used to hold the long limb of thread.
- *Step 2*: The short limb of the thread is crossed over the long limb.
- *Step 3*: The intersection point of thread should be pinched by left hand index finger and thumb. At the time of making intersection, surgeon should keep sufficient length of short limb to make it comfortably. It is important to remember that left hand is used only to hold the intersection point while the right hand will make the necessary hitches and loops.
- *Step 4*: The short limb is passed between the thread upward.
- *Step 5*: The short limb should be pulled from up by right hand to make first hitch.
- *Step 6*: The short limb is placed toward the left side and is passed between the two limbs upward to make a reverse hitch.
- *Step 7*: The short limb should encircle the thread from below upward and should be put in the first loop to lock it.

- Now hide the knot in the reducer with or without Maryland and push the knot sliding downward to the desired place where you want to tie by keeping the suture in the left hand and pulling the suture with the right hand.
- After tightening the knot, you can take a final square knot to secure.
- Introduce the scissors from the right port and cut the suture.
- You can again reuse the same suture needle to tie another knot.
- Weston knot is used in gynecological surgeries and also in arthroscopic surgeries. It can be used in situations where suture slides smoothly and freely through tissue and the anchoring device.
- Advantages of Weston knot are:
  - It is a relatively easy knot which can be tied outside, can slip easily into place, and tightly secured
  - It locks readily and is not bulky
  - No knot pusher needed
  - Can be used with the needle to take a bite
  - The suture needle is maintained, so it can be reused for taking another bite.

INTERRUPTED SUTURES

Interrupted Knots

Dundee Jamming loop knot is used to create interrupted sutures. For additional safety, a further hitch or two is recommended if it is to be used as an interrupted suture. More commonly interrupted intracorporeal sutures are made by the use of the surgeon's or the Tumble square knots.

Applications of Interrupted Sutures

Interrupted sutures have a multitude of uses. Simple examples are closure of the common bile duct after exploration and fundoplication.

Stapled Anastomosis

The use of disposable stapling guns has simplified a number of endoscopic procedures such as the division of vascular pedicles and gut anastomosis.

The following important points are emphasized:

- Port positions for stapling
- Stay sutures for tensioning
- Enterotomy positioning and size
- Positioning and angulations of the instrument prior to closure
- Checking suture line
- Complete closure of residual opening
- End-to-end anastomosis can also be carried out by stapling closed bowel ends side by side.

Clinical Applications

An anterior or posterior, side-to-side anastomosis of stomach and jejunum done laparoscopically can be a satisfactory palliative procedure. Likewise, a laparoscopic cholecystojejunostomy may be performed with stapler to relieve jaundice and itching in patients with inoperable pancreatic cancer.

Sutured Anastomosis

Sutured anastomosis can be carried out endoscopically, although the process is demanding in terms of skill and time. However, it is pertinent to note that staplers may not always be available, or appropriate, and even if a stapler is used, you require the skills to perform a sutured closure if the stapled anastomosis is not perfect.

Important points to remember are:

- Port positioning
- Use of communication with your assistant
- Positioning of sutures, especially at the corners
- Spacing the sutures (remember the magnification)
- Tensioning of sutures.

Direction of Suturing

It is important that you suture at the right height, ideally your elbows should be held adducted at right angles. Keep your wrists loose and remember that you have two hands that must manipulate to help each other. The choreography is as follows:

- The suturing line is started with a "starter knot" (surgeon's or Tumble square knot).
- The two needle holders must be kept in view and used in concert with each other.

- Passage from right to left through the tissue edges (bites consisting of entry and exit points) with dominant needle holder.
- The needle is picked up from the exit point by the passive needle holder (NH).
- It is transferred to dominant needle holder for the next bite if the orientation is correct. Otherwise, it is dropped and reorientated in the needle holder. Once the suture has passed through the two edges, the thread is pulled through, handing the suture one needle holder to the other.
- The distance between the suture bites must be approximately equal to the depth of the bites.

TECHNIQUES TO ASSIST IN CONTROL OF BLEEDING

Methods of Securing Hemostasis

Endoscopic surgery is controlled almost entirely by vision. Any loss of view will result in loss of control and a reduction in safety. Hemorrhage, even to a minor extent, tends to obscure the operative field and consequently to be avoided. This means that vessels of a size that in open surgery could be divided without particular attention need to be secured prior to division when working endoscopically. Dissection must be more meticulous to proceed smoothly and you must develop a disciplined approach.

Magnification of tissues by the endoscope may initially confuse an inexperienced endoscopic surgeon as to the severity of the bleeding. A moderate bleed can appear torrential but an inexperienced endoscopic surgeon is well-advised to convert if he have any doubt about his ability to control the situation quickly.

- Pressure on the area applied by grasping adjacent tissue and using this to overly and apply gentle pressure onto the area.
- Compression with pledget swab if the bleeding is not heavy until hemostasis is achieved by clipping or electrocoagulation and the sucker.
- Suction/irrigation to identify the bleeding point prior to securing it.
- Underrunning by suture if the bleeding point cannot be identified.
- Argon spray coagulation for raw bleeding areas.
- Occluding the vessel with graspers before clipping it.
- Application of fibrin and other glues or hemostatic agents.

Avoid Blind Coagulation

Control the initial bleeding and then take your time to identify the bleeding point. In anatomically crowded areas containing important structures, it may be advisable to allow time for the bleeding to stop by compression for 1 or 2 minutes. If bleeding cannot be controlled inside within 5 minutes, serious consideration should be given for conversion to open surgery. This period should be shorter if bleeding is massive or arterial.

Suction and Irrigation

The availability of suction and irrigation is as important for hemostasis in endoscopic surgery as gauze swabs are in open surgery. When bleeding does occur, irrigation can assist in visualization of the bleeding point and suction removes pooled blood and clears clots from the operative site. In addition, the irrigation activates Hageman factor and thus initiates spontaneous hemostasis.

Heparinized Hartmann's solution (1,000 units/500 mL bag) is ideal if clots are present. This solution is preferred to normal saline because of its lesser conductivity, an important consideration when using monopolar high frequency electrocautery. The heparin also reduces the stickiness of the instruments and thus improves handling, especially of suture and ligature materials. It also aids in removal of pooled blood. The bag of fluid is placed in a Fenwal pressure bag raised to 200 mm Hg and hung from a drip stand. As the contents of the bag are used, the pressure needs to be maintained. There are several pressurized irrigation systems available, some heat the irrigating fluid to body temperature, other provide pulse irrigation which is helpful from breaking up blood clots and cleaning the peritoneal gutters.

Suction and irrigation are also essential to deal with leakage from ultra-abdominal organs, e.g., bile leakage, bowel content, perforated ulcer, and appendicitis. In these acute emergency situations, laparoscopic abdominal lavage of the peritoneal quadrants is aided by shaking the patient from side to side and changing the position of the operating table (head up, head down, and sideways).

BIBLIOGRAPHY

1. Ali MR, Mowery Y, Kaplan B, DeMaria EJ. Training the novice in laparoscopy. Surg Endosc. 2002;16:1732-6.
2. Champion JK, Hunter J, Trus T, Laycock W. Teaching basic video skills as an aid in laparoscopic suturing. Surg Endosc. 1996;10:23-5.
3. Croce E, Olmi S. Intracorporeal knot-tying and suturing techniques in laparoscopic surgery: technical details. JSLS. 2000;4:17-22.
4. De Beer JF, Van Rooyen K, Boezaart AP. Nicky's knot: a new slip knot for arthroscopic surgery. Arthroscopy. 1998;14:109-10.
5. Derossis AM, Brothwell J, Sigman HH, Fried GM. The effect of practice on performance in a laparoscopic simulator. Surg Endosc. 1998;12:1117-20.
6. Dunkin BJ, Li Y, Marks JM, Ponsky JL. The "Yenni" knot: a simpler method of intracorporeal laparoscopic knot tying. J Am Coll Surg. 1997;185:492-3.
7. Faulkner H, Regehr G, Martin J, Reznick R. Validation of an objective structured assessment of technical skill for surgical residents. Acad Med. 1996;71:1363-5.
8. Figert PL, Park AE, Witzke DB, Schwartz RW. Transfer of training in acquiring laparoscopic skills. J Am Coll Surg. 2001;193:533-7.

9. Gallagher AG, McClure N, McGuigan J, Crothers I, Browning J. Virtual reality training in laparoscopic surgery: a preliminary assessment of minimally invasive surgical trainer virtual reality (MIST VR). Endoscopy. 1999;31:310-3.
10. Gaur DD. Laparoscopic suturing and knot tying: the Indian rope crick. J Endourol. 1998;12:61-6.
11. Grantcharov TP, Kristiansen VB, Bendix J, Bardram L, Rosenberg J, Funch-Jensen P. Randomized clinical trial of virtual reality simulation for laparoscopic skills training. Br J Surg. 2004;91:146-50.
12. Hamilton EC, Scott DJ, Fleming JB, Rege RV, Laycock R, Bergen PC, et al. Comparison of video trainer and virtual reality training systems on acquisition of laparoscopic skills. Surg Endosc. 2002;16:406-11.
13. Harold KL, Matthews BD, Backus CL, Pratt BL, Heniford BT. Prospective randomized evaluation of surgical resident proficiency with laparoscopic suturing after course instruction. Surg Endosc. 2002;16:1729-31.
14. Hasson HM, Kumari NV, Eekhout J. Training simulator for developing laparoscopic skills. JSLS. 2001;5:255-65.
15. Hay DL, Levine RL, Von Fraunhofer JA. Chromic gut pelviscopic loop ligature. Effect of the number of pulls on the tensile strength. J Reprod Med. 1990;5:260-2.
16. Inoue H, Kumagai Y, Ami K, Nishikage T, Baba H, Yoshida T, et al. A simple technique of using novel thread-holding and knot-pushing forceps for extracorporeal knot-tying. Surg Today. 2000;30:27-31.
17. Jones DB, Wu JS, Soper NJ. Laparoscopic Surgery, Principles and Procedures. St. Louis: Quality Medical Publishing; 1997. pp. 50-65.
18. Kadirkamanathan SS, Shelton JC, Hepworth CC, Laufer JG, Swain CP. A comparison of the strength of knots tied by hand and at laparoscopy. J Am Coll Surg. 1996;182:46-54.
19. Madan AK, Frantizdes CT, Shervin N, Tebbit CL. Assessment of individual hand performance in box trainers compared to virtual reality trainers. Am Surg. 2003;69:1112-4.
20. Madan AK, Frantzides CT. Substituting virtual reality trainers for inanimate box trainers does not decrease laparoscopic skill acquisition. JSLS. 2007;11:87-9.
21. Madan AK, Frantzides CT, Park WC, Tebbit CL, Kumari NVA, O'Leary PJ. Predicting baseline laparoscopic surgery skills. Surg Endosc. 2005;19:101-3.
22. Madan AK, Frantzides CT, Sasso L. Laparoscopic baseline ability assessment by virtual reality. J Laparoendosc Adv Surg Tech A. 2005;15:13-7.
23. Madan AK, Frantzides CT, Tebbit CL, Park WC, Kumari NVA, Shervin N. Evaluation of specialized laparoscopic suturing and tying devices. JSLS. 2004;8:191-3.
24. Madan AK, Frantzides CT, Tebbit CL, Quiros RM. Participant's opinions of laparoscopic trainers during basic laparoscopic training courses. Am J Surg. 2005;189:758-61.
25. Madan AK, Frantzides CT, Tebbit CL, Shervin N, Quiros R. Self-reported versus observed scores in laparoscopic skills training. Surg Endosc. 2005;19:670-2.
26. Martin JA, Regehr G, Reznick R, MacRae H, Murnaghan J, Hutchison C, et al. Objective structured assessment of technical skill (OSATS) for surgical residents. Br J Surg. 1997; 84:273-8.
27. Meilahn JE. The need for improving laparoscopic suturing and knot-tying. J Laparoendosc Surg. 1992;2:267.
28. Mori T, Hatano N, Maruyama S, Atomi Y. Significance of "hands-on training" in laparoscopic surgery. Surg Endosc. 1998;12:256-60.
29. Munz Y, Kumar BD, Moorthy K, Bann S, Darzi A. Laparoscopic virtual reality and box trainers: is one superior to the other? Surg Endosc. 2004;18:485-94.
30. Nathanson LK, Nathanson PK, Cushieri AL. Safety of vessel ligation in laparoscopic surgery. Endoscopy. 1991;23:206-9.
31. Keynes G, Pare A. The Apologies and Treatise of Ambroise Pare containing the Voyager Made into Divers Places with Many of his Writings Upon Surgery. London: Galcion Educational Books; 1951.
32. Pearson AM, Gallagher AG, Rosser JC, Satava RM. Evaluation of structured and quantitative training methods for teaching intracorporeal knot tying. Surg Endosc. 2002;16:130-7.
33. Pennings JL, Kenyon T, Swanstrom L. The knit stitch. An improved method of laparoscopic knot tying. Surg Endosc. 1995;9:537-40.
34. Peters JH, Fried GM, Swanstrom LL, Soper NJ, Sillin LF, Schirmer B, et al. Development and validation of a comprehensive program of education and assessment of the basic fundamentals of laparoscopic surgery. Surgery. 2004; 135:21-7.
35. Pietrafitta JJ. A technique of laparoscopic knot tying. J Laparoendosc Surg. 1992;2:273-5.
36. Reznick R, Regehr G, MacRae H, Martin J, McCulloch W. Testing technical skills via an innovative "bench station" examination. Am J Surg. 1997;173:226-30.
37. Roeder H. Die Technik der Mandelgesundungs bestrebungen. Artzl Rundschau Munchen. 1918;57:169-71.
38. Rosser JC, Murayama M, Gabriel NH. Minimally invasive surgical training solutions for the twenty-first century. Surg Clin North Am. 2000;80:1607-24.
39. Rosser JC, Rosser LE, Savalgi RS. Skill acquisition and assessment for laparoscopic surgery. Arch Surg. 1997;132: 200-4.
40. Rosser JC, Rosser LE, Savalgi RS. Objective evaluation of a laparoscopic surgical skill program for residents and senior surgeons. Arch Surg. 1998;133:657-61.
41. Scott DJ, Bergen PC, Rege RV, Laycock R, Tesfay ST, Valentine RJ, et al. Laparoscopic training on bench models: better and most cost-effective than operating room experience? J Am Coll Surg. 2000;191:272-83.
42. Sedlack JD, Williams VM, DeSimone J, Page D, Ghosh BC. Laparoscopic knot security. Surg Laparosc Endosc. 1996;6:144-6.
43. Semm K. Operative Manual for Endoscopic Abdominal Surgery. Chicago: Year Book Medical Publishers; 1987.
44. Seymour NE, Gallagher AG, Roman SA, O'Brien MK, Bansal VK, Andersen DK, et al. Virtual reality training improves operating room performance: results of a randomized, double-blinded study. Ann Surg. 2002;236:458-64.
45. Sharpe LA. A new device and method for extracorporeal knot tying in laparoscopic surgery. J Gynecol Surg. 1994;10: 27-31.
46. Swain CP, Kadirkamanathan SS, Gong F, Lal KC, Ratani RS, Brown GJ, et al. Knot tying at flexible endoscopy. Gastrointest Endosc. 1994;40:722-9.
47. Szold A. A novel technique for simple laparoscopic extracorporeal knot tying. J Am Coll Surg. 1997;184:523-4.
48. Tarn WW. Alexander the Great: Sources and Studies. Cambridge: Cambridge University Press; 1948. p. 262.
49. Tera H, Aberg C. Tensile strength of twelve types of knot employed in surgery, using different suture materials. Acta Chir Scand. 1976;142:1-7.
50. Youngblood PL, Srivastava S, Curet M, Heinrichs WL, Dev P, Wren SM. Comparison of training on two laparoscopic simulators and assessment of skills transfer to surgical performance. J Am Coll Surg. 2005;200:546-51.
51. Zimmer CA, Thacker JG, Powell DM, Bellian KT, Decker DG, Rodeheaver GT, et al. Influence of knot configuration and tying technique on the mechanical performance of sutures. J Emerg Med. 1997;9:107-13.

CHAPTER 10

Hand-assisted Laparoscopic Surgery

INTRODUCTION

In hand-assisted surgery, the surgeon can insert a hand through a small incision via a special pressurized sleeve. The surgeon makes a small incision in the abdomen and inserts his hand into the patient's body **(Figs. 1 and 2)**.

Hand-assisted laparoscopic surgery (HALS) devices allow for the introduction of the surgeon's nondominant hand into the peritoneal cavity without loss of the pneumoperitoneum. The use of hand-assisted techniques in difficult cases facilitates the surgical procedure and offers an interesting alternative to the purely laparoscopic approach.

Hand-assisted laparoscopic surgery allows for a reduction in the number of trocars compared to the purely laparoscopic approach. The proper placement of the hand-assisted device is one of the fundamental principles of HALS. The hand-assisted device should never be placed directly over the operative field. According to the principle of triangulation, the hand-assisted device is ideally placed in the same position as that of the nondominant operating trocar in the purely laparoscopic approach **(Fig. 3)**.

Hand is ideal for sensory perception and to guide the surgical instruments. Surgeon can manipulate with his other hand while observing the procedure on a monitor. With both a hand and laparoscopic instruments doing the work, the surgeon has more control over the operation and sense of depth and sensation of touch which cannot be gained through the lens of a camera. The large organ can be removed intact, making it possible to evaluate the cancer. The hand-assisted approach is also considered better for surgeons who are still learning laparoscopic techniques. HALS is the use of the nondominant hand intra-abdominally, together with the laparoscopic instruments in dominant hand.

The introduction of the surgeon's hand via the hand-assisted device allows for tactile feedback and complements the information obtained visually. HALS greatly facilitates mobilization of the organs and helps for identification of proper dissection plane, thus minimizing oozing and blood loss. HALS offers several real advantages during the procedure resulting in a significant time gain. This is especially true in obese patients as well as in cases of significant abdominal adhesions **(Fig. 4)**.

The size of the incision for placement of the hand cannula is determined by the size of the surgeon's glove. A retractor-protractor which is an open-ended plastic cylinder with a malleable ring at each end is then introduced into the abdominal cavity through the incision. This provides a seal for the skin wound both at the peritoneal and skin sites and keeps the incision open and also protects the

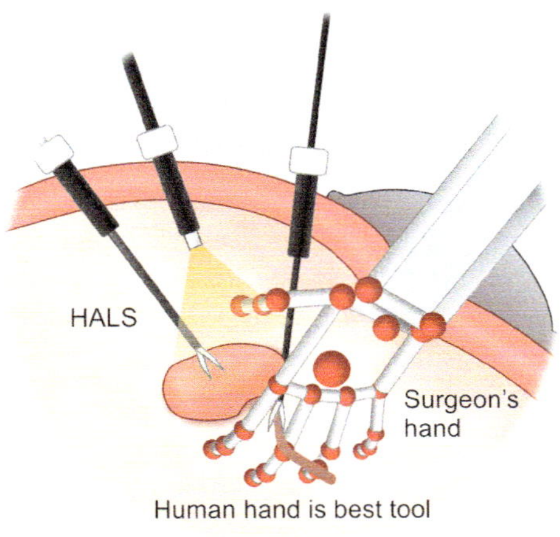

Fig. 1: Options before a laparoscopic surgeon. (HLAS: human-assisted laparoscopic surgery)

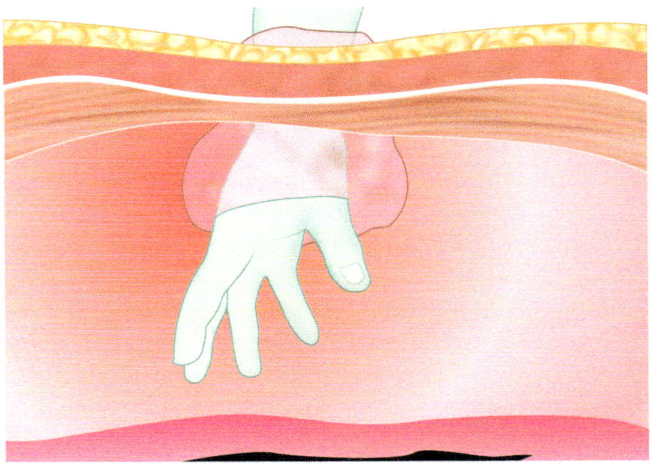

Fig. 2: Positioning through the abdominal wall.

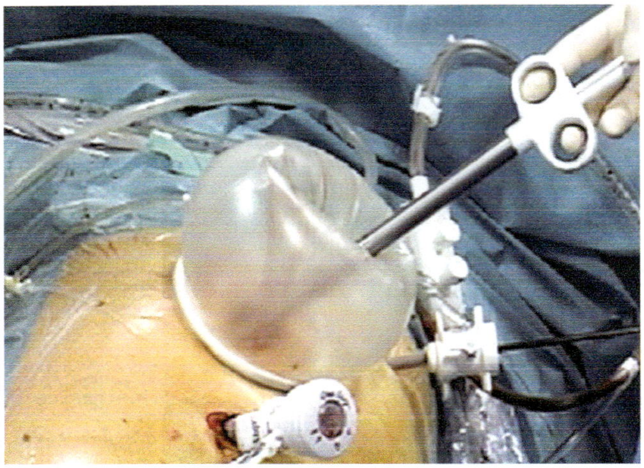

Fig. 3: Introduction of instruments.

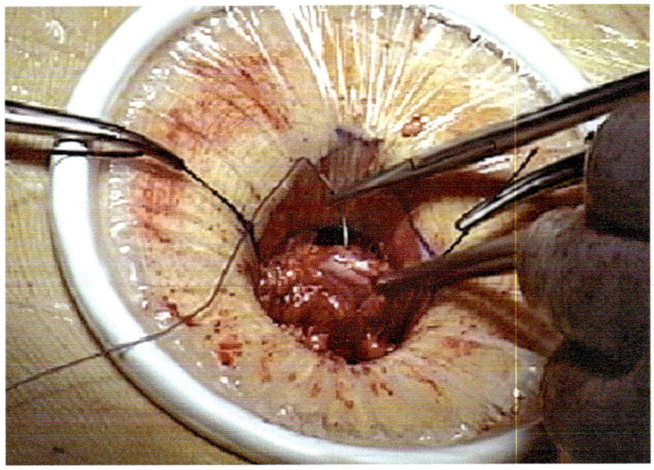

Fig. 4: Working through the port.

wound against contamination by bacteria and malignant cells. The pneumo-sleeve is fitted under hand cannula and manipulated to achieve the best possible angle for the surgeon's arm during dissection. The adhesive packing is removed and the flanges are secured to the skin. A one-way valve located in the sleeve's lumen prevents gas escaping from the abdomen **(Fig. 5)**.

An additional cover is placed on the surgeon's arm, which is impermeable to gas. The pneumo-sleeve is entered and secured to the surgeon's upper arm by means of a Velcro band to prevent gas escape. The hand is then placed through the hand cannula into the abdomen. HALS, open, and laparoscopic procedures are compared in **Table 1**.

Hand-assisted laparoscopic surgery is the use of the nondominant hand through a hand-port device. It is an important adjunctive tool with other laparoscopic instruments. The hand port will be fixed via a mini-laparotomy incision, aiming for a safe maintenance of intra-abdominal gas throughout the operative procedure. The main indication for HALS is in advanced and complex laparoscopic surgical procedures.

Rationale behind HALS is that laparoscopic surgery can be used for both simple and complex procedures.

Disadvantages of total laparoscopic surgery:

- Loss of direct tactile sensation
- Difficult hand-eye coordination
- Multiple times instrument change
- Conversion rate in complex abdominal procedures.
  "Hand-port" system allows surgeons the ability to insert a hand into the patient to gain a tactile sense during laparoscopic surgical procedures. This is a real improvement over previous techniques which precluded a surgeon from gaining information through touch. Commercially available to date and approved by the Food and Drug Administration (FDA) are Dexterity device, Intromit, Hand port, and Omniport. Omniport has been extensively studied by Europe University, Dundee University as well as being clinically applied with success in the repair of abdominal aortic aneurysms in Germany and the United States of America. Pneumoaccess bubble is one of the great advances by Cuschieri and Shapiro, allowing complete visual access with the hand inside and pneumoperitoneum safely maintained.

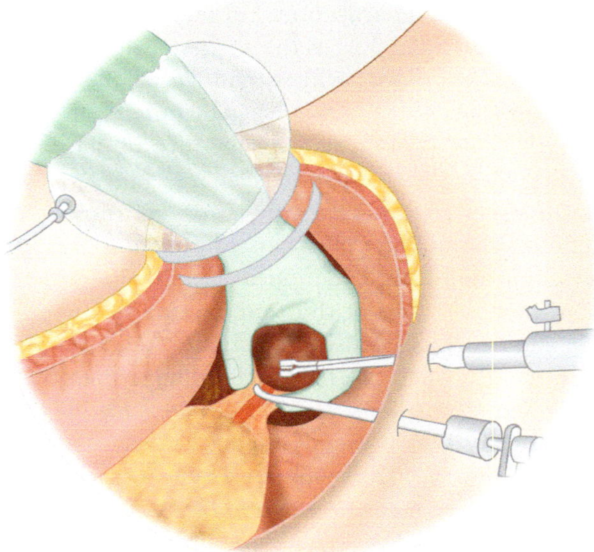

Fig. 5: Hand-assisted laparoscopic surgery.

HAND-PORT DEVICES

Devices connected to abdomen by adhesive flange:

- Dexterity (Inc., Roswell, GA, USA)
- IntroMit (Medtech Ltd., Dublin, Ireland).

Kissing balloon principle:

- Hand-port device (Smith-Nephew PLC, England).

Single-piece devices:

- LapDisc (Hakko Medical, Japan)
- Omniport (Advanced Surgical Concepts Ltd., Ireland).

TABLE 1: Comparison of hand-assisted laparoscopic surgery (HALS), open, and laparoscopic procedures.

Feature	*HALS*	*Open*	*Laparoscopic*
Tactile feedback	Yes (+++)	Yes (++++)	No
Minimal access	Yes (+)	No	Yes (++++)
Hand-eye coordination	Easy (+)	Easy (++++)	Difficult
Tissue retrieval	Easy (++)	Easy (++++)	Difficult
Postoperative recovery	Fast (++)	Slow	Fast (++++)
Operative time	More (+)	Less	More (++++)
Interior milieu	Yes (++)	No	Yes (++++)
Cancer surgery	Yes (++++)	Yes (++++)	No
Cosmetic	Yes (++)	No	Yes (++++)

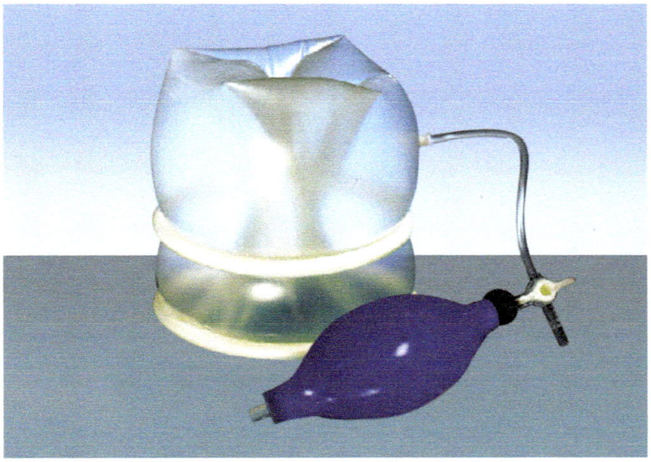

Fig. 6: Omniport inflated.

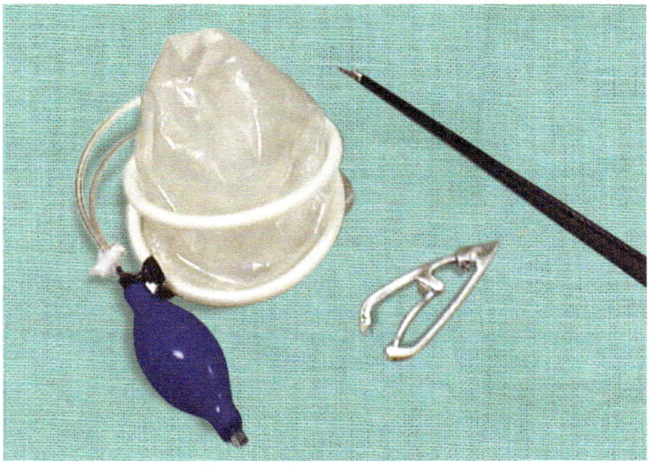

Fig. 7: Omniport deflated.

The IntroMit is a single-piece device that requires an adhesive to be secured to the body wall. There is no sleeve required and the device can be placed without a pneumoperitoneum.

In the hand-port system, the surgeon must wear a sleeve that attaches to the inflatable base of the device. Insertion or removal of the hand from the abdomen requires removal of the sleeve from the device, causing an immediate loss of pneumoperitoneum.

The GelPort is a three-piece device that uses a wound protecting sheath (inner ring), a wound retractor (outer ring) and a gel seal cap that affixes to the wound retractor. The seal that is created maintains pneumoperitoneum, even without the insertion of the surgeon's hand. Removal of the surgeon's hand from the abdominal cavity does not cause loss of pneumoperitoneum. Moreover, the gel seal cap can be pierced by a trocar or accessory instrument while maintaining a seal at the puncture site. The large surface area of this device requires an adequate area for application on the body wall and may not be ideal for lower-quadrant hand incisions in smaller patients. However, a unique benefit of this device is that it permits the insertion instruments through the gel seal cap even while the hand is inserted in the abdomen.

The Omniport is an inflatable device through which the surgeon can rapidly remove and reinsert the hand without losing pneumoperitoneum. The device also can be insufflated to maintain pneumoperitoneum without hand insertion, allowing an accessory trocar and instrument to be inserted through this device **(Figs. 6 to 8)**.

The LapDisc consists of inner and middle rings that are connected by a silicone membrane spanning the abdominal wall. A third outermost ring rotates on the middle ring and acts as an iris, which is tightened to seal the device around the surgeon's arm. There are no pieces that require assembly with this device and insertion is quick and simple. This device has the smallest diameter (12 cm) and can be placed on most abdominal walls without interfering with the placement of adjacent trocars **(Figs. 9A and B)**.

OMNIPORT

Omniport is preferred device because it is:

- Single
- Simple component
- Easy to insert
- Comfortable
- Efficient pneumatic seal.

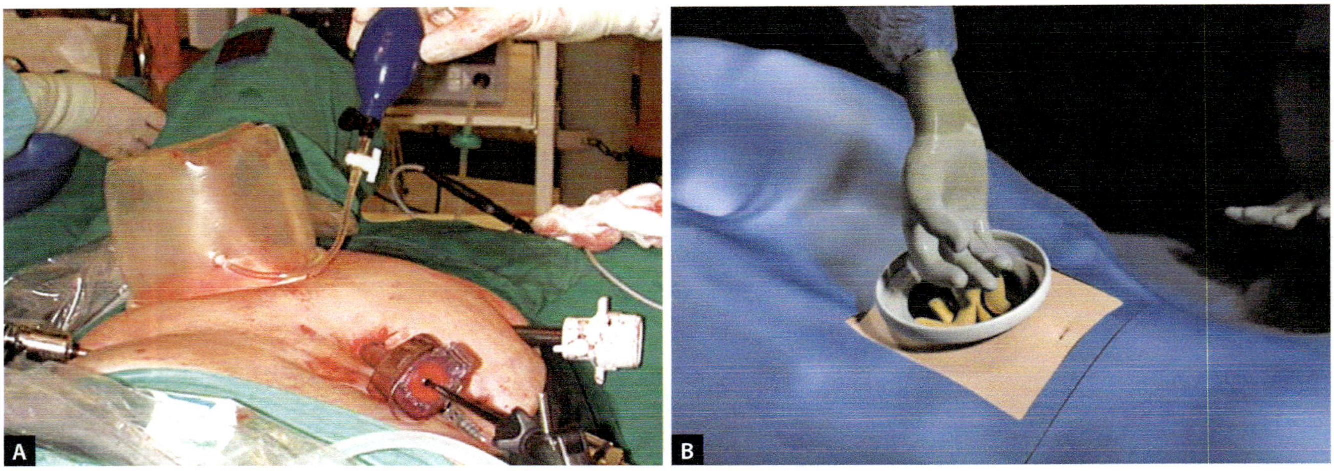

Figs. 8A and B: Hand-assisted laparoscopic surgery (HALS) with Omniport.

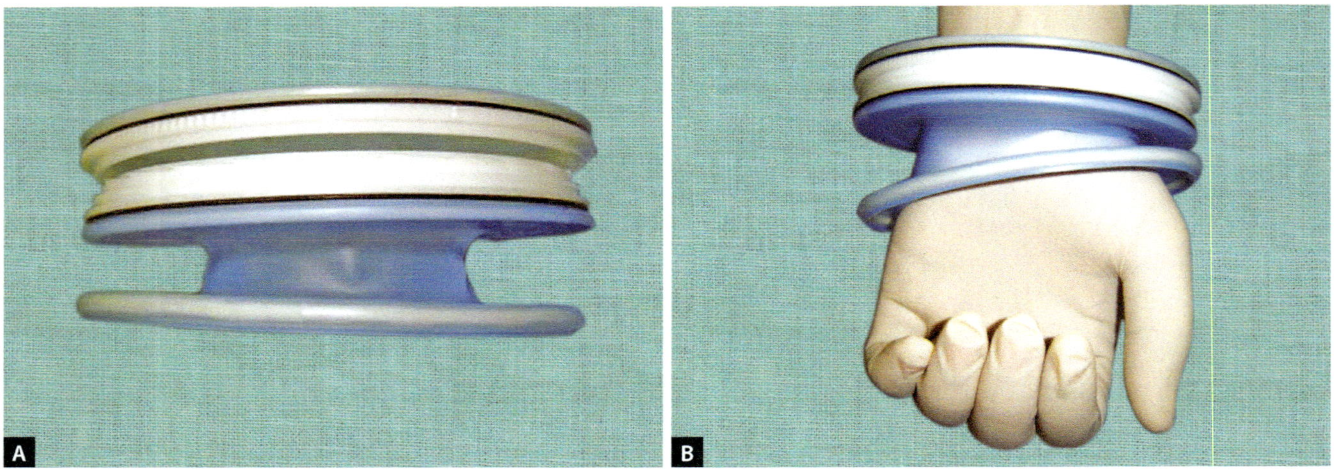

Figs. 9A and B: LapDisc.

INDICATIONS

Hand-assisted laparoscopic surgery is a new addition to minimal access surgery (MAS). It has a great potential. Many surgical operations, from the simplest to the very complicated, are greatly facilitated by the introduction of the hand into the laparoscopic arena. It is therefore purposefully designed in assisting the surgeon for complex intra-abdominal operation to be done with total laparoscopy. It stimulated many vascular surgeons throughout the world to reintroduce it into repair of complex and challenging abdominal vasculature. Nephrectomy, splenectomy, and colorectal surgeries are nicely performed through hand-assisted technique.

ADVANTAGES

- Restored tactile feedback
- Preserving the main idea of MAS
- A minilaparotomy hand port incision
- Reduced conversion rate in total laparoscopy
- Enhanced safety and efficiency allowing the completion of the operation with a hand inside
- Maintenance of the intra-abdominal pressure to facilitate the better view and magnification of laparoscopic telescope
- Improving the steep learning curve for inexperienced surgeons
- Promising reduced cost-benefit ratio.

LIMITATIONS

Limitations can be summarized as:

- Fatigue
- Possible impaired tactile feedback through a lengthy complex procedure
- Minor ergonomic restriction is due to the crowdedness of the hand with the instruments
- Not well accepted by patient and surgeons because there is already a minilaparotomy
- Cosmetically inferior than total laparoscopic surgery.

LAPDISC HAND ACCESS DEVICE

This essential product information sheet does not include all of the information necessary for selection and use of a device.

Indications

- The LapDisc hand access device is intended to provide extracorporeal extension of pneumoperitoneum and abdominal access for the surgeon during laparoscopic surgery.
- The LapDisc is indicated for use in laparoscopic procedures, where entry of the surgeon's hand may facilitate the procedure, and for extraction of large specimens.
- The LapDisc has application in colorectal, urological, and general surgical procedures. This indication for use includes the specific procedures which fall under these broad categories.

Contraindications

None known.

WARNINGS AND PRECAUTIONS

- Minimally invasive procedures should be performed only by persons having adequate training and familiarity with minimally invasive techniques, including laparoscopic, hand-assisted laparoscopic and open surgical procedures. Consult medical literature relative to techniques, complications, and hazards prior to performance of any minimally invasive procedure.
- Minimally invasive instruments may vary from manufacturer to manufacturer. When minimally invasive instruments and accessories from different manufacturers are employed together in a procedure, verify compatibility prior to initiation of the procedure.
- A thorough understanding of the principles and techniques involved in laser, electrosurgical, and ultrasonic procedures is essential to avoid shock and burn hazards to both patient and medical personnel and damage to the device or other medical instruments. Ensure that electrical insulation or grounding is not compromised. Do not immerse electrosurgical instruments in liquid unless they are designed and labeled to be immersed.

LD111-Precaution

- This device should not be used in patients with abdominal wall thickness >5 cm, or incisions <5 cm in length.
- Do not use the device where the incision length is >9 cm as loss of pneumoperitoneum may occur.

LD112-Precaution

- This device should be used in patients with abdominal wall thickness >5 cm and ≤9 cm.
- Do not use the device where the incision length is >9 cm as loss of pneumoperitoneum may occur.
- If pneumoperitoneum occurs:
  - Fully close the iris valve
  - Place damp gauze underneath the LapDisc, between the lower ring and the fascia, to stop the airflow.
- Do not allow sharp instruments such as forceps to come in contact with the silicone rubber sleeves as puncture or tearing may occur.
- Do not lay surgical instruments on the LapDisc or allow metal or sharp surgical instruments to come in contact with the LapDisc as this may weaken or damage the flexible silicone membranes.
- Sterile, water-soluble lubricant should be applied to the dorsum of the gloved hand prior to insertion through the LapDisc. Unlubricated hands may cause significant friction and tear the device.
- Do not remove the hand with the iris valve closed as it may tear the device.
- Do not overtighten the iris valve.
- Use caution when opening the iris valve when the abdomen is insufflated, as rapid loss of pneumoperitoneum may occur.
- After removing the instrument, inspect the site for hemostasis. If hemostasis is not present, appropriate techniques should be used to achieve hemostasis.
- Instruments or devices which come into contact with bodily fluids may require special disposal handling to prevent biological contamination.
- Dispose of all opened instruments whether used or unused. Do not resterilize the instrument. Resterilization may compromise the integrity of the device which may result in unintended injury.

FUTURE PROSPECT

There are general and specific limitations, awaiting multicenter prospective randomized trials in order to compare HALS in various major intra-abdominal procedures with the traditional open surgery **(Fig. 10)**. HALS can be used for all major complex abdominal surgeries such as:

- Splenectomy
- Nephrectomy
- Morbid obesity surgery
- Pancreatectomy
- Nissen fundoplication
- Esophagectomy
- Rectopexy
- Repair of abdominal aortic aneurysm.

Hand-assisted laparoscopic surgery is technically much easier than total laparoscopy in advanced abdominal procedures. It can help the beginning laparoscopic surgeon to practice such major operations.

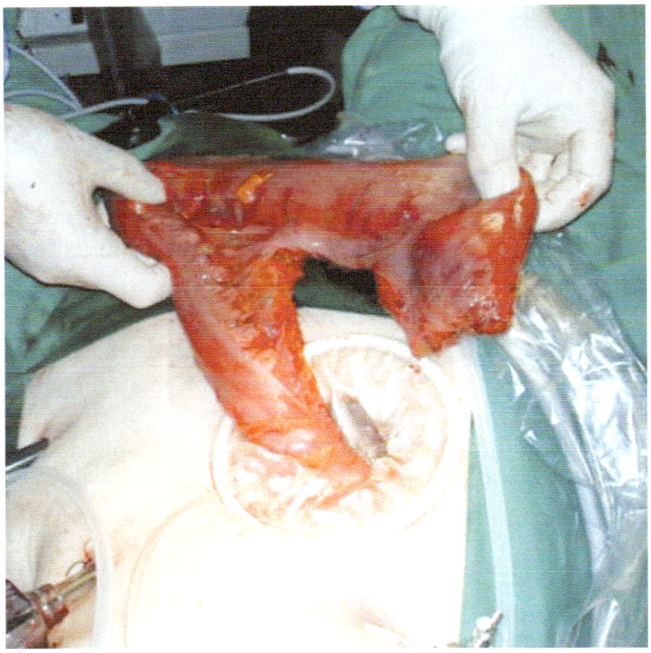

Fig. 10: Hemicolectomy with hand-assisted laparoscopic surgery.

BIBLIOGRAPHY

1. Antonetti MC, Killelea B, Orlando R III. Hand-assisted laparoscopic liver surgery. Arch Surg. 2002;137:407-12.
2. Ballaux KE, Himpens JM, Leman G, Van den Bossche MR. Hand-assisted laparoscopic splenectomy for hydatid cyst. Surg Endosc. 1997;11:942-3.
3. Bemelman WA, Ringers J, Meijer DW, de Wit CW, Bannenberg JJ. Laparoscopic assisted colectomy with the dexterity pneumosleeve. Dis Colon Rectum. 1996;39:S59-61.
4. Bemelman WA, Witt L, Busch OR, Gouma DJ. Hand-assisted laparoscopic splenectomy. Surg Endosc. 2000;14:997-8.
5. Bleier JI, Krupnick AS, Kreisel D, Song HK, Rosato EF, Williams NN. Hand-assisted laparoscopic vertical banded gastroplasty: early results. Surg Endosc. 2000;14:902-7.
6. Boland JP, Kuminsky RE, Tiley EH. Laparoscopic minilaparotomy with manipulation: the middle path. Minimal Invasive Surg. 1993;2:63-7.
7. Cuschieri A, Shapiro S. Extracorporeal pneumoperitoneum access bubble for endoscopic surgery. Am J Surg. 1995;170:391-4.
8. Cuschieri A. Laparoscopic hand-assisted surgery for hepatic and pancreatic disease. Surg Endosc. 2000;14:991-6.
9. Cuschieri A. Whither minimal access surgery: tribulations and expectations. Am J Surg. 1995;169:9-19.
10. Darzi A. Hand-assisted laparoscopic colorectal surgery. Semin Laparosc Surg. 2001;8:153-60.
11. Darzi A. Hand-assisted laparoscopic colorectal surgery. Surg Endosc. 2000;14:999-1004.
12. DeMaria EJ, Schweitzer MA, Kellum JM, Meador J, Wolfe L, Sugerman HJ. Hand-assisted laparoscopic gastric bypass does not improve outcome and increases costs when compared to open gastric bypass for the surgical treatment of obesity. Surg Endosc. 2002;16:1452-5.
13. Dunn DC. Digitally assisted laparoscopic surgery [letter]. Br J Surg. 1994;81:474.
14. Eijsbouts QA, de Haan J, Berends F, Sietses C, Cuesta MA. Laparoscopic elective treatment of diverticular disease: a comparison between laparoscopic assisted and resection-facilitated techniques. Surg Endosc. 2000;14:726-30.
15. Fadden PT, Nakada SY. Hand-assisted laparoscopic renal surgery. Urol Clin North Am. 2001;28:167-76.
16. Fong Y, Jarnagin W, Conlon K, DeMatteo R, Dougherty E, Blumgart LH. Hand-assisted laparoscopic liver resection: lessons from an initial experience. Arch Surg. 2000;135:854-9.
17. Gagner M, Gentileschi P. Hand-assisted laparoscopic pancreatic resection. Semin Laparosc Surg. 2001;8:114-25.
18. Gerhart CD. Hand-assisted laparoscopic transhiatal esophagectomy using the dexterity pneumo sleeve. JSLS. 1998;2:295-8.
19. Gerhart CD. Hand-assisted laparoscopic vertical banded gastroplasty: report of a series. Arch Surg. 2000;135:795-8.
20. Gill IS. Hand-assisted laparoscopy: con. Urology. 2001;58:313-7.
21. Glasgow RE, Swanstrom LL. Hand-assisted gastroesophageal surgery. Semin Laparosc Surg. 2001;8:135-44.
22. Gorey TF, Bonadio F. Laparoscopic-assisted surgery. Semin Laparosc Surg. 1997;4:102-9.
23. Gorey TF, O'Riordain MG, Tierney S, Buckley D, Fitzpatrick JM. Laparoscopic-assisted rectopexy using a novel hand-access port. J Laparoendosc Surg. 1996;6:325-8.
24. Gorey TF, Tierney S, Buckley D, O'Riordain MG, Fitzpatrick JM. Video-assisted Nissen's fundoplication using a hand access port. Minimal Invasive Ther. 1996;5:364-6.
25. Gorey TF, Tierney S, O'Riordain MG, Buckley D, Gibbons N, Fitzpatrick JM. Case report: combined hand-access with laparoscopic pneumoperitoneum in intraperitoneal adhesiolysis. Ir J Med Sci. 1996;165:297-8.
26. Gossot D, Meijer D, Bannenberg J, de Witt L, Jakimowicz J. La splenectomie laparoscopique revisitée. Ann Chir. 1995; 49:487-9.
27. HALS Study Group. Hand-assisted laparoscopic surgery vs standard laparoscopic surgery for colorectal disease. Surg Endosc. 2000;14:896-901.
28. Hanna GB, Elamass M, Cuschieri A. Ergonomics of hand-assisted laparoscopic surgery. Semin Laparosc Surg. 2001;8:92-5.
29. Hellman P, Arvidsson D, Rastad J. HandPort-assisted laparoscopic splenectomy in massive splenomegaly. Surg Endosc. 2000;14:1177-9.
30. Ichiara T, Nagahata Y, Nomura H, Fukumoto S, Urakawa T, Aoyama N, et al. Laparoscopic lower anterior resection is equivalent to laparotomy for lower rectal cancer at the distal line of resection. Am J Surg. 2000;179:87-8.
31. Iwase K, Higaki J, Yoon HE, Mikata S, Tanaka Y, Takahashi T, et al. Hand-assisted laparoscopic splenectomy for idiopathic thrombocytopenic purpura during pregnancy. Surg Laparosc Endosc Percutan Tech. 2001;11:53-6.
32. Jakimowicz, JJ. Will advanced laparoscopic surgery go hand-assisted? Surg Endosc. 2000;14:881-2.
33. Katkhouda N, Lord RV. Once more, with feeling: handoscopy or the rediscovery of the virtues of the surgeon's hand. Surg Endosc. 2000;14:985-6.
34. Katkhouda N, Mason RJ, Mavor E, Campos GM, Rivera RT, Hurwitz MB, et al. Laparoscopic finger-assisted technique (fingeroscopy) for treatment of complicated appendicitis. J Am Coll Surg. 1999;189:131-3.
35. Kawano T, Iwai T. Hand-assisted thoracoscopic esophagectomy using a new supportive approach. Surg Endosc. 2001;15(3):330.
36. Kercher KW, Matthews BD, Walsh RM, Sing RF, Backus CL, Heniford BT. Laparoscopic splenectomy for massive splenomegaly. Am J Surg. 2002;183:192-6.
37. Kevic MS. Hand-assisted laparoscopic surgery—HALS. JSLS. 2001;5:101-3.
38. Kim HB, Gregor MB, Boley SJ, Kleinhaus S. Digitally assisted laparoscopic drainage of multiple intra-abdominal abscesses. J Laparoendosc Surg. 1993;3:477-9.
39. Klinger PJ, Smith SL, Abendstein BJ, Hinder RA. Hand-assisted laparoscopic splenectomy for isolated splenic metastasis from

an ovarian carcinoma: a case report with review of the literature. Surg Laparosc Endosc. 1998;8:49-4.

40. Klingler PJ, Hinder RA, Menke DM, Smith SL. Hand-assisted laparoscopic distal pancreatectomy for pancreatic cystadenoma. Surg Laparosc Endosc. 1998;8:180-4.
41. Kuminsky RE, Tiley EH, Lucente FC, Boland JP. Laparoscopic staging laparotomy with intra-abdominal manipulation. Surg Laparosc Endosc. 1994;4:103-5.
42. Kurian NS, Patterson R, Andrei VE, Edye MB. Hand-assisted laparoscopic surgery: an emerging technique. Surg Endosc. 2001;15:1277-81.
43. Kurokawa T, Inagaki H, Sakamoto J, Nonami T. Hand-assisted laparoscopic anatomical left lobectomy using hemihepatic vascular control technique. Surg Endosc. 2002;15:300.
44. Kusminsky RE, Boland JP, Tiley EH, Deluca JA. Hand-assisted laparoscopic splenectomy. Surg Laparosc Endosc. 1995;5: 463-7.
45. Kusminsky RE, Boland JP, Tiley EH. Hand-assisted laparoscopic surgery [letter]. Dis Colon Rectum. 1996;39:111.
46. Litwin DE, Darzi A, Jakimowicz J, KellyJJ, Arvidsson D, Hansen P, et al. Hand-assisted laparoscopic surgery (HALS) with the HandPort system: initial experience with 68 patients. Ann Surg. 2000;231:715-23.
47. Lucarini L, Galleano R, Lombezzi R, Ippoliti M, Ajraldi G. Laparoscopic assisted Hartmann's reversal with the Dexterity pneumo sleeve. Dis Colon Rectum. 2000;43:1164-7.
48. Machi J, Oishi AJ, Mossing AJ, Furumoto NL, Oishi RH. Hand-assisted laparoscopic ultrasound-guided radiofrequency thermal ablation of liver tumors: a technical report. Surg Laparosc Endosc Percutan Tech. 2002;12:160-4.
49. Meijer DW, Gossot D, Jakimowicz JJ, De Wit LT, Bannenberg JJ, Gouma DJ. Splenectomy revised: manually assisted splenectomy with the dexterity device—a feasibility study in 22 patients. J Laparoendosc Adv Surg Tech A. 1999;9:507-10.
50. Meijer DW, Bannenberg JJ, Jakimowicz JJ. Hand-assisted laparoscopic surgery: an overview. Surg Endosc. 2000;14:891-5.
51. Memon MA, Fitzgibbons RJ. Hand-assisted laparoscopic surgery (HALS): a useful technique for complex laparoscopic abdominal procedures. J Laparoendosc Adv Surg Tech A. 1998;8:143-50.
52. Miura Y, Mitsuta H, Yoshihara T, Ohshiro Y, Okajima M, Asahara T. Gasless hand-assisted laparoscopic surgery for colorectal cancer: an option for poor cardiopulmonary reserve. Dis Colon Rectum. 2001;44:896-8.
53. Mooney MJ, Elliott PL, Galapon DB, James LK, Lilac LJ, O'Reilly MJ. Hand-assisted laparoscopic sigmoidectomy for diverticulitis. Dis Colon Rectum. 1998;41:630-5.
54. Naitoh T, Gagner M, Garcia-Ruiz A, Heniford BT, Ise H, Matsuno S. Hand-assisted laparoscopic digestive surgery provides safety and tactile sensation for malignancy or obesity. Surg Endosc. 1999;13:157-60.
55. Naitoh T, Gagner M. Laparoscopically assisted gastric surgery using the Dexterity pneumo sleeve. Surg Endosc. 1997;11: 830-3.
56. Neufang T, Post S, Markus P, Becker H. Manually assisted laparoscopic surgery—realistic evolution of the minimally invasive therapy concept? Initial experiences with the Endohand. Chirurg. 1996;67:952-8.
57. O'Reilly MJ, Saye WB, Mullins SG, Pinto SE, Falkner PT. Technique of hand-assisted laparoscopic surgery. J Laparoendosc Surg. 1996;6:239-44.
58. Ohki J, Nagai H, Hyodo M, Nagashima T. Hand-assisted laparoscopic distal gastrectomy with abdominal wall-lift method. Surg Endosc. 1999;13:1148-50.
59. Ou H. Laparoscopic-assisted mini-laparotomy with colectomy. Dis Colon Rectum. 1995;38:324-6.
60. Pelosi MA, Pelosi MA III, Eim J. Hand-assisted laparoscopy for megamyomectomy: a case report. J Reprod Med. 2000;45: 519-5.
61. Pelosi MA, Pelosi MA III, Eim J. Hand-assisted laparoscopy for pelvic malignancy. J Laparoendosc Adv Surg Tech A. 2000;10:143-50.
62. Pelosi MA, Pelosi MA III, Villalona E. Hand-assisted laparoscopic cholecystectomy at cesarean section. J Am Assoc Gynecol Laparosc. 1999;6:491-5.
63. Pietrabissa A, Boggi U, Moretto C, Ghilli M, Mosca F. Laparoscopic and hand-assisted laparoscopic live donor nephrectomy. Semin Laparosc Surg. 2001;8:161-7.
64. Pietrabissa A, Dario P, Ferrari M, Stefanini C, Menciassi A, Moretto C, et al. Grasping and dissecting instrument for hand-assisted laparoscopic surgery. Surg Endosc. 2002;16:1332-5.
65. Pietrabissa A, Moretto C, Carobbi A, Boggi U, Ghilli M, Mosca F. Hand-assisted laparoscopic low anterior resection: initial experience with a new procedure. Surg Endosc. 2002;16:431-5.
66. Posner MC, Alverdy J. Hand-assisted laparoscopic surgery for cancer. Cancer J. 2002;8:144-53.
67. Ren CJ, Salky B, Reiner M. Hand-assisted laparoscopic splenectomy for ruptured spleen. Surg Endosc. 2001;15:324.
68. Romanelli JR, Kelly JJ, Litwin DE. Hand-assisted laparoscopic surgery in the United States: an overview. Semin Laparosc Surg. 2001;8:96-103.
69. Romanelli JR, Litwin DE. Hand-assisted laparoscopic surgery: problems in general surgery. Probl Gen Surg. 2001;18:45-51.
70. Rudich SM, Marcovich R, Magee JC, Punch JD, Campbell DA, Merion RM, et al. Hand-assisted laparoscopic donor nephrectomy: comparable donor/recipient outcomes, costs, and decreased convalescence as compared to open donor nephrectomy. Transplant Proc. 2001;33:1106-7.
71. Ruiz-Deya G, Cheng S, Palmer E, Thomas R, Slakey D. Open donor, laparoscopic donor and hand-assisted laparoscopic donor nephrectomy: a comparison of outcomes. J Urol. 2001;166: 1270-4.
72. Schweitzer MA, Broderick TJ, Demaria EJ, Sugerman HJ. Laparoscopic assisted Roux-en-Y gastric bypass. J Laparoendosc Adv Surg Tech A. 1999;9:449-53.
73. Scoggin SD, Frazee RC, Snyder SK, Hendricks JC, Roberts JW, Symmonds RE, et al. Laparoscopic-assisted bowel surgery. Dis Colon Rectum. 1993;36:747-50.
74. Scott HJ, Darzi A. Tactile feedback in laparoscopic colonic surgery. Br J Surg. 1997;84:1004-5.
75. Shinchi H, Takao S, Noma H, Mataki Y, Iino S, Aikou T. Hand-assisted laparoscopic distal pancreatectomy with minilaparotomy for distal pancreatic cystadenoma. Surg Laparosc Endosc Percutan Tech. 2001;11:139-43.
76. Sjoerdsma W, Meijer DW, Jansen A, den Boer KT, Grimbergen CA. Comparison of efficiencies of three techniques for colon surgery. J Laparoendosc Adv Surg Tech A. 2000;10:47-53.
77. Southern Surgeons' Club Study Group. Handoscopic surgery: a prospective multicenter trial of a minimally invasive technique for complex abdominal surgery. Arch Surg. 1999;134:477-85.
78. Stifelman M, Nieder AM. Prospective comparison of hand-assisted laparoscopic devices. Urology. 2002;59:668-72.
79. Sundbom M, Gustavsson S. Hand-assisted laparoscopic bariatric surgery. Semin Laparosc Surg. 2001;8:145-52.
80. Sundbom M, Gustavsson S. Hand-assisted laparoscopic Roux-en-Y gastric bypass: early results. Obes Surg. 2000;10:420-27.
81. Tanimura S, Higashino M, Fukunaga Y, Osugi H. Hand-assisted laparoscopic distal gastrectomy with regional lymph node dissection for gastric cancer. Surg Laparosc Endosc Percutan Tech. 2001;11:155-60.
82. Targarona EM, Balague C, Cerdan G, Espert JJ, Lacy AM, Visa J, et al. Hand-assisted laparoscopic splenectomy (HALS) in cases

of splenomegaly: a comparative analysis with conventional laparoscopic splenectomy. Surg Endosc. 2002;16:426-30.

83. Targarona EM, Balague C, Trias M. Hand-assisted laparoscopic splenectomy. Semin Laparosc Surg. 2001;8:126-34.
84. Targarona EM, Gracia E, Garriga J, Martínez-Bru C, Cortés M, Boluda R, et al. Prospective, randomized trial comparing conventional laparoscopic colectomy with hand-assisted laparoscopic colectomy: applicability, immediate clinical outcome, inflammatory response and cost. Surg Endosc. 2002;16:234-9.
85. Targarona EM, Balague C, Trias M. Laparoscopic splenectomy for splenomegaly. Probl Gen Surg. 2002;19:58-64.
86. Van de Walle P, Blomme Y, Van Outrye L. Hand-assisted staging laparoscopy for suspected malignancies of the pancreas. Acta Chir Belg. 2002;102:183-6.
87. Vassallo C, Negri L, Della Valle A, Dono C, Martinotti R, Mussi P, et al. Divided vertical banded gastroplasty either for correction or as a first-choice operation. Obes Surg. 1999;9:177-9.
88. Wadstrom J, Lindstrom P. Hand-assisted retroperitoneoscopic living-donor nephrectomy: initial 10 cases. Transplantation. 2002;73:1839-41.
89. Watson DI, Davies N, Jamieson GG. Totally endoscopic Ivor Lewis esophagectomy. Surg Endosc. 1999;13:293-7.
90. Watson DI, Game PA. Hand-assisted laparoscopic vertical banded gastroplasty: initial report. Surg Endosc. 1997;11:1218-20.
91. Wolf JS Jr, Merion RM, Leichtman AB, Campbell DA Jr, Magee JC, Punch JD, et al. Randomized controlled trial of hand-assisted laparoscopic versus open surgical live donor nephrectomy. Transplantation. 2001;72:284-90.
92. Woods SD, Polglase AL. Laparoscopically assisted anterior resection for villous adenoma of the rectum. Aust NZJ Surg. 1993;63:146-8.
93. Yoshida T, Inoue H, Iwai T. Hand-assisted laparoscopic surgery for the abdominal phase in endoscopic esophagectomy for esophageal cancer: an alteration on the site of minilaparotomy. Surg Laparosc Endosc Percutan Tech. 2000;10:396-400.

CHAPTER 11

Tissue Retrieval Technique

INTRODUCTION

One of the limitations of minimal access surgery is difficulty in retrieval of tissue. Previously, surgeons were reluctant to perform many of the advanced surgical procedure due to this difficult procedure. New techniques for removing tissue have helped increase the number and types of laparoscopic surgeries that can be done laparoscopically. Recently, the Food and Drug Administration (FDA) recommends that surgeon should use tissue containment systems when using laparoscopic power morcellators, and that they ensure the laparoscopic power morcellator and tissue containment system are compatible. Legally, marketed laparoscopic power morcellation containment systems are intended to isolate and contain tissue that is considered benign. Based on testing and clinical data, use of a containment system confines morcellated tissue within the containment system.

Safe removal of tissue is an important consideration in laparoscopic surgery and applies to all specimens irrespective of whether they are thought to be benign or malignant. The importance of wound protection is shown by considering laparoscopic cholecystectomy for symptomatic gallstone disease. Most of the gallbladders at the time of retrieval can be squeezed out through an unprotected port wound. At the time of extraction exit wound must be of sufficient size, and wound protection should be used to ensure that there is no contact between the specimen and the abdominal wall during removal. We all know that the incidence of unsuspected gallbladder cancer is between 0.5 and 1% and there are reported cases of port site tumor nodules because of implantation of tumor cells after extraction of the gallbladder through an unprotected wound.

Tissue reduction enables extraction through small wounds but can be used only for benign specimens. Tissue reduction can be carried out by various techniques, including mechanical fragmentation and morcellation. It should be done inside a rip-proof bag whenever possible. This is essential for laparoscopic splenectomy to prevent implantation of splenic fragments on the serosal surfaces, which leads to splenosis **(Fig. 1)**.

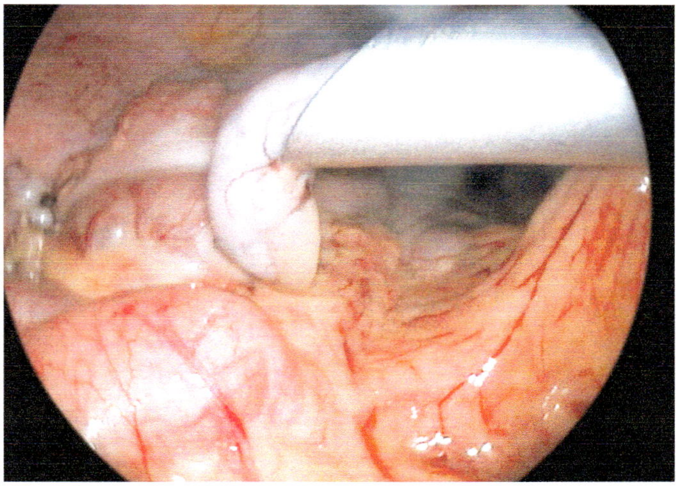

Fig. 1: Appendix hidden within cannula.

Most commonly the resected tissue should be hidden under port and then everything should come together with port. This technique is used for most of the small size organs such as appendix, gallbladder, small ovarian cyst, ectopic pregnancy, salpingectomy, small oophorectomy, etc.

ENDOBAGS

In some cases, the tissue to be removed is first encased in a specimen retrieval bag. These tissue retrieval bags are available in market and can be prepared by surgeon himself at the time of laparoscopic surgery **(Fig. 2A)**.

For infected tissue and in case of suspected carcinoma, tissue retrieval bag should be used. Many sizes of disposable tissue retrieval bags are available and hard rims of these retrieval bags are easy to negotiate inside the abdominal cavity **(Figs. 2B to D)**.

One can easily make the retrieval bag by tying and cutting the fingers of sterilized gloves. If the gloves used for the retrieval of tissue, it should be used carefully. It should not puncture while removing from the abdominal cavity **(Fig. 3)**.

The glove is kept stretched while one assistant will tie it in the middle **(Figs. 4A and B)**.

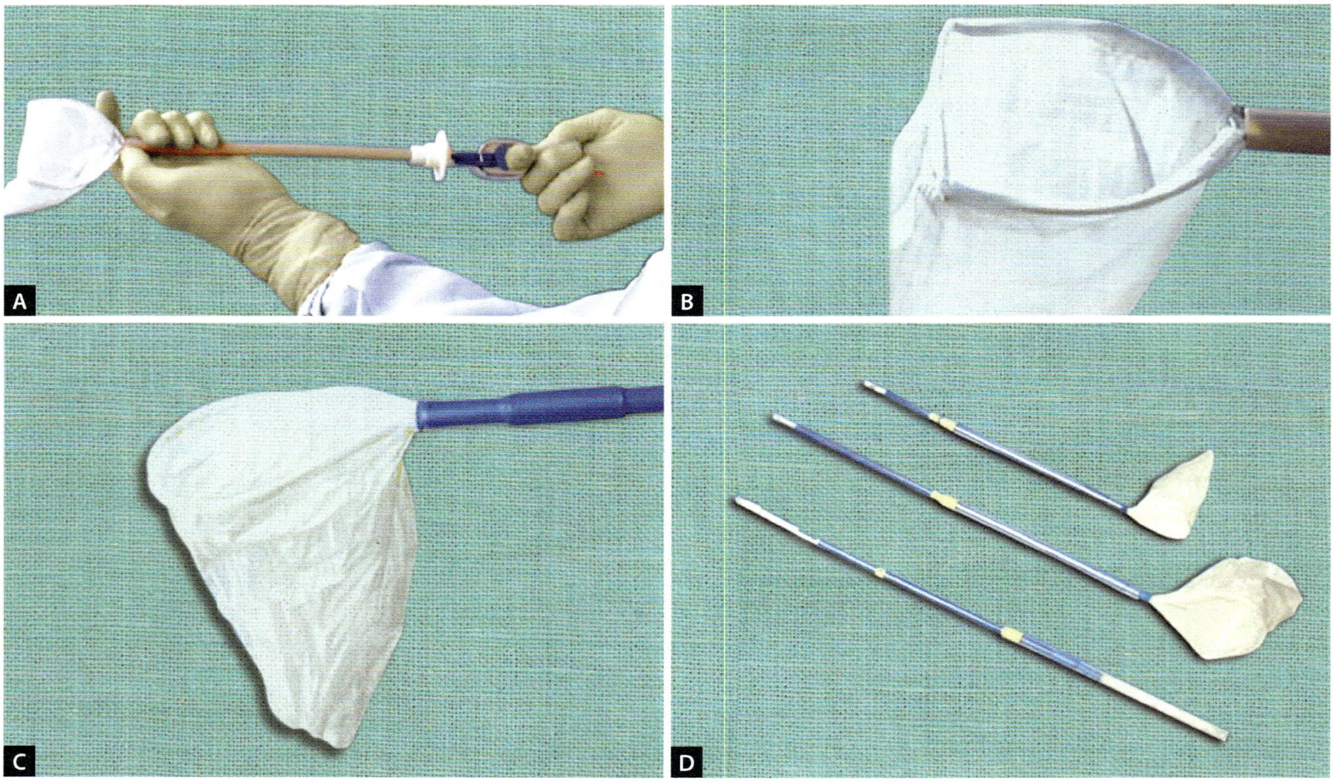

Figs. 2A to D: Disposable endobags.

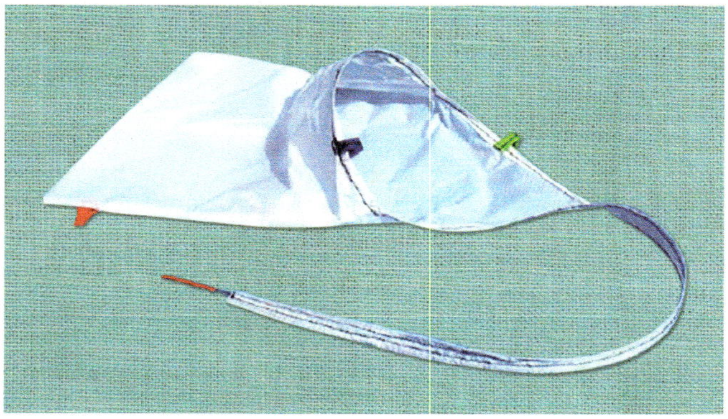

Fig. 3: Endobags.

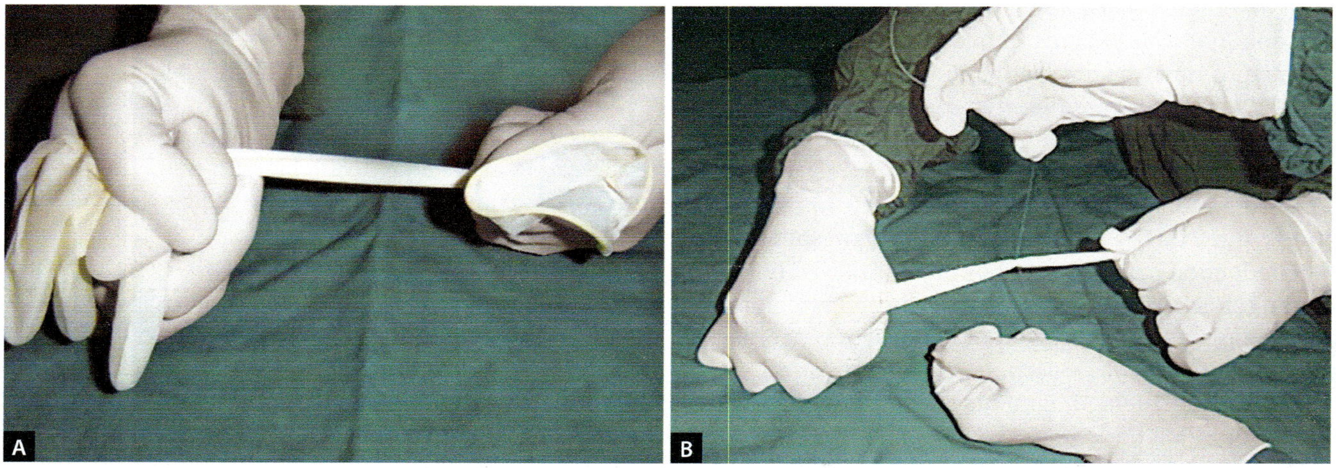

Figs. 4A and B: Making endobag with glove.

Keeping it stretched will create a good dumbbell after knotting and so there is no chance of slipping of knot inside the abdominal cavity **(Fig. 5)**.

The latex material used to manufacture gloves sometimes, react with human tissue and it can create a problem if the glove is punctured and a piece of latex is left inside human body. Most commonly this torn piece of gloves can be missed in the layers of abdominal wall **(Fig. 6)**.

At the time of introduction of glove endobag, it should be held by its cut end and kept stretched over the shaft of grasper to decrease its thickness **(Fig. 7)**.

The polythene covering of Ryle's tube can also be used as inexpensive readymade retrieval bag. This is sterilized and open at one end **(Figs. 8A and B)**.

These polythene bags can be used as excellent retrieval pouch if used carefully. The polythene bag has one demerit that sometime the edges are difficult to find out because it is transparent and secondly because it is thin and does not have elastic property like gloves so it slips easily after once held by grasper **(Figs. 9A to E)**.

Drawback of this self-made retrieval bag is that they do not have hard rim so it is difficult to manipulate inside the abdominal cavity.

These bags can be introduced inside the abdominal cavity through 10 mm ports. In special circumstances if there is difficulty is found, it can be introduced directly through the port wound after withdrawing the cannula.

Once the retrieval bag is inside, it should be positioned in free abdominal space and the rim of bag should be stabilized with nondominant hand and dominant hand should be used to put the specimen inside. Once the bag is inside the abdominal cavity both the edges of the retrieval bag should be lifted to displace the specimen into the base of the bag **(Figs. 10A and B)**. Condom can also be used for retrieving tissue. Lubricated condom should be avoided because it can cause tissue reaction.

To take the specimen out, surgeon should hide the mouth of retrieval bag inside the cannula by pulling it and then the cannula together with the neck of bag is pulled outside the abdominal cavity.

Once the neck of the bag is out, its opening is stretched by the help of assistant. Ovum forceps can be introduced inside to morcellate the tissue manually if there is difficulty in pulling the bag out **(Fig. 11)**.

COLPOTOMY

For large size gynecological tissue, colpotomy route is good for retrieval. Colpotomy can be done laparoscopically with the help of heal of hook. Counter pushing by other instruments is effective. Sponge over sponge-holding forceps is inserted in posterior vaginal fornix by one assistant and surgeon cuts the vaginal fascia between both the uterosacral ligaments with the heel of hook **(Fig. 12)**.

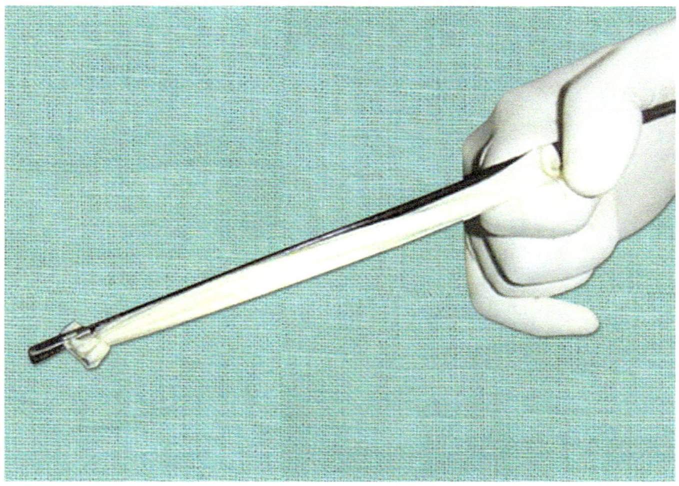

Fig. 6: Way of introducing endobag.

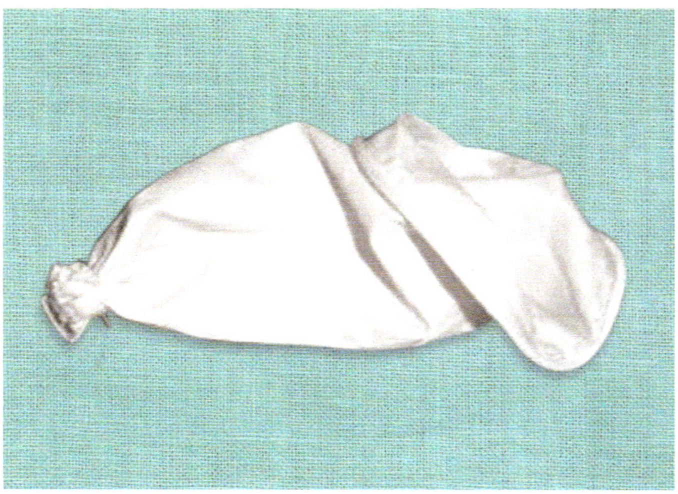

Fig. 5: Glove endobag.

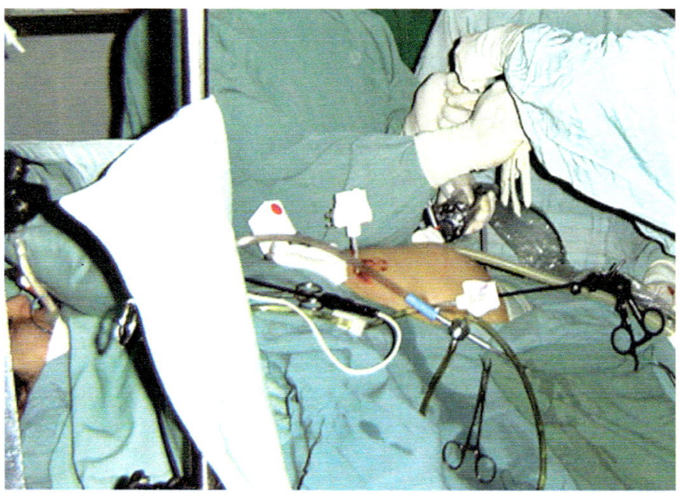

Fig. 7: Using glove endobag.

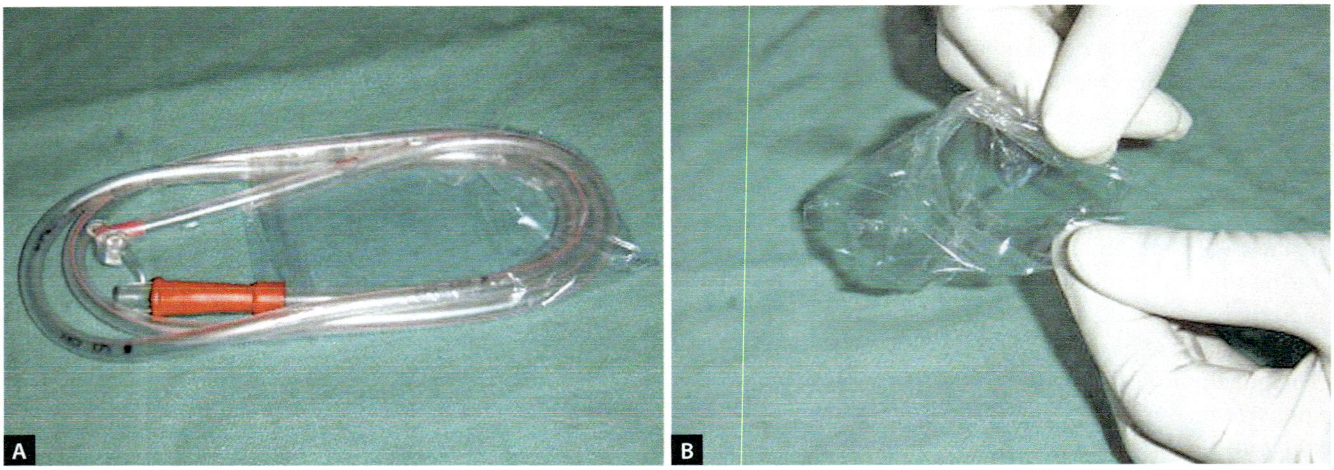

Figs. 8A and B: Polypropylene endobag.

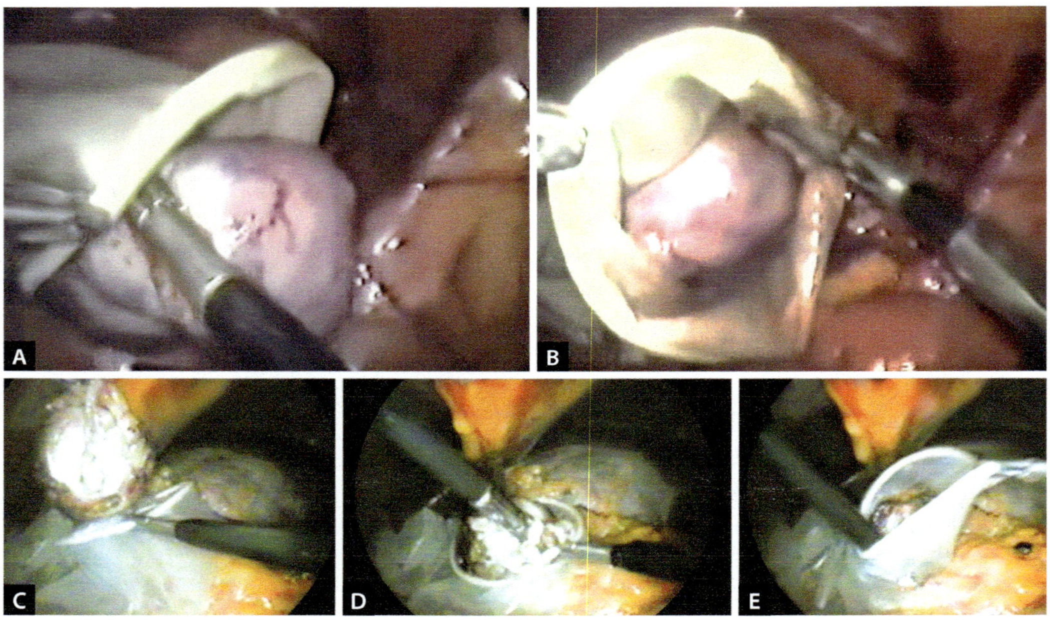

Figs. 9A to E: Introduction of tissue in endobag.

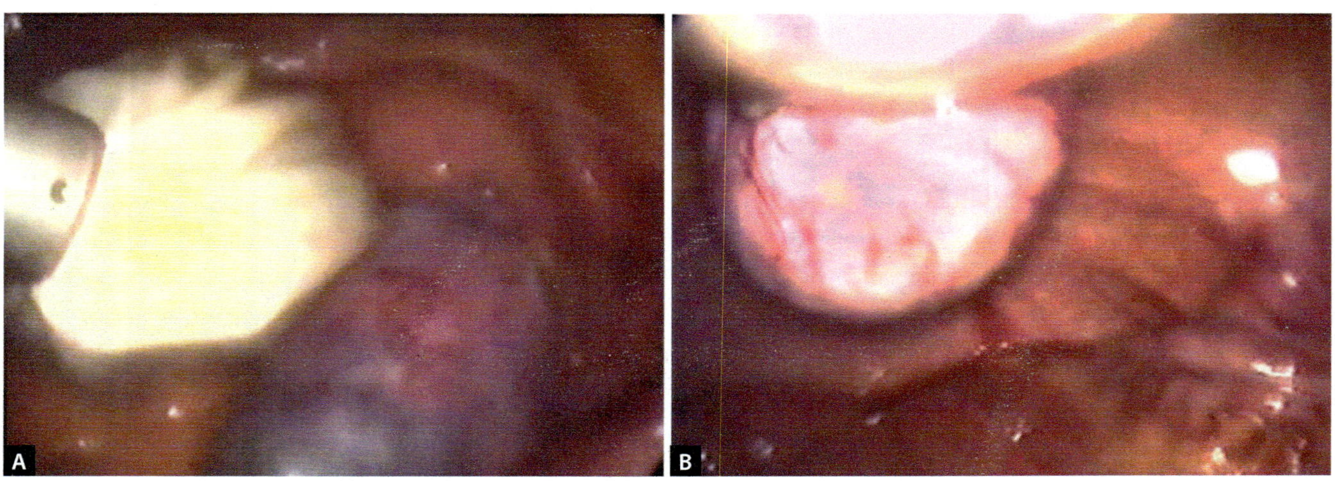

Figs. 10A and B: Neck of endobag pulled outside the abdominal wall.

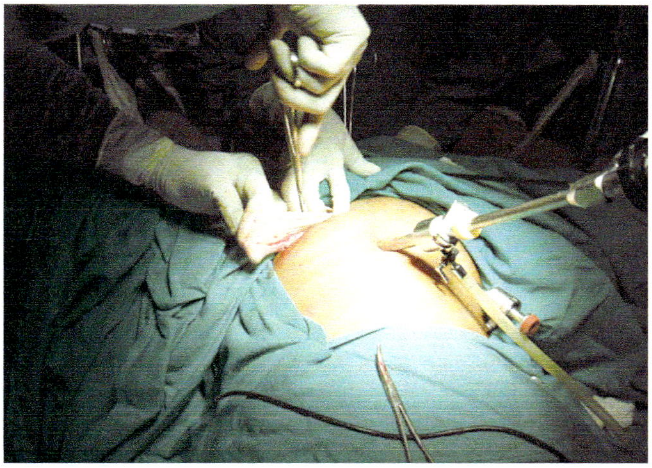

Fig. 11: Morcellation of tissue through endobag.

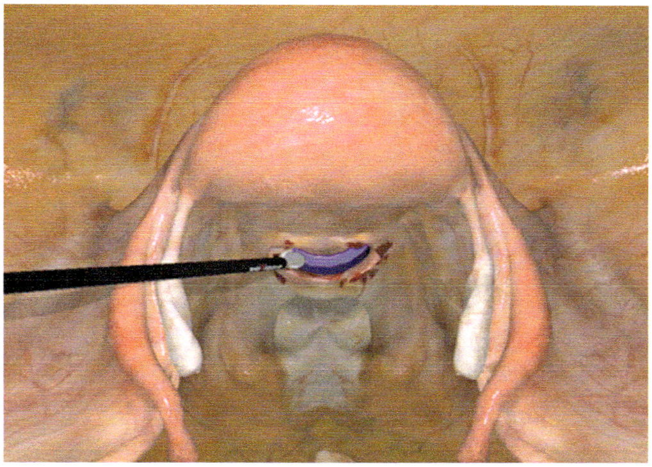

Figs. 12: Colpotomy.

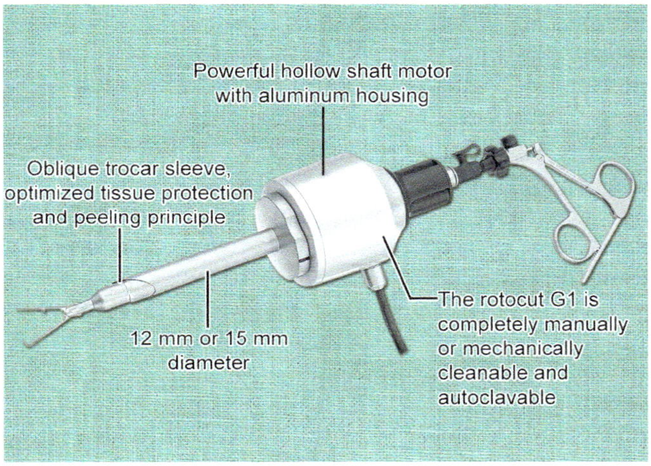

Fig. 13: Electrical morcellator.

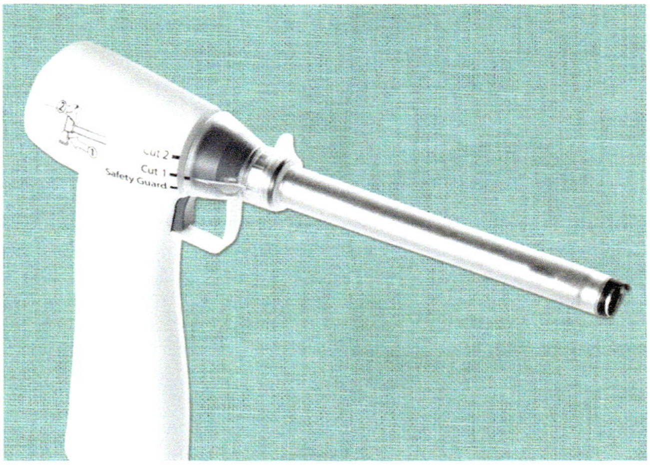

Fig. 14: Different type of morcellator.

HAND-ASSISTED LAPAROSCOPIC SURGERY

Hand-assisted technique was initially started keeping inside ease of tissue retrievals, wherein the surgeon uses his or her hand, inserted through the initial incision, to aid in the exploration, isolation, and removal of tissue.

Hand-assisted technique offers distinct advantages, the superior visualization afforded by the laparoscope and a tactile component that is important in many aspects of surgery and has allowed surgeons to apply a less invasive approach to surgeries that previously could not have been done laparoscopically.

Hand-assisted laparoscopy can also serve as a bridge between open surgery and straight laparoscopy, making it easier for surgeons to practice and learn the skills necessary for performing laparoscopic procedures.

MORCELLATOR

Use of morcellator is another way which facilitates grinding of solid tissue and then these can be taken out without any difficulty. Recently many companies have launched battery-operated morcellator. The morcellator is important instrument for tissue retrieval in myomectomy and splenectomy **(Fig. 13)**.

One of the early concerns about laparoscopic procedures in cancer patient was that they caused port site metastases, i.e., the appearance of recurrent tumor tissue at the site of trocar entry **(Fig. 14)**. Use of laparoscopic power morcellators allow for minimally invasive surgical procedures, which, when compared to open abdominal surgery, typically reduce the risk of infection, and shorten the postoperative recovery period. However, when used in myomectomy or hysterectomy procedures, there is an increased risk of spreading unsuspected cancer and benign tissue within the abdomen and pelvis. The risk of unsuspected cancer increases with age, particularly in women over 50 years of age.

Cancer surgery, however, poses some unique challenges that make the application of laparoscopic surgery in oncology more problematic. It is critically important in

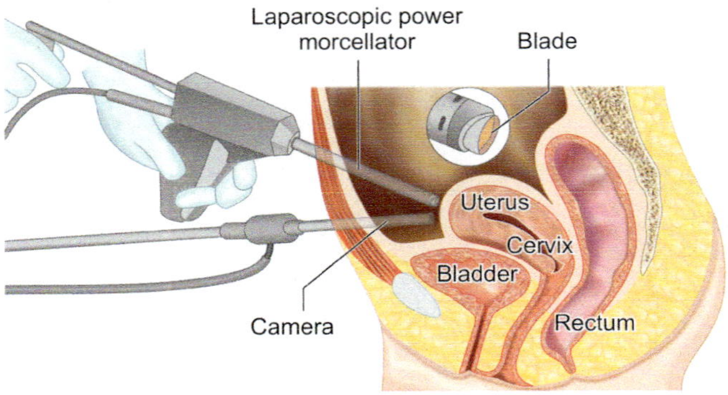

Fig. 15: Power morcellation of tissue.

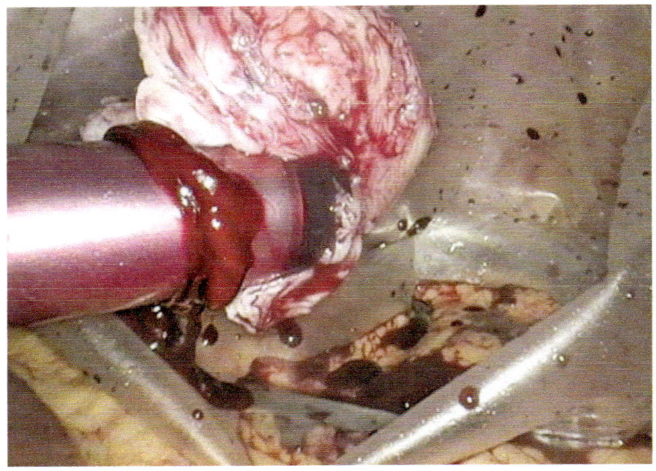

Fig. 16: Morcellation of tissue.

cancer that whole organs should be removed intact (en bloc) so that pathologists can properly examine them and measure and document the depths and margins of tumor invasion. A second concern for surgical oncologists is cell transfer or cell spillage. Diseased tissue must be removed without contaminating adjacent tissues and structures with cancer cells. Because of these concerns, tissue morcellation, a technique commonly used in noncancer laparoscopic surgery in which the tissue is divided into pieces so that it can be removed more easily should not be used for oncologic procedures. All the 10 mm or >10 mm defects should be closed properly to prevent any future possibility of hernia **(Figs. 15 and 16)**.

The suture passer should be used to pass the thread and then it should be tied externally.

Especially, designed port closure instruments are also available commercially.

If port is suddenly taken out, the chance of port site hernia and adhesion is much higher. It is a good practice to insert some blunt instrument while removing the last port out, to prevent entrapment of omentum or bowel content.

After closing the rectus sheath, the skin can be closed by intradermal, skin stapler or by any of the surgical skin glues available.

FDA Warnings about Power Morcellation (Fig. 15)

When laparoscopic power morcellators are used for myomectomy or hysterectomy in women with presumed uterine fibroids that are actually uterine sarcomas, the surgical procedure poses a risk of spreading cancerous tissue beyond the uterus, worsening a woman's chance of long-term survival. In April 2014, the FDA issued a statement discouraging use of laparoscopic power morcellation in hysterectomy for uterine fibroids; this was followed by a warning in November 2014 against use of uterine power morcellation because of risk for dissemination of malignant tissue. In response, many hospitals banned power morcellation. The FDA currently estimates that a hidden uterine sarcoma may be present in approximately 1 in 225 to 1 in 580 women undergoing surgery for uterine fibroids based on recent publications. The FDA also estimates that a leiomyosarcoma may be present in approximately 1 in 495 to 1 in 1,100 women undergoing surgery for uterine fibroids based on recent studies. Prior to 2014, the clinical community estimated uterine sarcomas to be present much less frequently, in as few as 1 in 10,000 women undergoing surgery for uterine fibroids.

Several studies show that using a laparoscopic power morcellator during gynecologic surgery in women with hidden uterine sarcomas is associated with lowering their chances of long-term survival without cancer. While these studies have limitations, women who have had fibroid surgery with a laparoscopic power morcellator later found to have a hidden uterine sarcoma, have lower disease-free survival, when compared to women who were treated with manual morcellation or without morcellation. MorSafe® is an innovative single-use disposable device intended to be used as a receptacle for benign tissue mass during gynecological procedures such as laparoscopic myomectomy or laparoscopic hysterectomy. The device has unique features to allow for quick deployment, insufflation, morcellation, and spill-proof withdrawal of the bag.

MorSafe® Tissue Isolator

MorSafe®, with its unique two port design, offers the surgeon superior visibility during the surgery compared to a single port approach **(Figs. 17A and B)**. Designed to fit and take the shape of the abdomen, it has been constructed utilizing a special tear-resistant material to prevent leakage. It also contains a special ring in the bag opening to allow the surgeon ultimate control of the bag opening and easy access to the interior of the bag during surgery.

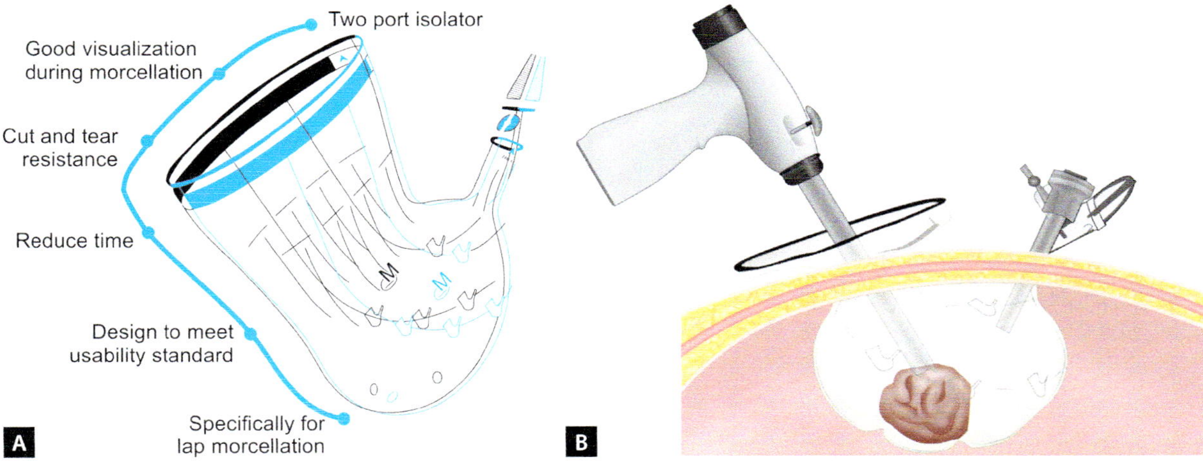

Figs. 17A and B: MorSafe® tissue isolator.

BIBLIOGRAPHY

1. Bach PB, Cramer LD, Warren JL, Begg CB. Racial differences in the treatment of early-stage lung cancer. N Engl J Med. 1999;341:1198-205.
2. Ballesta-Lopez C, Bastida-Vila X, Catarci M, Mato R, Ruggiero R. Laparoscopic Billroth II distal subtotal gastrectomy with gastric stump suspension for gastric malignancies. Am J Surg. 1996;171:289-92.
3. Begg CB, Cramer LD, Hoskins WJ, Brennan MF. Impact of hospital volume on operative mortality for major cancer surgery. JAMA. 1998;280:1747-51.
4. Bouvy ND, Marquet RL, Jeekel H, Bonjer HJ. Impact of gas (less) laparoscopy and laparotomy on peritoneal tumor growth and abdominal wall metastases. Ann Surg. 1996;224:694-701.
5. Callery MP, Strasberg SM, Doherty GM, Soper NJ, Norton JA. Staging laparoscopy with laparoscopic ultrasonography: optimizing resectability in hepatobiliary and pancreatic malignancy. J Am Coll Surg. 1997;185:33-9.
6. Charlson ME, Pompei P, Ales KL, MacKenzie CR. A new method of classifying prognostic comorbidity in longitudinal studies: development and validation. J Chron Dis. 1987;40:373-83.
7. Chew DK, Borromeo JR, Kimmelstiel FM. Peritoneal mucinous carcinomatosis after laparoscopic-assisted anterior resection for early rectal cancer: report of a case. Dis Colon Rectum. 1999;42:424-6.
8. Cox DR. Regression models and life-tables. J R Statist Soc (Ser B). 1972;34:187-220.
9. Cubiella J, Castells A, Fondevila C, Sans M, Sabater L, Navarro S, et al. Prognostic factors in nonresectable pancreatic adenocarcinoma: a rationale to design therapeutic trials. Am J Gastroenterol. 1999;94:1271-8.
10. DeMeester TR, Wang CI, Wernly JA, Pellegrini CA, Little AG, Klementschitsch P, et al. Technique, indications, and clinical use of 24-hour esophageal pH monitoring. J Thorac Cardiovasc Surg. 1980;79:656-70.
11. Dieter RA Jr, Kuzycz GB. Complications and contraindications of thoracoscopy. Int Surg. 1997;82:232-9.
12. Dorrance HR, Oien K, O'Dwyer PJ. Effects of laparoscopy on intraperitoneal tumor growth and distant metastases in an animal model. Surgery. 1999;126:35-40.
13. Drouard F, Delamarre J, Capron JP. Cutaneous seeding of gallbladder cancer after laparoscopic cholecystectomy. N Engl J Med. 1991;325:316.
14. Eadie LH, Seifalian AM, Davidson BR. Telemedicine in surgery. Br J Surg. 2003;90:647-58.
15. Fleshman JW, Nelson H, Peters WR, Kim HC, Larach S, Boorse RR, et al. Early results of laparoscopic surgery for colorectal cancer: retrospective analysis of 372 patients treated by Clinical Outcomes of Surgical Therapy (COST) Study Group. Dis Colon Rectum. 1996;39:S53-8.
16. Forde KA, Hulten L. Laparoscopy in colorectal surgery. Surg Endosc. 1996;10:1039-40.
17. Forster R, Storck M, Schafer JR, Honig E, Lang G, Liewald F. Thoracoscopy versus thoracotomy: a prospective comparison of trauma and quality of life. Langenbecks Arch Surg. 2002;387:32-6.
18. Freedman LS. Tables of the number of patients required in clinical trials using the logrank test. Stat Med. 1982;1:121-9.
19. Geer RJ, Brennan MF. Prognostic indicators for survival after resection of pancreatic adenocarcinoma. Am J Surg. 1993;165:68-72.
20. Giulianotti PC, Coratti A, Angelini M, Sbrana F, Cecconi S, Balestracci T, et al. Robotics in general surgery: personal experience in a large community hospital. Arch Surg. 2003;138:777-84.
21. Jacobi CA, Sabat R, Bohm B, Zieren HU, Volk HD, Müller JM. Pneumoperitoneum with carbon dioxide stimulates growth of malignant colonic cells. Surgery. 1997;121:72-8.
22. Jacobi CA, Wildbrett P, Volk T, Muller JM. Influence of different gases and intraperitoneal instillation of antiadherent or cytotoxic agents on peritoneal tumor cell growth and implantation with laparoscopic surgery in a rat model. Surg Endosc. 1999;13:1021-5.
23. Jones DB, Guo LW, Reinhard MK, Soper NJ, Philpott GW, Connett J, et al. Impact of pneumoperitoneum on trocar site implantation of colon cancer in hamster model. Dis Colon Rectum. 1995;38:1182-8.
24. Kalbfleisch JD, Prentice RL. The Statistical Analysis of Failure Time Data. New York, NY: John Wiley and Sons; 1980.
25. Kaplan EL, Meier P. Nonparametric estimation from incomplete observations. Am Stat Assoc. 1958;53:457-81.
26. Kumar A, Kumar S, Aggarwal S, Khilnani GC. Thoracoscopy: the preferred approach for the resection of selected posterior mediastinal tumors. J Laparoendosc Adv Surg Tech A. 2002;12:345-53.
27. Lacy AM, Garcia-Valdecasas JC, Pique JM, Delgado S, Campo E, Bordas JM, et al. Short-term outcome analysis of a randomized study comparing laparoscopic vs open colectomy for colon cancer. Surg Endosc. 1995;9:1101-5.

28. Mack MJ. Video-assisted thoracoscopy thymectomy for myasthenia gravis. Chest Surg Clin N Am. 2001;1:389-05.
29. Masaoka A, Yamakawa Y, Niwa H, Fukai I, Kondo S, Kobayashi M, et al. Extended thymectomy for myasthenia gravis patients: a 20-year review. Ann Thorac Surg. 1996;62:853-9.
30. Melfi FM, Menconi GF, Mariani AM, Angeletti CA. Early experience with robotic technology for thoracoscopic surgery. Eur J Cardiothorac Surg. 2002;21:864-8.
31. Milsom JW, Bohm B, Hammerhofer KA, Fazio V, Steiger E, Elson P. A prospective, randomized trial comparing laparoscopic versus conventional techniques in colorectal cancer surgery: a preliminary report. J Am Coll Surg. 1998;187:46-54.
32. Morgan JA, Ginsburg ME, Sonett JR, Morales DL, Kohmoto T, Gorenstein LA, et al. Advanced thoracoscopic procedures are facilitated by computer-aided robotic technology. Eur J Cardiothorac Surg. 2003;23:883-7.
33. Nagahiro I, Andou A, Aoe M, Sano Y, Date H, Shimizu N. Pulmonary function, postoperative pain, and serum cytokine level after lobectomy: a comparison of VATS and conventional procedure. Ann Thorac Surg. 2001;72:362-5.
34. Nifong LW, Chu VF, Bailey BM, Maziarz DM, Sorrell VL, Holbert D, et al. Robotic mitral valve repair: experience with the da Vinci system. Ann Thorac Surg. 2003;75:438-42.
35. Onnasch JF, Schneider F, Falk V, Mierzwa M, Bucerius J, Mohr FW. Five years of less invasive mitral valve surgery: from experimental to routine approach. Heart Surg Forum. 2002;5:132-5.
36. Onoda N, Ishikawa T, Yamada N, Okamura T, Tahara H, Inaba M, et al. Radioisotope-navigated video-assisted thoracoscopic operation for ectopic mediastinal parathyroid. Surgery. 2002;132:17-9.
37. Potosky AL, Riley GF, Lubitz JD, Mentnech RM, Kessler LG. Potential for cancer related health services research using a linked Medicare-tumor registry database. Med Care. 1993;31:732-48.
38. Poulin EC, Mamazza J, Schlachta CM, Gregoire R, Roy N. Laparoscopic resection does not adversely affect early survival curves in patients undergoing surgery for colorectal adenocarcinoma. Ann Surg. 1999;229:487-92.
39. Ramshaw BJ. Laparoscopic surgery for cancer patients. CA Cancer J Clin. 1997;47:327-50.
40. Romano PS, Mark DJ. Bias in the coding of hospital discharge data and its implications for quality assessment. Med Care. 1994;32:81-90.
41. Roviaro GC, Varoli F, Vergani C, Maciocco M. State of the art in thoracoscopic surgery: a personal experience of 2000 videothoracoscopic procedures and an overview of the literature. Surg Endosc. 2002;16:881-92.
42. Schmid T. Editorial to: main topics: robotic surgery. Eur Surg. 2002;34:155-7.
43. Schurr MO, Arezzo A, Buess GF. Robotics and systems technology for advanced endoscopic procedures: experiences in general surgery. Eur J Cardiothorac Surg. 1999;16(2):S97-105.
44. SEER Cancer Statistics Review, 1973–1997. Bethesda, MD: National Cancer Institute; 2000.
45. Sener SF, Fremgen A, Menck HR, Winchester DP. Pancreatic cancer: a report of treatment and survival trends for 100,313 patients diagnosed from 1985–1995, using the National Cancer Database. J Am Coll Surg. 1990;189:1-7.
46. Soper NJ, Brunt LM, Kerbl K. Medical progress: laparoscopic general surgery. N Engl J Med. 1994;330:409-19.
47. Takiguchi S, Matsuura N, Hamada Y, Taniguchi E, Sekimoto M, Tsujinaka M, et al. Influence of CO_2 pneumoperitoneum during laparoscopic surgery on cancer cell growth. Surg Endosc. 2000;14:41-4.
48. Tewari A, Peabody J, Sarle R, Balakrishnan G, Hemal A, Shrivastava A, et al. Technique of da Vinci robot-assisted anatomic radical prostatectomy. Urology. 2002;60:569-72.
49. Volz J, Koster S, Schaeff B, Paolucci V. Laparoscopic surgery: the effects of insufflations gas on tumor-induced lethality in nude mice. Am J Obstet Gynecol. 1998;178:793-5.
50. Wetscher GJ, Glaser K, Wieschemeyer T, Gadenstaetter M, Prommegger R, Profanter C. Tailored antireflux surgery for gastroesophageal reflux disease: effectiveness and risk of postoperative dysphagia. World J Surg. 1997;21:605-10.
51. Wexner SD, Cohen SM. Port site metastases after laparoscopic colorectal surgery for cure of malignancy. Br J Surg. 1995;82:295-8.
52. Whelan RL, Allendorf JD, Gutt CN, Jacobi CA, Mutter D, Dorrance HR, et al. General oncologic effects of the laparoscopic surgical approach. 1997 Frankfurt International Meeting of Animal Laparoscopic Researchers. Surg Endosc. 1998;12:1092-5.
53. Whelan RL, Lee SW. Review of investigations regarding the etiology of port site tumor recurrence. J Laparoendosc Adv Surg Tech A. 1999;9:1-16.
54. Bouvy ND, Giuffrida MC, Tseng LN, Steyerberg EW, Marquet RL, Jeekel H, et al. Effects of carbon dioxide pneumoperitoneum, air pneumoperitoneum, and gasless laparoscopy on body weight and tumor growth. Arch Surg. 1998;133:652-6.
55. Wittich P, Marquet RL, Kazemier G, Bonjer HJ. Port-site metastases after CO_2 laparoscopy. Is aerosolization of tumor cells a pivotal factor? Surg Endosc. 2000;14:189-92.
56. Wykypiel H, Wetscher GJ, Klaus A, Schmid T, Gadenstaetter M, Bodner J, et al. Robot-assisted laparoscopic partial posterior fundoplication with the DaVinci system: initial experiences and technical aspects. Langenbecks Arch Surg. 2003;387:411-6.
57. Yim AP. Thoracoscopic thymectomy: which side to approach? Ann Thorac Surg. 1997;64:584-5.

CHAPTER 12

Laparoscopic Port Closure Technique

INTRODUCTION

Minimal access surgery is a routine surgical practice due to its minimal invasive and associated advantages. It has a lot of advantages but not devoid of complication, one of the major concerned complication is the trocar site herniation (TSH). TSH is a serious complication often requiring emergency repair. If unattended, TSH can lead to small bowel strangulation and incarceration.

The literature says that preventative measures should be taken to avoid the occurrence of herniation at the portal site. Fascial closure has been recommended as a means of TSH prevention. One study reported a statistically higher frequency of hernia at 12 mm port site where the fascia was left open (8%) compared with those that were closed (0.22%) following laparoscopy. There is a consensus that all the port site ≥10 mm should be closed due to an increased risk of herniation. For smaller ports, fascial closure may not be necessary, except when manipulated extensively.

Trocar site herniation is also associated with other technical factors other than the port site. Port location is another factor. There are many reports suggesting that umbilical sites are at greater risk of herniation when compared to lateral port sites. This is due to weakness of the fascia and absence of supporting muscle in the area. Stretching or even extending the incision of a port site during specimen extraction has a great risk hernia development. Factors such as high body mass index (BMI) are patient-related risk factors that are associated with TSH. Here it is related to increase intra-abdominal pressure and increase abdominal wall thickness. Studies show that wound infection is a predisposing factor to hernia development. Therefore, closure of fascia is necessary for umbilical ports, ports sites that are stretched or enlarged for specimen retrieval, and trocar sites in obese patients.

Minimally invasive laparoscopic surgery has revolutionized the way surgery is performed for an increasing number of patients. Incisional hernia can occur after any abdominal surgery and laparoscopic surgery is not immune to this complication. The hernia that follows laparoscopy usually occurs through the larger ports (size >10 mm), especially the umbilicus.

Predisposing factors include:

- Previous laparoscopies
- Extensive manipulation during surgery
- Increased intra-abdominal pressure
- Obesity
- Use of sharp cutting-tip trocars
- Rapid abdominal deflation at the end of surgery
- Poor port removal techniques and defective closure of the abdominal fascia
- Wound extension
- Male sex
- Infection of the wound
- Pre-existing umbilical defects
- Postoperative chest infections
- Pre-existing diseases such as diabetes mellitus
- Connective tissue disorders
- Job profile of the patient (weight lifting).

Among all these factors, the single most important factor remains the improper closure of the fascial defects at the port sites and not using proper port closure instruments **(Figs. 1 to 3)**. The diagnosis is often delayed because most cases present late, and treatment might be instituted along other lines. Computed tomography scans are helpful in its diagnosis and will facilitate prompt treatment to avoid the grave consequence of bowel gangrene.

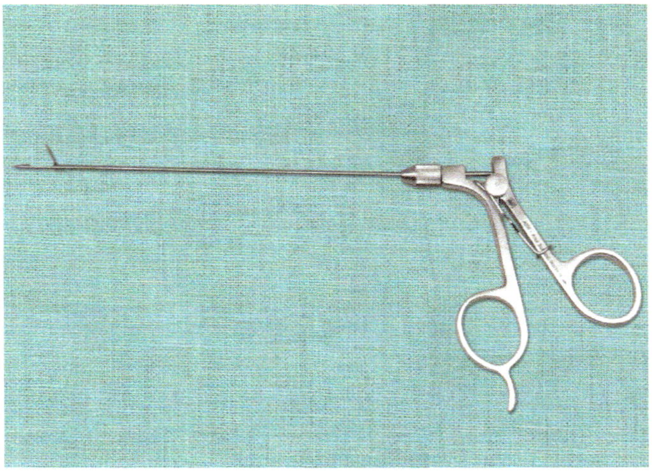

Fig. 1: Typical port closure needle.

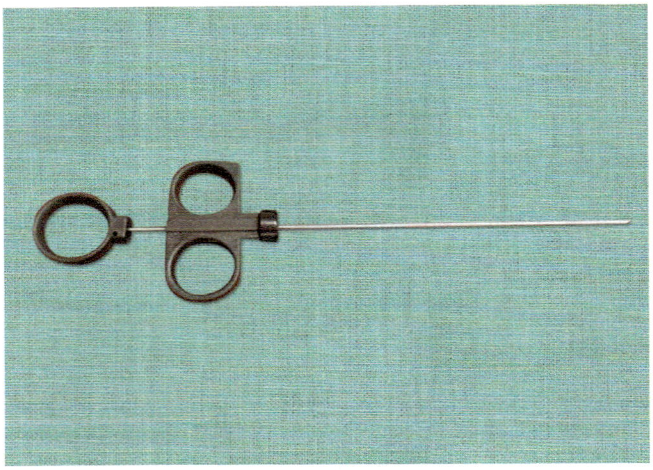

Fig. 2: Laparoscopic port closure Cobbler's needle.

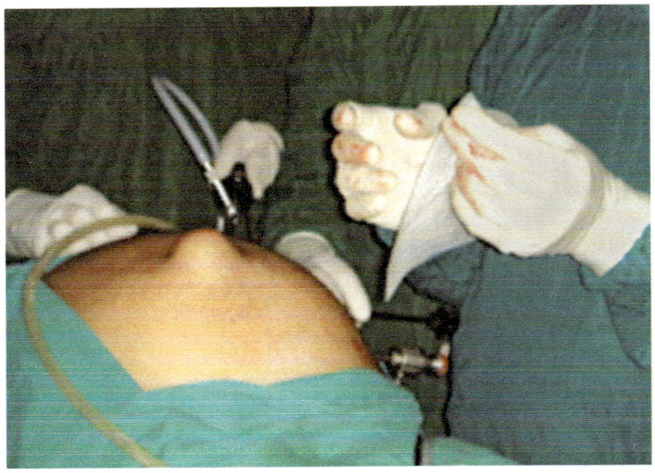

Fig. 3: Incisional hernia development due to improper closure of port should be repaired later by mesh.

While surgical techniques and instrumentation have made significant advances, it is usual that the surgical incision is closed using invasive suturing techniques or by the use of tapes or by the use of topical cyanoacrylate skin adhesives (TCAs) for closure of surgical wounds. The incidence of incisional hernia occurring at the port sites after laparoscopic surgery lies between 0.02 and 3.6% and usually remains unreported, until the development of complications.

Any port closure technique should have following characteristics:

- Effective (strong and secure) surgical wound closure
- Faster wound closure
- Better scar cosmesis
- Occlusive microbial wound dressing
- Less tissue trauma, reduced inflammatory reaction
- No requirement for suture/staple removal
- Easy to use/simple learning curve
- Reduced risk of needlestick injury—safety and costs
- Cost effective.

WITHDRAWAL OF INSTRUMENTS AND PORTS

Once the surgery is finished, all the instruments should be removed carefully under vision. All the accessory ports should be removed and the gas is removed by releasing the valve of 10 mm cannulas. The primary port should be taken out in the end **(Fig. 4)**.

If last port is suddenly withdrawn, sudden suction effect of cannula can pull the omentum or bowel inside the port wound, the chance of port-site hernia and adhesion is much higher in this case. It is a good practice to insert some blunt instrument or telescope inside the abdomen while removing the last cannula out over that instrument, to prevent inadvertent entrapment of omentum or bowel.

The access technique will result in breach in continuity of abdominal wall which need to be repaired at the end of surgery. All the 10 mm or >10 mm port should be repaired properly to prevent any future possibility of hernia. The rectus sheath should be sutured with Vicryl. Only one stitch is required in middle which will convert 10 mm wound into 5 mm. The 5 mm port wounds are not necessary to repair.

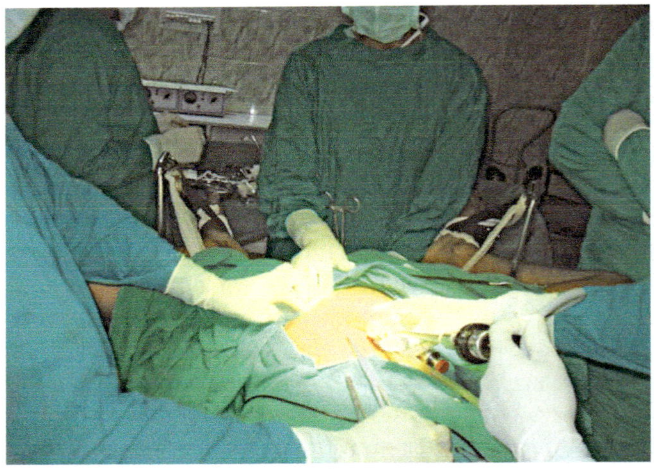

Fig. 4: The tip of telescope should be introduced in and cannula is pulled over telescope to prevent suction of omentum or bowel.

Laparoscopic Port Closure Instruments

Various types of port closure instruments are available. The suture passer is a convenient instrument for port closure. It is used to pass the thread on the side of cannula and then it is tied externally **(Figs. 5A to D)**.

Port Closure Needle

This is a simple instrument just like cobblers and it can be effectively used for closing the port. The tip of the instrument is blunt and the needle faces toward the fascia, so the chances of injury to the bowel are less with the use of this instrument **(Fig. 6)**.

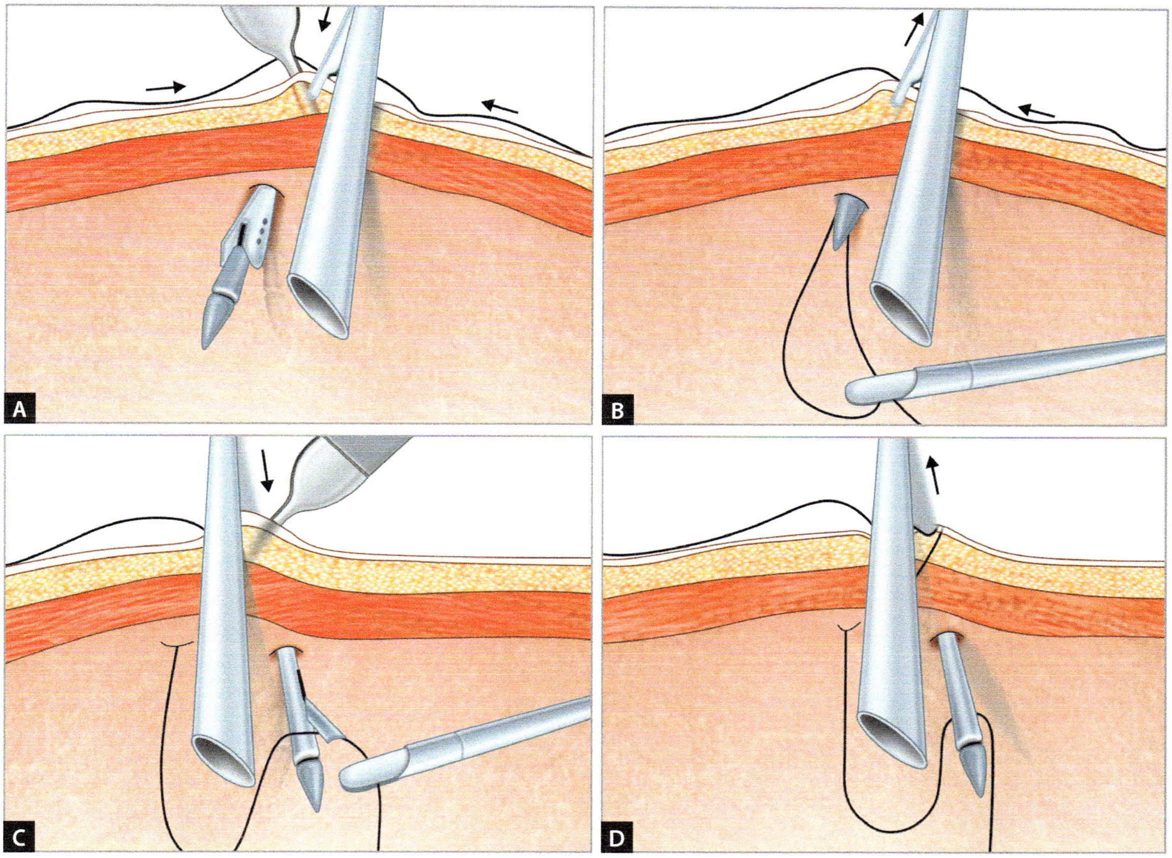

Figs. 5A to D: Port closure with the help of suture passer.

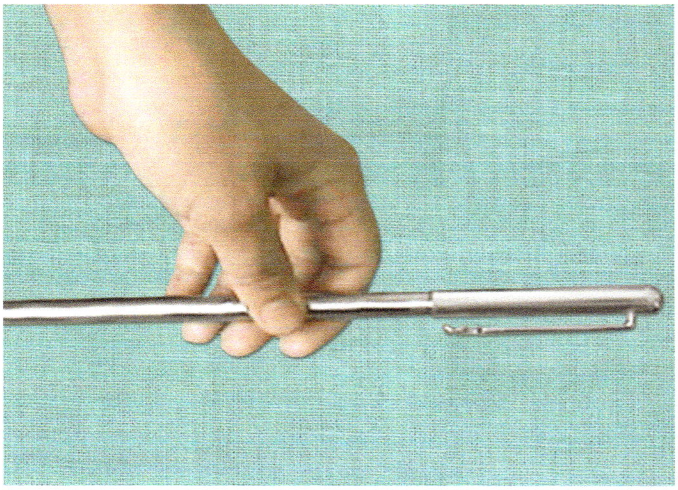

Fig. 6: Port closure needle.

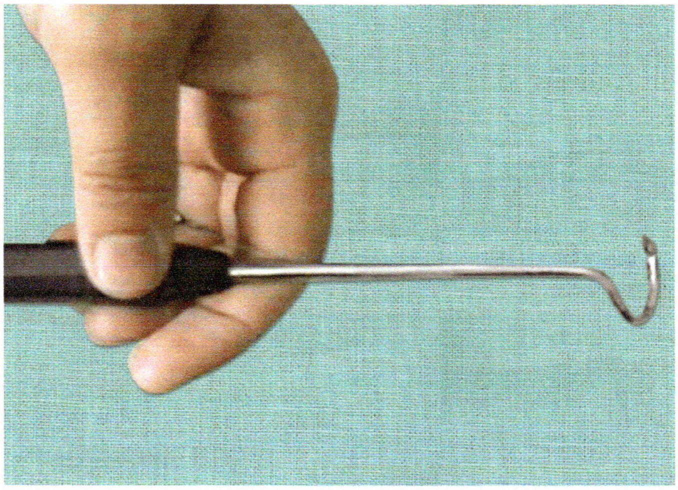

Fig. 7: Aneurysm needle.

Aneurysm needle can also be used for closing fascia. The advantage of this needle is that eye is at the tip and due to rigid structure there is no risk of bending or rotation of needle **(Fig. 7)**.

After closing the rectus sheath, the skin can be closed by intradermal, skin stapler or any of the surgical skin glues TCAs available **(Fig. 8)**.

New Laparoscopic Port Closure Instruments

Weck® EFx Shield Fascial Closure System (Figs. 9A and B)

The Weck® EFx Shield Fascial Closure System from Teleflex is the only shielded port closure device, providing enhanced sharps protection for uniform and consistent performance.

The EFx Shield® System is designed with speed and safety in mind. An array of enhanced features includes:
- Unique shielded wing design for enhanced sharps protection
- Intuitive wing deployment
- Innovative suture retrieval system for unassisted fascial closure.

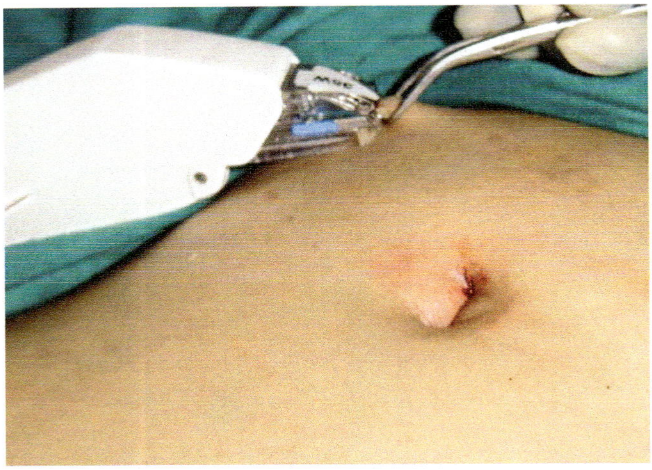

Fig. 8: Closure of skin wound by skin stapler.

NeatClose Automated Port Closure Device (Figs. 10A and B)

NeatStitch of Israel has come up with an automated port closure device known as NeatClose, where it also picked up both the Food and Drug Administration (FDA) and European approvals in the process. It is marketed to be an alternative to manual port closure, making it a speedy and efficient manner to help laparoscopic surgeon save time and money by lowering intraoperative costs. This system lets surgeons produce a watertight seal quickly, and it goes without saying that this would go a long way in aiding the recovery of a patient, never mind that one does not have Wolverine's healing factor. When inside the operating cavity, the surgeon can squeeze the handle leavers in order to release a couple of blunt needle guides, where said guides are specially positioned in a perpendicular manner to the

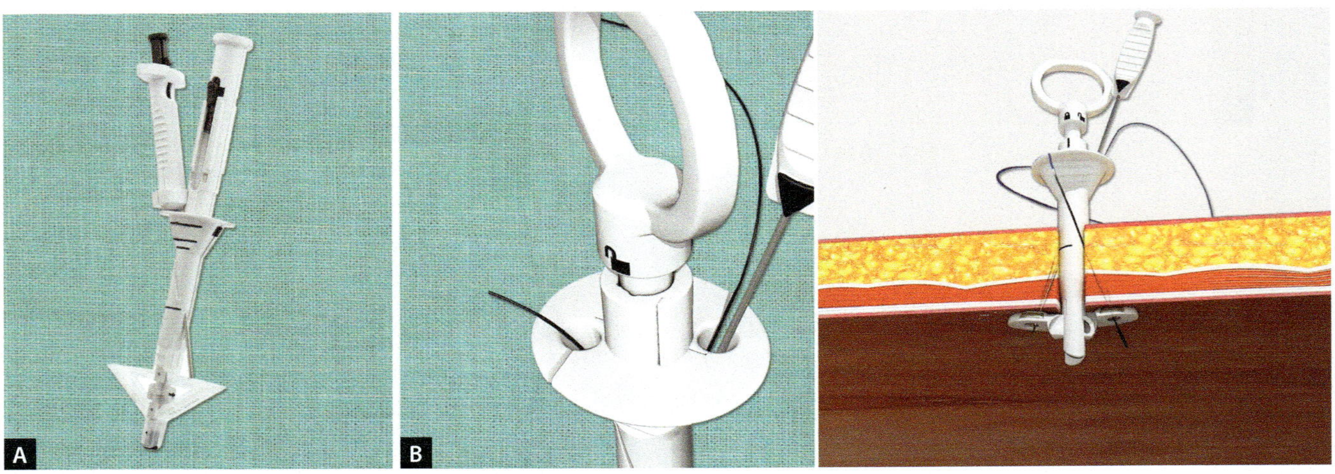

Figs. 9A and B: Weck® EFx Shield Fascial Closure System.

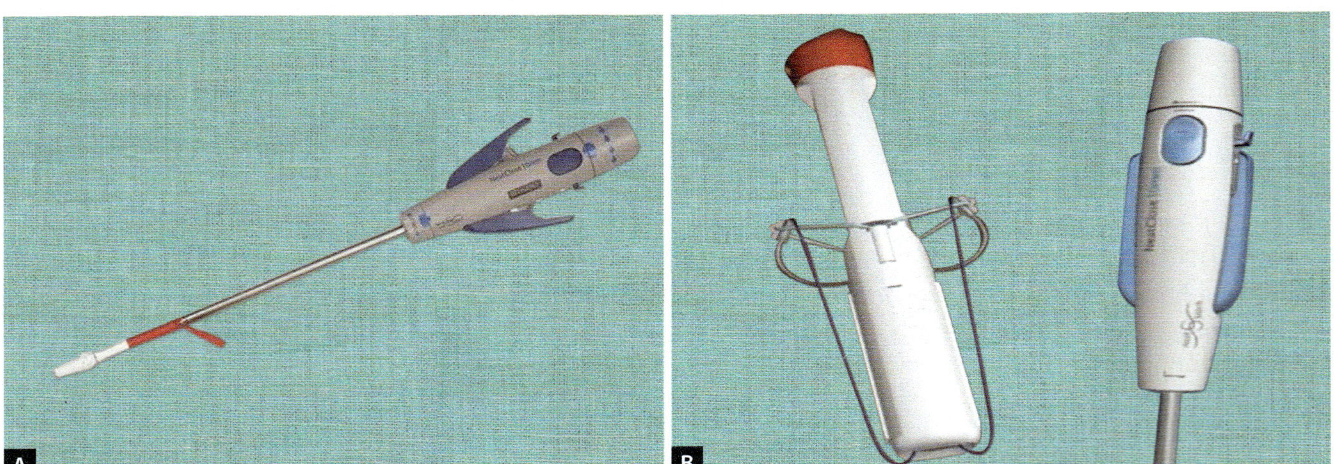

Figs. 10A and B: NeatClose automated port closure device.

port plane. With the activation button pressed, it will release the needles from the guide, via the tissue and back to the NeatClose cartridge. Once the system is pulled outside the port, you can be sure that a safe and efficient airtight seal is created, hence aiding the recovery of a patient for surgery quickly. Now we are still waiting for a painless method without the need for anesthesia.

Carter-Thomason CloseSure System—Port-site Closure (Figs. 11A and B)

Closing any trocar site is a simple, fast and safe procedure with the Carter-Thomason CloseSure System. The cone-shaped Pilot® Guide correctly angles the suture passer to achieve full-thickness closure. It closes the port including fascia and peritoneum (preventing Richter's hernias)—while maintaining pneumoperitoneum. The guide's unique design ensures precise placement of the suture passer for consistent, reproducible results on any body type.

VersaOne™ Fascial Closure System (Figs. 12 and 13)

Port-site hernias are serious complications across procedures and are a burden on patients, clinicians, and health systems. Appropriate port-site closure is considered to be one of the most critical factors for the prevention of port-site herniation. The VersaOne™ Fascial Closure System is a novel all-in-one device that serves as a trocar and fascial closure device to deliver consistent port-site closure and suture placement. The unique system features a special cannula that allows for defect closure without the need of additional devices.

As a result, the VersaOne™ Fascial Closure System:

- Provides procedure efficiency
- Eliminates the need to remove the trocar before closing
- Makes reinsufflation unnecessary—pneumoperitoneum can be maintained throughout the procedure
- Enables tissue layers to remain aligned.

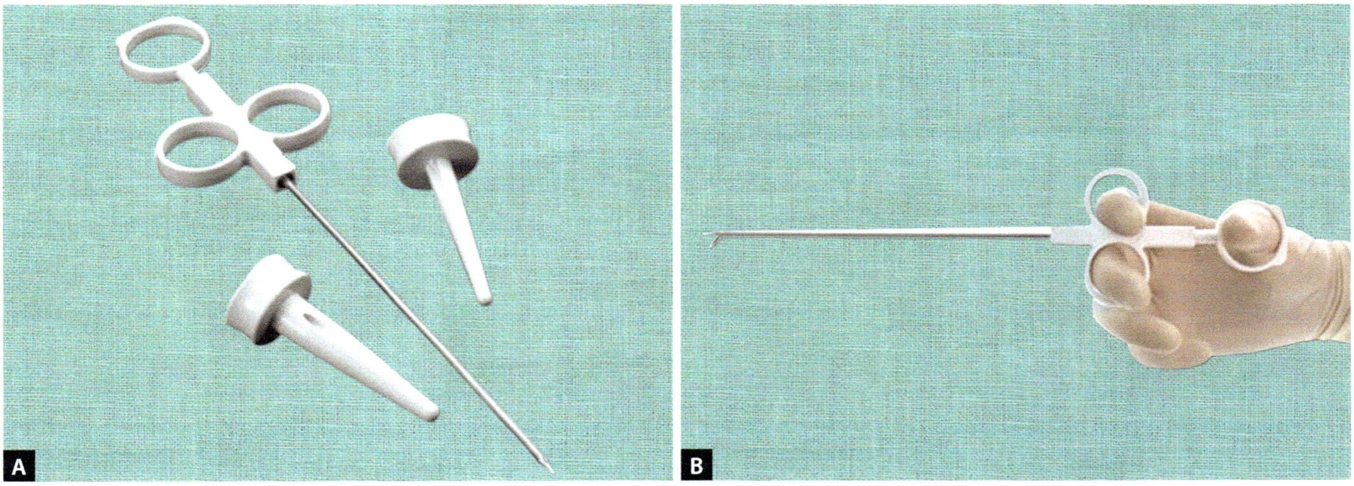

Figs. 11A and B: Carter-Thomason CloseSure System—port-site closure.

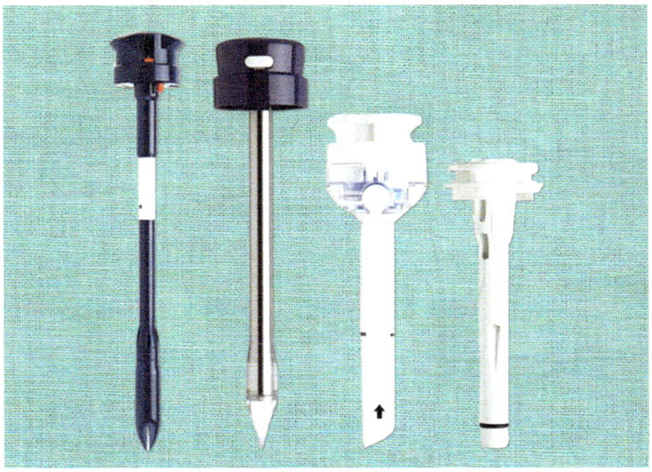

Fig. 12: VersaOne™ Fascial Closure System with its trocar.

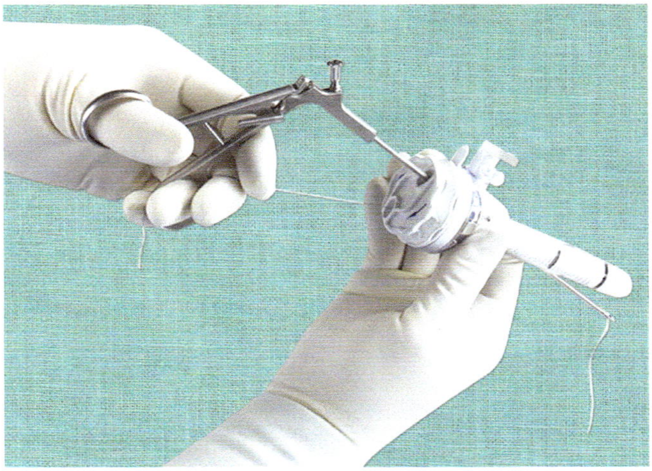

Fig. 13: VersaOne™ Fascial Closure System demonstrating insertion of suture.

There are a number of methods of post site closure but there is no gold standard. Use of traditional suturing techniques are difficult due to blind closure of the fascial defect. Varying degrees of success are achieved by modified hand suturing techniques. Finding the rectus sheath and suturing through the layers of a thicker abdominal wall through a relatively small hole is challenging particularly in the obese. In such cases, we need special instrument for efficient closure of the port site. Veress needle is an instrument that is commonly used for creating pneumoperitoneum but it has been used to close the port site efficiently under vision.

VERESS NEEDLE TECHNIQUE OF PORT CLOSURE

In 1983, Janos Veress of Hungary developed a specially designed spring-loaded needle. Interestingly, Veress did not promote the use of his needle for laparoscopy purposes. He used Veress needle for the induction of pneumothorax. But now Veress needle is the most important instrument today to create pneumoperitoneum. Veress needle consists of an outer cannula with a beveled needle point for cutting through tissues. Inside the cannula of Veress needle is an inner stylet, stylet is loaded with a spring forward in response to the sudden decrease in pressure encountered upon crossing the abdominal wall and entering the peritoneal cavity.

TECHNIQUE OF PORT CLOSURE BY VERESS NEEDLE (FIGS. 14 TO 25)

Occlude the port site with a finger so that the pneumoperitoneum is maintained and pass the Veress beside the finger through all the layers except the skin and subcutaneous tissue under vision. Maintenance of pneumoperitoneum is important as it is very difficult to close the port if vision is compromised.

Minimal access surgeries are the present and future of surgical procedures and no surgery is complete without port site closure. There are a lot of methods to close the port-site but no gold standard. This procedure with the Veress needle is safe, efficacious, and cost-effective.

One of the preventable complications is port-site incisional hernia (PIH), which could develop at any port site, most frequently at the midline, possibly because of the absence of supporting muscle. The incidence of PIH is variable from center to center, depending on several factors including surgical technique and of course surgical experience.

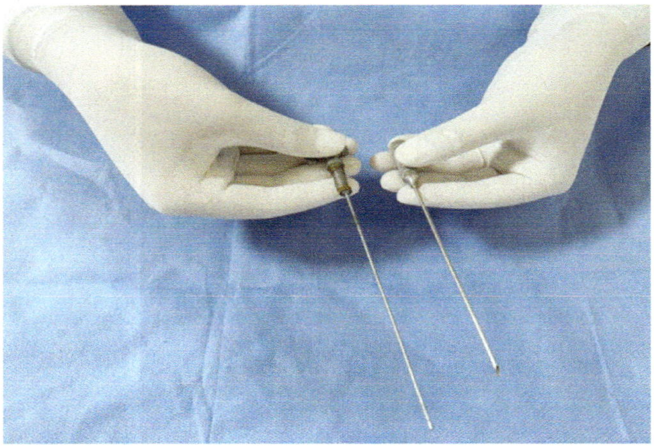

Fig. 14: Remove the stylet from the cannula.

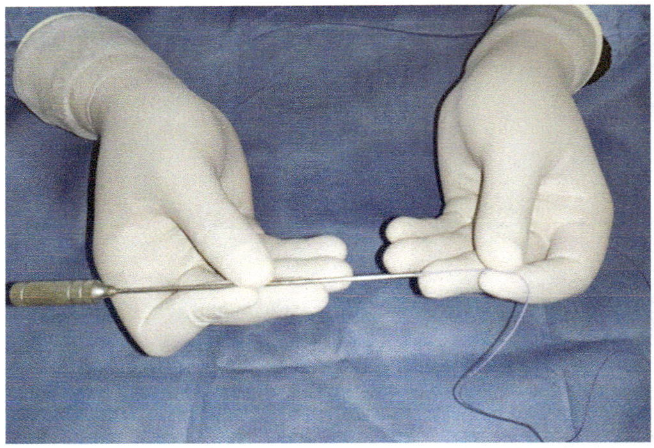

Fig. 15: Pass a suture material through the cannula from the tip.

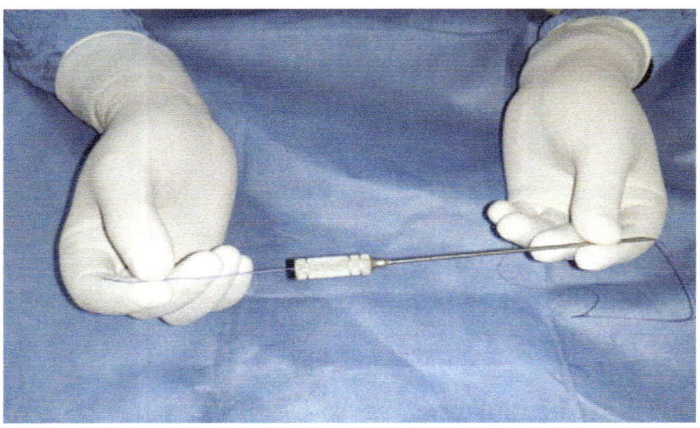

Fig. 16: Take suture out from the other end.

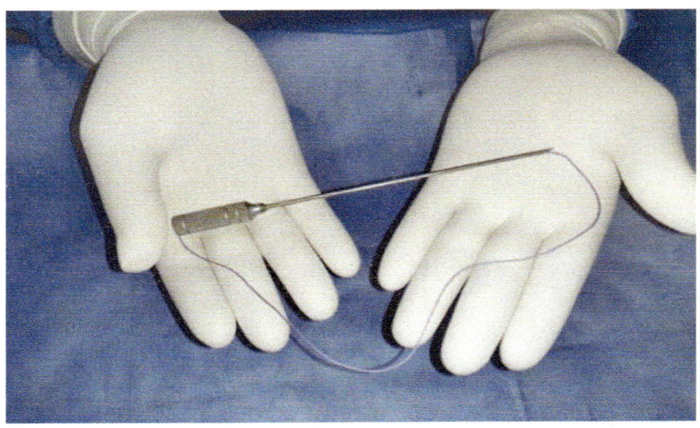

Fig. 17: Tie the loop and hide the knot in the cannula.

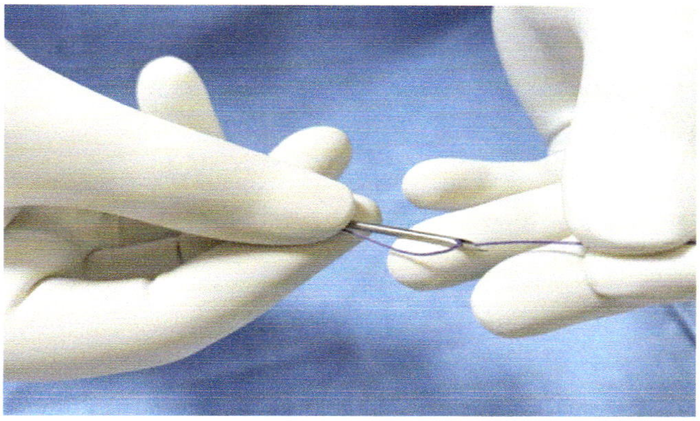

Fig. 18: Insert the suture material (that should close the port site) into the cannula tip about 2 cm deep and bend it so that it stays in place.

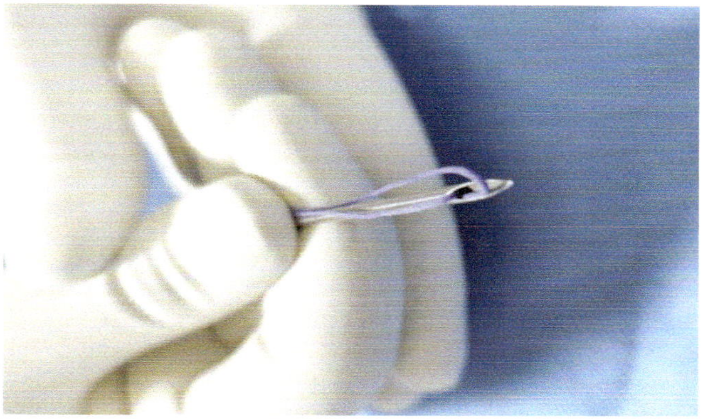

Fig. 19: Now Veress needle is ready for port closure.

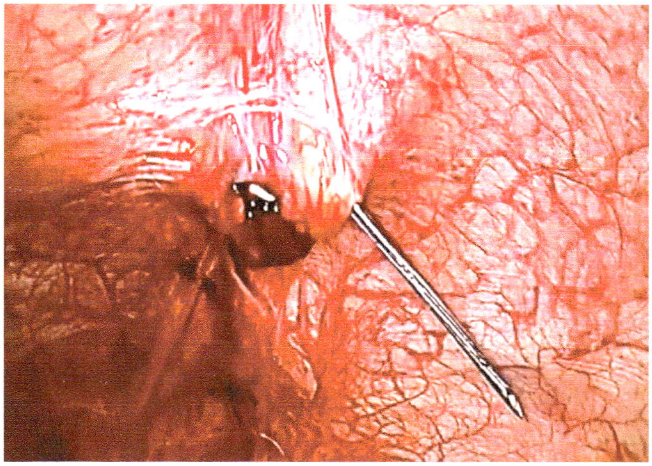

Fig. 20: Veress needle inserted with loop and tying suture on one side.

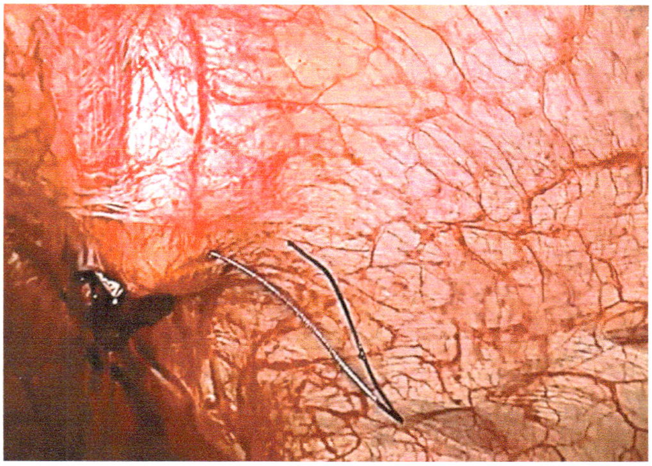

Fig. 21: Retract the Veress and the suture is automatically retained inside.

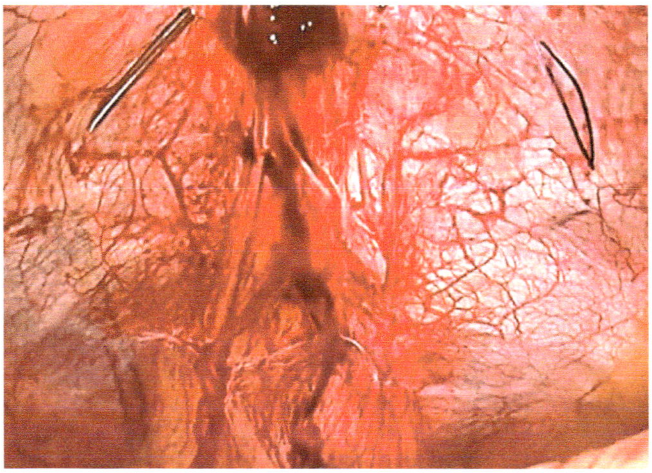

Fig. 22: Insert the Veress from the other side of the defect.

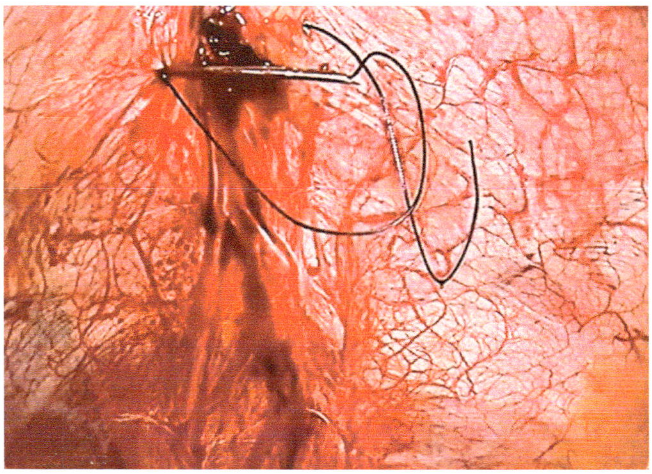

Fig. 23: Entangle the suture in the loop of the Veress.

The trocar diameter, trocar design, pre-existing fascial defects, tissue retrieval from the port site, and some operation and patient-related factors, direction of the port insertion, use of drain are the risk factors for development of PIH. In obese and bariatric patients because of larger preperitoneal space and elevated intra-abdominal pressure, the risk of formation of trocar site hernia is greater. Size of the port is another major risk factor and it is advisable to close the hole >5 mm at the fascia level.

The meticulous closure of the laparoscopic ports is important to prevent and reduce the chances of formation of PIH. Port-site closure by Veress needle is an efficient

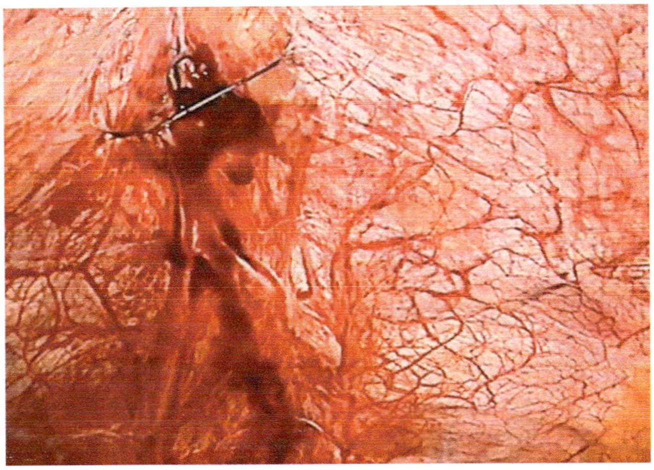

Fig. 24: Tighten the loop and retract the Veress along with the suture and tie the knot outside.

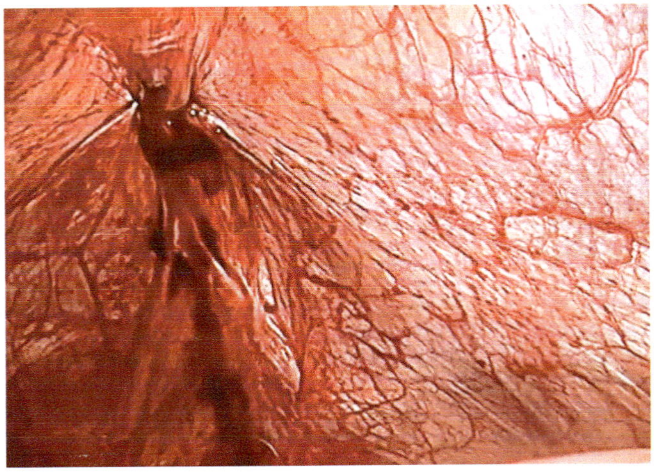

Fig. 25: Thus, the port site closed under vision and is safe procedure.

and safe technique done under vision and there is no need to buy additional equipment to close the port site thus cost effective.

The hernia may become evident at any time following laparoscopic surgery and the patient may either have an uncomplicated hernia, or may be afflicted with a variety of complications such as evisceration of the bowel or omentum and it may become a cause of significant morbidity. Meticulous closure of the fascia, avoidance of unnecessary wound extension, the use of nonabsorbable sutures when faced with defects >2 cm in size, completely defining the extent of any pre-existing hernia and repairing this at the time of port-site closure, are recommended to minimize the incidence of port-site hernia after laparoscopic surgery.

BIBLIOGRAPHY

1. Ahmad SA, Schuricht AL, Azurin DJ, Arroyo LR, Paskin DL, Bar AH, et al. Complications of laparoscopic cholecystectomy: the experience of a university-affiliated teaching hospital. J Laparoendosc Adv Surg Tech A. 1997;7:29-35.
2. Al-Haijar N, Duca S, Molnar G, Vasilescu A, Nicolescu N. Incidents and postoperative complications of laparoscopic cholecystectomies for acute cholecystitis. Rom J Gastroenterol. 2002;11:115-9.
3. Azurin DJ, Go LS, Arroyo LR, Kirkland ML. Trocar site herniation following laparoscopic cholecystectomy and the significance of an incidental preexisting umbilical hernia. Am Surg. 1995;61:718-20.
4. Baird DR, Wilson JP, Mason EM, Duncan TD, Evans JS, Luke JP, et al. An early review of 800 laparoscopic cholecystectomies at a university-affiliated community teaching hospital. Am Surg. 1992;58:206-10.
5. Bender E, Sell H. Small bowel obstruction after laparoscopic cholecystectomy as a result of a Maydl's herniation of the small bowel through a trocar site. Surgery. 1996;119:480.
6. Berthou JC, Charbonneau P. Elective laparoscopic management of sigmoid diverticulitis: results in a series of 110 patients. Surg Endosc. 1999;13:457-60.
7. Bhoyrul S, Payne J, Steffes B, Swanstrom L, Way LW. A randomized prospective study of radially expanding trocars in laparoscopic surgery. J Gastrointest Surg. 2000;4:392-7.
8. Boughey JC, Nottingham JM, Walls AC. Richter's hernia in the laparoscopic era: four case reports and review of the literature. Surg Laparosc Endosc Percutan Tech. 2003;13:55-8.
9. Bowrey DJ, Blom D, Crookes PF, Bremner CG, Johansson JL, Lord RV, et al. Risk factors and the prevalence of trocar site herniation after laparoscopic fundoplication. Surg Endosc. 2001;15:663-6.
10. Cadeddu MO, Schlachta CM, Mamazza J, Seshadri PA, Poulin EC. Soft-tissue images: trocar-site hernia after laparoscopic procedures. Can J Surg. 2002;45:9-10.
11. Callery MP, Strasberg SM, Soper NJ. Complications of laparoscopic general surgery. Gastrointest Endosc Clin N Am. 1996;6:423-44.
12. Chevallier JM, Zinzindohoue F, Elian N, Cherrak A, Blanche JP, Berta JL, et al. Adjustable gastric banding in a public university hospital: prospective analysis of 400 patients. Obes Surg. 2002;12:93-9.
13. Coda A, Bossotti M, Ferri F, Mattio R, Ramellini G, Poma A, et al. Incisional hernia and fascial defect following laparoscopic surgery. Surg Laparosc Endosc Percutan Tech. 2000;10:34-8.
14. Cottam DR, Gorecki PJ, Curvelo M, Weltman D, Angus LD, Shaftan G. Preperitoneal herniation into a laparoscopic port site without a fascial defect. Obes Surg. 2002;12:121-3.
15. Crist DW, Gadacz TR. Complications of laparoscopic surgery. Surg Clin North Am. 1993;73:265-89.
16. De Giuli M, Festa V, Denoye GC, Morino M. Large postoperative umbilical hernia following laparoscopic cholecystectomy: a case report. Surg Endosc. 1994;8:904-5.
17. Di Lorenzo N, Coscarella G, Lirosi F, Gaspari A. Port-site closure: a new problem, an old device. JSLS. 2002;6:181-3.
18. Dresel A, Kuhn JA, Westmoreland MV, Talaasen LJ, McCarty TM. Establishing a laparoscopic gastric bypass program. Am J Surg. 2002;184:617-20.
19. Duron JJ, Hay JM, Msika S, Gaschard D, Domergue J, Gainant A, et al. Prevalence and mechanisms of small intestinal obstruction following laparoscopic abdominal surgery: a retrospective multicenter study. Arch Surg. 2000;135:208-12.
20. Fear RE. Laparoscopy: a valuable aid in gynecologic diagnosis. Obstet Gynecol. 1968;31:297-309.
21. Fitzgibbons RJ Jr, Annibali R, Litke BS. Gallbladder and gallstone removal, open versus closed laparoscopy, and pneumoperitoneum. Am J Surg. 1993;165:497-504.
22. Freedman AN, Sigman HH. Incarcerated paraumbilical incisional hernia and abscess: complications of a spilled gallstone. J Laparoendosc Surg. 1995;5:189-91.

23. Hass BE, Schrager RE. Small bowel obstruction due to Richter's hernia after laparoscopic procedures. J Laparoendosc Surg. 1993;3:421-3.
24. Horgan PG, O'Connell PR. Subumbilical hernia following laparoscopic cholecystectomy. Br J Surg. 1993;80:1595.
25. Kadar N, Reich H, Liu CY, Manko GF, Gimpelson R. Incisional hernias after major laparoscopic gynecologic procedures. Am J Obstet Gynecol. 1993;168:1493-5.
26. Komuta K, Haraguchi M, Inoue K, Furui J, Kanematsu T. Herniation of the small bowel through the port site following removal of drains during laparoscopic surgery. Dig Surg. 2000;17:544-6.
27. Kopelman D, Schein M, Assalia A, Hashmonai M. Small bowel obstruction following laparoscopic cholecystectomy: diagnosis of incisional hernia by computed tomography. Surg Laparosc Endosc. 1994;4:325-6.
28. Kulacoglu IH. Regarding: small bowel obstruction and incisional hernia after laparoscopic surgery: should 5-mm trocar sites be sutured? J Laparoendosc Adv Surg Tech A. 2000;10:227-8.
29. Lafullarde T, Van Hee R, Gys T. A safe and simple method for routine open access in laparoscopic procedures. Surg Endosc. 1999;13:769-72.
30. Larson GM, Vitale GC, Casey J, Voyles CR. Multipractice analysis of laparoscopic cholecystectomy in 1,983 patients. Am J Surg. 1992;163:221-6.
31. Leibl BJ, Schmedt CG, Schwarz J, Kraft K, Bittner R. Laparoscopic surgery complications associated with trocar tip design: review of literature and own results. J Laparoendosc Adv Surg Tech A. 1999;9:135-40.
32. Li P, Chung RS. Closure of trocar wounds using a suture carrier. Surg Laparosc Endosc. 1996;6:469-71.
33. Liu CD, McFadden DW. Laparoscopic port sites do not require fascial closure when nonbladed trocars are used. Am Surg. 2000;66:853-4.
34. Lumley J, Stitz R, Stevenson A, Fielding G, Luck A. Laparoscopic colorectal surgery for cancer: intermediate to long-term outcomes. Dis Colon Rectum. 2002;45:867-72.
35. Maio A, Ruchman RB. CT diagnosis of post laparoscopic hernia. J Comput Assist Tomogr. 1991;15:1054-5.
36. Matter I, Nash E, Abrahamson J, Eldar S. Incisional hernia via a lateral 5-mm trocar port following laparoscopic cholecystectomy. Isr J Med Sci. 1996;32:790-1.
37. Matthews BD, Heniford BT, Sing RF. Preperitoneal Richter hernia after a laparoscopic gastric bypass. Surg Laparosc Endosc Percutan Tech. 2001;11:47-9.
38. Mayol J, Garcia-Aguilar J, Ortiz-Oshiro E, De-Diego Carmona JA, Fernandez-Represa JA. Risks of the minimal access approach for laparoscopic surgery: multivariate analysis of morbidity related to umbilical trocar insertion. World J Surg. 1997;21:529-33.
39. McMillan J, Watt I. Herniation at the site of cannula insertion after laparoscopic cholecystectomy. Br J Surg. 1993;80:915.
40. McMurrick PJ, Polglase AL. Early incisional hernia after use of the 12-mm port for laparoscopic surgery. Aust N Z J Surg. 1993;63:574-5.
41. Montz FJ, Holschneider CH, Munro MG. Incisional hernia following laparoscopy: a survey of the American Association of Gynecologic Laparoscopists. Obstet Gynecol. 1994;84:881-4.
42. Morrison CP, Wemyss-Holden SA, Iswariah H, Maddern GJ. Lateral laparoscopic port sites should all be closed: the incisional "spigelian" hernia. Surg Endosc. 2002;16:1364.
43. Nakajima K, Wasa M, Kawahara H, Hasegawa T, Soh H, Taniguchi E, et al. Revision laparoscopy for incarcerated hernia at a 5-mm trocar site following pediatric laparoscopic surgery. Surg Laparosc Endosc Percutan Tech. 1999;9:294-5.
44. Nassar AH, Ashkar KA, Rashed AA, Abdulmoneum MG. Laparoscopic cholecystectomy and the umbilicus. Br J Surg. 1997;84:630-3.
45. Ok E, Sozuer E. Intra-abdominal gallstone spillage detected during umbilical trocar site hernia repair after laparoscopic cholecystectomy: report of a case. Surg Today. 2000;30:1046-8.
46. Patterson M, Walters D, Browder W. Postoperative bowel obstruction following laparoscopic surgery. Am Surg. 1993;59:656-7.
47. Petrakis I, Sciacca V, Chalkiadakis G, Vassilakis SI, Xynos E. A simple technique for trocar site closure after laparoscopic surgery. Surg Endosc. 1999;13:1249-51.
48. Plaus WJ. Laparoscopic trocar site hernias. J Laparoendosc Surg. 1993;3:567-70.
49. Rabinerson D, Avrech O, Neri A, Schoenfeld A. Incisional hernias after laparoscopy. Obstet Gynecol Surv. 1997;52:701-3.
50. Ramachandran CS. Umbilical hernial defects encountered before and after abdominal laparoscopic procedures. Int Surg. 1998;83:171-3.
51. Reardon PR, McKinney G, Craig ES. The 2-mm trocar: a safe and effective way of closing trocar sites using existing equipment. J Am Coll Surg. 2003;196:333-6.
52. Reardon PR, Preciado A, Scarborough T, Matthews B, Marti JL. Hernia at 5-mm laparoscopic port site presenting as early postoperative small bowel obstruction. J Laparoendosc Adv Surg Tech A. 1999;9:523-5.
53. Rosen M, Ponsky J. Minimally invasive surgery. Endoscopy. 2001;33:358-66.
54. Sanz-Lopez R, Martinez-Ramos C, Nunez-Pena JR, Ruiz de Gopegui M, Pastor-Sirera L, Tamames-Escobar S. Incisional hernias after laparoscopic vs open cholecystectomy. Surg Endosc. 1999;13:922-4.
55. Schauer PR, Ikramuddin S, Gourash W, Ramanathan R, Luketich J. Outcomes after laparoscopic Roux-en-Y gastric bypass for morbid obesity. Ann Surg. 2000;232:515-29.
56. Schiller VL, Joyce PW, Sarti DA. Small-bowel obstruction due to hernia through the primary laparoscopic port: a complication of laparoscopic cholecystectomy. Am J Roentgenol. 1994;163:480-1.
57. Susmallian S, Ezri T, Charuzi I. Laparoscopic repair of access port site hernia after Lap-Band system implantation. Obes Surg. 2002;12:682-4.
58. Velasco JM, Vallina VL, Bonomo SR, Hieken TJ. Post laparoscopic small bowel obstruction: rethinking its management. Surg Endosc. 1998;12:1043-5.
59. Voyles CR, Petro AB, Meena AL, Haick AJ, Koury AM. A practical approach to laparoscopic cholecystectomy. Am J Surg. 1991;161:365-70.
60. Wagner M, Farley GE. Incarcerated hernia with intestinal obstruction after laparoscopic cholecystectomy. Wis Med J. 1994;93:169-71.
61. Waldhaussen JH. Incisional hernia in a 5-mm trocar site following pediatric laparoscopy. J Laparoendosc Surg. 1996;6 (Suppl 1):S89-90.
62. Wallace DH, O'Dwyer PJ. Clinical experience with open laparoscopy. J Laparoendosc Adv Surg Tech A. 1997;7:285-8.
63. Williams MD, Flowers SS, Fenoglio ME, Brown TR. Richter hernia: a rare complication of laparoscopy. Surg Laparosc Endosc. 1995;5:419-21.

SECTION

2 Laparoscopic General Surgical Procedures

- Laparoscopic Cholecystectomy
- Laparoscopic CBD Exploration
- Laparoscopic Appendicectomy
- Laparoscopic Repair of Inguinal Hernia
- Laparoscopic Repair of Ventral Hernia
- Laparoscopic Repair of Hiatus Hernia
- Laparoscopic Repair of Duodenal Perforation
- Laparoscopic Fundoplication
- Laparoscopic Bariatric Surgery
- Laparoscopic Splenectomy
- Laparoscopic Management of Hepaticopancreatic Diseases
- Diagnostic Laparoscopy
- Laparoscopic Small Bowel Surgery
- Laparoscopic Colorectal Surgery
- Laparoscopic Adhesiolysis

CHAPTER 13

Laparoscopic Cholecystectomy

INTRODUCTION

Laparoscopic surgery has undergone rapid development in recent years. Laparoscopic cholecystectomy was first performed in 1985. Since the introduction of laparoscopic cholecystectomy into general practice in 1990, it has rapidly become the dominant procedure for gallbladder surgery. By the end of the decade, laparoscopic cholecystectomy had spread throughout the world. The importance of laparoscopic cholecystectomy was the cultural change it engendered rather than the operation it replaced. In terms of technique, laparoscopic cholecystectomy is now the gold standard for the treatment of symptomatic gallstone disease. It is most commonly performed minimal access surgery by general surgeons' worldwide. In Europe and America, 98% of all the cholecystectomy is performed by laparoscopy. The credit of popularizing minimal access surgery goes to laparoscopic cholecystectomy. This is most popular and most accepted minimal access surgical procedure worldwide. Laparoscopic surgery has expanded from gallbladder surgery to virtually every operation in the abdominal cavity.

INDICATIONS (FIG. 1)

- Cholelithiasis
- Mucocele gallbladder
- Empyema gallbladder
- Cholesterolosis
- Typhoid carrier

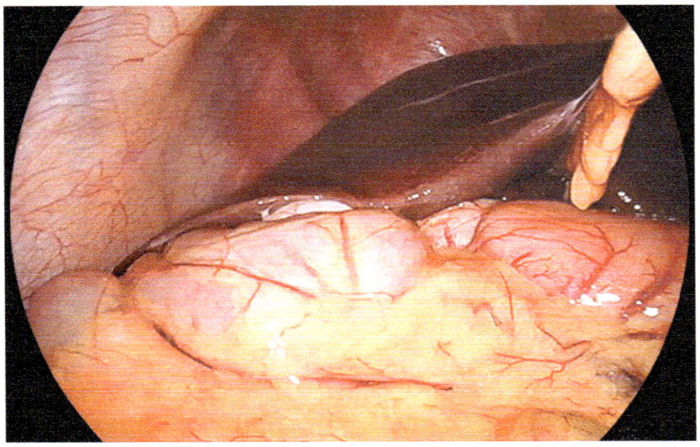

Fig. 1: Appearance of fundus of gallbladder in first look.

- Porcelain gallbladder
- Acute cholecystitis (calculous and acalculous)
- Adenomatous gallbladder polyps
- As part of other procedures, viz., Whipple's procedure.

CONTRAINDICATIONS

- Hemodynamic instability
- Uncorrected coagulopathy
- Generalized peritonitis
- Severe cardiopulmonary disease
- Abdominal wall infection
- Multiple previous upper abdominal procedures
- Late pregnancy

The general anesthesia and the pneumoperitoneum required as part of the laparoscopic procedure do increase the risk in certain groups of patients. Contraindications to laparoscopic cholecystectomy are primarily related to anesthetic concerns and include diffuse peritonitis with hemodynamic compromise and uncontrolled bleeding disorders. Most surgeons would not recommend laparoscopy in those with pre-existing disease conditions. Patients with severe cardiac diseases and chronic obstructive pulmonary disease (COPD) should not be considered a good candidate for laparoscopy. The laparoscopic cholecystectomy may also be more difficult in patients who have had previous upper abdominal surgery. The elderly may also be at increased risk for complications with general anesthesia combined with pneumoperitoneum. Relative contraindications are dependent on the surgeon's judgment and experience but include patients with previous extensive abdominal surgery, cirrhosis with portal hypertension, severe cardiopulmonary disease, active cholangitis, and morbid obesity.

ADVANTAGES OF LAPAROSCOPIC APPROACH

- Cosmetically better outcome
- Less tissue dissection and disruption of tissue planes
- Less pain postoperatively
- Low intraoperative and postoperative complications in experienced hand
- Early return to work.

TIMING OF SURGERY

The optimal timing of surgery will depend upon the patient's overall medical condition and underlying diagnosis.

- *Acute cholecystitis*: Patients with acute cholecystitis, who are surgical candidates, should undergo cholecystectomy as soon as they are fully resuscitated, and the most qualified surgeon is available. Early cholecystectomy has been associated with improved patient outcomes compared with interval cholecystectomy.
- *Gallstone pancreatitis*: Patients with gallstone pancreatitis have a high risk of recurrence within 30 days of their attack and therefore should undergo cholecystectomy during their index hospitalization after their symptoms resolve.
- *Obstructive jaundice*: A history of pancreatitis or jaundice raises the likelihood of common bile duct (CBD) stones. Patients with isolated obstructive jaundice with or without cholangitis should either have their CBD cleared with urgent endoscopic retrograde cholangiopancreatography (ERCP) preoperatively or with cholangiography and laparoscopic common duct exploration at the time of surgery. If ERCP is successful, the patient should electively be scheduled for cholecystectomy.
- *Medical comorbidities*: Identification of bleeding diatheses and poor cardiopulmonary reserve will help to identify patients who may not tolerate pneumoperitoneum or will have higher likelihood for conversion to open operation. In patients with multiple comorbidities or acute medical problem, a trial of antibiotics with consideration for a percutaneous cholecystostomy tube with delayed laparoscopic cholecystectomy in 6–8 weeks may be preferable.

PREOPERATIVE INVESTIGATIONS

Apart from routine preoperative investigations, in fit patients, the only investigations needed are ultrasound examination. Although practiced in some centers, intravenous cholangiography may not be confirmative and is attended with the risk of anaphylactic reactions.

Laboratory Testing

Laboratory testing in patients being evaluated for acute cholecystitis typically includes a complete blood count, liver enzymes, amylase, and lipase.

Elevations in the serum total bilirubin and alkaline phosphatase concentrations are *not* common in uncomplicated cholecystitis, since biliary obstruction is limited to the gallbladder; if present, they should raise concerns about complicating conditions such as cholangitis, choledocholithiasis, or Mirizzi's syndrome. However, mild elevations have been reported even in the absence of these complications and may be due to the passage of small stones, sludge, or pus.

For young, otherwise healthy patients with gallstones but no evidence of pericholecystic inflammation or bile duct dilation, additional preoperative laboratory testing is not routinely necessary, unless a new clinical event has occurred, such as significant pain, fever, or jaundice, or the physical examination suggests that an abnormality is present. An electrocardiogram or chest radiograph is obtained as appropriate.

For patients with complicated biliary tract disease, abnormal tests (e.g., liver function tests, amylase, and lipase) should be repeated to serve as a baseline for postoperative comparison. Coagulation tests are not routinely needed but may be obtained, if there is a reason to believe an abnormality may be present.

Imaging

Ultrasonography (US) of the right upper quadrant establishes the diagnosis of gallstones or abnormalities of the gallbladder wall. The US may also demonstrate CBD dilatation, stones, or evidence of acute inflammation of the gallbladder. Nuclear cholescintigraphy may be useful in cases in which the diagnosis remains uncertain after US.

Magnetic resonance cholangiopancreatography (MRCP) may be useful to evaluate the common duct in patients with mild elevations of their transaminases or mild CBD dilatation on US.

Endoscopic Retrograde Cholangiopancreatography

If a patient has a dilated CBD, CBD stones, or jaundice, consideration should be given to a preoperative ERCP with clearing of the stones followed by laparoscopic cholecystectomy. In the absence of frank jaundice or cholangitis, mild abnormalities of liver enzymes and/or bile duct dilation may also be managed effectively with intraoperative evaluation of the CBD, rather than preoperative ERCP.

Patient Position

Patient is operated in the supine position with a steep head-up and left tilt. This typical positioning of laparoscopic cholecystectomy should be achieved once the pneumoperitoneum has been established. The patient is then placed in reverse Trendelenburg's position and rotated to the left to give maximal exposure to the right upper quadrant.

Position of Surgical Team (Fig. 2)

The surgeon stands on the left side of the patient with the scrub nurse-camera holder-assistant. One assistant stands right to the patient and should hold the fundus-grasping forceps.

Tasks Analysis

- Preparation of the patient
- Creation of pneumoperitoneum
- Insertion of ports
- Diagnostic laparoscopy
- Dissection of visceral peritoneum
- Dissection of Calot's triangle
- Clipping and division of cystic duct and artery
- Dissection of gallbladder from liver bed
- Extraction of gallbladder and any spilled stone
- Irrigation and suction of operating field
- Final diagnostic laparoscopy
- Removal of the instrument with complete exit of CO_2
- Closure of wound.

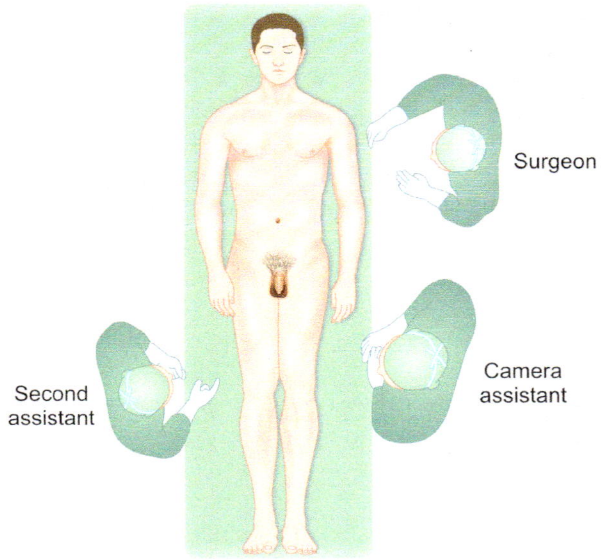

Fig. 2: Position of surgical team.

Port Location (Figs. 3A to C)

Four ports are used—optical (10 mm), one 5 mm, one 10 mm operating, and one 5.0 mm assisting port. The optical port is at or near the umbilicus and routinely a 30° laparoscope is used. Some surgeons who have started laparoscopy earlier are more comfortable with 0° telescope. The laparoscope is inserted through a 10-mm umbilical port and the abdominal cavity is explored for any obvious abnormalities. The secondary ports are then placed under direct visualization with the laparoscope. The surgeon places a 10-mm trocar in the midline and left to the falciform ligament at the epigastrium. Two 5-mm ports, one subcostal trocar in the right upper quadrant and another 5 mm trocar, lower, near the right anterior axillary line, are placed.

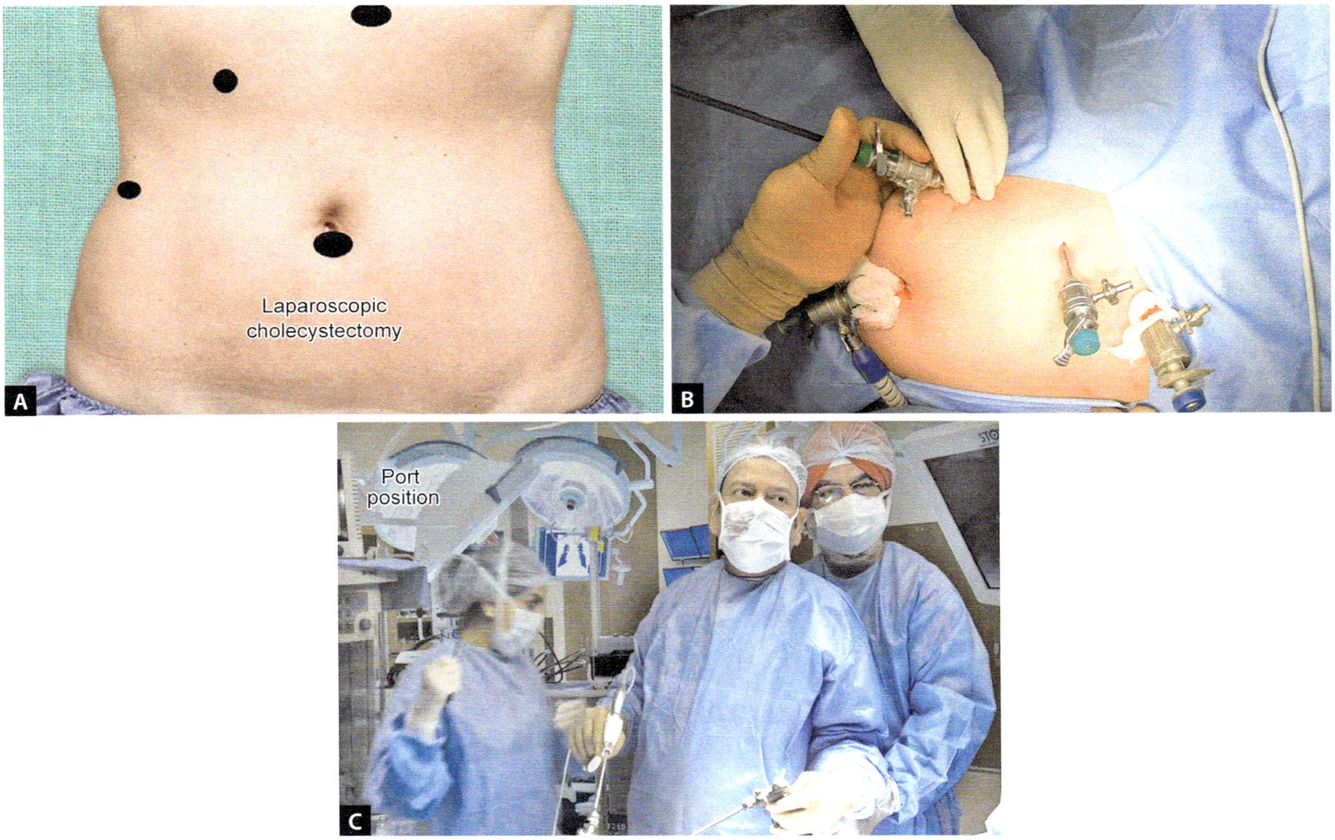

Figs. 3A to C: (A) Ideal port position for laparoscopic cholecystectomy; (B and C) Port position of cholecystectomy.

LAPAROSCOPIC ANATOMY (FIG. 4)

Laparoscopic view of the right upper quadrant on first look will demonstrate primarily the subphrenic spaces, abdominal surface of diaphragm, and diaphragmatic surface of the liver. The fundus of the gallbladder can be seen popping from the inferior surface of liver. The falciform ligament is seen as a prominent dividing point between left subphrenic space and the right subphrenic space. As the gallbladder is elevated and retracted toward the diaphragm, adhesion to the omentum or duodenum and transverse colon is seen.

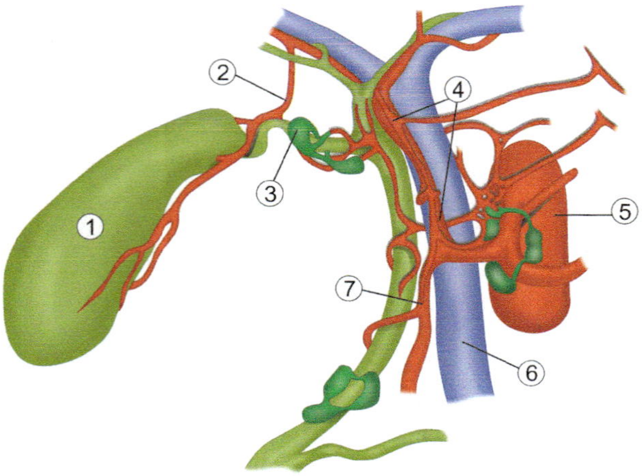

Fig. 4: Topographic anatomy of gallbladder: (1) Gallbladder; (2) Cystic artery; (3) Mscagni lymph node; (4) Proper hepatic artery; (5) Abdominal aorta; (6) Portal vein; (7) Gastroduodenal artery.

Exposure of Gallbladder and Cystic Pedicle (Figs. 5A to D)

A grasper is used through the right lower 5-mm trocar to grasp the gallbladder fundus and retract it up over the liver edge to expose the entire length of the gallbladder. If there are adhesions to the gallbladder, they will need to be taken down using blunt and sharp dissection. With the entire gallbladder visualized, a second grasper is inserted through the other right upper quadrant trocar to grasp the gallbladder infundibulum and retract it up and to the right to expose the triangle of Calot.

Careful evaluation of the anatomy reveals whether it is partially intrahepatic, on a mesentery, or possesses a Phrygian cap or any other odd shape. Hartmann's pouch should be identified and seen to be funnel down to continue as tubular structure, the cystic duct. It is important to identify Hartmann's pouch clearly, because most of the laparoscopic surgeons clip and divide the cystic duct, high on its termination at Hartmann's pouch, rather than attempting to trace the cystic duct's junction with the CBD. Dissection of the junction of cystic duct with the CBD increases the chance of traction injury and bleeding from small vessels and lymphatic.

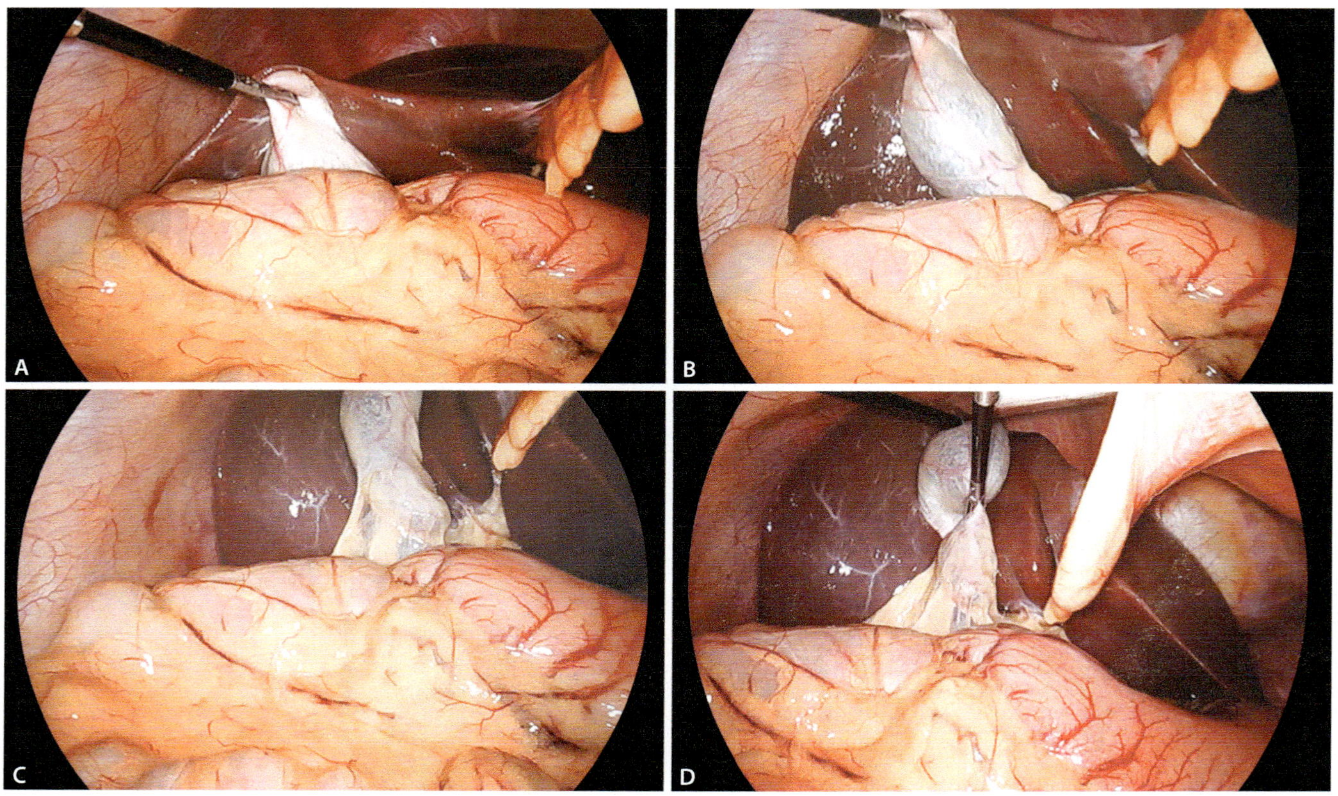

Figs. 5A to D: Proper traction for exposure of cystic pedicle.

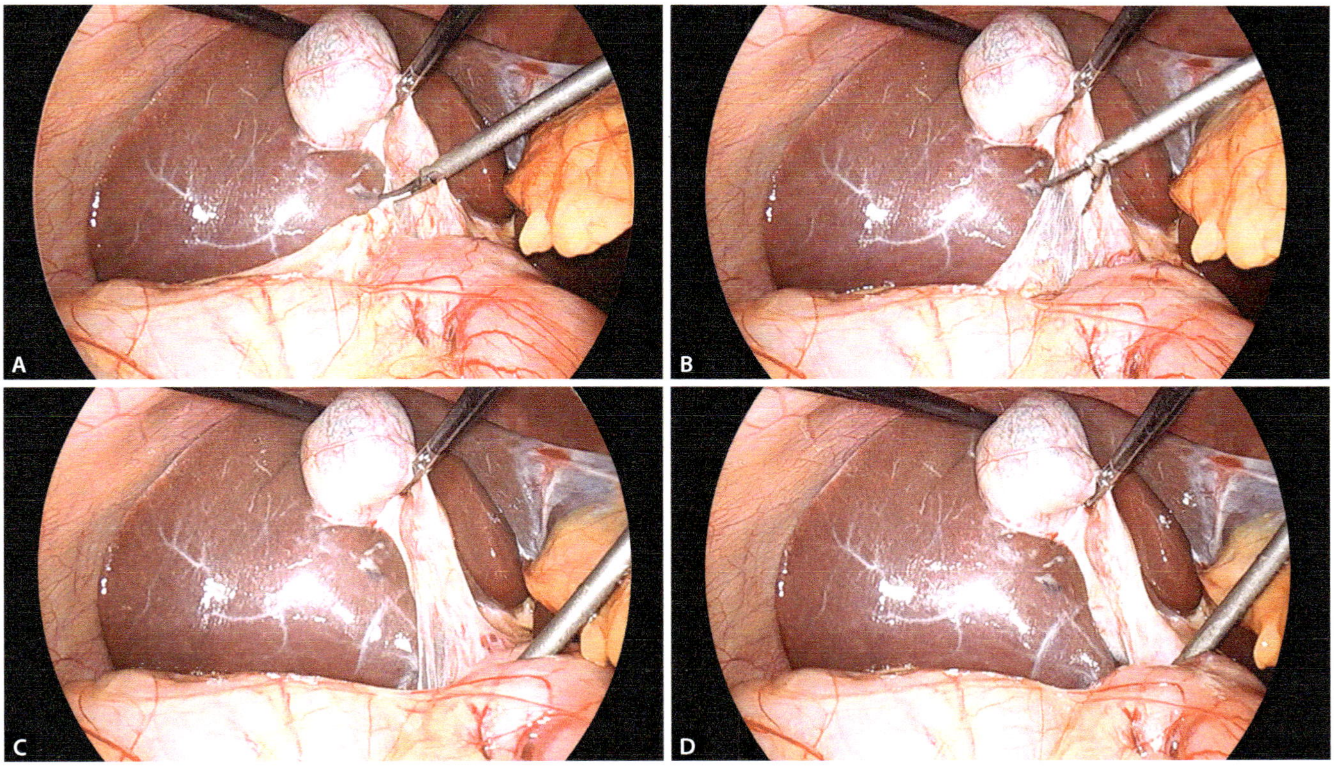

Figs. 6A to D: Clearing adhesions by hook.

Cystic artery can be seen, if attention is given, as it runs along the surface of gallbladder. A lymph node may be seen anterior to the cystic artery. The cystic artery gives off a small artery that supplies the cystic duct. This tiny twig often avulsed and bleeds at the time of creating window between artery and duct. This bleeding stops when the cystic duct is clipped.

Adhesiolysis (Figs. 6A to D)

Any adhesion should be cleared from the gallbladder. The surgeon uses a dissector through the epigastric trocar to tear the peritoneal attachments from the infundibulum. The attachments are taken down from high on the gallbladder, beginning laterally in order to help avoid injury to the CBD. Sharp dissection may be carried out with the help of scissors attached with monopolar current. At the time of separating adhesion, surgeon should try to be as near as possible toward gallbladder. The cystic pedicle is a triangular fold of peritoneum containing the cystic duct and artery, the cystic node, and a variable amount of fat. It has a superior and an inferior leaf, which are continuous over the anterior edge formed by the cystic duct **(Fig. 7)**. An important consideration is the frequent anomalies of the structures contained between the two leaves (15–20%). The normal configuration is for an anterior cystic duct with the cystic artery situated posterosuperiorly and arising from the right hepatic artery usually behind the CBD.

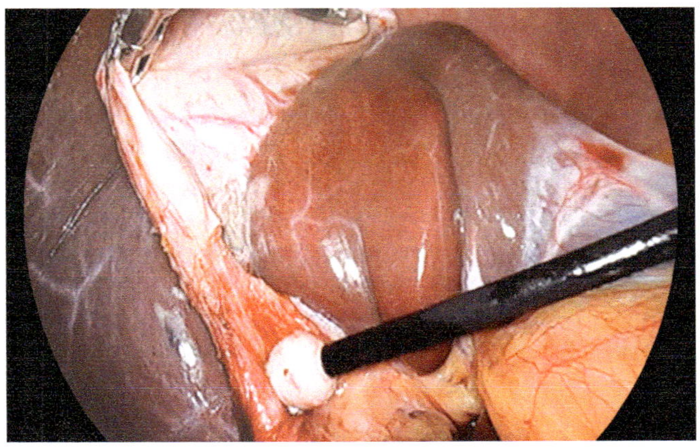

Fig. 7: Pledget can be used for adhesiolysis.

Dissection of Cystic Pedicle (Figs. 8A to D)

The dissection of the cystic pedicle can be carried out with two-handed technique. The dissection should be started with anteromedial traction by left hand grasper placed on the anterior edge of Hartmann's pouch. The anteromedial traction by left hand will expose the posterior peritoneum. The peritoneum of the posterior leaf of the cystic pedicle is divided superficially as far back as the liver. Posterior leaf is better to dissect before anterior leaf because it is relatively less vascular and the bleeding, if any, will not soil the anterior peritoneum; whereas if anterior peritoneum is tackled first, it may make the dissection area of posterior peritoneum filled

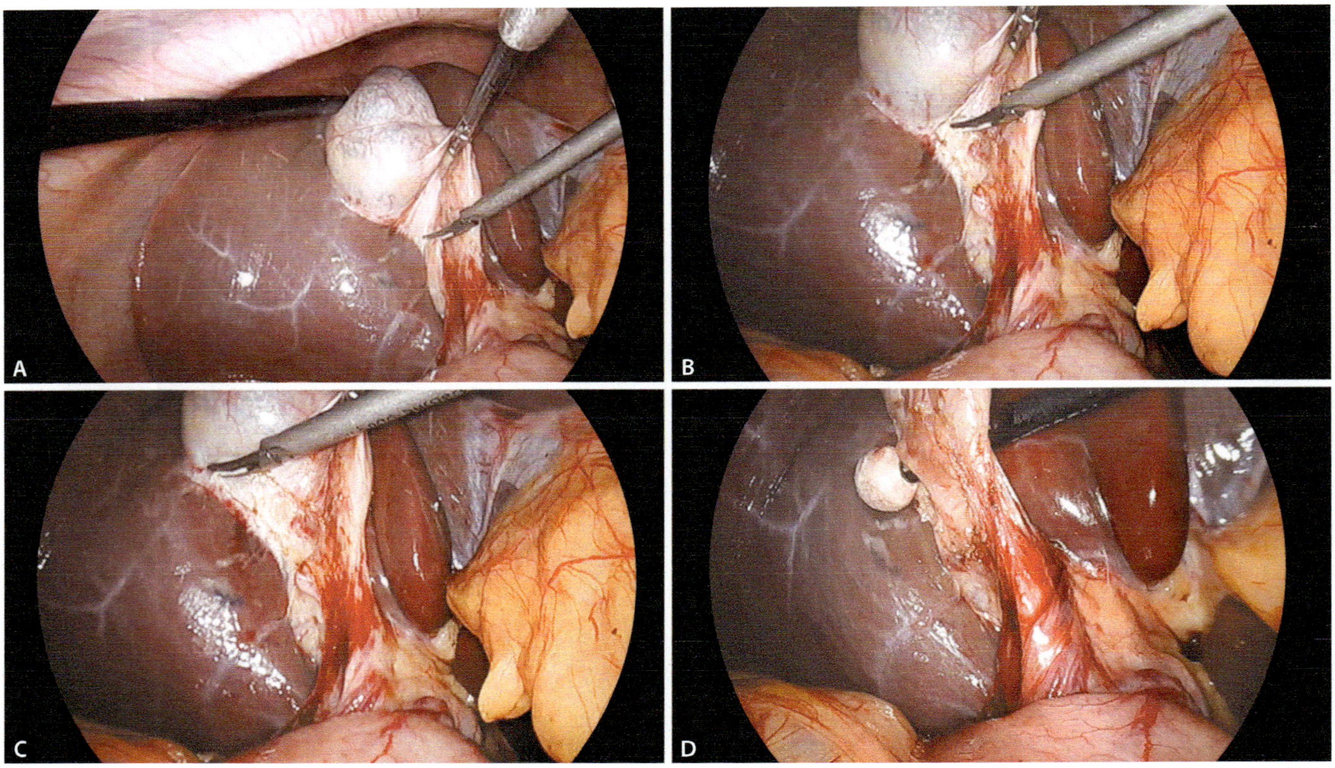

Figs. 8A to D: Dissection of cystic pedicle.

with blood making dissection of this area difficult. Once the visceral peritoneum is dissected, a pledget mounted securely in a pledget holder is used for blunt dissection.

Critical View of Safety

Anterior and posterior dissection continues with alternating inferolateral and superomedial retraction of the neck until the gallbladder is dissected away from the liver, creating a "window" crossed by two structures—the cystic duct and artery. This is the "critical view of safety (CVS)" that should be achieved prior to clipping or dividing any tubular structures.

There is no need to dissect down to the cystic duct–CBD junction unless the cystic duct is very short. The cystic artery should be dissected in a similar fashion. Calot's node, or the cystic duct lymph node, is usually encountered adjacent and anterior to the artery and can be a useful landmark.

The surgeon should be aware of certain anatomic variations in order to avoid misidentification of structures. A common anomaly is the right hepatic artery looping onto the infundibulum and being mistaken for the cystic artery. A short cystic duct is also seen quite frequently and could drain into the right hepatic duct, the common duct, or a low-lying aberrant right sectoral duct. In the presence of severe, acute, or chronic inflammation, or with a large stone in the neck of the gallbladder, the infundibulum may be "tethered" to the hepatic duct, which may lead the surgeon to misidentify the CBD for the cystic duct.

Separation of Cystic Duct from Artery (Figs. 9A to D)

Once the cystic duct is visualized, the dissector can be used to create a window in the triangle of Calot between the cystic duct and cystic artery. This window should be created high near the gallbladder-cystic duct junction to avoid injury to the common duct.

The separation of the cystic duct anteriorly from the cystic artery behind can be performed by a Maryland's grasper by gently opening the jaw of Maryland between the duct and artery. The opening of the jaw of Maryland dissector should be in the line of duct never at right angle to avoid injury of artery behind. Sufficient length of the cystic duct and artery on the gallbladder side should be mobilized so that three clips can be applied.

The electrosurgical hook may be inserted into the window and hooked around the cystic duct. With an up and down movement, the hook is used to clear as much tissue as possible from the duct nearer to the cystic duct–gallbladder junction. Tissue that is not dissected free from the duct is retracted by the hook away from all structures and is divided using active cutting current. Depending on the length of the duct, it is usually not necessary to dissect it all the way down to its junction with the CBD. In a similar fashion, the hook can be used to isolate the cystic artery for a length that is adequate enough to clip it.

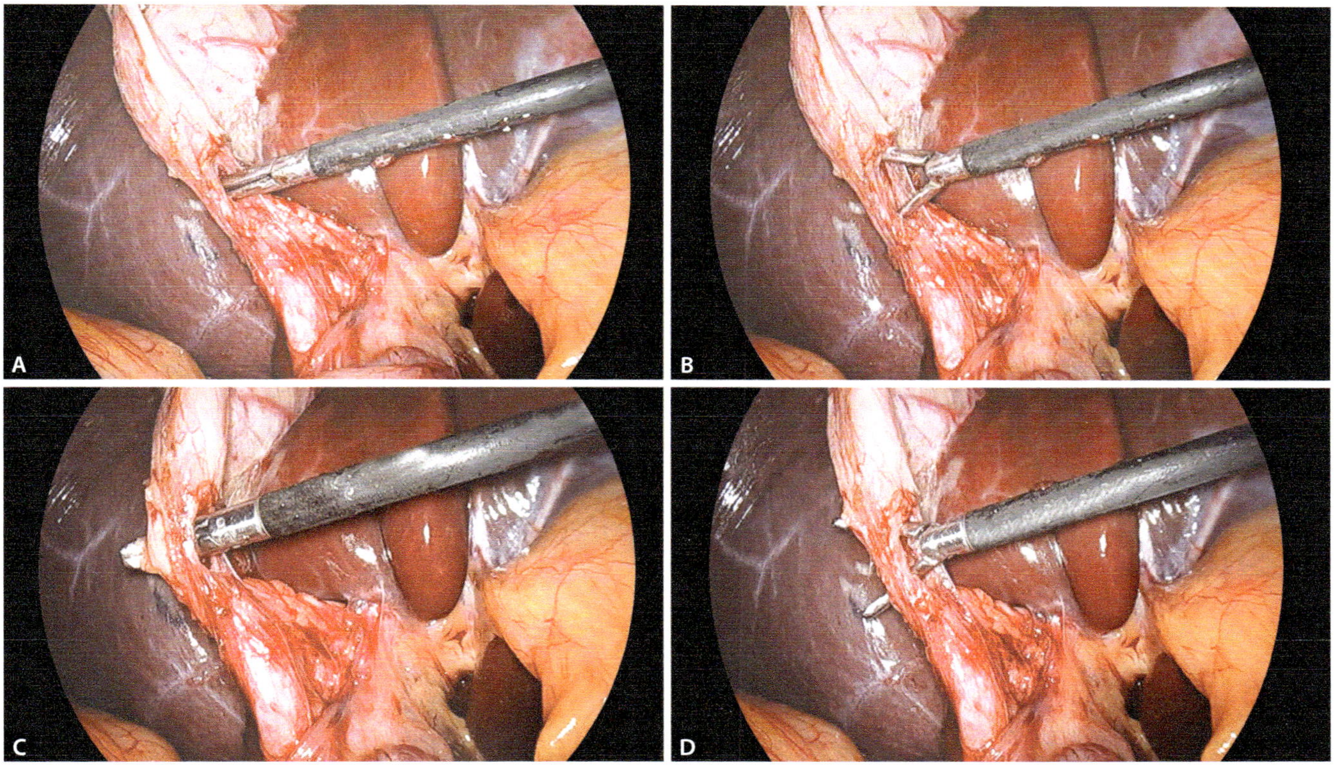

Figs. 9A to D: Cystic duct is separated from artery by creating a window.

Clipping and Division of Cystic Artery (Figs. 10A to D)

The cystic artery is clipped and then divided by harmonic scalpel **(Figs. 10I and J)**. Two clips are placed proximally on the cystic artery and one clip is applied distally. The artery is then grasped with a duckbill grasper on the gallbladder wall and then divided between second and third clip.

Clipping and Division of Cystic Duct (Figs. 10E to L)

After isolating the cystic duct and artery, the clipper is introduced through the epigastric port and at least two clips are placed on the proximal side of the cystic duct. Care is taken not to place the clips too low because retraction can tent up the CBD or cause it to be obstructed. Another clip is placed on the gallbladder side of the cystic duct, leaving enough distance between the clips to divide it. In a similar fashion, clips are placed on the cystic artery, two proximally and one on the gallbladder side of the artery. The harmonic scalpel are then used through the epigastric port to divide the cystic duct and artery between the clips. Both the jaw of scissors should be under vision.

Intraoperative Cholangiogram (Figs. 11A and B)

In many institutions, routine intraoperative cholangiogram (IOC) is performed. Routine cholangiogram decreases the risk of CBD injury in case of difficult anatomy. If a cholangiogram is to be performed, the cystic duct is isolated and occluded with a clip, which is placed high on the duct at its junction with the gallbladder. This will avoid leakage of contents from the gallbladder when the duct is opened. The scissors are used to incise the duct.

The opening in the cystic duct is made on the anterosuperior aspect. Correct alignment of the cystic duct and infusion of saline facilitates insertion of ureteric catheter to perform cholangiography. Insertion is difficult, if the opening in the cystic duct is made too close to the gallbladder. The dissector is used to spread the incision to adequately dilate it for introduction of the cholangiogram catheter. The catheter is introduced through one of the 5-mm port. It is secured by either inflating a balloon or placing a clip to hold it in place. The catheter is then flushed with saline to ensure appropriate placement. All instruments are removed and a dynamic cholangiogram with real-time fluoroscopy is performed. The contrast medium should be injected slowly during screening and the patient should be in a slight Trendelenburg's position with the table rotated slightly to the right. It is essential that the entire biliary tract be outlined.

When the cholangiogram is completed, the catheter is removed, and two clips are placed proximally on the duct. The duct is then divided. Surgeon should ligate or clip cystic duct when he is sure up to the point of absolute certainness.

The main advantages of intraoperative cholangiography during cholecystectomy are:

- Detection of CBD stone
- Reduction of the incidence of residual CBD stone
- Delineation of the biliary anatomical variations at risk for bile duct injury

Intraoperative cholangiogram is a highly sensitive tool for detecting choledocholithiasis, with an overall accuracy of

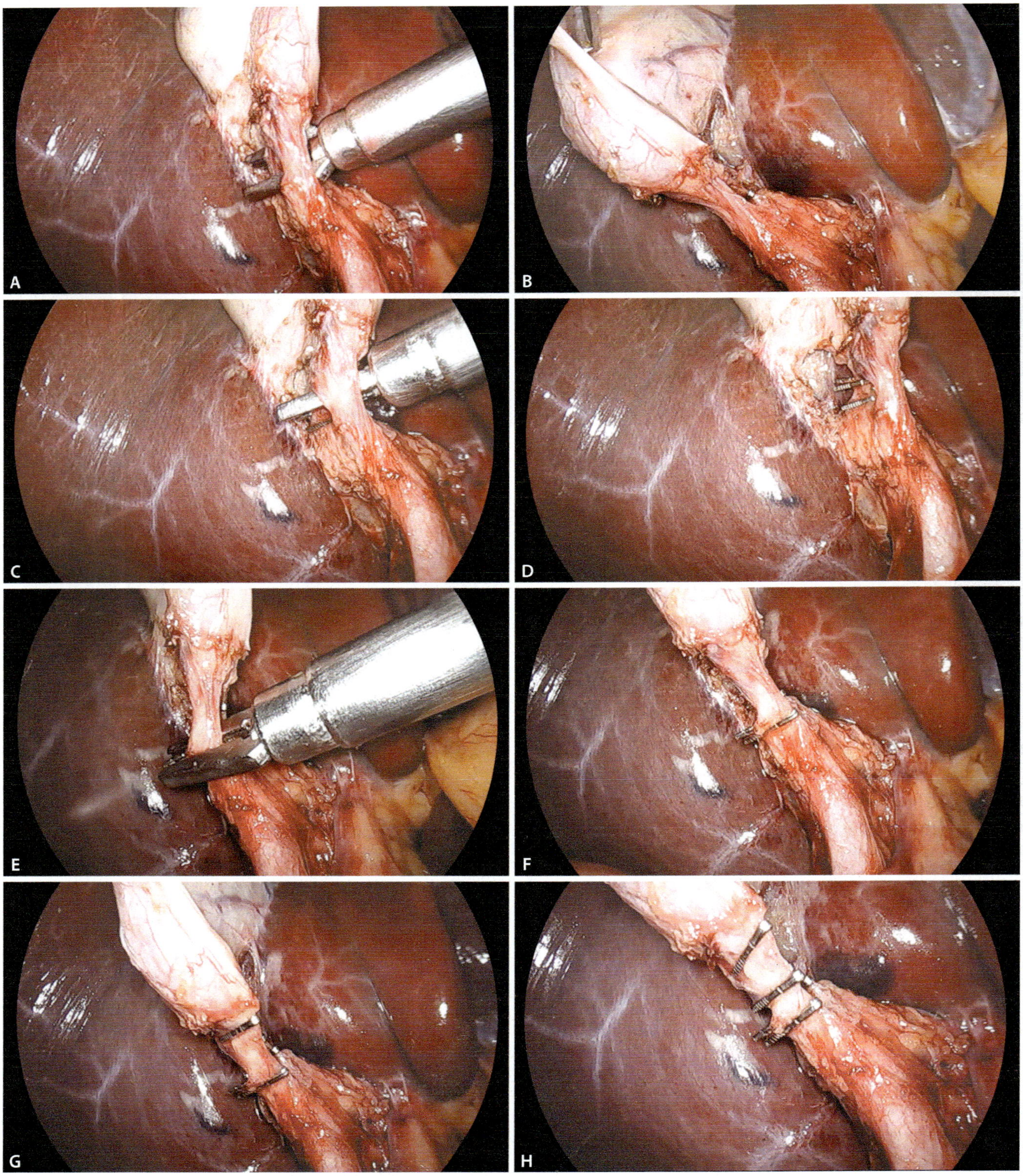

Figs. 10A to H

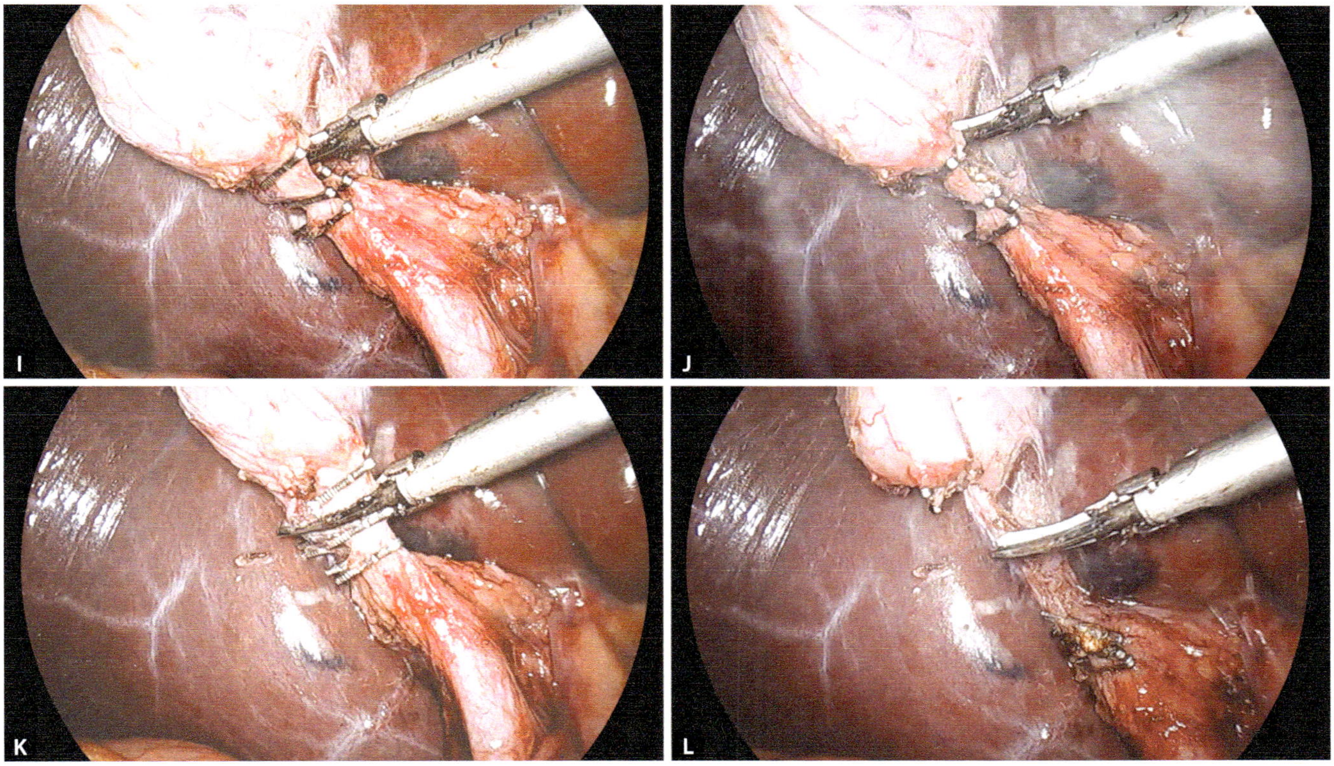

Figs. 10I to L

Figs. 10A to L: Cystic duct and artery are clipped and divided.

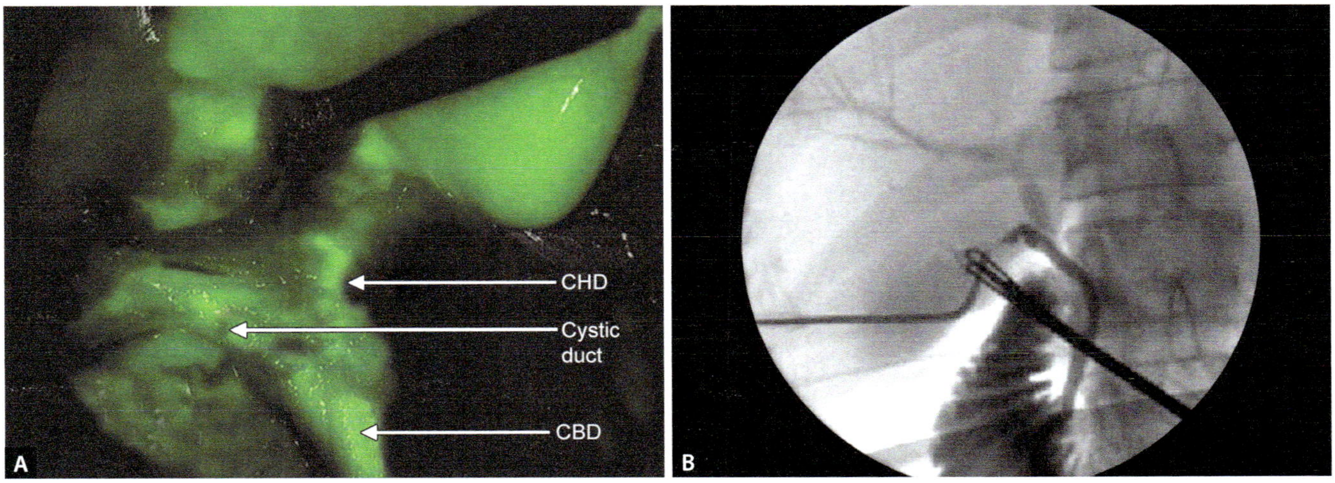

Figs. 11A and B: Intraoperative cholangiogram.
(CBD: common bile duct; CHD: common hepatic duct)

95%. Routine intraoperative cholangiography can diagnose unsuspected CBD stone in 1–14% (average 5%) of patients without indications for ductal exploration.

The failure of laparoscopic IOC is due to:

- The narrowness of the cystic duct
- Cystic duct rupture
- Obstructive cystic valves
- Impacted cystic stones
- Dye extravasation from cystic duct perforation

With increased experience, successful laparoscopic IOC can be achieved in 90–99% of cases, a rate similar to that of IOC during open cholecystectomy.

Intraoperative Ultrasonography

If there is any concern for choledocholithiasis (elevated bilirubin and dilated duct) or uncertain anatomy, the CBD should be imaged intraoperatively. This should occur after the first clip is placed on the cystic duct. IOC or laparoscopic ultrasound (LUS) may be performed. Many studies focused on the role of intraoperative US in laparoscopic cholecystectomy. Intraoperative US is technically demanding, but is as accurate as IOC (88–100%) for screening CBD stone.

The advantages of intraoperative US over IOC are:

- Speedy
- Safer
- Multiple time use
- Economical

The greater sensitivity of intraoperative US examination concerned mainly small stones or debris in the CBD.

The disadvantages of intraoperative US is that it is impossible to provide extended views of the intrahepatic and extrahepatic biliary tree, difficult to show passage of contrast into the duodenum and to identify bile duct injuries.

Ligation of Cystic Duct

Although the majority of surgeons opt for clipping the cystic duct, before dividing it, this technique, though quick, is intrinsically unsound, as internalization of the metal clip inside the CBD over the ensuing months is well documented. There is report of internalization of clip and subsequent stone formation after many years. The internalized clip becomes covered with calcium bilirubinate pigment. For this reason, to tie the cystic duct using a catgut Roeder external slip knot should be done.

Dissection of Gallbladder from Liver Bed (Fig. 12)

The assistant places continual cephalad traction on the gallbladder fundus while the surgeon alternates medial and lateral anteroposterior traction on the infundibulum with the left hand grasper. The electrosurgical hook or harmonic scalpel is used with cautery through the epigastric port to dissect the gallbladder from the bed of the liver. Using a grasper, the gallbladder is first retracted right to expose and dissect the medial side of the attachment. The gallbladder is then retracted to the left and the lateral side is dissected. Using this back-and-forth action, the hook is used to dissect the gallbladder off the bed from inferior to superior until it is 90% removed from the liver. Holding the remaining portion of the gallbladder attached to the liver, the dissection bed and the clipped structures are evaluated and any active bleeding is stopped using heal of the hook or spatula.

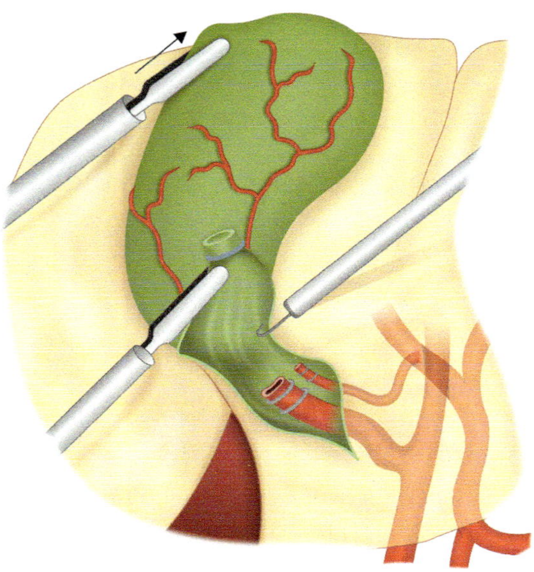

Fig. 12: Separation of gallbladder from gallbladder bed.

Gallbladder should be separated from the liver through the areolar tissue plane binding the gallbladder to the Glisson's capsule lining the liver bed **(Fig. 13)**. The actual separation can be performed with scissors with electrosurgical attachment or electrosurgical hook knife. Pledget can be used to remove the gallbladder from liver bed once a good plane of dissection is found. Perforation of the gallbladder during its separation is a common complication, which is encountered in 15% of cases.

One should be careful at the time of dissection and if there is spillage of stone, each stone should be removed from the peritoneal cavity to avoid abscess formation in future.

Extraction of Gallbladder (Figs. 14A to D)

The gallbladder is now freed from the liver and placed on top of the liver. The patient is returned to the supine position and the area of dissection and the upper right quadrant are irrigated and suctioned until clear. The gallbladder is extracted through the 11-mm epigastric operating port with the help of gallbladder extractor. The specimen can also be retrieved through the subxiphoid (epigastric) port site. We generally prefer epigastric port for removal of uncomplicated gallbladder. We feel that the subxiphoid site may be better for specimen extraction, as the subxiphoid site has a lower likelihood of hernia formation. Many surgeons use umbilical port for withdrawal of gallbladder. The umbilical incision

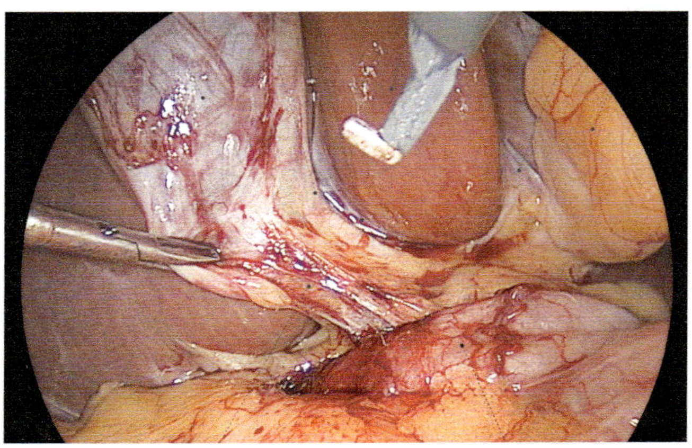

Fig. 13: Glisson's capsule lining the liver bed.

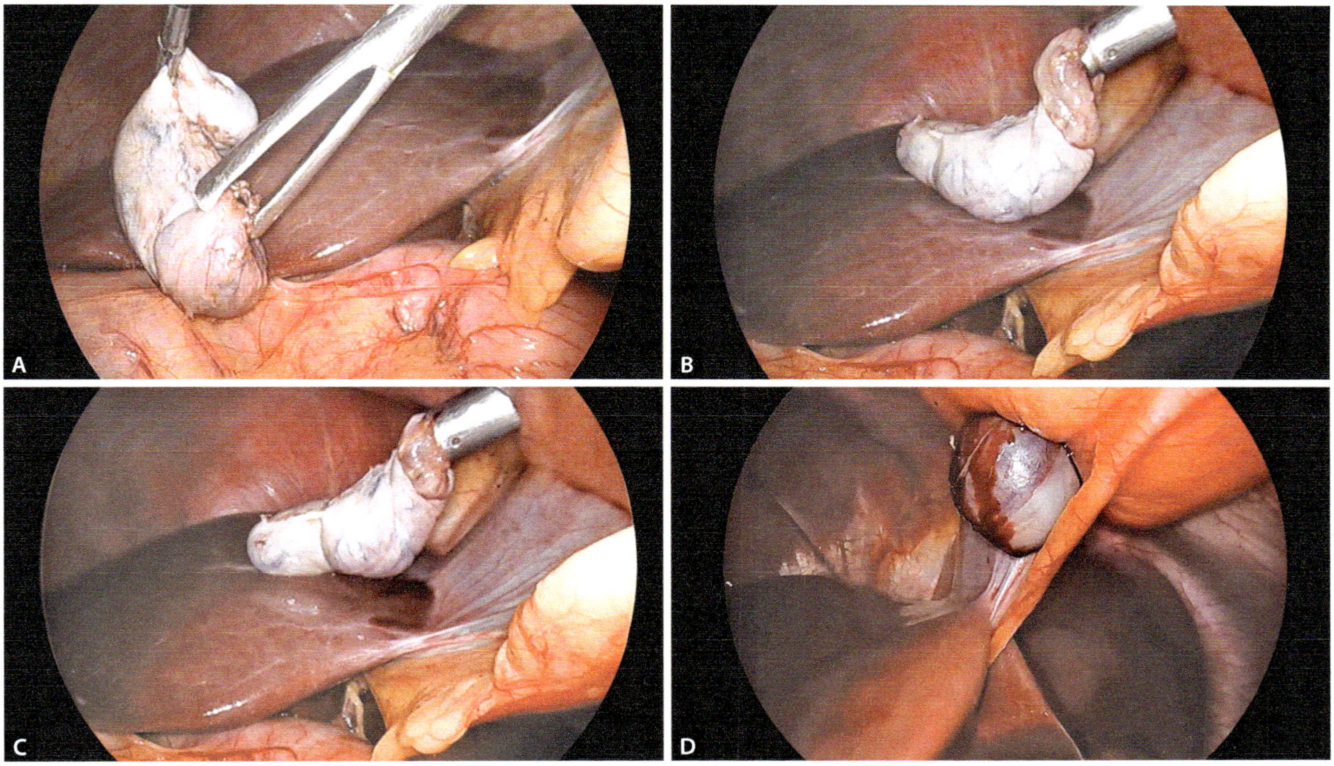

Figs. 14A to D: Extraction of gallbladder.

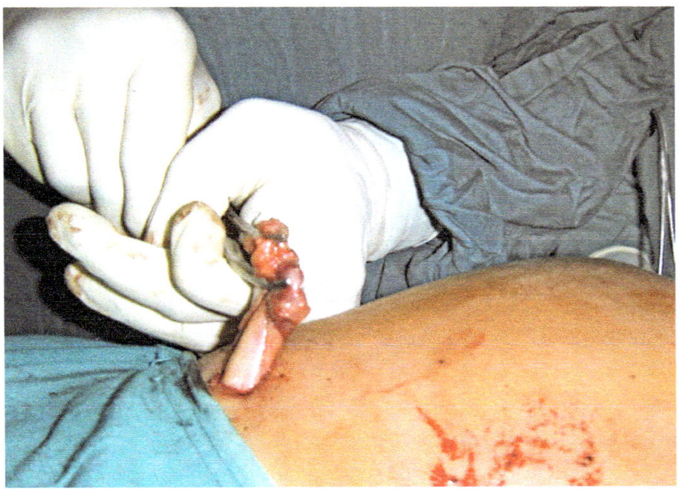

Fig. 15: Extraction of gallbladder by gentle pull from outside.

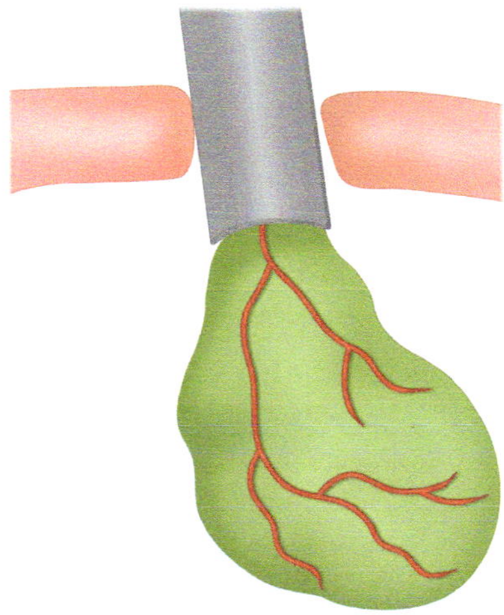

Fig. 16: Extraction of gallbladder by hiding the neck in cannula.

has no muscle layers and is easy to extend with minimal pain and cosmetic sequelae. If gallbladder is removed through the umbilical port, the laparoscope is placed through the epigastric port and the gallbladder is visualized on the dome of the liver. A large grasper with teeth is placed through the umbilical port and used to grasp the gallbladder along the edge of the clipped cystic duct stump. The gallbladder is then exteriorized through the umbilical incision where it is held into position with a clamp **(Fig. 15)**.

First, the neck of the gallbladder should be engaged in the cannula and then cannula will withdraw together with neck of gallbladder held within the jaw of gallbladder extractor **(Fig. 16)**.

Once the port with the neck of the gallbladder is out, the neck is grasped with the help of a blunt hemostat and it should be pulled out with screwing.

If gallbladder is of small size, it will come without much difficulty, otherwise small incision should be given over the

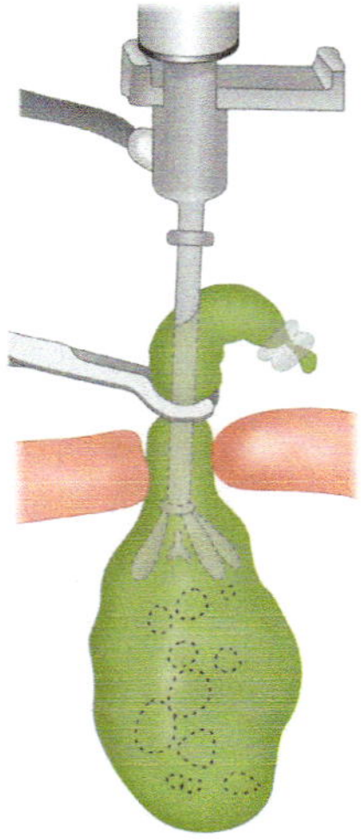

Fig. 17: Suction of bile to extract gallbladder.

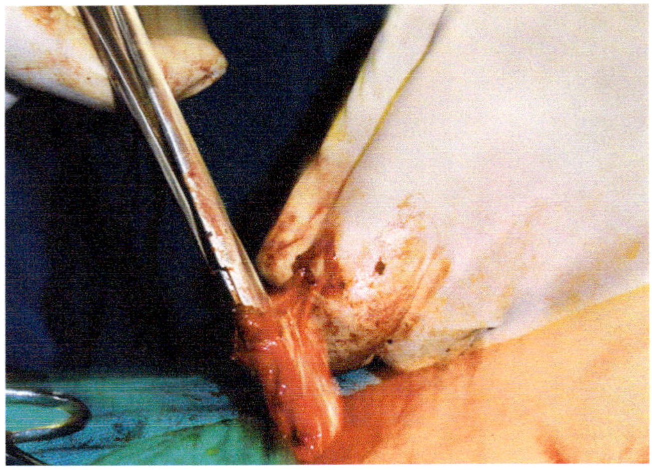

Fig. 18: Stone should be taken out to reduce volume of gallbladder.

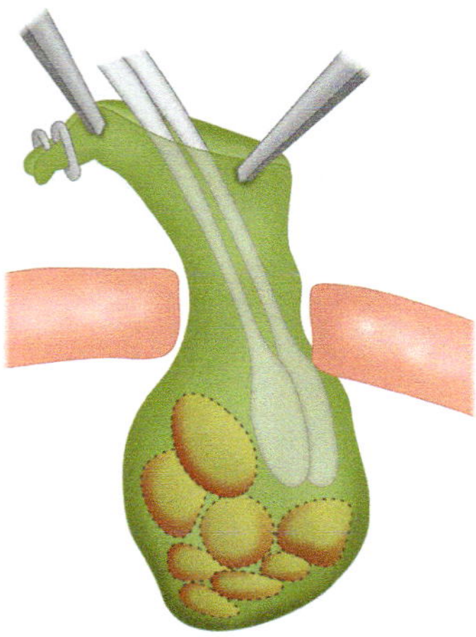

Fig. 19: Stone may be crushed to reduce volume of gallbladder.

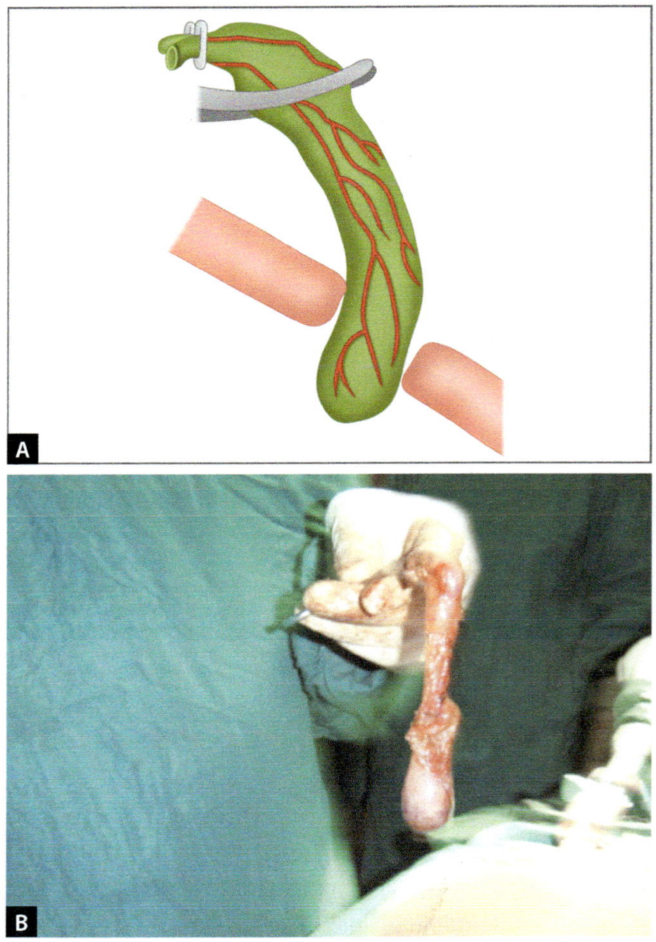

Figs. 20A and B: Once the gallbladder is empty, gentle pull from outside will facilitate its extraction.

neck of the gallbladder and suction irrigation instrument should be used to suck all the bile to facilitate easy withdrawal **(Figs. 17 and 18)**.

Sometimes big stones will not allow easy passage of gallbladder and in these situations, ovum forceps should be inserted inside the lumen of gallbladder through the incision of its neck and all the stone should be crushed **(Fig. 19)**. When ovum forceps is used to remove the big stones from the gallbladder, care should be taken that gallbladder should be held loose to have room for forceps, otherwise it will perforate and all the stone may spill out **(Figs. 20A and B)**.

Extraction inside a bag is recommended as a safeguard against stone loss and contamination of the exit wound **(Figs. 21 and 22)**.

Gallbladder Perforation during Laparoscopic Cholecystectomy

During the dissection of the gallbladder, the laparoscopic surgeon may enter the gallbladder inadvertently, causing spillage of bile and/or stones. The hole in the gallbladder can be closed by incorporating it within the grasping forceps or may be sutured closed to prevent further spillage. The bile should be suctioned and irrigated. Bile spillage, when not

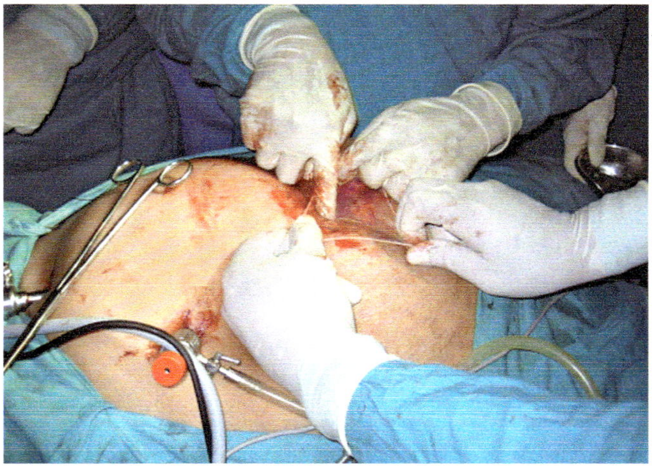

Fig. 21: The spilled stone and torn gallbladder can be taken out with the help of endobag.

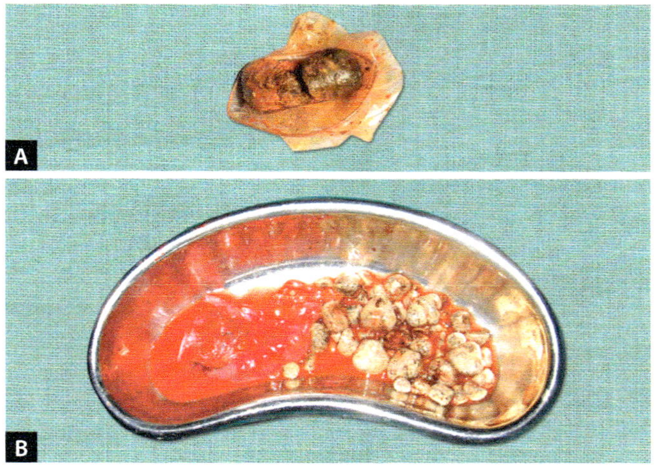

Figs. 22A and B: Extracted spilled stone and torn gallbladder.

accompanied by stone spillage and promptly evacuated, has not been shown to increase postoperative infections.

Ending of the Operation

The instrument and then ports are removed. Telescope should be removed leaving gas valve of umbilical port open to let out all the gas. At the time of removing umbilical port, telescope should be again inserted and umbilical port should be removed over the telescope to prevent any entrapment of omentum. The wound is then closed with suture. Vicryl should be used for rectus and unabsorbable intradermal or stapler for skin. A single suture is used to close the umbilicus and upper midline fascial opening. Many laparoscopic surgeons routinely leave this fascial defect without ill defect. Some surgeons like to inject local anesthetic agent over port site to avoid postoperative pain. Sterile dressing over the wound should be applied.

Since the first laparoscopic cholecystectomy was performed, it has met with widespread acceptance as a standard procedure using four trocars. The fourth (lateral) trocar is used to grasp the fundus of the gallbladder so as to expose Calot's triangle. It has been argued that the fourth trocar is not necessary in most cases. The three-port technique is as safe as the standard four-port. The main advantages of the three-port technique are that it causes less pain, is less expensive, and leaves fewer scars. The three-port cholecystectomy should be performed by experienced laparoscopic surgeon because left hand movement is very important in this surgery. Bimanual skill and correct interpretation of anatomy is a must before proceeding for this technique. Three-port cholecystectomy is possible by the experienced laparoscopic surgeons.

Mini-laparoscopic Cholecystectomy

Mini-laparoscopy uses instruments that are thinner than the standard instruments (<3 versus 5–10 mm). These instruments are either placed through special low-friction trocars of small diameters (2–4 mm). Although mini-laparoscopic cholecystectomy requires the same four incisions as standard cholecystectomy, three of the incisions are smaller and therefore less invasive to the patient. The remaining umbilical incision has a standard size of 5–10 mm, which permits the use of a standard laparoscope and specimen extraction. About 10% of attempted mini-laparoscopic cholecystectomies require conversion, most often to standard laparoscopic cholecystectomy rather than open surgery.

Laparoscopic Cholecystectomy in Acute Cholecystitis

Impaction of a stone in the cystic duct will result in bile stasis in the gallbladder. Acute cholecystitis results from inflammation of the mucosa of the gallbladder, which may secondarily become infected. This inflammation can then evolve to hydrops of the gallbladder and gallbladder abscess. Complications such as necrosis, perforation, phlegmon, or peritonitis can result, if surgical intervention is not done in timely manner.

In certain cases, acute cholecystitis can be acalculous, especially in diabetic patients or in the immediate postoperative period following other surgical interventions. In the elective setting, a laparoscopic cholecystectomy has become the standard of care; the laparoscopic approach to acute cholecystitis remains controversial. In past publications, acute cholecystitis was considered as a relative or absolute contraindication to a laparoscopic approach. The laparoscopic approach to acute cholecystitis is preferred in practice by a large number of experienced teams. Nowadays, laparoscopic approach is considered safe, if the intervention is performed in a timely fashion. If laparoscopy is considered in acute attack, a conversion rate of 20% demonstrates that the procedure is only pursued when felt to be safe.

Laparoscopic cholecystectomy can be done safely in the setting of acute or gangrenous cholecystitis and should be done as soon as possible to fall within the "golden period" within 72 hours when edema is the primary manifestation of the inflammation. If the patient presents in a delayed fashion (>72 hours from onset of symptoms), the surgery can be performed if there are no contraindications to an open procedure, as conversion is a significant risk. In the face of acute cholecystitis with multiple comorbidities, it may be preferable to treat with intravenous antibiotics and possibly percutaneous drainage, with subsequent laparoscopic cholecystectomy 6–8 weeks later.

- Acute cholecystitis is distinguished from biliary colic by the presence of at least two of the following signs:
    - Right upper quadrant pain lasting for more than 24 hours
    - Fever more than 37°C
    - The presence of a palpable distended tender gallbladder
    - Elevation of the WBC count >11,000/mm^3
    - Ultrasonographic findings demonstrating thickening of the gallbladder wall > 4 mm
    - Pericholecystic fluid collection in ultrasound

The studies have concluded that the ideal time for the surgical intervention is within 48–72 hours of the appearance of symptoms.

Laparoscopic cholecystectomy, when performed early, leads to reduction in:

- Operative difficulty
- Conversion rate
- Operative time

One of the major determining factors is the conversion rate, an indicator of the actual difficulty of the procedure. Numerous studies have demonstrated a significantly lower conversion rate when the laparoscopic cholecystectomy is performed within the first 72 hours of the onset of symptoms as opposed to a delayed procedure after this period. In case of an interval cholecystectomy following medical therapy, it must be performed within a period of 8–12 weeks. It is demonstrated that interval cholecystectomy is associated with a higher morbidity rate than in early intervention.

Laparoscopic Cholecystectomy during Pregnancy

There is a strong association between pregnancy and gallstones. In the past, elective laparoscopic cholecystectomy for symptomatic gallstones was deferred as much as possible until after pregnancy. For patients with severe biliary colic, however, waiting until after pregnancy can lead to repeated hospitalizations and complications. Laparoscopic cholecystectomy is relatively contraindicated during pregnancy due to the potentially adverse side effects on the fetus. However, when complications arise, a surgical intervention becomes mandatory. This intervention should be ideally performed during the second trimester of pregnancy where the operative risks are considered to be the lowest. Laparoscopic cholecystectomy during pregnancy has been reported in many series of randomized controlled trials, with no specific complications related to the laparoscopic approach. When laparoscopic surgery is performed in pregnant patients, the trocars need to be placed higher in the abdomen due to the enlarged uterus. The CO_2 insufflation should be kept at the lowest possible pressure while maintaining an adequate working space. If CBD imaging is necessary, LUS should be used in place of IOC to limit radiation exposure.

Single Incision Laparoscopic Cholecystectomy

Single incision laparoscopic (SILS) cholecystectomy uses one rather than multiple skin incisions for trocar placement. Through a single skin incision typically made periumbilically, multiple trocars are placed through one or more fascial punctures. SILS has been most widely used in gallbladder surgery and has been extensively studied in comparison with standard laparoscopic cholecystectomy. Overall, SILS offers little benefit over standard laparoscopic surgery. A 2017 meta-analysis of 37 trials comparing SILS with conventional laparoscopic cholecystectomy showed that SILS is associated with better cosmesis, body image, and wound satisfaction and less postoperative pain, but a slightly longer operative time and a higher conversion rate. Additionally, the risk of incisional hernia is four times higher after SILS than after conventional laparoscopic cholecystectomy.

POSTOPERATIVE CARE

Most of the patients can be discharged 6 hours after the surgery or on the next day. The patient who has urinary retention, prolonged nausea, more pain, or difficulty in walking can be discharged after bowel sound. Three doses broad-spectrum antibiotic should be administered. First dose infused 1 hour before surgery, second and third should be administered on consecutive days. Few patients may complain pain over tip of shoulder after laparoscopic surgery. This is due to irritation of diaphragm from CO_2. Tramadol hydrochloride is advised in these patients. Most of the patients are able to resume their normal day-to-day activity within 48–72 hours after surgery. Generally, the patient can return to their sedentary work within a week. The patient should have no activity restriction unless the umbilical incision was particularly large. Then, limited heavy lifting for a few weeks is advisable. Most patients are able to return to work within 1 week. Patients follow-up in clinic 2–4 weeks after their operation.

Postcholecystectomy Syndrome

Postcholecystectomy syndrome is a complex of heterogeneous symptoms including persistent abdominal pain and dyspepsia that recur and persist after cholecystectomy. In a prospective cohort study, only 60% of patients reported complete relief of abdominal pain at 12 weeks after cholecystectomy for uncomplicated symptomatic cholelithiasis. Treatment for postcholecystectomy syndrome is tailored to the specific cause of the symptoms. Diagnosis of the underlying problem causing postcholecystectomy syndrome usually requires imaging to look for retained or recurrent stones or identify a bile duct leak, stricture, or transection. This can be accomplished in most cases with ultrasound and/or computed tomography (CT) scanning followed by direct cholangiography or MRCP. MRCP provides a noninvasive alternative to direct cholangiography for evaluation of the biliary tract.

Robotic Cholecystectomy

Robot-assisted cholecystectomy has also been performed. Compared with conventional laparoscopic cholecystectomy, robotic cholecystectomy has not been found to be more effective or safer than for benign gallbladder diseases but incurs longer operative time and higher cost. The use of robotic-assisted extended cholecystectomy for gallbladder cancer is currently being evaluated.

Cholecystectomy by Natural Orifice Transluminal Endoscopic Surgery

Transgastric or transvaginal cholecystectomy has been performed with natural orifice transluminal endoscopic surgery (NOTES). Compared with conventional surgery, NOTES offers true scarless cholecystectomy, which has the potential of minimizing postoperative patient discomfort. However, as an emerging technology, NOTES still faces many technical challenges. Currently, the transgastric cholecystectomy is no longer performed; only a few international centers continue to offer transvaginal cholecystectomy.

COMPLICATIONS OF LAPAROSCOPIC CHOLECYSTECTOMY

Early Complications

- Common bile duct injury
- Bile leak
- Injury to viscera
- Hemorrhage
- Retained stones and abscess formation.

Late Complications

- Biliary strictures
- Cystic duct clip stones.

Laparoscopic Cholecystectomy and CBD Injury

Incidence of iatrogenic CBD injury is 0.12% and 0.55% during open and laparoscopic cholecystectomy, respectively.

Common Causes of CBD Injury

- Misinterpretation of anatomy—70%
- Technical errors
- Risk factors
- Surgeon operates on image rather than reality.

Visual psychological studies have shown that laparoscopic surgeon works on snap interpretation by brain and success or disaster depends on whether snaps are right or wrong. Snap interpretation will be wrong, if there is eyeball degradation. Surgeon should not dissect the cystic duct, if there is lack of initial identification and memory of key structure to the point of absolute certainty **(Figs. 23A and B)**. Most important technical error is hilar bleeding and frantic attempts are made to control bleeding by electrosurgery. This frantic attack can catch the CBD and will be injured.

In case of bleeding, surgeon should first apply pressure and if it does not stop, he should take suction irrigation

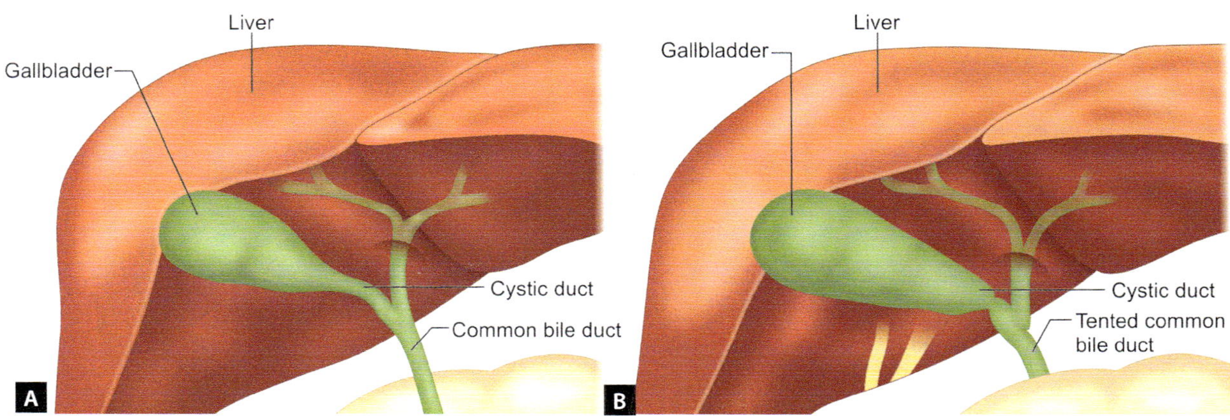

Figs. 23A and B: Testing of common bile duct.

and atraumatic grasper to find out exact point of bleeding. Electrosurgery should be used only when bleeding point is identified.

Types of CBD Injury

Bismuth classification:

- Type 1—CBD stump >2 cm
- Type 2—CBD stump <2 cm
- Type 3—hilar, right, and left duct confluence intact
- Type 4—hilar, separation of right and left ducts
- Type 5—injury to aberrant right duct ± CBD injury

If complication of CBD injury is recognized intraoperatively, reconstructive surgery should be performed same time if surgeon has sufficient experience. For high complete transaction, Roux-en-Y hepaticojejunostomy is preferred. For lower complete injuries, primary suture repair over T-tube is better but long end of T-tube must not be exteriorized from same site. For partial injuries, insertion of T-tube and Roux-en-Y serosal patch should be thought.

Strategy to Handle Complication Recognized Postoperatively

- USG + ERCP + MRCP
- Fluid + electrolyte + systemic antibiotic
- Conservative treatment and biliary drainage for 6 weeks by ERCP stent insertion or
- PTBD (percutaneous transhepatic biliary drainage), if endoscopic stent application is not possible
- *After several weeks*: Reconstructive surgery
- Roux-en-Y choledocoduodenostomy or hepato-jejunostomy

All the variation of cystic duct and artery should be memorized to avoid inadvertent injury of CBD.

The variation in cystic artery and hepatic duct is shown in **Figures 24A to D**.

How to avoid injury?

- Try to memorize initial anatomy of Calot's triangle
- A large distended gallbladder should be aspirated and lifted rather than grasped
- Anterolateral traction is better than fundus pull to avoid tenting of CBD
- Avoid meticulous dissection by energized instrument
- Better to do skeletonization through pledget
- During detachment of gallbladder from liver bed, maintain plane of adipose tissue
- Use suction irrigation frequently.

Tenting of the CBD should always be kept in mind at the time of dissection to avoid injury.

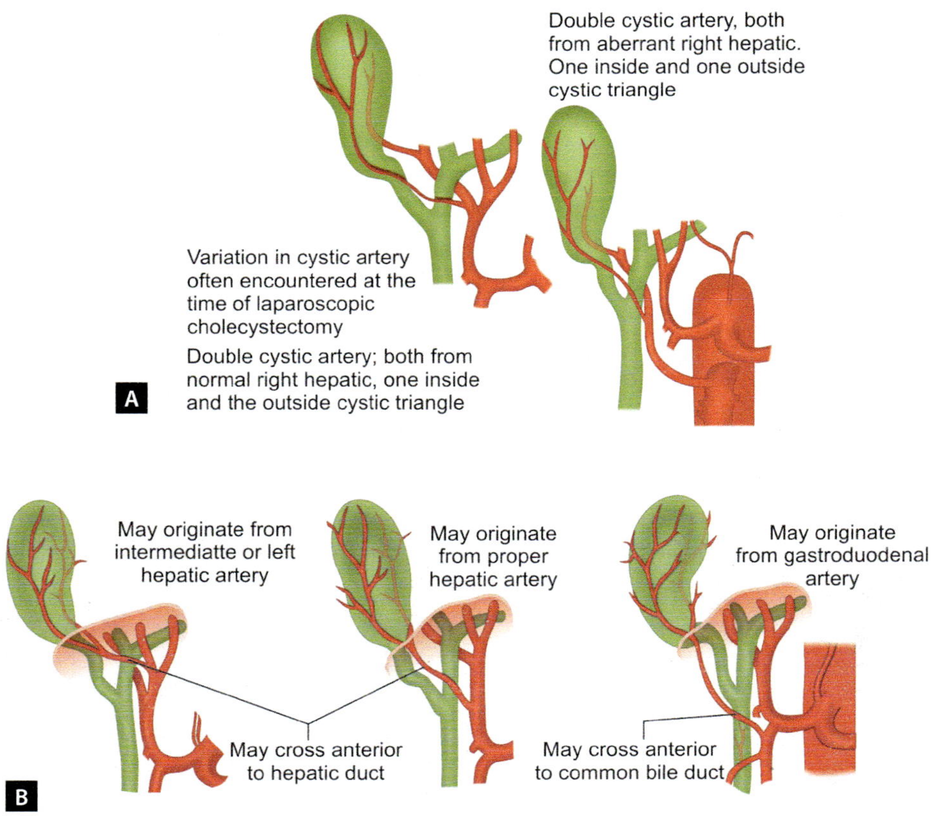

Figs. 24A and B

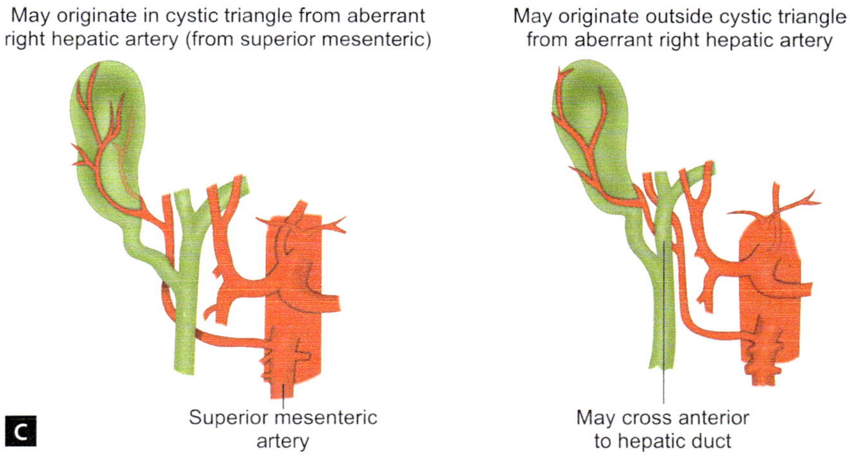

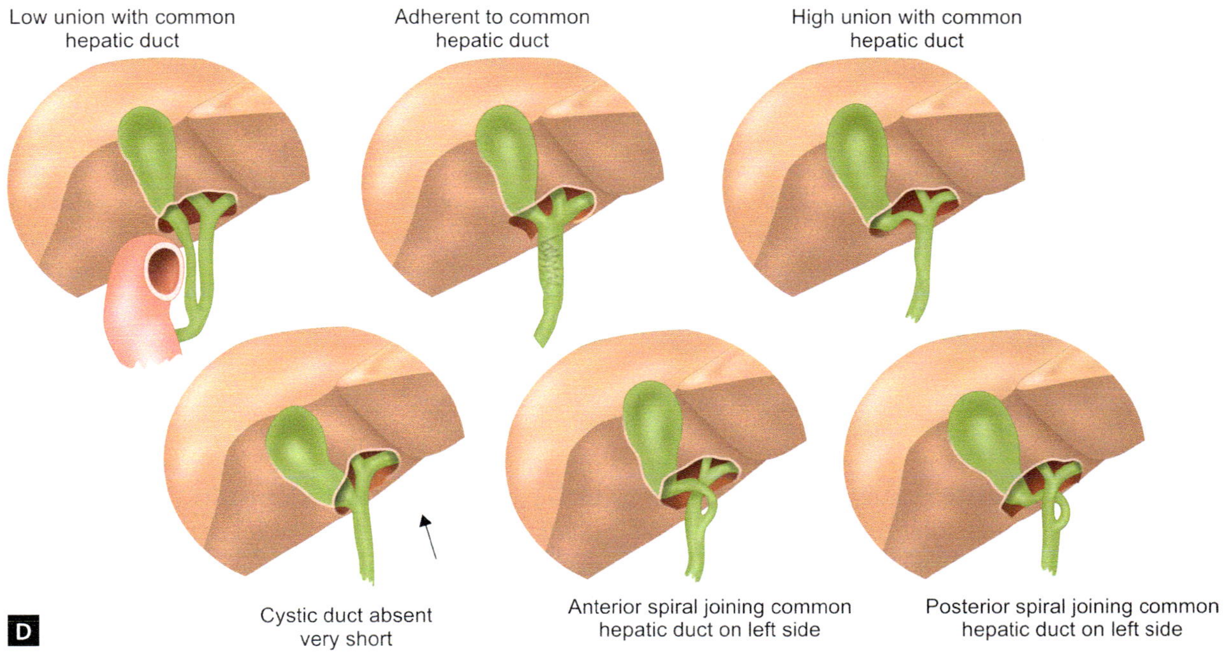

Figs. 24C and D

Figs. 24A to D: Variation in cystic artery and hepatic duct.

LAPAROSCOPIC CHOLECYSTECTOMY WITH REAL-TIME NEAR-INFRARED FLUORESCENT CHOLANGIOGRAPHY

Sometimes, there are certain mistakes that can happen during laparoscopic cholecystectomy procedure. The most common mistake is usually the misidentification of the extrahepatic bile duct anatomy, which can lead to bile duct injury. At World Laparoscopy Hospital, now we have started using indocyanine green (ICG) during laparoscopic cholecystectomy **(Fig. 25)**. However, there is something that can be down about the mistake, or basically, the mistake can be avoided. In order to avoid the mistake, it requires the doctor to use a technique or tools that will enhance or promote the easier recognition of the biliary anatomy

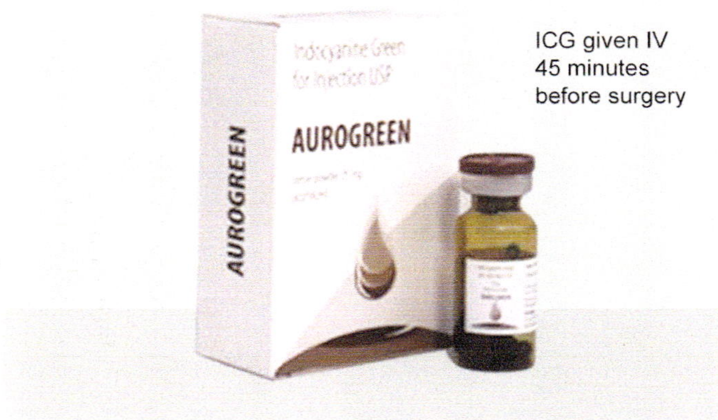

Fig. 25: Indocyanine green (ICG) used in laparoscopic cholecystectomy.

in the intraoperative procedure by use of near-infrared fluorescence cholangiography or imaging.

According to various studies on the use of the near-infrared cholangiography in laparoscopic cholecystectomy, the report showed that there was positive and successful intraoperative identification of the extrahepatic bile ducts. This reduced the likelihood of causing an injury to the bile ducts. This is, however, unlike the conventional imaging; whose results are usually not highly successful.

Understanding Laparoscopic Cholecystectomy

Laparoscopic cholecystectomy is one of the most performed procedures in various countries. The procedure itself is usually associated with bile duct injury due to a poor intraoperative identification of the extrahepatic bile ducts. However, that complication is usually rare and actually it is associated with an incidence of 0.3–0.7%. However, it should be noted that when the mistake happens and there happens to be a bile duct injury, it can lead to various complications such as lower quality of life, morbidity, and mortality that are clinically relevant, and extra costs.

Often an injury to the bile duct leads to leakage of bile and abdominal sepsis, which can lead to the obstruction or blockage of bile duct with obstructive jaundice. This will eventually lead to orthotopic liver transplantation.

This complication should be detected as early as possible; however, if it is detected when it is late or has really advanced, it can be difficult to manage the bile ducts injuries since they will have caused severe damage, which progresses to biliary peritonitis, multiorgan failure, sepsis, and eventually death. Therefore, you need to understand that this is a condition that can be fatal, if not detected and managed early enough. As earlier mentioned, the intraoperative misidentification of the bile ducts anatomy is usually the main cause of bile ducts injury.

Fluorescence cholangiography can help to reduce the risk of the bile duct, by helping to improve the orientation of the anatomy during laparoscopic cholecystectomy **(Fig. 26)**. When the doctor can identify the relevant anatomical structure, he is able to perform the operation easily without making any mistakes that can be costly and fatal to the patient. However, given this advantage, the procedure is yet to be adopted across the globe due to several reasons. One of the reasons is that the procedure takes times, involves exposure to radiation, and requires additional practitioners. Additionally, the ability to clearly identify the relevant anatomical structure or interpret an IOC clearly to some extent depends on the expertise of the surgeon.

Understanding Real-time Infrared Cholangiography

On the other hand, real-time infrared fluorescent cholangiography required is often performed after the intravenous injection of ICG is viewed as a better and new technique for easier recognition of the biliary anatomy **(Fig. 27)**. One is not exposed to radiation and the procedure does not require any additional manpower. This makes it easy and actually a real-time and a flexible technique to use during laparoscopic cholecystectomy. Since the procedure is able to provide real-time visual or identification of the bile duct relevant anatomy, the outcome of the surgery can be improved leading to almost 100% success rates in various patients.

According to a clinical study, results showed that infrared cholangiography provided an improved and real-time identification of the extrahepatic bile ducts during the phase of CVS dissection. The identification was faster, in fact, up to 10 minutes of earlier identification of the cystic duct and the CBD was recorded. One of the best things about this procedure is that the liver is able to quickly and exclusively clear ICG that is often intravenously administered before the technique is put into action. Still, according to the clinical study, it was established that the real-time identification of the hepatic and cystic arteries was obtained after a repeated dose of intravenous injection of ICG.

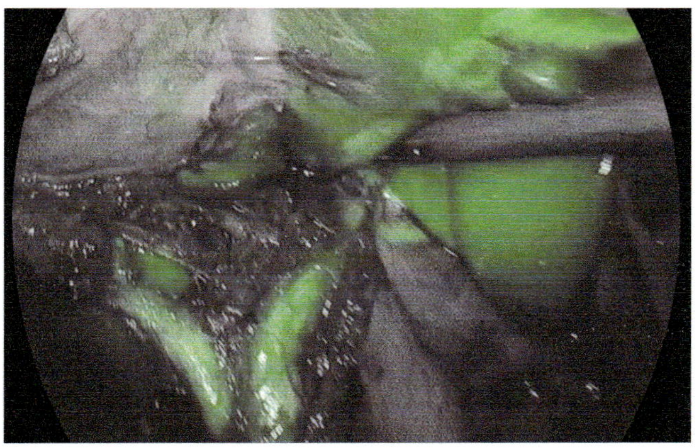

Fig. 26: Indocyanine green fluorescence cholangiography.

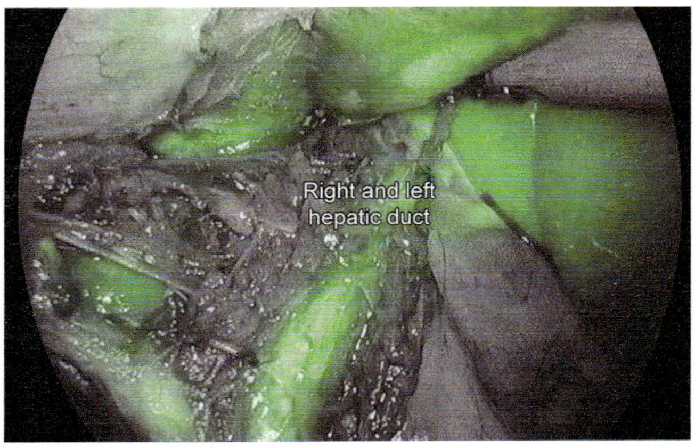

Fig. 27: Recognition of the biliary anatomy.

Indocyanine Green

Indocyanine green is also known as the fluorescent dye. As earlier mentioned, the liquid is usually injected intravenously; it is actually the one that helps to light the path for better and real-time identification of the biliary anatomy during the laparoscopic cholecystectomy.

The near-infrared fluorescent cholangiography is usually performed using, as its name goes, a fluorescent imaging system that is usually used together with a laparoscope. The system must have a lighting system that provides light for both infrared and xenon rays. To perform this cholangiography technique, the ICG must be administered at least 45 minutes before the procedure. This dye has been used for quite some time now, in fact, since 1956. Today, it is widely being used in almost every hospital for surgical and various clinical purposes.

Indocyanine green is able to provide better visualization of the biliary anatomy when it is illuminated by the infrared light, which makes it manifest fluorescence. When this happens the practitioner is able to clearly and in real time identify all the relevant biliary anatomy, thus enabling one to perform laparoscopic cholecystectomy better without causing injury to the bile ducts.

Therefore, ICG acts as an imaging agent, which is sterile, water-soluble, and has a peak spectral absorption averaging at 805 nm in blood plasma or simply the blood. Since it is exclusively eliminated by the liver, it does not undergo enterohepatic recirculation. It only stays in the bile for about 8 minutes after injection. The removal of ICG depends on several factors, including the blood flow of the liver, biliary excretion, and parenchymal cellular function.

Sometimes, fluorescence may not be detected 45 minutes after the injection of ICG. Therefore, when this happens, the second dose of 2.5 mg of ICG can be administered intravenously also. A second injection of ICG can also be given if there is anything regarding perfusion that cannot be clearly understood during the surgery.

Exploration of the Biliary Anatomy

Practitioners always report their experience with real-time near infrared cholangiography using ICG. Most of the times when it comes to laparoscopic cholecystectomy, feasibility and safety of the technique are usually well reported.

The reports are quite interesting when it comes to robot single-site cholecystectomy (RSSC) where the ICG is still administered before the surgery and the biliary anatomy can be analyzed before any dissection is made. This is quite different for cholangiography requiring extensive dissection of the cystic duct. Therefore, using ICG during RSSC can help to analyze the extrahepatic biliary anatomy better and this could help to reduce the bile duct injury due to the misinterpretation of the biliary anatomy. However, there are no data to prove this statement.

Other Advantages of Real-time Near-infrared Fluorescent Cholangiography

Near-infrared fluorescent cholangiography improves the ability to analyze and identify the relevant biliary anatomic structure in a quick manner; therefore, it can help to reduce the time used in performing the procedure. Quicker assessment of the extrahepatic biliary anatomy is what is needed during laparoscopic cholecystectomy. The technique is usually able to shorten the operative time due to the fact there is no need to bring on board additional equipment and manpower, especially the radiology personnel for an X-ray.

The technique also serves as a good teaching tool for practitioners who are able to identify the relevant extrahepatic structures in almost every patient. This helps them become more experienced with the procedure, which makes it easier for them to perform future procedures.

The technique does not require any X-ray, therefore, no one is exposed to radiation. The ICG that is used is usually safe and does not cause any adverse reactions in patients. It is exclusively removed by the liver even before it undergoes enterohepatic recirculation. It is also a cost-effective technique that can help the patients to save some of their money that would otherwise have been used, if the technique was not used.

However, near-infrared fluorescent technique comes with some limitations. The common one is that it lacks the standardization of the fluorescence imaging systems. This is quite a drawback for this technique because standardization is needed for the determination of the objective assessments during any fluorescence-guided surgery like the laparoscopic cholecystectomy. The differences in fluorescence cholangiography make it difficult for the comparisons between fluorescence cholangiography studies.

CONCLUSION

The real-time near-infrared fluorescence cholangiography is new and better technology that can help with the identification of the vital biliary anatomy. Several studies have been done on the technique and have been proven to be good for laparoscopic cholecystectomy. It helps to reduce the risk of the bile duct injury by proving clear vision of the vital extrahepatic structures. The reduced risk helps to avoid various complications that can arise from the injury of the bile duct, which sometimes can be fatal to a patient.

BIBLIOGRAPHY

1. Airan M, Appel M, Berci G, Coburg AJ, Cohen M, Cuschieri A, et al. Retrospective and prospective multi-institutional laparoscopic cholecystectomy study by the Society of American Gastrointestinal Endoscopic Surgeons. Surg Endosc. 1992;6:169-76.
2. Barkum AN, Barkun JS, Fried GM, Ghitulescu G, Steinmetz O, Pham C, et al. Useful predictors of bile duct stones in patients undergoing laparoscopic cholecystectomy. Ann Surg. 1994; 220:32-9.

3. Bartlett DL, Fong Y, Fortner JG, Brennan MF, Blumgart LH. Long-term results after resection for gallbladder cancer: implications for staging and management. Ann Surg. 1996;224:639-46.
4. Berci G, Morgenstern L. Laparoscopic management of common bile duct stones. Surg Endosc. 1994;8:1168-75.
5. Berrevoet E, Biglari M, Sinove Y, De Baardemaeker L, Troisi R, de Hemptinne B. Outpatient laparoscopic cholecystectomy in Belgium: what are we waiting for? Acta Chir Belg. 2006;106:537-40.
6. Branum G, Schmitt C, Baillie J, Suhoclri P, Baker M, Davidoff A, et al. Management of major biliary complications after laparoscopic cholecystectomy. Ann Surg. 1993;217:532-41.
7. Calik A, Topaloglu S, Topcu S, Turkyilmaz S, Kucuktulu U, Piskin B. Routine intraoperative aspiration of gallbladder during laparoscopic cholecystectomy. Surg Endosc. 2007;21(9):1578-81.
8. Callagham J. Twenty-five years of gallbladder surgery in a small rural hospital. Am J Surg. 1995;169:313-5.
9. Champault A, Vons C, Dagher I, Amerlinck S, Franco D. Low-cost laparoscopic cholecystectomy. Br J Surg. 2002;89:1602-7.
10. Chijiiwa K, Nakano K, Ueda J, Noshiro H, Nagai E, Yamaguchi K, et al. Surgical treatment of patients with T2 gallbladder carcinoma invading the subserosal layer. J Am Coll Surg. 2001;192:600-7.
11. Clavies PA, Sanabria JR, Strasberg SM. Proposed classification of complications of surgery with examples of utility in cholecystectomy. Surgery. 1992;111:518-6.
12. Cleary SP, Dawson LA, Knox JJ, Gallinger S. Cancer of the gallbladder and extrahepatic bile ducts. Curr Probl Surg. 2007;44:396-482.
13. Coburn NG, Cleary SP, Tan JC, Law CH. Surgery for gallbladder cancer: a population-based analysis. J Am Coll Surg. 2008; 207:371-82.
14. Cullen DJ, Apolone G, Greenfiled S, Guadagnoli E, Cleary P. ASA physical status and age predict morbidity after three surgical procedures. Ann Surg. 1994;220:3-9.
15. Davies MG, O'Broin E, Mannion C, McGinley J, Gupta S, Shine MF, et al. Audit of open cholecystectomy in a district general hospital. Br J Surg. 1992;79:314-6.
16. de Aretxabala XA, Roa IS, Burgos LA, Araya JC, Villaseca MA, Silva JA, et al. Curative resection in potentially resectable tumours of the gallbladder. Eur J Surg. 1997;163:419-26.
17. Deziel DJ, Millikan KW, Economou SG, Doolas A, Ko ST, Airan MC. Complications of laparoscopic cholecystectomy: a national survey of 4,292 hospitals and an analysis of 77,604 cases. Am J Surg. 1993;165:9-14.
18. Deziel DJ. Complications of cholecystectomy. Surg Clin N Am. 1994;74:809-23.
19. Dixon E, Vollmer CM Jr, Sahajpal A, Cattral M, Grant D, Doig C, et al. An aggressive surgical approach leads to improved survival in patients with gallbladder cancer: a 12-year study at a North American Center. Ann Surg. 2005;241:385-94.
20. Driessen PJHA, Pradhan GN. Laparoscopic cholecystectomy in a small rural hospital. CJRM. 2000;5:70-3.
21. Escarce JJ, Shea JA, Chen W, Qian Z, Schwartz JS. Outcomes of open cholecystectomy in the elderly: a longitudinal analysis of 21,000 cases in the prelaparoscopic era. Surgery. 1995;117:156-64.
22. Fong Y, Heffernan N, Blumgart LH. Gallbladder carcinoma discovered during laparoscopic cholecystectomy: aggressive reresection is beneficial. Cancer. 1998;83:423-7.
23. Fried GM, Clas D, Meakins JL. Minimally invasive surgery in the elderly patient. Surg Clin North Am. 1994;74:375-87.
24. Galandiuk S, Mahid SS, Polk Jr HC, Turina M, Rao M, Lewis JN. Differences and similarities between rural and urban operations. Surgery. 2006;140:589-96.
25. Ganey JB, Johnson PA Jr, Prillaman PE, McSwain GR. Cholecystectomy: clinical experience with a large series. Am J Surg. 1986;151:352-7.
26. Gilliland TM, Traverso LW. Modern standards for comparison of cholecystectomy with alternative treatments for symptomatic cholelithiasis with emphasis on long-term relief of symptoms. Surg Gynecol Obst. 1990;170:39-44.
27. Girometti R, Brondani G, Cereser L, Como G, Pin MD, Bazzocchi M, et al. Post-cholecystectomy syndrome: spectrum of biliary findings at magnetic resonance cholangiopancreatography. Br J Radiol. 2010;83:351.
28. Gupta A, Agarwal PN, Kant R, Malik V. Evaluation of fundus first laparoscopic cholecystectomy. JSLS. 2004;8:255-8.
29. Hainsworth PJ, Rhodes M, Gompertz RHK, Armstrong CP, Lennard TWJ. Imaging of the common bile duct in patients undergoing laparoscopic cholecystectomy. Gut. 1994;35:991-5.
30. Haynes JH, Guha SC, Taylor SG. Laparoscopic cholecystectomy in a rural family practice: the Vivian, LA, experience. J Fam Pract. 2004;53:205-8.
31. Herzog U, Messmer R, Sutter M, Tondeffi R. Surgical treatment for cholelithiasis. Surg Gynecol Obstet. 1992;175:238-42.
32. Jatzko GR, Lisborg PH, Pertl AM, Stettner HM. Multivariate comparison of complications after laparoscopic cholecystectomy and open cholecystectomy. Ann Surg. 1995;221:381-6.
33. Kondo S, Nimura Y, Hayakawa N, Kamiya J, Nagino M, Uesaka K. Extensive surgery for carcinoma of the gallbladder. Br J Surg. 2002;89:179-84.
34. Kumar TS, Saklani AP, Vinayagam R, Blackett RL. Spilled gallstones during laparoscopic cholecystectomy: a review of literature. Postgraduate Med J. 2004;80:77-9.
35. Lamberts MP, Den Oudsten BL, Gerritsen JJ, Roukema JA, Westert GP, Drenth JPH, et al. Prospective multicentre cohort study of patient-reported outcomes after cholecystectomy for uncomplicated symptomatic cholecystolithiasis. Br J Surg. 2015;102:1402-9.
36. Leeder PC, Matthews T, Krzeminska K, Dehn TC. Routine day-case laparoscopic cholecystectomy. Br J Surg. 2004;91:312-6.
37. Macintyre IM, Wilson RG. Laparoscopic cholecystectomy. Br J Surg. 1993;80:552-9.
38. Mayol J, Alvarez Fernandez-Represa J. Imaging of the common bile duct (Letter). Gut. 1994;35:1773.
39. Mayol J, Tamayo FJ, Ortiz-Oshiro E, Ortega Lopez D. Resultados de la colecistectomia laparoscopica en pacientes ancianos. Or Esp. 1995;55:45-7.
40. Mayol J, Vincent-Hamelin E, Sarmiento JM, Oshiro EO, Diaz-Gonzalez J, Tamayo FJ, et al. Pulmonary embolism following laparoscopic cholecystectomy: report of two cases and review of the literature. Surg Endosc. 1994;8:214-7.
41. McSherry CK, Glenn F. The incidence and causes of death following surgery for non-malignant biliary tract disease. Ann Surg. 1980;191:271-5.
42. McSherry CK. Laparoscopic management of common bile duct stone [Editorial]. Surg Endosc. 1994;8:1161-2.
43. Mrozowicz A, Polkowski W. Initial three years' experience with laparoscopic cholecystectomy in a district hospital: evaluation of early results and operative measures. Ann Univ Mariae Curie Sklodowska [Med]. 2004;59:26-31.
44. Muhe E. Die erste Cholezystektomie durch das Laparoskop. Langeb Arch Klin Chir. 1986;369:804.
45. Nakamura S, Sakaguchi S, Suzuki S, Muro H. Aggressive surgery for carcinoma of the gallbladder. Surgery. 1989;106:467-73.
46. Nakeeb A, Tran KQ, Black MJ, Erickson BA, Ritch PS, Quebbeman EJ, et al. Improved survival in resected biliary malignancies. Surgery. 2002;132:555-63.
47. Nimura Y, Hayakawa N, Kamiya J, Maeda S, Kondo S, Yasui A, et al. Hepatopancreatoduodenectomy for advanced carcinoma of the biliary tract. Hepatogastroenterology. 1991;38:170-5.

48. Parkar RB, Thagana NG, Baraza R, Otieno D. Experience with laparoscopic surgery at the Aga Khan Hospital, Nairobi. East Afr Med J. 2003;80:44-50.
49. Patel SC, Bhatt JR. Laparoscopic cholecystectomy at the Aga Khan Hospital, Nairobi. East Afr Med J. 2000;77:194-8.
50. Reddick EJ, Olsen DO. Laparoscopic laser cholecystectomy. Surg Endosc. 1989;3:131-3.
51. Shirai Y, Yoshida K, Tsukada K, Muto T. Inapparent carcinoma of the gallbladder. An appraisal of a radical second operation after simple cholecystectomy. Ann Surg. 1992;215:326-31.
52. Smith N, Max MH. Gallbladder surgery in patients over 60: is there an increased risk? South Med J. 1987;80:472-4.
53. Southern Surgeons group. A prospective analysis of 1518 laparoscopic cholecystectomies. N Engl J Med N. 1991;324:1073-8.
54. Tan JT, Suyapto DR, Neo EL, Leong PS. Prospective audit of laparoscopic cholecystectomy experience at a secondary referral centre in South Australia. ANZ J Surg. 2006;76:335-8.
55. Taylor OM, Sedman PC, Jones BM, Royston CM, Arulampalam T, Wellwood J. Laparoscopic cholecystectomy without operative cholangiogram: 2038 cases over 5-year period in two district general hospitals. Ann R Coll Surg Engl. 1997;79:376-80.
56. Todoroki T, Kawamoto T, Takahashi H, Takada Y, Koike N, Otsuka M, et al. Treatment of gallbladder cancer by radical resection. Br J Surg. 1999;86:622-7.
57. Vagenas K, Karamanakos SN, Spyropoulos C, Panagiotopoulos S, Karanikolas M, Stavropoulos M. Laparoscopic cholecystectomy: a report from a single center. World J Gastroenterol. 2006; 12:3887-90.
58. van Dijk AH, Wennmacker SZ, de Reuver PR, Latenstein CSS, Buyne O, Donkervoort SC, et al. Restrictive strategy versus usual care for cholecystectomy in patients with gallstones and abdominal pain (SECURE): a multicentre, randomised, parallel-arm, non-inferiority trial. Lancet. 2019;393:2322.
59. Voyles CR, Sanders DL, Hogan R. Common bile duct evaluation in the era of laparoscopic cholecystectomy. 1050 cases later. Ann Surg. 1994;219:744-52.
60. Wakai T, Shirai Y, Hatakeyama K. Radical second resection provides survival benefit for patients with T2 gallbladder carcinoma first discovered after laparoscopic cholecystectomy. World J Surg. 2002;26:867-71.
61. Wang SJ, Fuller CD, Kim JS, Sittig DF, Thomas CR Jr, Ravdin PM, et al. Prediction model for estimating the survival benefit of adjuvant radiotherapy for gallbladder cancer. J Clin Oncol. 2008;26:2112-7.
62. Wherry DC, Marohn MR, Malanoski MP, Hetz SP, Rich NM. An external audit of laparoscopic cholecystectomy in the steady state performed in medical treatment facilities of the Department of Defense. Ann Surg. 1996;224:145-54.
63. Williams Jr LF, Chapman WC, Bonau RA, McGee Jr EC, Boyd RW, Jacobs JK. Comparison of laparoscopic cholecystectomy with open cholecystectomy in a single center. Am J Surg. 1993;165:459-65.
64. Wittgen CM, Andrus JP, Andrus CH, Kaminski DL. Cholecystectomy. Which procedure is best for the high-risk patient? Surg Endosc. 1993;7:395-9.
65. Yamaguchi K, Chijiiwa K, Shimizu S, Yokohata K, Tsuneyoshi M, Tanaka M. Anatomical limit of extended cholecystectomy for gallbladder carcinoma involving the neck of the gallbladder. Int Surg. 1998;83:21-3.
66. Yamashita Y, Kurohiji T, Kakegawa T. Evaluation of two training programs for laparoscopic cholecystectomy: incidence of major complications. World J Surg. 1994;18:279-85.

CHAPTER 14

Laparoscopic CBD Exploration

INTRODUCTION

Laparoscopic exploration of the common bile duct (CBD) is performed either for the diagnosis or the treatment of CBD stones. CBD stones demonstrated by laparoscopic intraoperative cholangiography (IOC) or laparoscopic ultrasonography (LUS) are extracted either through the cystic duct or through choledochotomy. An alternative for the treatment of CBD stones is to perform an endoscopic sphincterotomy either before, during, or after laparoscopic cholecystectomy.

The main advantages of IOC during cholecystectomy are:

- Detection of CBD stone
- Reduction of the incidence of residual CBD stone
- Delineation of the biliary anatomical variations at risk for bile duct injury

Intraoperative cholangiogram is a highly sensitive tool for detecting choledocholithiasis, with an overall accuracy of 95%. Routine IOC can diagnose unsuspected CBD stone in 1–14% (average 5%) of patients without indications for ductal exploration.

INTRAOPERATIVE CHOLANGIOGRAPHY

Techniques of Cholangiography

Cholangiograms obtained during laparoscopy are usually performed after catheterization of the cystic duct through a cholangioclamp (Storz Endoscopy, USA), or inserting a catheter through a hollow gasketed needle pinned through the abdominal wall along the right subcostal margin. Difficulties in catheterization of the small cystic duct have led to consider cholecystocholangiography by direct puncture of the gallbladder as an alternative to cystic duct cholangiography. Cystic duct cholangiography is clearly better than cholecystocholangiography, and fluoroscopic imaging should be the standard for IOC. Until now, no specific clinically significant complications directly attributable to laparoscopic IOC have been reported.

Expected success rates for laparoscopic IOC are in a 90–100% range. Inability to cannulate a narrow cystic duct is the main cause of failure. When performed after clipping (but not cutting), the anatomical structures identified by careful dissection such as the cystic artery and the cystic duct, a correctly interpreted IOC allows the detection of the most frequently reported cause of CBD injury, i.e., mistaken identification of a narrow main bile duct in place of the cystic duct.

LAPAROSCOPIC ULTRASONOGRAPHY

Several studies on LUS have been published and conclusions of these studies favor LUS as compared to IOC. LUS is performed with a higher success rate, in less time, with better specificity, but with less precision with regard to the delineation of biliary tree anatomy. LUS is of little, if any, helps in the diagnosis or prevention of bile duct injuries. While detection of smaller stones by LUS should increase its sensitivity, most of these stones are reputed to be flushed out through the sphincter and therefore the question arises if such small stones require any treatment at all. Specificity of LUS is higher (less false positives) than of IOC. When IOC and LUS were combined, there is chance of less than 1% of false positives. The question that comes to mind is whether LUS should be a screening test, and IOC performed only in case of doubt or should IOC be the screening test, and LUS used only when IOC is of doubtful value? IOC performs better than LUS to delineate the entire biliary tree, from the intrahepatic tree to the pancreatic portion of the CBD. Injection of saline into the biliary tree enhanced the images obtained by LUS, especially in the distal portion of the bile duct.

Criteria for Routine Intraoperative Cholangiography

Preoperative Factors

- Failed endoscopic retrograde cholangiography ± sphincterotomy
- Ultrasonographic findings
- CBD size (>6 mm)
- Choledocholithiasis
- History of jaundice or pancreatitis
- Elevated bilirubin, alkaline phosphatase, and transaminases

Intraoperative Factors

- Unclear anatomy
- Conversion to open cholecystectomy
- Dilated cystic duct over 4 mm

LAPAROSCOPIC EXTRACTION OF COMMON BILE DUCT STONES

Once detected during laparoscopic IOC, laparoscopic extraction of CBD stones is a logical extension of the procedure. Laparoscopic exploration of the CBD can be performed either through the cystic duct or by laparoscopic choledochotomy. A critical evaluation of the retrospective and prospective series on laparoscopic CBD exploration published since 1989 shows that both procedures are feasible and safe. Any comparisons between the two techniques would be fallacious because of their obviously different indications. Nonetheless, whenever feasible, laparoscopic transcystic CBD exploration best fulfills the expectancy of mini-invasive approach. Laparoscopic management of CBD stones is considered as technically difficult and demanding, requiring advanced laparoscopic skills as well as expensive endoscopic and radiological equipment. Endoscopic sphincterotomy is commonly proposed preoperatively as the alternative to surgery for CBD stones. Endoscopic sphincterotomy is indicated in patients with severe cholangitis for urgent drainage of infected bile, and in patients with retained stones after cholecystectomy. In open conventional surgery, controlled studies have not shown that ES, performed prior to surgery in patients with CBD stones in situ, was superior to single-step surgical management.

In case of preoperative diagnosis of CBD stone, options for management include:

- Preoperative endoscopic retrograde cholangiopancreatography (ERCP) and endoscopic sphincterotomy followed by laparoscopic cholecystectomy
- Conventional open CBD exploration
- Laparoscopic CBD exploration

Today, most of the laparoscopic surgeons prefer the "single-stage" laparoscopic approach to choledocholithiasis. None of the randomized trials published to date concluded superiority of endoscopic treatment alone or associated with surgery as compared to first-line surgical treatment. Immediate postoperative mortality was 2.6% in the endoscopic group as opposed to 1% in the surgical group. In global analysis, the rate of major and minor complications were respectively 8% and 10% after endoscopy followed by surgery, and 8% and 15% after surgery alone.

Study of European Association for Endoscopic Surgery (Table 1)

Choledocholithiasis is found in approximately 10–20% of patients who undergo open cholecystectomies. In the era of laparoscopic cholecystectomies, the prevalence of CBD stones averages 6% (range: 3–10%). The incidence of choledocholithiasis increases over the age of 60 years. To achieve a maximal benefit to risk ratio, radiological investigations of the CBD should be restricted to patients with high suspicion of CBD stones, as determined by preoperative predictive scoring.

TABLE 1: Study of European Association for Endoscopic Surgery (EAES).

	LCBDE	*(ERC ± ES) + LC*	*p*
Patients (N)	133	136	
With CBD	109 (82%)	99 (73%)	
Failed ERCP ± ES		23 (17%)	
Stone clearance		82/98 (84%)	NS
Successful LCBDE	92/109 (84%)	12/17 (71%)	
Conversions	14 (13%)	5 (5%)	NS
Postoperative ES	3		
Complications	21/133	17/136	NS
Deaths	0	2	
Hospital stay (range)	6.4 (4.2–12)	9 (5.5–14)	<0.05

(ES: endoscopic sphincterotomy; LC: laparoscopic cholecystectomy; ERCP: endoscopic retrograde cholangiopancreaticography; LCBDE: laparoscopic common bile duct exploration; NS: nonsignificant)

Diagnostic and therapeutic choices in cholelithiasis must be considered conjointly. Data gathered from randomized trials have demonstrated that endoscopic sphincterotomy, as an additional procedure to surgery, does not improve the clinical results in patients fit for primary single-stage surgical treatment, whether performed laparoscopically or not. Discussions regarding the optimal way to treat patients with demonstrated CBD stones could lead to endless debate. Due to marginal differences between the endoscopic and surgical techniques, the number of patients needed to show any significant difference in terms of morbidity, mortality, or clearance rates would be enormous and therefore unrealistic. Cholangitis, jaundice, and CBD stones, as demonstrated on percutaneous ultrasonography, are the only reliable preoperative indicators available with predictive value of CBD stones better than 50%. Severe cholangitis is an unquestionable indication for urgent endoscopic drainage, regardless of whether the CBD can be cleared of associated stones or not. The notorious insufficiencies of all other preoperative indicators for CBD stones should lead to a requiem for preoperative invasive diagnostic procedures, both in terms of risk, benefits, and costs.

Laparoscopic common bile duct exploration (LCBDE) can be performed via the cystic duct (transcystic approach) or an incision in the CBD (choledochotomy approach). In general, small distal stones are best suited for transcystic removal, while large or proximal stones may require a choledochotomy approach. All surgeons undertaking laparoscopic cholecystectomy must be able to perform an IOC. When IOC demonstrates CBD stones, appropriate treatment is decided according to available equipment and skills. Transcystic clearance of CBD stones is successful in at least two of three patients. In case of large (>20 mm) stones or other potential difficulties as regards postoperative endoscopic sphincterotomy such as a periampullary diverticulum, conversion to open surgery is indicated in case of failed laparoscopic CBD exploration. In the other cases, the available data do not allow any formal conclusions regarding the alternative between advanced laparoscopic biliary explorations and postoperative endoscopic sphincterotomy. The potential risk of reoperation in case of failed postoperative endoscopic sphincterotomy might be more theoretical than practical. In one decision analysis, assessing different approaches to using ERC in patients undergoing laparoscopic cholecystectomy, postoperative ERC was associated with less costs and morbidity, but laparoscopic CBD exploration was not considered in the study design. Last, before embarking on a more invasive laparoscopic CBD exploration policy for small stones, irretrievable by the transcystic approach, surgeons must remember that asymptomatic migration does exist, even if the definitive fate of small CBD stones remains unknown at the present time. The potential security afforded by temporary biliary drainage still has to be balanced with its unavoidable morbidity.

PROCEDURE

Patient Position

Patient is operated in the supine position with a steep head-up and left tilt. This typical positioning of laparoscopic choledochotomy should be achieved once the pneumoperitoneum has been established **(Fig. 1)**.

Port Position

The standard four-port configuration for laparoscopic cholecystectomy is used. A fifth port should be used later between the right midclavicular and epigastric port just below the subcostal margin for inserting the choledochoscope.

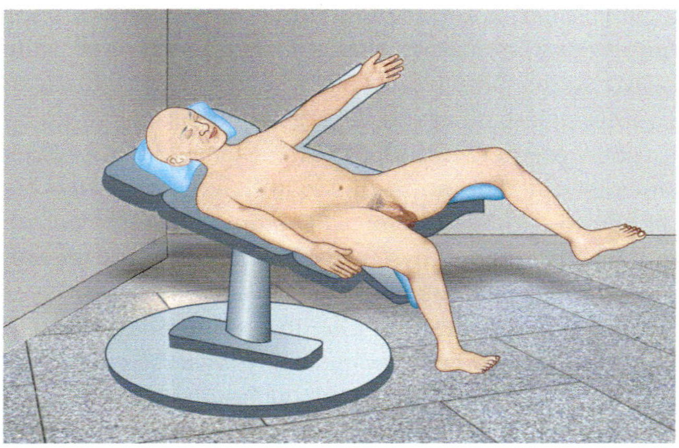

Fig. 1: Patient position for laparoscopic choledochotomy.

The fundus of the gallbladder should be retracted toward the right shoulder and the Hartmann's pouch should be retracted anterolaterally toward right anterior-superior iliac spine. Dissection began onto the neck of the gallbladder and continued proximally until the junction of gallbladder with the cystic duct is clearly defined. Dissection should be continued proximally onto the cystic duct until there was adequate length to perform cholangiogram.

Cystic duct should be milked toward the gallbladder to dislodge any cystic duct stone into the gallbladder. Single titanium clip should be applied on the gallbladder side of cystic duct to prevent any back slippage of gallstone into the CBD and to prevent biliary spillage into the operative field.

A small nick in the cystic duct should be given with the help of hook scissors or microscissors. Intraoperative cholangiogram should be performed using a ureteric catheter (4–5 Fr) or an infant feeding tube (no. 5–6), which is passed through the cystic duct into the CBD. After the insertion of the catheter, a titanium clip should be applied loosely to prevent any back leakage of the contrast medium. Digital C-arm fluoroscopy provided the real-time imaging of the biliary tree. In cases where the cystic duct could not be cannulated, contrast was directly injected into the CBD through a 24-Fr lumbar puncture needle percutaneously.

On cholangiogram, surgeon must look for any filling defect—its size, site, number of bile duct stones, and free passage of contrast into the duodenum and for any anatomical variation of the biliary tree.

Transcystic or transcholedochal approach to remove CBD stones should be decided on the following factors **(Table 2)**.

Common bile duct stone should be extracted with the help of Dormia basket/balloon catheter, irrigation/suctioning, or by simply manipulating bile duct using blunt forceps. After retrieving the stones, the cystic duct stump was closed with clips or extracorporeal knots and the gallbladder was removed in the usual manner.

For transcholedochal exploration after opening up of the Calot's triangle, the anterior surface of the CBD should be dissected carefully and choledochotomy should be performed by a longitudinal incision with the help of endoscopic knife just below the insertion of the cystic duct into the bile duct **(Figs. 2A to D)**. Before giving incision with knife, mild coagulation of serosal surface of CBD can help in preventing oozing **(Figs. 3A to D)**. The single large stone can be retrieved by spontaneous evacuation while incising the bile duct, blunt instrumental pressure with atraumatic forceps can facilitate its easy removal **(Figs. 4A to D)**.

In case of multiple stones Dormia basket, Fogarty balloon catheter or irrigation and suction can be used to remove the stone **(Figs. 5 and 6)**.

TABLE 2: Transcystic versus transcholedochal approach for removal of common bile duct (CBD) stone.

Criteria	*Findings*		*Transcystic approach*	*Transcholedochal approach*	*Any of these approach*
Diameter of cystic duct	<3 mm			Recommended	
Diameter of cystic duct	>3 mm		Recommended	Recommended	Recommended
CBD diameter	<7 mm		Recommended		
CBD diameter	>7 mm		Recommended	Recommended	Recommended
Large stone (>6 mm)				Recommended	
Number of stone	<4		Recommended	Recommended	Recommended
Number of stone	>4			Recommended	
Stone location	Proximal			Recommended	
Stone location	Distal				Recommended
Junction of cystic duct with CBD	Right lateral				Recommended
Junction of cystic duct with CBD	Left lateral or	posterior		Recommended	
Stone impacted in ampulla	Yes				Recommended
Severe inflammation of CBD	Yes		Recommended		
Laparoscopic suturing	Good				Recommended

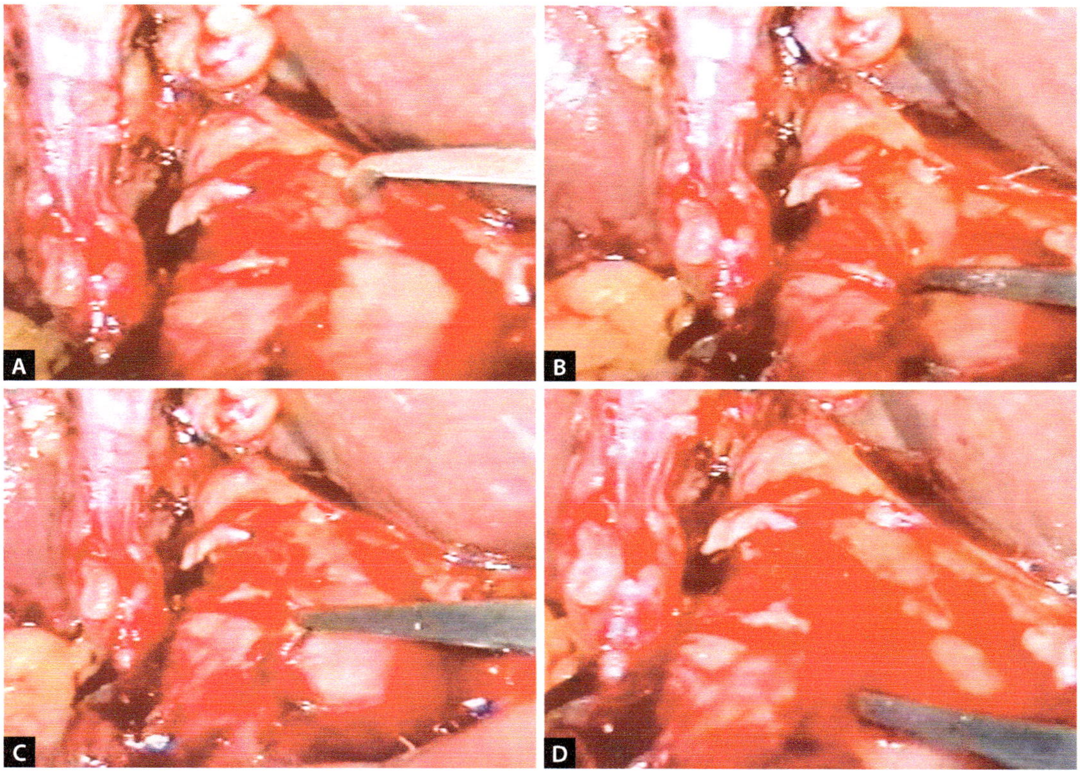

Figs. 2A to D: Endo-knife used to explore common bile duct (CBD).

Completion cholangiography or choledochoscopy must be performed to assess any remaining stone. Some surgeons use 5.5-Fr bronchoscope for this purpose but ideally choledochoscope will give more flexibility.

Once all the stone is removed, choledochotomy should be closed over a T-tube with interrupted Vicryl suture **(Figs. 7 to 9)**. In case of single stone, primary closure of CBD after assessing the clearance of the CBD can be tried. After bile duct closure, cholecystectomy should be performed in the usual manner. An intrahepatic nasogastric tube drain should be used routinely in this surgery, which is usually removed on days 3–4 as the output decreased below 30 mL/day.

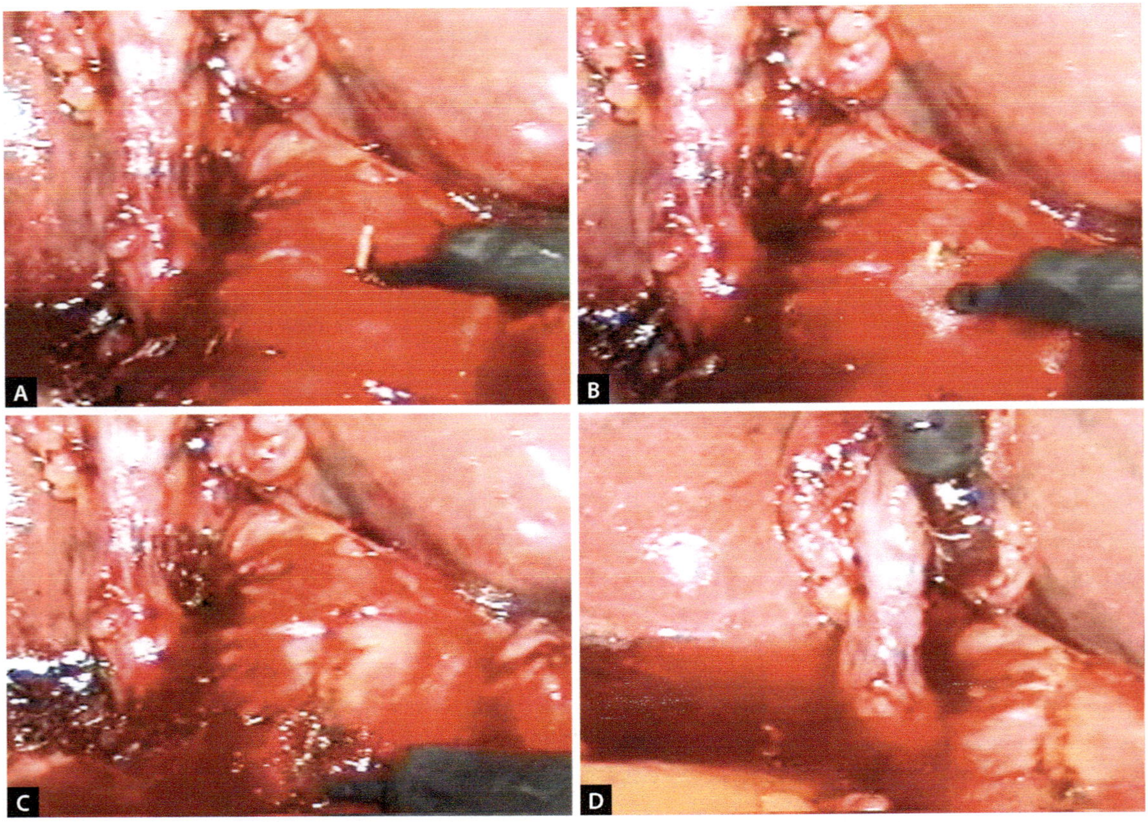

Figs. 3A to D: Mild coagulation current applied over serosal surface of common bile duct.

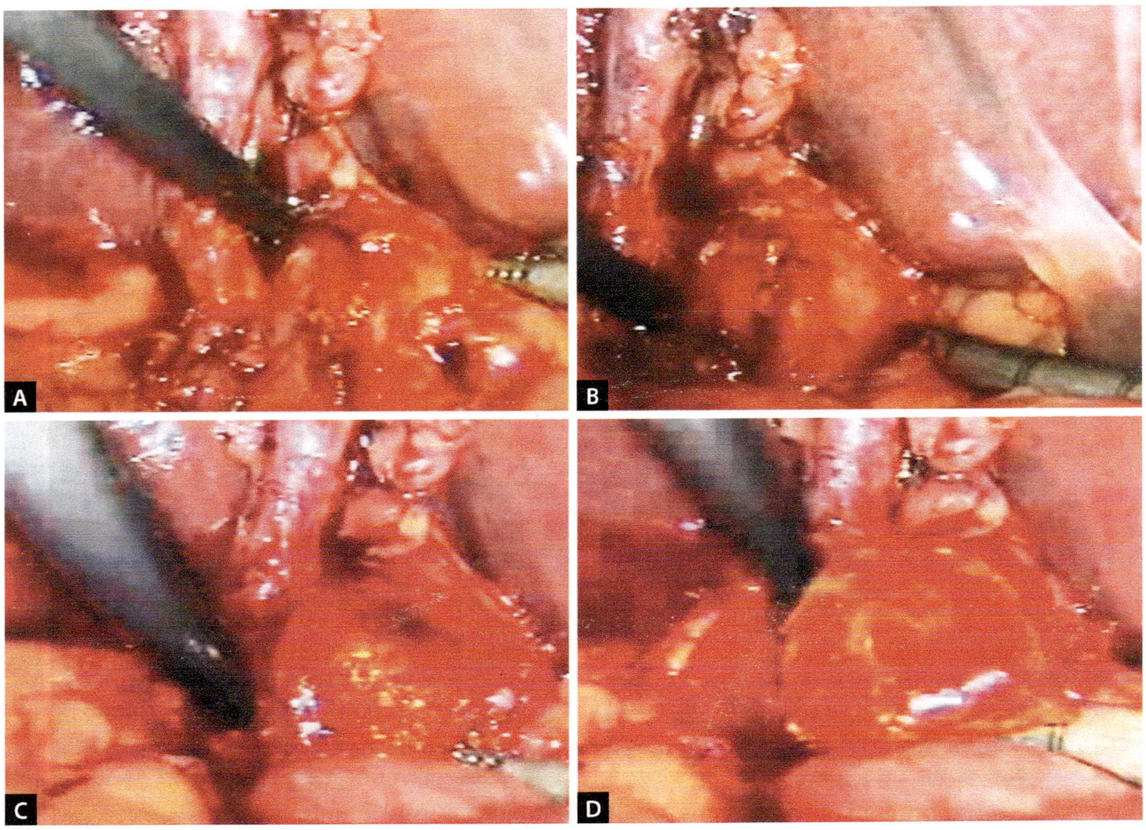

Figs. 4A to D: Bigger single stone can be extracted by milking.

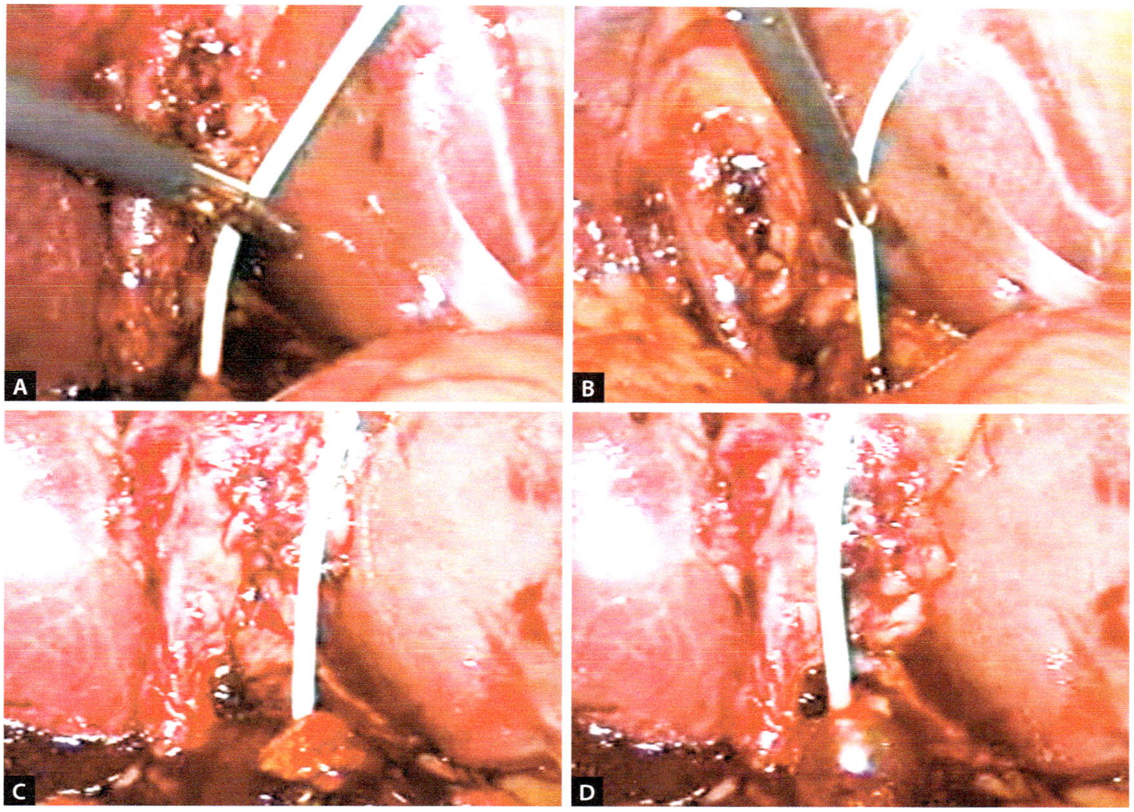

Figs. 5A to D: Fogarty catheter used to extract stone.

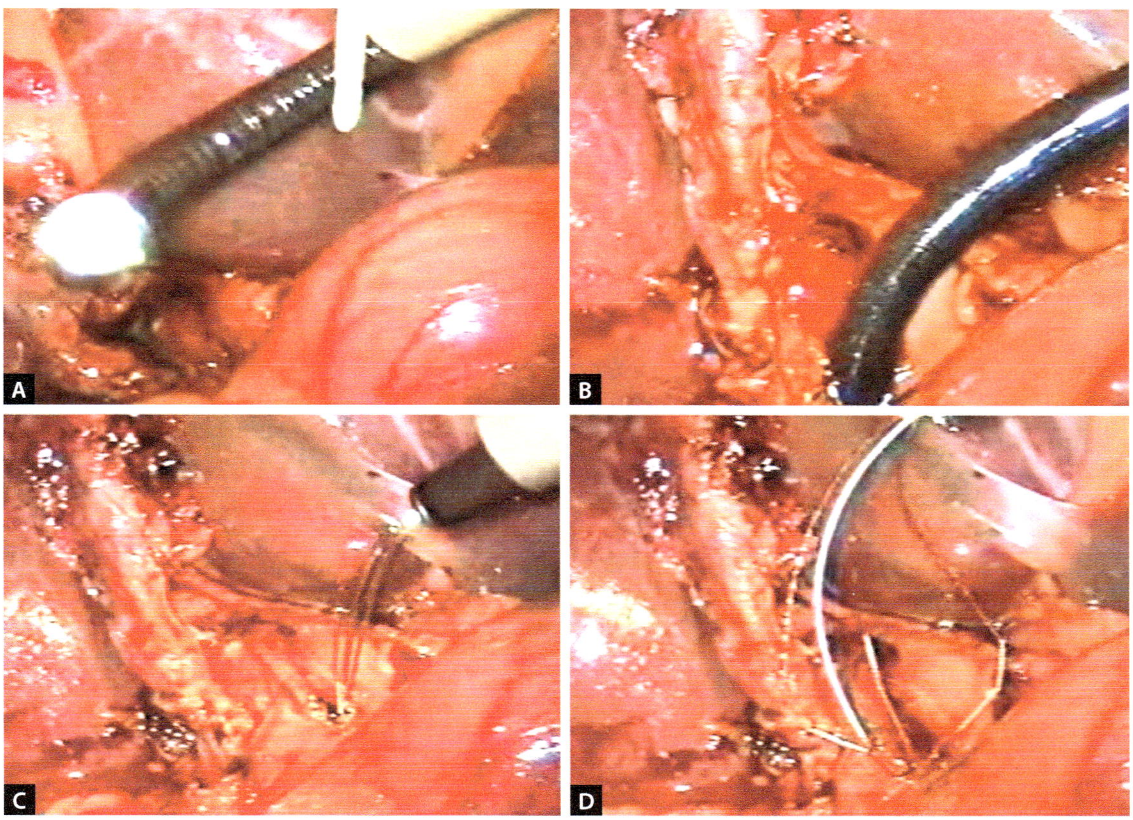

Figs. 6A to D: Choledochoscope with Dormia basket is used to extract stone.

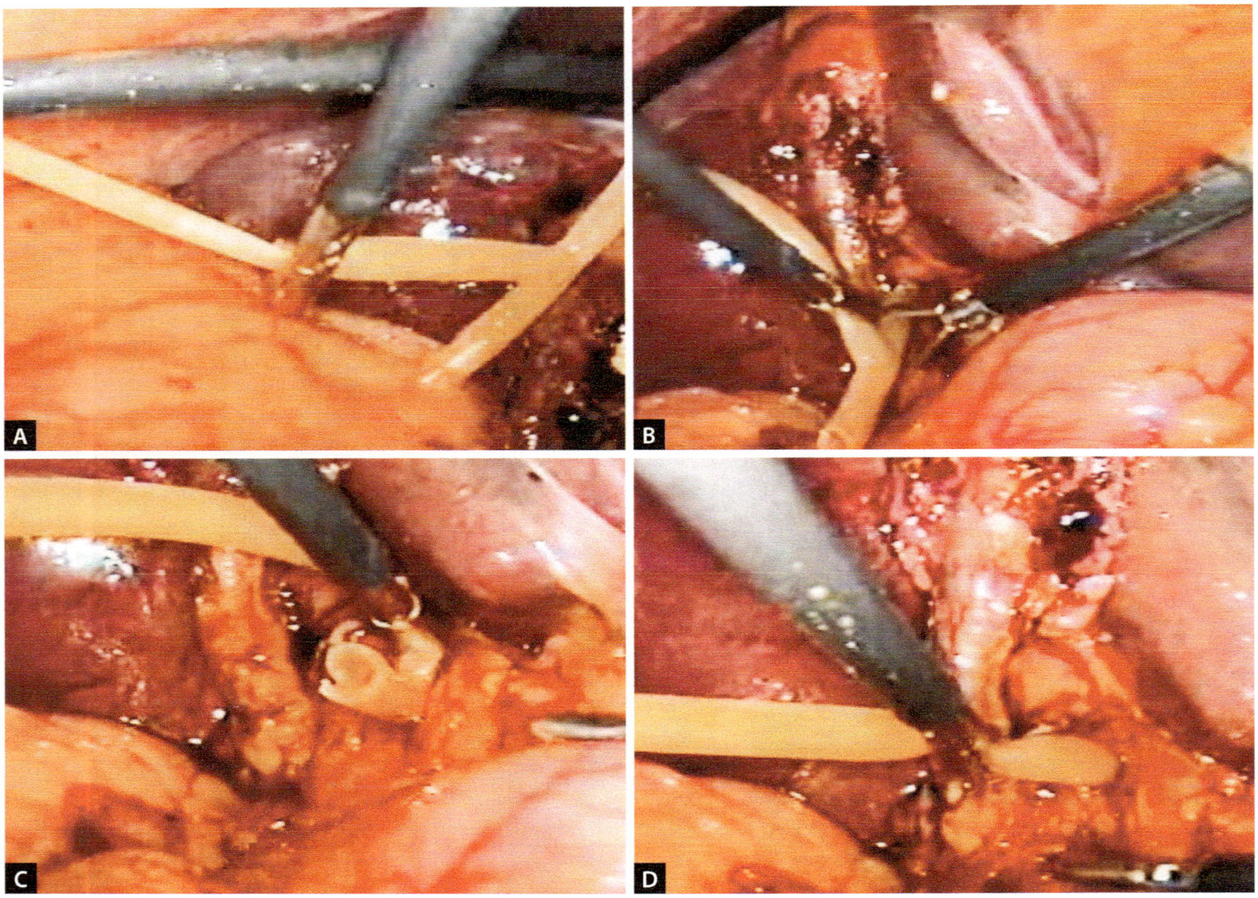

Figs. 7A to D: Introduction of T-tube.

T-tube Management

If a T-tube has been placed, a T-tube cholangiogram is performed 24–48 hours postoperatively. If the initial T-tube cholangiogram shows biliary obstruction or retained stones, the T-tube is left open for 1–2 weeks. If a repeat T-tube cholangiogram shows persistent stone or biliary obstruction, ERCP or interventional radiologic procedure via the T-tube is required to clear the duct. A normal T-tube cholangiogram and liver function tests (LFTs) should be ascertained prior to T-tube removal. In patients with a T-tube, the drain should be kept until a T-tube cholangiogram shows no biliary leak or stenosis. In patients without a T-tube, the drain may be removed after LFTs normalize without bilious drain output; alternatively, an HIDA scan can also be obtained to access the biliary anatomy prior to drain removal.

COMPLICATIONS

Common complications after laparoscopic exploration are:

- Bile duct leak
- Persistent stones
- Impacted stones
- Bile duct stricture
- Pancreatitis

Most of the complications are same as found in open CBD exploration. Bile may leak from the cystic duct orifice, cystic duct-CBD junction, or the CBD itself. It occurs in 2–16% of cases. Stones persist in the CBD in 0–5% of patients after surgical CBD exploration. Rarely, severely impacted stones are encountered. Strictures of the bile duct are a long-term complication of CBD exploration that occurs in 0–0.8% of cases. Impacted stones are difficult to remove with Fogarty balloon catheters or wire baskets. Pancreatitis occurs in 0–3% of patients following CBD exploration due to reflux of contrast into the pancreatic duct or ampullary obstruction by stones, edema, or blood clots. In the latter case, ERCP may be required to relieve the obstruction. According to data from the American College of Surgeons National Surgical Quality Improvement Program (ACS NSQIP) database, laparoscopic CBD exploration has significantly lower mortality (0.25 vs. 5.5%), surgical site infection rate (1.2 vs. 10%), and overall morbidity rate (3.7 vs. 22%) compared with open CBD exploration. However, the increased morbidity and mortality associated with open exploration may be a reflection of underlying comorbidities or more complicated disease requiring an open approach.

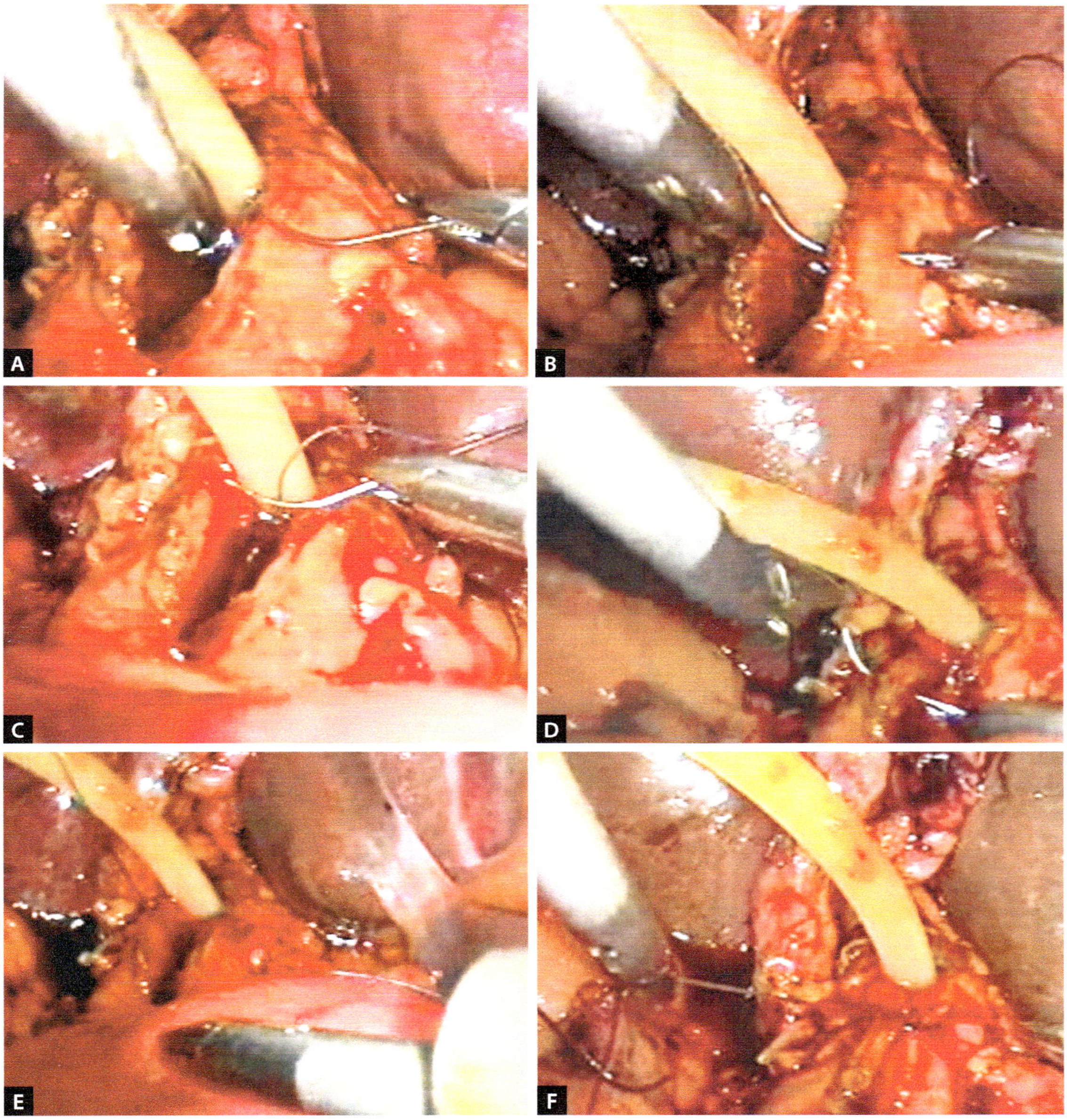

Figs. 8A to F: T-tube is fixed with intracorporeal interrupted surgeons knot.

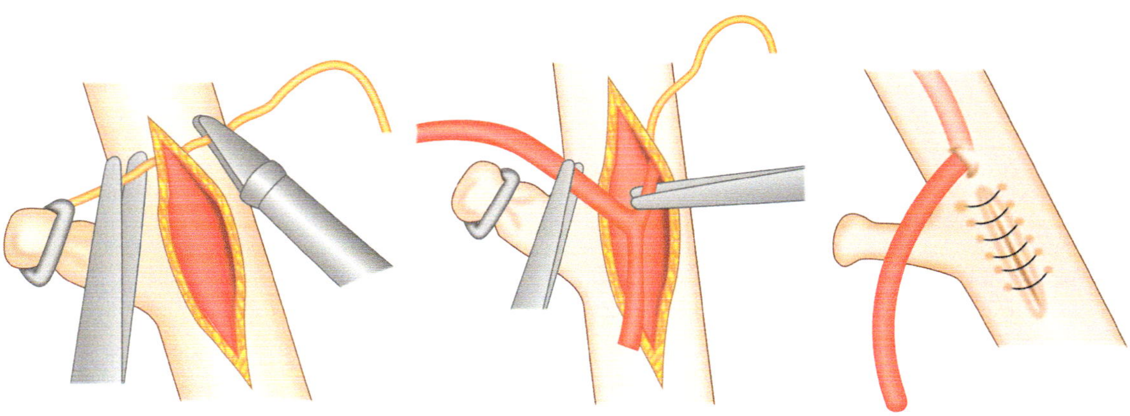

Fig. 9: Diagrammatic representation of T-tube fixation with intracorporeal interrupted surgeons knot.

BIBLIOGRAPHY

1. Altman DG. Practical Statistics for Medical Research. London, England: Chapman and Hall; 1992.
2. Anciaux ML, Pelletier G, Attali P, Meduri B, Liguory C, Etienne JP. Prospective study of clinical and biochemical features of symptomatic choledocholithiasis. Dig Dis Sci. 1986;31:449-53.
3. Bansal VK, Misra MC, Rajan K, Kilambi R, Kumar S, Krishna A, et al. Single-stage laparoscopic common bile duct exploration and cholecystectomy versus two-stage endoscopic stone extraction followed by laparoscopic cholecystectomy for patients with concomitant gallbladder stones and common bile duct stones: a randomized controlled trial. Surg Endosc. 2014;28:875.
4. Barkun AN, Barkun JS, Fried GM, Ghitulescu G, Steinmetz O, Pham C, et al. Useful predictors of bile duct stones in patients undergoing laparoscopic cholecystectomy. Ann Surg. 1994; 220:32-9.
5. Bates T, Ebbs SR, Harrison M, A'Hern RP. Influence of cholecystectomy on symptoms. Br J Surg. 1991;78:964-7.
6. Behan M, Kazam E. Sonography of the common bile duct: value of the right anterior oblique view. Am J Roentgenol. 1978;130:701-9.
7. Bhargava S, Vashisht S, Kakaria A, Tandon RK, Berry M. Choledocholithiasis: an ultrasonic study with comparative evaluation with ERCP/PTC. Australas Radiol. 1988;32:220-6.
8. Clemets D, Aslan S, Wilkins WE. Common bile duct gallstones, anicteric presentation in the elderly: under-recognized but important. Postgrad Med J. 1990;66:878-9.
9. Cooperberg PL, Li D, Wong P, Cohen MM, Burhenne HJ. Accuracy of common hepatic duct size in the evaluation of extrahepatic biliary obstruction. Radiology. 1980;135:141-4.
10. Cotton PB. Endoscopic retrograde cholangiopancreatography and laparoscopic cholecystectomy. Am J Surg. 1993;165:474-8.
11. Cuscheri A, Croce E, Faggioni A, Jakimowicz J, Lacy A, Lezoche E, et al. EAES ductal stone study. Surg Endosc. 1996;10:1130-5.
12. DePaula AL, Hashiba K, Bafatto M. Laparoscopic management of choledocholithiasis. Surg Endosc. 1994;8:1399-1403.
13. Diehl AK, Sugarek NJ, Todd KH. Clinical evaluation for gallstone disease: usefulness of symptoms and signs in diagnosis. Am J Med. 1990;89:29-33.
14. Dorman JP, Franklin ME Jr, Glass JL. Laparoscopic common bile duct exploration by choledochotomy: an effective and efficient method of treatment of choledocholithiasis. Surg Endosc. 1998;12:926-8.
15. Edwin B, Rosseland ARR, Trondsen E. Prophylactic endoscopic sphincterotomy as treatment. Hepatogastroenterology. 1993; 40:550-5.
16. Ferzli GS, Hurwitz JB, Massaad AA, Piperno B. Laparoscopic common bile duct exploration: a review. J Laparoendosc Surg. 1996;6:413-19.
17. Gigot JF, Navez B, Etienne J, Cambier E, Jadoul P, Guiot P, et al. A stratified intraoperative surgical strategy is mandatory during laparoscopic common bile duct exploration for common bile duct stones. Surg Endosc. 1997;11:722-8.
18. Gilliland TM, Traverso LW. Modern standards for comparison of cholecystectomy with alternative treatments for symptomatic cholelithiasis with emphasis on long-term relief of symptoms. Surg Gynecol Obstet. 1990;170:39-44.
19. Graham SM, Flowers JL, Scott TR. Laparoscopic cholecystectomy and common bile duct stones. Ann Surg. 1993;1:61-7.
20. Gross BH, Harter LP, Gore RM, Callen PW, Filly RA, Shapiro HA, et al. Ultrasonic evaluation of common bile duct stones: prospective comparison with endoscopic retrograde cholangiography. Radiology. 1983;146:471-4.
21. Hand DJ. Discrimination and Classification. New York, NY: John Wiley and Sons; 1976.
22. Hauer-Jensen M, Karesen R, Nygaard K, Solheim K, Amlie E, Havig O, et al. Predictive ability of choledocholithiasis indicators: a prospective evaluation. Ann Surg. 1985;202:64-8.
23. Hauer-Jensen M, Karesen R, Nygaard K, Solheim K, Amlie E, Havig O, et al. Consequences of routine preoperative cholangiography during cholecystectomy for gallstone disease: a prospective, randomized study. World J Surg. 1986;10: 996-1002.
24. Houdart R, Perniceni T, Darne B, Salmeron M, Simon JF. Predicting common bile duct lithiasis: determination and prospective validation of a model predicting low risk. Am J Surg. 1995;170:38-43.
25. Hunt DR, Reiter L, Scott AJ. Preoperative ultrasound measurement of bile duct diameter: basis for selective cholangiography Aust N Z J Surg. 1990;60:189-92.
26. Hunt DR, Scott AJ. Changes in bile duct diameter after cholecystectomy: a 5-year prospective study. Gastroenterology. 1989;97:1485-8.
27. Hunter JG. Laparoscopic transcystic common bile duct exploration. Am J Surg. 1992;163:53-8.
28. Jennrich RI. Stepwise discriminant analysis. In: Enslein K, Ralston A, Wilf H (Eds). Statistical Methods for Digital Computers. New York, NY: John Wiley and Sons; 1979.
29. Jorgensen T. Abdominal symptoms and gallstone disease: an epidemiological investigation. Hepatology. 1989;9:856-60.
30. Kelly TR. Gallstone pancreatitis: the timing of surgery. Surgery. 1980;88:345-50.
31. Lacaine F, Corlette MB, Bismuth H. Preoperative evaluation of the risk of common bile duct stones. Arch Surg. 1980;115: 1114-6.
32. Larson GM, Vitale GC, Casey J, Evans JS, Gilliam G, Heuser L, et al. Multi-practice analysis of laparoscopic cholecystectomy in 1,983 patients. Am J Surg. 1991;163:221-6.
33. Liberman MA, Phillips EH, Carroll BJ, Fallas MJ, Rosenthal R, Hiatt J. Cost-effective management of complicated choledocholithiasis: laparoscopic transcystic duct exploration or endoscopic sphincterotomy. J Am Coll Surg. 1996;182:488-94.
34. Mjaaland O, Raeder J, Aaseboe V, Trondsen E, Buanes T. Outpatient laparoscopic cholecystectomy, patient satisfaction and safety: prospective study of 200 patients. Br J Surg. 2007;31:1010-5.
35. Naude GP, Stabile BE, Bongard FS. Antegrade laparoscopic common bile duct stone removal using a balloon-tipped embolectomy catheter. J Am Coll Surg. 1997;184:655-7.
36. Neoptolemos JP, Carr-Locke DL, Fossard DP. Prospective randomized study of preoperative endoscopic sphincterotomy versus surgery alone for common bile duct stones. BMJ. 1987;294:470-4.
37. Neuhaus H, Feussner H, Ungeheuer A, Hoffmann W, Siewert JR, Classen M. Prospective evaluation of the use of endoscopic retrograde cholangiography prior to laparoscopic cholecystography. Endoscopy. 1992;24:745-9.
38. Niederau C, Sonnenberg A, Mueller J. Comparison of the extrahepatic bile duct size measured by ultrasound and by different radiographic methods. Gastroenterology. 1984;87:615-21.
39. Noble H, Tranter S, Chesworth T, Norton S, Thompson M. A randomized, clinical trial to compare endoscopic sphincterotomy and subsequent laparoscopic cholecystectomy with primary laparoscopic bile duct exploration during cholecystectomy in higher risk patients with choledocholithiasis. J Laparoendosc Adv Surg Tech A. 2009;19:713.
40. O'Connor HJ, Bartlett RJ, Hamilton I, Ellis WR, Watters JK, Lintott DJ, et al. Bile duct calibre: the value of ultrasonic and cholangiographic measurement in the postcholecystectomy patient. Gut. 1984;25:A576.

41. Onken J, Brazer S, Eisen G, et al. Accurate prediction of choledocholithiasis. In: Program and abstracts of the American Association for the Study of Liver Disease, American Gastroenterological Association, American Society for Gastrointestinal Endoscopy, and Society for Surgery of the Alimentary Tract group conference; May 15–18, 1994; New Orleans, La. Abstract 699.
42. Pan L, Chen M, Ji L, Zheng L, Yan P, Fang J, et al. The safety and efficacy of laparoscopic common bile duct exploration combined with cholecystectomy for the management of cholecysto-choledocholithiasis: an up-to-date meta-analysis. Ann Surg. 2018;268:247.
43. Pasanen P, Partanen K, Pikkarainen P, Alhava E, Pirinen A, Janatuinen E. Ultrasonography, CT, and ERCP in the diagnosis of choledochal stones. Acta Radiol. 1992;33:53-6.
44. Patwardhan RV, Smith OJ, Farmelant MH. Serum transaminase levels and cholescintigraphic anomalies in acute biliary tract obstruction. Arch Intern Med. 1987;147:1249-53.
45. Petelin JB. Clinical results of common bile duct exploration. Endosc Surg Allied Technol. 1993;1:125-9.
46. Petelin JB. Laparoscopic approach to common duct pathology. Am J Surg. 1993;165:487-91.
47. Phillips E, Daykhovsky L, Carroll B, Gershman A, Grundfest WS. Laparoscopic cholecystectomy: instrumentation and technique. J Laparoendosc Surg. 1990;1:3-15.
48. Phillips EH, Berci G, Carroll B, Daykhovsky L, Sackier J, Paz-Partlow M. The importance of intraoperative cholangiography during laparoscopic cholecystectomy. Am Surg. 1990;56:792-5.
49. Phillips EH, Rosenthal RJ, Carroll BJ, Fallas MJ. Laparoscopic transcystic-duct common bile duct exploration. Surg Endosc. 1994;8:1389-94.
50. Poh BR, Ho SP, Sritharan M, Yeong CC, Swan MP, Devonshire DA, et al. Randomized clinical trial of intraoperative endoscopic retrograde cholangiopancreatography versus laparoscopic bile duct exploration in patients with choledocholithiasis. Br J Surg. 2016;103:1117.
51. Poulose BK, Arbogast PG, Holzman MD. National analysis of in-hospital resource utilization in choledocholithiasis management using propensity scores. Surg Endosc. 2006;20:186.
52. Reiss R, Deutsch AA, Nudelman I, Kott I. Statistical value of various clinical parameters in predicting the presence of choledochal stones. Surg Gynecol Obstet. 1984;159:273-6.
53. Robertson GSM, Jagger C, Johnson PRV, Rathbone BJ, Wicks AC, Lloyd DM, et al. Selection criteria for preoperative endoscopic retrograde cholangiography in the laparoscopic era. Arch Surg. 1996;131:89-94.
54. Ros E, Zambon D. Postcholecystectomy symptoms: a prospective study of gallstone patients before and two years after surgery. Gut. 1987;28:1500-4.
55. Roslyn JJ, Binns GS, Hughes EF, Saunders-Kirkwood K, Zinner MJ, Cates JA. Open cholecystectomy: a contemporary analysis of 42,474 patients. Ann Surg. 1993;218:129-37.
56. Rosseland AR, Osnes M. Biliary concrements: the endoscopic approach. World J Surg. 1989;13:178-85.
57. Rosseland AR, Solhaug JH. Early or delayed endoscopic papillotomy (EPT) in gallstone pancreatitis. Ann Surg. 1984;199:165-7.
58. Roush TS, Traverso LW. Management and long-term follow-up of patients with positive cholangiograms during laparoscopic cholecystectomy. Am J Surg. 1995;169:484-7.
59. Saltzstein EC, Peacock JB, Thomas MD. Preoperative bilirubin, alkaline phosphatase and amylase levels as predictors of common duct stones. Surg Gynecol Obstet. 1982;154:381-4.
60. Santo PD, Kazarian KK, Rogers JF, Bevins PA, Hall JR. Prediction of operative cholangiography in patients undergoing elective cholecystectomy with routine liver function chemistry. Surgery. 1985;98:7-11.
61. Sauerbrei EE, Cooperberg PL, Gordon P, Li D, Cohen MM, Burhenne HJ. The discrepancy between radiographic and sonographic bile duct measurements. Radiology. 1980;137:751-5.
62. Schultz LS, Kamel M, Graber JN, Hickok DF. Four-year outcome data for 400 laparoscopic cholecystectomy patients: recognition of persistent symptoms. Int Surg. 1994;79:205-8.
63. Sgourakis G, Karaliotas K. Laparoscopic common bile duct exploration and cholecystectomy versus endoscopic stone extraction and laparoscopic cholecystectomy for choledocholithiasis. A prospective randomized study. Minerva Chir. 2002;57:467.
64. Stefanini P, Carboni M, Patrassi N, L origa P, De Bernardinis G, Negro P. Factors influencing the long-term results of cholecystectomy. Surg Gynecol Obstet. 1974;139:734-8.
65. Stiegman GV, Goff JS, Mansour A, Pearlman N, Reveille RM, Norton L. Precholecystectomy endoscopic cholangiography and stone removal is not superior to cholecystectomy, cholangiography, and common bile duct exploration. Am J Surg. 1992;163:227-30.
66. Stoker ME. Common bile duct exploration in the era of laparoscopic surgery. Arch Surg. 1995;130:265-9.
67. Taylor TV, Armstrong CP, Rimmer S, Lucas SB, Jeacock J, Gunn AA. Prediction of choledocholithiasis using a pocket microcomputer. Br J Surg. 1988;75:138-40.
68. Trondsen E, Edwin B, Reiertsen O, Fagertun H, Rosseland AR. Selection criteria for endoscopic retrograde cholangiography (ERCP) in patients with gallstone disease. World J Surg. 1995;19:852-7.
69. Vander Velpen GC, Shimi SM, Cuschieri A. Outcome after cholecystectomy for symptomatic gallstone disease and effect of surgical access: laparoscopic vs open approach. Gut. 1993;34:1448-51.
70. Voyles CR, Petro AB, Meena AL, Haick AJ, Koury AM. A practical approach to laparoscopic cholecystectomy. Am J Surg. 1991;161:365-70.
71. Wegge C, Kjaergaard J. Evaluation of symptoms and signs of gallstone disease in patients admitted with upper abdominal pain. Scand J Gastroenterol. 1985;20:933-6.
72. Welbourn CRB, Mehta D, Armstrong CP, Gear MWL, Eyre-Brook IA. Selective preoperative endoscopic retrograde cholangiography with sphincterotomy avoids bile duct exploration during laparoscopic cholecystectomy. Gut. 1995;37:576-9.

CHAPTER 15 Laparoscopic Appendicectomy

INTRODUCTION

Appendicitis was first recognized as a disease entity in the 16th century and was called perityphlitis. McBurney first described its clinical findings in 1889. Laparoscopic appendectomy in expert hands is now quite safe and effective and considered as an excellent alternative for patients with acute appendicitis. Acute appendicitis is the most common abdominal surgical emergency in the world, with a lifetime risk of 8.6% in males and 6.9% in females. First successful laparoscopic appendicectomy was performed by Semm in 1982. Although open appendectomy preceded it by almost 100 years, laparoscopic appendectomy has overtaken its open counterpart in popularity. Although laparoscopic appendicectomy can be performed in all groups of patients, surgeons agree that for women of childbearing age, laparoscopic appendectomy is unquestionably the method of choice. Perforation is found in 13–20% of patients who present with acute appendicitis. Perforation rate is higher among men (18% men versus 13% women) and older adults.

LAPAROSCOPIC ANATOMY

The appendix is derived from a cecal diverticulum of the fetus. The appendix is generally within 1.7 cm of the ileocecal junction. Its length varies from 2 to 20 cm, average 9 cm **(Fig. 1)**. Most of the time when telescope is introduced through umbilicus, appendix is hidden behind the cecum.

The anterior tenia coli of the cecum is an important landmark, which leads to cecum **(Figs. 2 and 3)**. The triangular mesoappendix tethers the appendix posteriorly, which contains appendicular artery and veins. The appendicular artery is a branch of the ileocolic artery.

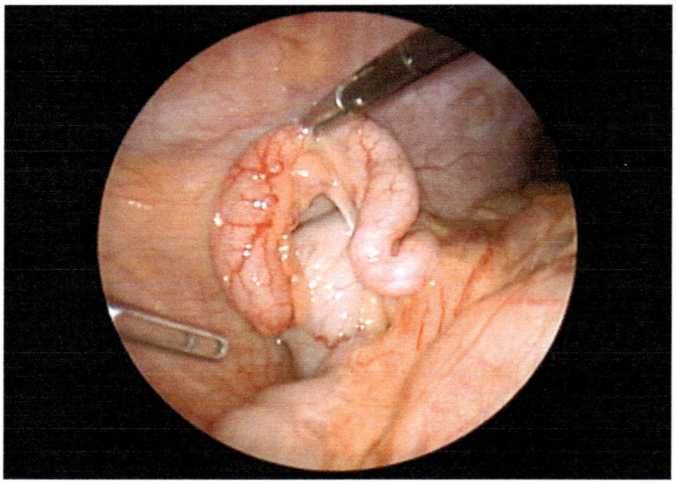

Fig. 1: Normal laparoscopic view of appendix.

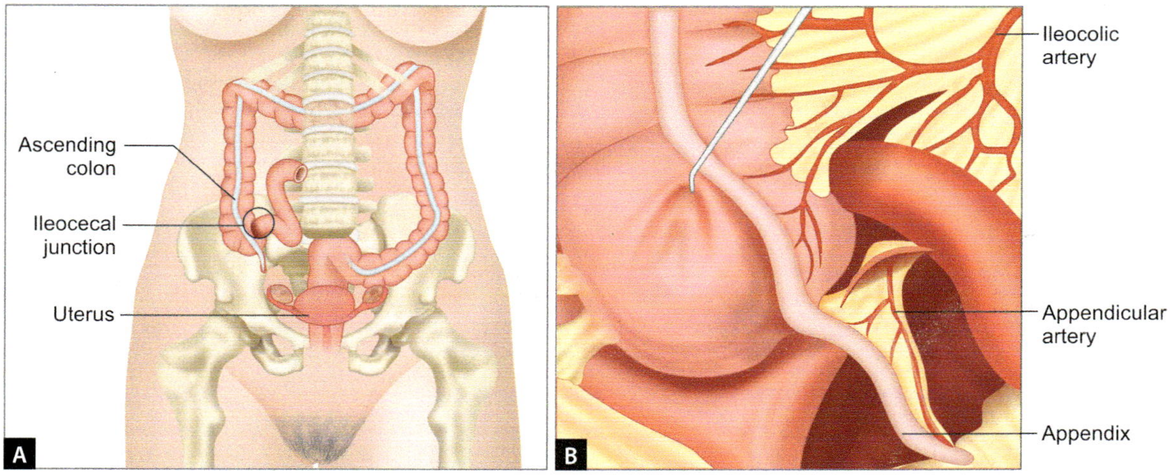

Figs. 2A and B: Anatomic position of appendix.

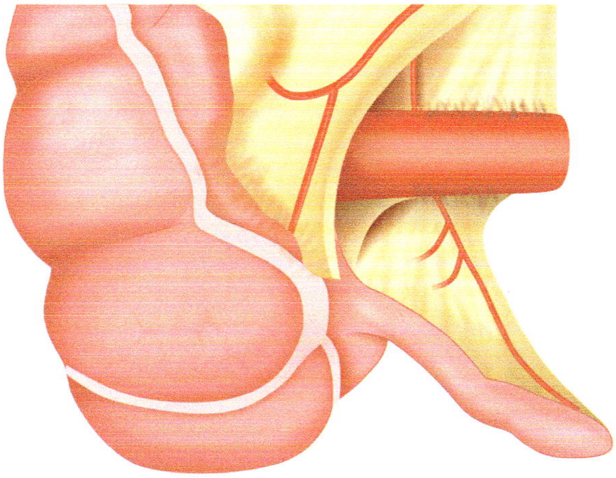

Fig. 3: Normal appendix.

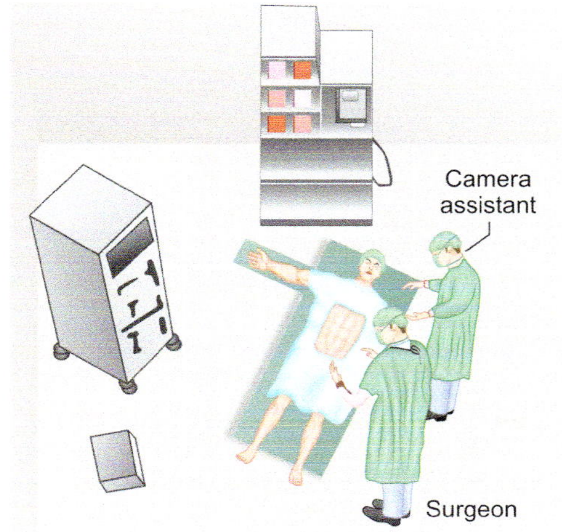

Fig. 4: Patient position and setup of operating team.

TABLE 1: Indications of laparoscopic and open appendectomy.

Laparoscopic appendectomy	*Open appendectomy*
• Female of reproductive age group • Female of premenopausal group • Suspected appendicitis • High working class • Previous lower abdominal surgery • Obese patients • Disease conditions such as cirrhosis of liver and sickle cell disease • Immunocompromised patients	• Complicated appendicitis • COPD or cardiac disease • Generalized peritonitis • Hypercoagulable sites • Stump appendicitis after previous incomplete appendicectomy

(COPD: chronic obstructive pulmonary disease)

Laparoscopic exposure of the appendix is facilitated by gently pulling the cecum upward.

The base of the appendix must be visualized carefully to avoid leaving a remnant of appendix at the time of laparoscopic appendicectomy. Exposures of retrocecal appendix require mobilization of right colon. The peritoneal reflection is incised, and the cecum is pulled medially to visualize retrocecal appendix.

Advantage of Laparoscopic Appendectomy

Thorough exposure of the peritoneal cavity is possible.

Indications

Indications of laparoscopic and open appendectomy are described in **Table 1**.

Relative Contraindications

- Complicated appendicitis
- Stump appendicitis (develops after previous incomplete appendectomy)
- Poor risk for general anesthesia
- Some cases of previous extensive pelvic surgery.

The general anesthesia and the pneumoperitoneum required as part of the laparoscopic procedure do increase the risk in certain groups of patients. Most surgeons would not recommend laparoscopic appendectomy in those with pre-existing disease conditions. Patients with moderate cardiac diseases and chronic obstructive pulmonary disease (COPD) should not be considered a good candidate for laparoscopy. The laparoscopic appendectomy may also be more difficult in patients who have had previous lower abdominal surgery. The elderly may also be at increased risk for complications with general anesthesia combined with pneumoperitoneum.

Patient Position

In the laparoscopic approach, an orogastric tube is typically placed to decompress the stomach. The bladder can be decompressed either with a Foley catheter or by having the patient void immediately prior to entering the operating room. The patient is in supine position, arms tucked at the side. The surgeon stands on the left side of the patient with the camera-holder assistant **(Fig. 4)**. For maintaining coaxial alignment, surgeon should stand near left shoulder and monitor should be placed near right hip facing toward surgeon. In females, the lithotomy position should be preferred because there may be necessity to use uterine manipulator in difficult diagnosis **(Figs. 5A and B)**.

Port Position

Various port placements have been advocated for laparoscopic appendectomy. These methods share the principle of triangulation of instrument ports to ensure adequate visualization and exposure of the appendix **(Figs. 6A and B)**.

- Total three trocars should be used
- Two 10-mm, umbilical and left lower quadrant (LLQ) trocars
- One 5 mm right upper quadrant (RUQ) trocar
- The RUQ trocar can be moved below the bikini line in females.

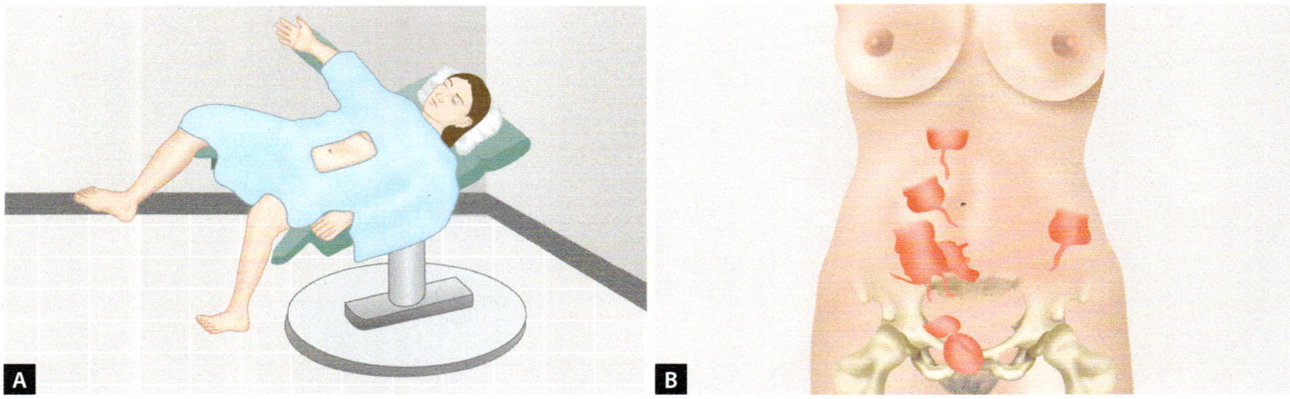

Figs. 5A and B: (A) Patient position in female; (B) Variation in position of appendix.

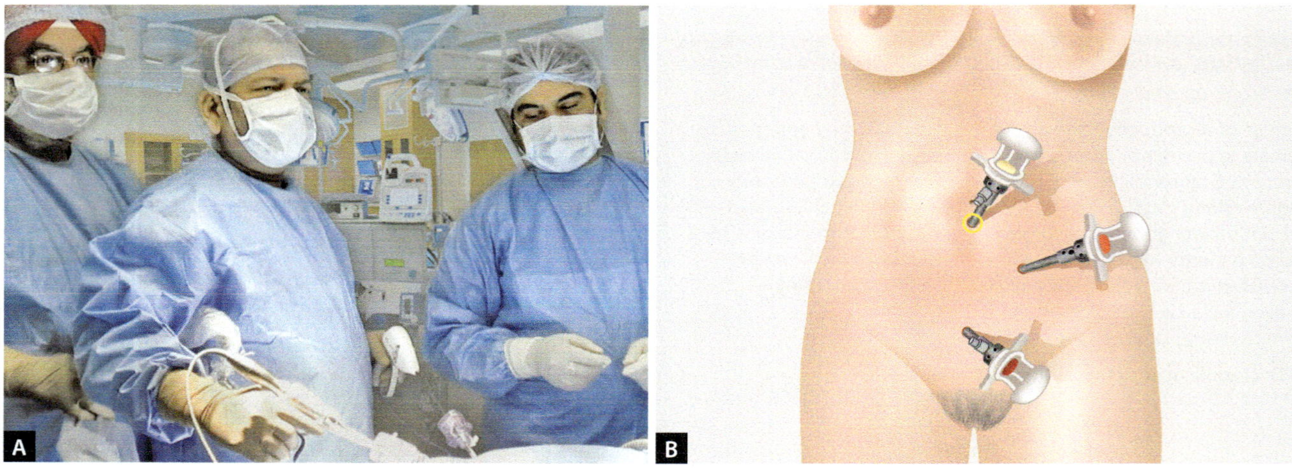

Figs. 6A and B: (A) Position of surgical team in appendectomy; (B) Port position in appendicectomy.

Alternative Port and Theater Setup

In beauty conscious females, for cosmetic reason, the baseball diamond concept of port position can be altered from contralateral to ipsilateral port and three ports should be placed in such a way so that the two 5-mm ports will be below bikini line. Access should be performed by 10 mm umbilical port. Once the telescope is inside, one 5-mm port should be placed in left iliac fossa below the bikini line under vision. Second 5-mm port should be placed in right iliac fossa, just mirror image of left port. After fixing all the ports in position, one another 5-mm telescope is introduced through left iliac fossa and surgery should be performed through umbilical port (for right hand) and left iliac fossa port (for left hand) **(Fig. 7)**. In this alternative port position, 60° manipulation angle cannot be achieved and it is ergonomically difficult for surgeon, but patient gets cosmetic benefit.

This alternative port position for laparoscopic appendicectomy should not be performed in case of retrocecal appendix or perforated appendix **(Fig. 5B)**.

Alternative port position in beauty conscious female is shown in **Figure 7**.

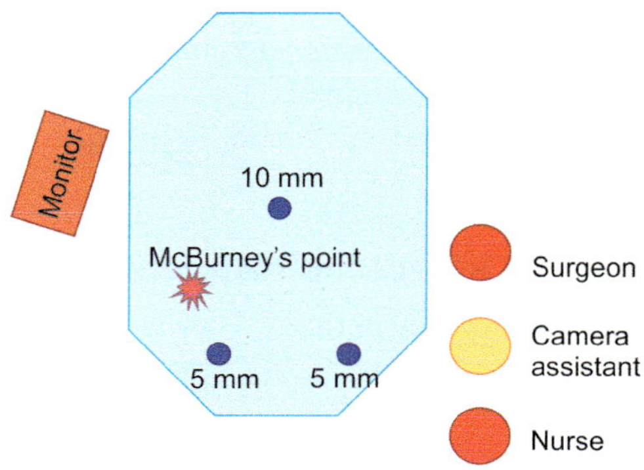

Fig. 7: Alternative port position.

OPERATIVE TECHNIQUES

Pneumoperitoneum is created in the usual fashion. Three ports are used. An atraumatic grasper (Endo Babcock or Dolphin Nose Grasper) is inserted via the RUQ port, if contralateral ports are used, and through the suprapubic port, if ipsilateral port is used. The cecum is retracted upward toward the liver. In most cases, this maneuver will elevate the appendix in the optical field of the telescope.

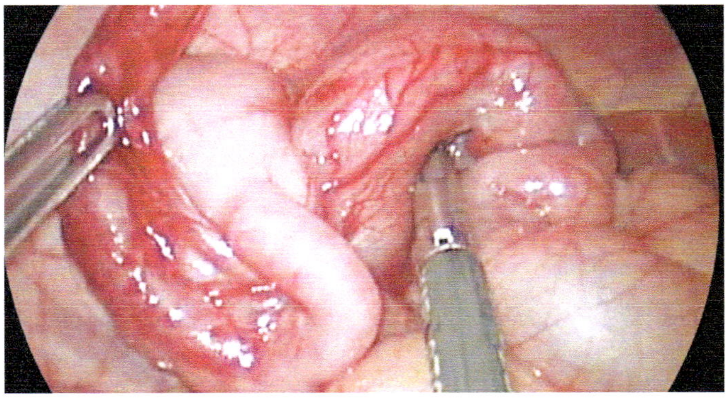

Fig. 8: Retraction of appendix.

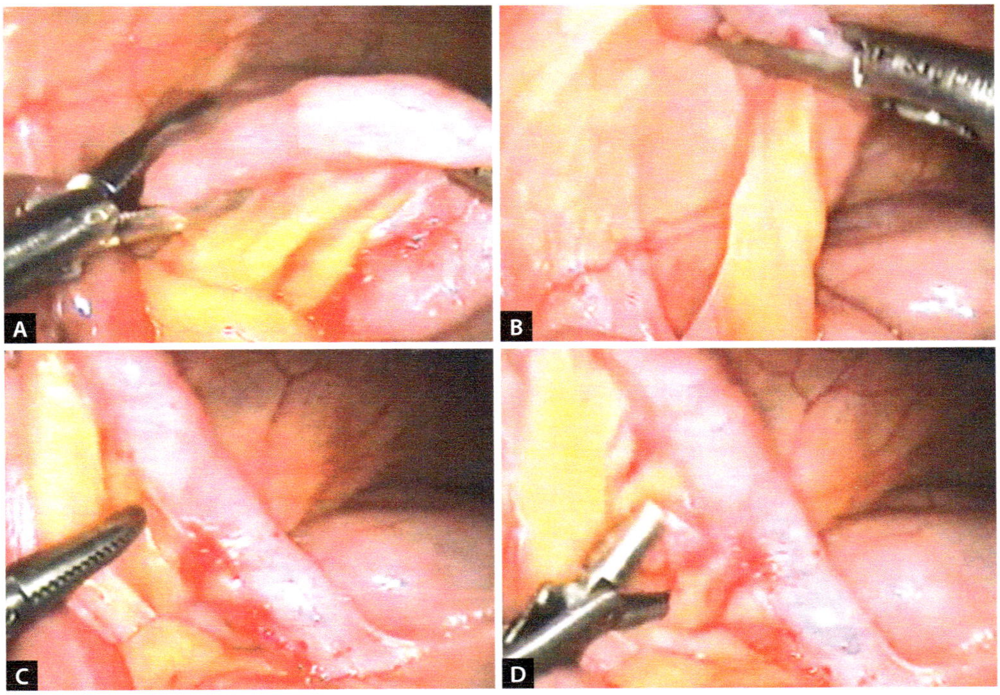

Figs. 9A to D: Retraction of appendix and creation of a window over mesoappendix.

Retraction of Appendix

Once the diseased appendix is identified, any adhesions to surrounding structures can be lysed with a combination of blunt and sharp dissection. If a retrocecal appendix is encountered, division of the lateral peritoneal attachments of the cecum to the abdominal wall often improves visualization. The appendix is grasped at its tip with a 5-mm claw grasper via the RUQ trocar. It is held in upward position. After the pelvis is inspected, the appendix is identified, mobilized, and examined properly **(Figs. 8 and 9)**. Periappendiceal or pericecal adhesions are lysed using either bipolar or harmonics and scissors. LLQ grasper is used to create a mesenteric window behind the base of the appendix.

A dolphin nose grasper or Maryland dissector is used to create a mesenteric window under the base of the appendix. The window should be made as close as possible to the base of the appendix and should be approximately 1 cm in size **(Fig. 10)**.

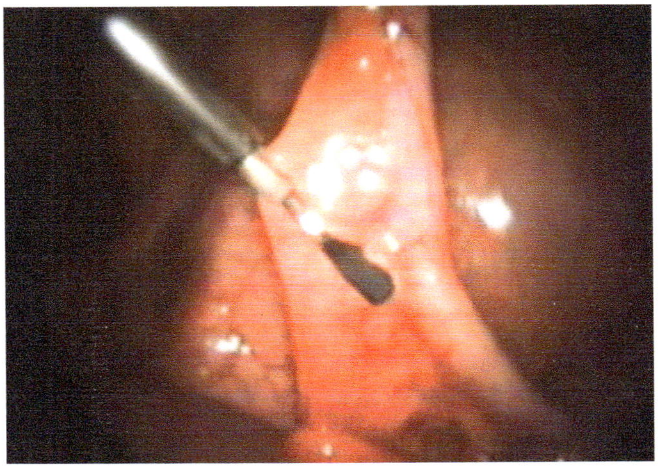

Fig. 10: Window in mesoappendix.

The appendiceal artery, or mesoappendix containing it, can be divided sharply between hemostatic clips, with a laparoscopic gastrointestinal anastomosis (GIA) stapler, monopolar cautery, or one of the advanced vessel ligation devices such as ultrasonic scalpel or LigaSure **(Figs. 11 and 12)**.

Extracorporeal knotting can be performed (Roeder's, Mishra, Meltzer, or Tayside knot) for mesoappendix as well as appendix. Two endoloop sutures are passed sequentially through one of the 5-mm ports and pushed around the base of appendix on top of each other at a distance of 3–5 mm. A third endoloop suture can be applied 6 mm distal to the second suture so that surgeon will cut between second and third knot **(Figs. 13A to F)**. If harmonic scalpel is used, only one extracorporeal knot can be used at the base of appendix and then it is cut with the harmonic scalpel 6 mm away from the knot. Harmonic will seal the appendicular end preventing any spillage.

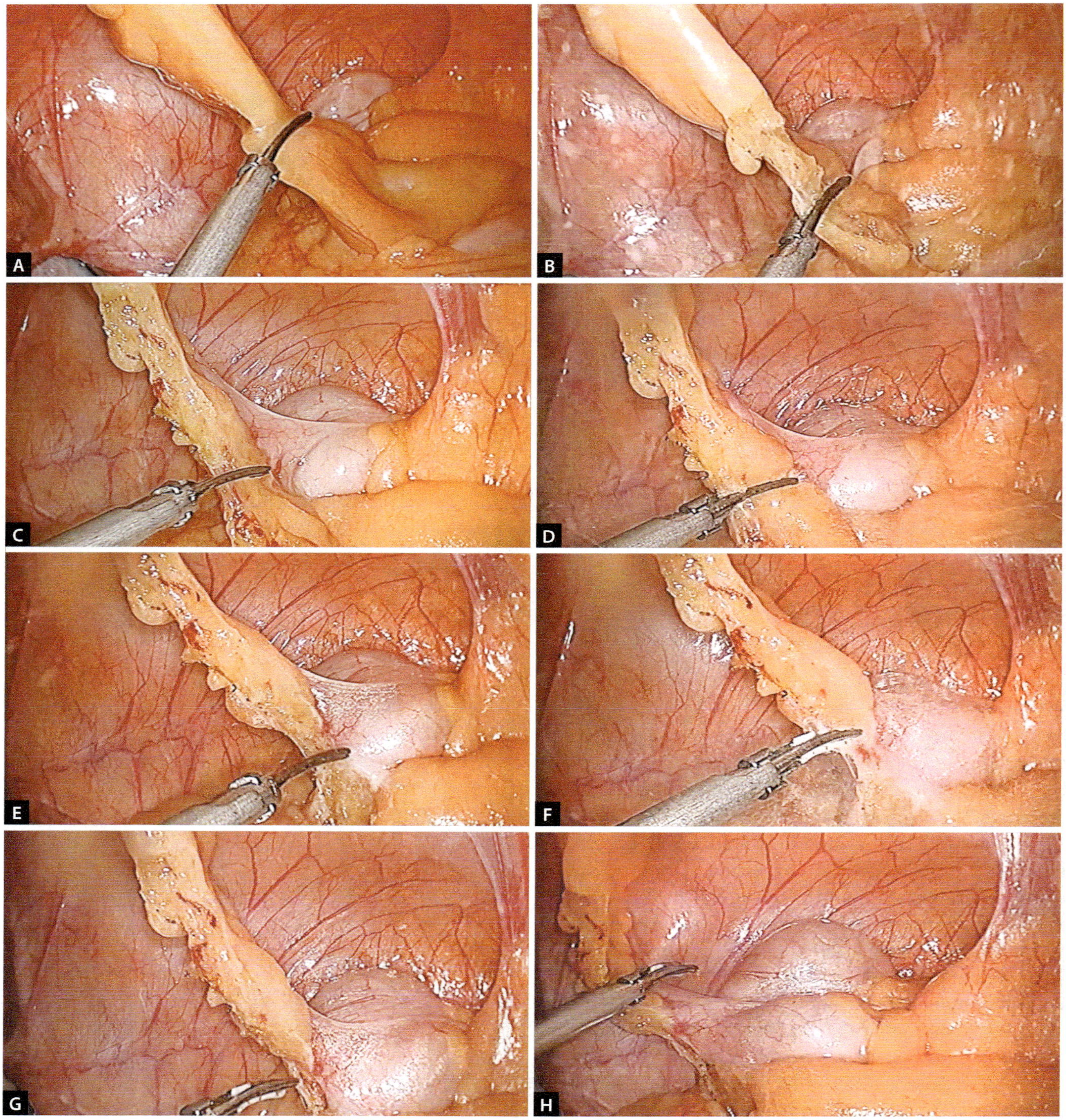

Figs. 11A to H: Successive dissection of mesoappendix by harmonic scalpel.

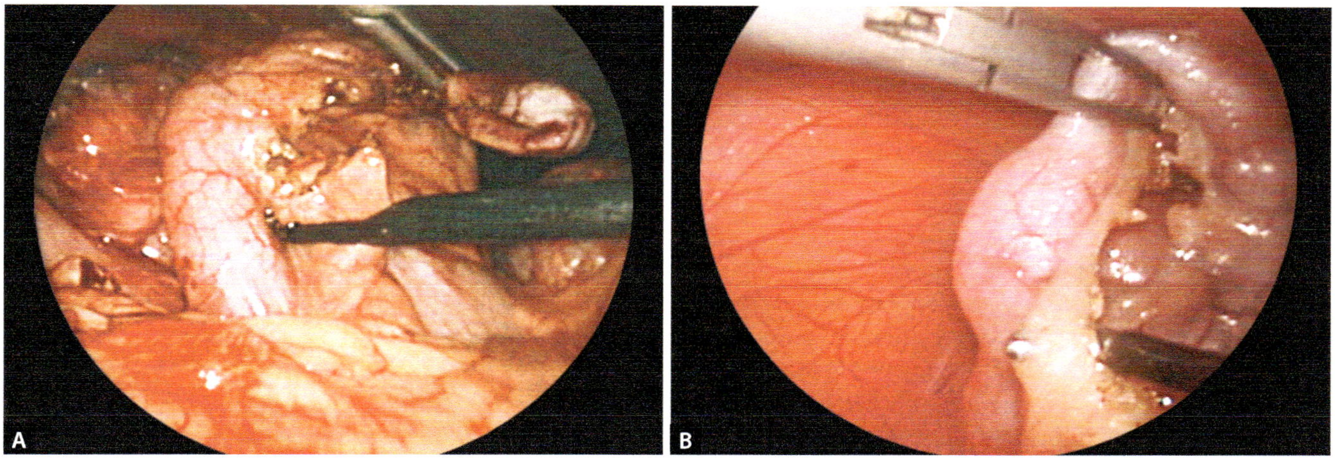

Figs. 12A and B: Dissection of mesoappendix by monopolar hook.

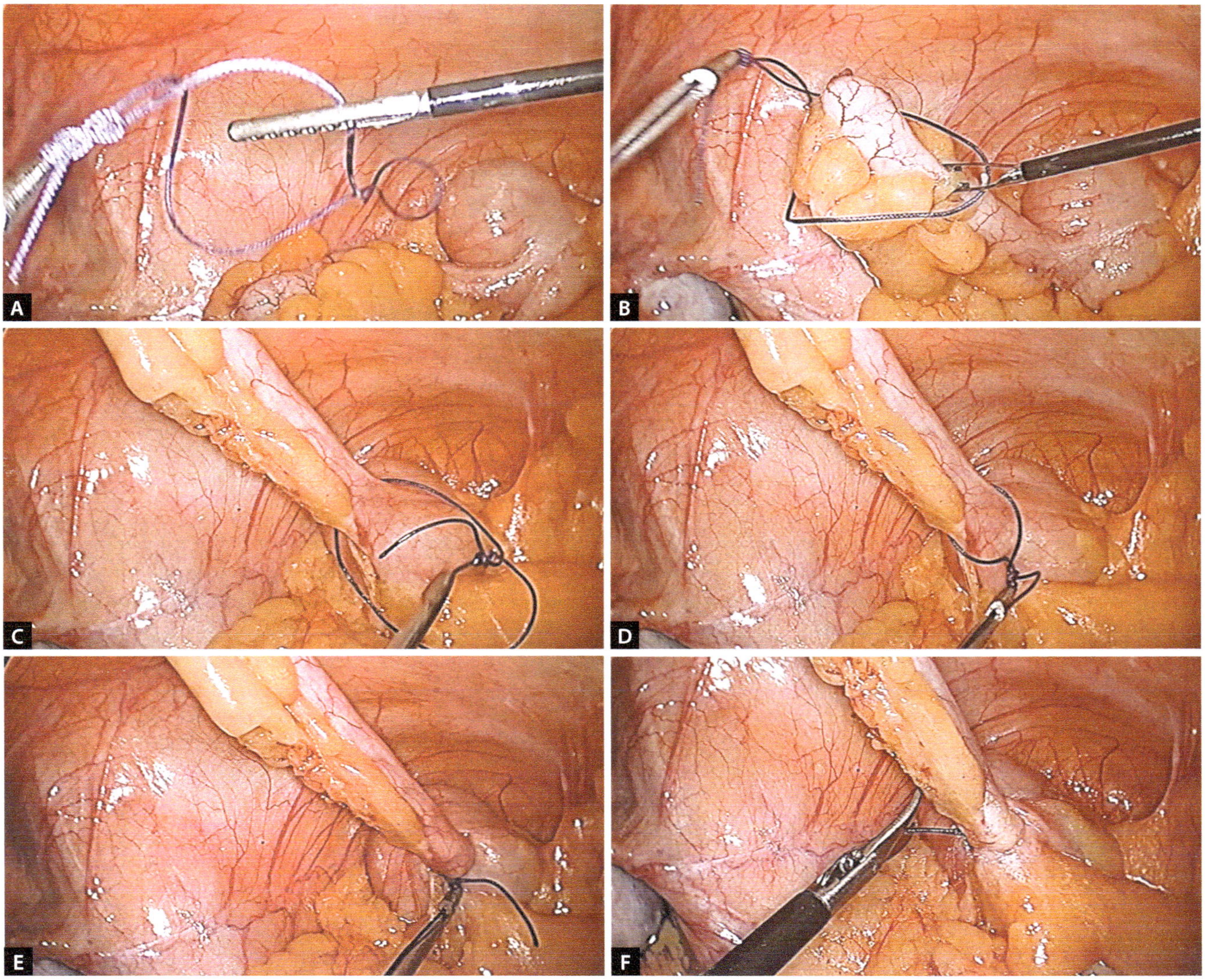

Figs. 13A to F: Tying Roeder's, Meltzer's, or Mishra's knot over appendix.

The Aesculap DS Titanium Ligation Clips can also be used sometimes to secure the proximal or distal portion of the appendix. The luminal portion of the appendiceal stump is sterilized with electrosurgery to prevent spillage and contamination of peritoneal cavity. In case of perforated appendix with peritonitis, Betadine can be applied over the stump of appendix and thorough suction and irrigation is performed either by normal saline or by Ringer's lactate solution.

After extracting the appendix out of abdominal cavity, surgeon should examine the abdomen for any possible bowel injury or hemorrhage.

Stapler Appendicectomy

The stapling devices make laparoscopic appendectomy simpler and faster. The Multifire stapler is introduced though a 12-mm port. The appendix may be transacted by inserting an ENDO GIA instrument via the RUQ trocar (blue cartridge, 3.5), closing it around the base of the appendix and firing it. For perforated appendicitis with or without an intra-abdominal abscess, a drain is left in the RLQ and pelvis **(Figs. 14A to C)**. In stapler appendicectomy, the appendix is cleared to its attachment with the cecum, and the appendiceal base is divided using a laparoscopic GIA stapler, taking care not to leave a significant stump. It is sometimes necessary to include part of the cecum within the stapler to ensure that the staples are placed in healthy, uninfected tissue.

Extracorporeal knot (Meltzer, Roeder, or Tayside knot) should be preferred over stapler, depending on the surgeon's expertise.

Extraction of Appendix

The appendix can be removed from the abdomen with the help of grasping forceps placed through one of the 10-mm ports. However, this may contaminate both the cannula and instrument. Alternatively, an endoloop suture, which was tied last, can be used instead of grasping forceps to pull the appendix out.

Abdomen should be examined for any possible bowel injury or hemorrhage. All the instruments should be removed carefully. The wound should be closed with suture. Use Vicryl for rectus and unabsorbable intradermal or stapler for skin. Adhesive sterile dressing should be applied over the wound.

POSTOPERATIVE CARE AFTER APPENDECTOMY

Patients may be discharged once they tolerate a regular diet, usually in 2 days. Three to five days of intravenous or oral antibiotics is recommended for perforated appendicitis after appendectomy. Patients with perforated appendicitis often develop an ileus postoperatively regardless of the surgical approach. Thus, diet should only be advanced as the clinical situation warrants.

RISK FACTORS IN LAPAROSCOPIC APPENDECTOMY

The mortality associated with appendicitis is low but can vary by geographic locations. In developed countries, the mortality rate is between 0.09 and 0.24%. In developing countries, the mortality rate is higher, between 1 and 4%. Overall complication rates of 8.2–31.4%, wound infection rates of 3.3–10.3%, and pelvic abscess rates of 9.4% have been reported following appendectomy.

Missed Diagnosis

There is report also of mucinous cystadenoma of the cecum missed at laparoscopic appendectomy. Less than 1% of all patients with suspected acute appendicitis are found to have an associated malignant process. During conventional appendectomy, through a laparotomy incision, the cecum and the appendix are easily palpated, and an obvious mass can be detected and properly managed at the time of appendectomy. The inability to palpate any mass is an inherent inadequacy of laparoscopic surgery.

Bleeding

Bleeding may occur from the mesoappendix, omental vessels, or retroperitoneum. Bleeding is usually recognized intraoperatively via adequate exposure, lighting, and suction. It is recognized postoperatively by tachycardia, hypotension, decreased urine output, anemia, or other evidence of hemorrhagic shock.

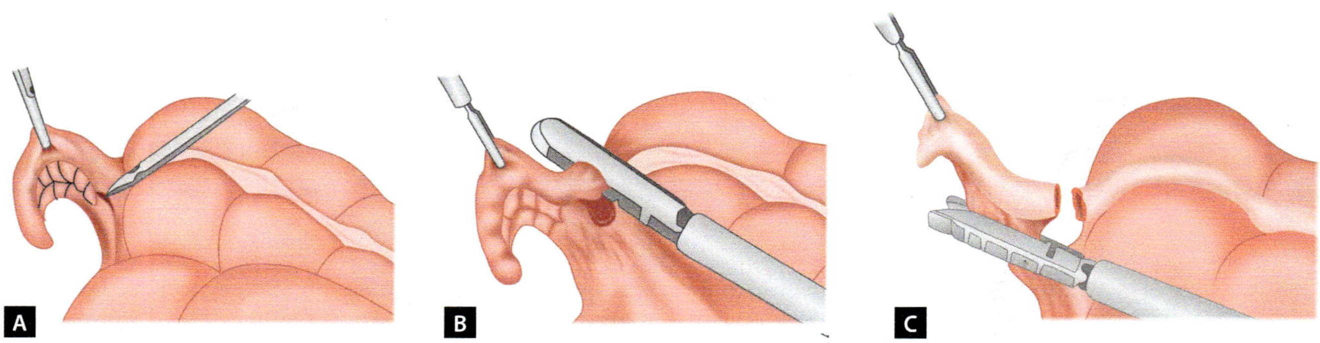

Figs. 14A to C: Stapler appendicectomy.

Visceral Injury

Risk of accidental burns is higher with monopolar system because electricity seeks the path of least resistance, which may be adjacent bowel. In a bipolar system since the current does not have to travel through the patient, there is little chance of injury to remote viscera. In laparoscopic appendectomy, only bipolar current should be used. Laparoscopists should also routinely explore the rest of the abdomen.

Wound Infection

Proper tissue retrieval technique is required to prevent wound infection after appendectomy.

If ensues, it is recognized by erythema, fluctuation, and purulent drainage from port sites. The absence of wound infections after laparoscopic appendectomy can be attributed to the practice of placing the appendix in a sterile bag or into the trocar sleeve prior to removal from the abdomen. The regular use of retrieval bag is a very good practice for preventing infection of the wound.

Incomplete Appendectomy

If surgeon is not experienced, he/she is likely to leave the stump of the appendix too long. There is a report of intra-abdominal abscess formation due to retained fecalith after laparoscopic appendectomy. It is important that the surgeons performing laparoscopic appendectomy should remove fecalith if found, and the stump of appendix should not be big enough to contain any remaining fecalith. Incomplete appendectomy is a result of ligation of the appendix too far from the base.

It may lead to recurrent appendicitis, which presents with symptoms and signs of appendicitis even after laparoscopic appendectomy.

Some surgeons prefer stapling of the appendiceal stump for laparoscopic appendectomy for the treatment of all forms of appendicitis **(Figs. 14 and 15)**. But most of the surgeons now agree that ligation of the appendectomy stump is the best approach **(Figs. 16 to 18)**. There is report of slippage of clip, residual appendicitis followed by abscess formation after using clip for appendiceal stump. The ligation should be performed by using endoloop, an intracorporeal surgeon's knot, or done extracorporeally using a Meltzer's knot or Tayside knot. The security of the knot is essential. It is influenced by the proper port location and experience of the surgeon.

Leakage of Purulent Exudates

It is usually seen intraoperatively while dissecting appendix. Copious irrigation and suction followed by continued antibiotics can prevent this complication until patient is afebrile with a normal white blood cell count. Retrieval bag should be used to prevent the spillage of infected material from the appendiceal lumen.

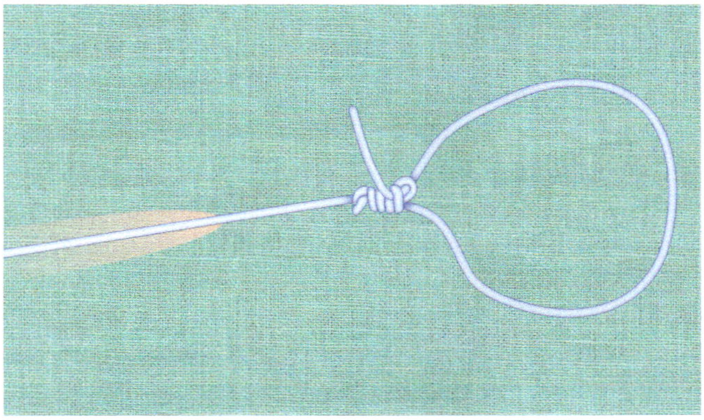

Fig. 16: Roeder's knot at the time of appendicectomy.

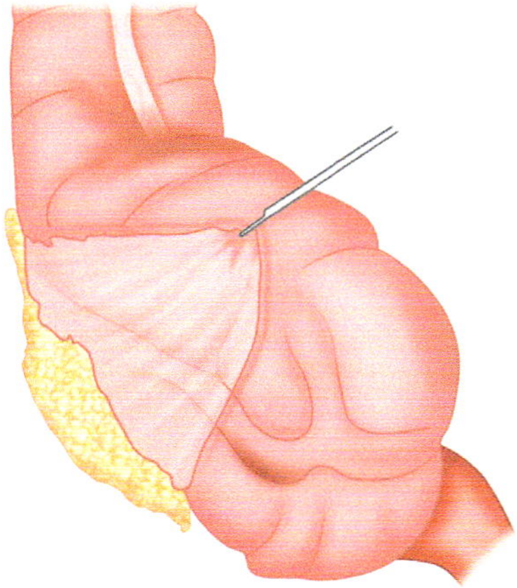

Fig. 15: Retrocecal appendix.

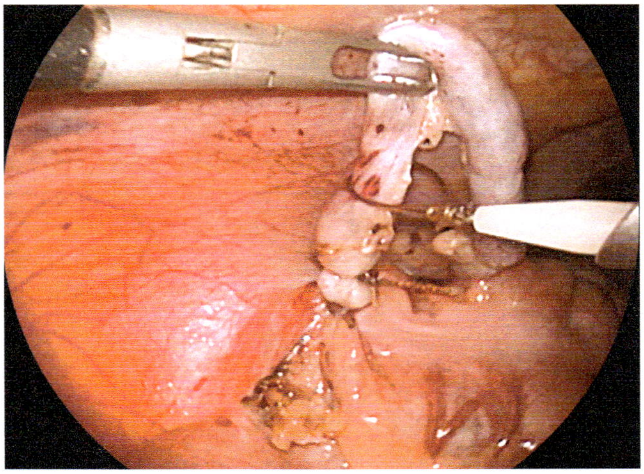

Fig. 17: Three Roeder's or Meltzer's knots over appendix.

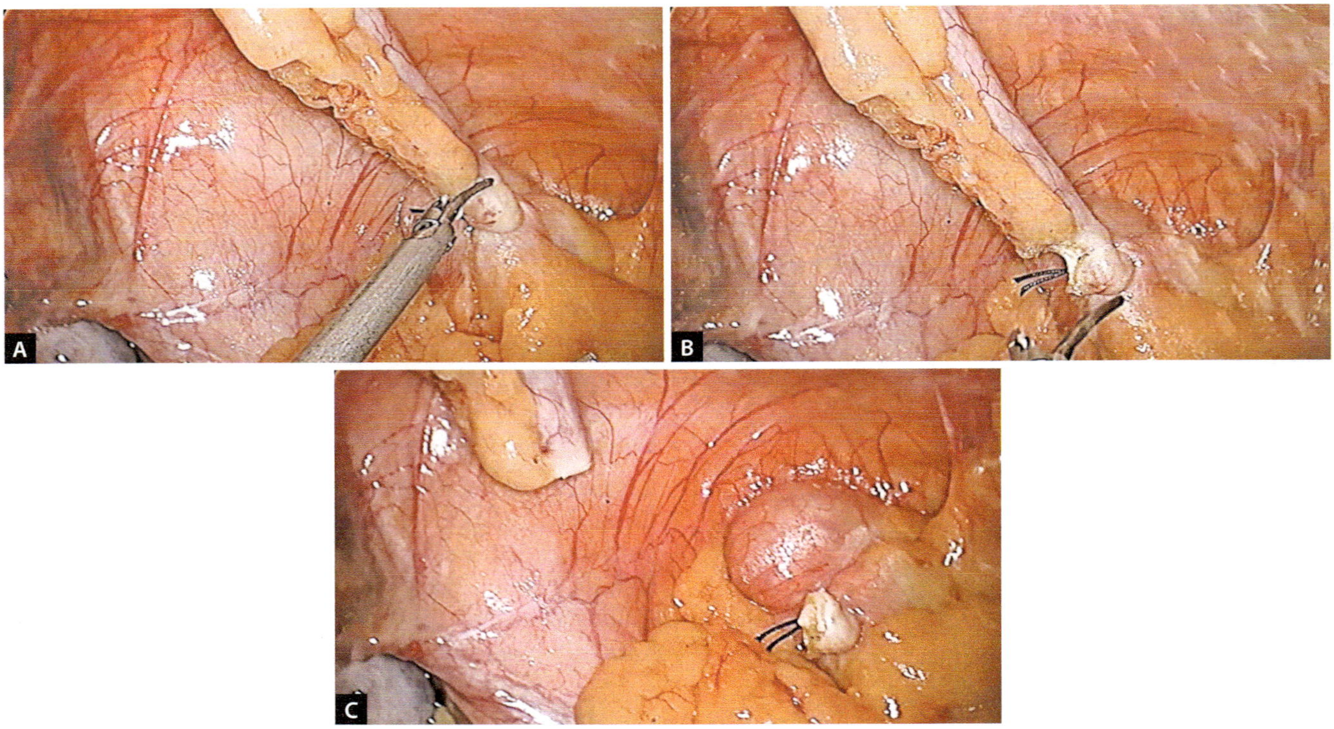

Figs. 18A to C: Amputation of appendix with harmonic scalpel.

Intra-abdominal Abscess

This postoperative morbidity is recognized by prolonged ileus, sluggish recovery, rising leukocytosis, spiking fevers, tachycardia, and rarely a palpable mass. After confirmation of the intra-abdominal abscess, drainage of pus followed by antibiotic therapy is essential. Rarely, laparotomy may be required.

Hernia

Trocar site hernia as visible or palpable bulge is sometimes encountered. Possible occult hernia is manifested by pain or symptoms of bowel obstruction.

Laparoscopic-assisted Appendectomy

It has been described for cases in which the proper endoscopic instruments and sutures are unavailable. The laparoscope facilitates the diagnosis of acute appendicitis and a grasper is passed through an accessory trocar located just over the McBurney's point. The tip of the appendix is grasped and then pulled along with cannula and grasper **(Figs. 19 and 20)**. Once the appendix is exteriorized, the routine appendectomy is performed through this small abdominal incision. This procedure usually takes less time than total laparoscopic appendectomy, but it has more incidence of incomplete appendectomy.

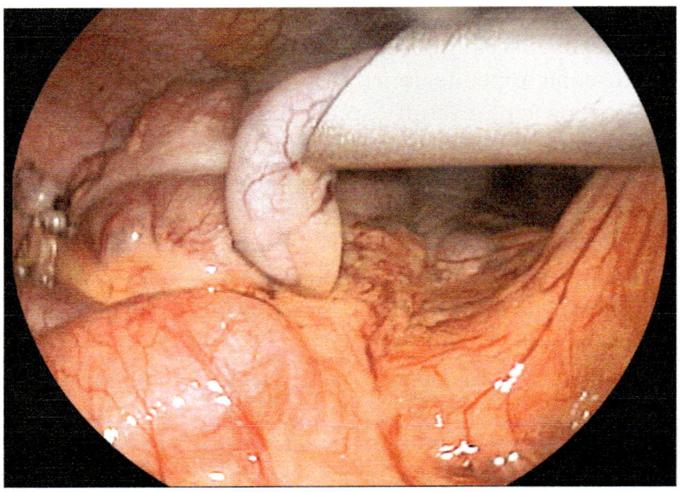

Fig. 19: Amputated appendix inside the cannula.

Perforated Appendix

Perforation of the appendix can cause intraperitoneal dissemination of pus and fecal material and generalized peritonitis. These patients are typically quite ill and may be septic or hemodynamically unstable, thus requiring preoperative resuscitation. The diagnosis is not always appreciated before exploration.

For patients who are septic or unstable, and for those who have perforation of the appendix or generalized peritonitis, emergency appendectomy is required, as well as drainage and irrigation of the peritoneal cavity. Emergency appendectomy in this setting can be accomplished open or laparoscopically; the choice is determined by surgeon preference with consideration of patient condition and local resources.

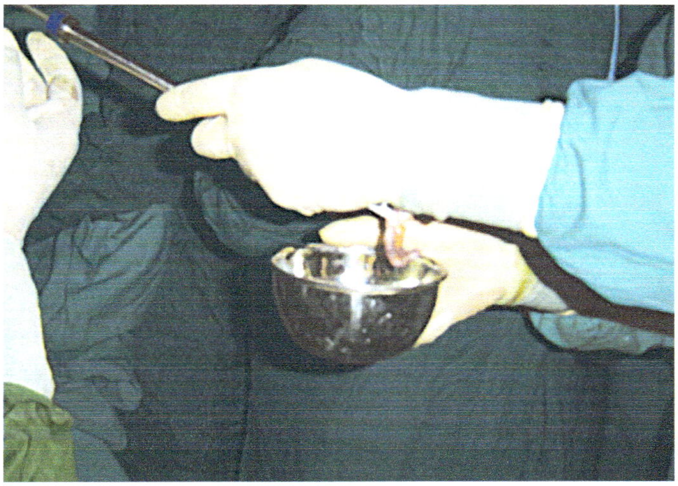

Fig. 20: Appendix hidden in cannula is ejected out.

DISCUSSION

Laparoscopic appendectomy has gained lot of attention around the world. However, the role of laparoscopy for appendectomy, one of the most common indications, remains controversial. Several controlled trials have been conducted, of which some are in favor of laparoscopy, and others not. There is also diversity in the quality of the randomized controlled trials. The main variable in these trials are following parameters:

- Number of patients in trial
- Withdrawal of cases
- Exclusion of cases
- Blinding
- Intention to treat analysis
- Publication biases
- Local practice variation
- Prophylactic antibiotic used
- Follow-up failure.

Without proper attention to the detail of all the parameters, it is very difficult to draw a conclusion. It has been found that there is a hidden competition between laparoscopic surgeons and the surgeons who are still doing conventional surgery, and this competition influences the result of study. One should always think of laparoscopic surgery and open procedures as being complimentary to each other.

A successful outcome requires greater skills from the operator. The results of many comparative studies have shown that outcome of laparoscopic appendectomy was influenced by the experience and technique of the operator. Minimal access surgery requires different skills and technological knowledge. With a clear diagnosis of complicated appendicitis, the skill and experience of the surgeon should be considered for the selection of operating method. Surgeons should perform the procedure with which they are more comfortable.

Laparoscopic appendectomy is equally safe and can provide less postoperative morbidity in experienced hands, as in open appendectomy. Most cases of acute appendicitis can be treated laparoscopically. Laparoscopic appendectomy is a useful method for reducing hospital stay, complications, and early return to normal activity. With better training in minimal access surgery now available, the time has arrived for it to take its place in the surgeon's repertoire. As surgeons gained more experience with the technique, laparoscopic appendectomy became feasible for patients with perforated appendicitis undergoing immediate surgery.

BIBLIOGRAPHY

1. Addiss DG, Shaffer N, Fowler BS, Tauxe RV. The epidemiology of appendicitis and appendectomy in the United States. Am J Epidemiol. 1990;132:910-25.
2. Alexander F, Magnuson D, DiFiore J, Jirousek K, Secic M. Specialty versus generalist care of children with appendicitis: an outcome comparison. J Pediatr Surg. 2001;36:1510-13.
3. Azzie G, Salloum A, Beasley S, Maoate K. The complication rate and outcomes of laparoscopic appendicectomy in children with perforated appendicitis. Pediatr Endosurgery Innovative Techniques. 2004;8:19-23. [online] Available from: http://www.liebertonline.com/doi/abs/10.1089/109264104773513098. [Last accessed June, 2020].
4. Banieghbal B, Al-Hindi S, Davies MRQ. Laparoscopic appendectomy with appendix mass in children. Pediatr Endosurgery Innovative Techniques. 2004;8:25-30. [online] Available from: http://www.liebertonline.com/doi/abs/10.1089/109264-104773513106. [Last accessed June, 2020].
5. Beldi G, Muggli K, Helbling C, Schlumpf R. Laparoscopic appendectomy using endoloops: a prospective, randomized clinical trial. Surg Endosc. 2004;18:749-50.
6. Blewett CJ, Krummel TM. Perforated appendicitis: past and future controversies. Semin Pediatr Surg. 1995;4:234-8.
7. Bova R, Meagher A. Appendicitis in HIV-positive patients. Aust N Z J Surg. 1998;68:337.
8. Bratton SL, Haberkern CM, Waldhausen JH. Acute appendicitis risks of complications: age and medical insurance. Pediatrics. 2000;106:75-8.
9. Charfi S, Sellami A, Affes A, Yaïch K, Mzali R, Boudawara TS, et al. Histopathological findings in appendectomy specimens: a study of 24,697 cases. Int J Colorectal Dis. 2014;29:1009.
10. Chen C, Botelho C, Cooper A, Hibberd P, Parsons SK. Current practice patterns in the treatment of perforated appendicitis in children. J Am Coll Surg. 2003;196:212-21.
11. Ciarrocchi A, Amicucci G. Laparoscopic versus open appendectomy in obese patients: a meta-analysis of prospective and retrospective studies. J Minim Access Surg. 2014;10:4-9.
12. David IB, Buck JR, Filler RM. Rational use of antibiotics for perforated appendicitis in childhood. J Pediatr Surg. 1982;17:494-500.
13. Fleming FJ, Kim MJ, Messing S, Gunzler D, Salloum R, Monson JR, et al. Balancing the risk of postoperative surgical infections: a multivariate analysis of factors associated with laparoscopic appendectomy from the NSQIP database. Ann Surg. 2010;252:895-900.
14. Flum DR, Steinberg SD, Sarkis AY, Wallack MK. Appendicitis in patients with acquired immunodeficiency syndrome. J Am Coll Surg 1997;184:481.
15. Guller U, Hervey S, Purves H, Muhlbaier LH, Peterson ED, Eubanks S, et al. Laparoscopic versus open appendectomy:

outcomes comparison based on a large administrative database. Ann Surg. 2004;239:43-52.
16. Harrell AG, Lincourt AE, Novitsky YW, Rosen MJ, Kuwada TS, Kercher KW, et al. Advantages of laparoscopic appendectomy in the elderly. Am Surg. 2006;72:474-80.
17. Heiss K. Victim or player: pediatric surgeons deal with quality improvement and the information age. Semin Pediatr Surg. 2002;11:3-11.
18. Himal HS. Minimally invasive (laparoscopic) surgery. Surgical Endosc. 2002;16:1647-52.
19. Horattas MC, Guyton DP, Wu D. A reappraisal of appendicitis in the elderly. Am J Surg. 1990;160:291.
20. Horwitz JR, Custer MD, May BH, Mehall JR, Lally KP. Should laparoscopic appendectomy be avoided for complicated appendicitis in children? J Pediatr Surg. 1997;32:1601-3.
21. Hui TT, Major KM, Avital I, Hiatt JR, Margulies DR. Outcome of elderly patients with appendicitis: effect of computed tomography and laparoscopy. Arch Surg. 2002;137:995.
22. Ikeda H, Ishimaru Y, Takayasu H, Okamura K, Kisaki Y, Fujino J. Laparoscopic vs open appendectomy in children with uncomplicated and complicated appendicitis. J Pediatr Surg. 2004;39:1680-5.
23. Kanona H, Al Samaraee A, Nice C, Bhattacharya V. Stump appendicitis: a review. Int J Surg. 2012;10:425-8.
24. Kokoska ER, Silen ML, Tracy TF, Dillon PA, Cradock TV, Weber TR. Perforated appendicitis in children: risk factors for the development of complications. Surgery. 1998;124:619-26.
25. Krisher SL, Browne A, Dibbins A, Tkacz N, Curci M. Intra-abdominal abscess after laparoscopic appendectomy for perforated appendicitis. Arch Surg. 2001;136:438-41.
26. Lintula H, Kokki H, Vanamo K, Antila P, Eskelinen M. Laparoscopy in children with complicated appendicitis. J Pediatr Surg. 2002;37:1317-20.
27. Lintula H, Kokki H, Vanamo K, Valtonen H, Mattila M, Eskelinen M. The costs and effects of laparoscopic appendectomy in children. Arch Pediatr Adolesc Med. 2004;158:34-7.
28. Lintula H, Kokki H, Vanamo K. Single-blind randomized clinical trial of laparoscopic vs open appendicectomy in children. Br J Surg. 2001;88:510-4.
29. Lund DP, Murphy EU. Management of perforated appendicitis in children: a decade of aggressive treatment. J Pediatr Surg. 1994;29:1130-4.
30. Martin LC, Puente I, Sosa JL, Bassin A, Breslaw R, McKenney MG, et al. Open vs laparoscopic appendectomy: a prospective randomized comparison. Ann Surg. 1995;222:256-62.
31. Merhoff AM, Merhoff GC, Franklin ME. Laparoscopic vs open appendectomy. Am J Surg. 2000;179:375-8.
32. Moraitis D, Kini SU, Annamaneni RK, Zitsman JL. Laparoscopy in complicated pediatric appendicitis. JSLS. 2004;8:310-13.
33. Nathaniel J, Soper L, Brunt M, Kerbl K. Laparoscopic general surgery. N Eng J Med. 1994;330:409-19.
34. Newman K, Ponsky T, Kittle K, Dyk L, Throop C, Gieseker K, et al. Appendicitis 2000: variability in practice, outcomes, and resource utilization at thirty pediatric hospitals. J Pediatr Surg. 2003;38:372-9.
35. Nguyen NT, Zainabadi K, Mavandadi S, Paya M, Stevens CM, Root J, et al. Trends in the utilization and outcomes of laparoscopic vs open appendectomy. Am J Surg. 2004;188:813-20.
36. Paajanen H, Kettunen J, Kostiainen S. Emergency appendectomies in patients over 80 years. Am Surg. 1994;60:950.
37. Phillips S, Walton JM, Chin I, Farrokhyar F, Fitzgerald P, Cameron B. Ten year experience with pediatric laparoscopic appendectomy: are we getting better? J Pediatr Surg. 2005;40:842-5.
38. Pittman-Waller VA, Myers JG, Stewart RM, Dent DL, Page CP, Gray GA, et al. Appendicitis: why so complicated? Analysis of 5755 consecutive appendectomies. Am Surg. 2000;66:548-54.
39. Reich H. Laparoscopic bowel injury. Surg Laparosc Endosc. 1992;2:74-8.
40. Rymer B, Forsythe RO, Husada G. Mucocoele and mucinous tumours of the appendix: a review of the literature. Int J Surg. 2015;18:132.
41. Schrenk P, Woisetschlager R, Rieger R, Wayand W. Mechanism, management, and prevention of laparoscopic bowel injuries. Gastrointest Endosc. 1996;43:572-4.
42. Siddharthan RV, Byrne RM, Dewey E, Martindale RG, Gilbert EW, Tsikitiset VL, et al. Appendiceal cancer masked as inflammatory appendicitis in the elderly, not an uncommon presentation (Surveillance Epidemiology and End Results (SEER)-Medicare Analysis). J Surg Oncol. 2019;120:736-9.
43. Simpson J, Humes D, Speake W. Appendicitis. Clin Evid BMJ. 20076;2007:0408. [online] Available from: www.clinicalevidence.com/ceweb/conditions/dsd/0408/0408_keymessages.jsp. [Last accessed June, 2020].
44. Tang E, Ortega AE, Anthone GJ, Beart RW Jr. Intra-abdominal abscesses following laparoscopic and open appendectomies. Surg Endosc. 1996;10:327-8.
45. Tannoury J, Abboud B. Treatment options of inflammatory appendiceal masses in adults. World J Gastroenterol. 2013;19:3942.
46. Utpal De. Laparoscopic versus open appendicectomy: an Indian perspective. J Minimal Access Surg. 2005;1:15-20.
47. Vernon AH, Georgeson KE, Harmon CM. Pediatric laparoscopic appendectomy for acute appendicitis. Surg Endosc. 2003;18:75-9.
48. Voyles C, Tucker R. A better understanding of monopolar electrosurgery and laparoscopy. In: Brooks D (Ed). Current Techniques in Laparoscopy. Philadelphia, Pa: Current Medicine; 1994. pp. 1-10.
49. Voyles CR, Tucker RD. Education and engineering solutions for potential problems with laparoscopic monopolar electrosurgery. Am J Surg. 1992;164:57-62.
50. Wagner M, Aronsky D, Tschudi J, Metzger A, Klaiber C. Laparoscopic stapler appendectomy: a prospective study of 267 consecutive cases. Surg Endosc. 1996;10:895-9.
51. Watters JM, Blakslee JM, March RJ, Redmond ML. The influence of age on the severity of peritonitis. Can J Surg. 1996;39:142.
52. Whitney TM, Macho JR, Russell TR, Bossart KJ, Heer FW, Schecter WP. Appendicitis in acquired immunodeficiency syndrome. Am J Surg. 1992;164:467-70.
53. Yong JL, Law WL, Lo CY, Lam CM. A comparative study of routine laparoscopic versus open appendectomy. JSLS. 2006;10:188-92.

CHAPTER 16

Laparoscopic Repair of Inguinal Hernia

INTRODUCTION

Inguinal hernia results from a hole or defect in the muscles, through which the peritoneum protrudes, forming the sac **(Figs. 1 to 5)**. Inguinal herniorrhaphy is one of the most common operations that general surgeons perform. Minimally invasive surgical approaches are increasingly popular because they offer the potential for less postoperative pain and a quick return to normal activities. Laparoscopic herniorrhaphy is being done at a time when laparoscopic cholecystectomy has shown definite benefits over the open technique. Laparoscopic repair of inguinal and femoral hernia is no exception, with laparoscopic approach. The laparoscopic approach to inguinal hernia repair is theoretically possible in nearly all inguinal hernias. However, the precise role of laparoscopy in inguinal hernia repair remains somewhat controversial given the increased costs and greater technical demands.

Ger in 1982 attempted minimal access groin hernia repair by closing the opening of an indirect inguinal hernial sac using Michel clips. Bogojavlensky in 1989 modified the technique by intracorporeal suture of the deep ring after plugging a polypropylene mesh (PPM) into the sac. Toy and Smoot in 1991 described a technique of intraperitoneal onlay mesh (IPOM) placement, where an intra-abdominal piece of polypropylene or expanded polytetrafluoroethylene (e-PTFE) was stapled over the myopectineal orifice without dissection of the peritoneum.

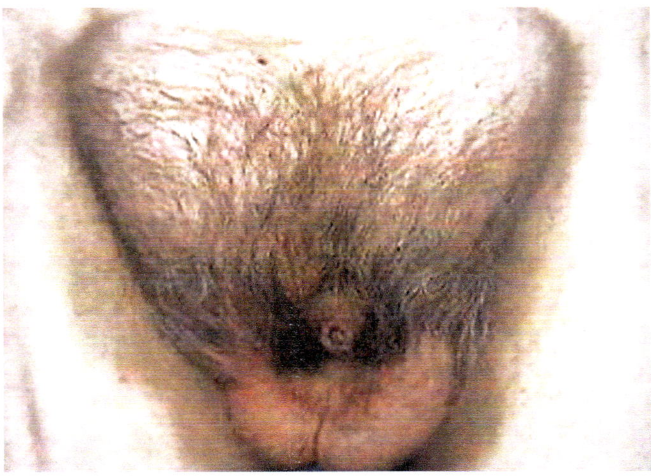

Fig. 1: Bilateral direct hernia.

The present day techniques of laparoscopic hernia repair evolved from Stoppa concept of preperitoneal reinforcement of fascia transversalis over the myopectineal orifice with its multiple openings by a prosthetic mesh. In the early 1990s, Arregui and Doin described the transabdominal preperitoneal (TAPP) repair, where the abdominal cavity is first entered, peritoneum over the posterior wall of the inguinal canal is incised to enter into the avascular preperitoneal plane which is adequately dissected to place a large (15 × 10 cm) mesh over the hernial orifices. After fixation of the mesh, the peritoneum is carefully sutured or stapled. TAPP approach has the advantage of identifying missed additional direct or femoral hernia during the first operation itself.

Around the same time, Phillips and McKernan described the totally extraperitoneal (TEP) technique of endoscopic hernioplasty where the peritoneal cavity is not breached and the entire dissection is performed bluntly in the extraperitoneal space with a balloon device or the tip of the laparoscope itself. An advanced knowledge of the posterior anatomy of the inguinal region is imperative. Once the dissection is complete, a 15 × 10 cm mesh is stapled in place over the myopectineal orifice. It appears to be the most common endoscopic repair today.

In both these repairs, the mesh in direct contact with the fascia of the transversalis muscle in the preperitoneal space, allows tissue in growths leading to the fixation of the mesh as opposed to being in contact to the peritoneum as in IPOM repair where it is prone to migrate.

TOTALLY EXTRAPERITONEAL REPAIR

Totally extraperitoneal repair is performed in the preperitoneal space and was developed to avoid the risks associated with entering the peritoneal cavity **(Fig. 2A)**. The surgeon develops a space between the peritoneum and the anterior abdominal wall so that the peritoneum is never violated. In experienced hands and smaller direct hernia, this approach has the advantage of eliminating the risk of intra-abdominal adhesion formation.

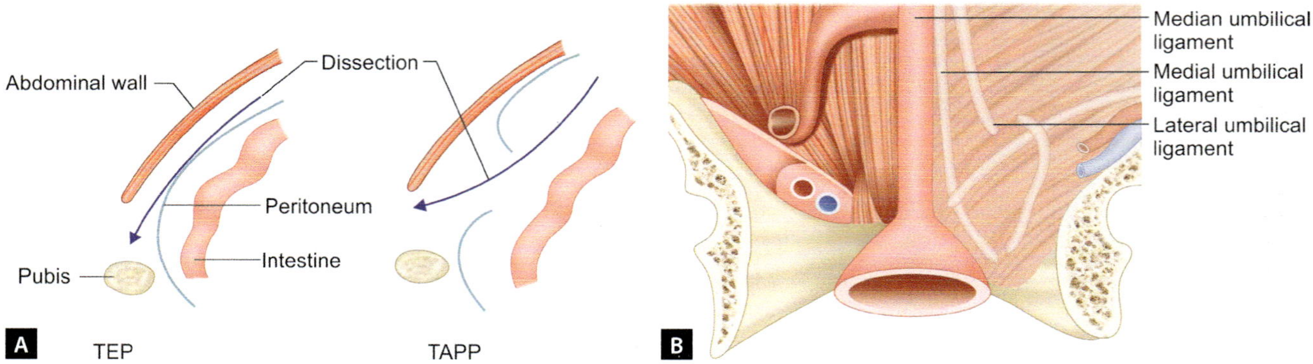

Figs. 2A and B: (A) Totally extraperitoneal (TEP) versus transabdominal preperitoneal (TAPP) hernia repair; (B) Diagrammatic representation of ligaments.

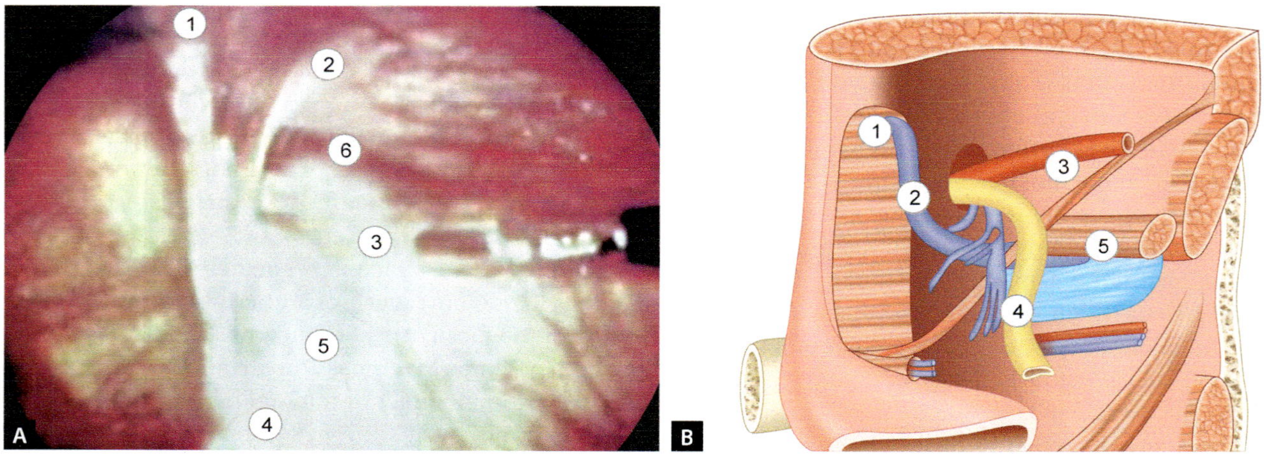

Figs. 3A and B: Important landmarks in laparoscopic hernia repair: (1) Medial umbilical ligament; (2) Inferior epigastric vessels; (3) Spermatic vessels; (4) Vas deferens; (5) External iliac vessels in "triangle of doom"; (6) Indirect defect.

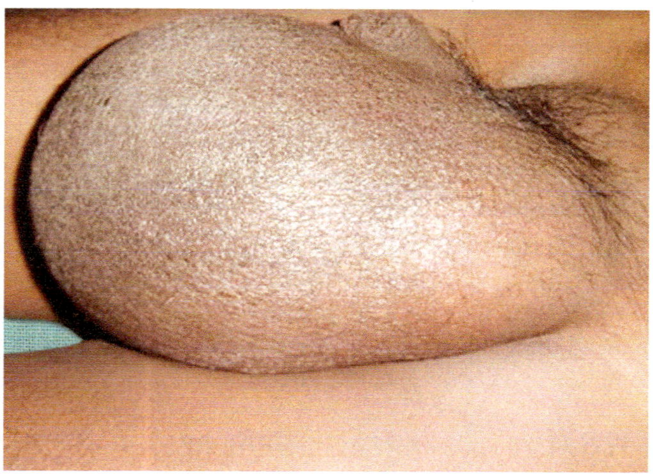

Fig. 4: Left side indirect hernia.

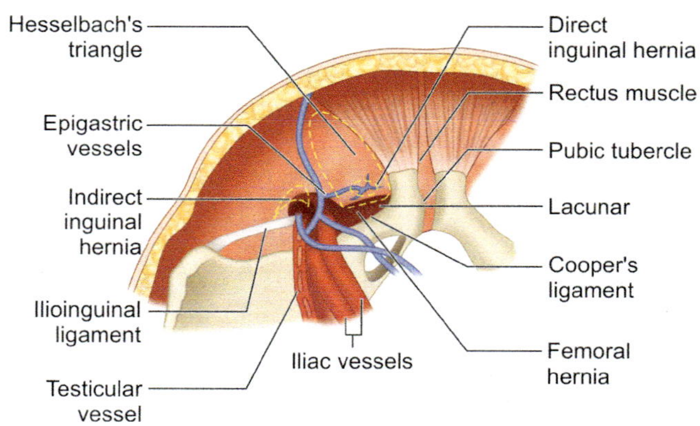

Fig. 5: Triangle of doom.

TRANSABDOMINAL PREPERITONEAL REPAIR

Transabdominal preperitoneal repair involves the placement of mesh in a preperitoneal position, but peritoneal incision is given after entering in abdominal cavity, which is covered by peritoneum to keep the mesh away from the bowel **(Fig. 2A)**. Because TAPP is performed transabdominally, it has a larger working space than TEP, with ready access to both groins, and can be attempted in patients with prior lower abdominal surgery. However, TAPP rarely results in injuries to adjacent intra-abdominal organs, adhesions resulting in intestinal obstruction, or bowel herniation.

For patients in whom the TEP technique is not appropriate or fails due to inability to develop the preperitoneal space, conversion to a TAPP approach can be performed. On occasion, conversion to an open surgical approach may be necessary. Larger hernias, especially huge scrotal hernias, are probably best repaired open. In female patients with indirect inguinal hernia, a TAPP approach may be easier. Indirect inguinal hernia sacs are frequently much more intimately attached to the round ligament in women than are indirect sacs to the cord structures in males.

LAPAROSCOPIC ANATOMY

A clear understanding of the anatomy of the groin and its anatomic approaches is important for successful laparoscopic hernia repair. In the lower abdomen, there are five peritoneal folds or ligaments which are seen through the laparoscope in umbilicus. These ligaments are generally overlooked at the time of open surgery.

One Median Umbilical Ligament

In the midline, there is median umbilical ligament which extends from the mid of urinary bladder up to the umbilicus. Median umbilical ligament is obliterated urachus **(Fig. 2B)**.

Two Medial Umbilical Ligament One on Either Side

The paired medial umbilical ligament is obliterated umbilical artery except where the superior vesical arteries are found in the pelvic portion. The medial umbilical ligaments are the most prominent fold of the peritoneum. Sometimes, it hangs down and obscures the vision of lateral pelvic wall. These ligaments are important landmarks for the lateral extent of the urinary bladder **(Figs. 3A and B)**.

Two Lateral Umbilical Ligaments

Lateral to the medial umbilical ligament, the less prominent paired lateral umbilical fold contains the inferior epigastric vessels. The inferior epigastric artery is lateral border of Hesselbach's triangle and hence is a useful landmark for differentiating between direct and indirect hernia. Any defect lateral to the lateral umbilical ligament is in direct hernia and medial to it is direct inguinal hernia **(Fig. 4)**.

The femoral hernia is below and slightly medial to the lateral inguinal fossa, separated from it by the medial end of the iliopubic tract internally and the inguinal ligament externally.

Important landmarks for extraperitoneal hernia dissection include the musculoaponeurotic layers of the abdominal wall, the bladder, Cooper's ligament, and the iliopubic tract. The inferior epigastric artery and vein, the gonadal vessels, and vas deferens should also be recognized. The space of Retzius lies between the vesicoumbilical fascia posteriorly and the posterior rectus sheath and pubic bone anteriorly. This is the space first entered in extraperitoneal repair of hernia.

Three dangerous areas where stapling and electrosurgery should be avoided are described below.

Triangle of Doom (Fig. 5)

The triangle of doom is defined by vas deferens medially, spermatic vessels laterally, and external iliac vessels inferiorly. This triangle contains external iliac artery and vessels, the deep circumflex iliac vein, the genital branch of genitofemoral nerve, and, hidden by fascia, the femoral nerve. Staple should not be applied in this triangle otherwise chances of mortality are there if these great vessels are injured.

Triangle of Pain

Triangle of pain is defined as spermatic vessel medially, the iliopubic tract laterally, and inferiorly the inferior edge of skin incision. This triangle contains lateral femoral cutaneous nerve and anterior femoral cutaneous nerve of thigh. The staple in this area should be less because nerve entrapment can cause neuralgia.

Circle of Death

This is also called as corona mortis and refers to vascular ring form by the anastomosis of an aberrant obturator artery with the normal obturator artery arising from a branch of the internal iliac artery. At the time of laparoscopic hernia if this vessel is torn, both ends of vessel can bleed profusely, because both arise from a major artery.

The surgeon should remember these anatomic landmarks and the point of mesh fixation should be selected superiorly, laterally, and medially.

INDICATIONS OF LAPAROSCOPIC REPAIR OF HERNIA

The indications for performing a laparoscopic hernia repair are essentially the same as repairing the hernia conventionally. There are, however, certain situations where laparoscopic hernia repair may offer definite benefit over conventional surgery to the patients. These include:

- Bilateral inguinal hernias
- Recurrent inguinal hernias

In recurrent hernia, surgery failure rate is as high as 25–30%, if again repaired by open surgery. The distorted anatomy after repeated surgery makes it more prone to recurrence and other complications such as ischemic orchitis. In recurrent hernia, the laparoscopic approach offers repair through the inner healthy tissues with clear anatomical planes and thus, a lower failure rate. In laparoscopic bilateral repair with three ports technique, there is simultaneous access to both sides without any additional trocar placement. Even in patients with clinically unilateral defect after entering inside the abdominal cavity, there is 20–50% incidence of a contralateral asymptomatic hernia being found which can be repaired, simultaneously, without any additional morbidity of the patient.

CONTRAINDICATIONS OF LAPAROSCOPIC REPAIR OF HERNIA

- Nonreducible, incarcerated inguinal hernia
- Prior laparoscopic herniorrhaphy
- Massive scrotal hernia
- Prior pelvic lymph node resection
- Prior groin irradiation
- Inability to tolerate general anesthesia (GA)
- Prior pelvic surgery in the preperitoneal space
- Incarcerated inguinal hernia
- Large scrotal hernia
- Ascites
- Active infection

ADVANTAGES OF LAPAROSCOPIC APPROACH

- Tension-free repair that reinforces the entire myopectineal orifice
- Less tissue dissection and disruption of tissue planes
- Three ports are adequate for all type of hernias.
- Less pain postoperatively
- Low intraoperatively and postoperative complications
- Early return to work

DISADVANTAGES OF OPEN METHOD

- Requires 4–6 inches of incision at the groin
- Generally very painful, because of muscle spasm
- Considerable postoperative swelling of tissues in groin, around the wound
- Requires cutting through the skin, fat, and good muscles in order to gain access for repair, which in itself causes damage
- Frequent complications of wound hematomas, wound infection, scrotal hematomas, and neuroma
- Usually takes 6–8 weeks for recovery.
- Sometimes long-term disability may follow, e.g., neuralgia, neuroma, and testicular ischemia.
- Whether a flat mesh or a plug is used from the front, they do not hold themselves in place; what holds them in place are stitches, so the strength of the repair still depends on the stitches, not so much on the mesh or plug.
- Bilateral inguinal hernias require two incisions, doubling the pain; or two operations.
- Recurrent inguinal hernias are very difficult to operate open, and more liable to complications.
- The size of mesh used in open methods is limited by natural fusion of muscles.
- All meshes and plugs shrink with time, and this works against all open methods.

Any method of repair must achieve two fundamental goals—removal of the sac from the defect and durable closure of the defect. In addition, the ideal method should achieve these with the least invasion, pain, or disturbance of normal anatomy. Laparoscopic repair in expert hands is now quite safe and effective, and is an excellent alternative for patients with inguinal hernia. It is confusing that laparoscopic repair is more complex and is not widely available. The public needs to be educated as to its advantages. All surgeons agree that for bilateral or recurrent inguinal hernias, laparoscopic repair is unquestionably the method of choice. The argument against its use for unilateral or primary inguinal hernias is unfounded if it is the best for bilateral or recurrent hernias.

TYPES OF LAPAROSCOPIC HERNIA REPAIR

Many techniques were used to repair hernia such as:

- Simple closure of the internal rings
- Plug and patch repair
- IPOM repair
- TAPP mesh repair
- TEP repair

The technique of TAPP repair was first described by Arregui in 1991. In the TAPP repair, the peritoneal cavity is entered, the peritoneum is dissected from the myopectineal orifice, mesh prosthesis is secured, and the peritoneal defect is closed. This technique has been criticized for exposing intra-abdominal organs to potential complications, including small bowel injury and obstruction.

The TEP repair maintains peritoneal integrity, theoretically eliminating these risks while allowing direct visualization of the groin anatomy, which is critical for a successful repair. The TEP hernioplasty follows the basic principles of the open preperitoneal giant mesh repair, as first described by Stoppa in 1975 for the repair of bilateral hernias.

Both approaches (TAP or TEP) are acceptable, and one approach may be preferred over the other under specific clinical circumstances. TAPP was the original approach, and TEP evolved to minimize some of the problems associated with TAPP, but TEP repair is technically more challenging because of the limited working space, which may explain higher conversion rates. TAPP approach is more popular and commonly used procedure all over the world for inguinal hernia repair. Although surgeons should learn both techniques, they should use the technique with which they are most familiar.

Patient Selection

The GA and the pneumoperitoneum required as part of the laparoscopic procedure do increase the risk in certain groups of patients. Most surgeons would not recommend laparoscopic hernia repair in those with pre-existing disease conditions. Patients with cardiac diseases and chronic obstructive pulmonary disease (COPD) should not be considered good candidates for laparoscopy. The laparoscopic hernia repair may also be more difficult in patients who have had previous lower abdominal surgery. The elderly may also be at increased risk for complications with GA combined with pneumoperitoneum.

If the patient is young or the hernia is small, it does not matter how the hernia is repaired. Many surgeons agree that for bilateral or recurrent inguinal hernias, laparoscopic repair is unquestionably the method of choice.

Laparoscopic surgery is not recommended for big irreducible and incarcerated hernia. Hernia repair like many other laparoscopic procedures should not be performed under local anesthesia. Small direct hernia can be performed under spinal anesthesia if TEP is planned, but best anesthesia for laparoscopic hernia repair is GA.

TRANSABDOMINAL PREPERITONEAL REPAIR OF INGUINAL HERNIA

As with most laparoscopic procedures, the peritoneal cavity is entered during TAPP hernia repair. The major advantage of the TAPP approach to groin hernias is that all three hernia defects (direct, indirect, and femoral) are well visualized and in close proximity to each other, allowing easy repair of any type of groin hernia.

Position of Surgical Team and Patient

Surgeon stands toward the opposite side of the hernia, near the shoulder. Camera assistant should stand either right to the patient or on the opposite side of the patient **(Fig. 6)**. The patient is usually placed in 15–20° of Trendelenburg position to improve exposure of the hernia defect, which is particularly important with TAPP hernia repair to move the small bowel or omentum away from the area of dissection.

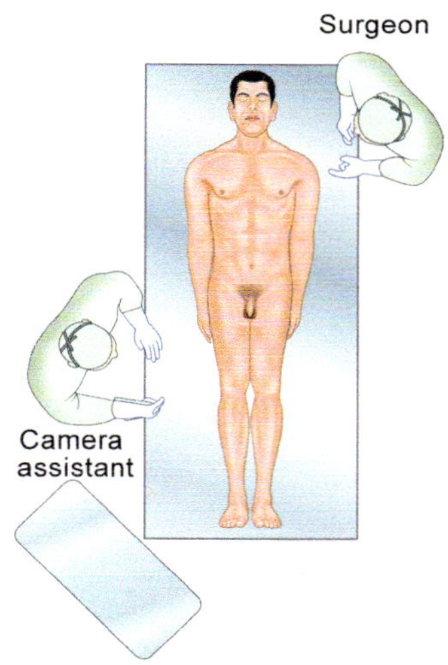

Fig. 6: Position of surgeon in right-sided hernia.

Port Position

The position of port in a laparoscopic repair of transabdominal hernia repair should be again according to baseball diamond concept **(Figs. 7A to C)**. Please refer Chapter 6: Abdominal Access Techniques.

The telescopic port should be in umbilicus. A 30° telescope is a better choice for laparoscopic hernia surgery. A 10 mm umbilical port is used. Two other ports, usually 10 mm for dominant hand and 5 mm for nondominant hand, are placed lateral to the umbilicus **(Figs. 8A to C)**. In a left-sided hernia, the right lateral port should be in right iliac fossa and left port in left hypochondrium so that both the instruments should make a manipulation angle of 60°. In right-sided hernia surgery, right port should move up toward hypochondrium and left port will come down to make the triangle.

PROCEDURE OF TRANSABDOMINAL PREPERITONEAL REPAIR

After access, diagnostic laparoscopy is performed to rule out any adhesion or other intra-abdominal lesion. All the important anatomical landmarks of hernia surgery are identified with the help of telescope and one atraumatic grasper. The important landmarks of laparoscopic hernia repair are the pubic bone and inferior epigastric vessels. The defect should be seen carefully and if any content is present inside the sac, it should be reduced gently **(Figs. 9A to D)**. A sliding hernia of colon should be carefully reduced because chances of perforation of large bowel are more than other viscus so the assistant should reduce the hernia by pressing it from outside. Any adhesion between bowel and omentum should be divided carefully using harmonic scalpel or bipolar and scissors.

The next step of TAPP repair of hernia is the creation of preperitoneal space. Many surgeons like to do hydrodissection to create this preperitoneal space just by injecting normal saline into preperitoneal space. Some surgeons think that it is easy to create preperitoneal space with sharp dissection as well. The peritoneum is cut at a distance of minimum 4 cm lateral to the outer margin of deep ring at 2 o'clock position if the hernia is right side and 10 o'clock position for the left side of hernia. Medial dissection of peritoneal incision should continue up to medial umbilical ligament **(Figs. 9E and F)**. Going medial to medial umbilical ligament is risky because there is risk of injury of the urinary bladder. The flap

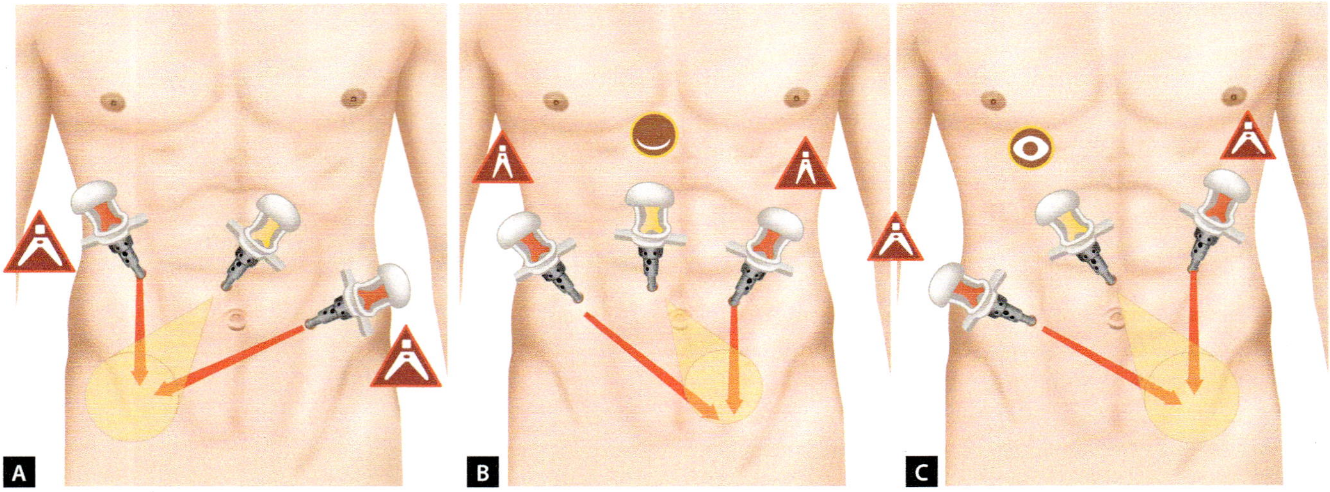

Figs. 7A to C: (A) Port position of right-sided hernia; (B) Port position of bilateral hernia; (C) Port position of left-sided hernia.

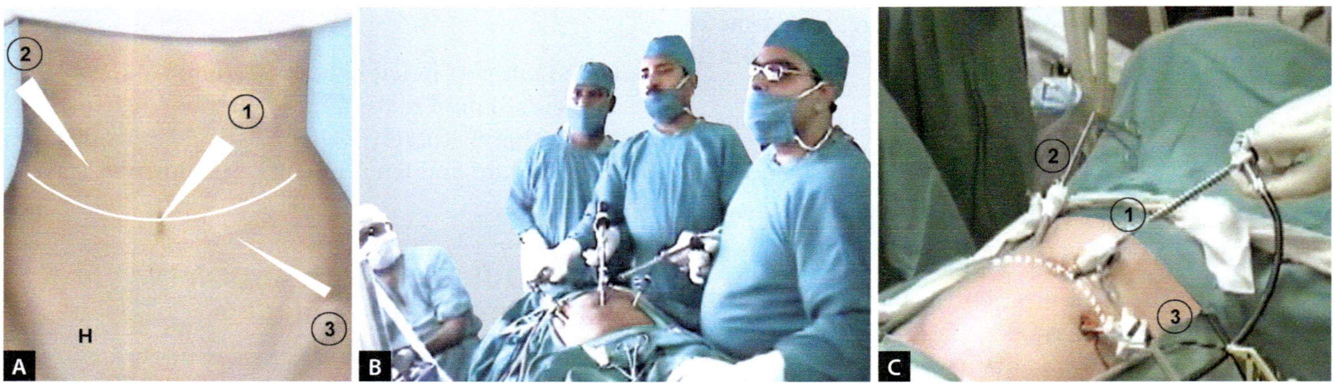

Figs. 8A to C: (A) Port position of right-sided hernia; (B) Port position of surgical team; (C) Port position right hernia (1—Camera; 2 and 3—Instruments).

of peritoneum is separated from above downward as soon as it reaches the site of internal ring, the hernia sac will be encountered.

Dissection should be started with opening the peritoneum lateral to the medial umbilical fold in order to identify Cooper's ligament. Stoppa's parietalization technique should be used for dissection of the spermatic cord from the peritoneum by separating the elements of the spermatic cord from the peritoneum and peritoneal sac **(Figs. 10A to E)**.

In case of indirect defect, the hernial sac has to be either gently dissected free or inverted or else if it is completely adhered with the transversalis fascia and cord structures, it can be transected. Surgeons should use both blunt and sharp dissection and the sac is dissected off the anterior abdominal wall. After being reduced partially, it is ligated using an endoloop and then transected with scissors. In case of bilateral hernias, the procedure is repeated on the other side. The vas and spermatic vessels also need to be separated from the sac. The next step is separation of the sac from cord structures and dissection for creation of proper lateral space for the placement of mesh. Lateral limit of dissection is the anterosuperior iliac spine, while inferior limit laterally is the psoas muscle. Dissection should be avoided in the "triangle of doom" which is bounded medially by the vas deferens and laterally by the gonadal vessels. A large hernial sac creates multiple planes and it is easy for the beginners to get disoriented with sac, vas, and vessel. The best way to avoid this confusion is that surgeon should keep himself as close as possible to the outer surface of peritoneum. If the spermatic vessels are injured accidentally, it can be clipped. Even if the testicular vessel is injured, the testes will get the blood supply from collateral vessels developed through cremasteric vessels.

In direct hernias, the creation of preperitoneal space is comparatively easy as there is no chance of injury of spermatic vessels and vas. The bulge in the transversalis fascia may be repaired by suturing or stapling.

The tacker application and application of electrosurgery should be done very carefully in the triangle of doom, triangle of pain, and trapezoid of disaster. In case of massive complete indirect scrotal hernias, no attempt should be made to reduce the sac completely as it may increase the risk of testicular nerve injury and hematoma formation.

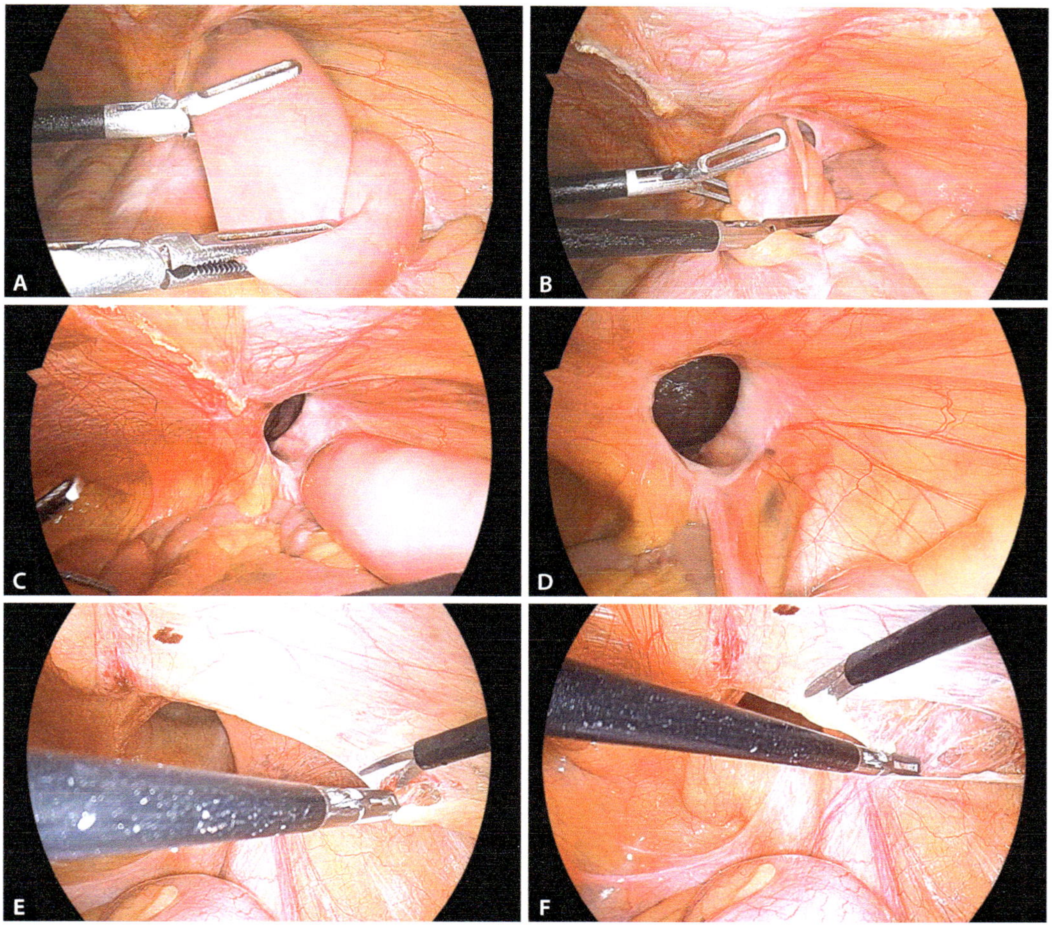

Figs. 9A to F: (A to D) Reduction of the content of hernia sac; (E and F) Incision over peritoneum.

Placement of the Mesh

Mesh is a necessary element of laparoscopic inguinal hernia repair to provide a tension-free hernia repair, which is the recommended method. Preformed mesh that conforms to the preperitoneal space is available and is preferred by some surgeons over a flat piece of mesh that needs to be trimmed to accommodate the patient's anatomy.

Criteria for laparoscopic mesh are as follows:

- Nonabsorbable
- Adequate size
- Adequate memory

Polypropylene woven mesh (e.g., Marlex, Prolene, and SurgiPro) has been used in laparoscopic inguinal hernia repair and is preferred over other prosthetic materials. e-PTFE is another material that is also used extensively for incisional hernias, but it has not been used for the laparoscopic inguinal and femoral hernia repair, except for the IPOM technique. PPM is commercially available in light, medium, or heavy weight. Light weight mesh is associated with a lower incidence of chronic groin pain, groin stiffness, and foreign body sensations without any increased risk for hernia recurrence.

A Prolene mesh of appropriate size, usually 15 × 15 cm should be taken and one corner of mesh should be tailored **(Fig. 11)**. Mesh is placed inside the abdominal cavity through 10 mm port. Mesh should be rolled and loaded backward in this port. If surgery is being performed by 10 mm port only the port should be removed and rolled mesh should be introduced though the port wound directly **(Fig. 12)**. After introduction of mesh, it is unrolled when it reaches in the peritoneal cavity. The mesh is fixed medially over the Cooper's ligament and pubic bone using a tacker or anchor **(Figs. 13A and B)**. The tailored corner of the mesh should be positioned inferomedially. No lateral slit should be made in the mesh and it should not be fixed lateral to cord structures to prevent injury to lateral cutaneous nerve of thigh. The mesh in this position covers the direct, indirect, and femoral defects. It is essential that mesh should extend below the pubic tubercle so that it covers the femoral orifice. Mesh should also extend medially to cover all the possible orifices of hernia. Laterally mesh should project at least 2–3 cm beyond the margin of deep ring. If mesh is not of appropriate size, the chances of recurrence increase. Sometimes, the surgeon may be disoriented and mesh is placed with its long axis vertical

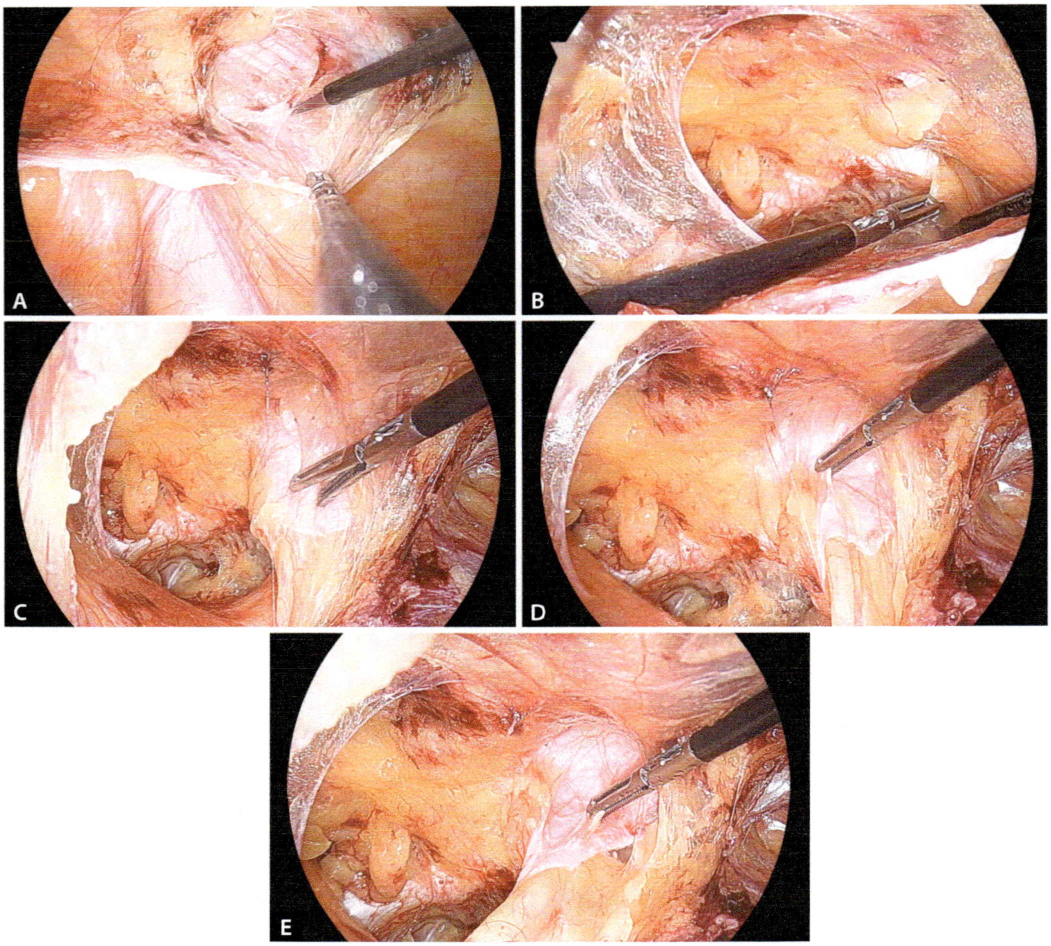

Figs. 10A to E: Creation of preperitoneal space.

instead of transverse. If the mesh is cut at one of the corners, chances of this disorientation are minimum.

Implant for Fixing Mesh

Many preloaded devices are available for fixing mesh in hernia surgery. Mesh is fixed medially over the Cooper's ligament and pubic bone using an implant.

Currently, three popular brands of implants to fix the mesh are available. These are Tacker, Protack, and Anchor. The comparative chart of these implants is shown in **Table 1**.

After adjusting the mesh properly, it should be fixed by stapling first its middle part three fingers above the superior limit of the internal ring. With mesh duly stapled, pneumoperitoneum is reduced to 9 mm Hg. It is important to avoid pricking of the inferior epigastric artery or the testicular vessels. Intracorporeal suturing can also be used for fixation of mesh if surgeon has sufficient suturing skill.

After fixing the mesh properly, the peritoneum flap is replaced over the mesh. It is important that mesh should be completely covered by the peritoneum. Ideally, peritoneum should be opposed by overlap fashion and peritoneum defect is closed either by staples or by continuous suturing and Aberdeen termination **(Figs. 14A and B)**.

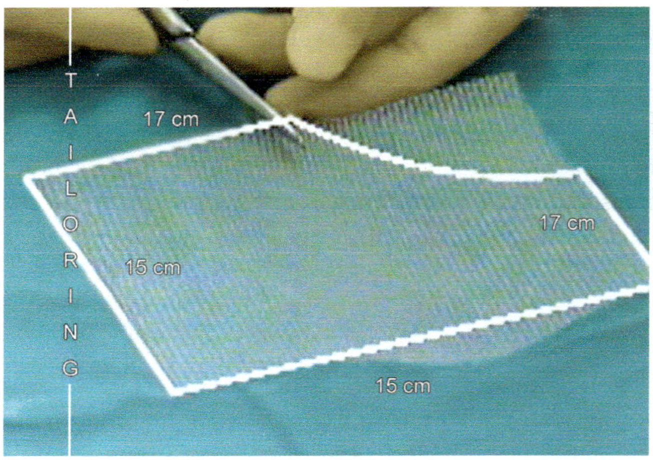

Fig. 11: Cutting the corner of mesh.

Repair of Bilateral Inguinal Hernia

In laparoscopic surgery, postoperative recovery of bilateral hernia is same as that of unilateral hernia. The technique of bilateral laparoscopic repair of hernia is same as that of unilateral hernia. Patients with bilateral hernia are good candidates of laparoscopy. The two sides may be repaired using two meshes, but single long mesh also can be used and is pushed across from one side behind the bladder, and across the inguinal orifice on the opposite side. The size of the mesh for bilateral hernia should be 30 × 15 cm **(Fig. 15)**. Surgeon should avoid twisting of the mesh. After placing the mesh in bilateral hernia surgery, it should look just like a bow tie.

Repair of Recurrent Inguinal Hernia

Recurrent laparoscopic hernia after open surgery is better to be repaired laparoscopically, because external anatomy is disrupted and open repair has more chances of recurrence. Laparoscopy is method of choice for recurrent hernia. The defect is usually direct and more than one in recurrent hernia.

The result of laparoscopic repair is excellent even in case of multiple hernias.

Laparoscopic Hernia in Children

Laparoscopy has been tried in small children. Only closure of ring and herniotomy is possible in pediatric age group. The sac is simply inverted and tied internally. Care should be taken that the vas or vessels should not be caught in the ligature **(Figs. 16A and B)**.

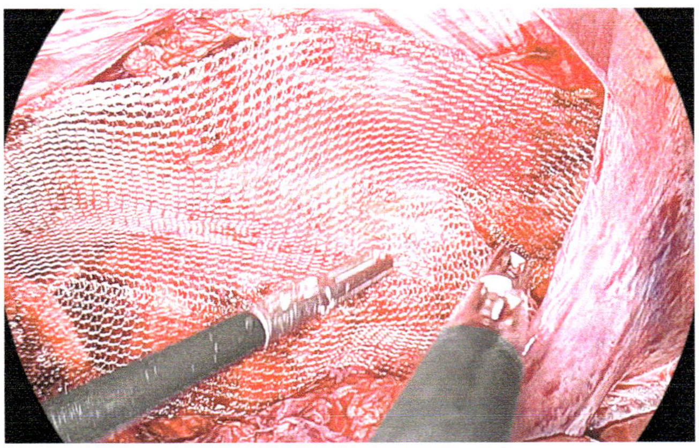

Fig. 12: Introduction of mesh in preperitoneal space.

Ending of the Operation

At the end of surgery, the abdomen should be examined for any possible bowel injury or hemorrhage. The entire instrument should be removed followed by all the ports. Each port should be removed under direct observation through telescope. Ports larger than 10 mm should be sutured. Telescope should be removed at last after releasing all the gas keeping in mind that last port should not be pulled without putting telescope or any blunt instrument in, to prevent entrapment of bowel or omentum and formation of omental or intestinal adhesion. Wound should be closed with suture, especially 10 mm wound.

TOTALLY EXTRAPERITONEAL HERNIA REPAIR

The technique of TEP repair of inguinal hernia was described even before the TAPP technique; however, technical difficulties of working in closed space and anatomy with very limited working space hindered its popular acceptance. The effectiveness of this type of repair has been well established by the open operation of Stoppa.

ADVANTAGES OF TOTALLY EXTRAPERITONEAL REPAIR

- Pneumoperitoneum is not required.
- Less chance of dangerous vessel injury or bowel injury
- The view of groin is better for dissection around the neck of the sac.
- Continuity of peritoneum is not breached so it need not be closed.

DISADVANTAGES OF PREPERITONEAL REPAIR

- The identification of correct plane of dissection is difficult.

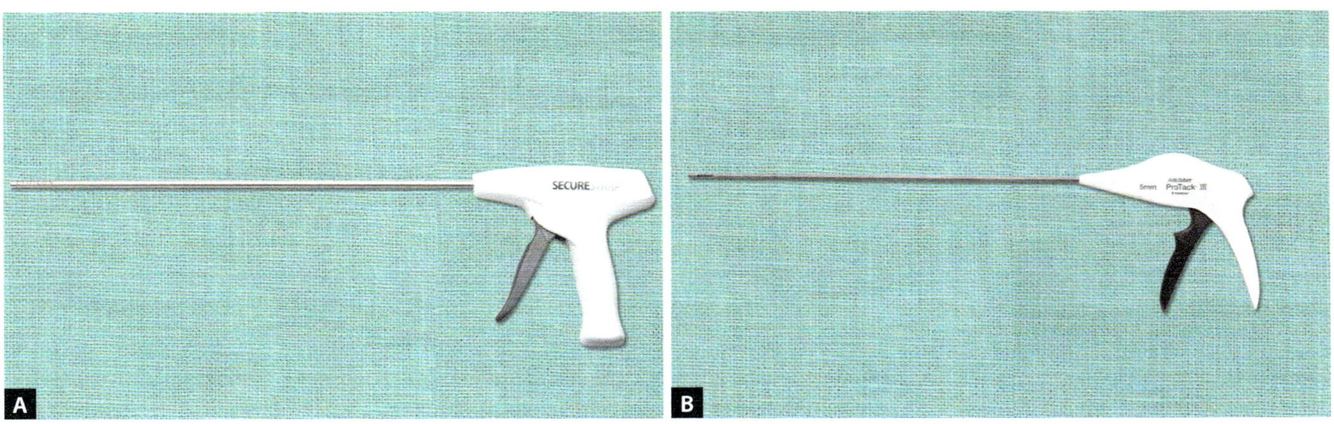

Figs. 13A and B: (A) Hernia secure trap Ethicon stapler; (B) Hernia tacker from Covidien.

TABLE 1: Comparison of ESS Endoanchor, Tyco Protack, and Tyco Tacker.

Feature	*ESS Endoanchor*	*Tyco Protack*	*Tyco Tacker*
Number of implants	20	30	20
Geometry of implant	Anchor	Helical fastener	Helical fastener
Implant material	Nitinol	Titanium	Titanium
Implant length	5.9 mm	3.8 mm	3.6 mm
Implant width	6.7 mm	4 mm	3.4 mm
Port size required	5 mm	5 mm	5 mm
Shaft length	360 mm	356 mm	356 mm
Trigger fire orientation	Release to deploy	Depress to deploy	Depress to deploy

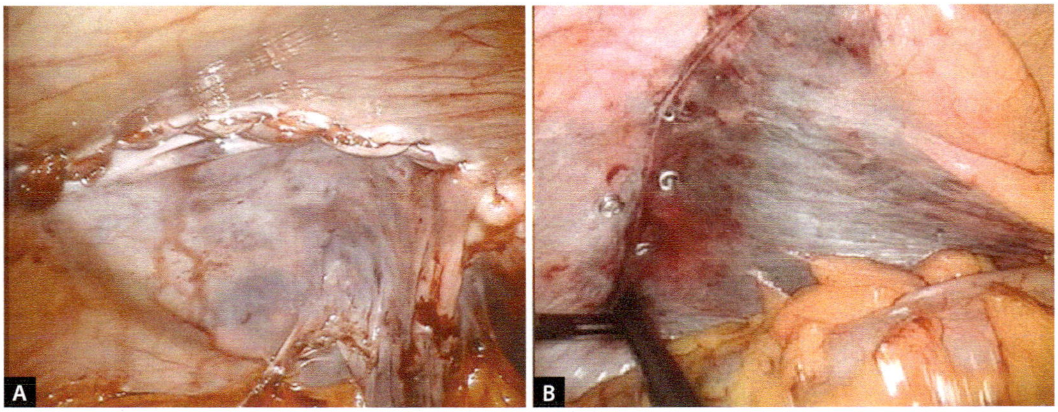

Figs. 14A and B: (A) Closure of peritoneum by suturing; (B) Closure of peritoneum by tacker.

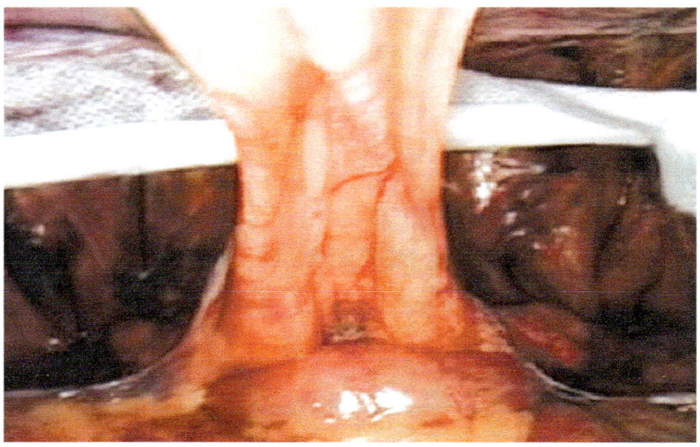

Fig. 15: Introduction of mesh for bilateral hernia.

- The landmarks of hernia dissection can only be identified when they are encountered.
- Reduction of content of sac is difficult to ensure.
- Sliding hernia is difficult to recognize from outside of the sac.
- If the sac gets accidentally cut, it is difficult to close it again.
- In recurrent hernia, extensive adhesion makes the dissection difficult because peritoneum may be adherent to the under surface of the scar.
- There is always a chance of breach of peritoneum continuity and this will reduce the view.
- Four ports generally are necessary for bilateral hernia surgery. Whereas, in TAPP only three ports are sufficient.

Preparation of the Patient

Preparation of the patient in totally preperitoneal hernia repair is same as of the transabdominal hernia repair. Knowledge of the anatomy of the abdominal wall muscle and recognition of the transition zone that occur at the arcuate line of Douglas is very important for totally preperitoneal hernia repair.

Approach to Preperitoneal Space

In TEP repair of hernia, the main concern is to make an extraperitoneal space. The extraperitoneal space is made possible by the fact that the peritoneum in suprapubic region can easily be separated from anterior abdominal wall, thereby creating enough space for dissection.

A 2 cm longitudinal skin incision is made just below the umbilicus 1 cm lateral to the midline on the side of hernia **(Figs. 17A and B)**. The incision is deepened down to reach up to the anterior rectus sheath. All the subcutaneous fat is cleared and the rectus is opened under direct vision. Two-stay

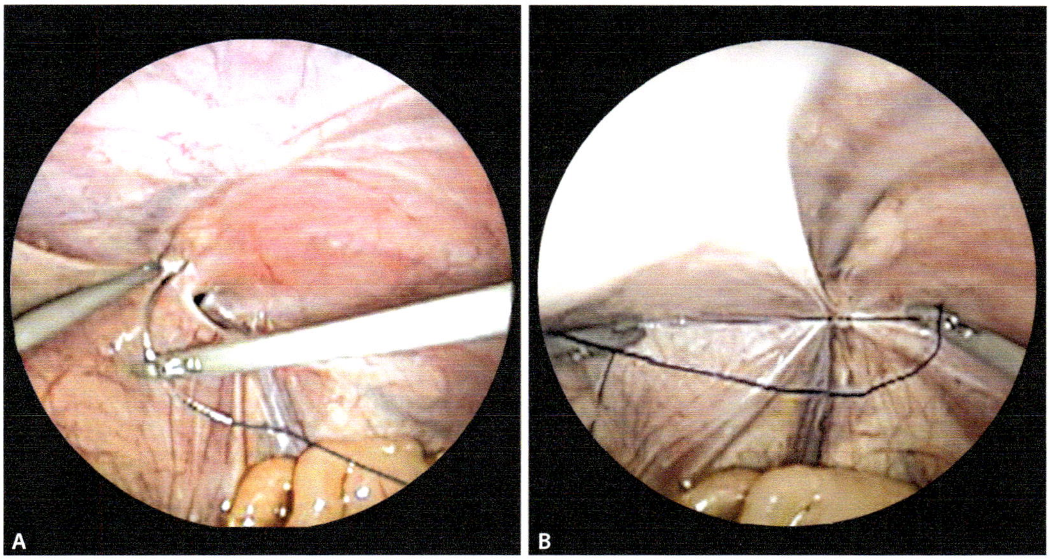

Figs. 16A and B: Closure of defect with intracorporeal suturing in pediatric age.

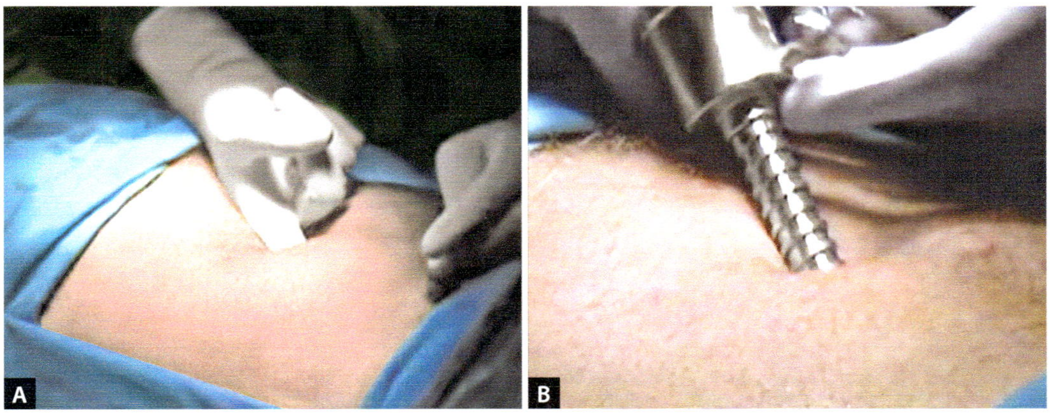

Figs. 17A and B: Access technique of totally extraperitoneal hernia repair.

suture on each leaf of rectus sheath is placed and the rectus muscle is retracted by two retractors downward toward symphysis pubis in an oblique fashion; we should never cross the posterior fascia of the rectus muscle while dissecting.

By finger or swab toward the hernia, dissection should performed carefully, and preperitoneal space will be found below the arcuate line of Douglas.

Insertion of Port

A balloon dissector should be introduced with telescope and balloon is inflated for further dissection of the preperitoneal space. An 11 mm port is introduced without its sharp tip with a laparoscope of 30°. A small preperitoneal pocket is created by manipulating laparoscope in sweeping manner.

If balloon dissector is not available, the glove finger can be tied around the suction irrigation instrument and can be used to create some preperitoneal space **(Figs. 18A and B)**.

Sweeping Movement of Telescope

Once the telescope is placed properly, a 10 mm port is inserted under direct view approximately halfway between the symphysis pubis and the umbilicus **(Figs. 19A to D)**. Another 5 mm port should be placed two fingers below and medial to the right anterior iliac spine. If the secondary port site is not seen clearly through the telescope, one can infiltrate the port site with local anesthetic and look for the tip of the needle internally **(Fig. 20)**. This will insure the exact placement of port and allow the tip of trocar to be seen by telescope at the time of insertion.

Dissection of Preperitoneal Space and Cord Structures in TEP Repair

In TEP repair of hernia, Stoppa parietalization technique is used for dissection of the spermatic cord from the peritoneum by separating the elements of the spermatic cord from the peritoneum and peritoneal sac should be done **(Fig. 21)**.

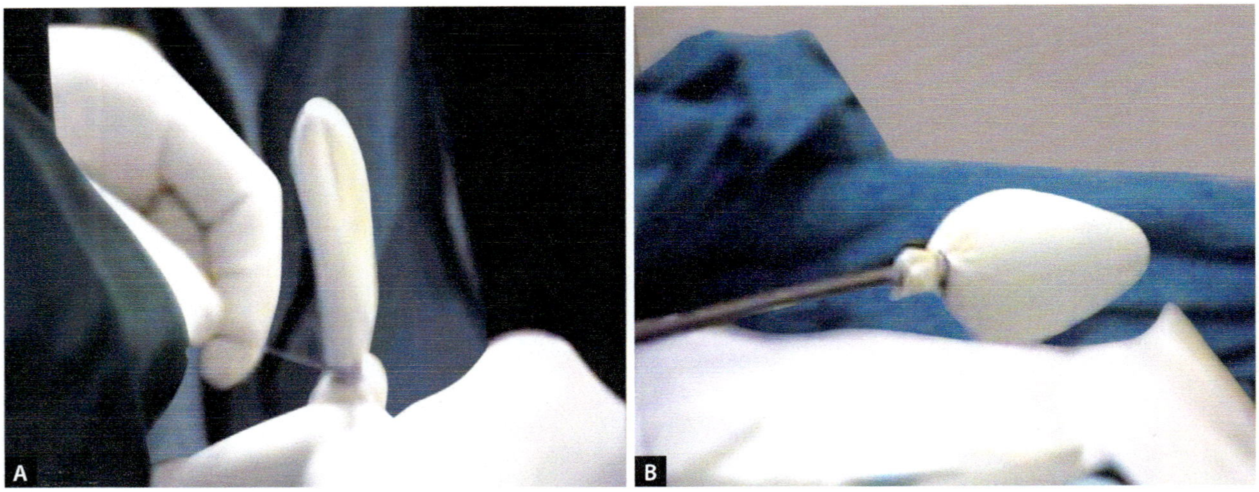

Figs. 18A and B: Making balloon dissection with finger of gloves.

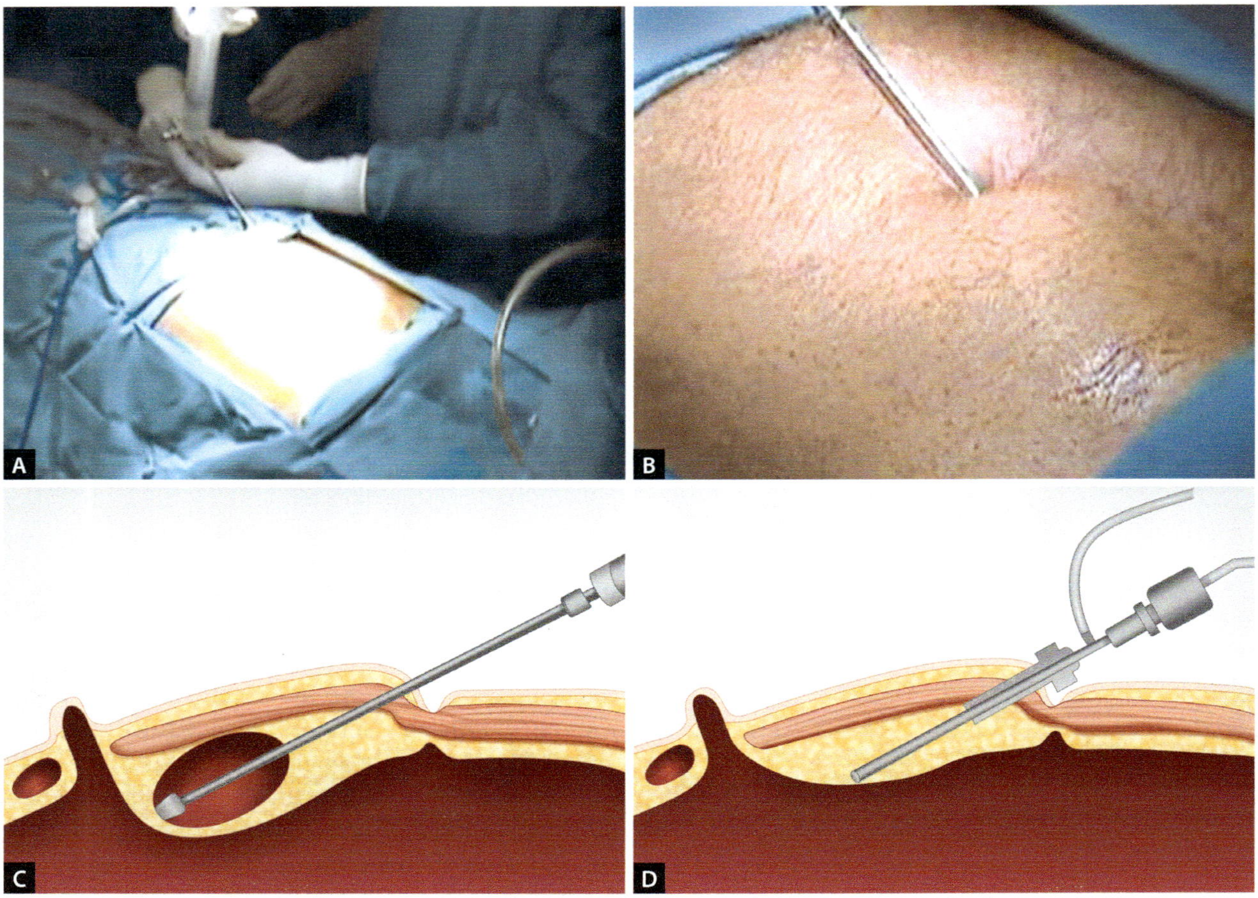

Figs. 19A to D: Balloon dissection.

The dissection is started by tracing the inferior epigastric vessels toward the deep ring. The upper border of the hernia sac is readily recognized because indirect hernia is lateral to the inferior epigastric vessels and direct hernia is medial to it.

As the inguinal region is approached, the dissection is continued all around the sac to encircle the neck. The surgeon should try to remain close to peritoneum and dissection continues medially to separate vas from the sac. Under the neck of the sac, care should be taken to avoid injury of iliac vessels.

In case of direct inguinal hernia, the dissection is carried out from above downward and progressed medially to the

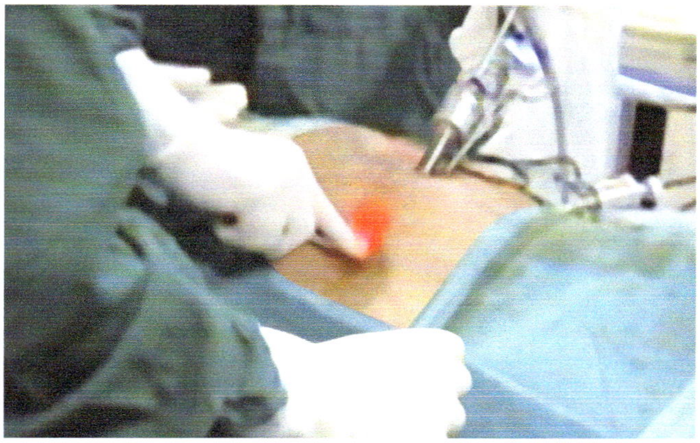

Fig. 20: Introduction of secondary port.

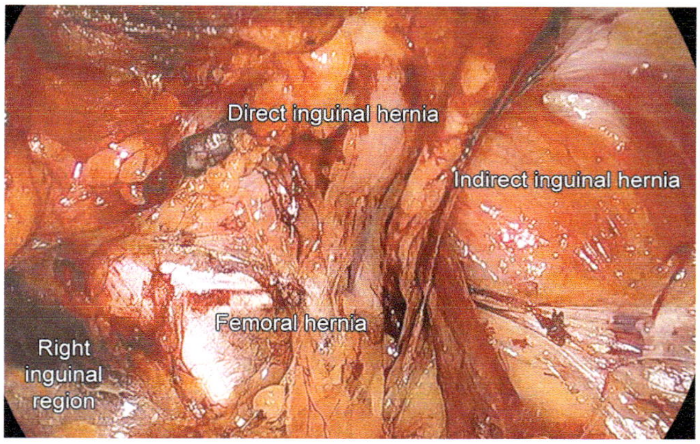

Fig. 21: Dissection of preperitoneal space.

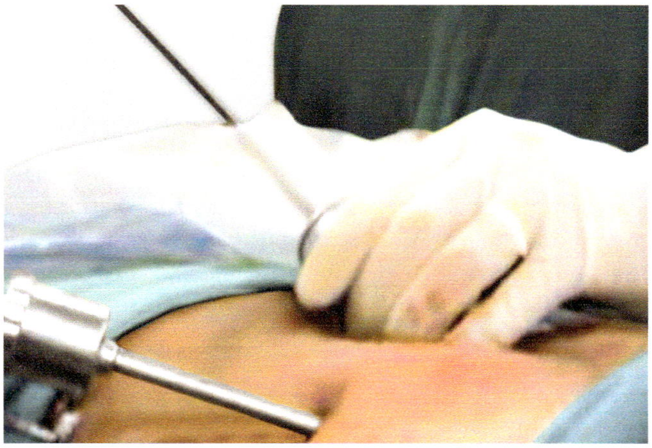

Fig. 22: Introduction of mesh.

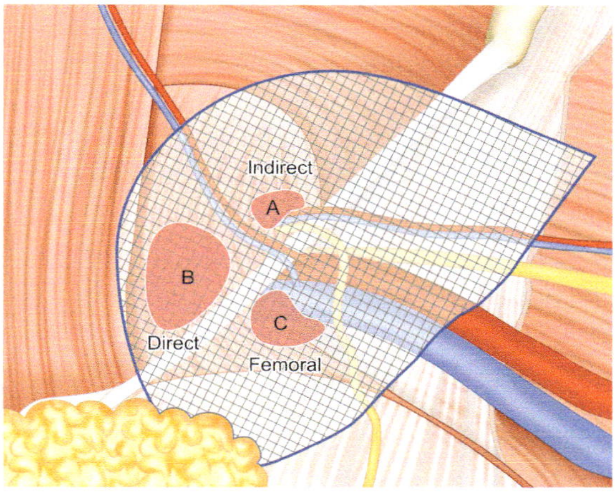

Fig. 23: Placement of mesh.

inferior epigastric vessels. The direct sac is freed from the transversalis fascia. Dissection should be continued until the peritoneum has reached the iliac vessels inferiorly.

Care should be taken that any hole in peritoneum is not made, otherwise it will be difficult to maintain good working space because the gas will escape into the abdominal cavity increasing the intra-abdominal pressure. If the hole is made accidentally, it should be identified and enlarged as this will equalize the pressure on both sides of peritoneum and allows the peritoneum to drop back down due to gravity. A venting 5 mm port or Veress needle can be placed in the right upper quadrant at Palmer's point to decompress the abdominal cavity.

The technique of insertion of mesh in TEP repair of hernia is same as that of transabdominal preperitoneal. Mesh of appropriate size usually 15 × 15 cm is used and rolled and loaded backward in one of the port.

Mesh should be fixed by stapling first in its middle part, three fingers above the superior limit of the internal ring **(Figs. 22 and 23)**. In TEP repair, some surgeons do not use staple, because peritoneum is not breached and once the gas from the preperitoneal space is removed, it will hold the mesh in its proper position. In 1–2% of cases of TEP, conversion to open or TAPP may be necessary due to large peritoneal tear making the vision difficult or in the cases where content is not reduced completely.

Ending of the Operation

At the end of the surgery, the abdomen should be examined for any possible bowel injury or hemorrhage. The entire instrument should be removed and then all the ports. Generally, vicryl is used for rectus and stapler for skin. Adhesive sterile dressing should be applied over the wound.

LAPAROSCOPIC REPAIR OF FEMORAL HERNIA

Laparoscopic repair of femoral hernia is same as that of laparoscopic direct or indirect hernia. It can be performed by both TAPP and TEP methods. In case of laparoscopic femoral hernia repair, the sac should be carefully excised because rigid femoral ring makes it difficult to mobilize the sac. The dissection should be done very carefully because there is increased risk of injury of abnormal obturator artery on the lateral side of the sac. The femoral hernia defect is

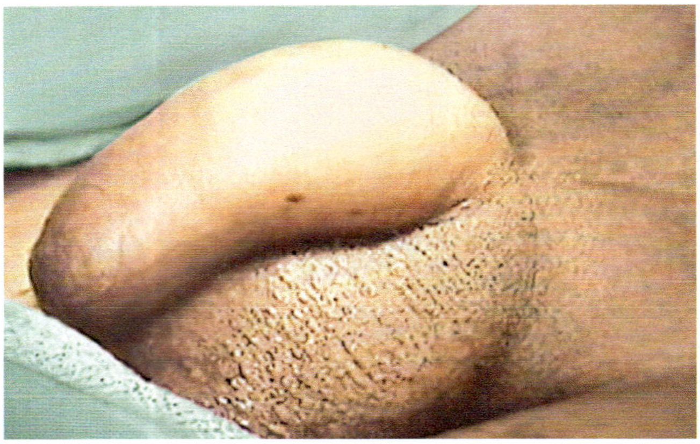

Fig. 24: Postoperative scrotal hematoma.

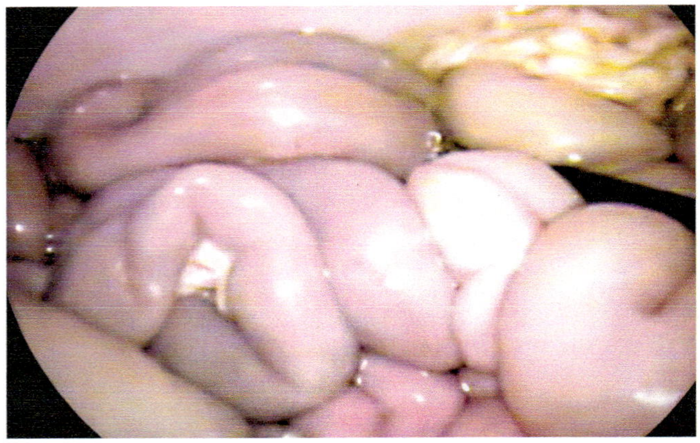

Fig. 25: Perforation bowel during hernia surgery.

between the iliopubic tract and pubic ramus and can be easily identified. Repair of the femoral canal should be done by approximating iliopubic tract to the Cooper's ligament by Prolene stitches.

COMPLICATIONS OF LAPAROSCOPIC HERNIA REPAIR

Like any other laparoscopic procedures, several complications have been recorded during the learning curve. The major problems include:

- Recurrence
- Neurovascular injury
- Urinary tract injury
- Injury to vas
- Testicular complications
- Problems due to mesh

The mechanism of recurrence can be related to lack of understanding of the difficult laparoscopic anatomy, wrong hernia repair technique, or the wrong prosthesis. These include incomplete dissection without proper pocket formation, missed sac, migration of mesh due to small sized mesh which may be prone to get displaced once fixed, inadequate fixation with rolling up of the mesh, and hematoma formation leading to infection.

The complication of laparoscopic hernia repair can be summarized as follows:

- *Immediate*: Visceral injury, vascular injury, and injury to vas and spermatic vessels **(Fig. 24)**
- *Late*: Bowel adhesions to mesh, intestinal obstruction, fistulization, orchitis, testicular atrophy, nerve entrapment, and incisional hernia recurrence **(Fig. 25)**.

Relative Contraindications for Laparoscopic Approach

- Obesity with body mass index (BMI) > 30
- Significant chest disease
- Patient on anticoagulants
- Adhesions
- Massive hernias
- Pregnancy
- Unfit for GA

Inguinal Hernia Repair in Pediatric Patients

Small children gain little benefit from laparoscopic hernia repair as inguinal skin crease incision used in the herniotomy is one of best incisions as far as cosmesis is concerned. It is hardly visible after a few months. Also, it is covered by underwear. Compared to this, three stab incisions, however small, are in the visible area.

Inguinal Hernia Repair in Obese Patients

Operations in patients with BMI above 27 may be difficult for less experienced surgeons, particularly when trying to encircle an indirect sac. Patients with BMI of above 30 should be encouraged to lose weight or should even be turned down for the laparoscopic approach. They are incidentally more likely to develop recurrence after even an open hernia repair. It is also easy for the laparoscopic surgeon to become disoriented when the patient is very obese.

Inguinal Hernia Repair in Recurrence

Generally, the short-term recurrence rate of laparoscopic inguinal hernia repair is reported to be <5%.

In both the open and laparoscopic repair procedures, the aim is to cover the whole inguinofemoral area by a preperitoneal prosthetic mesh, so that recurrences should not occur. When they do occur, recurrences must be regarded as technical failures. Recurrences after laparoscopic repair most often result from using too small a mesh, or not using staples to fix the mesh. Most recurrences after laparoscopic hernia repair occurred medially, and the technique was needed modifications. The mesh is now placed at least until the midline, and occasionally hernia staples are used when an adequate overlap (2 cm) cannot be achieved medially. The TEP technique is now used more often, allowing for better visual control in the medial part of the operating field.

Operating Time

Operating times of surgical techniques varies between surgeons and also vary considerably between centers. It reduces with experience and comparison between laparoscopic and open surgery is subject to bias due to pre-existing familiarity with open techniques. It is less important to the patient than a successful operation. The time taken to perform the surgery can have cost implications. The operative time to perform unilateral primary inguinal repair has frequently been reported as longer for laparoscopic compared to open repair, however, the mean difference in 36 of 37 randomized trials is 14.81 minutes. These differences disappear in bilateral and recurrent hernia repairs.

Postoperative Pain and Amount of Narcotics Used

The open tension-free mesh repair is found to cause less postoperative pain than open nonmesh repairs; however, most randomized trials assessing postoperative pain between open tension-free repairs and laparoscopic repairs report less pain in the laparoscopic groups. In many cases, this also results in less analgesia being consumed by the patient.

Complication Rates

Complications in endoscopic inguinal hernia surgery are more dangerous and more frequent than those of open surgery, especially in inexperienced hands and hence are best avoided. It is possible to avoid most of these complications if one follows a set of well-defined steps and principles of endoscopic inguinal hernia surgery.

Complications of laparoscopic repair of inguinal hernia can be divided into:
- Intraoperative
- Postoperative

INTRAOPERATIVE COMPLICATIONS AND PRECAUTION

During Creation of Preperitoneal Space

This is the most important step for beginners.
- A wide linea alba may result in breaching the peritoneum; in such a situation, it is best to close the rectus and incise the sheath more laterally.
- Improper placement of balloon trocar causing dissection of muscle fibers
- Entry into peritoneum causing pneumoperitoneum
- Rupture of balloon in preperitoneal space
- The Hassan trocar must snugly fit into the incision to avoid CO_2 leak.

To avoid these, one must ensure that the balloon is made properly and the correct space is entered by retracting the rectus muscle laterally to visualize the posterior rectus sheath. Also, the balloon trocar is inserted gently, parallel to the abdominal wall, to avoid puncturing the peritoneum. The balloon must be inflated slowly with saline to ensure smooth and even distention and prevent its rupture.

Precautions During Port Placement

The trocars should be short and threaded in proportion to the less workspace and to ensure a snug fit, respectively. The skin incisions should be just adequate to grip the trocar and prevent its slipping. The patient should empty their bladder before surgery as the suprapubic trocar could injure a filled bladder. The pressure in the preperitoneal space must be such as to offer sufficient resistance during trocar insertion to avoid puncturing the peritoneum.

Correct Identification of the Anatomical Landmarks

The next most important and crucial step in any hernia surgery is the correct identification of anatomical landmarks. This is difficult for beginners as the anatomy is different from that seen in open surgery. The first most important step is to identify the pubic bone. Once this is seen, the rest of the landmarks are traced keeping this as a reference point. One is advised to keep away from the triangle of doom, which contains the iliac vessels, and to avoid placing tacks in the triangle of pain laterally.

Bladder Injuries

Bladder injury most commonly occurs during port placement, dissecting a large direct sac or in a sliding hernia. It is mandatory to empty the bladder prior to an inguinal hernia repair to avoid a trocar injury. It is advisable that beginners catheterize the bladder during the initial part of their learning curve. The diagnosis is evident when one sees urine in the extraperitoneal space. Repair is done with vicryl in two layers and a urinary catheter inserted for 7–10 days.

Bowel Injuries

Bowel injury is rare during hernia surgery. It can occur when reducing large hernias, inadvertent opening of peritoneum causing the bowel to come into the field of surgery, and in reduction of sliding hernias. Injury is best avoided in such circumstances by opening the hernial sac as close as possible to the deep ring. The initial studies showed a higher incidence, especially with TAPP, but gradually it has decreased over time.

Vascular Injury

This is one of the most common injuries occurring in hernia repair and often a reason for conversion. The various sites where it can occur is rectus muscle vessel injury during trocar insertion; inferior epigastric vessel injury; bleeding from venous plexus on the pubic symphysis; aberrant obturator vein injury; testicular vessel injury; and the most disastrous of all, iliac vessels, which requires an emergency conversion to control the bleeding and the immediate services of a vascular surgeon to repair the same. Most of the other bleedings can be controlled with cautery or clips. Careful dissection and adherence to the principles of surgery will help in avoiding most of these injuries.

Injury to Vas Deferens

Injury occurs while dissecting the hernia sac from the cord structures. The injury causes an eventual fibrotic narrowing of the vas. A complete transaction of the vas needs to be repaired in a young patient. An injury to the vas is best avoided and this may be done by identifying before dividing any structure near the deep ring or floor of the extraperitoneal space. Also, the separation of cord structures from the hernial sac must be gentle and direct; grasping of vas deferens with forceps must be avoided.

Pneumoperitoneum

It is a common occurrence in TEP which every surgeon should be prepared to handle. Putting the patient in Trendelenburg position and increasing the insufflation pressures to 15 mm Hg helps. If the problem still persists, a Veress needle can be inserted at Palmer's point.

POSTOPERATIVE COMPLICATIONS

Seroma/Hematoma Formation

It is a common complication after laparoscopic hernia surgery, the incidence being in the range of 5–25% **(Fig. 24)**. They are especially seen after large indirect hernia repair. Most resolve spontaneously over 4–6 weeks. A seroma can be avoided by minimizing dissection of the hernia sac from the cord structures, fixing the direct sac to pubic bone and fenestrating the transversalis fascia in a direct hernia. Some surgeons put in a drain if there is excessive bleeding or after extensive dissection.

Urinary Retention

This complication after hernia repair has a reported incidence of 1.3–5.8%. It is usually precipitated in elderly patients, especially if symptoms of prostatism are present. These patients are best catheterized prior to surgery and catheter removed the next day morning.

Vascular Injury

The incidence of vascular injury has been documented to be about 0.5–1% and inferior epigastric artery is one of the most commonly traumatized.

- *Injury to iliac vessels*: Chances of mortality
- *Inferior epigastric vessel*: Hematoma
- *Iliopubic vein and artery which traverse the lacunar ligament*: Hematoma
- *Injury to spermatic vessels*: Postoperative scrotal hematoma

Nerve Entrapment and Injury

The lateral cutaneous nerve of thigh and the femoral branch of genitofemoral nerve are the two nerves vulnerable to trauma due to indiscriminate placement of staplers lateral to the spermatic cord on the iliopubic tract.

- Injury of lateral cutaneous nerve injury
- *Most common nerve injured is lateral femoral cutaneous nerve (2%)*: Hyperesthesia or paresthesia of upper aspect of thigh and hip.
- If pain starts days after the surgery, it will recover within 2–4 weeks (or percutaneous steroid).
- If pain starts within 24 hours of surgery, there is permanent nerve damage.
- Cryotherapy with destruction of sensory branch is indicated.
- Lifelong numbness

Nerve entrapment should be avoided in laparoscopic repair of hernia:

- Genitofemoral nerve injury
- *Genitofemoral nerve injury (1%)*: Hyperesthesia or paresthesia of scrotum
- Not significant
- With time, it will subside.

Other Complications

- Migration of mesh
- Rejection of mesh (rare)
- Bowel adhesion

Complete transaction of vas requires immediate anastomosis. Other complications include testicular pain, orchitis, epididymitis, swelling due to seromas, or hematoma. The treatment is supportive and incidence of all these complications is similar to that in conventional surgery.

After some experience, most cases of inguinal hernia can be treated laparoscopically. Several prospective randomized trials comparing open versus laparoscopic repair have reported better outcomes following laparoscopic repair. Reduced postoperative pain, earlier return to work, and fewer complications and less chance of recurrences for the laparoscopic approach are some of the crucial advantages. Although the procedural cost for laparoscopic hernia repair is more compared to conventional repair but overall expense for open repair is high if we calculate number of working days lost and medications taken into consideration. Data is now available which documents the TEP repair to have distinct advantage over the TAPP repair in terms of lesser postoperative complications and lower recurrence rate. TAPP has been stated to violate the peritoneal cavity with all its known possible complication of pneumoperitoneum, vessel, or bowel injury. There is no doubt that the laparoscopic hernia repair is a proven technique and will become more popular over a period of time.

Neuralgias

The incidence of this complication is reported to be between 0.5 and 4.6% depending on the technique of repair.

The intraperitoneal onlay mesh method had the highest incidence of neuralgias in one study and was hence abandoned as a form of viable repair. The commonly involved nerves are lateral cutaneous nerve of thigh, genitofemoral nerve, and intermediate cutaneous nerve of thigh **(Figs. 26A and B)**. They are usually involved by mesh-induced fibrosis or entrapment by a tack. The complication is prevented by avoiding fixing the mesh lateral to the deep inguinal ring in the region of the triangle of pain, safe dissection of a large hernial sac, and no dissection of fascia over the psoas.

Testicular Pain and Swelling

It occurs due to excessive dissection of a sac from the cord structures, especially a complete sac. The reported incidence is of 0.9–1.5%, and most are transient. Orchitis was found in a small number of patients but did not lead to testicular atrophy.

Mesh Infection and Wound Infection

Wound infection rates are very low. Mesh infection is a very serious complication and care must be taken to maintain strict aseptic precautions during the entire procedure. Any endogenous infection must be treated with an adequate course of antibiotics prior to surgery.

Recurrence

It is the most important endpoint of any hernia surgery. It requires a proper and thorough knowledge of anatomy and a thorough technique of repair to help keep the recurrence in endoscopic repair to a minimum.

POSTOPERATIVE RECOVERY

Marked variations are seen in postoperative recovery due to patient motivation, postoperative advice, and definition of "normal activity," existing comorbidity, and local "culture." Nevertheless all trials reporting this as an endpoint of study show a significant improvement in the laparoscopic group, with no real difference between the TAPP and TEP groups. This is estimated to equate to an absolute difference of about 7 days in terms of time off work.

RECURRENCE

Recurrence rates are low with the use of mesh and not significantly different between open or laparoscopic techniques.

CAUSES OF RECURRENCE IN LAPAROSCOPIC INGUINAL HERNIA REPAIR

The factors involved in mesh dislocation or failure are insufficient size, wrong/defective material, incorrect placement, immediate or very early displacement by folding, lifting by a hematoma or urinary retention, missed cord lipomas and herniation through the keyhole (mesh slit), late displacement by insufficient scar tissue ingrowth, mesh protrusion, collagen disease, or pronounced shrinkage. Despite the correct and stable mesh position, there is still a limited risk of a late sliding of the retroperitoneal fat under/in front of the mesh into the enlarged inner ring.

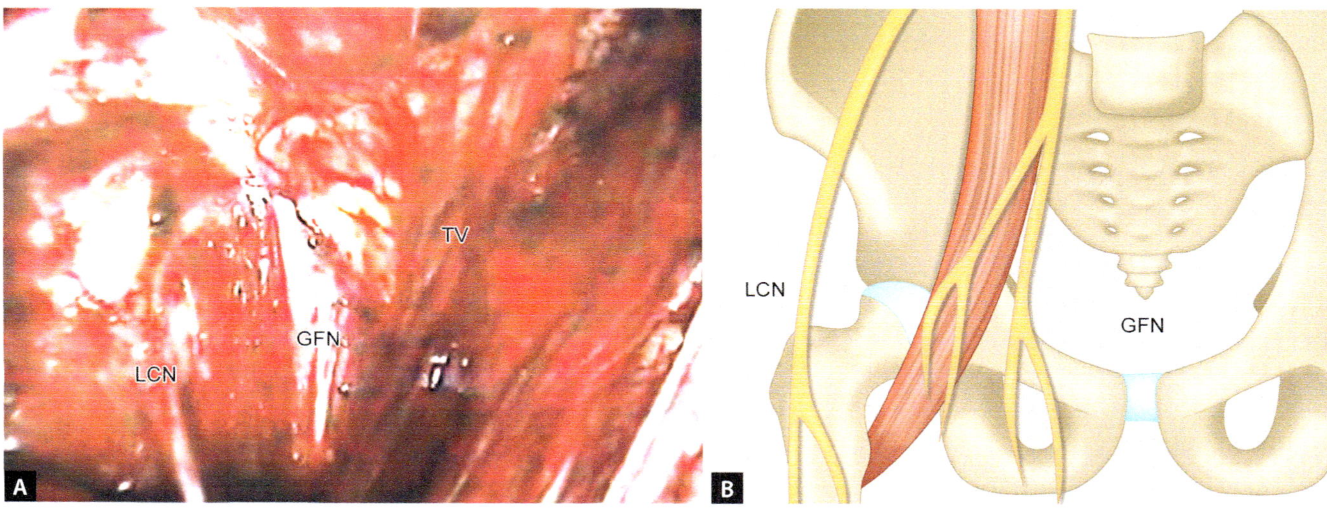

Figs. 26A and B: Anatomical landmarks.
(GFN: genitofemoral nerve, LCN: lateral cutaneous nerve; TV: testicular vessel)

Leibl in 2000 advised to avoid slitting of the mesh and increase its size to reduce the recurrence rate. Generous dissection of preperitoneal space is required to eliminate potential herniation through the slit or strangulation of the cord structures completely and also reduces the risk of genitofemoral neuropathy.

Mesh Size

The mesh size should be adequate to cover the entire myopectineal orifice. The established size in 2006 is 15 × 10 cm per unilateral hernia, with minor deviations.

Mesh Material

The mechanical strength of available meshes exceeds the intra-abdominal peak pressures and by far even the light weight meshes are strong enough for inguinal repair. Aachen group made an important contribution for understanding the interaction of the living tissue with the implanted mesh material. The negative impact of pronounced shrinkage of the traditional heavy weight meshes was recognized as an important factor promoting recurrence. Schumpelick introduced the logical trend of the use of light weight meshes. The new macroporous compound meshes present both the successful reduction of the overall foreign body amount and the preservation of mesh elasticity after the scar tissue ingrowths, due to very limited shrinkage and reduced bridging effect.

Fixation of the Mesh

In the early years of laparoscopic hernia repairs, a strong fixation seemed to be the most important factor in prevention of recurrence. With growing size of the mesh and true macroporous materials being used, the belief in strength reduced and gave way to the concern of acute/chronic pain possibly caused by fixation. The controversy of fixing or nonfixing the mesh is currently under scrutiny.

Technical Experience

The long learning curve of endoscopic repairs presents the potential risk of technical errors leading to unacceptable rise of recurrence rate. This fact highlights the need for structured well-mentored teaching, a high level of standardization of the procedure and rigorous adherence to the principles of laparoscopic hernia repair. The impact of experience on the recurrence rate was in both extremes well documented.

Collagen Status

Inborn or acquired abnormalities in collagen synthesis are associated with higher incidence of hernia formation and recurrences.

Other Factors

The negative effect on healing in hernia repair is often related with malnutrition, obesity, steroids, type II diabetes, chronic lung disease, jaundice, radiotherapy, chemotherapy, oral anticoagulants, smoking, heavy lifting, malignancy, and anemia. Laparoscopic inguinal hernia repair offers excellent results in experienced hands.

Bilateral Assessment and Treatment

Up to 30% of patients with a unilateral hernia will subsequently develop a further hernia on the contralateral side. Also, when examined at operation, 10–25% are found to have an occult hernia on the contralateral side. Both laparoscopic approaches allow assessment and treatment of the contralateral side at the same operation without the need for further surgical incisions, very little further dissection, and minimal additional postoperative pain. In open surgery, a further large incision is required in the opposite groin. This considerably impairs postoperative mobility and increases the likelihood of more admitted days in the hospital. Some surgeons advocate routine repair of the contralateral side during laparoscopic repair.

Cost Effectiveness

It is suggested that laparoscopic hernia repair is more expensive to perform than open hernia repair. The primary reason for this relates to the cost of extra equipment used for the laparoscopic repair with secondary costs attributed to perceived increases in operating time for the laparoscopic procedure. From the Indian perspective, various factors come into play when analyzing the cost implications of laparoscopic repair of inguinal hernia. In most hospitals, except the larger corporate ones, the theater time is charged on a per-case basis rather than by the hour. Thus, increase in the operating time, particularly during the learning curve, does not necessarily mean additional expense for the patient. If the surgeon were to adopt cost-containment strategies such as use of reusable laparoscopic instruments (which is more or less the norm in India) as against disposable ones, use of indigenous balloons devices rather than commercially available ones, sparing use of fixation devices, and reliance on sutures for fixation of the mesh, the cost of the laparoscopic hernia repair should be comparable to the open repair. It is likely that many surgeons are already practicing these strategies and passing on the benefits of laparoscopic repair to their patients.

Learning Curve

This period represents the developmental and learning curve for the consultant and the senior registrars. There have been some modifications of the technique as difficulties have been recognized. There is steep learning curve for laparoscopic repair. Initially, everyone used to fix mesh with staples, but nowadays many surgeons are using sutures for it. As experience increases, our ability to recognize finer structures and to keep within the correct tissue planes improves. This has been associated with lower minor-complication rates and higher percentage of pain-free recoveries.

RECOMMENDATIONS

The important points to be kept in mind during the surgery are:

- After dissecting direct sac, all peritoneal adhesions around the margin of the defect should be meticulously lysed.
- Always search for an indirect sac, even if a direct hernia has been reduced.
- Reflect the peritoneum off the cord completely.
- Place an adequate size mesh to cover the myopectineal orifice completely, preferably the size of 15 × 15 cm.
- The lower margin of the mesh must be comfortably placed—medially in the retropubic space and laterally over the psoas muscle.
- Perform a two-point fixation of the mesh on the medial aspect over the Cooper's ligament.
- Avoid cutting of the mesh over the cord. This weakens the mesh and provides a potential site for recurrence.
- Ensure adequate hemostasis prior to placing the mesh.
- The most important factor is the adequate training and learning of the right technique.

BIBLIOGRAPHY

1. Aasvang E, Kehlet H. Chronic postoperative pain: the case of inguinal herniorrhaphy. Br J Anaesth. 2005;95(1):69-76.
2. Abrahamson J. Etiology and pathophysiology of primary and recurrent groin hernia formation. Surg Clin North Am. 1998;78(6):953-72.
3. Amid PK, Shulman AG, Lichtenstein IL, Kotsifopoulos N, Stavrou A, Antonopoulos C, et al. Open "tension free" repair of inguinal hernias: the Lichtenstein technique. Eur J Surg. 1996;162(6):447-53.
4. Barkun JS, Wexler MJ, Hinchey EJ, Thibeault D, Meakins JL. Laparoscopic verus open inguinal herniorrhaphy: preliminary results of a randomized controlled trial. Surgery. 1995;118(4):703-10.
5. Bay-Nielsen M, Nilsson E, Nordin P, Kehlet H, Swedish Hernia Data Base the Danish Hernia Data Base. Chronic pain after open mesh and sutured repair of indirect inguinal hernia in young males. Br J Surg. 2004;91(10):1372-6.
6. Bay-Nielsen M, Perkins FM, Kehlet H, Danish Hernia Database. Pain and functional impairment 1 year after inguinal herniorrhaphy: a nationwide questionnaire study. Ann Surg. 2001;233(1):1-7.
7. Beets GL, Dirksen CD, Go PM, Geisler FE, Baeten CG, Kootstra G. Open or laparoscopic preperitoneal mesh repair for recurrent inguinal hernia: a randomized controlled trial. Surg Endosc. 1999;13(4):323-7.
8. Bessell JR, Baxter P, Riddell P, Watkin S, Maddern GJ. A randomized controlled trial of laparoscopic extraperitoneal hernia repair as a day surgical procedure. Surg Endosc. 1996;10(5):495-500.
9. Burney RE, Jones KR, Coon JW, Blewitt DK, Herm A, Peterson M. Core outcomes measures for inguinal hernia repair. J Am Coll Surg. 1997;185(6):509-15.
10. Callesen T, Bech K, Kehlet H. Prospective study of chronic pain after groin hernia repair. Br J Surg. 1999;86(12):1528-31.
11. Canonico S, Santoriello A, Campitiello F, Fattopace A, Corte AD, Sordelli I, et al. Mesh fixation with human fibrin glue (Tissucol) in open tension-free inguinal hernia repair: a preliminary report. Hernia. 2005;9(4):330-3.
12. Champault G, Rizk N, Catheline JM, Turner R, Boutelier P. Inguinal hernia repair: totally preperitoneal laparoscopic approach versus Stoppa operation. Randomized trial of 100 cases. Surg Laparosc Endosc. 1997;7(6):445-50.
13. Cunningham J, Temple WJ, Mitchell P, Nixon JA, Preshaw RM, Hagen NA. Cooperative hernia study. Pain in the postrepair patient. Ann Surg. 1996;224(5):598-602.
14. Damamme A, et al. Evaluation me´dico-e´conomique de la cure de hernie inguinale: Shouldice vs laparoscopie. Ann Chir 52: 11-16 29. Fuchsja 'ger N, Feichter A, Kux M. Die Lichtenstein-Plug Methode sur Reparation von Rezidivleistenhernien: Indikation, Technik und Ergebnisse. Ch. 1995;66:409-12.
15. EU Hernia Trialists Collaboration. Repair of groin hernia with synthetic mesh: meta-analysis of randomized controlled trials. Ann Surg. 2002;235(3):322-32.
16. Gerber S, Hammerli PA, Glattli A. Laparoscopic transabdominal preperitoneal hernioplasty. Evaluation of complications due to transabdominal approach. Chirurg. 2000;71(7):824-8.
17. Glassow F. Inguinal hernia repair. Am J Surg. 1976;131:306-11.
18. Grant AM, EU Hernia Trialists Collaboration. Open mesh versus non-mesh repair of groin hernia: meta-analysis of randomised trials based on individual patient data [corrected]. Hernia. 2000;6(3):130-6.
19. Heikkinen T, Haukipuro K, Leppälä J, Hulkko A. Total costs of laparoscopic and Lichtenstein inguinal hernia repairs: a randomized prospective study. Surg Laparosc Endsoc. 1997;7(1):1-5.
20. Helbling C, Schlumpf R. Sutureless Lichtenstein: first results of a prospective randomised clinical trial. Hernia. 2003;7(2):80-4.
21. Herzog U, Kocher T. Leistenhernienchirurgie in der Schweiz 1994: eine Umfrage an 142 Ausbildungskliniken in der Schweiz [Surgery of inguinal hernia in Switzerland in 1994: a survey of 142 teaching clinics in Switzerland]. Chirurg. 1996;67:921-6.
22. Hidalgo M, Castillo MJ, Eymar JL, Hidalgo A. Lichtenstein inguinal hernioplasty: sutures versus glue. Hernia. 2005;9(3):242-4.
23. Hofbauer C, Andersen PV, Juul P, Qvist N. Late mesh rejection as a complication to transabdominal preperitoneal laparoscopic hernia repair. Surg Endosc. 1998;12(9):1164-5.
24. Hyryla ML, Sintonen H. The use of health services in the management of wound infection. J Hosp Infect. 1994;26(1):1-14.
25. International Association for the Study of Pain. Classification of chronic pain. Descriptions of chronic pain syndromes and definitions of pain terms. Prepared by the International Association for the Study of Pain Subcommittee on Taxonomy. Pain Suppl. 1986;3:S1-S226.
26. Kald A, Anderberg B, Carlsson P, Park PO, Smedh K. Surgical outcome and cost-minimisation-analysis of laparoscopic and open hernia repair: a randomised prospective trial with one year follow-up. Eur J Surg. 1997;163(7):505-10.
27. Kingsnorth AN, Gray MR, Nott DM. Prospective randomized trial comparing the Shouldice and plication darn for inguinal hernia. Br J Surg. 1992;79(10):1068-70.
28. Kumar S, Wilson RG, Nixon SJ, Macintyre IM. Chronic pain after laparoscopic and open mesh repair of groin hernia. Br J Surg. 2002;89(11):1476-9.
29. Laparoscopic groin hernia trial group laparoscopic versus open repair of groin hernia: a randomised comparison.

The MRC Laparoscopic Groin Hernia Trial Group. Lancet. 1999;354(9174):185-90.

30. Lawrence K, McWhinnie D, Goodwin A, Doll H, Gordon A, Gray A, et al. Randomised controlled trial of laparoscopic versus open repair of inguinal hernia repair: early results. Br Med J. 1995;311(7011):981-5.
31. Lichtenstein IL, Shulman AG, Amid PK. The tension-free repair of groin hernias. In: Nyhus LM (Ed). Philadelphia: Hernia Lippincott; 1995. pp. 237-49.
32. Liem MS, Halsema JA, van der Graaf Y, Schrijvers AJ, van Vroonhoven TJ. Cost-effectiveness of extraperitoneal laparoscopic inguinal hernia repair: a randomized comparison with conventional herniorrhaphy. Ann Surg. 1997;226(6):668-76.
33. Liem MS, van der Graaf Y, van Steensel CJ, Boelhouwer RU, Clevers GJ, Meijer WS, et al. Comparison of conventional anterior surgery and laparoscopic surgery for inguinal hernia repair. N Engl J Med. 1997;336(22):1541-7.
34. Lorenz H, Trede M. Oral communication at the surgical week in Mexico City. TAPP vs Shouldice. Surg Week, August 1997.
35. Lowham AS, Filipi CJ, Fitzgibbons RJ, Stoppa R, Wantz GE, Felix EL, et al. Mechanisms of hernia recurrence after preperitoneal mesh repair: traditional and laparoscopic. Ann Surg. 1997;225(4):422-31.
36. Maddern GJ, Rudkin G, Bessell JR, Devitt P, Ponte L. A comparison of laparoscopic and open hernia repair as a day surgical procedure. Surg Endosc. 1994;8(12):1404-8.
37. McCormack K, Scott NW, Go PM, Ross S, Grant AM. Laparoscopic techniques versus open techniques for inguinal hernia repair. Cochrane Database Syst Rev. 2003;(1):CD001785.
38. Memon MA, Cooper NJ, Memon B, Memon MI, Abrams KR. Meta-analysis of randomized clinical trials comparing open and laparoscopic inguinal hernia repair. Br J Surg. 2003;90(12):1479-92.
39. Mikkelsen T, Werner MU, Lassen B, Kehlet H. Pain and sensory dysfunction 6 to 12 months after inguinal herniotomy. Anesth Analg. 2004;99(1):146-51.
40. Mixter CG, Meeker LD, Gavin TJ. Preemptive pain control in patients having laparoscopic hernia repair: a comparison of ketorolac and ibuprofen. Arch Surg. 1998;133(4):432-7.
41. Nilsson E, Haapaniemi S, Gruber G, Sandblom G. Methods of repair and risk for reoperation Swedish hernia surgery from 1992 to 1996. Br J Surg. 1998;85(12):1686-91.
42. Nordin P, Bartelmess P, Jansson C, Svensson C, Edlund G. Randomized trial of Lichtenstein versus Shouldice hernia repair in general surgical practice. Br J Surg. 2002;89(1):45-9.
43. Nyhus LM, Klein MS, Rogers FB. Inguinal hernia. Curr Probl Surg. 1991;28(6):401-50.
44. Payne JH Jr, Grininger LM, Izawa MT, Podoll EF, Lindahl PJ, Balfour J. Laparoscopic or open inguinal herniorraphy? A randomized prospective trial. Arch Surg. 1994;129(9):973-81.
45. Poobalan AS, Bruce J, King PM, Chambers WA, Krukowski ZH, Smith WC. Chronic pain and quality of life following open inguinal hernia repair. Br J Surg. 2001;88(8):1122-6.
46. Poobalan AS, Bruce J, Smith WC, King PM, Krukowski ZH, Chambers WA. A review of chronic pain after inguinal herniorrhaphy. Clin J Pain. 2003;19(1):48-54.
47. Rotman N, Hay JM, Lacaine F, Fagniez PL. Prophylactic antibiotherapy in abdominal surgery: first vs third-generation cephalosporins. Arch Surg. 1989;124(3):323-7.
48. Rutkow IM. The recurrence rate in hernia surgery: how important is it? Arch Surg. 1995;130(6):575-6.
49. Salcedo-Wasicek MD, Thirlby RC. Postoperative course after herniorrhaphy: a case-controlled comparison of patients receiving workers compensation vs patients with commercial insurance. Arch Surg. 1995;130(1):29-32.
50. Sales JP, Lorand I, Gayral F. Pratiques Françaises enmatie're de cure de hernie inguinale. Etude des donne´es. PMSI National 1997. In: Congre's de l'Association Françaises de Chirurgie. Paris., October. 1999;2000:4-5.
51. Schrenk P, Woisetschläger R, Rieger R, Wayand W. Prospective randomized trial comparing postoperative and return to physical activity after transabdominal preperitoneal, total preperitoneal and Shouldice techniques for inguinal hernia repair. Br J Surg. 1996;83(11):1563-6.
52. Shulman AG, Amid PK, Lichtenstein IL. The safety of mesh repair for primary inguinal hernia: results of 3,019 operations from five diverse surgical sources. Am Surg. 1992;58(4):255-7.
53. Simons MP, Hoitsma HFW, Mullan FJ. Primary inguinal hernia repair in the Netherlands. Eur J Surg. 1995;161(5):345-8.
54. Southern Surgeons Club. A prospective analysis of 1518 laparoscopic cholecystectomies. N Engl J Med. 1991;324(16): 1073-8.
55. Stoker DL, Spiegelhalter DJ, Singh R, Wellwood JM. Laparoscopic versus open inguinal hernia repair: randomized prospective trial. Lancet. 1994;343(8908):1243-5.
56. Striffeler H, Zufferey S, Schweizer W. Quality control after introduction of a new hernia technique. Barwell transversal fasciaplasty. Helv Chir Acta. 1993;59(5-6):771-4.
57. Taylor SG, O'Dwyer PJ. Chronic groin sepsis following tension-free inguinal hernioplasty. Br J Surg. 1999;86(4):562-5.
58. Topart P, Vandenbroucke F, Lozach P. Tisseel versus tack staples as mesh fixation in totally extraperitoneal laparoscopic repair of groin hernias: a retrospective analysis. Surg Endosc. 2005;19(5):724-7.
59. Vogt DM, Curet MJ, Pitcher DE, Martin DT, Zucker KA. Preliminary results of a prospective randomized trial of laparoscopic only versus conventional inguinal herniorrhaphy. Am J Surg. 1995;169:84-90.
60. Vrijland WW, van den Tol MP, Luijendijk RW, Hop WC, Busschbach JJ, de Lange DC, et al. Randomized clinical trial of nonmesh versus mesh repair of primary inguinal hernia. Br J Surg. 2002;89(3):293-7.
61. Wellwood J, Sculpher MJ, Stoker D, Nicholls GJ, Geddes C, Whitehead A, et al. Randomised controlled trial of laparscopic versus open mesh repair for inguinal hernia: outcome and cost. Br Med J. 1998;317(7151):103-10.
62. Wilson MS, Deans GT, Brough WA. Prospective trial comparing Lichtenstein with laparoscopic tension-free mesh repair of inguinal hernia. Br J Surg. 1995;82(2):274-7.
63. Wright DM, Kennedy A, Baxter JN, Fullarton GM, Fife LM, Sunderland GT, et al. Early outcome after open versus extra-peritoneal tension-free hernioplasty: a randomized clinical trial. Surgery. 1996;119(5):552-7.
64. Zieren J, Zieren HU, Jacobi CA, Wenger FA, Muller JM. Prospective randomized study comparing laparscopic and open tension-free inguinal hernia repair with Shouldice's operation. Am J Surg. 1998;175(4):330-3.

CHAPTER 17

Laparoscopic Repair of Ventral Hernia

INTRODUCTION

Ventral hernias refer to fascial defects of the anterolateral abdominal wall through which intermittent or continuous protrusion of abdominal tissue or organs may occur **(Fig. 1)**. They are either congenital or acquired. In adults, more than 80% of ventral hernias result from previous surgery, hence the term incisional hernias. They have been reported to occur after 0–26% of abdominal procedures. Although these hernias mostly become clinically manifest between 2 and 5 years after surgery, studies have shown that the process starts within the first postoperative month. They are said to occur as a result of a biomechanical failure of the acute fascial wound coupled with clinically relevant impediments to acute tissue repair and normal support function of the abdominal wall.

Historically, incisional hernias have been repaired with either primary suture techniques or placement of a variety of prosthetic materials. Before the 1960s, most ventral hernias were repaired primarily with suture and a few with metallic meshes. Even with some modifications, recurrence rates with the primary suture repair ranged from 24 to 54%. The introduction of polypropylene mesh (PPM) repair by Usher in 1958 opened a new era of tension-free herniorrhaphy. Recurrence rates with prosthetic mesh significantly decreased down to 10–20%. Subsequently, it was realized that the placement and fixation of the mesh was more crucial in determining the outcome of the repair. The concept of placement of the mesh in the preperitoneal, retromuscular position with a wide overlap of at least 5 cm over the hernia defect in all directions was introduced in the late 1980s. The refinement of this method decreased the recurrence rates to as low as 3.5% making it to be declared as the standard of care of ventral hernias. However, implantation of the mesh by open techniques requires wide dissection of soft tissue contributing to an increase in wound infection and wound-related complications.

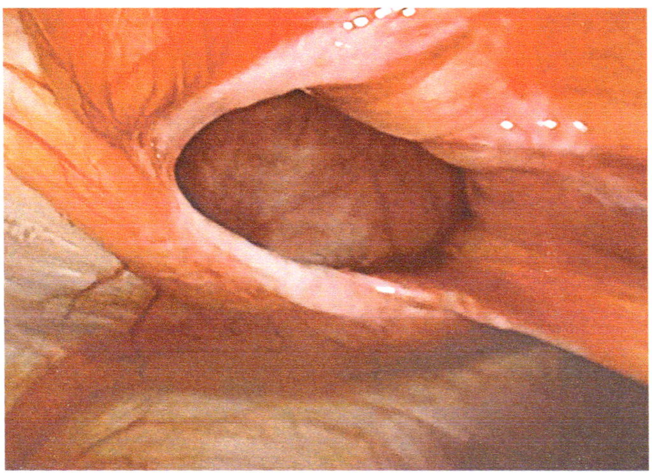

Fig. 1: Laparoscopic view of ventral hernia.

The treatment of ventral hernias (primary and incisional) represents an underappreciated challenge for surgeons. Ventral hernia results from a weakness in the musculoaponeurotic layer of the anterior abdominal wall. This type of hernia has root of development during the embryonic growth such as omphalocele, gastroschisis, and congenital umbilical hernia.

Recently, the ventral hernias are reported more due to iatrogenic factors. Even after laparoscopic surgery, if the 10-mm port is not repaired properly, there is always a chance of ventral hernia (incisional hernia) development. Obviously, the initial closure is the most important factor, since faulty technique will universally lead to development of herniation. There are other associated co-morbid conditions, which may encourage the creation of incisional herniation. These include intra-abdominal sepsis or wound infection, morbid obesity, steroid use, previous use of the incision, hematoma formation, and respiratory compromise with increased cough. Other factors include duration of the operation, crossing incisions, ineffective wound drainage, and excessive wound tension. Two other important variables include nutritional aspects as well as presence of cancer, which reduce the overall ability for wound healing and collagen deposition in the wound.

The repair of incisional and ventral hernias continues to be a surgical challenge. Reports published in the medical literature indicate 3–13% of laparotomy patients develop incisional hernias. Moreover, clinical studies indicate that the traditional, or open, technique to repair large abdominal wall defects is associated with recurrence rates ranging from 25 to 49%.

Among the noniatrogenic ventral hernias, divarication of rectus abdominis, umbilical, paraumbilical, spigelian, and epigastric are more common. In 1992, a successful series of laparoscopic incisional hernia repairs was reported in the medical literature. Since then, the technique has been refined and has grown in acceptance within the surgical community.

The laparoscopic technique for ventral hernia repair involves the placement of a tension-free prosthetic bridge across the musculofacial defect rather than attempting to approximate the edge of defect. The hernia defect is covered by appropriate size of mesh, once the content of the sac is reduced. Most of the time, sac content is omentum. Sometime omentum is adhered so strongly that electrosurgical dissection with the help of bipolar is essential. Recently, many newer types of meshes are available in which polytetrafluoroethylene (PTFE) and polypropylene are more popular. There was always a fear of bowel adhesion and fistulization with use of PPM but the clinical evidence of thousands of surgeries has suggested that the omental adhesion is expected but bowel adhesion is not common and intraperitoneal placement of PPM is quite safe.

Almost all types of ventral hernia can be repaired by minimal access surgical approach. Hernias like multiple defects (Swiss cheese hernias) are greatly benefited by this approach as all defects get directly visualized and appropriately covered by single mesh.

Contraindication of laparoscopic repair of ventral hernia is very large hernia with huge protrusion of skin, which is thin enough. Skin folds mandate correction by abdominoplasty. Dense intra-abdominal adhesions are also a relative contraindication of laparoscopic repair of ventral hernia. Ventral hernias with an associated acute moderate-to-high grade gastrointestinal tract obstruction can be difficult to repair with minimally invasive techniques. Distended bowel can easily be injured with trocar placement or manipulation with laparoscopic instruments, which could further complicate the repair, if mesh is used. Definitive treatment of ventral hernias in patients with an infected mesh and associated complications, such as enteric fistulas, often requires abdominal wall reconstruction with component separation techniques and sublay mesh placement. Intraperitoneal permanent mesh placement is generally not recommended in infected or contaminated fields, and intraperitoneal placement of biologic or bioabsorbable meshes may be associated with significantly increased rates of complications and recurrences.

LAPAROSCOPIC ANATOMY

Ventral hernia develops due to structural weakness of the abdominal wall. The muscle and fascia that span the space between costal margin superiorly, the spine and muscles of the back posteriorly, and the pelvis inferiorly support the abdominal wall by giving strength. The parietal peritoneum in ventral hernia extends into the defect to form the sac. Adhesions to adjacent viscera must be divided to define the defect. Large ventral hernias with a defect width >8–10 cm or with greater than one-half of the abdominal viscera being outside of the boundary of the abdomen, which is called loss of domain, are difficult to repair without using advanced techniques such as component separation.

OPERATIVE PROCEDURES

Commonly used techniques:

- Transabdominal preperitoneal repair (TAPP)
- Transabdominal retromuscular repair
- Transabdominal partially extraperitoneal repair (TAPE)
- Enhanced view totally extraperitoneal repair (eTEP)
- Endoscopic mini/less open sublay technique/repair (EMILOS)
- Robotic transabdominal preperitoneal repair (rTAPP)

The optimal operative management of primary ventral hernia and incisional hernia is still debatable. No single treatment has been able to tackle all ventral and incisional hernias. LeBlanc and Booth in 1993 first reported application of intraperitoneal onlay mesh (IPOM) for ventral and incisional hernia. It is a relatively straightforward procedure, which in comparison to open mesh repair has been found to reduce chances of surgical site and mesh infection. However, the technique requires expensive fixation devices, which may cause acute and chronic pain.

- *Transabdominal preperitoneal repair*: It refers to the laparoscopic ventral hernia and incisional hernia repair whereby mesh is placed in the preperitoneal space, similar to TAPP and total extraperitoneal repair (TEP) for inguinal hernia repair. It involves use of a transabdominal preperitoneal approach and can be used for midline and lateral hernias.
- *The eTEP approach*: It has been described previously for inguinal hernia repair. In ventral hernia repair, it relies on initiation of dissection in one retrorectus space and then crossover to the contralateral retrorectus space. The initial port setup and point of crossover depends on the location of defect. Patients with long midline laparotomy scar are a relative contraindication to this technique.
- *Endoscopic mini/less open sublay repair technique*: This technique is basically a reversed TEP procedure, which has been designed for midline, epigastric, umbilical, or incisional hernia with coexisting rectal diastasis. It utilizes the original MILOS concept (mini/less open sublay), which has been introduced by Reinpold. A large mesh (20 × 30) is implanted in the retromuscular space via a small skin incision (2–8 cm) without any fixation.
- *Robotic transabdominal preperitoneal repair robotic approach*: It is an emerging minimal access technique,

which utilizes set principles of open as well as conventional laparoscopic techniques. The popularity of this technique is growing in the west, attributed to its enhanced precision, 3D vision, and surgeon ergonomics. The robotic platform allows exploration of the individual abdominal wall layers and subsequent mesh placement in a preperitoneal, retromuscular, and onlay position.

Patient Position

Acutely incarcerated or strangulated ventral hernias require urgent repair. Chronic symptomatic ventral hernias may be repaired electively assuming there are no medical contraindications. Chronic ventral hernias with minimal or no symptoms may be watched, if the patient wishes to avoid surgical repair. Patient should be clearly informed that laparoscopic repairs will not help cosmetically, if the skin is lax and hanging loosely. Bowel preparation is a good practice to have more room inside the abdominal cavity to handle instruments. After anesthesia, nasogastric tube is required to deflate the stomach completely because in most of the cases, access made through left hypochondrium. Splenohepatomegaly is absolute contraindication of the access through left hypochondrium. In general, both arms should be tucked with all pressure points padded. Patients should be secured to the bed with straps to allow the bed to be steeply tilted into reverse Trendelenburg or Trendelenburg positions when necessary, depending on the location of the hernia.

Position of Surgical Team

Surgeon stands left to the patient with camera operator on his left or right side depending upon the location of ventral hernia **(Fig. 2)**. If ventral hernia is below the umbilicus, the camera operator stands right to the surgeon. If the defect is above umbilicus, camera operator should stand left to the surgeon. Monitor should be placed opposite to surgeon and instrument trolley should be toward the leg of the patient.

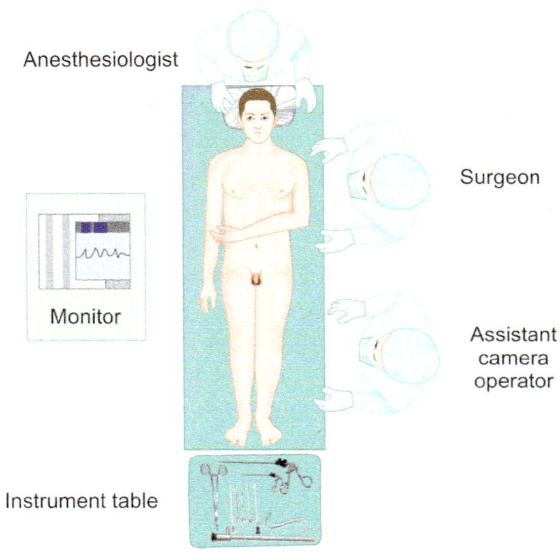

Fig. 2: Operating room setup in ventral hernia repair.

Port Position

Technique of laparoscopic repair of ventral hernia is quite simple. First pneumoperitoneum is created at a site away from the defect. Three-port techniques are used for laparoscopic repair of ventral hernia. The first step in performing laparoscopic repair of ventral hernia is gaining access to the free peritoneal cavity. A site distant from any prior incision and the hernia defect is chosen. Typically, this is in the right upper quadrant (RUQ) or left upper quadrant (LUQ) **(Figs. 3 to 7)**. The absence of incisions in these locations does not necessarily guarantee the absence of adhesions to viscera. While many approaches for access to the peritoneal cavity have been described, including blind insufflation and specialty trocars, open access in the fashion of Hasson is by far the safest alternative.

Once the pneumoperitoneum is created, all other ports are placed according to baseball diamond concept. The most preferred site of access is left hypochondrium in most midline and lower abdominal defects.

Most of the surgeons prefer optical trocar in the left subcostal location, lateral to the midclavicular line (Palmer's point). We generally go over the costal margin called Mishra's point and during access, pull the abdominal wall caudally to bring it subcostal **(Fig. 4)**. First access should be preferably through left hypochondria, if Veress needle technique is used and then two other ports should be made so that proper triangle is formed. The distance between two ports should not be less than 5 cm **(Fig. 3)**.

The telescope will first enter through left hypochondriac port but once dissection starts, the telescope will come in the middle, so that the angle between two working ports will become 60°. The 10-mm 30° telescope is better to view anterior abdominal wall **(Fig. 7)**.

Achieving free access to the peritoneal cavity represents the greatest risk to the patient. For most ventral incisional

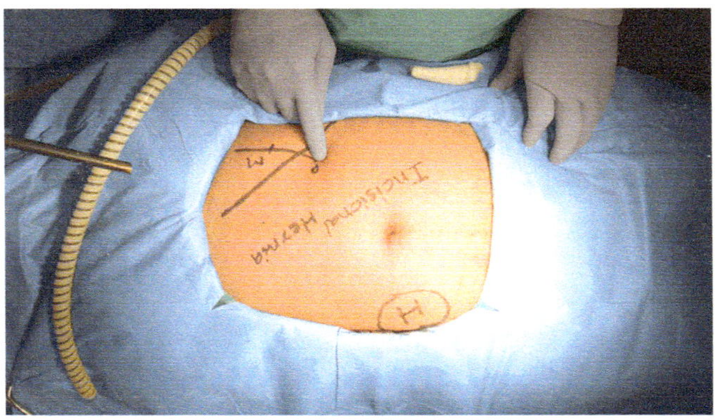

Fig. 3: Palmer's point is used for access.

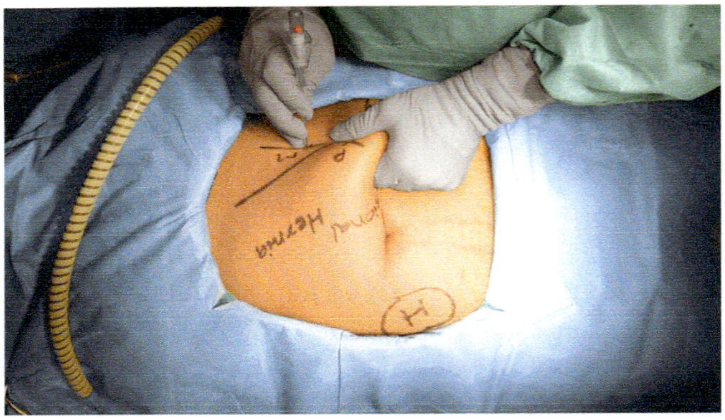

Fig. 4: Veress needle introduction through Palmer's point.

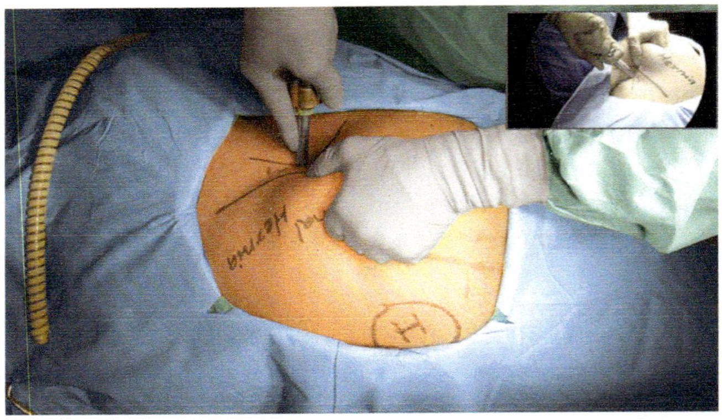

Fig. 5: Palmer's point is used for trocar introduction.

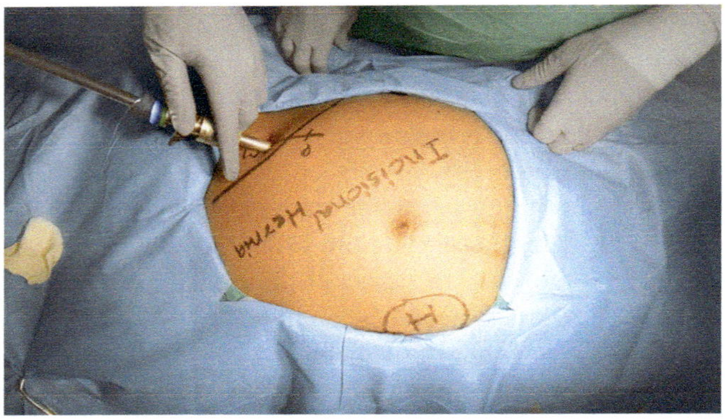

Fig. 6: Telescope is introduced to check any adhesion.

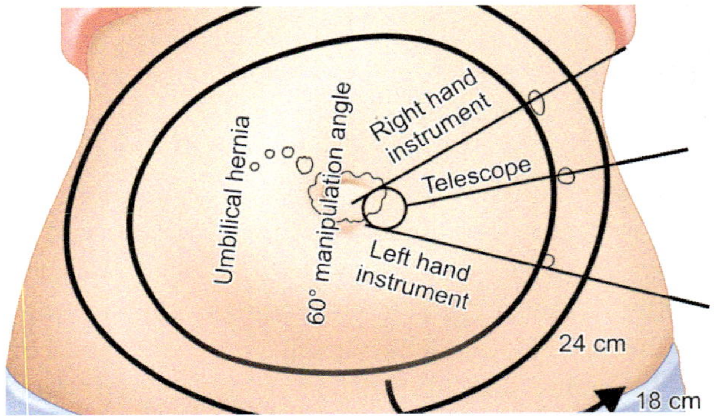

Fig. 7: Secondary ports are introduced.

hernia repairs, adhesiolysis is required to make room for subsequent mesh insertion, manipulation, and fixation. The difficulty of adhesiolysis is unpredictable, and the presence of PPM should be a red flag indicating the potential for the presence of dense and difficult to dissect adhesions, often involving the bowel. All maneuvers performed as part of the lysis of adhesions must be done under direct vision. This is best carried out by sharp dissection utilizing bimanual palpation of the anterior abdominal wall, placing the adhesions under variable degrees of tension **(Figs. 8 and 9)**.

There is significant risk in extensive blunt dissection, as the bowel may be fixed at several points placing it at risk for unrecognized perforation with the tip of dissecting instruments. In spite of the enthusiasm for different energy sources, these are best avoided. As in open cases, dissection should be carried out at the avascular junction of the adhesions and the anterior abdominal wall. Ligating clips or the limited application of an energy source can be used when significant bleeding from vessels is encountered. In the majority of cases, even this is unnecessary. The risk of monopolar cautery is well known, but there is also risk of thermal injury by direct contact with ultrasonic or radio frequency dissection instruments. Ultrasonic dissector should be preferred over monopolar. If bowel is incarcerated, cold scissor dissection should be preferred rather than energy. This is particularly true in the poorly visualized area behind adhesions.

If omentum is adhered with the anterior abdominal wall, it should be dissected after applying bipolar or extracorporeal knot **(Figs. 10A and B)**. It is critical that all adhesions to the anterior abdominal wall be released to allow adequate patch placement and fixation.

Once adhesiolysis has been completed, the exact extent of the defect can be directly evaluated. The defects are carefully drawn onto the skin of the anterior abdominal **(Figs. 11A to C)**. In the case of multiple defects, the area drawn should include all of the defects. We have transformed now to repairing the entire area of a previous incision as opposed to simply repairing a single defect. There have been a number of patients who have presented later in follow-up and are discovered to have a new hernia, outside the area of previous repair. In open surgery, these may have unknowingly simply been considered recurrences. If there is any difficulty in delineating the margins of the defect, a spinal needle can be passed perpendicular to the anterior abdominal wall and through the margins of the defect.

The selection of size of mesh is important to prevent recurrence of hernia and it should be sufficiently big so that approximately 4 cm healthy margin of defect of hernia should be covered all around. Recently, new hybrid mesh has been introduced with absorbable material on one side and unabsorbable prolene on the other. These meshes are better than prolene because adhesions are less likely to develop due to absorbable material toward the bowel.

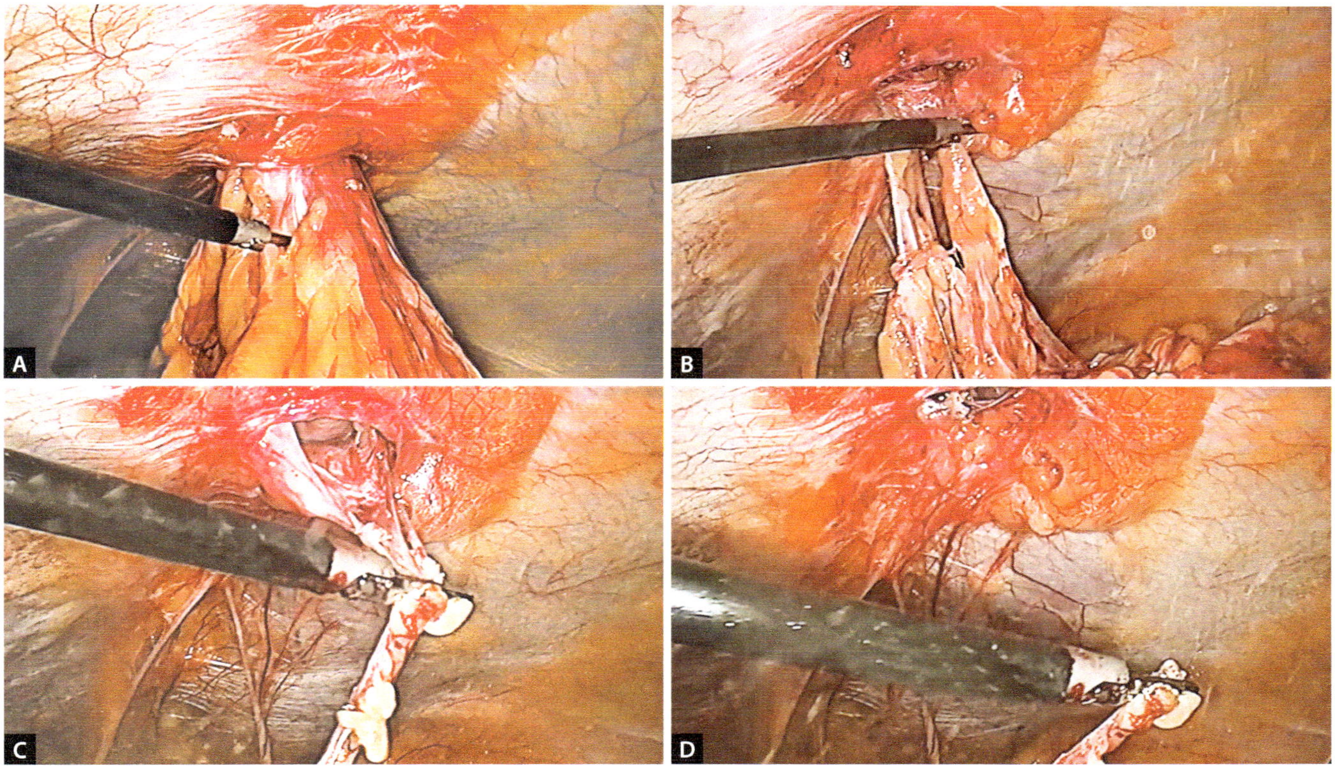

Figs. 8A to D: Any adhesion should be removed with bipolar and scissors.

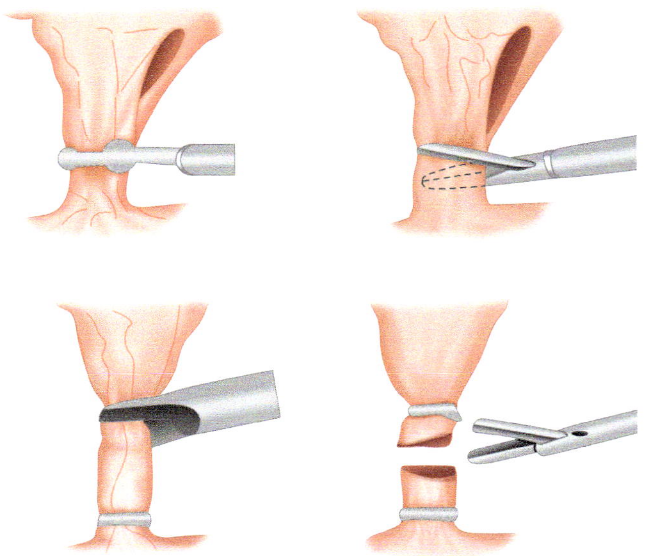

Fig. 9: Bipolar can be used safely in case of adhesion with omentum.

The mesh is fixed along margins and around the ring of defect of rectus to ensure a close approximation of mesh to abdominal wall. Care should be taken that mesh should not be corrugated and it should be in proper contact with anterior abdominal wall. Tacker, Protack, or Endo anchor can be used to fix the mesh. Fibrin glue has been used to fix the mesh, but less frequently. Because of a higher-than-expected recurrence rate at 1 year (26% fibrin sealant versus 6% tacks) in a trial of umbilical hernia repairs, this technique should be avoided until further studies demonstrate safety and efficacy. After fixing the mesh, greater omentum is spread like an apron in-between the bowel and mesh **(Figs. 12A and B)**. Some adhesions of mesh with omentum are always expected in this technique. Very high epigastric hernias close to the costal margin are best managed by leaving an overhang of mesh draped over the diaphragm without fixation. Fixation with tacks to the diaphragm should be avoided, as it has been associated with serious complications such as lung and cardiac injuries (tamponade). If patient is mobilized early and newer generations of meshes are used, the long-term complication of adhesions is very less with this technique.

Loosely held mesh hanging through the anterior abdominal wall will definitely increase the chances of adhesions with bowel. Tacker should be used to fix the mesh in position. Recently, a technique of using prolene suture to fix the mesh with anterior abdominal wall is being used with the help of suture passer or looping technique with the help of Veress needle cannula (transfascial suture). The main idea of this method is to reduce the cost of surgery, but there is increased chance of infection and adhesions with this method. We also lack any long-term randomized controlled trial (RCT) to prove the outcome of this external suture technique to fix the mesh in ventral hernia repair. Meshes can be fixated to the anterior abdominal wall with transfascial sutures, tacks, or a combination of the two. If no transfascial sutures are placed, two rows of permanent tacks

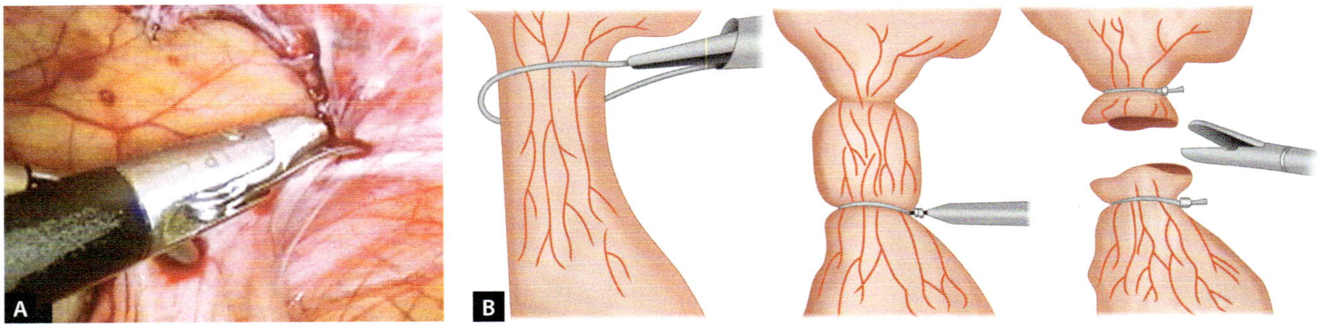

Figs. 10A and B: Extracorporeal knot can be used in case of adhesion with omentum.

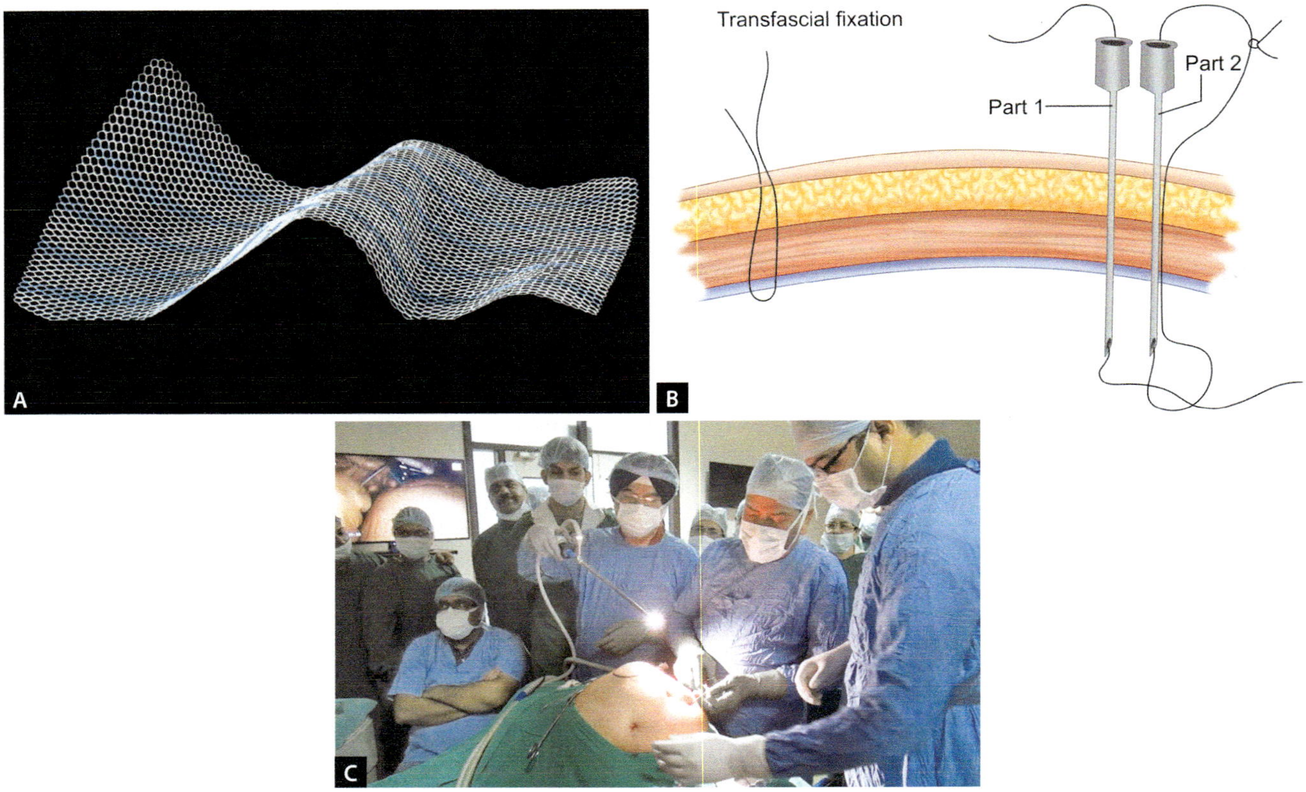

Figs. 11A to C: (A) Appropriate size of mesh should be used to prevent recurrence; (B) Transfascial fixation of the mesh with suture inside view; (C) Transfascial fixation of the mesh outside view.

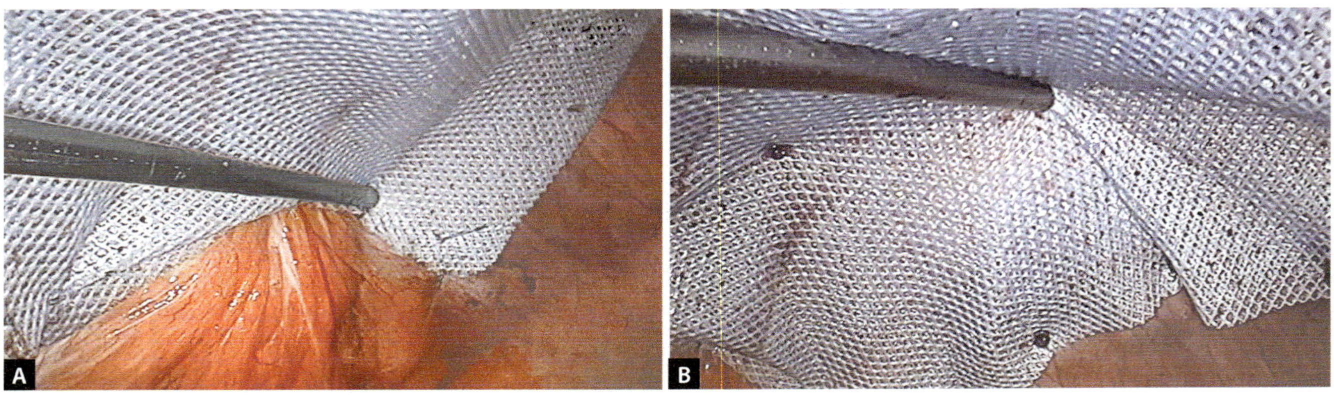

Figs. 12A and B: Fixation of mesh can be accomplished outer and inner crowning.

should be used to fixate the mesh; if transfascial sutures are used, one or two rows of either absorbable or permanent tacks may be placed at the surgeon's discretion.

To place transfascial sutures, multiple small "stab" incisions are made in the skin at locations that correspond to those of the previously placed sutures on the mesh **(Figs. 11B and C)**. A transcutaneous laparoscopic suture-passing device is advanced through the stab wound into the peritoneum. The assistant uses a laparoscopic grasper to feed each end of the sutures into the jaws of the awaiting suture passing device, which, when closed, brings the suture through the abdominal wall. Once all the sutures are brought through the abdominal wall, the peritoneal cavity is desufflated and the sutures are tied. The peritoneal cavity is then reinsufflated to a lower pressure (8 mm Hg), and the mesh is examined laparoscopically to ensure appropriate coverage of fascial defect as well as appropriate apposition to the abdominal wall. The mesh is then additionally fixated utilizing single or double rows (outer and inner crowning) of absorbable or permanent tacks, per surgeon preference. If transfascial sutures are not utilized, the stay stitch on the mesh is generally brought through the abdominal wall at the center of the hernia fascial defect to facilitate mesh fixation with a double crown of permanent tacks. Other commercially available mesh positioning devices are available but may be difficult to place.

CHOICE OF MESH IN VENTRAL HERNIA

Synthetic Materials

A variety of synthetic polymeric meshes were developed in the second half of the 20th century, which revolutionized the hernia repair. Meshes can be categorized in terms of weight, pore size, material, fiber type, and flexibility. Heavyweight meshes tend to form a dense scar plate and are best suited to applications where mechanical stability is a factor. Lightweight meshes are formed from thin fibers and are designed to flex with normal physiological movement. They form a flexible scar and may cause less discomfort than heavyweight meshes. Fibers may be monofilament or multifilament, and the gaps between the fibers, known as pores, can vary depending on the design.

In general, a smaller pore size reduces the ability of the mesh to be incorporated into the body's own tissues, which may a desirable quality, if the mesh is to be used around delicate bowel tissue, to avoid unwanted adhesions. Meshes of the same material may differ between manufacturers in terms of weight, flexibility, shrinkage, and potential for adhesion formation. With these meshes, abdominal wall defects could be repaired without undue tension on the sutured tissue, decreasing the high recurrence rates of abdominal wall hernia repair.

Sir Francis Usher introduced woven monofilament PPM in 1958. It was modified to a knitted mesh in 1962 so that the mesh would not unravel when it was cut. PPM gained widespread popularity over the next 30 years and several types of PPM are commercially available today. Polyester mesh was also introduced in the 1950s in Europe. Rives and Stoppa employed polyester mesh in their landmark article describing a preperitoneal technique of ventral hernia repair in 1989. The technique described by Rives and Stoppa has become the standard by which all abdominal wall incisional hernia repairs are measured. PPM and polyester mesh revolutionized abdominal wall repair because the meshes did not deteriorate with age, were pliable, and would stretch, allowing for more even load distribution. Nevertheless, the large interstices in polypropylene and polyester mesh promoted adhesion formation when the mesh came into contact with the visceral abdominal cavity. Reported complications included small bowel obstruction, erosion, and fistulization.

Expanded polytetrafluoroethylene (ePTFE), initially used as a vascular prosthesis, was adapted for abdominal wall incisional hernia repair in 1983 by WL Gore and Associates and modified several times in the 1990s. Unlike the polypropylene and polyester meshes that preceded it, ePTFE is microporous and select products are uniquely designed with pores measuring 3 μ on the visceral side facing the abdominal cavity and 22 μ facing the abdominal wall. This design promotes fibroblastic and vascular ingrowth from the abdominal wall 22 μ side, but inhibits tissue attachment to the material on 3 μ side when exposed to the intra-abdominal cavity. There are no reports of fistulization or small bowel obstructions due to adhesions from ePTFE material.

Synthetic meshes, made of materials such as ePTFE and polypropylene, are used most of the time for repair of hernia. The repair process for these materials is based on scar formation in and around the mesh. The advantage of using these materials is that they generally do not react with the human tissue. They are strong and do not tear easily, are readily available, inexpensive, and have a long history of being used for soft tissue replacements.

However, use of synthetic materials is not without problems. As a foreign material, body may react to its presence by growing around it (encapsulation) in an attempt to exclude it from body. In the process, tissue forms a capsule of rigid, fibrous scar tissue around the synthetic material. The rigid capsule could affect the function and the esthetic outcome of the repair. Furthermore, foreign bodies such as synthetic materials increase the risk of infection when implanted in the body. As part of the foreign body response, the repair site may be subjected to inflammation, infection, and pain.

Surgisis

It is porcine intestinal submucosa and specifically designed as a surgical graft for hernia and abdominal body wall

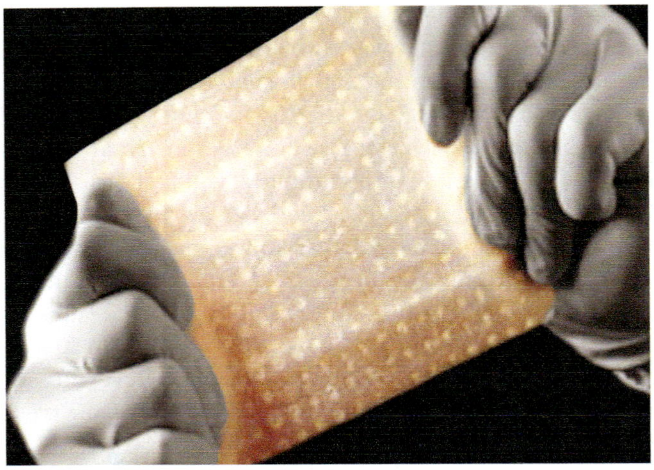

Fig. 13: Surgisis.

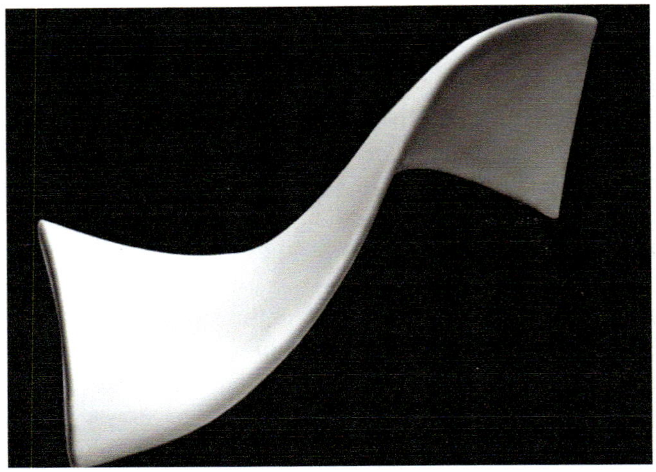

Fig. 14: AlloDerm.

repair **(Fig. 13)**. Surgisis® Gold™ combines strength with flexibility in a naturally occurring graft material that allows for hernia repair without the need for a permanent synthetic prosthesis. Surgisis® Gold™ supports the surgical site while the body's natural healing process replaces the graft with new host tissue. It is collagen biomatrix, naturally occurring and acellular with 18 months shelf-life.

AlloDerm

It is biological dermal matrix from processed donated human tissue **(Fig. 14)**. AlloDerm is processed from donated human skin. The tissue goes through a cell removal process while retaining the important biochemical and structural components. AlloDerm is, thus, acellular human tissue. Since AlloDerm is derived from human tissue, there may be a concern that it might harbor disease-carrying viruses. Tissue donors are screened and tested for transmissible diseases including HIV, hepatitis, and syphilis before tissue processing. AlloDerm has been utilized in more than 750,000 implants and grafts to date, without any reported incidence of viral disease transmission to a patient. AlloDerm repairs damaged tissue by providing a foundation for new tissue regeneration. The skin components preserved in AlloDerm contain the information that will help your own tissue to grow into the AlloDerm after placement at the repair site.

Proceed Mesh

It is soft PPM covered with polydioxanone (PDS) and oxidized regenerated cellulose fabric **(Fig. 15)**.

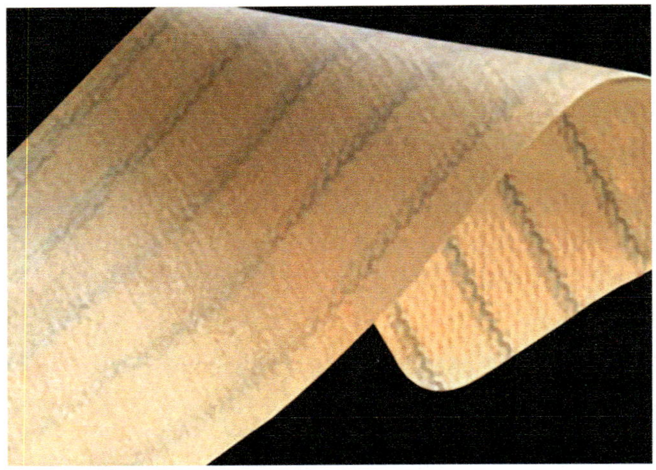

Fig. 15: Proceed mesh.

Titanized Polypropylene Mesh

Despite the vast selection of mesh for hernia repair available, nearly all synthetic meshes for hernia surgery continue to use one or other of three basic materials—polypropylene, polyester, and ePTFE. These are used in combination with each other or with a range of additional materials such as titanium, omega-3, monocryl, PVDF, and hyaluronate. Titanized mesh is a lightweight, monofilamentous PPM with a weight of 45 g/m^2 and a pore size of 3.0 mm. The polypropylene filaments are coated with titanium dioxide. In the tetanized mesh, the polypropylene filaments are coated with a few layers of atomic titanium using what is known as the PACVD (plasma-activated chemical vapor deposition) technique **(Fig. 11)**.

Polyurethane-covered Mesh

Polyurethane-coated mesh has a permeable peritoneal side (white color) in polyester for excellent fibroblast colonization and rapid tissue fixation; and a nonabsorbable and nonadherent (blue color) smooth side in polyurethane allowing fluid transfer and contact with viscera. The dual-side mesh is equipped with sutures and has a visual mark printed on polyester for easy transfascial mesh centering in IPOM inguinal hernia surgery.

Biological Mesh

Biological meshes, derived from animal tissues such as porcine skin or bovine pericardium, can be a useful alternative to synthetic fabrics under certain circumstances. Such products are expensive, and can stretch out over time, but offer significantly reduced susceptibility to infection relative to synthetic products. A fully synthetic long-term absorbable mesh made from a combination of fast and slow absorbing fibers has also been developed. The basic concept behind the development of these types of materials is that—they provide proper environment for the population of native cells, generation of connective tissue which ultimately leads to the replacement of defective tissue present in the hernia defect. Although biological meshes show great promise in repairing hernia, currently surgeons are hesitant to opt for this over synthetic mesh materials. Because the connective tissue formed by these materials is only 70–80% strong, emphasizing the inherent defect of their native tissue. Therefore, there is a greater chance for the recurrence of hernia upon usage of these meshes.

PREPERITONEAL REPAIR OF VENTRAL HERNIA

This technique is also called inlay technique of laparoscopic ventral hernia repair. The peritoneum is incised and preperitoneal space is created in this technique. The sac of the hernia is excised nicely. It can give some extra flap of peritoneum for successful overlapping of both the edges. In this technique, margin of defect is sutured intracorporeally to decrease the gap. Pressing the abdominal wall on both the side from outside will help to obliterate the space in this hernia surgery. Either intracorporeal stitches or external mattress sutures can be used to fix the mesh to the musculofacial defect. Once the mesh is fixed, the peritoneum is sutured using Vicryl to cover the mesh. This method of laparoscopic ventral hernia repair (LVHR) is same as that of open surgery and it is supposed that formation of adhesion is less.

MINIMALLY INVASIVE COMPONENT SEPARATION

In laparoscopic ventral hernia repair, it is often difficult to achieve primary fascial closure in patients with large fascial defects (width >8–12 cm) without a relaxing incision. In open ventral hernia repair, component separation is the most commonly used technique to achieve midline fascial closure. Laparoscopic and robotic-assisted component separation techniques have been described, which can be used to facilitate primary fascial closure in laparoscopic ventral hernia repair. The increasing popularity of minimally invasive techniques, particularly robotic techniques, for abdominal wall reconstruction has led to increased use of robotic posterior component separation techniques. The complication rates of minimally invasive component separation techniques are more challenging than those of traditional open component separation techniques.

EXTENDED TOTALLY EXTRAPERITONEAL REPAIR FOR VENTRAL HERNIAS

Enhanced view TEP approaches for laparoscopic repairs of incisional and ventral hernias have been described in many recent case series. Extended totally extraperitoneal repair is a novel technique that was first introduced by Jorge Daes in 2012 to address difficult inguinal hernias. The principle is to create a larger space than what is done in TEP to tackle large groin hernias. Purported advantages include the ability to place wide pieces of mesh in the retrorectus/retromuscular spaces. It may also help to facilitate minimally invasive primary fascial closure in the cases of large fascial defects requiring posterior (transversus abdominis) component release techniques.

COMPLICATIONS

- Bowel adhesion
- Fistulization
- Nerve injury
- Vascular injury
- Seroma
- Infection and cellulitis
- Recurrence
- Pain

Multiple studies have documented that open hernioplasty has significant morbidity. Leber reported a 27% long-term complication rate with open repair, among them being infection, hematoma and seroma, chronic sinus tract formation, mesh extrusion, fistula formation as well as soft tissue problems such as nonhealing wound. White reported 34% of 250 open ventral hernia repairs had wound-related complications. The complications of the open repair mainly relate to the type of mesh that is most commonly used (polypropylene and polyester meshes). In addition, the wide dissection of soft tissue that is required for a Stoppa-type retrorectus repair or a Chevrel-type anterior repair leads to the many wound-related problems.

Some patients will develop a fluid collection, what is commonly called a seroma, between the mesh and the abdominal wall. Many of these are not apparent to the patient or the surgeon but some are evident and can be bothersome to the patient. Complications from these seromas have been reported in many studies. Most surgeons do not aspirate these fluid collections for fear of infecting the prosthesis. However, the author has freely aspirated the seromas, if they are large or if they are bothersome to the patient. The author has never seen an infection of the prosthesis from aspiration of these fluid collections if full aseptic precautions are taken.

Probably, the most dreaded complication that has been seen is bowel injury. Enterotomy is a well-documented complication and commonly occurs and can be readily visualized and handled through an incision. Laparoscopy presents a whole new situation with respect to enterotomy.

Prevention is the first line of defense. Lysis of adhesions is well visualized due to the magnification and high-intensity light source inherent in the laparoscopic technique. It is very important that energy sources be used very sparingly if at all during lysis of adhesions. If a surgeon enters the proper planes, there is very little bleeding and thus low need for energy sources. Inappropriate use of energy sources is a common cause of unrecognized enterotomy. Monopolar cautery has the problem of current spread, and it is easy to coagulate one area and see the current spread to the adjacent area instantaneously. For this reason, monopolar cautery should not be used adjacent to the bowel. The ultrasonic or radio frequency dissection instruments are "sold" with the supposed advantage that there is minimal thermal spread unlike monopolar cautery. Although this may be true, the tip remains very hot and any touching of viscera can cause a burn that may not be apparent during the operation. It is only after several hours, either that night or the next day, when the tissue sloughs, that is when the enterotomy presents itself. We do not recommend the use of ultrasonic or radio frequency dissection instruments for this reason. The most important thing to remember is that if lysis of adhesions involving the intestine is not safe, i.e., the surgeon cannot see well or the surgeon cannot determine if an enterotomy has occurred, the patient should be opened! Deaths have been reported from laparoscopic incisional hernioplasty due to bowel injuries that have not been perceived during surgery and only become apparent postoperatively. By the time, the diagnosis is made, the patients are generally septic, and may succumb to this complication.

DISCUSSION

Initially described in 1992, laparoscopic repair of incisional hernias has evolved from an investigational procedure to one that can safely and successfully be used to repair ventral hernias. The well-established benefits of laparoscopy repair are less postoperative pain, reduced hospital stay and recovery time, low complication and recurrence rates based on numerous reports, meta-analysis, and few randomized trials. Conventionally, the LVHR entails the intraperitoneal placement and fixation of the prosthetic mesh. Many alternative techniques have been tried in few studies and propose to be an advancement of the conventional approach.

Despite its significant prevalence and associated morbidity, there is little in the way of evidence-based guidelines regarding the timing and method of repair of ventral and particularly, incisional hernias. Several large studies on LVHR have been reported. This technique has proven to be a safe and feasible alternative to open mesh repair. Although many are retrospective series and a few comparative studies, only two completed randomized trials comparing open versus laparoscopic mesh repair have been published. Based on these studies, LVHR has been found to have shorter operating time depending on the surgeon's experience, shorter hospital stay, and lower complication rates especially wound and mesh infections and lower recurrence rate during the follow-up period. This evidence has led to the suggestion that now; it would be unethical to conduct a prospective RCT comparing LVHR and open approach.

Laparoscopic ventral hernia repair techniques are based on the fundamental principles of the open preperitoneal repair described by Stoppa and Rives. The placement of a large mesh in the preperitoneal location allows for an even distribution of forces along the surface area of the mesh, which may account for the strength of the repair and the decreased recurrence associated with it. The repair capitalizes on the physics of Pascal's principle of hydrostatics by using the forces that create the hernia defect to hold the mesh in place. For this, to attain maximum effect, there has to be a wide mesh overlap over the defect and adequate, secure fixation. In the open approach, attaining an overlap of 3–5 cm requires extensive soft tissue dissection, with the resultant increase in wound complications. Larger defects should require more overlap and smaller ones theoretically less. The laparoscopic approach not only allows clear definition of the defect margins but also the identification of additional defects that may not have been clinically apparent preoperatively.

Both the inlay and onlay placements of prosthetic mesh embrace these fundamental principles of hernia repair. The onlay and the transabdominal inlay methods allow for adequate diagnostic laparoscopy to clearly define the margins and the number of the hernia defects including the occult ones.

MESH PLACEMENT AND FIXATION

One of the critical technical points that significantly impacts on any method of hernia mesh repair is adequate mesh fixation. The mesh is held in position by sutures and/or staples, clips, tacks, intra-abdominal pressure, and later by fibrinous growth. The most widespread technique in onlay approach involves fixation of mesh with tacks and transabdominal permanent sutures. Some surgeons have tried to reduce the operating and possibly postoperative discomfort by reducing or eliminating the use of sutures. The physics of mesh fixation does not support the sole placement of tacks. Majority of the meshes used are about 1-mm thick. A perfectly placed tack can be expected to penetrate only 2 mm beyond the mesh thus tacks will not give the same holding strength as full-thickness abdominal wall suture. Furthermore, the mesh is placed against the peritoneum, so any ingrowth is most likely into the peritoneum and not into the fascia.

Detachment of tacks has also been an attributing factor to some recurrence of hernias. Postoperative recurrence of ventral hernia repair is reported to be as high as 13% when only a stapling, clipping, or the tacking device is used for mesh fixation. Proper use of the transfascial fixation sutures in combination with staples decreased the recurrence rate to as low as 2%. Therefore, the current recommendation for mesh fixation is that a transfascial suture should be placed at a distance of 5 cm each along the perimeter of the mesh and tacking devices be used to affix the edge of the mesh at 1-cm intervals. The preperitoneal approach mesh fixation differs in that, there is immediate and continued fixation by the intact peritoneal sac and whether tacks or sutures or both are used, they fix the mesh directly onto the fascia. The primary concern of the peritoneal flap in the inlay technique is to achieve secure fixation of the mesh to the underlying fascia. The fibrinous ingrowth is from the fascia and not the peritoneum. Furthermore, the preperitoneal positioning confers with the original design of Stoppa.

Perhaps the most compelling advantage of the preperitoneal placement of the mesh in the inlay approach is the avoidance of direct interaction between the mesh and the intra-abdominal viscera. Contact of the viscera with foreign material such as the prosthesis may lead to an inflammatory response and adhesion formation, which can induce chronic pain, intestinal obstruction, enterocutaneous fistula, and infertility. In addition, adhesions complicate any future intra-abdominal surgery. The peritoneal covering also allows the use of conventional meshes, which have been associated with intense inflammatory response and adhesion formation by some workers. The choice of the mesh used in LVHR may be the most contentious issue, particularly when financial cost is a major consideration.

The biomaterials available for ventral hernia repair have undergone many changes over the last several years. There are new products that have either been recently introduced or are in developmental stages. All seek to achieve two goals—rapid and permanent ingrowth into the body wall and diminution of the risk of intestinal adhesions while maintaining its tensile strength. The visceral side should be smooth, nonerosive antiadhesive, and not easily susceptible to infection. This visceral barrier should be present for at least 1 week because this is the time frame in which adhesions form. The ventral side should be macroporous allowing for fibroblast in growth and a foreign body reaction may be necessary for incorporation and high-tensile strength.

Polypropylene (prolene) mesh, introduced by Sir Francis Usher in 1958 and modified in 1962, has gained widespread popularity and several types are commercially available today. Polyester mesh was introduced in Europe in the 1950s. Stoppa used the polyester mesh in their landmark article describing preperitoneal repair of ventral hernia in 1989. Prolene mesh is currently the most widely used because it is relatively inexpensive, easy to handle, has a memory (allows them to regain the original shape), and is firmly incorporated in the abdominal wall due to its ability to induce an intense inflammatory reaction. A 2–5% fistula rate has been reported with PPM used intra-abdominally leading to the suggestion that great care must be taken to separate it from the bowel, if it has to be used at all. However, some studies do not support this view. Bingener found no association of visceral adhesion when prolene was used with adequate omental interposition between it and the bowel. In another study involving 136 patients, Vrijland concluded that enterocutaneous fistula appears to be very rare after prolene mesh repair regardless of intraperitoneal placement, omental coverage, or closing the peritoneum.

A study comparing the biomaterials used in LVHR found polyester to have the highest incidence of infection, fistulization, and recurrence. The ePTFE has the longest history in the use for these hernias repair. The original description of the procedure used an early generation of the ePTFE product. The current product has one smooth surface with 3 μ ePTFE interstices, while the other side has 22 μ interstices to facilitate fibroblastic ingrowth for firm fixation. Other modifications of this product involve incorporation of antimicrobials on the visceral surface. All of the composite prostheses have ePTFE and prolene or polyester but differ in the number and attachment of them together. There are no reports of intestinal fistulization or obstruction with ePTFE though it has also been found to induce inflammation and fibrosis in laboratory animals.

However, the use of synthetic materials is not without problems. As a foreign material, the repair site is subjected to inflammation, susceptibility to infection and pain as a foreign body response. Encapsulation could affect the elastic function of the abdominal wall and esthetic outcome of the repair. This has stimulated the search for natural biological prostheses such as surgisis, collagen, glycosaminoglycans from porcine intestinal submucosa, and AlloDerm. The financial cost to clinical benefit ratio for use of the substantially expensive composite meshes is unquantified and is likely to remain, as such because, given the widespread acceptance of composite products, a randomized, clinical comparison with prolene is unlikely to occur. Therefore, in selected circumstances, it may be acceptable to use a simple mesh, if this can be excluded from the bowel by tissue interposition be it omentum or peritoneum. A composite mesh should be considered as the current standard of care.

The extraperitoneal placement of the prostheses would in principle diminish the intra-abdominal complications associated with formation of adhesions. It would also allow the safe use of the conventional meshes such as prolene, which has high intrinsic tensile strength, good memory, and is cheaper. In addition, the peritoneal coverage over the entire mesh provides additional security of fixation and a better mechanical advantage. As such, it can be seen as an advance over the onlay approach. However, the placement is technically demanding as evidenced by the high-iatrogenic peritoneal tears in the largest series and it may not be feasible in the scarred abdomen of incisional and recurrent hernias, which constitute the bulk and seems to benefit most, from LVHR. Thus, the issue of limitation of patient population among the technical feasibility and adequacy of defect coverage are issues of great concern before the method is accepted as an additional procedure for LVHR.

The good results and the attributed safety of LVHR are based on the large number of studies mainly utilizing the intraperitoneal approach. The generalization of the procedure has resulted in multiple variations of techniques. Overall, fewer complications are reported after LVHR than after open mesh repair, especially in relation to wound and mesh infection. The efficacy of the inlay approach as an advancement of the conventional repair needs to be evaluated in terms of the several specific complications that are of particular relevance in laparoscopic procedures.

BOWEL INJURY

Probably the most dreaded complication is bowel injury, and particularly if it is missed intraoperatively. It is a potentially lethal complication. The overall incidence of bowel injury does not differ significantly between open repair and laparoscopic repair and is generally low with either approach (1–5% when serosal injuries are included). Pneumoperitoneum may hinder the recognition of bowel injury at the time of operation. There have also been reports of late bowel perforation secondary to thermal injury with laparoscopic repair.

Minimizing the use of electrocauterization and ultrasonic dissection markedly reduces the risk of bowel injury. The visualization afforded by the pneumoperitoneum places adhesions between the abdominal wall and the bowel under tension. The high-intensity light source and the magnification inherent in the laparoscopy facilitate identification of the least vascularized planes. As far as possible, direct grasping, the bowel should be avoided preferring simply to push it or to grasp the adhesions themselves to provide countertraction. External pressure on the hernia may also help. Larger vessels in the omentum or adhesions are controlled with clips. Some degree of oozing from the dissected areas is tolerated; such oozing almost always settles down without specific hemostatic measures.

ADHESION (FIG. 16)

In cases of dense adhesions, it is preferable to divide the sac or the fascia rather than risk injury to bowel **(Fig. 1)**. Densely, adherent PPM is best excised along with the abdominal wall rather than attempting to separate it from the serosa of the bowel. If bowel injury is suspected, immediate and thorough inspection should be carried out. It may be difficult or impossible to find the exact site of injury later once the bowel has been released and freed of its attachments. Once the injury is recognized, it is the surgeon's level of comfort with laparoscopic suture repair that determines the best approach. With minimal spillage of bowel contents, the injury may be treated with either laparoscopic repair or open repair; the latter usually can be carried out through a mini-laparotomy over the injured area. Whether the mesh prosthesis is put primarily or later depends on the degree of contamination. More significant bowel injuries necessitate conversion to open repair. Missed injuries manifest postoperatively mandating re-exploration with occasional removal of the mesh and immediate recurrence of the hernia.

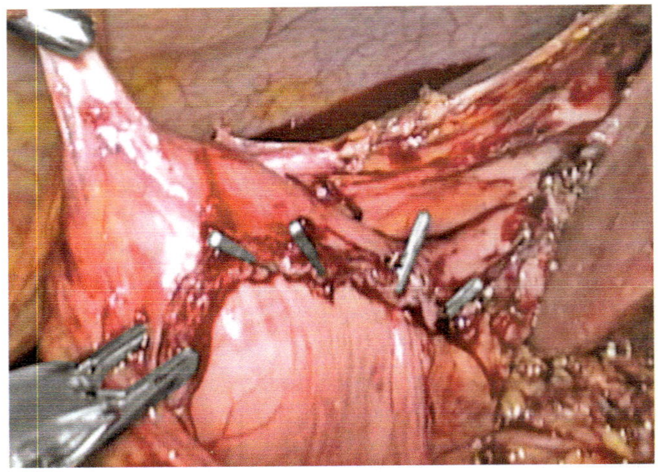

Fig. 16: Adhesiolysis for adhesion developed during previous intraperitoneal onlay mesh (IPOM).

CELLULITIS

Compared with open ventral hernia repair, laparoscopic repair causes fewer surgical site infections, both superficial and deep. About 2–4% of patients develop abdominal wall cellulitis after laparoscopic ventral hernia repair as a result of either infection or inflammatory response to the prosthetic mesh. Postoperative cellulitis can be treated with antibiotics.

SEROMA

Seroma formation is one of the most commonly reported complications in LVHR, though it is not unique to laparoscopy **(Figs. 17A and B)**. It is a swelling-like mass that occurs immediately after operation in virtually all patients, but disappears after a few weeks. Most seromas develop above the mesh and within the retained hernia sac. The mean incidence of seroma in reported series at a range of 4–8 weeks is 11.4%. In the largest multi-institutional trial, seromas that were clinically apparent for more than 8 weeks were considered a complication and occurred in 2.6% cases. Regardless of whether they are aspirated under sterile conditions or allowed to resolve, they rarely cause long-term morbidity. Aspiration may increase the risk

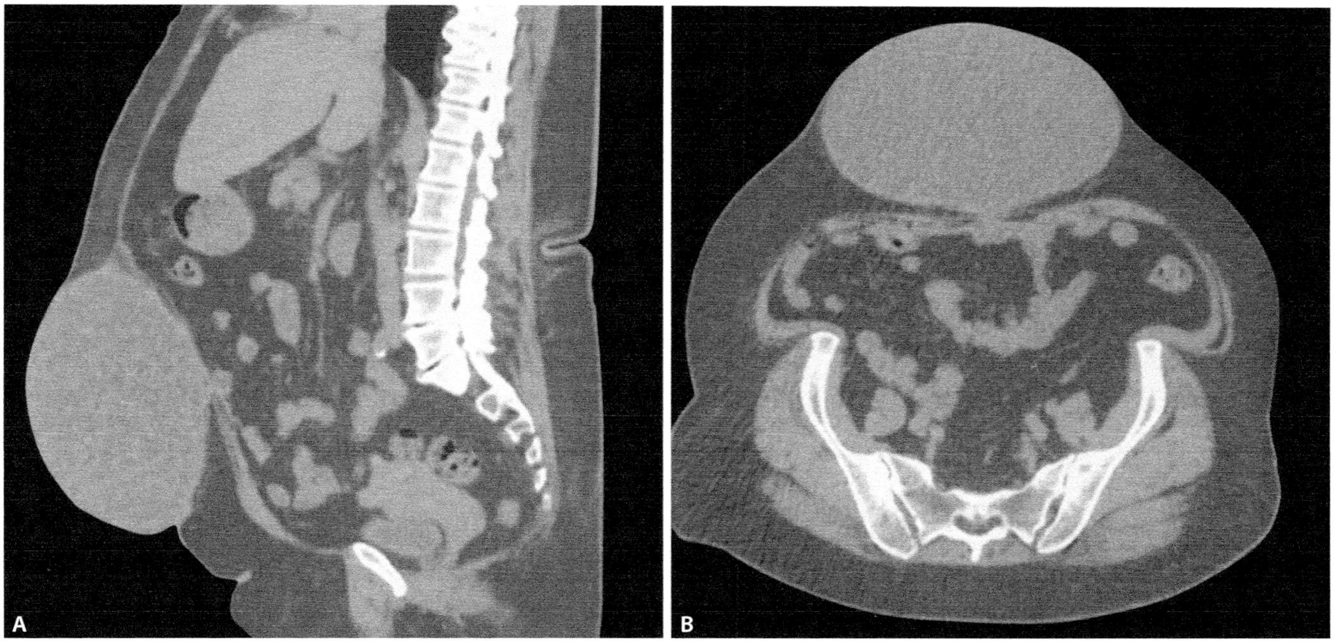

Figs. 17A and B: Seroma developed after ventral hernia repair.

of mesh infection but is recommended if they enlarge or persist before they reach their extremes. Patients sometimes mistake a tense seroma for recurring incisional hernia, but appropriate preoperative discussion should provide them with significant reassurance on this point.

Although Feldman suggests that seroma formation is not related to a particular type of mesh, Carbanjo and Heniford reported a higher incidence of seroma formation with ePTFE than prolene-based meshes. The low incidence in the latter meshes has been attributed to the large pores of the prolene-based meshes that allow more efficient resorption of wound secretions into the abdominal cavity than ePTFE meshes. The dissection of the preperitoneal space during the inlay method may lead to more seroma formation. This is supported by the fact that—in the classical description of the onlay technique, it is emphasized that no attempts should be made to reduce or resect the hernia sac. This has been established to be unnecessary and to increase the incidence of seroma formation. The peritoneum interposed barrier between the mesh and the abdominal cavity may hinder the direct drainage of this fluid regardless of the mesh used. Thus based on these facts, it seems plausible that the problem of seroma formation is expected to be higher in the inlay than the conventional onlay approach.

POSTOPERATIVE PAIN

After LVHR, about 5% of patients complain of persistent pain and point tenderness at the transabdominal suture site, which usually resolves spontaneously within 6–8 weeks. If it does not, injection of local anesthetic into the area around the painful suture has good results. Since missed enterotomy is a grave concern in LVHR, particularly after a difficult adhesiolysis, correct interpretation of the significance of postoperative pain is an important issue. Whether or not to relaparoscope a patient who experiences severe pain remains an important issue. A possible explanation of the common type of pain may be that—the transabdominal suture entraps an intercostal nerve, as it courses through the abdominal muscles. Local muscle ischemia may be another possibility. As such, it is an unavoidable adverse outcome of either approach so long as there is suture fixation of the prosthetic mesh. Whether it can be avoided by not using suture in the preperitoneal approach has to be weighed against the clinical benefit ratio of such a repair.

INFECTION (FIGS. 18A TO C)

One of the greatest benefits of LVHR is the reduction in wound and mesh infections. In a detailed analysis of wound complications from a pooled data of forty-five published series involving 5,340 patients, Pierce reported wound infection rates of 4.6–8 times fold higher in open versus LVHR. The number of mesh infections was also significantly higher with open approaches. Wound problems are strongly linked with soft tissue dissection required for retromuscular placement of large pieces of mesh. The intraperitoneal approach obviates the need of this dissection that potentially devascularizes the fascia and causes hematoma formation, both of which contribute to infection. Although the incidence of mesh infection is very low, the consequences are severe. Infections of prolene meshes can be managed locally with surgical drainage and excision of exposed, unincorporated segments but that of ePTFE require removal in most cases

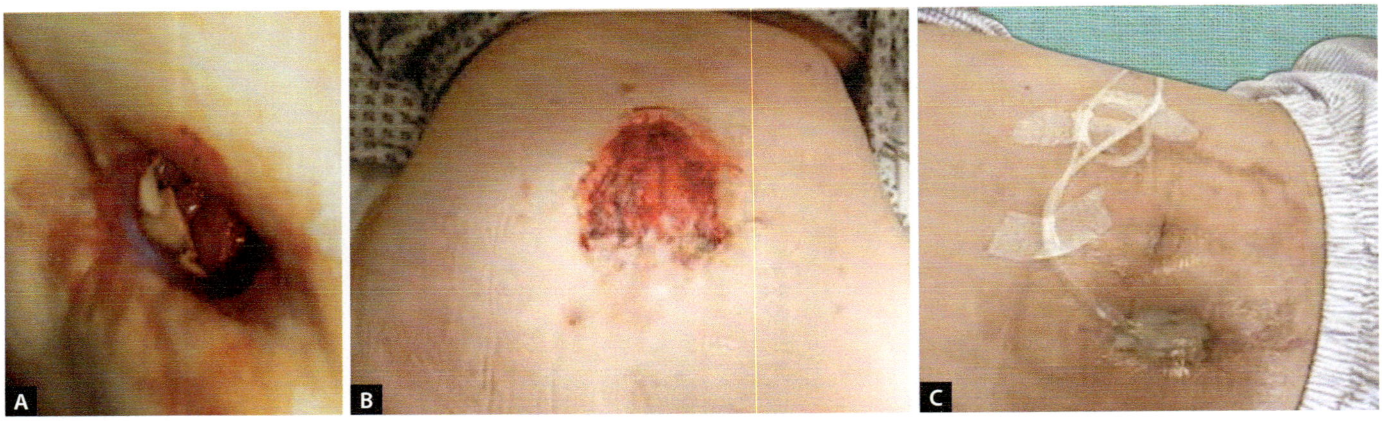

Figs. 18A to C: Infection developed after ventral hernia repair.

due to its relatively low incorporation onto the body wall. Removal of the mesh results in return of the defect and its added morbidity. An analysis of all series with more than 50 patients indicated a mesh infection rate of 0.6% cellulitis of the trochar sites that resolved on antibiotics alone in 1.1% and an overall wound and mesh complications of 1.7%. This has led to the widely perceived conclusion that the most compelling argument for LVHR is the minimization of soft tissue dissection and the associated reduction in the morbidity of local wound complications and potential infection of the implanted mesh. The high mesh infection rate reported in the inlay approach could be related to the extensive dissection of the peritoneal flap.

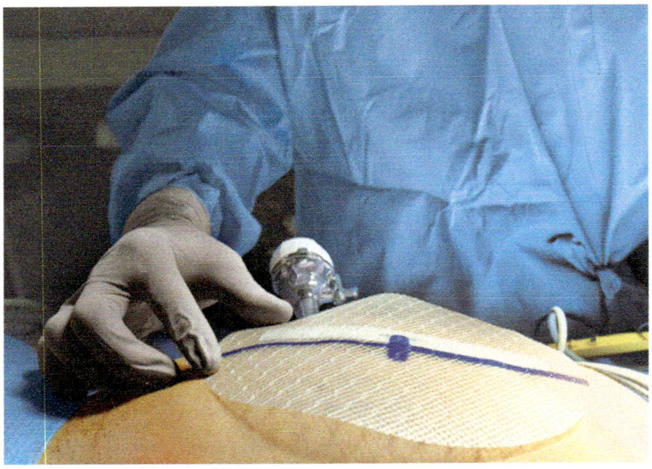

Fig. 19: Appropriate size of mesh is necessary to prevent recurrence.

RECURRENCE

The ultimate measure of the effectiveness of hernia surgery is the recurrence rate. Recurrence rates after LVHR range from 1.1 to 13%, whereas those after the open repairs ranged from 25 to 49%. In a multicenter series of 850 cases, the recurrence rate after a mean follow-up period of 20 months was 4.7%. The average recurrence rates using the onlay approach are approximately 4.2%, although rates as high as 17% have been reported. The critical technical points related with recurrence are inadequate mesh fixation particularly with sutures and prostheses that overlap the defect by less than 2–3 cm. Other factors associated with high recurrence rates include postoperative complications, previous repairs, missed hernias as in the "Swiss cheese" defects, longer operating time, and obesity. The surgeon's level of experience plays a significant role in patient outcome, as demonstrated by a group that compared the outcomes for their first 100 laparoscopic incisional hernia repair patients, with those for their second 100. Recurrence rates after a mean follow-up period of 36 months dropped from 9% in the first 100 patients to 4% in the second 100. Small size of Mesh is also one of the factors of recurrence so the mesh should be at least 12 cm + defect size **(Fig. 19)**. In addition, the second set of patients were an average of 9 years older, had a higher percentage of recurrent hernias, and exhibited more comorbidities, yet despite these added challenges, operating time was not lengthened, length of stay was similarly short, and the complication rate was no different. A multivariate analysis of these variables indicated that prior failed hernia and increased estimated blood loss predicted recurrence, while the other variables included—body mass index, defect size, and the size of the mesh did not have a positive correlation.

Although the results of large randomized trials are not available yet, the recent evidence to date suggests that the conventional onlay laparoscopic approach to the repair of ventral hernias is highly promising. The proposed laparoscopic preperitoneal placement of prostheses seems to negate most of the positive attributes of LVHR in most ways. This technique may be advantageous in small primary hernias in a highly selected patients' population. However, the widespread application of this approach or even the possibility of it being entered into a randomized trial appears dismal in the prevailing evidence, and in the patients' population that usually present with this structural disability.

BIBLIOGRAPHY

1. Alonso J, Ferrer M, Gandek B, Ware JE Jr, Aaronson NK, Mosconi P, et al. Health-related quality of life associated with chronic conditions in eight countries: results from the International Quality of Life Assessment (IQOLA) Project. Qual Life Res. 2004;13:283-98.
2. Anthony T, Bergen PC, Kim LT, Henderson M, Fahey T, Rege RV, et al. Factors affecting recurrence following incisional herniorrhaphy. World J Surg. 2000;24:95-101.
3. Berger D, Bientzle M, Muller A. Postoperative complications after laparoscopic incisional hernia repair. Incidence and treatment. Surg Endosc. 2002;16:1720-3.
4. Bergner L, Hallstrom AP, Bergner M, Eisenberg MS, Cobb LA. Health status of survivors of cardiac arrest and of myocardial infarction controls. Am J Public Health. 1985;75:1321-3.
5. Birgisson G, Park AE, Mastrangelo MJ Jr, Witzke DB, Chu UB. Obesity and laparoscopic repair of ventral hernias. Surg Endosc. 2001;15:1419-22.
6. Bower CE, Reade CC, Kirby LW, Roth JS. Complications of laparoscopic incisional ventral hernia repair: the experience of a single institution. Surg Endosc. 2004;18:672-5.
7. Bradley JF 3rd, Williams KB, Wormer BA, Tsirline VB, Walters AL, Sing RF, et al. Preliminary results of surgical and quality of life outcomes of Physiomesh in an international, prospective study. Surg Technol Int. 2012;22:113.
8. Brahmbhatt R, Martindale R, Liang MK. Jumping the gun? Evaluating the evidence for synthetic mesh in contaminated hernia repairs. J Am Coll Surg. 2014;218:498-9.
9. Brook RH, Ware JE Jr, Rogers WH, Keeler EB, Davies AR, Donald CA, et al. Does free care improve adults' health? Results from a randomized controlled trial. N Engl J Med. 1983;309:1426-34.
10. Bucknall TE, Cox PJ, Ellis H. Burst abdomen and incisional hernia: a prospective study of 1,129 major laparotomies. BMJ. 1982;284:931-3.
11. Carbajo MA, del Martin Olmo JC, Blanco JI, de la CC, Toledano M, Martin F, et al. Laparoscopic treatment vs open surgery in the solution of major incisional and abdominal wall hernias with mesh. Surg Endosc. 1999;13:250-2.
12. Carbonell AM, Criss CN, Cobb WS, Novitsky YW, Rosen MJ. Outcomes of synthetic mesh in contaminated ventral hernia repairs. J Am Coll Surg. 2013;217:991-8.
13. Cassar K, Munro A. Surgical treatment of incisional hernia. Br J Surg. 2002;89:534-45.
14. Chowbey PK, Sharma A, Khullar R, Mann V, Baijal M, Vashistha A. Laparoscopic ventral hernia repair. J Laparoendosc Adv Surg Tech. 2000;10:79-84.
15. Costanza MJ, Heniford BT, Arca MJ, Gagner M. Laparoscopic repair of recurrent ventral hernias. Am Surg. 1998;64:1121-7.
16. Darehzereshki A, Goldfarb M, Zehetner J, Moazzez A, Lipham JC, Mason RJ, et al. Biologic versus nonbiologic mesh in ventral hernia repair: a systematic review and meta-analysis. World J Surg. 2014;38:40-50.
17. Deerenberg EB, Verhelst J, Hovius SER, Lange JF. Mesh expansion as the cause of bulging after abdominal wall hernia repair. Int J Surg Case Rep. 2016;28:200-3.
18. DeMaria EJ, Moss JM, Sugerman HJ. Laparoscopic intraperitoneal polytetrafluoroethylene (PTFE) prosthetic patch repair of ventral hernia. Prospective comparison to open prefascial polypropylene mesh repair. Surg Endosc. 2000;14:326-9.
19. Department of Health (2002). Day surgery: operational guide. [online] Available from http://www.doh.gov.uk/daysurgery/2002 [Last accessed June, 2020].
20. Eid GM, Mattar SG, Hamad G, Cottam DR, Lord JL, Watson A, et al. Repair of ventral hernias in morbidly obese patients undergoing gastric bypass should not be deferred. Surg Endosc. 2004;18:207-10.
21. Goodney PP, Birkmeyer CM, Birkmeyer JD. Short-term outcomes of laparoscopic and open ventral hernia repair: a meta-analysis. Arch Surg. 2002;137:1161-5.
22. Groene SA, Prasad T, Lincourt AE, Augenstein VA, Sing R, Heniford BT. Prospective, multi-institutional surgical and quality-of-life outcomes comparison of heavyweight, midweight, and lightweight mesh in open ventral hernia repair. Am J Surg 2016;212:1054-62.
23. Healthcare Commission (2004). Day surgery. [online] Available from www.healthcarecommission.org.uk/acutehospitalportfolio. [Last accessed June, 2020].
24. Heniford BT, Park A, Ramshaw BJ, Voeller G. Laparoscopic repair of ventral hernias: nine years' experience with 850 consecutive hernias. Ann Surg. 2003;238:391-9; discussion 391-400.
25. Holzman MD, Purut CM, Reintgen K, Eubanks S, Pappas TN. Laparoscopic ventral and incisional hernioplasty. Surg Endosc. 1997;11:32-5.
26. IQOLA Project Group. Translating functional health and well-being: International Quality of Life Assessment (IQOLA) Project Studies of the SF-36 Health Survey. J Clin Epidemiol. 1998;51:891-1214.
27. Itani KM, Neumayer L, Reda D, Kim L, Anthony T. Repair of ventral incisional hernia: the design of a randomized trial to compare open and laparoscopic surgical techniques. Am J Surg. 2004;188:22S-9S.
28. Jenkinson C, Lawrence K, McWhinnie D, Gordon J. Sensitivity to change of health status measures in a randomized controlled trial: comparison of the COOP charts and the SF-36. Qual Life Res. 1995;4:47-52.
29. Koc M, Aslar AK, Yoldas O, Ertan T, Kilic M, Gocmen E. Comparison of quality-of-life outcomes of Stoppa vs bilateral Lichtenstein procedure. Hernia. 2004;8:53-5.
30. Koehler RH, Voller G. Recurrences in laparoscopic incisional hernia repairs a personal series and review of literature. JSLS. 1999;3:293-304.
31. Korolija D, Sauerland S, Wood-Dauphinee S, Abbou CC, Eypasch E, Caballero MG, et al. Evaluation of quality of life after laparoscopic surgery: evidence-based guidelines of the European Association for Endoscopic Surgery. Surg Endosc. 2004;18:879-97.
32. Kroese LF, Kleinrensink GJ, Lange JF, Gillion JF, Club H. External validation of the european hernia society classification for postoperative complications after incisional hernia repair: a cohort study of 2,191 patients. J Am Coll Surg. 2018;226:223-9.e1.
33. Kurth BM, Ellert U. The SF-36 questionnaire and its usefulness in population studies: results of the German Health Interview and Examination Survey, 1998. Soz Praventivmed. 2002; 47:266-77.
34. Leber GE, Garb JL, Alexander AI, Reed WP. Long-term complications associated with prosthetic repair of incisional hernias. Arch Surg. 1998;133:378-82.
35. LeBlanc KA, Booth WV. Laparoscopic repair of incisional abdominal hernias using expanded polytetrafluoroethylene: preliminary findings. Surg Laparosc Endosc. 1993;3:39-41.
36. LeBlanc KA, Elieson MJ, Corder JM 3rd. Enterotomy and mortality rates of laparoscopic incisional and ventral hernia repair: a review of the literature. JSLS. 2007;11:408-14.
37. Majumder A, Winder JS, Wen Y, Pauli EM, Belyansky I, Novitsky YW. Comparative analysis of biologic versus synthetic mesh outcomes in contaminated hernia repairs. Surgery. 2016;160:828-38.
38. Manning WG, Newhouse JP, Ware JE Jr. The status of health in demand estimation; or beyond excellent, good, fair, and poor. In: Fuchs VR (Ed). Economic aspects of health. University of Chicago Press, Chicago. 1982;143-84.
39. Mayor S. Day surgery facilities in England are underused. BMJ. 2005;331:130.

40. McHorney CA, Ware JE Jr, Lu JF, Sherbourne CD. The MOS 36-item Short-Form Health Survey (SF-36): III. Tests of data quality, scaling assumptions, and reliability across diverse patient groups. Med Care. 1994;32:40-66.
41. McHorney CA, Ware JE Jr, Raczek AE. The MOS 36-Item Short-Form Health Survey (SF-36): II. Psychometric and clinical tests of validity in measuring physical and mental health constructs. Med Care. 1993;31:247-63.
42. Mitura K, Skolimowska-Rzewuska M, Garnysz K. Outcomes of bridging versus mesh augmentation in laparoscopic repair of small and medium midline ventral hernias. Surg Endosc. 2017;31:382-8.
43. Moreno-Egea A, Carrillo-Alcaraz A, Soria-Aledo V. Randomized clinical trial of laparoscopic hernia repair comparing titanium-coated lightweight mesh and medium-weight composite mesh. Surg Endosc. 2013;27:231-9.
44. Moreno-Egea A, Castillo JA, Girela E, Canteras M, Aguayo JL. Outpatient laparoscopic incisional/ventral hernioplasty: our experience in 55 cases. Surg Laparosc Endosc Percutan Tech. 2002;12:171-4.
45. Mudge M, Hughes LE. Incisional hernia: a 10-year prospective study of incidence and attitudes. Br J Surg. 1985;72:70-1.
46. Novitsky YW, Cobb WS, Kercher KW, Mathews BD, Sing RF, Heniford TB. Laparoscopic ventral hernia repair in obese patients. Arch Surg. 2006;141:57-61.
47. Park A, Birch DW, Lovrics P. Laparoscopic and open incisional hernia repair: a comparison study. Surgery. 1998;124:816-21.
48. Quintana JM, Cabriada J, Arostegui I, Lopez de Tejada I, Bilbao A. Quality-of-life outcomes with laparoscopic vs open cholecystectomy. Surg Endosc. 2003;17:1129-34.
49. Raftopoulos I, Vanuno D, Khorsand J, Kouraklis G, Lasky P. Comparison of open and laparoscopic prosthetic repair of large ventral hernias. JSLS. 2003;7:227-32.
50. Raftopoulos I, Vanuno D, Khorsand J, Ninos J, Kouraklis G, Lasky P. Outcome of laparoscopic ventral hernia repair in correlation with obesity, type of hernia, and hernia size. J Laparoendosc Adv Surg Tech A. 2002;12:425-9.
51. Ramshaw BJ, Esartia P, Schwab J, Mason EM, Wilson RA, Duncan TD, et al. Comparison of laparoscopic and open ventral herniorrhaphy. Am Surg. 1999;65:827-31.
52. Reynvoet E, Deschepper E, Rogiers X, Troisi R, Berrevoet F. Laparoscopic ventral hernia repair: is there an optimal mesh fixation technique? A systematic review. Langenbecks Arch Surg. 2014;399:55-63.
53. Schoenmaeckers EJ, Wassenaar EB, Raymakers JT, Rakic S. Bulging of the mesh after laparoscopic repair of ventral and incisional hernias. JSLS. 2010;14:541-6.
54. Sharma A, Khullar R, Soni V, Baijal M, Kapahi A, Najma K. Iatrogenic enterotomy in laparoscopic ventral/incisional hernia repair: a single center experience of 2,346 patients over 17 years. Hernia. 2013;17:581-7.
55. Sugerman HJ, Kellum JM Jr, Reines HD, De Maria EJ, Newsome HH, Lowry JW. Greater risk of incisional hernia with morbidly obese than steroid dependent patients and low recurrence with prefascial polypropelene mesh. Am J Surg. 1996;171:80-84 2297.
56. Tandon A, Pathak S, Lyons NJ, Nunes QM, Daniels IR, Smart NJ. Meta-analysis of closure of the fascial defect during laparoscopic incisional and ventral hernia repair. Br J Surg. 2016;103:1598-1607.
57. Thaler K, Dinnewitzer A, Mascha E, Arrigain S, Weiss EG, Nogueras JJ, Wexner SD. Long-term outcome and health-related quality of life after laparoscopic and open colectomy for benign disease. Surg Endosc. 2003;17:1404-8.
58. Turner-Bowker DM, Bayliss MS, Ware JE Jr, Kosinski M. Usefulness of the SF-8 Health Survey for comparing the impact of migraine and other conditions. Qual Life Res. 2003;12:1003-12.
59. Velanovich V. Laparoscopic vs open surgery: a preliminary comparison of quality-of-life outcomes. Surg Endosc. 2000; 14:16-21.
60. Ware JE Jr, Sherbourne CD. The MOS 36-Item Short-Form Health Survey (SF-36). I. Conceptual framework and item selection. Med Care. 1992;30:473-83.

CHAPTER 18

Laparoscopic Repair of Hiatus Hernia

INTRODUCTION

The esophageal hiatus is an elliptical opening in the diaphragmatic muscular portion. The crura of diaphragm originate from the anterior surface of the first four lumbar vertebrae on the right and L2–L3 on the left to insert anteriorly into the transverse ligament of the central portion of diaphragm.

Hiatal hernia is an opening in the diaphragm through which stomach or omentum is forced into the chest cavity. A hiatus hernia can exist without any symptom.

ANATOMY AND PHYSIOLOGY OF THE GASTROESOPHAGEAL JUNCTION

Distal esophagus is anchored to the diaphragm by the phrenoesophageal membrane, formed by the fused endothoracic and endoabdominal fascia **(Fig. 1)**. Phrenoesophageal membrane inserts circumferentially into the esophageal musculature, very close to the squamocolumnar junction, which resides within the diaphragmatic hiatus.

This configuration in lower esophagus altered during swallow-initiated peristalsis. With contraction of the esophageal longitudinal muscle, the esophagus shortens and the phrenoesophageal membrane is stretched; its elastic recoil is then responsible for pulling the squamocolumnar junction back to its normal position following each swallow. Gastroesophageal (GE) junction serves to minimize GE reflux and antegrade propulsive function.

Severe stress of swallowing, as well as that associated with abdominal straining and episodes of vomiting, subjects the phrenoesophageal membrane to substantial wear and tear and in due course of time make it a plausible target of age-related degeneration. Repetitive tonic contraction of the esophageal longitudinal muscle induced by GE reflux and mucosal acidification is also a potential source of stress on the phrenoesophageal membrane.

Type I or Sliding Hernia

A type I or sliding hiatus hernia is characterized by the displacement of the GE junction above the diaphragm. GE junction migrates above the esophageal hiatus. It is the most common type of hiatus hernia (80%). This results in loss of the cardiac angle of His and commonly incompetence of the cardioesophageal junction. The symptoms and complications of this type of hernia are those which are consequence of GE reflux and reflux esophagitis (chronic blood loss, stricture, Barrett's epithelium, etc.).

Type II, III, IV: Paraesophageal Hernias

Paraesophageal hernia is a true hernia with a hernia sac and is characterized by an upward dislocation of the gastric fundus through a defect in the phrenoesophageal membrane. True paraesophageal hernia is characterized by normally positioned GE junction and an intrathoracically migrated stomach. The fundus of the stomach rotates in front of the esophagus and herniates through the hiatus into

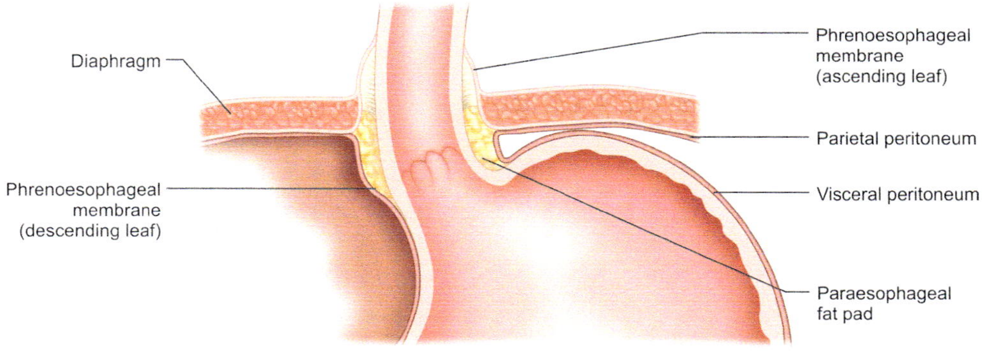

Fig. 1: Phrenoesophageal membrane.

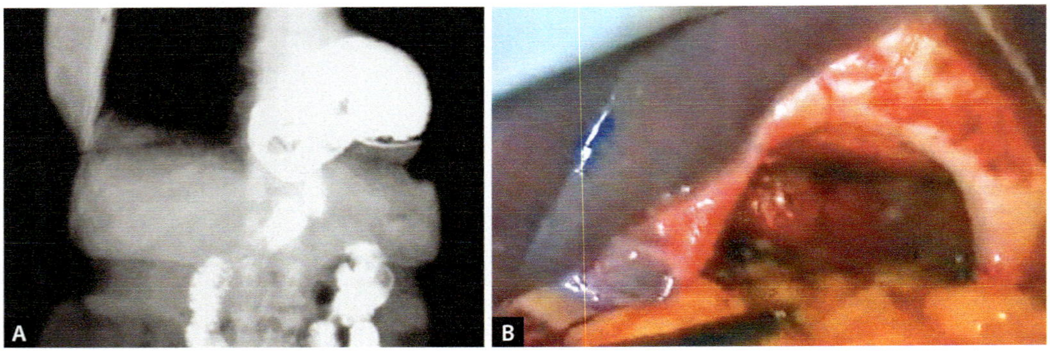

Figs. 2A and B: Hiatus hernia.

the mediastinum **(Figs. 2A and B)**. As the cardioesophageal junction remains in situ within the abdomen, cardiac incompetence and reflux are not usually encountered. These hernias account for 8–10% of cases and is found predominantly in the elderly patients. These types of hernias are prone to incarceration and strangulation with infarction and perforation of the stomach.

Type II hernia results from a localized defect in the phrenoesophageal membrane where the gastric fundus serves as a lead point of herniation, while the GE junction remains fixed to the preaortic fascia and the median arcuate ligament.

Type III hernias have elements of both types I and II hernias and are characterized by both the GE junction and the fundus herniating through the hiatus. The fundus lies above the GE junction.

Type IV hiatus hernia is associated with a large defect in the phrenoesophageal membrane and is characterized by the presence of organs other than the stomach in the hernia sac. It may contain colon, spleen, pancreas, or small intestine.

Mixed Hernia

Mixed hernias are those with both sliding and paraesophageal component. This resembles a large paraesophageal hernia, but GE junction is also herniated above the diaphragm. Mixed hernias have features and complications of both types I and II hernias. It is found in 10% of patients.

There are rare instances of post-traumatic herniation of the stomach through the hiatus and these must be differentiated from traumatic rupture of diaphragm. In majority of cases, the development of hiatus hernia is spontaneous. Gallstone and colonic diverticular disease are commonly present in patients with a hiatus hernia (Saint's triad).

Symptoms of Type II Hiatus Hernia

- Typical heartburn (47%)
- Dysphagia (35%)
- Epigastric pain (26%)
- Vomiting (23%)
- Anemia (21%)
- Barrett's epithelium (13%)
- Aspiration (7%).

Symptomatic gastroesophageal reflux disease (GERD) is frequently associated with finding of a sliding hernia. A number of procedures such as Nissen fundoplication and its modification (the Toupet procedure), Hill procedure, and Belsey transthoracic repair have been described for its management. Nissen fundoplication is, however, the simplest and most effective. Success has been achieved in performing laparoscopically these procedures of Nissen fundoplication, Hill repair, and Toupet procedure as well as thoracoscopic Belsey Mark IV. Laparoscopic Nissen fundoplication shows the most progress and has the potential of becoming gold standard. It offers the opportunity for correction of the underlying anatomical and functional defect associated with GERD with lessened discomfort and hospitalization.

The indications are:
- Severe heartburn
- Refractory to medical therapy—symptoms present even 12 weeks after therapy
- Noncompliance with therapy
- Development of complications such as aspiration
- A type of hiatal hernia where the stomach is at risk of getting stuck in the chest or twisting on itself (paraesophageal hernia)
- Bleeding
- Barrett's mucosa
- Stricture.

Relative contraindications include:
- Previous hiatal or upper abdominal surgery
- Morbid obesity with left hepatomegaly
- Shortened esophagus
- Aperistalsis of esophagus (achalasia, scleroderma, and end-stage GERD).

Appropriate preoperative evaluation of esophago-gastric junction is essential prior to performing laparoscopic fundoplication. Failure of surgery to control symptoms occurs in up to 10% of cases. It is a reflection that antireflux surgery has been inadvertently utilized for unrecognized cardiac, hepatobiliary, or other esophageal and gastric etiologies.

PREOPERATIVE EVALUATION

Preoperative investigation can be divided into mandatory and selective tests.

Mandatory

- Endoscopy upper gastrointestinal (UGI) with/without biopsy
- Esophageal manometry.

Selective

- Barium swallow
- 24 hours pH monitoring
- Gastric studies.

OPERATIVE MANAGEMENT OF HIATUS HERNIA

Surgical repair of an asymptomatic type I hiatal hernia is not indicated. Management of patients with a symptomatic sliding hiatus hernia consists of management of GERD. Most common is laparoscopic fundoplication, which is discussed separately in fundoplication chapter of this book.

Surgical repair is indicated in patients with a symptomatic paraesophageal hernia. Paraesophageal hernias can be repaired transabdominally or transthoracically. Transabdominal repairs can be performed open or laparoscopically. Emergent repair is required in patients with a gastric volvulus, uncontrolled bleeding, obstruction, strangulation, perforation, and respiratory compromise secondary to a paraesophageal hernia. Reoperation for a symptomatic paraesophageal hernia presents a significant technical challenge, especially if mesh has been placed at the time of the initial operation. These procedures should be performed by very experienced surgeons.

Port Position

The patient is positioned supine on the operating table, and the surgeon works from the right side or many surgeons prefer position of the surgeon in between the legs of the patient with the assistant on the left **(Fig. 2C)**.

A laparoscopic paraesophageal hernia repair (PEHR) usually requires placement of five ports in the following positions:

- The first port, used for the laparoscope, is placed approximately 14 cm distal to the xiphoid process and 3 cm to the left of the midline.
- The second and third ports, used for stomach and liver retractors, are placed lateral to the first port in the left and right midclavicular line.
- The last two ports, used for the surgeon's dissection and suturing instruments, are placed approximately 6 cm from midline under the costal margins.

Four 5 mm and one 10 mm laparoscopic ports are placed in the upper abdomen **(Fig. 2D)**. Positioning of liver retractor is shown in **Figure 2E**.

The dissection of the hernia sac begins with gentle reduction of the stomach and any other organs from the hernia sac.

- Dissection of the hernia sac requires great care to avoid injury to adjacent organs such as mediastinal pleura, pericardium, and aortic adventitia, which could cause bleeding or pneumothorax.
- An incarcerated stomach, if present, can be friable and should be handled with care.
- The dissection of the hernia sac is performed within the plane between the hernia sac and the adjacent tissues.
- The peritoneal covering of the crus on the abdominal side is preserved when dividing the gastrohepatic omentum from the right crus of the diaphragm.
- A drain is placed around the esophagus to facilitate the dissection of the posterior portion of the hernia sac. Using gentle upward traction on the Penrose drain, the dissection begins at the right crus and proceeds posteriorly to the left crus.
- The hernia sac must be completely removed from the mediastinum.
- Injury or transection of the vagal nerves should be avoided to reduce the risk of delayed gastric emptying.

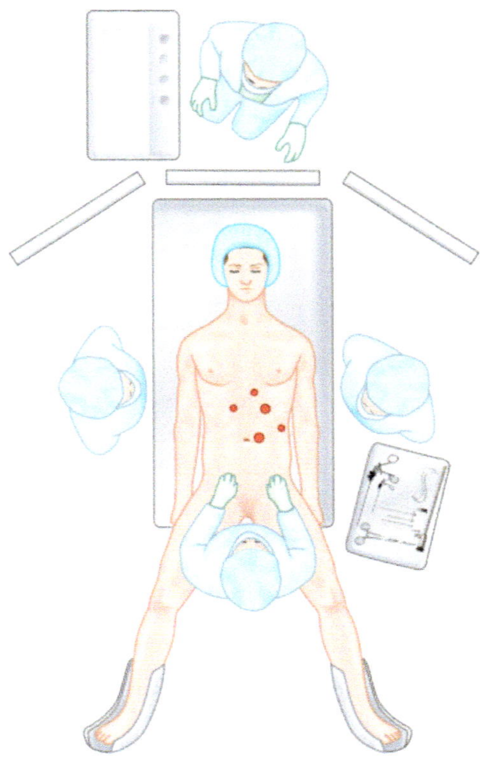

Fig. 2C: Position of surgical team during hiatus hernia surgery.

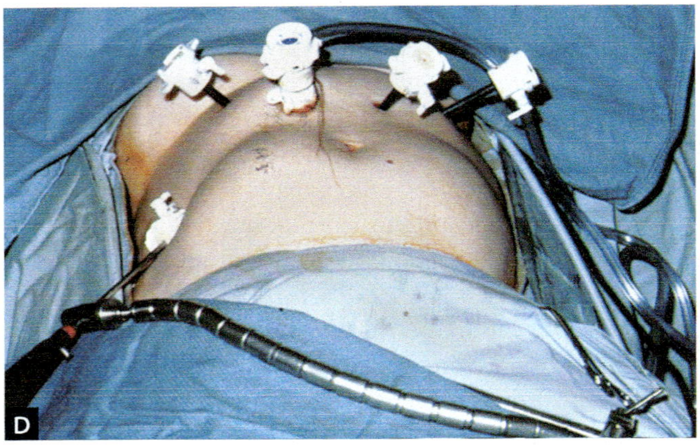

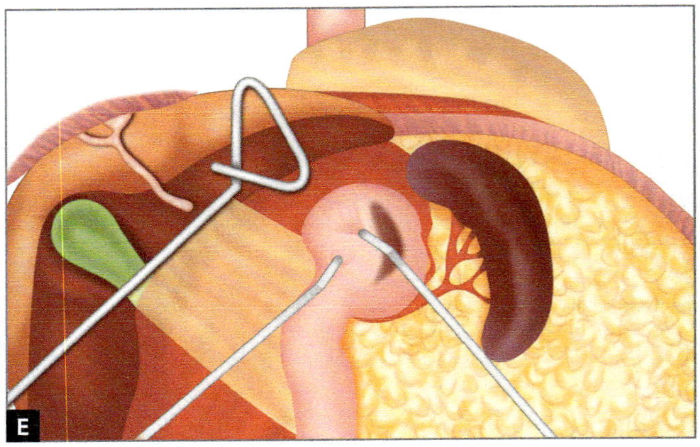

Figs. 2D and E: (D) Port position in hiatus hernia; (E) Liver retractor.

- Dividing the short gastric vessels will increase mobilization of the stomach, facilitate a fundoplication, and improve exposure of the operative site.

Esophageal Mobilization

At least 3–5 cm of esophagus must be mobilized inside the abdomen to ensure adequate intra-abdominal length for fixation **(Fig. 3)**. In order to prevent reherniation, a proper PEHR requires the complete dissection and removal of the hernia sac from the mediastinum, rather than the mere reduction of hernia contents from the sac.

The use of electrocautery should be limited when mobilizing the esophagus since the potential risk of cautery damage to the esophagus is high. A sling should be used to give downward traction of esophagus **(Figs. 4A and B)**.

The esophagus must be mobilized to the level of the aortic arch or until ≥4 cm of intra-abdominal esophagus has been freed without tension. If adequate intra-abdominal esophageal length cannot be achieved with esophageal mobilization alone, an esophageal-lengthening procedure such as Collis gastroplasty may be required. Although shortened esophagus is not common. Short esophagus is found in <1% of patients. The failure to lengthen a shortened esophagus can lead to hernia recurrence as it produces tension on the repair. Collis procedure entails the creation of a gastric tube by vertically stapling the proximal stomach from the angle of His, parallel to a large bougie placed along the lesser curvature of the stomach. The newly created gastric tube becomes an extension or elongation of the native esophagus such that the new esophagogastric junction can be located intra-abdominally.

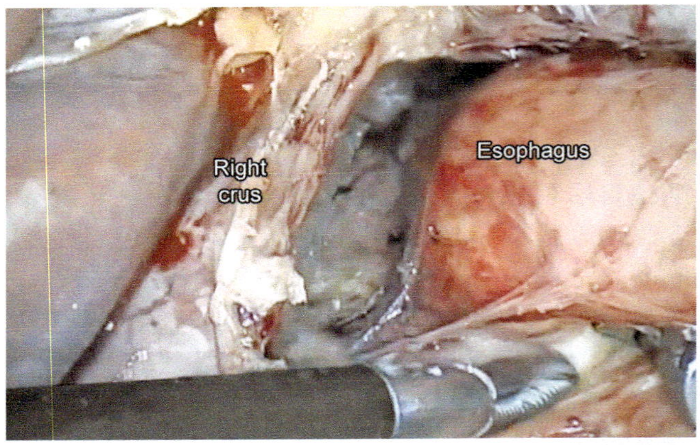

Fig. 3: Esophageal mobilization.

Closure of Hiatal Defect

The crura are approximated with 2–3 nonabsorbable sutures of No. Zero **(Figs. 5A to D)**. The short gastric vessels are routinely divided along the upper one-third of stomach using harmonic scalpel. After complete dissection of the esophagus, the pillars of the crura of the diaphragm are closed inferiorly and posteriorly to the esophagus. The repair of crura must be tension free and can be performed as a primary suture repair or with mesh in case of giant hernia. We suggest against the routine use of mesh during PEHR. Routine use of mesh should be avoided. Both permanent and biologic meshes have been shown to be effective in reducing recurrences in separate randomized trials. Mesh should be used selectively during PEHR because mesh can cause serious complications such as intraluminal mesh erosion, esophageal stenosis, dense fibrosis, and the need for reoperations (e.g., esophagectomies, partial and total gastrectomies, and esophageal stent placement).

Fundoplication

After the closure of hiatal defect, Nissen fundoplication should be performed, except in patients with severe preoperative dysphagia **(Figs. 6A and B)**, for whom we perform a partial fundoplication to minimize the potential for worsening dysphagia postoperatively. The detail of the steps of laparoscopic fundoplication can be found in the fundoplication chapter of this book.

Postoperatively, a chest X-ray is obtained in the recovery room to exclude a pneumothorax. Patients are kept on clear liquids on the day of surgery and soft diet the

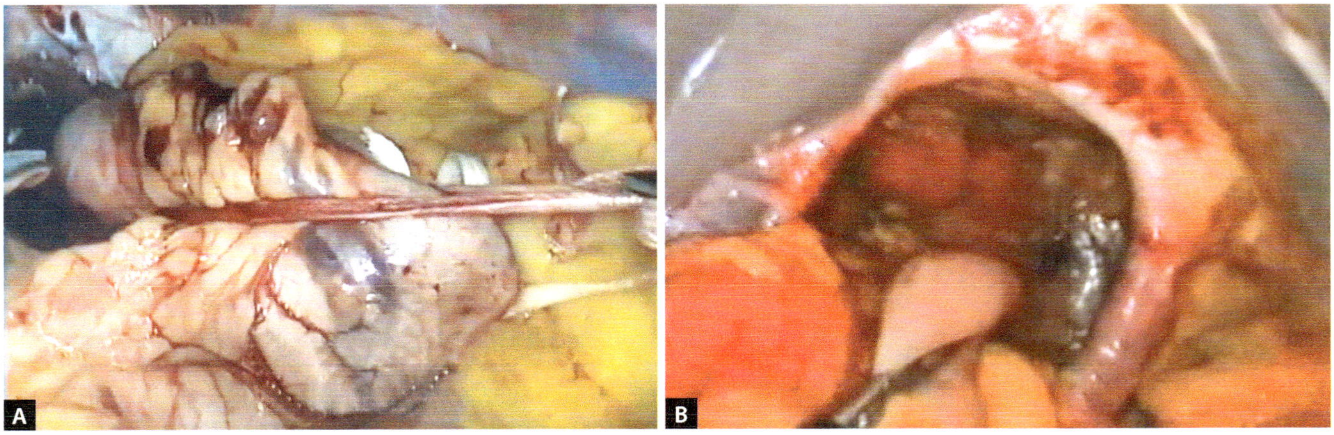

Figs. 4A and B: (A) Use of sling to give downward traction to esophagus; (B) Pulling the content of hernia sac.

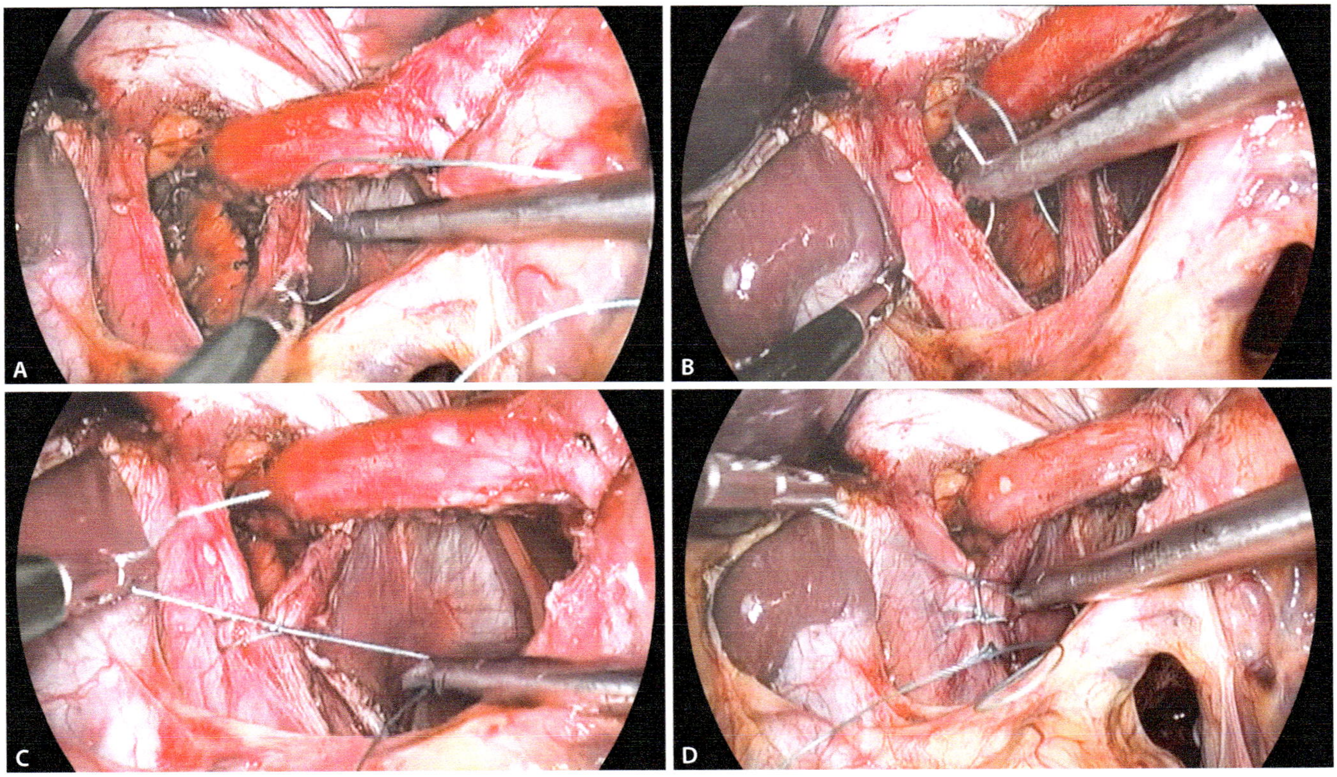

Figs. 5A to D: Crural approximation by suturing.

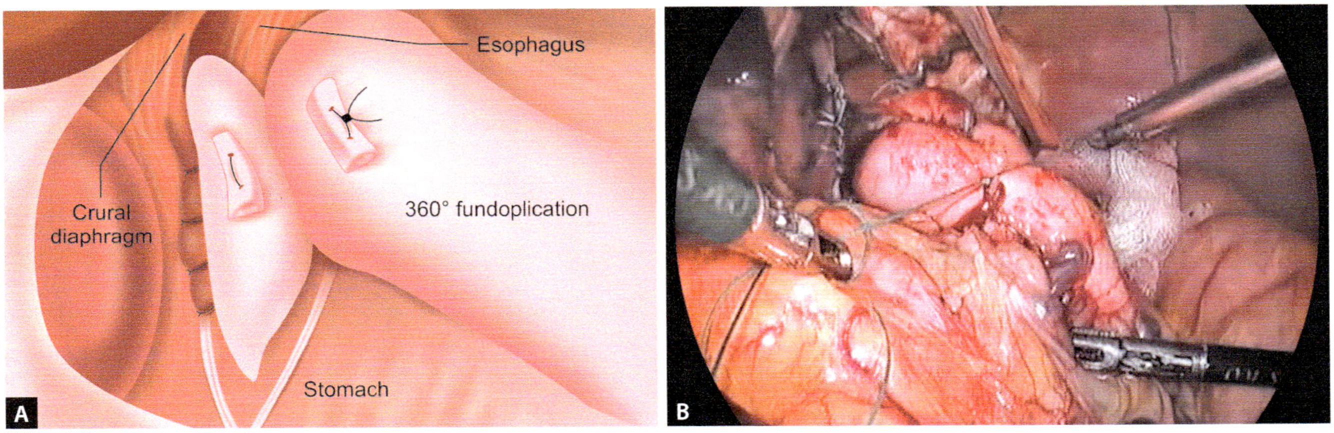

Figs. 6A and B: Nissen fundoplication after repair of hernia.

following day. Average length of stay is 2 days. Intraoperative complications may include injury to visceral organs, bleeding, pneumothorax, and vagal injury. Postoperative complications include wrap slippage. An anterior gastropexy can be used to reduce the risk of gastric reherniation into the thoracic cavity. The stomach can be fixated to the abdominal wall with sutures or percutaneous endoscopic gastrostomy (PEG) tubes depending upon whether a primary repair of paraesophageal hernia has been performed.

OPERATIVE PROCEDURE OF GIANT PARAESOPHAGEAL HERNIA

After exposing the hiatus, the herniated stomach is reduced into the abdomen using atraumatic graspers in a "hand-over-hand" fashion **(Figs. 4A and B)**. Dissection is started for exposing the right and left crura of the diaphragm and mobilizing the esophagus. Sling is applied to retract the esophagus, which facilitate mobilization of esophagus posteriorly **(Fig. 7)**. Once the dissection is complete, appropriate size of mesh should be taken and sutured from below the level of esophagus to repair the defect **(Figs. 8A to I)**.

Barium swallow study on the first postoperative day should be performed to assess for possible esophageal leak and early hernia recurrence and to evaluate gastric emptying and motility. Patients with a long-standing paraesophageal hernia often have delayed gastric emptying after the repair, mediated by possible mechanisms of an atrophic gastric musculature or vagal neurapraxia from the dissection. If the barium swallow study shows an adequate repair, patients are started on a clear liquid diet and advanced to soft solids as tolerated.

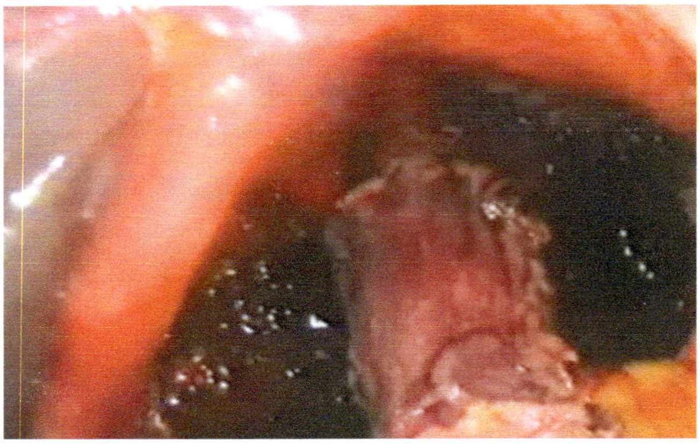

Fig. 7: Mobilization of esophagus.

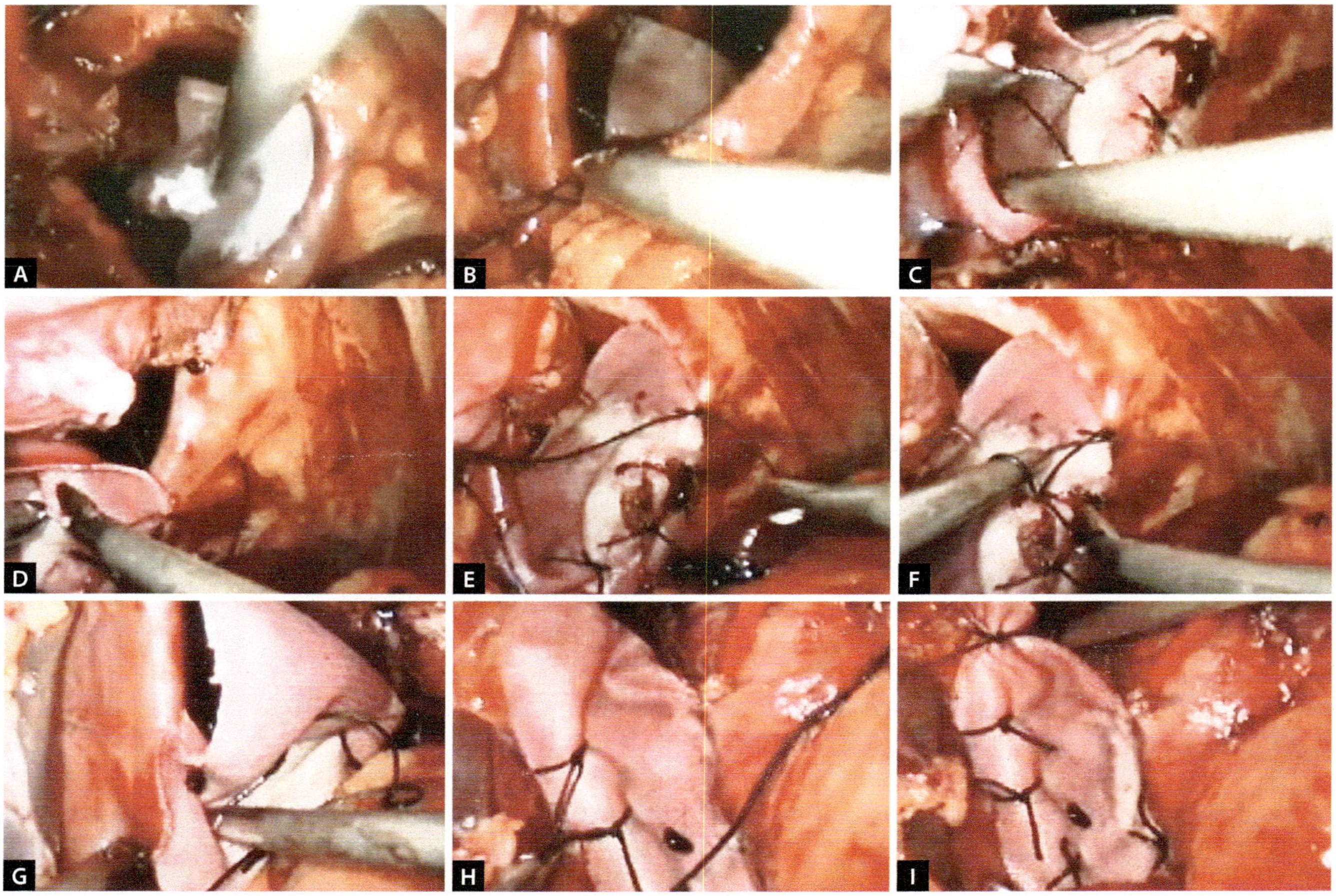

Figs. 8A to I: Fixation of mesh in paraesophageal hiatus hernia.

The overall mortality and morbidity rates associated with laparoscopic PEHR are 1.7 and 0.8%, respectively. The reported major complications include pneumonia (4.0%), pulmonary embolism (3.4%), heart failure (2.6%), and postoperative leak (2.5%). The mortality and morbidity rates are higher in patients who are ≥70 years of age, those who require emergency surgery, and those who have one or more comorbid illnesses.

RECOMMENDATIONS TO AVOID COMPLICATION

- Ports should be placed high on the abdomen since much of the stomach will be up in the mediastinum.
- Compression stockings and subcutaneous heparin should be used to prevent deep venous thrombosis.
- Intra-abdominal pressures <15 mm Hg should be used.
- Prefer the bipolar for mobilization of the anterior GE fat pad.
- It is important to remove the hernia sac from the mediastinum while avoiding entry into the pleural spaces.
- Stomach should be handled gently with graspers—the chronically herniated stomach has a tendency to perforate relatively easily.
- At the end of surgery, perforations or leaks during dissection should be watched carefully.

BIBLIOGRAPHY

1. Allison PR. Reflux esophagitis, sliding hiatus hernia and the anatomy of repair. Surg Gynecol Obstet. 1951;92(4):419-31.
2. Anvari M, Allen C. Postprandial bloating after laparoscopic Nissen fundoplication. Can J Surg. 2001;44(6):440-4.
3. Awad ZT, Puri V, LeBlanc K, Stoppa R, Fitzgibbons Jr RJ, Iqbal A, et al. Mechanisms of ventral hernia recurrence after mesh repair and a new proposed classification. J Am Coll Surg. 2005;201(1):132-40.
4. Basso N, Rosato P, De LA, Genco A, Rea S, Neri T. "Tension free" hiatoplasty, gastrophrenic anchorage, and 360 degrees fundoplication in the laparoscopic treatment of paraesophageal hernia. Surg Laparosc Endosc Percutan Tech. 1999;9(4):257-62.
5. Benjamin SB, Kerr R, Cohen D, Motaparthy V, Castell DO. Complications of the Angelchik antireflux prosthesis. Ann Intern Med. 1984;100(4):570-5.
6. Booth MI, Jones L, Stratford J, Dehn TC. Results of laparoscopic Nissen fundoplication at 2–8 years after surgery. Br J Surg. 2002;89(4):476-81.
7. Carlson MA, Condon RE, Ludwig KA, Schulte WJ. Management of intrathoracic stomach with polypropylene mesh prosthesis reinforced transabdominal hiatus hernia repair. J Am Coll Surg. 1998;187(3):227-30.
8. Casabella F, Sinanan M, Horgan S, Pellegrini CA. Systematic use of gastric fundoplication in laparoscopic repair of paraesophageal hernias. Am J Surg. 1996;171(5):485-9.
9. Catarci M, Gentileschi P, Papi C, Carrara A, Marrese R, Gaspari AL, et al. Evidence-based appraisal of antireflux fundoplication. Ann Surg. 2004;239(3):325-37.
10. Champion JK, Rock D. Laparoscopic mesh cruroplasty for large paraesophageal hernias. Surg Endosc. 2003;17(4):551-3.
11. Coluccio G, Ponzio S, Ambu V, Tramontano R, Cuomo G. Dislocation into the cardial lumen of a PTFE prosthesis used in the treatment of voluminous hiatal sliding hernia, a case report. Minerva Chir. 2000;55(5):3410-5.
12. Edelman DS. Laparoscopic paraesophageal hernia repair with mesh. Surg Laparosc Endosc. 1995;5(1):32-7.
13. Frantzides CT, Madan AK, Carlson MA, Stavropoulos GP. A prospective, randomized trial of laparoscopic polytetrafluoroethylene (PTFE) patch repair vs simple cruroplasty for large hiatal hernia. Arch Surg. 2002;137(6):649-52.
14. Gajbhiye R, Quraishi AH, Mahajan P, Warhadpande M. Dysphagia due to transmural migration of polypropylene mesh into esophagus. Indian J Gastroenterol. 2005;24(5): 226-7.
15. Geha AS, Massad MG, Snow NJ, Baue AE. A 32-year experience in 100 patients with giant paraesophageal hernia: the case for abdominal approach and selective antireflux repair. Surgery. 2000; 128(4):623-30.
16. Granderath FA, Kamolz T, Schweiger UM, Pointner R. Impact of laparoscopic Nissen fundoplication with prosthetic hiatal closure on esophageal body motility: results of a prospective randomized trial. Arch Surg. 2006;141(7):625-32.
17. Granderath FA, Schweiger UM, Kamolz T, Asche KU, Pointner R. Laparoscopic Nissen fundoplication with prosthetic hiatal closure reduces postoperative intrathoracic wrap herniation: preliminary results of a prospective randomized functional and clinical study. Arch Surg. 2005;140(1):40-8.
18. Hashemi M, Peters JH, DeMeester TR, Huprich JE, Quek M, Hagen JA, et al. Laparoscopic repair of large type III hiatal hernia: objective follow-up reveals high recurrence rate. J Am Coll Surg 2000;190(5):553-60; discussion. 560-1.
19. Hergueta-Delgado P, Marin-Moreno M, Morales-Conde S, Reina-Serrano S, Jurado-Castillo C, Pellicer-Bautista F, et al. Transmural migration of a prosthetic mesh after surgery of a paraesophageal hiatal hernia. Gastrointest Endosc. 2006;64(1):120; discussion 121.
20. Hill LD. An effective operation for hiatal hernia: an eight year appraisal. Ann Surg. 1967;166(4):681-92.
21. Hill LD. Incarcerated paraesophageal hernia. A surgical emergency. Am J Surg. 1973; 126(2):286-91.
22. Ireland AC, Holloway RH, Toouli J, Dent J. Mechanisms underlying the antireflux action of fundoplication. Gut. 1993;34(3):303-8.
23. Johnson JM, Carbonell AM, Carmody BJ, Jamal MK, Maher JW, Kellum JM, et al. Laparoscopic mesh hiatoplasty for paraesophageal hernias and fundoplications: a critical analysis of the available literature. Surg Endosc. 2006;20(3):362-6.
24. Johnsson F, Holloway RH, Ireland AC, Jamieson GG, Dent J. Effect of fundoplication on transient lower oesophageal sphincter relaxation and gas reflux. Br J Surg. 1997;84(5):686-9.
25. Kauten JR, Mansour KA. Complications of the Angelchik prosthesis in the management of gastroesophageal reflux. Am Surg. 1986;52(4):208-13.
26. Kemppainen E, Kiviluoto T. Fatal cardiac tamponade after emergency tension-free repair of a large paraesophageal hernia. Surg Endosc. 2000;14(6):593.
27. Khajanchee YS, O'Rourke RW, Lockhart B, Patterson EJ, Hansen PD, Swanstrom LL. Postoperative symptoms and failure after antireflux surgery. Arch Surg. 2002;137(9):1008-13.
28. Kulich KR, Malfertheiner P, Madisch A, Labenz J, Bayerdorffer E, Miehlke S, et al. Psychometric validation of the German translation of the Gastrointestinal Symptom Rating Scale (GSRS) and Quality of Life in Reflux and Dyspepsia (QOLRAD) questionnaire in patients with reflux disease. Health Qual Life Outcomes. 2003;1:62.
29. Leeder PC, Smith G, Dehn TC. Laparoscopic management of large paraesophageal hiatal hernia. Surg Endosc. 2003; 17(9):1372-5.
30. Lilly MP, Slafsky SF, Thompson WR. Intraluminal erosion and migration of the Angelchik antireflux prosthesis. Arch Surg. 1984;119(7):849-53.

31. Lord RV, Kaminski A, Oberg S, Bowrey DJ, Hagen JA, Demeester SR, et al. Absence of gastroesophageal reflux disease in a majority of patients taking acid suppression medications after Nissen fundoplication. J Gastrointest Surg. 2002;6(1):3-9.
32. Luketich JD, Nason KS, Christie NA, Pennathur A, Jobe BA, Landreneau RJ, et al. Outcomes after a decade of laparoscopic giant paraesophageal hernia repair. J Thorac Cardiovasc Surg 2010; 139(2):395-404.
33. Mainie I, Tutuian R, Agrawal A, Adams D, Castell DO. Combined multichannel intraluminal impedance-pH monitoring to select patients with persistent gastro- oesophageal reflux for laparoscopic Nissen fundoplication. Br J Surg. 2006;93(12): 1483-7.
34. Matthews BD, Mostafa G, Carbonell AM, Joels CS, Kercher KW, Austin C, et al. Evaluation of adhesion formation and host tissue response to intra- abdominal polytetrafluoroethylene mesh and composite prosthetic mesh. J Surg Res. 2005;123(2):227-34.
35. Matthews BD, Pratt BL, Pollinger HS, Backus CL, Kercher KW, Sing RF, et al. Assessment of adhesion formation to intra-abdominal polypropylene mesh and polytetrafluoroethylene mesh. J Surg Res. 2003;114(2): 126-32.
36. Müller-Stich BP, Linke GR, Borovicka J, Marra F, Warschkow R, Lange J, et al. Laparoscopic mesh-augmented hiatoplasty as a treatment of gastroesophageal reflux disease and hiatal hernias—preliminary clinical and functional results of a prospective case series. Am J Surg, 2008;195(6):749-56.
37. Narbona-Arnau B, Olavarietta L, Lioris JM, Narbona-Calvo B. Reflujo gastroesofagico hernia hiatal. Rehabilitacion quirurgica del musculo esofagico mediante pexia con el ligamento redondo. Resultados (1143 operados en 15 anos). Bol Soc Val Digest, 1980.
38. Novitsky YW, Harrell AG, Cristiano JA, Paton BL, Norton HJ, Peindl RD, et al. Comparative evaluation of adhesion formation, strength of ingrowth, and textile properties of prosthetic meshes after long-term intra- abdominal implantation in a rabbit. J Surg Res. 2007;140(1):6-11.
39. Oelschlager BK, Barreca M, Chang L, Pellegrini CA. The use of small intestine submucosa in the repair of paraesophageal hernias: initial observations of a new technique. Am J Surg. 2003;186(1):4-8.
40. Oelschlager BK, Pellegrini CA, Hunter J, Soper N, Brunt M, Sheppard B, et al. Biologic prosthesis reduces recurrence after laparoscopic paraesophageal hernia repair: a multicenter, prospective, randomized trial. Ann Surg. 2006;244(4):481-90.
41. Perdikis G, Hinder RA, Filipi CJ, Walenz T, McBride PJ, Smith SL, et al. Laparoscopic paraesophageal hernia repair. Arch Surg. 1997;132(6):586.
42. Pitcher DE, Curet MJ, Martin DT, Vogt DM, Mason J, Zucker KA. Successful laparoscopic repair of paraesophageal hernia. Arch Surg. 1995;130(6):590-6.
43. Purkiss SF, Argano VA, Kuo J, Lewis CT. Oesophageal erosion of an Angelchik prosthesis: surgical management using fundoplication. Eur J Cardiothorac Surg. 1992;6(9):517-8.
44. Roman S, Poncet G, Serraj I, Zerbib F, Boulez J, Mion F. Characterization of reflux events after fundoplication using combined impedance-pH recording. Br J Surg. 2006;94(1): 48-52.
45. Rydberg L, Ruth M, Lundell L. Does oesophageal motor function improve with time after successful antireflux surgery? Results of a prospective, randomised clinical study. Gut. 1997;41(1):82-6.
46. Rydberg L, Ruth M, Lundell L. Mechanism of action of antireflux procedures. Br J Surg. 1999;86(3):405-10.
47. Schauer PR, Ikramuddin S, McLaughlin RH, Graham TO, Slivka A, Lee KK, et al. Comparison of laparoscopic versus open repair of paraesophageal hernia. Am J Surg. 1998;176(6): 659-65.
48. Shulman AG, Amid PK, Lichtenstein IL. The safety of mesh repair for primary inguinal hernias: results of 3,019 operations from five diverse surgical sources. Am J Surg. 1992;58(4):255-7.
49. Sifrim D, Holloway R, Silny J, Tack J, Lerut A, Janssens J. Composition of the postprandial refluxate in patients with gastroesophageal reflux disease. Am J Gastroenterol. 2001;96(3): 647-55.
50. Skinner DB, Belsey RH. Surgical management of esophageal reflux and hiatus hernia. Long-term results with 1,030 patients. J Thorac Cardiovasc Surg. 1967; 53(1):33-54.
51. Spechler SJ. The management of patients who have "failed" antireflux surgery. Am J Gastroenterol. 2004;99(3):552-61.
52. Stylopoulos N, Gazelle GS, Rattner DW. Paraesophageal hernias: operation or observation? Ann Surg. 2002;236(4):492-500.
53. Targarona EM, Bendahan G, Balague C, Garriga J, Trias M. Mesh in the hiatus: a controversial issue. Arch Surg. 2004;139(12):1286-96.
54. Tew S, Ackroyd R, Jamieson GG, Holloway RH. Belching and bloating: facts and fantasy after antireflux surgery. Br J Surg. 2000;87(4):477-81.
55. Trus TL, Bax T, Richardson WS, Branum GD, Mauren SJ, Swanstrom LL, et al. Complications of laparoscopic paraesophageal hernia repair. J Gastrointest Surg. 1997;1(3): 221-7; discussion 228.
56. Tutuian R, Castell DO. Multichannel intraluminal impedance: general principles and technical issues. Gastrointest Endosc Clin N Am. 2005;15(2):257-64.
57. van der Peet DL, Klinkenberg-Knol EC, Alonso Poza A, Sietses C, Eijsbouts QA, Cuesta MA. Laparoscopic treatment of large paraesophageal hernias: both excision of the sac and gastropexy are imperative for adequate surgical treatment. Surg Endosc. 2000;14(11):1015-8.
58. Varga G, Cseke L, Kalmar K, Horvath OP. Prevention of recurrence by reinforcement of hiatal closure using ligamentum teres in laparoscopic repair of large hiatal hernias. Surg Endosc. 2004;18(7):1051-3.
59. Wildi SM, Tutuian R, Castell DO. The influence of rapid food intake on postprandial reflux: studies in healthy volunteers. Am J Gastroenterol. 2004;99(9):1645-51.
60. Zaninotto G, Costantini M, Anselmino M, Boccu C, Bagolin F, Polo R, et al. Excessive competence of the lower oesophageal sphincter after Nissen fundoplication: evaluation by three-dimensional computerised imaging. Eur J Surg. 1995;161(4):241-6.
61. Zerbib F, des Varannes SB, Roman S, Pouderoux P, Artigue F, Chaput U, et al. Normal values and day- to-day variability of 24-h ambulatory oesophageal impedance-pH monitoring in a Belgian-French cohort of healthy subjects. Aliment Pharmacol Ther. 2005;22(10):1011-21.

CHAPTER 19

Laparoscopic Repair of Duodenal Perforation

INTRODUCTION

Perforation is a life-threatening complication of peptic ulcer disease. Intestinal perforation can present acutely or in an indolent manner like abscess or intestinal fistula formation. A confirmatory diagnosis is made primarily using abdominal imaging studies. Duodenal perforation is a common complication of duodenal ulcer. The first clinical description of perforated duodenal ulcer was made by Crisp in 1843. Laparoscopic treatment of perforated duodenum was first reported by Mouret in 1989.

Perforated duodenal ulcer is mainly a disease of young men but because of increasing smoking in women and use of nonsteroidal anti-inflammatory drug (NSAID) in all the age group, nowadays, it is common in all adult population. In Western society, it is a problem seen mainly in elderly women due to smoking, alcohol, and use of NSAID. Majority of patients of perforated duodenal ulcers are *Helicobacter pylori (H. pylori)* positive.

Diagnosis is made clinically and confirmed by the presence of pneumoperitoneum on radiographs **(Figs. 1A and B)**. Additional studies may be indicated as a means to further investigate a suspected perforation in a specific organ. Other imaging studies include endoscopy (upper, lower), esophagography, upper gastrointestinal series, ultrasound, contrast enema, and dye studies. Nonoperative management is successful in patients identified to have a spontaneously sealed perforation proven by water-soluble contrast gastroduodenogram. For most of the patient of perforation of duodenal ulcer, the preferred treatment is its immediate surgical repair. The traditional management of perforated duodenal ulcer was Graham patch plication described in 1937. Laparoscopic repair of duodenal perforation by Graham patch plication is an excellent alternative approach.

Operative management consists of the time-honored practice of omental patch closure, but now same can be done by laparoscopic methods. The practice of addition of acid-reducing procedures is currently being debated, though it continues to be recommended in high-risk patients. Laparoscopic approaches to closure of duodenal perforation are now being applied widely and may become the gold standard in the future, especially in patients with <10 mm perforation size presenting within the first 24 hours of onset of pain. The role of *H. pylori* in duodenal ulcer perforation is controversial and more studies are needed to answer this question, though recent indirect evidence suggests that eradicating *H. pylori* may reduce the necessity for adding acid-reducing procedures and the associated morbidity.

Perforated duodenal ulcer is a surgical emergency. Laparoscopic repair of duodenal perforation is a useful

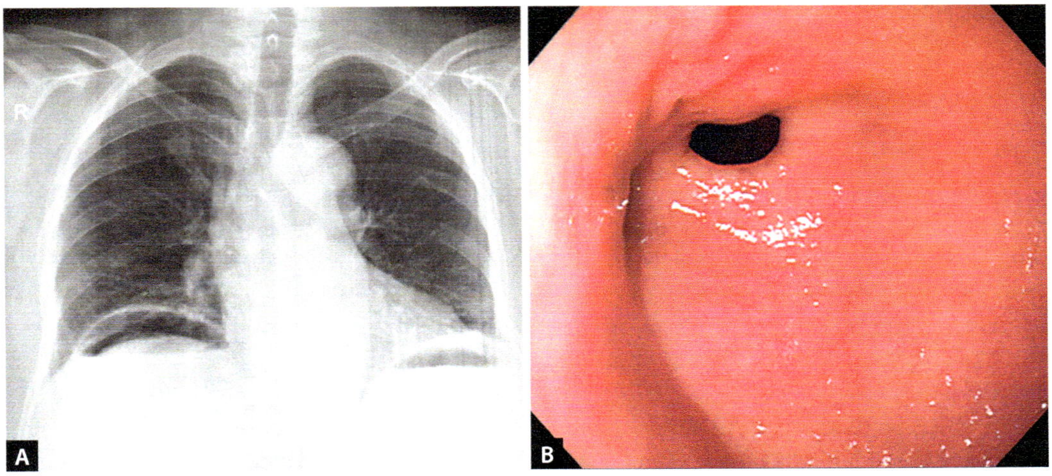

Figs. 1A and B: (A) Gas under diaphragm revealing perforation; (B) Endoscopic finding of duodenal perforation.

method for reducing hospital stay, complications, and return to normal activity. In many elegantly designed and meticulously executed prospective randomized trial, the laparoscopic approach in the management of perforated peptic ulcer disease has been compared to the open approach. Studies validate that laparoscopic approach is safe, feasible, and with morbidity and mortality comparable to that of the open approach. With better training in minimal access surgery now available, the time has arrived for it to take its place in the surgeon's repertoire.

ADVANTAGES OF LAPAROSCOPIC APPROACH

- Cosmetically better outcome
- Less tissue dissection and disruption of tissue planes
- Less pain postoperatively
- Low intraoperative and postoperative complications
- Early return to work.

The main tasks of this operation consist of:

- Preparation of the patient
- Creation of pneumoperitoneum
- Insertion of ports
- Diagnostic laparoscopy and locating the perforation
- Cleaning the abdomen
- Closure of the perforation with an omental patch
- Irrigation and suction of operating field
- Final diagnostic laparoscopy for any bowel injury or hemorrhage
- Removal of the instrument with complete exit of carbon dioxide (CO_2)
- Closure of wound.

Patient Selection

Duodenal perforation is a surgical emergency. If the patient condition is otherwise stable and peritonitis is diagnosed within 12 hours of onset, it is possible to repair the perforation by laparoscopic method. After 12 hours, chemical peritonitis will give way to bacterial peritonitis, with severe sepsis and then the laparoscopic repair is not advisable.

OPERATIVE TECHNIQUE

Patient Position

The patient is placed on the operating table with the legs in stirrups, the knees slightly bent, and the hips flexed approximately 10°. The operating table is tilted head up by approximately 15° **(Figs. 2A and B)**. Compression bandage is used on leg during the operation to prevent thromboembolism. The surgeon stands between the patient's legs. The first assistant, whose main task is to position the video camera, sits on the patient's left side. The instrument trolley is placed on the patient's left allowing the scrub nurse to assist with placing the appropriate instruments in the operating ports. Television monitors are positioned on either side of the top end of the operating table at a suitable height for surgeon, anesthetist, and assistant to see the procedure.

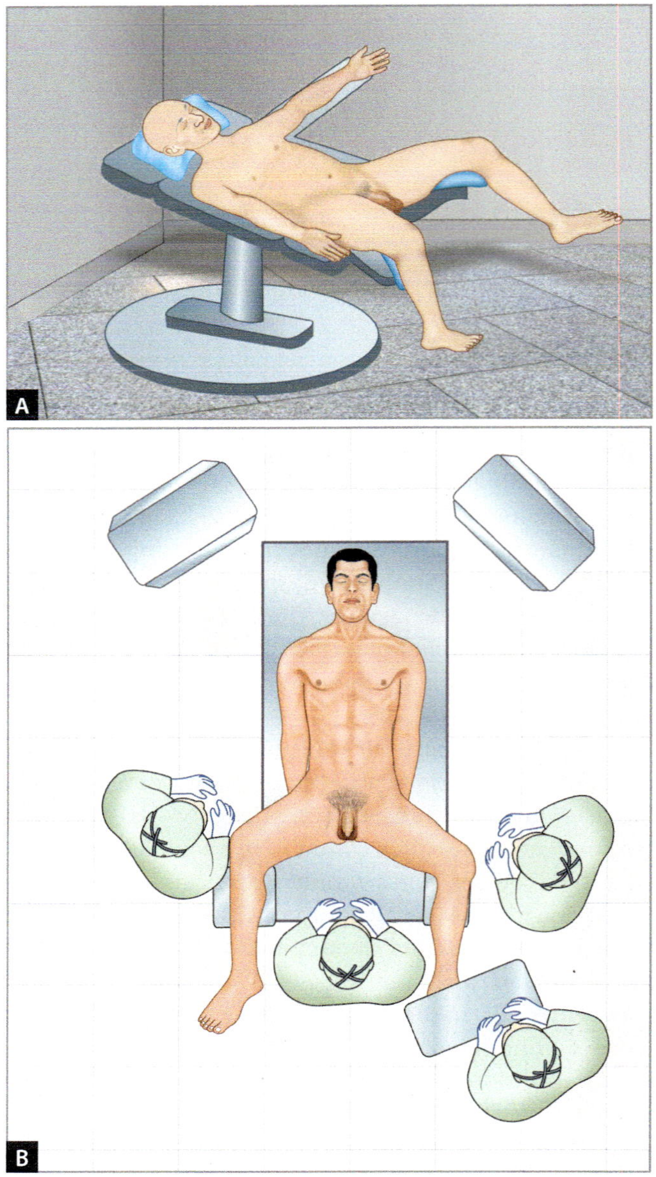

Figs. 2A and B: Position of patient for laparoscopic repair of duodenal perforation.

Anesthesia

General endotracheal anesthesia is used. Each patient is injected in the preinduction phase with 60 mg intramuscular (IM) contramal, intravenous (IV) metronidazole or tinidazole, and with 2 g of cefizox IV. The H_2-receptor antagonist like ranitidine injection is also advisable.

Creation of Pneumoperitoneum

- Check Veress needle before insertion
- Check Veress needle tip spring
- Confirm that gas connection is functioning

- Ensure flushing with saline (does not block that needle)
- Make a small incision just above the umbilicus
- Lift up abdominal wall and gently insert Veress needle till a feeling of giving way and two click sound
- Confirm position of needle by saline drop tests
- Connect CO_2 tube to needle and confirm quadromanometric indicators
- Switch off gas when desired pneumoperitoneum is created and remove the Veress needle.

Port Location

Four ports are then inserted, using the triangulation concept, to form a diamond shape. The surgeon usually stands between the legs of patient. A 10 mm camera port is placed in the umbilicus; this position will vary according to the build of the patient. A 5 mm port is inserted in the right upper quadrant 8–10 cm from the midline. A 5 mm port is placed in the left upper quadrant and another 5 mm port is placed in the right subxiphoid region **(Fig. 3)**.

The patient is placed in reverse Trendelenburg's position, with the first assistant to the right and a second assistant to the left. The surgeon thus works comfortably with two hands, triangulated with the cameras.

Locating the Perforation

The gallbladder, which usually adheres to the perforation, is retracted by the surgeon's left hand and moved upward. The gallbladder is passed to the assistant using the subxiphoid port which is placed to the right of the falciform ligament. The exposed area is checked and the perforation is usually clearly identified as a pinpoint hole on the anterior aspect of the duodenum.

Cleaning the Abdomen

Whole abdomen should be irrigated and aspirated with about 10 L of saline mixed with antibiotics. Each quadrant is cleaned methodically, starting at the right upper quadrant, going to the left, moving down to the left lower quadrant, and then finally over to the right. Special attention should be given to the vesicorectal pouch. Fibrous membranes are removed as much as possible, since they might contain bacteria.

Closure of the Perforation with an Omental Patch

A flappy piece of omental flap should be taken and the assistant holds the omentum patch just over the perforation using both the hands **(Figs. 4A to C)**. Intracorporeal knot together with omental patch should be applied to seal the perforation. The perforation is closed by intracorporeal stitches (simple closure by 3/0 Vicryl on Ski needle) and re-enforced by a pedicle omental graft **(Figs. 5A to F)**. This should be followed by a complete lavage of the peritoneal cavity with an ample amount of warm physiological saline. Always insert the omental patch in the knot rather than tail of the knot to hold the omentum because with the latter, a small space remains between the knots. Do not use extracorporeal knotting because this exerts tension on the friable tissue.

Ending of the Operation

At the end of the procedure, the abdomen should be examined for any possible bowel injury or hemorrhage. The instruments and then the ports should be removed. Telescope should be removed leaving gas valve of umbilical port open to let out all the gas. Closure of the wound is done with suture, Vicryl for rectus, and unabsorbable intradermal or stapler for skin. Adhesive sterile dressing over the wound should be applied. Patient may be discharged after 3 days.

Oral intake can be started after 48 hours, starting with clear fluids. They all are prescribed the triple therapy regimen, which consisted of clarithromycin and amoxicillin for 10 days, in addition to omeprazole for 14 days. This

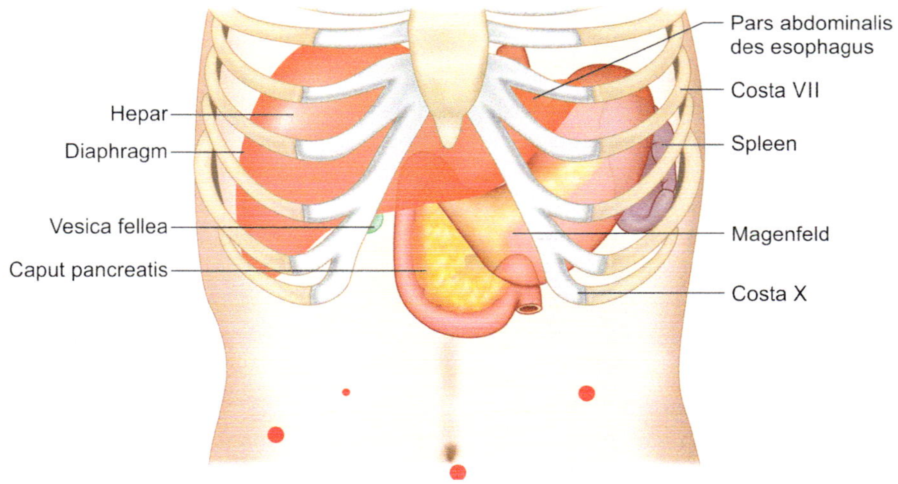

Fig. 3: Port position for laparoscopic repair of duodenal perforation.

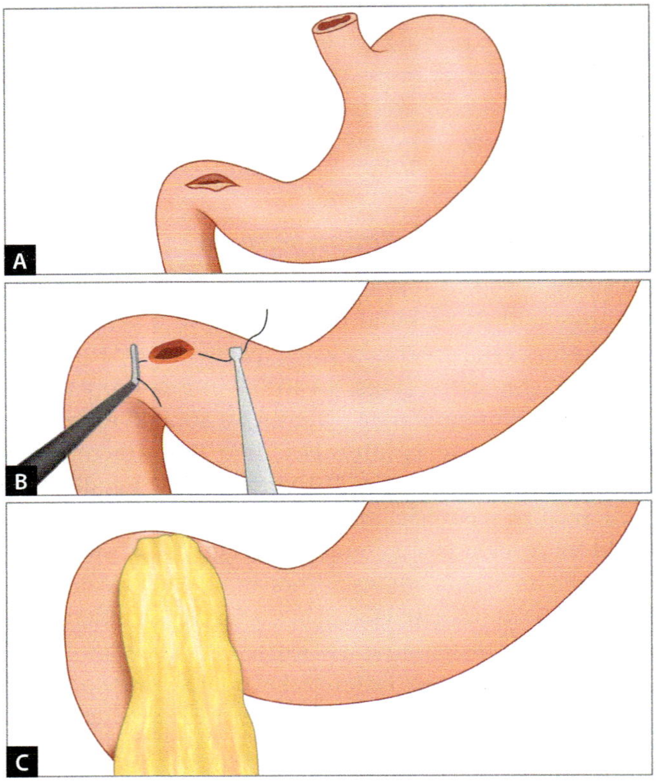

Figs. 4A to C: Closure of perforation with omental patch.

should be followed by gastroduodenoscopy after 2 months. All patients should be followed on an outpatient basis for at least 6 months and most (66%) of them for up to 2 years.

DISCUSSION

The incidence of perforated duodenal perforation remains the same. Operative treatment of perforated duodenal ulcer consists of time-honored practice of omental patch closure, but now this can be done by laparoscopic method. Laparoscopic approaches to closure of duodenal perforation are now being applied widely and may become the gold standard in the future, especially in patient with <10 mm perforation size presented within the first 24 hours of onset of pain. Perforated duodenal ulcer is a surgical emergency. Urgent simple closure of the perforation with omental patching is widely applied for the vast number of these patients; the consensus is to perform simple closure alone without any definite procedures, especially in patients with poor surgical risks and severe peritonitis. Various laparoscopic techniques have been advocated for closing the perforation by intra- and extracorporeal knots, sutureless techniques, holding the omental patch by fibrin glue or sealing with a gelatin sponge, stapled patch closure, or gastroscopically aided management in the perforation. Many surgeons have reported patient with sealed perforation and have been managed by peritoneal lavage and drainage only.

LAPAROSCOPIC CLOSURE OF PERFORATION OFFERS IMPORTANT ADVANTAGES

- Decreased postoperative pain
- Less abdominal wall complication
- Better visualization and ability to carry out a thorough peritoneal lavage
- Cosmetically better outcome
- Lower intraoperative and postoperative complications
- Early return to work
- Early mobilization
- Lower mortality
- It is as safe and effective as open surgery
- Patients subjective well-being was better after laparoscopic repair of perforated duodenal ulcer.

Laparoscopic duodenal ulcer perforation closure was performed in 30 patients. The interval before surgical intervention from the onset of perforation ranged between 20 and 36 hours. Perforation closure with Graham's patch omentoplasty was performed in all cases. In three patients, posterior truncal vagotomy and anterior highly selective vagotomy were combined with perforation closure. Oral fluid was permitted in second postoperative day (POD) in 21 patients and others on third and fourth POD. Postoperative morbidity was very minimal. Two patients had trocar site infection. All the patients were discharged between 5th and 7th POD.

Though the management of peptic ulceration has reduced the incidence of perforated peptic ulcer, it remains a challenging disease for the surgeons since it is an emergency procedure. The proper management of this complication of peptic ulcer disease has generated a lot of discussion; laparoscopic surgical treatment of perforated peptic ulcer is an attractive alternative for conventional treatment because of the absence of complications as compared to conventional surgery for patients who develop perforation in the setting of *H. pylori* infection. Eradication of infection may prevent ulcer recurrence.

Those patients who tolerate insult and whose ulcer was sealed may be adopted for nonoperative therapy. However, decision of nonoperative therapy is difficult and can be done only after evaluation by and close consultation with an experienced surgeon. If nonoperative treatment is chosen, then the patient requires frequent clinical examinations so the operative therapy can be done at the first sign of clinical deterioration. A variety of laparoscopic techniques have been described. A combined laparoscopic-endoscopic method was described, also mini-laparoscopy was described. Intracorporeal suturing was better than extracorporeal knotting because the latter one is liable to cut through tissues. The choice between combining definitive treatment and simple closure is still a matter of controversy. The choice depends on certain factors including age, fitness, and status of peritoneal cavity. The definitive surgical procedure of

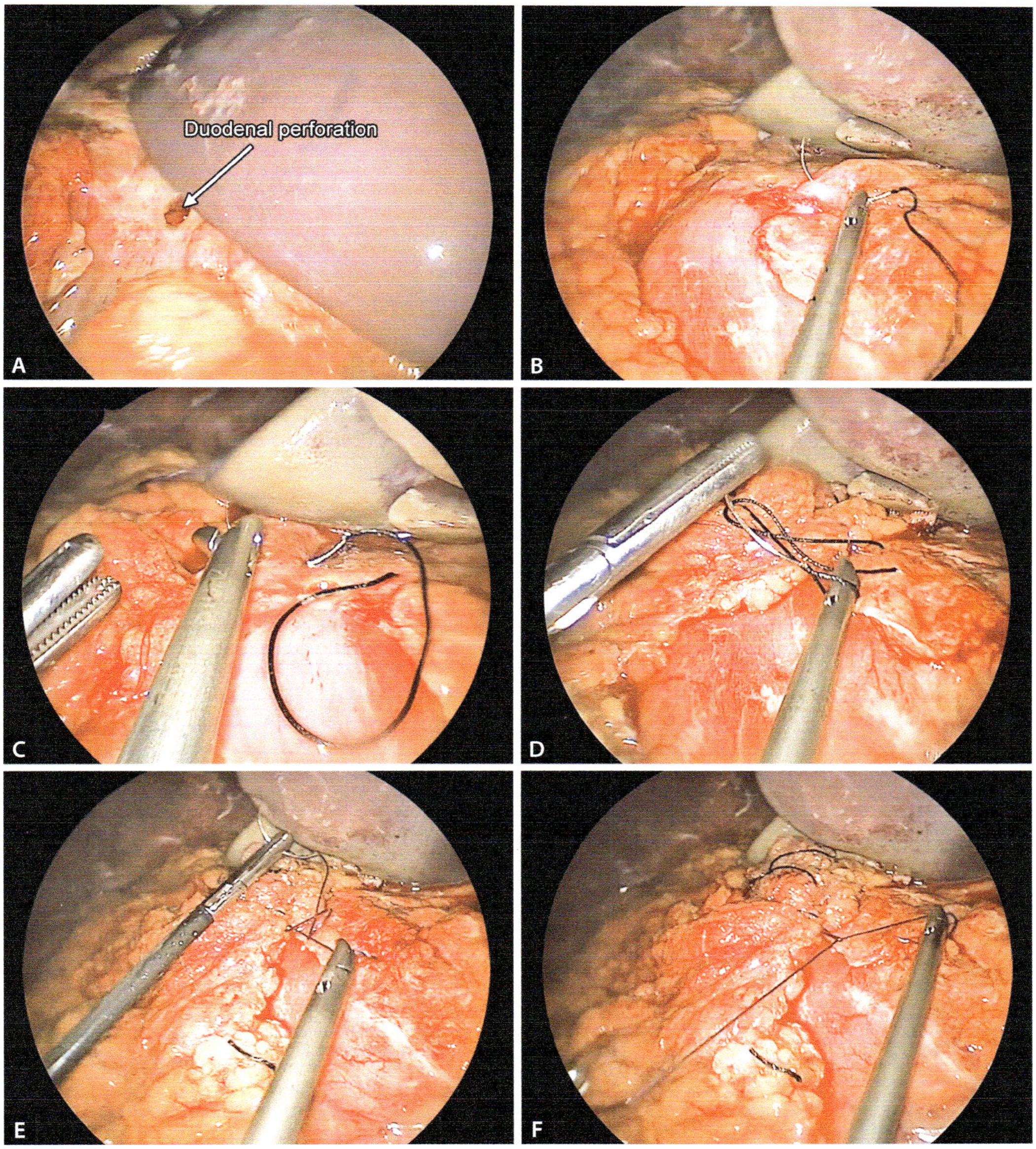

Figs. 5A to F: Closure of perforation with omental patch.

choice in perforated duodenal ulcer is patch closure and highly selective vagotomy. Although this procedure has low mortality and morbidity, it is technically demanding and requires experienced surgeon to ensure adequate vagotomy.

In this series, 30 cases of perforated duodenal perforation, three were treated with combined definitive treatment. Older patients with septic shock and generalized peritonitis should better be served by conventional surgery. Open conversion may be required, especially in the presence of certain high-risk factors as:

- Inadequate ulcer localization
- Posterior location of gastric ulcer
- Pancreatic infiltration (penetrating ulcer)
- Localized abscess formation.

It been shown that the age, presence of concomitant disease and length of free air, or fluid collection in abdominal CT scan correlate with conversion in meta-analysis of 13 publication comprising 658 patients comparing open versus laparoscopic closure of perforated duodenal perforation, it was found that postoperative pain was lower after laparoscopic repair than open repair supported by significant reduction in postoperative analgesic requirement after laparoscopy repair, meta-analysis demonstrated a significant reduction in wound infection after laparoscopic repair as compared with open. But, a significant higher reoperation rate was observed after laparoscopic perforated duodenal repair. Laparoscopic perforated duodenal repair is a safe and reliable procedure associated with short operating time, less postoperative pain, reduced chest complication, shorter postoperative hospital stay, and earlier returns to normal daily activity than conventional open repair. Operative time is also shorter and morbidity also lowers in laparoscopic repair of perforated duodenal ulcer. Also, low mortality, better cosmetic outcome with laparoscopic repair, and postoperative adhesions and incision hernia were lower in comparing with open method. Laparoscopic repair is as safe and effective as open repair. The patient's subjective well-being was better after laparoscopic repair. Laparoscopy provides better vision of peritoneal cavity and allows early mobilization.

The incidence of perforated peptic ulcer disease has decreased nowadays with vast improvement in medical therapy. However, minimal invasive surgery still has a significant role to play in treatment of complicated disease. It decreases hospital stay and overall recovery period as compared to open surgery, regardless of the preference of the individual surgeon. Our result has shown that the laparoscopic surgery may become the gold standard for surgical treatment of complicated peptic ulcer disease.

Laparoscopic closure of duodenal ulcer perforation is an attractive alternative to conventional surgery with the benefits of minimally invasive surgery such as parietal wall integrity, cosmetic benefits, and early subjective postoperative comfort and rehabilitation.

BIBLIOGRAPHY

1. Andersen IB, Bonnevie O, Jørgensen T, Sørensen TI. Time trends for peptic ulcer disease in Denmark, 1981-1993. Analysis of hospitalization register and mortality data. Scand J Gastroenterol. 1998;33:260-6.
2. Canoy DS, Hart AR, Todd CJ. Epidemiology of duodenal ulcer perforation: a study on hospital admissions in Norfolk, United Kingdom. Dig Liver Dis. 2002;34:322-7.
3. Crofts TJ, Park KG, Steele RJ, Chung SS, Li AK. A randomized trial of nonoperative treatment for perforated peptic ulcer. N Engl J Med. 1989;320:970-3.
4. Darby CR, Berry AR, Mortensen N. Management variability in surgery for colorectal emergencies. Br J Surg. 1992;79:206-10.
5. Dawson EJ, Paterson-Brown S. Emergency general surgery and the implications for specialisation. Surgeon. 2004;2:165-70.
6. Dunkley AS, Eyers PS, Vickery CJ, Welbourn CR, Chester JF. The emergency general surgeon: a new career pathway. Bull Royal Coll Surg Engl. 2007;89:32-6.
7. Lau JY, Sung JJ, Lam YH, Chan AC, Ng EK, Lee DW, et al. Endoscopic retreatment compared with surgery in patients with recurrent bleeding after initial endoscopic control of bleeding ulcers. N Engl J Med. 1999;340:751-6.
8. Leontiadis GI, Sharma VK, Howden CW. Proton pump inhibitor treatment for acute peptic ulcer bleeding. Cochrane Database Syst Rev. 2006;25:CD002094.
9. Lunevicius R, Morkevicius M. Systematic review comparing laparoscopic and open repair for perforated peptic ulcer. Br J Surg. 2005;92:1195-207.
10. Mercer SJ, Knight JS, Toh SK, Walters AM, Sadek SA, Somers SS. Implementation of a specialist-led service for the management of acute gallstone disease. Br J Surg. 2004;91:504-8.
11. Noguiera C, Silva AS, Santos JN, Silva AG, Ferreira J, Matos E, et al. Perforated peptic ulcer: main factors of morbidity and mortality. World J Surg. 2003;27:782-7.
12. Paimela H, Oksala NK, Kivilaakso E. Surgery for peptic ulcer today. A study on the incidence, methods and mortality in surgery for peptic ulcer in Finland between 1987 and 1999. Dig Surg. 2004;21:185-91.
13. Post PN, Kuipers EJ, Meijer GA. Declining incidence of peptic ulcer but not of its complications: a nation-wide study in The Netherlands. Aliment Pharmacol Ther. 2006;23:1587-93.
14. Qvist P, Arnesen KE, Jacobsen CD, Rosseland AR. Endoscopic treatment and restrictive surgical policy in the management of peptic ulcer bleeding. Five years' experience in a central hospital. Scand J Gastroenterol. 1994;29:569-76.
15. Read TE, Myerson RJ, Fleshman JW, Fry RD, Birnbaum EH, Walz BJ, et al. Surgeon specialty is associated with outcome in rectal cancer treatment. Dis Colon Rectum. 2002;45:904-14.
16. Ripoll C, Bañares R, Beceiro I, Menchén P, Catalina MV, Echenagusia A, et al. Comparison of transcatheter arterial embolization and surgery for treatment of bleeding peptic ulcer after endoscopic treatment failure. J Vasc Interv Radiol. 2004;15:447-50.
17. Thomsen RW, Riis A, Munk EM, Nørgaard M, Christensen S, Sørensen HT. 30-day mortality after peptic ulcer perforation among users of newer selective COX-2 inhibitors and traditional NSAIDs: a population-based study. Am J Gastroenterol. 2006;101:2704-10.
18. Tu JV, Austin PC, Johnston KW. The influence of surgical specialty training on the outcomes of elective abdominal aortic aneurysm surgery. J Vasc Surg. 2001;33:447-52.
19. Zorcolo L, Covotta L, Carlomagno N, Bartolo DC. Toward lowering morbidity, mortality, and stoma formation in emergency colorectal surgery: the role of specialization. Dis Colon Rectum. 2003;46:1461-7.

CHAPTER 20 Laparoscopic Fundoplication

INTRODUCTION

Gastroesophageal reflux disease (GERD) is defined as the failure of the antireflux barrier, allowing abnormal reflux of gastric contents into the esophagus. It is a condition which develops when the reflux of stomach contents causes troublesome symptoms and complications. It is a mechanical disorder which is caused by a defective lower esophageal sphincter (LES), a gastric-emptying disorder, or failed esophageal peristalsis. Gastroesophageal reflux is one of the most common digestive symptoms. Exposure of the esophageal mucosa to acid, enzymes, and other digestive secretions leads to acute and chronic inflammations, with pain, and ulceration or stricture formation if untreated.

Heartburn occurs in 5–45% of adults in Western countries, depending on the frequency of symptoms, 30–45% suffer from symptoms once a month and 5–10% everyday. The majority of patients suffering from GERD experience minor symptoms for which they do not seek medical attention. Age does not seem to have an impact on the frequency of GERD symptoms, and no causal factor has been identified. Esophagitis due to reflux occurs in approximately 2% of the global population. It is the most frequent form of lesion detected on upper gastrointestinal (GI) endoscopy, occurring more frequently than gastric ulcers or duodenal ulcers. GERD is often a chronic ailment. After a 5–10-year follow-up, about two-thirds of patients complain of persistent symptoms requiring occasional or continuous treatment.

PATHOPHYSIOLOGY

The pathophysiology of GERD is multifactorial, although it is usually due to the weakening of the anatomical or functional gastroesophageal barrier located at the esophagogastric junction. Injury to the esophageal mucosa by acid-peptic gastric secretions, while secondary to this weakening, plays a major role in the development of GERD symptoms and lesions. In fact, suppressing the gastric acid secretion, which is the usual treatment of this ailment, leads to the disappearance of symptoms and healing of lesions in almost all cases. GERD is, therefore, acid-dependent.

Symptoms

- Heartburn (retrosternal burning)
- Regurgitation
- Pain
- Respiratory symptoms

Diagnostic Test

- Endoscopy
- Barium swallow
- Esophageal transit +/– manometry
- pH monitoring

Treatment of Gastroesophageal Reflux Disease

Medical therapy is the first line of management. Lifestyle modification and medications are the first-line treatment for GERD. Surgical management is generally reserved for patients who have persistent symptoms or develop complications despite optimal medical therapy. Esophagitis will heal in approximately 90% of cases with intensive medical therapy. However, symptoms recur in >80% of cases within 1 year of drug withdrawal. Since, it is a chronic condition, medical therapy involving acid suppression and/or promotility agents may be required for the rest of patient's life. Despite the fact that current medical management is very effective for the majority, a small number of patients do not get complete relief of symptoms. Currently, there is increasing interest in the surgical management of GERD.

The goal of surgical therapy is to recreate an antireflux barrier. Surgical management of GERD focuses on restoring a physiologic equivalent to the normal LES. It is the only treatment capable of changing the natural history of GERD. This interest in surgical therapy has been renewed with the advent of laparoscopic surgery.

Indications for Surgical Treatment

Currently, there is increasing interest in the surgical management of GERD. There are a number of reasons for this. Despite the fact that current medical management is very effective for the majority, a small number of patients do not get complete relief of symptoms. Secondly, some patients, particularly those who are in their 20s or 30s, face the prospect of a lifetime of continuous proton-pump inhibitor (PPI) therapy with the possible risk of, as yet, unknown side effects. In addition, the laparoscopic approach with its benefits of reduced operative trauma and less time off work has become a more common place. As a consequence, general practitioners and gastroenterologists are more convinced to refer patients with disabling symptoms for surgical treatment. Antireflux surgery is most often performed to control GI symptoms such as heartburn and regurgitation that are refractory to medical therapy. It may also be performed for non-GI symptoms such as chronic cough, laryngeal disease, and asthma. If there is solid objective evidence to attribute such symptoms to reflux. The GI symptoms are also referred to as typical symptoms and the non-GI symptoms as atypical symptoms. The gold standard antireflux operation is undoubtedly the Nissen type of total fundoplication and many studies have affirmed its effectiveness in controlling acid reflux. However, new symptoms after fundoplication such as gas bloat and dysphagia, which probably result from a hypercompetent LES produced by the Nissen operation, are common.

Concerning the indication for surgery, a distinction between heartburn and regurgitation symptoms is considered an important factor (medical treatment appears to be more effective for heartburn than for regurgitation). Even after successful medical acid suppression, the patient can have recurrent symptoms of epigastric pain and retrosternal pressure as well as food regurgitation due to an incompetent cardia, insufficient peristalsis, or a large hiatal hernia.

Surgical therapy should be considered in individuals with documented GERD who are:

- Refractory to medical management
- Associated with hiatus hernia
- Intolerance to postpartum hemorrhage (PPH) or H_2-receptors
- Not compliant to medical therapy
- Have complications of GERD, e.g., Barrett's esophagus, stricture, and grade 3 or 4 esophagitis
- Atypical symptoms such as asthma, hoarseness, cough, chest pain, and aspiration

Study has shown those patients resistant to antisecretory treatment are not good candidates for antireflux surgery.

PREOPERATIVE EVALUATION

All the patients should have endoscopy, standard pH testing, esophageal manometry, and barium esophagram be performed before antireflux surgery. Nonstandard pH testing or gastric-emptying study may be required for some patients.

Upper Gastrointestinal Endoscopy

Esophageal and gastric endoscopy should be performed to assess the esophageal and gastric mucosa for signs of malignancy prior to proceeding with an antireflux procedure. Patients with endoscopic findings of severe (Los Angeles grade C or D) esophagitis, biopsy-proven Barrett's esophagus ≥1 cm, or a benign peptic stricture are good candidates for fundoplication surgery.

Esophageal pH Testing

Esophageal pH monitoring is the gold standard technique for the detection of gastroesophageal reflux in adults and children. Patients with typical symptoms of GERD should undergo standard pH testing. Patients with atypical symptoms may require nonstandard pH testing, such as one with dual pH probe or impedance in order to document proximal and/or nonacidic reflux.

Standard pH Testing

Ambulatory pH testing is the gold standard for diagnosing pathologic GERD. Prior to antireflux surgery, all patients with nonerosive GERD, including those with Los Angeles grade A or B, esophagitis, and those with short-segment (<1 cm) Barrett's esophagus, should undergo standard pH testing to document abnormal distal esophageal acid exposure. An abnormal pH test in a PPI-dependent patient with typical symptoms predicts successful outcomes with antireflux surgery. Standard pH testing can be done via a transnasal catheter for 24 hours or a wireless pH system for 48 hours after the patient has been off acid suppression for 7 days.

Multichannel Intraluminal Impedance Testing

Multichannel intraluminal impedance (MII) is a catheter-based method to detect intraluminal bolus movement within the esophagus. MII is performed in combination with manometry or pH testing. Combined MII and pH (MII-pH) testing can detect both acid and nonacid gastroesophageal reflux. It should be recognized that this testing is somewhat controversial and interpretation is operator-dependent.

Dual pH Probe

Despite other available and seemingly superior technologies such as impedance testing, the current "gold standard" diagnosis of extraesophageal reflux continues to be 24-hour dual pH probe monitoring. This procedure involves placing a catheter through the nose and into the esophagus. Two sensors, proximally and distally located within the catheter, detect the pH level or acidity in the distal esophagus and hypopharynx. Extraesophageal reflux is diagnosed when stomach contents are shown to flow upward from the stomach to the distal esophagus, and subsequently to the proximal esophagus and into the hypopharynx. Measurements of pH are recorded to a small, portable device that is worn on a belt during the study.

Esophageal Manometry

Esophageal manometry is the most reliable way to assess LES competence and esophageal peristalsis. Overall, the LES is incompetent in about 60% of patients with GERD, while transient relaxation of a competent LES is the cause of GERD in the remaining 40%. Manometry assesses esophageal peristalsis as well and occasionally provides alternative diagnoses, such as scleroderma or achalasia, for which antireflux surgery may be contraindicated. Manometric findings may influence the surgical approach such as partial instead of complete fundoplication for those with weak peristalsis.

Barium Esophagram

Barium esophagram can demonstrate esophageal length, presence, and size of any hiatal hernia, presence of any esophageal diverticulum or stricture, and the extent of reflux with provocation.

Gastric-emptying Study

A 4-hour gastric-emptying study should be performed when the history of a patient with GERD symptoms suggests gastric outlet obstruction or gastroparesis with significant nausea, repeated vomiting, severe bloating or postprandial fullness, or retained food in the stomach after overnight fast.

METHODS OF FUNDOPLICATION

There is no one best operation for all patients with GERD. Currently available antireflux procedures include:

- Endoscopic radiofrequency treatment (Stretta)
- Endoscopic transoral incisionless fundoplication (TIF)
- Laparoscopic magnetic sphincter augmentation (LINX)
- Laparoscopic Hill gastropexy
- Laparoscopic partial fundoplication
- Laparoscopic Nissen fundoplication (NF)

Laparoscopic fundoplication is a safe procedure and can provide less postoperative morbidity in experienced hands. Fundus of the stomach, which is on the left of the esophagus and main portion of the stomach, is wrapped around the back of the esophagus until it is once again in front of this structure. The portion of the fundus that is now on the right side of the esophagus is sutured to the portion on the left side to keep the wrap in place. The fundoplication resembles a buttoned shirt collar. The collar is the fundus wrap and the neck represents the esophagus imbricated into the wrap. This has the effect of creating a one-way valve in the esophagus to allow food to pass into the stomach, but prevent stomach acid from flowing into the esophagus and thus prevent GERD.

Laparoscopic fundoplication is a useful method for reducing hospital stay, complications, and early return to normal activity.

TYPES OF FUNDOPLICATION SURGERY

Laparoscopic fundoplication has become the standard surgical method of treating GERD. Although Nissen total fundoplication is the most commonly performed procedure, partial fundoplication, either anterior or posterior, is becoming more acceptable because of a suggested lower risk of long-term side effects **(Fig. 1)**.

The 360° Nissen fundoplication has been the standard operation for gastroesophageal reflux, but is associated with substantial rates of "gas bloat," gagging, and dysphasia **(Fig. 2)**.

Toupet fundoplication (TF), a 270° posterior wrap, has fewer complications, and its outcome in compared with Nissen fundoplication, is favorable both in children as well as adults **(Fig. 3)**.

Although Nissen total fundoplication is the most commonly performed procedure, partial fundoplication, either anterior or posterior, is becoming more acceptable because of lower risk of long-term complication. Dor in 1962 described anterior fundoplication as an antireflux operation for patients who had a Heller myotomy for achalasia. In the 1970s, Watson developed an operation for patient suffering from GERD.

Most surgeons believe that the TF, a 270° posterior wrap, originally described in conjunction with myotomy for achalasia, has fewer complications, and its long-term outcome in comparison with NF is favorable both in children as well as adults.

The main tasks of this operation consist of:

- Preparation of the patient
- Creation of pneumoperitoneum and insertion of ports
- Diagnostic laparoscopy and dissection of visceral peritoneum

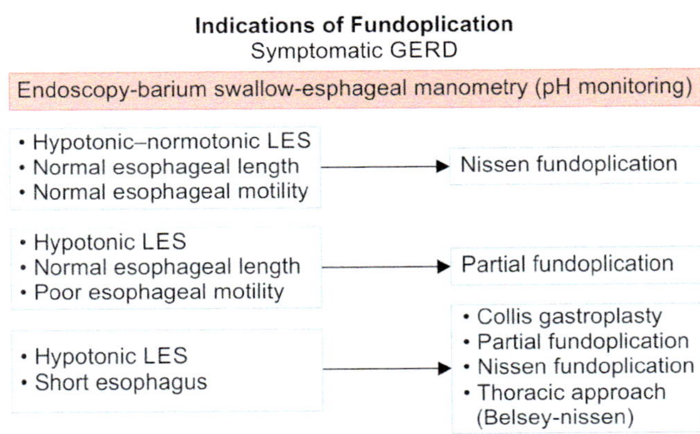

Fig. 1: Selection of type of fundoplication.
(GERD: gastroesophageal reflux disease; LES: lower esophageal sphincter)

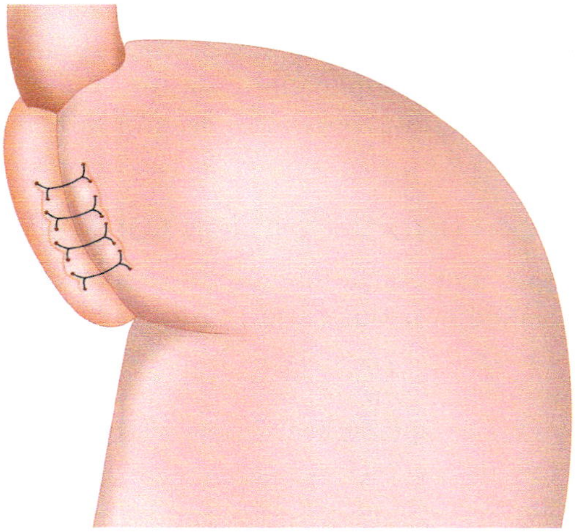

Fig. 2: Nissen fundoplication.

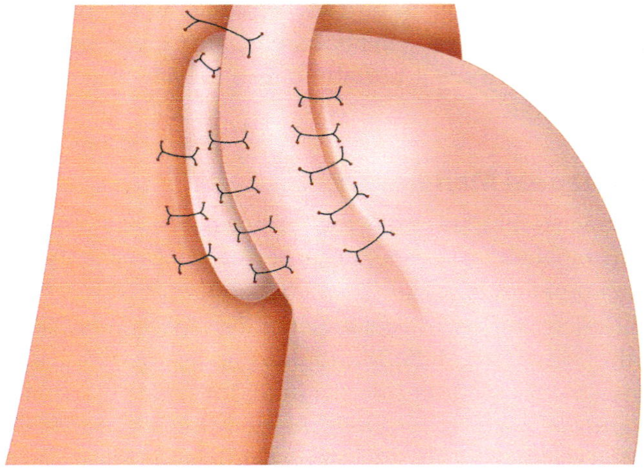

Fig. 3: Toupet fundoplication (TF), a 270° wrap.

- Mobilization of 5 cm of intra-abdominal esophagus
- Fundus pull from below the esophagus
- Insertion of posterior sutures to tighten the crural opening
- Fixation of fundus to the left crura
- Fixation of the fundus with the right crura
- Fixation of the fundus with esophagus. Inspection of tightness of fundoplication
- Irrigation and suction of operating field
- Final diagnostic laparoscopy for any bowel injury or hemorrhage
- Removal of the instrument with complete exit of CO_2. Closure of wound.

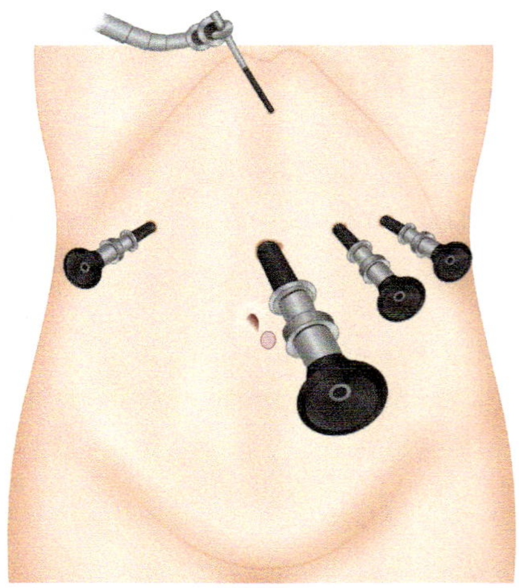

Fig. 4: Laparoscopic fundoplication port position.

PATIENT SELECTION

Many patients have symptoms palliated by lifestyle such as diet and exercise, others by simple medication, and some by strong medication such as PPI. A certain proportion of patients have refractory or long-term symptoms, and operation can be considered in this group of patients. As reflux symptoms are frequent and variable, it is wise to obtain both ambulatory 24 hours pH-metry and esophageal motility studies prior to surgery. Upper GI endoscopies should be performed in all patients.

OPERATIVE TECHNIQUE

The original fundoplication as described by Rudolph Nissen in 1956 involved passage of the gastric fundus behind the esophagus to encircle the distal 5 cm of the esophagus. In contemporary surgical practice, fundoplication is performed laparoscopically in most patients. Compared with open transabdominal or transthoracic fundoplication, laparoscopic fundoplication demonstrates comparable safety, efficacy in symptom relief, and patient satisfaction.

Patient Position

The patient is placed on the operating table with the legs in stirrups, the knees slightly bent, and the hips flexed approximately 10°. The operating table is tilted head up by approximately 15°. Compression bandage is used on leg during the operation to prevent thromboembolism. The surgeon stands between the patient's legs. The first assistant, whose main task is to position the video camera, sits on the surgeon's left side. The instrument trolley is placed on the patient's left allowing the scrub nurse to assist with placing the appropriate instruments in the operating ports.

Television monitors are positioned on either side of the top end of the operating table at a suitable height for surgeon, anesthetist, and assistant to see the procedure.

Port Position

The 10-mm camera (port 1) is placed in the midline approximately 5 cm above the umbilicus; this position will vary depending on the build of the patient **(Fig. 4)**. After inserting the camera, a 5-mm port (2) is inserted in the right upper quadrant 8–10 cm from the midline. A port (3), with a variable 5–10 mm size, is placed in the left upper quadrant—a mirror image of the one on the patient's right.

This allows both 5 mm and 10 mm instruments to be used through the same cannula without changing ports. A further 5-mm port (4) is positioned in the left anterior axillary line immediately below the costal margin. This port is mainly used for a forceps which will hold the tape encircling the esophagus **(Fig. 5)**. Liver retraction used to be one of the more problematic aspects of laparoscopic fundoplication. In our experience, these difficulties have been largely overcome by the use of the Nathanson liver retractor. Alternate port position in laparoscopic fundoplication is shown in **Figures 6A and B**.

Tissue Dissection and Mobilization

Mobilization of Stomach

The fundus part of the stomach is mobilized nicely along with the gastroesophageal junction by anteromedial traction. The short gastric vessels are separated with the help of a bipolar or harmonic scalpel which aids in further mobilization of the fundus of the stomach through the earlier formed posterior window. Care must be taken not to injure the spleen which is adjacent to the stomach.

Mobilization of Esophagus

Dissection starts at the avascular portion of the lesser omentum above the hepatic branch of the vagus. The dissection is continued carefully up to the hiatus, which can be seen through the defect created. An opening is created in the lesser omentum, above the hepatic branch of vagus to allow better access to the hiatus **(Figs. 7A to H)**.

The right crus is dissected using electrosurgery and scissors to identify the plane between the crus and surrounding loose areolar tissues. The loose areolar tissue around the esophagus is exposed and secures the bleeding from any blood vessels visible during mobilization of esophagus. Always remember not to injure the esophageal wall and vagal fibers when dissecting this area around esophagus. The space between the hiatus and the anterior aspect of esophagus is developed using fine dissection by scissors to divide blood vessels crossing this space.

Lesser Sac Opened

The posterior aspect of the left crus is identified as it meets the right crus and dissection of its surface commences, especially the peritoneal covering over the margin of right crus is dissected down to the fundus from the diaphragm known as Rossetti dissection technique. Dissection of the posterior aspect of the left crus is done by lifting the intra-abdominal esophagus forward with a blunt instrument. A sling is fed into the jaws of the grasping forceps and then pulled round behind the esophagus **(Fig. 8)**.

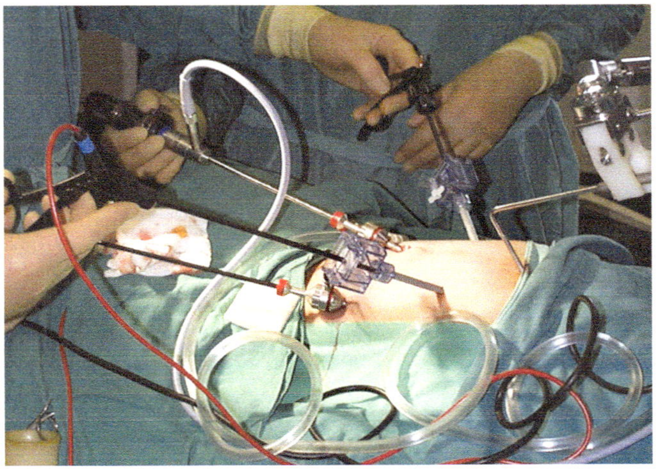

Fig. 5: Port position in fundoplication.

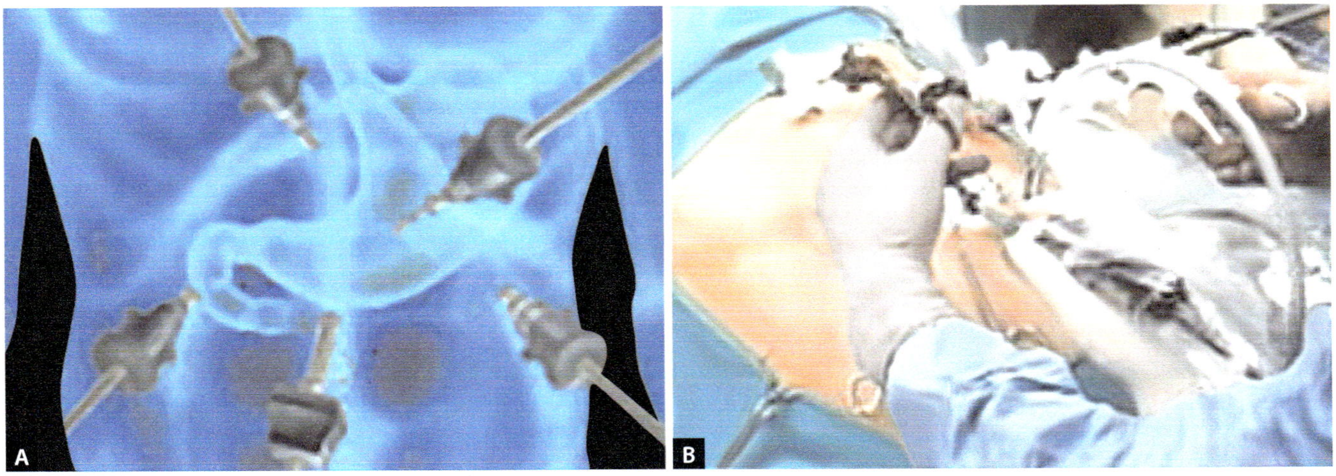

Figs. 6A and B: Alternative port position in laparoscopic fundoplication.

Sling is passed through a separate punctured wound from abdominal wall without port. A grasping forceps is inserted through one of the port to hold the sling so that the esophagus can be manipulated. Dissection surroundings of esophagus in the posterior mediastinum should for approximately 5–6 cm. Mobilization of the esophagus and stomach should be sufficient enough to have a good floppy fundus for wrap (**Fig. 9**).

The next step is to pull the fundus from behind the esophagus to form a wrap.

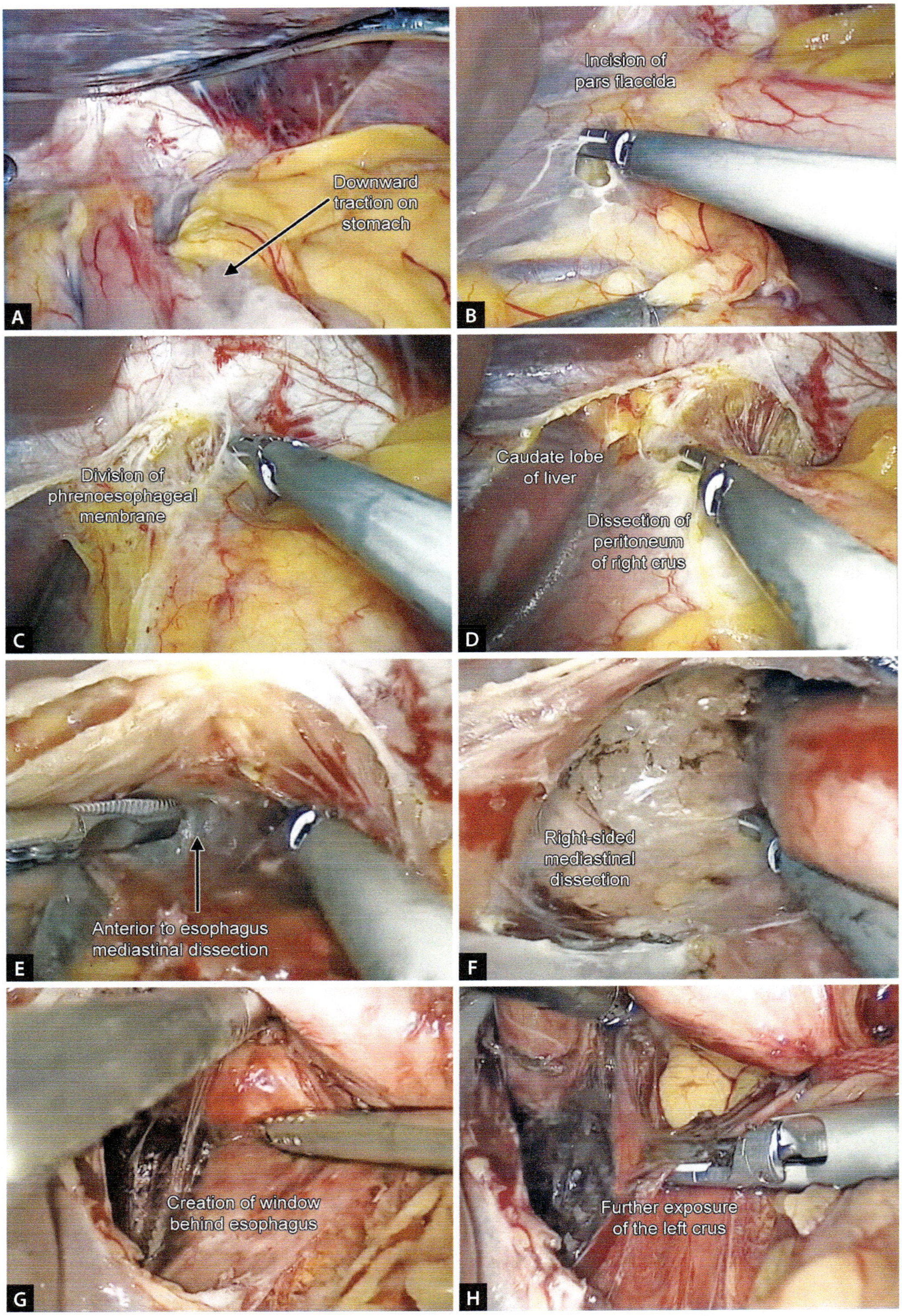

Figs. 7A to H: Mobilization of esophagus.

Fundus Pull

After mobilizing the fundus nicely, the tip of the fundus is pulled by one of the grasper introduced through below and right side of the esophagus **(Figs. 10 and 11)**.

The mobilization of stomach should be adequate to give a floppy fundus for plication otherwise patient may develop dysphagia. One stay suture may be applied to the fundus to hold it in place or one of the grasper may be used to keep it pulled. The next step is crural repair.

Crural Approximation

A posterior crural repair should be performed by approximating the right and left pillar of the left crus with sutures. Crura should be approximated behind the esophagus using two or three sutures of 2/0 braided polyamide on a 30-mm needle using tumble square knot or surgeon's knot. A further one or two sutures are inserted in the same way, at about 1 cm intervals and tied. It is important not to make the crural opening too tight since this will produce dysphagia **(Figs. 12A to D)**.

Further three sutures are then positioned at approximately 1 cm intervals to the posterior fundus and the right crus. The sling used for esophageal retraction is removed. A 50–60 French bougie should be placed in the stomach along the lesser curvature to calibrate the tightness of the fundoplication.

Fundoplication

By using an atraumatic grasper in the left hand, the posterior wall of the fundus is held through the opening made behind the esophagus. The posterior wall of fundus is pulled gently and at the same time, the extra-anterior wall is pushed back to avoid crowding of tissue within the window. By serial movements of pulling posterior wall forward and pushing anterior wall back, a sufficient amount of wrap is made around the esophagus, this can be ascertained by seeing the "buttock sign." The wrap made by both posterior and anterior walls of fundus should not be too tight. A Floppy Nissen's is made by doing the "shoe shine" maneuver. Suture material used is nonabsorbable sutures such as Dacron, silk, or polypropylene. Approximately 5 cm of mobilized esophagus should be prepared for fundal wrap.

First suture is taken with full thickness of anterior wall of fundus, and full thickness of posterior wall of fundus is taken. Intracorporeal surgeon's knot are used for plicating the stomach on to the esophagus, though "tumble square knots" can also be used.

Two sutures are taken above the first knot at a distance of 1 cm between each knot, involving full thickness of anterior wall of fundus, partial muscular layer of esophagus, and full thickness posterior wall of fundus. In the above suture, wall of esophagus is sandwiched between walls of fundus. Taking full thickness of esophagus in above sutures should be avoided as it may cause a complication of perforation of

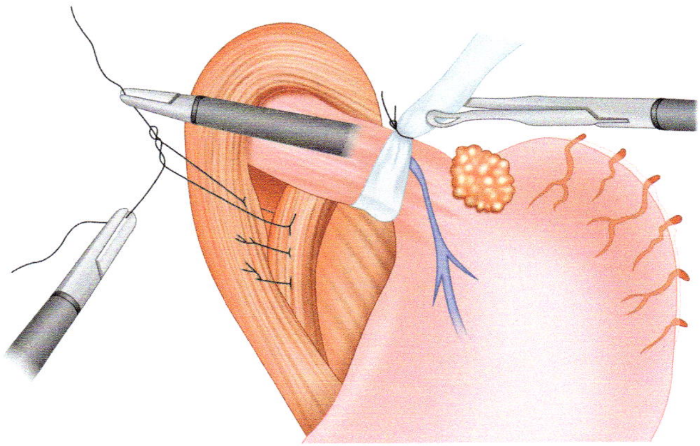

Fig. 9: Sling application around esophagus for proper exposure of crura.

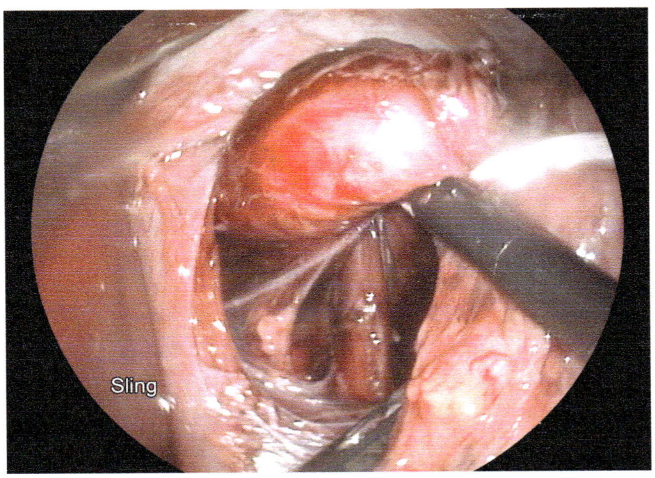

Fig. 8: Sling insertion.

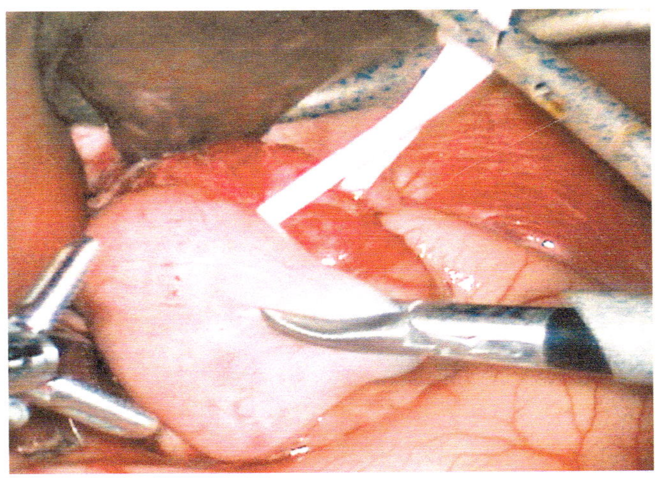

Fig. 10: Mobilized fundus of stomach is pulled from behind the esophagus.

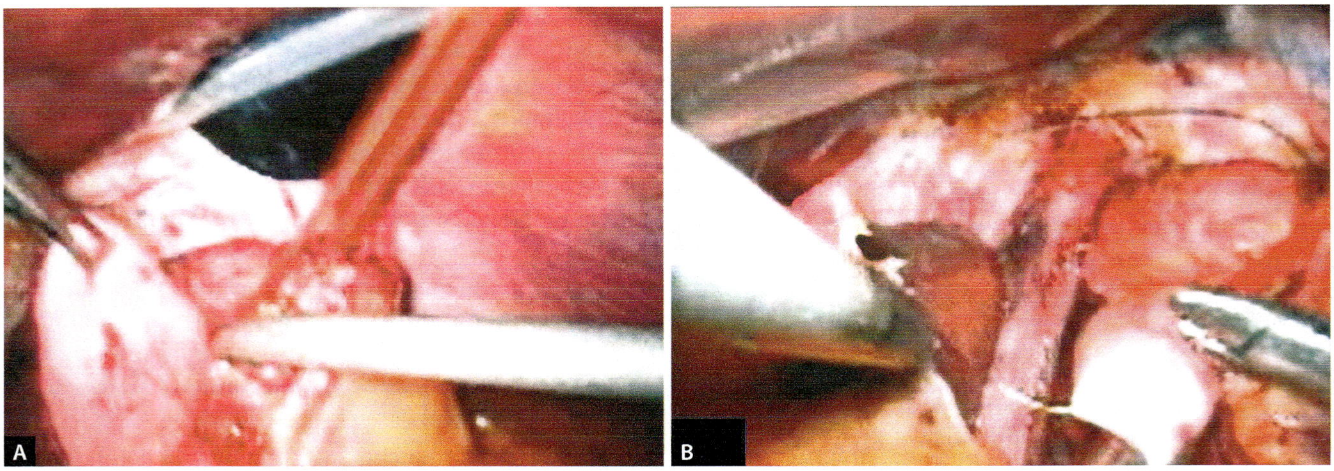

Figs. 11A and B: Fundus of stomach is pulled from behind the esophagus.

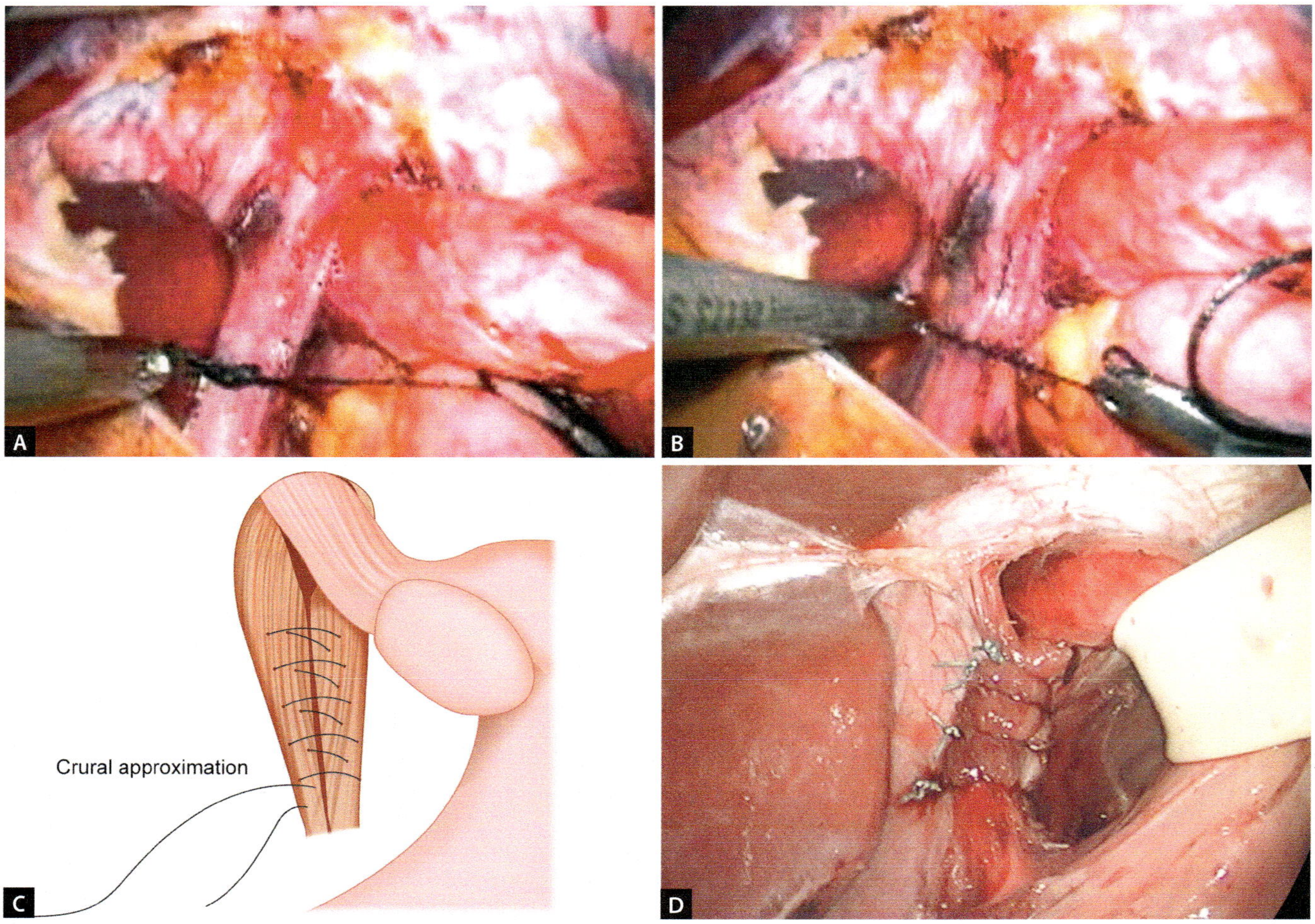

Figs. 12A to D: Approximation of crura.

esophagus. Two sutures are taken below the first knot at a distance of 1 cm between each knot in similar manner. Most surgeons would perform a wrap of 2–3 cm **(Figs. 13A to C)**.

Ending of the Operation

Abdomen should be examined for any possible bowel injury or hemorrhage. The instrument and then port should be removed carefully. Remove telescope leaving gas valve of umbilical port open to let out all the gas. Close the wound with suture. Use vicryl for rectus and unabsorbable intradermal or stapler for skin. Apply adhesive sterile dressing over the wound.

Patient may be discharged 2 days after operation, if everything goes well. Long-term observational studies of

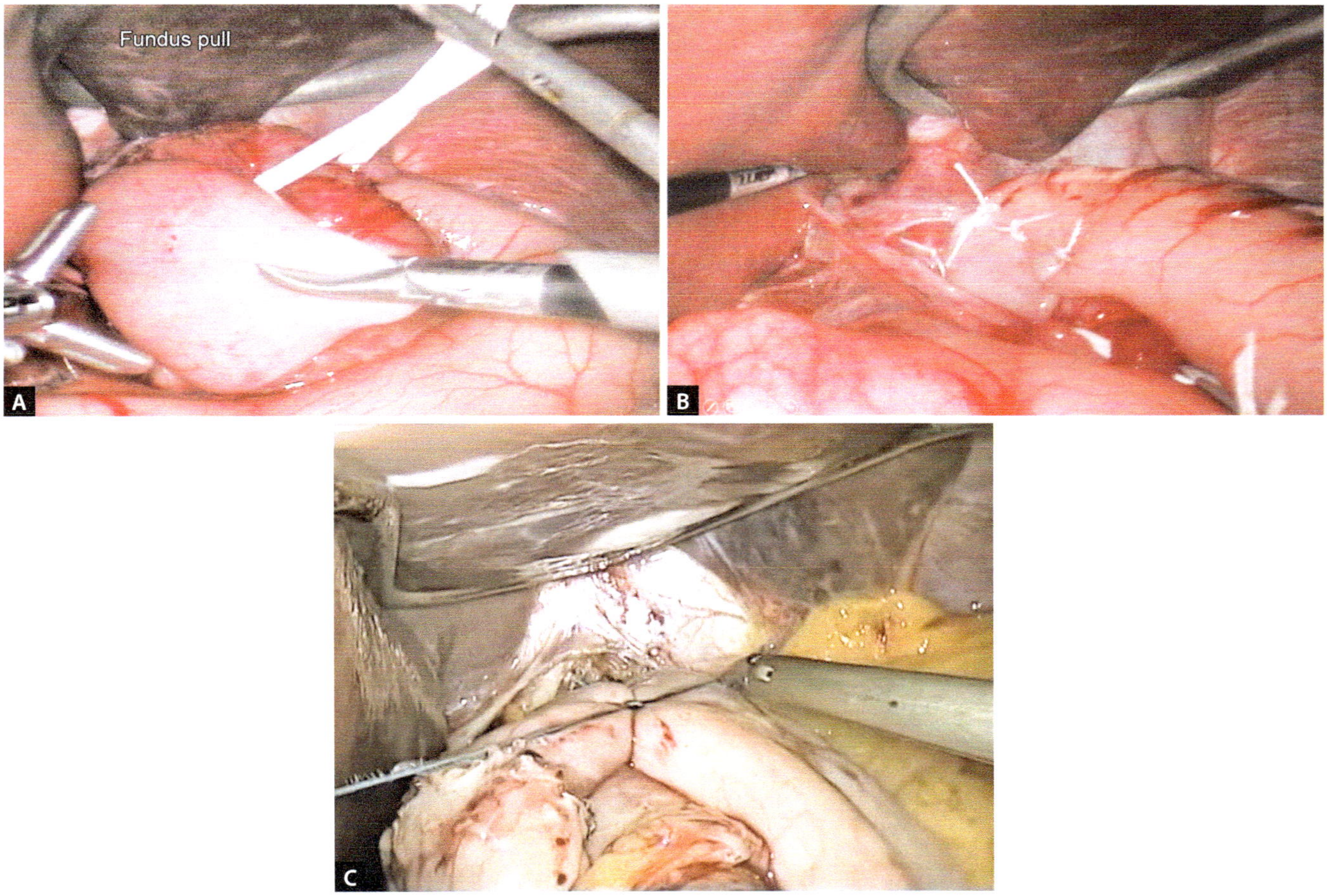

Figs. 13A to C: Fixation of wrap by intracorporeal sutures.

laparoscopic fundoplication performed by experienced operators generally report that 90–95% of adult patients are satisfied with the results of their surgery. The patient may have slight dysphagia initially but usually resolves after 6 weeks. The patient having any complain of dysphagia should be examined endoscopically after 3–4 weeks of operation. Dysphagia that persists for >12 weeks requires evaluation, which typically begins with a barium swallow to assess the anatomic placement of the fundoplication. In case of tight plication endoscopic dilatation technique, bougie or guidewire dilation should be done. Endoscopic dilatation procedure is well tolerated and produces good results. Patients who have a 360° fundoplication may be candidates for revision to a partial fundoplication, if dysphagia persists and effective barium tablet passage cannot be established despite dilation.

Symptoms of gas bloat syndrome can be elicited in a significant number of patients after fundoplication. Symptoms tend to lessen over time in most patients. In patients with severe persistent symptoms despite the medical treatment approaches, pyloroplasty, pyloric Botox injection, and pneumatic pyloric dilatation are options in select patients who have documented gastroparesis.

Long-term mortality of laparoscopic fundoplications is very low. The reported 30-day surgical mortality rate of laparoscopic fundoplication is <0.1–0.2%. The most commonly reported acute complications for laparoscopic fundoplications are gastric or esophageal injury, splenic injury or splenectomy, pneumothorax, bleeding, pneumonia, fever, wound infections, bloating, and dysphagia. Major acute complications are uncommon. In a study of 2,655 patients, 4.1% had a complication within 30 days of surgery, including 1.1% infection, 0.9% bleeding, and 0.9% esophageal perforation.

Rossetti–Nissen Fundoplication

A common modification is a 360° fundic wrap without division of the short gastric vessels is called Rossetti–Nissen fundoplication. However, most surgeons prefer to divide the short gastric vessels to allow for greater freedom of mobilization and reduced concern about torque on the fundoplication which is hard to measure and also facilitate lower esophageal relaxation.

Partial Fundoplications

A partial 270° posterior wrap, TF is used for patients with severe associated motor abnormalities. A partial 180° anterior wrap (Dor) has also been described. Based on currently available data, the choice of anterior versus posterior or partial versus complete NF should be left to the individual surgeon.

Hill Gastropexy

The Hill procedure involves imbrication of the anterior and posterior collar sling muscular fibers at the level of the gastroesophageal junction around the esophagus with tethering of the complex to the median arcuate ligament and closure of the diaphragm. Intraoperative manometry is used to achieve a desired LES pressure. This operation can also be used in a patient with a small stomach because of prior gastric resection. In a randomized trial, laparoscopic Hill gastropexy and laparoscopic Nissen fundoplication yielded similar and both excellent outcomes at 1-year follow-up. In a single-center retrospective study with a median follow-up of 18.5 years, 85% of patients who underwent Hill gastropexy reported good to excellent symptomatic outcomes and quality of life.

Magnetic Sphincter Augmentation (LINX Device)

In 2012, the US Food and Drug Administration (FDA) approved the LINX reflux management system as a treatment for GERD **(Figs. 14A and B)**. The device works by augmenting the LES with a ring made up of a series of rare earth magnets. The magnets have sufficient attraction to increase the LES closure pressure but permit food passage with swallowing.

Eligible patients must demonstrate typical GERD symptoms, an abnormal pH study, partial response to daily PPI therapy, and absence of a large hiatal hernia (>3 cm) or severe esophagitis. Patients who have allergies to titanium, stainless steel, nickel, or iron should not receive a LINX prosthesis. Patients who have the LINX device need to consult their surgeon before undergoing magnetic resonance imaging (MRI). A new version of LINX considered "MR Conditional" in a MRI system up to 1.5 Tesla (1.5 T) is now available. Scanning under different conditions may interfere with the magnetic strength and function of the device.

Laparoscopic magnetic sphincter augmentation device has been compared with laparoscopic Nissen fundoplication in several meta-analyses. Clinical control of reflux was comparable after the two procedures in both the short and longer term. In the longer term, there was less gas bloat associated with LINX than fundoplication. Presently, however, there is insufficient evidence that would allow surgeons to choose between the two procedures.

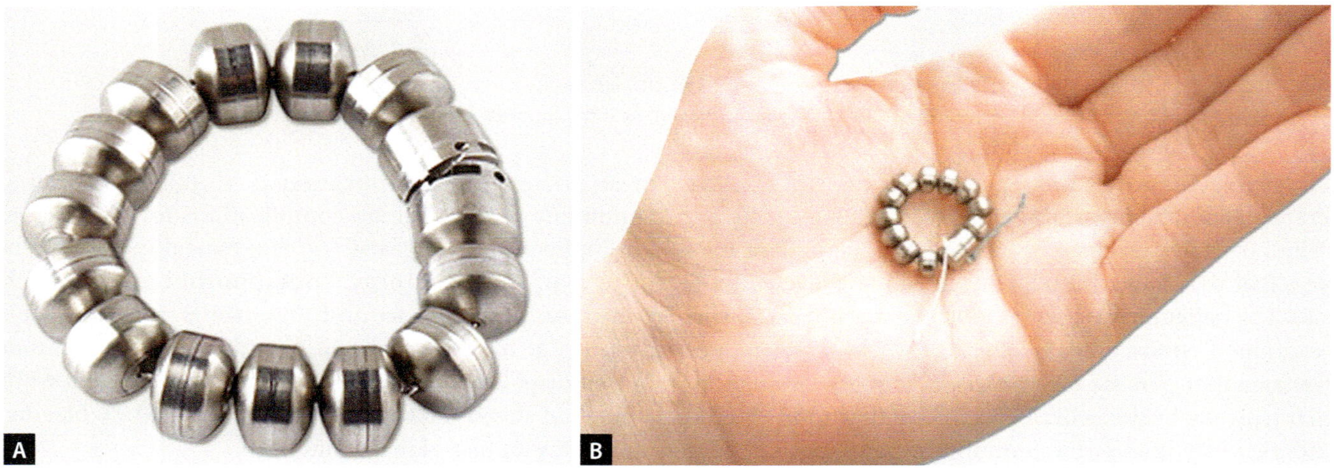

Figs. 14A and B: LINX sphincter augmentation system.

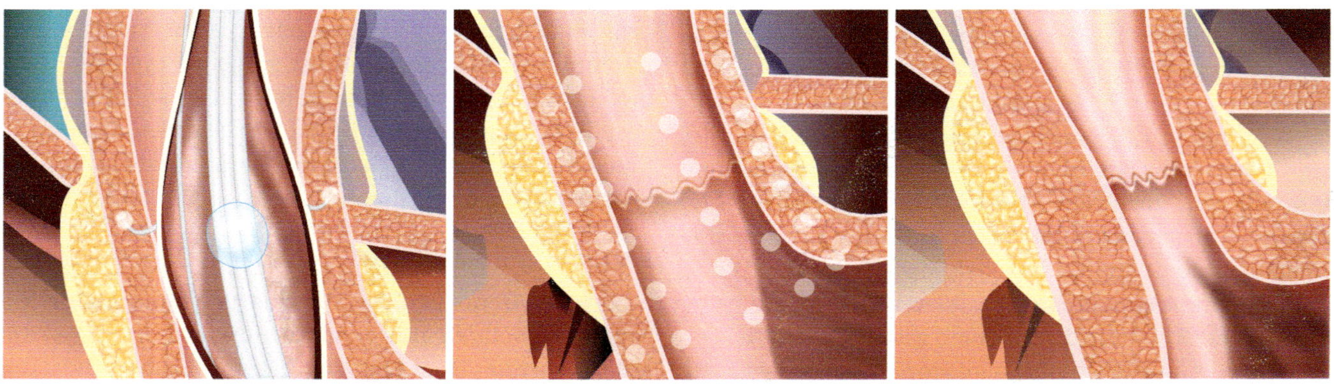

Fig. 15: Stretta therapy as a treatment option for gastroesophageal reflux disease (GERD).

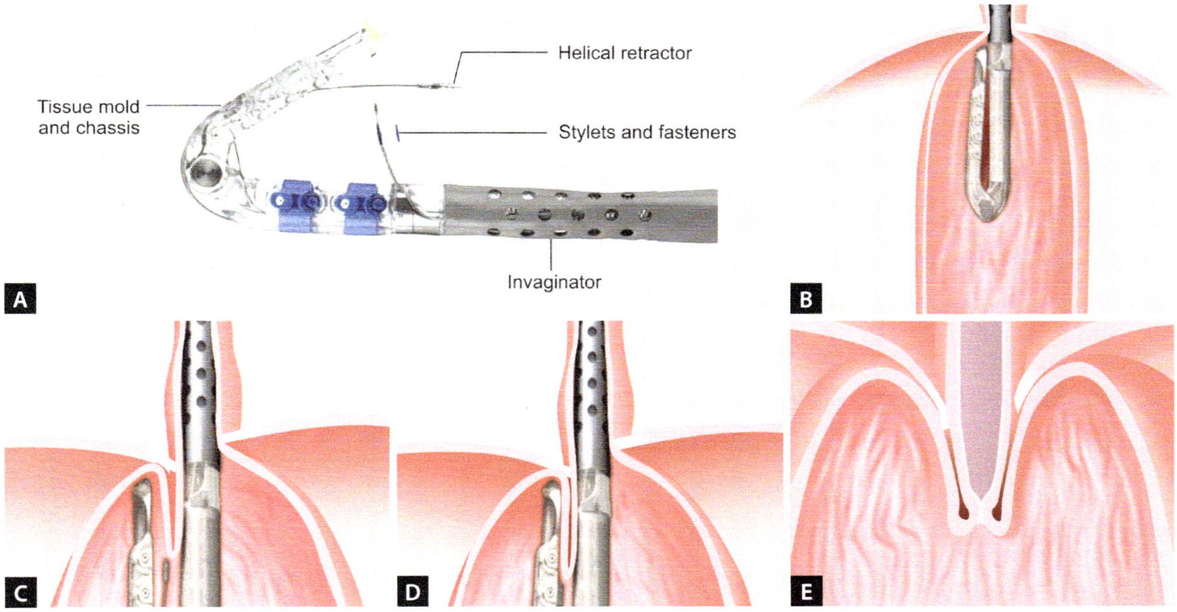

Figs. 16A to E: Transoral incisionless fundoplication (TIF).

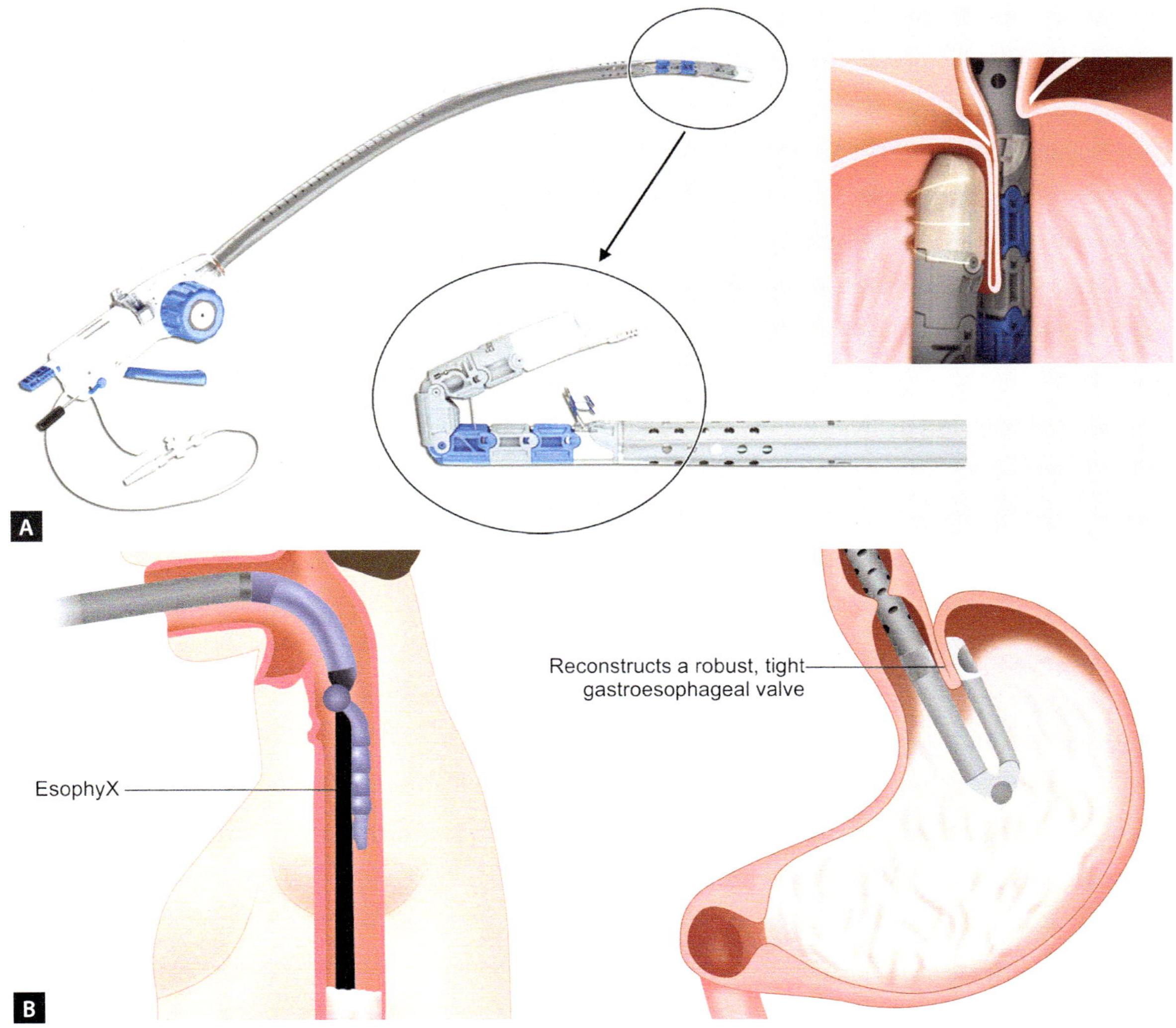

Figs. 17A and B: EsophyX device for transoral incisionless fundoplication (TIF).

Stretta Endoscopic Procedure

The Stretta procedure is the most widely studied endoscopic antireflux procedure. The specialized catheter is placed with endoscopic assistance over a guidewire. Using monopolar energy, a series of 56 treatments is delivered across five levels. Stretta is rated as effective therapy in patients with a lower esophageal pressure of at least 8 mm Hg and hiatal hernia <3 cm. The energy heats the tissue, ultimately causing it to swell and stiffen; the way this works was not understood as of 2019, but it was thought that perhaps the heat causes local inflammation, collagen deposition, and muscular thickening of the LES and that it may disrupt the nerves there **(Fig. 15)**.

Transoral Incisionless Fundoplication

Transoral incisionless fundoplication is an endoscopic procedure performed under general anesthesia to create a full-thickness serosa-to-serosa plication **(Figs. 16A to E)**. TIF creates 3–5 cm in length and 200–300° in circumference partial fundoplication. TIF can be performed in patients with typical GERD symptoms, no or only low-grade erosive esophagitis (grades A and B), and no or only small hiatal hernia (≤2 cm). TIF is contraindicated in patients with high-grade erosive esophagitis, Barrett's esophagus, atypical and extraesophageal symptoms of GERD, scleroderma, or other esophageal pathology or surgery. The EsophyX device has been CE marked for the market and FDA approved for the United States market for TIF procedures **(Figs. 17A and B)**.

Transoral incisionless fundoplication has been compared with PPI therapy in several randomized trials. In the latest trial (TEMPO), 63 patients with GERD refractory to PPI received TIF versus maximum standard dose PPI therapy. At 6 months, both regurgitation and extraesophageal symptoms were eliminated in more TIF than PPI patients (62 vs. 5%); 90% of TIF patients were off PPIs. After 6 months, all patients in the PPI (control) group elected to cross-over to TIF. At 3 years, 90% and 88% of patients reported elimination of troublesome regurgitation and all atypical symptoms, respectively. Although TIF is associated with fewer postoperative adverse effects such as gas bloating and dysphagia compared with surgical fundoplication, the durability of TIF is less certain than that of surgery.

For most patients undergoing surgical treatment for GERD, laparoscopic NF is a better option. This procedure appears to be the most effective and durable amongst all the procedures but is also associated with the greatest potential for dysphagia, difficulty in vomiting, and gas bloating. Patients with decreased esophageal motility or morbid obesity may benefit from an alternative procedure. For an individual patient, the best procedure may be the procedure in which the surgeon is most skilled.

BIBLIOGRAPHY

1. Akinola E, Rosenkrantz TS, Pappagallo M, McKay K, Hussain N. Gastroesophageal reflux in infants <32 weeks gestational age at birth: lack of relationship to chronic lung disease. Am J Perinatol. 2004;21(2):57-62.
2. Anvari M, Bamehriz F. Outcome of laparoscopic Nissen fundoplication in patients with body mass index >or= 35. Surg Endosc. 2006;20(2):230-4.
3. Augood C, MacLennan S, Gilbert R, Logan S. Cisapride treatment for gastroesophageal reflux in children. Cochrane Database Syst Rev. 2003;(4):CD002300.
4. Boyce PM, Talley NJ, Burke C, Koloski NA. Epidemiology of the functional gastrointestinal disorders diagnosed according to Rome II criteria: an Australian population-based study. Int Med J. 2006;36(1):28-36.
5. Bredenoord AJ, Weusten BL, Smout AJ. Symptom association analysis in ambulatory gastroesophageal reflux monitoring. Gut. 2005;54(12):1810-7.
6. Cameron BH, Blair GK, Murphy JJ III, Fraser GC. Morbidity in neurologically impaired children after percutaneous endoscopic versus Stamm gastrostomy. Gastrointest Endosc. 1995;42(1):41-4.
7. Cezard JP. Managing gastroesophageal reflux disease in children. Digestion. 2004;69(1):3-8.
8. Chicella MF, Batres LA, Heesters MS, Dice JE. Prokinetic drug therapy in children: a review of current options. Ann Pharmacother. 2005;39(4):706-11.
9. Chitkara DK, Fortunato C, Nurko S. Esophageal motor activity in children with gastroesophageal reflux disease and esophagitis. J Pediatr Gastroenterol Nutr. 2005;40(1):70-5.
10. Chung DH, Georgeson KE. Fundoplication and gastrostomy. Semin Pediatr Surg. 1998;7(4):213-9.
11. Colletti RB, Di Lorenzo C. Overview of pediatric gastroesophageal reflux disease and proton pump inhibitor therapy. J Pediatr Gastroenterol Nutr. 2003;37(1):S7-S11.
12. Corey KE, Schmitz SM, Shaheen NJ. Does a surgical antireflux procedure decrease the incidence of esophageal adenocarcinoma in Barrett's esophagus? A meta-analysis. Am J Gastroenterol. 2003;98(11):2390-4.
13. Costantini M, Crookes PF, Bremner RM, Hoeft SF, Ehsan A, Peters JH, et al. Value of physiologic assessment of foregut symptoms in a surgical practice. Surgery. 1993;114(4):780-6.
14. Craig WR, Hanlon-Dearman A, Sinclair C, Taback S, Moffatt M. Metoclopramide, thickened feedings, and positioning for gastroesophageal reflux in children under two years. Cochrane Database Syst Rev. 2004;(4):CD003502.
15. Curry JI, Lander TD, Stringer MD. Review article: erythromycin as a prokinetic agent in infants and children. Aliment Pharmacol Ther. 2001;15(5):595-603.
16. D'Alessio MJ, Arnaoutakis D, Giarelli N, Villadolid DV, Rosemurgy AS. Obesity is not a contraindication to laparoscopic fundoplication. J Gastrointest Surg. 2005;9(7):949-54.
17. Davidson GP, Omari TI. Pathophysiological mechanisms of gastroesophageal reflux disease in children. Curr Gastroenterol Rep. 2001;3(3):257-62.
18. Downing TE, Sporn TA, Bollinger RR, et al. Pulmonary histopathology in an experimental model of chronic aspiration is independent of acidity. Exp Biol Med (Maywood). 2008;233(10):1202-12.
19. El-Serag HB, Sweet S, Winchester CC, Dent J. Update on the epidemiology of gastro-oesophageal reflux disease: a systematic review. Gut. 2014;63(6):871-80.
20. Esposito C, Langer JC, Schaarschmidt K, Mattioli G, Sauer C, Centonze A, et al. Laparoscopic antireflux procedures in the management of gastroesophageal reflux following esophageal atresia repair. J Pediatr Gastroenterol Nutr. 2005;40(3):349-51.

21. Eubanks TR, Omelanczuk P, Richards C, Pohl D, Pellegrini CA. Outcomes of laparoscopic antireflux procedures. Am J Surg. 2000;179(5):391-5.
22. Farrell TM, Richardson WS, Halkar R, Lyon CP, Galloway KD, Waring JP, et al. Nissen fundoplication improves gastric motility in patients with delayed gastric emptying. Surg Endosc. 2001;15(3):271-4.
23. Franco MT, Salvia G, Terrin G, Spadaro R, De Rosa I, Iula VD, et al. Lansoprazole in the treatment of gastroesophageal reflux disease in childhood. Dig Liver Dis. 2000;32(8):660-6.
24. Fraser J, Watson DI, O'Boyle CJ, Jamieson GG. Obesity and its effect on outcome of laparoscopic Nissen fundoplication. Dis Esophagus. 2001;14(1):50-3.
25. Galvani C, Fisichella PM, Gorodner MV, Perretta S, Patti MG. Symptoms are a poor indicator of reflux status after fundoplication for gastroesophageal reflux disease. Arch Surg. 2003;138(5):514-9.
26. Georgeson K. Personal experience with laparoscopic fundoplication in children. Birmingham, AL: Elsevier; 2005.
27. Georgeson KE. Laparoscopic fundoplication and gastrostomy. Semin Laparosc Surg. 1998;5(1):25-30.
28. Gilger MA, Yeh C, Chiang J, Dietrich C, Brandt ML, El-Serag HB. Outcomes of surgical fundoplication in children. Clin Gastroenterol Hepatol. 2004;2(11):978-84.
29. Gold BD. Outcomes of pediatric gastroesophageal reflux disease: in the first year of life, in childhood, and in adults ...oh, and should we really leave *Helicobacter pylori* alone? J Pediatr Gastroenterol Nutr. 2003;37(1):S33-9.
30. Gregersen H, Drewes AM. Functional findings in irritable bowel syndrome. World J Gastroenterol. 2006;12(18):2830-8.
31. Gwee K, Chua ASB. Functional dyspepsia and irritable bowel syndrome, are they different entities and does it matter? World J Gastroenterol. 2006;12(17):2708-12.
32. Hassall E. Decisions in diagnosing and managing chronic gastroesophageal reflux disease in children. J Pediatr. 2005;146(3 Suppl):S3-12.
33. Hassall E. Wrap session: Is the Nissen slipping? Can medical treatment replace surgery for severe gastroesophageal reflux disease in children? Am J Gastroenterol. 1995;90(8):1212-20.
34. Hatch KF, Daily MF, Christensen BJ, Glasgow RE. Failed fundoplications. Am J Surg. 2004;188(6):786-91.
35. Jamieson GG, Duranceau A. What is a Nissen fundoplication? Surgery. 1984;159(6):591-3.
36. Jamieson JR, Stein HJ, DeMeester TR, Bonavina L, Schwizer W, Hinder RA, et al. Ambulatory 24-h esophageal pH monitoring: normal values, optimal thresholds, specificity, sensitivity, and reproducibility. Am J Gastroenterol. 1992;87(9):1102-11.
37. Jesch NK, Schmidt AI, Strassburg A, Gluer S, UreBM. Laparoscopic fundoplication in neurologically impaired children with percutaneous endoscopic gastrostomy. Eur J Pediatr Surg. 2004;14(2):89-92.
38. Johanson JF. Epidemiology of esophageal and supraesophageal reflux injuries. Am J Med. 2000;108 Suppl 4a:99S.
39. Jones R, Canal DF, Inman MM, Rescorla FJ. Laparoscopic fundoplication: a three-year review. Am Surg. 1996;62(8):632-6.
40. Katz PO, Gerson LB, Vela MF. Guidelines for the diagnosis and management of gastroesophageal reflux disease. Am J Gastroenterol. 2013;108(3):308-28.
41. Khajanchee YS, O'Rourke RW, Lockhart B, Patterson EJ, Hansen PD, Swanstrom LL. Postoperative symptoms and failure after antireflux surgery. Arch Surg. 2002;137(9):1008-14.
42. Klauser AG, Schindlbeck NE, Muller-Lissner SA. Symptoms in gastroesophageal reflux disease. Lancet. 1990;335(8683):205-8.
43. Langer JC. The failed fundoplication. Semin Pediatr Surg. 2003;12(2):110-17.
44. Lazarchik DA, Frazier KB. Dental erosion and acid reflux disease: an overview. Gen Dent. 2009;57(2):151-6.
45. Lindquist SG, Kirchhoff M, Lundsteen C, Pedersen W, Erichsen G, Kristensen K, et al. Further delineation of the 22q13 deletion syndrome. Clin Dysmorphol. 2005;14(2):55-60.
46. Liu DC, Somme S, Mavrelis PG, Hurwich D, Statter MB, Teitelbaum DH, et al. Stretta as the initial antireflux procedure in children. J Pediatr Surg. 2005;40(1):148-51; discussion 151-42.
47. Lord RVN, Kaminski A, Oberg S, Bowrey DJ, Hagen JA, DeMeester SR, et al. Absence of gastroesophageal reflux disease in a majority of patients taking acid suppression medications after Nissen fundoplication. J Gastrointest Surg. 2002;6(1):3-9.
48. Ludemann R, Watson DI, Jamieson GG, Game PA, Devitt PG. Five-year follow-up of a randomized clinical trial of laparoscopic total versus anterior 180° fundoplication. Br J Surgery. 2005;92(2):240-3.
49. Madan A, Minocha A. Despite high satisfaction, majority of gastroesophageal reflux disease patients continue to use proton pump inhibitors after antireflux surgery. Aliment Pharmacol Ther. 2006;23(5):601-5.
50. Maddern GJ. The reproducibility of esophageal manometry. Dis Esophagus. 1991;4(2):95-9.
51. Maret-Ouda J, Konings P, Lagergren J, Brusselaers N. Antireflux surgery and risk of esophageal adenocarcinoma: a systematic review and meta-analysis. Ann Surg. 2016;263(2):251-7.
52. Mattioli G, Sacco O, Repetto P, Pini Prato A, Castagnetti M, Carlini C, et al. Necessity for surgery in children with gastroesophageal reflux and supraesophageal symptoms. Eur J Pediatr Surg. 2004;14(1):7-13.
53. Ollyo JB, Lang F, Fontolliet CH, Monnier P. Savary-Miller's new endoscopic grading of reflux esophagitis: a simple, reproducible, logical, complete and useful classification. Gastroenterology. 1990;89:A100.
54. Papasavas PK, Keenan RJ, Yeaney WW, Caushaj PF, Gagne DJ, Landreneau RJ. Effectiveness of laparoscopic fundoplication in relieving the symptoms of gastroesophageal reflux disease (GERD) and eliminating antireflux medical therapy. Surg Endosc. 2003;17(8):1200-5.
55. Patterson EJ, Davis DG, Khajanchee Y, Swanstrom LL. Comparison of objective outcomes following laparoscopic Nissen fundoplication versus laparoscopic gastric bypass in the morbidly obese with heartburn. Surg Endosc. 2003;17(10):1561-5.
56. Patti MG. An evidence-based approach to the treatment of gastroesophageal reflux disease. JAMA Surg. 2016;151(1):73-8.
57. Post JC, Ze F, Ehrlich GD. Genetics of pediatric gastroesophageal reflux. Curr Opin Allergy Clin Immunol. 2005;5(1):5-9.
58. Quigley EMM. Changing face of irritable bowel syndrome. World J Gastroenterol. 2006;12(1):1-5.
59. Ravelli AM, Milla PJ. Vomiting and gastroesophageal motor activity in children with disorders of the central nervous system. J Pediatr Gastroenterol Nutr. 1998;26(1):56-63.
60. Rothenberg SS. Laproscopic redo-Nissen fundoplication in infants and children. Surg Endosc. 2006;20(10):1518-20.
61. Rothenberg SS. The first decade's experience with laparoscopic Nissen fundoplication in infants and children. J Pediatr Surg. 2005;40(1):142-6; discussion 147.
62. Rudolph CD. Supraesophageal complications of gastroesophageal reflux in children: challenges in diagnosis and treatment. Am J Med. 2003;115(Suppl 3A):150S-6S.
63. Sages (2010). Guidelines for surgical treatment of gastroesophageal reflux disease (GERD). Society of American Gastrointestinal and Endoscopic Surgeons (SAGES). [online] Available from: https://www.sages.org/publications/guidelines/guidelines-for-surgical-treatment-of-gastroesophageal-reflux-disease-gerd/. [Last accessed August, 2020).
64. Schier F. Indications for laparoscopic antireflux procedures in children. Semin Laparosc Surg. 2002;9(3):139-45.

65. Shay S, Tutuian R, Sifrim D, Vela M, Wise J, Balaji N, et al. Twenty-four hour ambulatory simultaneous impedance and pH monitoring: a multicenter report of normal values from 60 healthy volunteers. Am J Gastroenterol. 2004;99(6):1037-43.
66. Smith CD, McClusky DA, Rajad MA, Lederman AB, Hunter JG. When fundoplication fails: redo? Ann Surg. 2005;241(6):861-71.
67. Spechler SJ, Lee E, Ahnen D, Goyal RK, Hirano I, Ramirez F, et al. Long-term outcome of medical and surgical therapies for gastroesophageal reflux disease: follow-up of a randomized controlled trial. JAMA. 2001;285(18):2331-8.
68. Spechler SJ. The management of patients who have "failed" antireflux surgery. Am J Gastroenterol. 2004;99(3):552-61.
69. Spence GM, Watson DI, Jamieson GG, Lally CJ, Devitt PG. Single center prospective randomized trial of laparoscopic Nissen versus anterior 90° fundoplication. J Gastrointest Surg. 2006;10(5):698-705.
70. Spiroglou K, Xinias I, Karatzas N, Karatza E, Arsos G, Panteliadis C. Gastric emptying in children with cerebral palsy and gastroesophageal reflux. Pediatr Neurol. 2004;31(3):177-82.
71. Spitz L, McLeod E. Gastroesophageal reflux. Semin Pediatr Surg. 2003;12(4):237-40.
72. Stein HJ, DeMeester TR. Who benefits from antireflux surgery? World J Surg. 1992;16(2):313-9.
73. Stylopoulos N, Rattner DW. The history of hiatal hernia surgery: from Bowditch to laparoscopy. Ann Surg. 2005;241(1):185-93.
74. Sydorak RM, Albanese CT. Laparoscopic antireflux procedures in children: evaluating the evidence. Semin Laparosc Surg. 2002;9(3):133-38.
75. Thomson M, Fritscher-Ravens A, Hall S, Afzal N, Ashwood P, Swain CP. Endoluminal gastroplication in children with significant gastroesophageal reflux disease. Gut. 2004;53(12):1745-50.
76. Vaezi MF, Richter JE. Role of acid and duodenogastroesophageal reflux in gastroesophageal reflux disease. Gastroenterology. 1996;111:1192-9.
77. Vakil N, van Zanten SV, Kahrilas P, Dent J, Jones R, Global Consensus Group. The Montreal definition and classification of gastroesophageal reflux disease: a global evidence-based consensus. Am J Gastroenterol. 2006;101(8):1900-20.
78. Vandenplas Y, Hassall E. Mechanisms of gastroesophageal reflux and gastroesophageal reflux disease. J Pediatr Gastroenterol Nutr. 2002;35(2):119-36.
79. Watson DI, Jamieson GG, Lally C, Archer S, Bessell JR, Booth M, et al. Multicenter prospective double blind randomized trial of laparoscopic Nissen versus anterior 90 degree partial fundoplication. Arch Surg. 2004;139(11):1160-7.
80. Watson DI, Jamieson GG, Pike GP, Davies N, Richardson M, Devitt PG. Prospective randomized double-blind trial between laparoscopic Nissen fundoplication and anterior partial fundoplication. Br J Surg. 1999;86(1):123-30.
81. Yadlapati R, Vaezi MF, Vela MF, Spechler SJ, Shaheen NJ, Richter J, et al. Management options for patients with GERD and persistent symptoms on proton pump inhibitors: recommendations from an expert panel. Am J Gastroenterol. 2018;113(7):980-6.
82. Zaninotto G, Attwood SE. Surgical management of refractory gastro-oesophageal reflux. Br J Surg. 2010;97(2):139-40.
83. Zeid MA, Kandel T, el-Shobary M, Talaat AA, Fouad A, el-Enien AA, et al. Nissen fundoplication in infants and children: a long-term clinical study. Hepatogastroenterology. 2004;51(57):697-700.

CHAPTER 21

Laparoscopic Bariatric Surgery

INTRODUCTION

Obesity has become a major health problem in the last few decades. Obesity is the most prevalent chronic disease of the 21st century. The World Health Organization (WHO) has identified obesity as one of the five leading health risks in developed countries. WHO has reported that over a billion people are overweight and that 300 million are clinically obese with a projection of 3 million deaths annually worldwide. In the United States, 65% of adult Americans are overweight and 31% are clinically obese. Fourteen percent of American children and adolescents are obese. Bariatric surgery is now considered the only valid therapeutic option for morbidly obese patients but can be associated with significant risk, especially in patients affected by life-threatening comorbidities. Morbid obesity [defined as a body mass index (BMI) > 40 kg/m^2] affects 4.7% of Americans and these numbers are rapidly rising. For these patients, surgery represents the most effective treatment. However, failure is frequent issue and selection of correct surgery is of paramount importance for success.

Among various bariatric procedures, laparoscopic sleeve gastrectomy (LSG) has rapidly gained popularity to become most frequently performed worldwide. The sleeve gastrectomy is a restrictive form of weight loss surgery in which approximately 85% of the stomach is removed leaving a cylindrical or sleeve-shaped stomach with a capacity ranging from about 60 to 150 cc. Stomach is reduced to about 15% of its original size, by surgical removal of a large portion of the stomach along greater curvature **(Fig. 1)**. The open edges are then attached together with the help of stapler to form a sleeve or tube with a banana shape **(Figs. 2A and B)**. The procedure permanently reduces the size of the stomach. The procedure is performed either open or laparoscopically and is not reversible.

Laparoscopic sleeve gastrectomy is a relatively new option originally published by Marceau et al. Unlike many other forms of bariatric surgery, the outlet valve and the nerves to the stomach remain intact and, while the stomach is drastically reduced in size, although its function is preserved. Again, unlike other forms of surgery such as the Roux-en-Y gastric bypass (RYGB), the sleeve gastrectomy is not reversible.

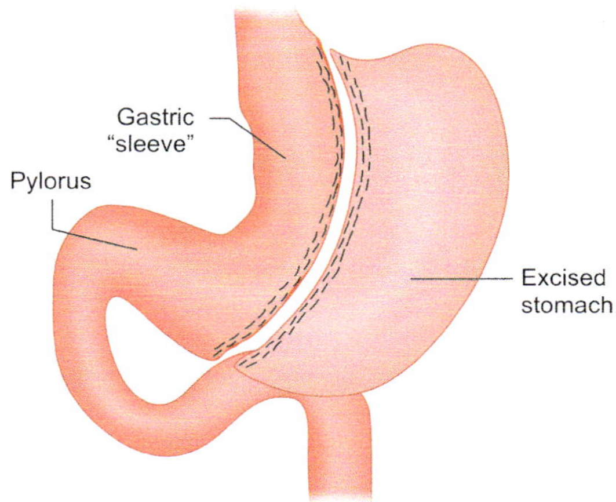

Fig. 1: Sleeve gastrectomy.

Because the new stomach continues to function normally there are far fewer restrictions on the foods which patients can consume after surgery, although the quantity of food that can be eaten will be considerably reduced. This is seen by many patients as being one of the great advantages of the sleeve gastrectomy, as is the fact that the removal of the majority of the stomach also results in the virtual elimination of hormone (ghrelin) produced within the stomach which stimulate hunger.

GHRELIN HORMONE

Ghrelin got its name from the word "ghre" from the Proto-Indo-European language, meaning to grow. Scientists did not go purposefully looking for a substance that stimulated appetite. Indeed the discovery of ghrelin occurred when scientists were investigating drugs that stimulated the release of growth hormone from the anterior pituitary gland. They came across some drugs that, rather than acting on the growth hormone releasing hormone receptor, were acting on an unknown receptor located in the hypothalamus and pituitary, these drugs were called growth hormone secretagogues. It was concluded that the body had a second pathway for the induction of growth hormone secretion.

Ghrelin was identified as being the natural legend for these receptors causing secretion of growth hormone in

1999 by the Japanese scientist Masayasu Kojima. During Kojima's investigations, they found that although ghrelin's receptors were in the brain, ghrelin was surprisingly identified in the human stomach and circulating in the blood leading to the conclusion that it was released from the stomach, from where it then traveled in the blood and acted on the brain.

Ghrelin is a hormone produced mainly by P/D1 cells lining the fundus of the human stomach and epsilon cells of the pancreas that stimulates hunger **(Figs. 2A and B)**. Ghrelin levels increase before meals and decrease after meals. It is considered as the counterpart of the hormone leptin, *produced by adipose tissue, which induces satiation when present at higher levels.* In some bariatric procedures, the level of ghrelin is reduced in patients, thus causing satiation before it would normally occur. Ghrelin is also produced in the hypothalamic arcuate nucleus, where it stimulates the secretion of growth hormone from the anterior pituitary gland. Receptors for ghrelin are expressed by neurons in the arcuate nucleus and the ventromedial hypothalamus. Once the high amount of ghrelin is secreted the patient feels intense hunger **(Fig. 3)**. Apart from hunger,

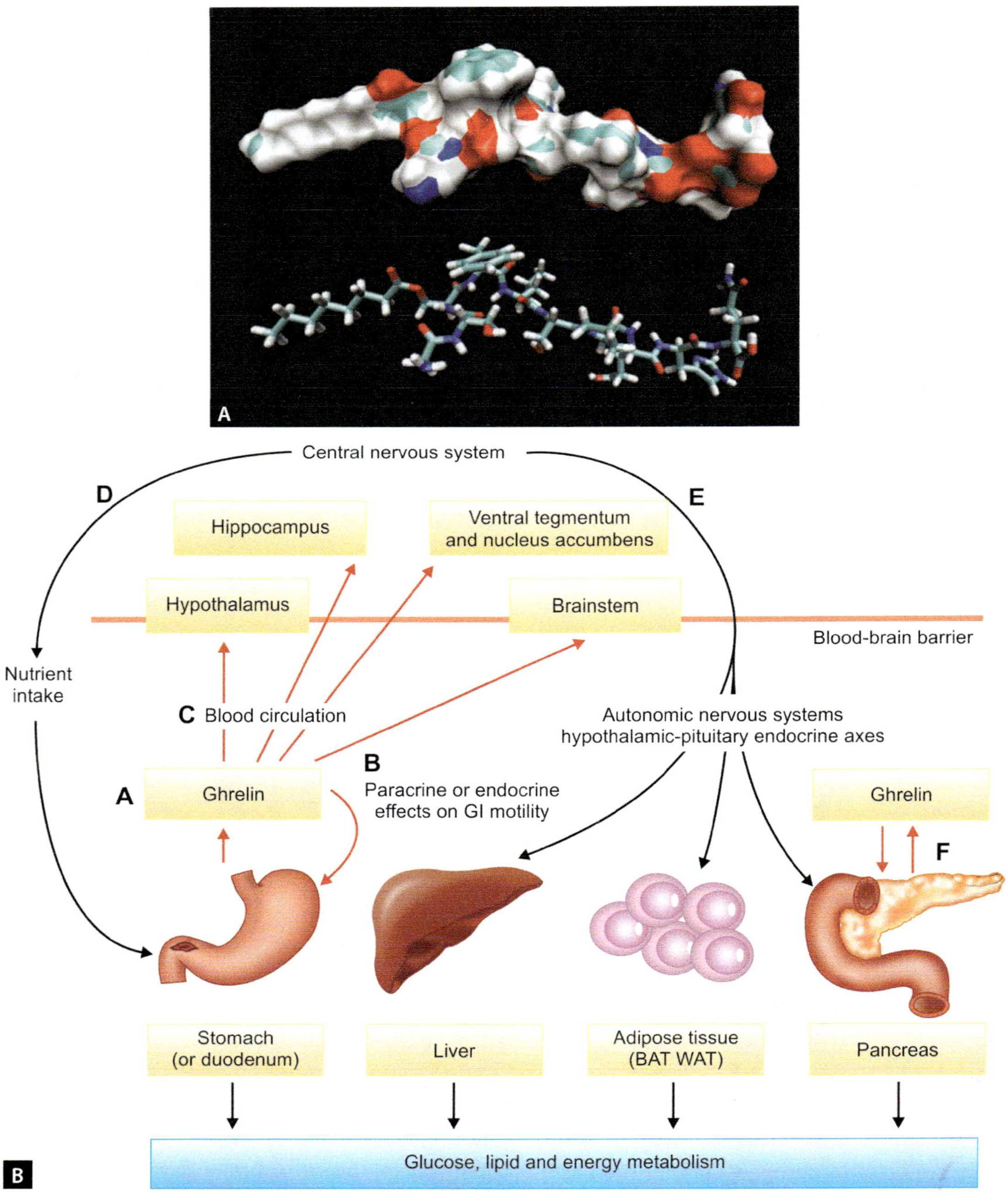

Figs. 2A and B: (A) Ghrelin hormone; and (B) Role of ghrelin in glucose and lipid metabolism. (BAT: brown adipose tissue; GI: gastrointestinal; WAT: white adipose tissue)

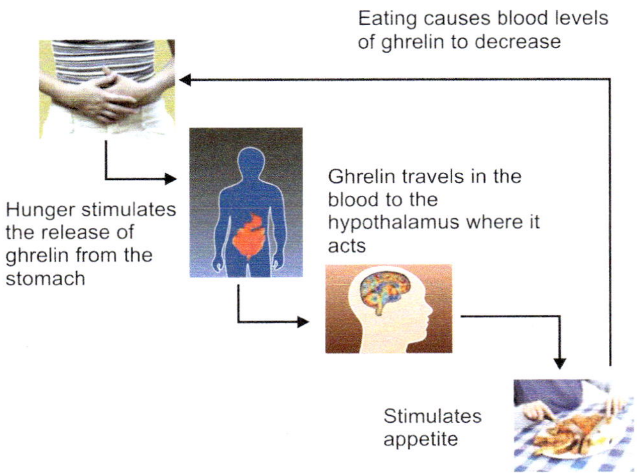

Fig. 3: Mode of action of ghrelin.

ghrelin plays a significant role in neurotrophy, particularly in the hippocampus, and is essential for cognitive adaptation to changing environments and the process of learning.

Ghrelin has emerged as the first circulating hunger hormone. Ghrelin and synthetic ghrelin mimetic increase food intake and increase fat mass by an action exerted at the level of the hypothalamus. They activate cells in the arcuate nucleus that include the orexigenic neuropeptide Y (NPY) neurons. Ghrelin-responsiveness of these neurons is both leptin- and insulin-sensitive. Ghrelin also activates the mesolimbic cholinergic-dopaminergic reward link, a circuit that communicates the hedonic and reinforcing aspects of natural rewards, such as food, as well as of addictive drugs, such as ethanol **(Fig. 3)**.

Ghrelin levels in the plasma of obese individuals are lower than those in leaner individuals. Recently, Scripps research scientists have developed an anti-obesity vaccine, which is directed against the hormone ghrelin. The vaccine uses the immune system, specifically antibodies, to bind to selected targets, directing the body's own immune response against them. This prevents ghrelin from reaching the central nervous system, thus producing a desired reduction in weight gain.

Obesity is the result of multifactorial changes involving both genetic and environmental factors. The physiopathology of obesity from the point of view of intake regulation has led to numerous experimental studies aimed at identifying new forms of regulation. These new forms of regulation are not only found in the secretion of ghrelin from gastrointestinal system but also in the adipose tissue (via the metabolism of leptin and insulin) and the central nervous system to finally produce the relevant orexigenic or anorexigenic effect.

GLUCAGON-LIKE PEPTIDE

Glucagon-like peptide 1 (GLP-1) is a 30-amino-acid peptide mainly secreted by the small intestine L cells after contact of food. This hormone increases insulin secretion on one end and slows gastric emptying and intestinal motility on the other. GLP-1 is increased after LSG, and it is postulated that increased levels of GLP-1 contribute to weight loss by improving glucose metabolism, reducing hunger, and increasing satiety. Although GLP-1 has been shown to slow gastric emptying, the gastric emptying time accelerated after LSG (47.6 ± 23.2 vs. 94.3 ± 15.4 minutes) in one study. It is likely that more than one mechanism is in play when determining the gastric transit time after LSG. LSG has also been shown to alter the levels of glucose-dependent insulinotropic peptide (GIP), bile acids, and leptin, the clinical significance of which is still under investigation.

INDICATIONS OF SLEEVE GASTRECTOMY

Similar to other bariatric operations, LSG is indicated in all patients meeting the 1991 National Institutes of Health (NIH) consensus conference criteria. These criteria include:

- Body mass index ≥40 kg/m^2 with or without any associated comorbidities.
- Body mass index between 35 and 40 kg/m^2 with at least one serious weight-related comorbidity, including but not limited to diabetes, obstructive sleep apnea, hypertension, and coronary artery disease.
- Body mass index between 30 and 35 kg/m^2 with uncontrollable type 2 diabetes or metabolic syndrome.

Besides being a primary bariatric operation, LSG has also been used as a bridging procedure in super morbid obese patients (BMI of 50 kg/m^2 and above) before biliopancreatic diversion with duodenal switch (BPDDS). Additionally, LSG is also a good revisional procedure for patients who fail laparoscopic adjustable gastric banding (AGB).

Laparoscopic sleeve gastrectomy is safe for patients with diabetes, metabolic syndrome, and inflammatory bowel disease. LSG is also an effective treatment for type 2 diabetes. Finally, LSG has been safely performed in both adolescents and older adult patients. LSG can also be offered to high-risk patients such as those with child's A or B liver cirrhosis, and those awaiting kidney, liver, or heart transplant, with the goals of improving eligibility for transplant through weight loss and improving future graft function. As an example, between 2006 and 2016, the number of patients with end-stage kidney disease undergoing bariatric surgery increased ninefold, and the use of LSG increased.

ADVANTAGES OF SLEEVE GASTRECTOMY

Some authors described LSG as a stand-alone procedure with good results with respect to excessive weight loss (EWL) and lower plasma ghrelin levels **(Figs. 4A and B)**. Also, there are numerous reports of morbidly obese patients who underwent LSG as a first step before an intended malabsorptive procedure and lost their excessive weight after LSG, so that further surgery was not necessary. This is important because the disadvantages of the malabsorptive

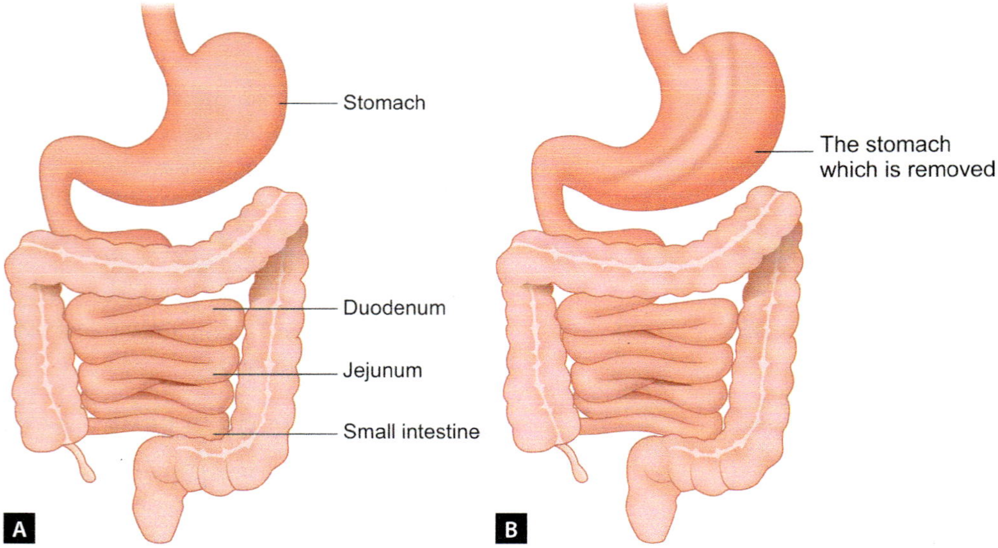

Figs. 4A and B: Before and after sleeve gastrectomy.

procedure are avoided. Perhaps the greatest advantage of the gastric sleeve lies in the fact that it does not involve any bypass of the intestinal tract and patients do not, therefore, suffer the complications of intestinal bypass such as intestinal obstruction, anemia, osteoporosis, and vitamin and protein deficiency. It also makes it a suitable form of surgery for patients who are already suffering from anemia, Crohn's disease and a variety of other conditions that would place them at high risk for surgery involving intestinal bypass. Sleeve gastrectomy can be performed laparoscopically without much problem in patients who are extremely overweight and this accounts for the rising popularity of the LSG.

DISADVANTAGES OF SLEEVE GASTRECTOMY

Perhaps the main disadvantage of this form of surgery is that it does not always produce the reduction in weight which people would wish for and, in the longer term, can result in weight regain. This is indeed true of any form of purely restrictive surgery, but is perhaps especially true in the case of the sleeve gastrectomy. Because the procedure requires stapling of the stomach, patients do run the risk of leakage and of other complications directly related to stapling. In addition, as with any surgery, patients run the risk of additional complications such as postoperative bleeding, small bowel obstruction, pneumonia and even death. The risk of encountering any of these complications is, however, extremely small and varies from about 0.5 and 1%. Having said this, the risk of death from this form of surgery at about 0.25% is extremely small.

CONTRAINDICATIONS OF SLEEVE GASTRECTOMY

Absolute contraindications to LSG include prohibitive anesthesia risks, severe uncontrolled psychiatric illnesses (including certain eating disorders such as malignant hyperphagia), and coagulopathy. Barrett's esophagus and uncontrolled severe gastroesophageal reflux disease (GERD) are relative contraindications to LSG. Some surgeons do not perform LSG in the presence of Barrett's esophagus, for fear that a sleeve gastrectomy would preclude a future gastric pull-up procedure, which may be required if Barrett's esophagus progresses to esophageal cancer. Others do not consider Barrett's esophagus a contraindication to LSG. Hiatal hernia without esophagitis is not a contraindication to LSG. Performing LSG in patients with known GERD is controversial. RYGB is a better surgical option of weight loss than LSG in patients with severe GERD.

SURGICAL TECHNIQUE

The patient is positioned in a modified reverse Trendelenburg position with the right arm away from the body. The abdomen is prepared and draped in the customary fashion. Ports are placed in the given order (1–5) according to base ball diamond concept as shown in **Figures 5A and B**.

After exploration of the abdomen and the anterior wall of the stomach, the liver is retracted via fifth port **(Fig. 6)**. The first step is to identify the pylorus by visualizing the prepyloric vein of Mayo and palpating with laparoscopic instruments. The pylorus is a crucial landmark because gastric transection typically begins 6 cm from the pylorus. Dissection should be started with dissection of the short gastric vessels to the point of the angle of His, using either the harmonic scalpel (Ethicon Endo-Surgery) or LigaSure™. The greater omentum is then separated from the greater curvature under protection of the gastroepiploic arcade **(Fig. 7)**. A complete mobilization of the greater curvature ensures that a sizable portion of the posterior fundus is not left behind during gastric transection.

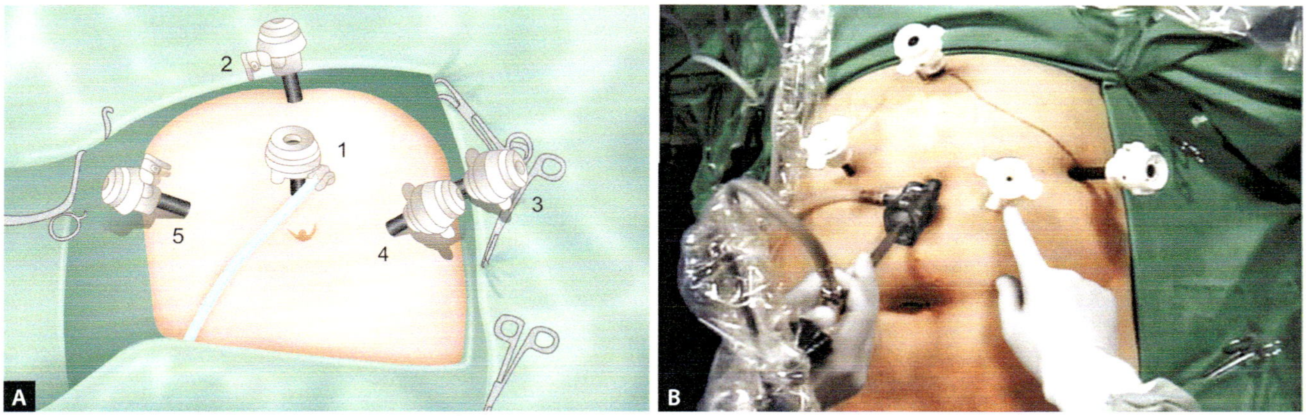

Figs. 5A and B: Port position for laparoscopic sleeve gastrectomy.

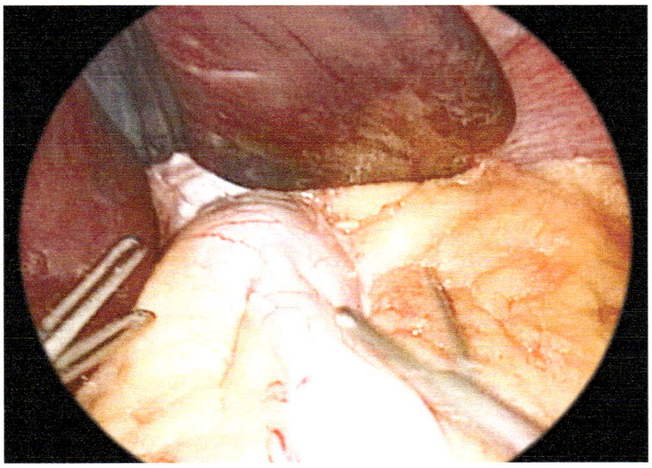

Fig. 6: Exposure of stomach up to angle of HIS.

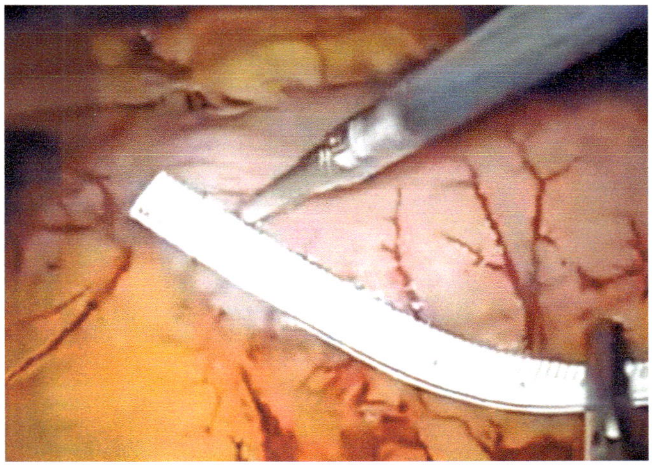

Fig. 7: 6 cm of stomach toward the pylorus is left.

At this point, surgeon should assess the hiatus for hernias. Any large hiatal hernia should be repaired using standard laparoscopic techniques. The blood supply to the lesser curvature (i.e., left gastric artery) must be preserved since it will become the sole blood supply to the sleeve after gastric transection.

A 36-Fr tube is then positioned along the lesser curvature of stomach as the leading structure for the stapling line to follow. Although experts agree on the need for calibrating the sleeved stomach with a bougie, the optimal size of such a bougie is still debated. According to a survey of 863 surgeons with a cumulative experience of 520,230 procedures, the majority of experts used a bougie size of 36 French.

After freeing the omentum, staple should be applied along the greater curvature strictly along the stomach tube using a 60-mm Endo-GIA, Ethicon Endo-Surgery or Auto Suture **(Figs. 8A and B)**. The starting point is 7–8 cm prepyloric to the point of the angle of His. Typically, 4–5 staple lines are needed **(Figs. 9A to C)**. Different types of staplers are available in the market. As the gastric transection proceeds, the height of the staples may need to be adjusted according to the thickness of the tissue. In general, most experts would not use staples with closed height <2.0 mm to transect the antrum (the thicker part of the stomach) or staples with closed height <1.5 mm to transect the rest of the stomach (thinner parts).

While transecting the stomach, the surgeon must avoid twisting the staple line along the longitudinal axis and avoid narrowing the sleeve, particularly at the level of the incisura angularis. A twisted or narrowed sleeve can cause distal obstruction, which is responsible for the majority of the occurrences and persistence of staple line leaks in the proximal sleeve.

The dissected part of the stomach is withdrawn from the abdomen at port number 3 and the staple line is overstitched by absorbable intracorporeal suturing. This is done not to prevent insufficiency in the staple line but rather to prevent staple line bleeding. It is possible to overstitch only areas of bleeding between the staples, and not the whole staple line. When performing the last stapler firing, it is important to avoid stapling too close to the gastroesophageal junction, which may result in ischemia and postoperative leak.

Like most of the bariatric surgery operations, currently there are multiple variations in the technique for the LSG.

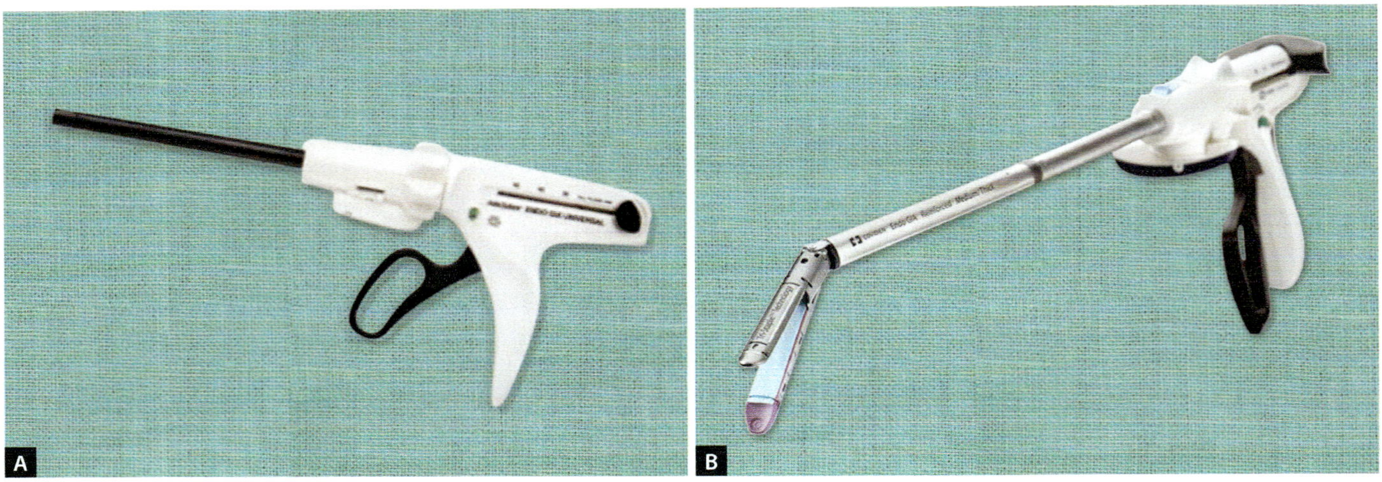

Figs. 8A and B: Laparoscopic Endo-GIA stapler.

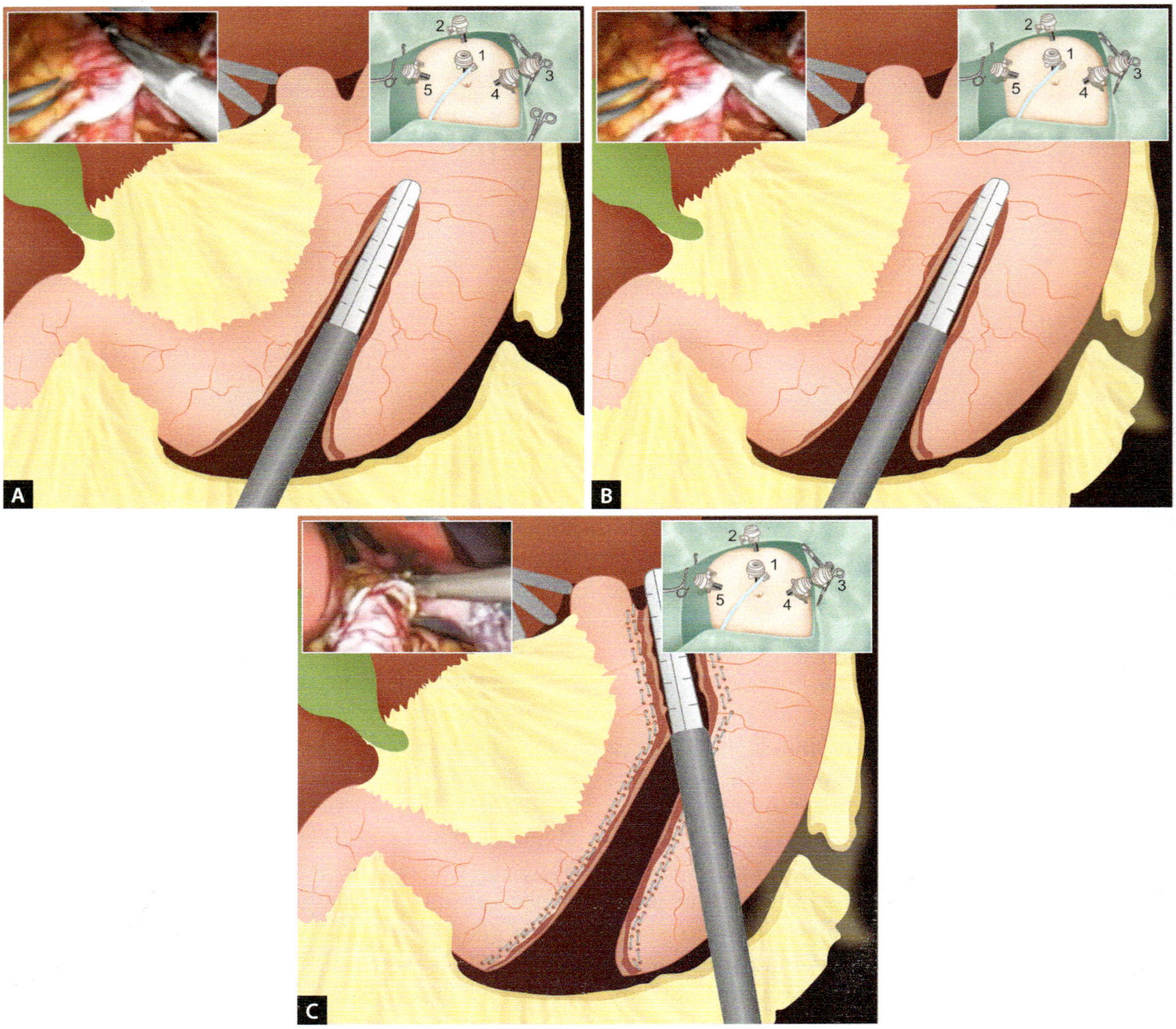

Figs. 9A to C: (A) After dissecting the greater omentum from the greater curvature, a 34-Fr stomach tube is placed along the lesser curvature. The first staple line is then set strictly along the stomach. The starting point of the dissection of the greater curvature is about 7–8 cm prepyloric; (B) The second staple line is set strictly and continued along the stomach tube; and (C) Finishing of the gastric sleeve with the third staple line. The greater curvature is resected to the point of the angle of His.

Some of these variations are: the size of bougie (determines the size of the pouch) beside which the Endo-GIA staplers are placed to divide the stomach, the level at which the surgeons start the division in the central area. Many surgeons leave most of the antrum for its pumping, emptying action and also to avoid the possibility of leak from this thick-walled tough area, and whether to reinforce or not reinforce this long staple line.

Five or six ports are used for LSG and the surgeon standing between the patient's legs. An open technique could be used for the first port, establishing a pneumoperitoneum of 15 mm Hg. Then, two right ports, one left port, and a midline ports are usually sufficient **(Figs. 5A and B)**. The right subcostal trocar is used to insert the fan retractor for the liver. The camera should be placed high between the umbilicus and xiphoid. Initial decompression of the stomach with nasogastric tube (NGT) is preferable. Some surgeons commence the LSG with an opening through the gastrocolic ligament to lesser sac, and the posterior stomach wall is visualized and fine adhesions to the pancreas are divided and the lesser sac totally freed using harmonic scalpel, LigaSure™, or coagulation hook. The left side of the gastroesophageal junction should be cleared off fat to avoid later compromise of the stapling during creation of the sleeve **(Figs. 10A to D)**. Left crus should be exposed completely.

Majority of surgeons start the dissection 6 cm proximal to the pylorus, but some European surgeons start the dissection closer to the pylorus. If the dissection starts too close to the pylorus, the antrum will not empty properly and its pumping mechanism will be defective, thus postoperative nausea may occur. The linear Endo-GIA stapler is generally introduced through a right trocar toward the left shoulder and leaves about 1 cm of fat pad along the lesser curvature (3 cm width). This assures adequate blood supply on the lesser curvature for the sleeve. Transaction of the stomach should be started 6 cm proximal to the pylorus and then the anesthesiologist inserts a 36–40-Fr bougie down to pylorus if the LSG is intended as the sole operation, but if only as a preliminary step before duodenal switch, then instead a 60-Fr bougie is used. Kueper et al. considered using a 34-Fr bougie in their study, which results in a pouch of 100 mL. The sleeve is started at the lower end of the crow's foot. The procedure requires 5–6 firings of the linear cutting stapler (60 mm long, 4.8 mm staple-height, and green cartridge) to divide the entire stomach **(Figs. 11A to H)**. It is important to remove

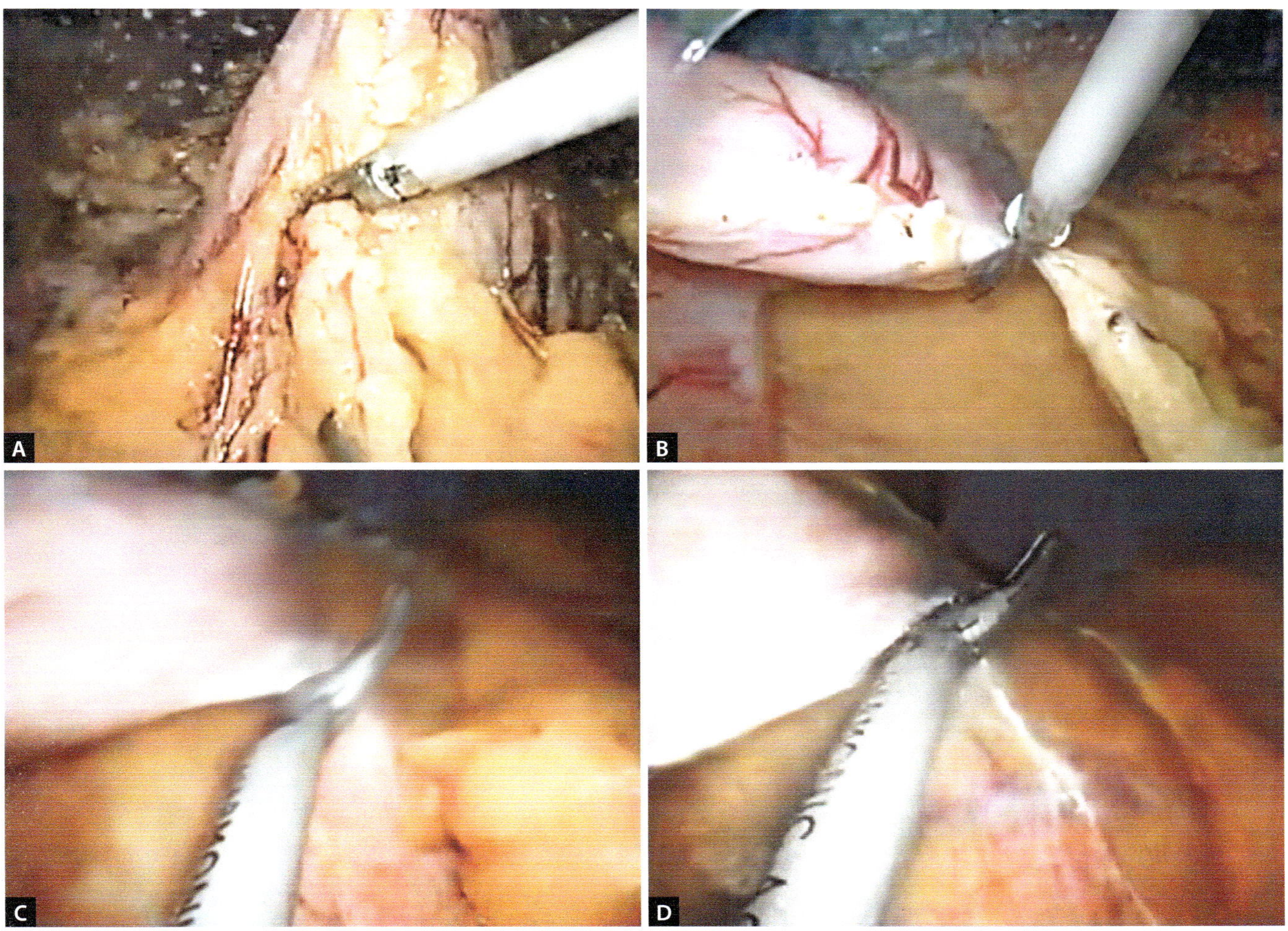

Figs. 10A to D: Dissection and mobilization of stomach along the greater curvature outside the epiploic arcade.

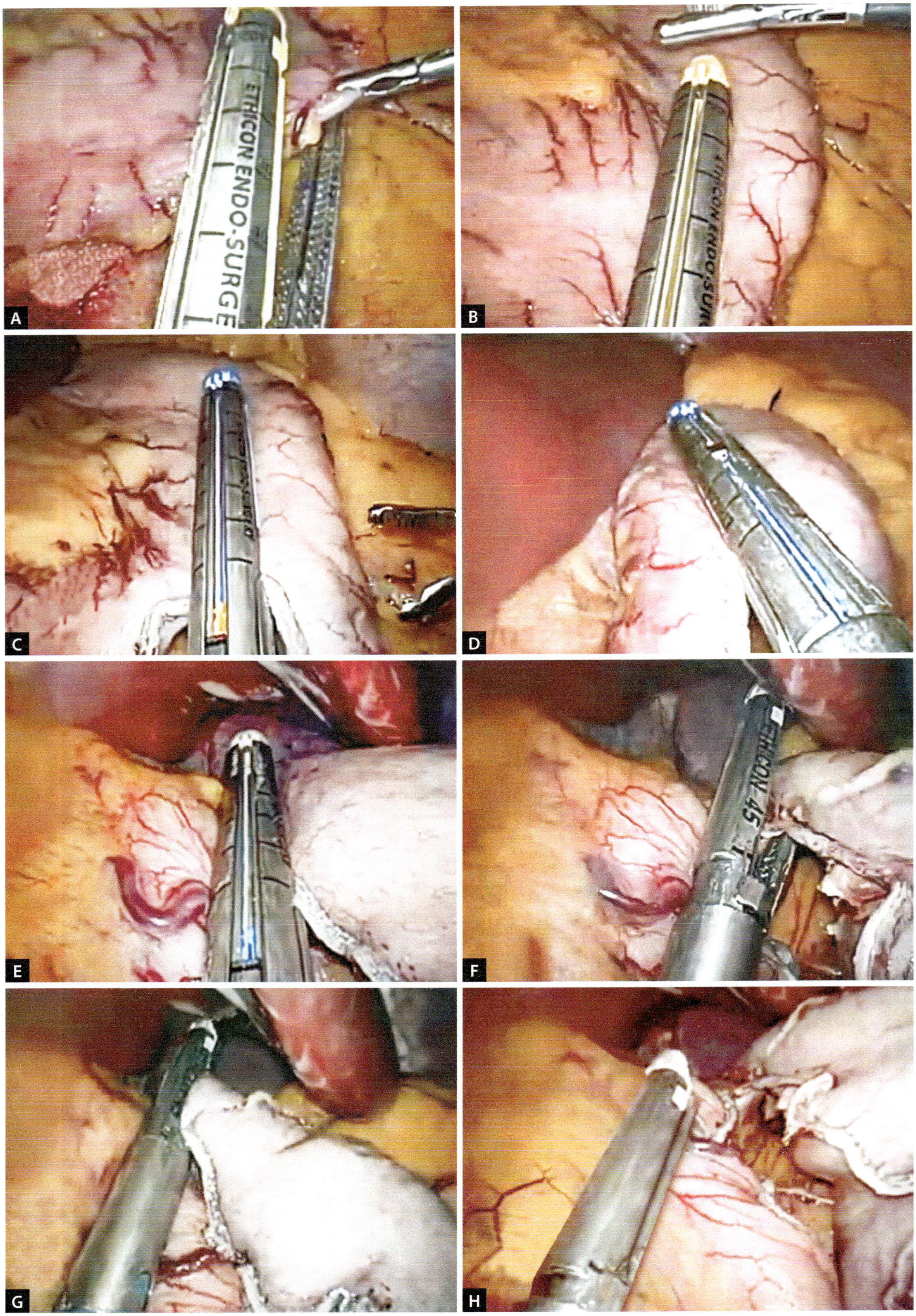

Figs. 11A to H: Gastrectomy with the help of Endo-GI stapler.

all of the fundus to avoid regain of weight. The vagus nerves anteriorly and posteriorly are preserved for normal gastric emptying.

Many surgeons recommend reinforcing the staple line to reduce the risk of bleeding and leak. This can be accomplished by using a buttressing material at the time of stapler firing or by oversewing the staple line. A combination of buttressing and oversewing, however, increased staple line leak rate compared with either method alone in one study was done and there was no significant difference. Oversewing should be done with the bougie still in place to avoid excessive imbrication and narrowing of the sleeve lumen.

The resected greater curvature could be extracted in a bag via epigastric or right paramedian port-site after being dilated to two-finger diameter. The typical specimen has the shape of a comma or banana with the fundus at the top. After dividing the stomach, most surgeons use over sewing of the staple-line by continuous or interrupted absorbable sutures to prevent bleeding and leak.

Intraoperative testing through an 18-Fr Argyle tube with diluted methylene blue or air under saline using a gastroscope, with concurrent compression of prepyloric area is a complementary step. A Gastrografin swallow is ordered by many surgeons on the second postoperative day, or others perform this study only if there is a problem. A liquid diet may be commenced on the first postoperative day.

POSTOPERATIVE CARE

Most patients are admitted for overnight observation after LSG, especially if they have a history of obstructive sleep apnea. Postoperative nausea is the most common complaint and should be treated with scheduled doses of intravenous antiemetics such as ondansetron, with other antiemetics, such as prochlorperazine and scopolamine patch, provided as needed for breakthrough symptoms. Minimizing narcotic use by liberal use of local anesthetic infiltration, transverse abdominis plane (TAP) blocks, and intravenous acetaminophen also contributes to the reduction of postoperative nausea and early discharge.

A clear liquid diet is usually started in the morning after the procedure. If the patient tolerates that, they can be advanced to a full liquid diet within 24 hours. Once the patient tolerates a liquid diet and their pain is controlled with oral pain medications, they can be discharged home with instructions to only take crushed or liquid medications and a full liquid diet for 2 weeks

A postoperative contrast study is performed after LSG to detect leak by some surgeons but not others. Because most leaks from LSG occur late after patient discharge, routine contrast studies on postoperative day 1 have a very low yield of detecting leaks.

RISKS AND COMPLICATIONS OF THE SLEEVE GASTRECTOMY

As with all forms of weight loss surgery, the vertical gastrectomy does carry risk and these will clearly vary from one patient to the other. In modern series, the overall mortality rate of LSG is approximately 0–1.2%; the overall morbidity rates range from 0 to 17.5%.

Complications include:

- Bleeding to 15%
- Gastric leakage and fistula 1.0%
- Strictures 0.26–4%
- Deep vein thrombosis 0.5%
- Nonfatal pulmonary embolus 0.5%
- Postoperative bleeding 0.5%
- Splenectomy 0.5%
- Acute respiratory distress 0.25%
- Pneumonia 0.2%
- Death 0.25%

BLEEDING AFTER SLEEVE GASTRECTOMY

Postoperative bleeding after LSG has been described in up to 15% of cases. It can occur within the lumen of the stomach, intra-abdominally, or at the trocar/incision sites. In a retrospective study of over 175,000 LSGs performed from 2015 to 2016, 0.6% were complicated by postoperative bleed. Bleeding after LSG was associated with higher rates of complications, readmission, reoperation, and mortality at 30 days. With bleeding, the mortality rate increased over 10-fold from 0.07 to 0.99%. In multivariate analysis, bleeding was associated with patient factors such as older age, prior cardiac procedure, hypertension, renal insufficiency, therapeutic anticoagulation, diabetes, obstructive sleep apnea, as well as technical factors such as larger bougie size and longer operative length. Staple-line reinforcement or oversewing and higher BMI were protective against bleeding

LEAK AFTER SLEEVE GASTRECTOMY

Although LSG does not involve an anastomosis, it is more susceptible to a leak than RYGB (2.4 vs. 0.7%) because of a long staple line and high intraluminal pressure. As explained above, the high luminal pressure is generated by a narrow-sleeved stomach sealed between an intact pylorus and lower esophageal sphincter. Leaks that occur after LSG are also less likely to close spontaneously because of the high luminal pressure. Other etiologies, besides a high intraluminal pressure, that also contribute to staple line leaks include ischemia, hematoma formation, and staple misfiring. Besides (rare) manufacturing issues, staple misfiring can be due to improper use of the stapler or improper selection of the staple height. When choosing staple cartridges, surgeons must be aware of the progressive decrease in the thickness of the gastric wall from the antrum to the fundus and adjust the staple height accordingly. In unstable patient with a contained or uncontained symptomatic leak requires immediate reoperation. In stable patients with leak, endoluminal stenting is a valid treatment option for an acute proximal leak that has failed conservative therapy. Stenting has limited efficacy for chronic leaks. After 30 days, the likelihood of a leak to seal by means of exclusion via stent is very low. In stable patients with a proximal leak, the surgeon should wait at least 12 weeks before reoperating to allow the body to heal and avoid thick adhesions. Surgical options include revising the sleeve and converting to RYGB. When revising the sleeve, the surgeon should oversew the leak with a bougie in place to avoid a stricture. Converting to RYGB is a valid treatment option that is usually reserved as the last resort for patients with chronic proximal leaks. It converts a high-pressure system (LSG with distal obstruction) to a lower-pressure system (RYGB), which promotes healing of the leak/fistula.

Although sleeve strictures have been reported in 0.26–4% of LSG operations, <1% result in symptoms that require endoscopic or surgical intervention. A stricture can manifest acutely, early after surgery, or more chronically. Although strictures can occur anywhere along the long staple line, they are most often located at the level of the incisura angularis for anatomic reasons. Patients with an acute stricture who do not respond to conservative management require early surgical reintervention. Laparoscopy could demonstrate kinking of the gastric tube, a tight suture, or a compressing hematoma. Patients with chronic strictures often present with mild symptoms that mimic acid reflux. Such patients can be initially managed with proton pump inhibitors. Those who fail medical management or develop severe symptoms are candidates for further endoscopic or surgical interventions. Endoscopy is a good initial treatment for short-segment strictures, most of which can be dilated with balloons. Multiple treatments in 4- to 6-week intervals are sometimes needed to treat the stricture and improve patient symptoms.

WEIGHT LOSS

"Durable" weight loss is the one most important gain of bariatric surgery operations, and it is the parameter by which success or failure of weight-reducing techniques is measured. Success of treatment has been defined as weight loss >50% of excess weight, maintaining or even losing further after surgery **(Table 1)**.

TABLE 1: Outcome of published series on sleeve gastrectomy.

S. No.	*Author*	*No. of patients*	*Average preoperative BMI*	*Bougie (Fr)*	*FU (Months)*	*Weight loss (%)*
1.	Weiner et al. (2007)	A = 25	61.6	NR	60	62% at 12 ms
		B = 32	60.8	44	60	C > B > A
		C = 63	60.3	32	60	Significantly
2.	Skrekas (2008)	93	46.86 ± 6.48	36	12.51 ± 4.15	58.32± 16.54%
3.	Dapri et al. (2007)	A = 20	42.5	34	12	48.3%
		B = 20	47	34	12	49.5%
4.	Lee et al. (2007)	216	49 ± 11	32		
5.	Melissas et al. (2007)	23	47.2 ± 4.8	34	12	33.1%
6.	Hamoui et al. (2006)	118	55		24	47.3%
7.	Langer et al. (2006) (Sleeve dilatation)	23	48.5 ± 6.9	48	12	56%
8.	Quesada (2008)	15	54	38	6	44%
9.	Baltasar (2006) (Re-sleeve)	2	46, 42			
10.	Cottam et al. (2006) (Initial, high-risk)	126	65.3 ± 0.8	48	12	46%
11.	Vidal et al. (2007) (Effect of LSG on DM)	35		48		NR
12.	Silecchia, et al. (2006)	41; superobese ≥ 2 major comorbidities	57.3 ± 6.5	48	22.2± 7.1	NR
13.	DePaula et al. (2008) (Effect of LSG as initial to two different procedures on DM with BMI ≤ 35	39	23.4–34.9	NR	7	22%
14.	Madhala et al. (2007) (Technique)	25	44 ± 2	50	4	22.7%
15.	Till et al. (2008) (LSG in morbid obese children)	4 (≤14.5 years)	48.4	40	12	23%
	Total	**707**	**MEAN = 57.76**	**MEAN = 43.7Fr.**	**Mean = 14.5 months**	**Mean= 40%**

(BMI: body mass index; DM: diabetes mellitus; LSG: laparoscopic sleeve gastrectomy)

The percentage weight loss after LSG in 707 morbidly obese patients included in the reviewed series is 40% (a mean) after a mean follow-up of 14 months **(Table 1)**.

Effect on Associated Comorbidities

Laparoscopic sleeve gastrectomy had been carried out for super obese patients with multiple severe comorbidities and in at least 50% of the patients; there was marked improvement of the comorbidities especially diabetes mellitus which got marked benefit in 50–57%.

Complications Review

In one of the reviewed series (n = 707), there are 17 major complications with an incidence of 2.4%. One should consider the heterogeneity of the patient's population where those with high risk and multiple severe comorbidities are included. One death due to gastric leakage reported with 11 gastric leakage, four renal failures, and one stenosis. GERD occurs in too many cases but most of the patients improve gradually on conservative management. Bleeding from the suture line was reported rarely and could be managed conservatively in most of the cases.

Laparoscopic Sleeve Gastrectomy as Initial Step for Super Obese and High-risk Patients

In two studies, LSG was used as a planned initial step and entertained over other major final technique due to super obesity with poor general condition in an attempt to minimize the risk in this subgroup of patients. During the post-LSG follow-up, the authors found the second stage operation is only needed in 5% in one study and 39% in the others **(Table 2)**.

TABLE 2: Main complications of LSG in the reviewed published series.

S. No.	*Author*	*No. of patients*	*Main complications*	*Recommendations*
1.	Weiner (2007)	120	Reflux symptoms, severe esophagitis	
2.	Skrekas (2008)	93	Four cases of gastric leak, three managed conservatively	More suitable for intermediate morbidly obese patients with BMI between 40 and 50 kg/m^2
3.	Dapri et al. (2007)	20 + 20	One early leak. One late leak, one stenosis	Better mobilize the stomach than resect it
4.	Lee et al. (2007)	23	Two leaks	Recommended for BMI < 50 kg/m^2
5.	Melissas et al. (2007)	23	Eight GERD; only one persisted	The term restrictive may not be applicable to the LSG
6.	Hamoui et al. (2006)	118	One death due to gastric leakage	Out of 118 super obese patients, only six requested second stage duodenal switch
7.	Langer et al. (2006)	23	One severe GERD, one renal failure	Sleeve dilatation does not necessarily lead to weight gain
8.	Quesada (2008)	15	-	LSG is best option in the presence of adhesions
9.	Baltasar (2006)	2	-	Re-LSG is achievable with minimal complication
10.	Cottam et al. (2006) (Initial, high-risk)	126 (+9.3 comorbidities in each; mean)	-	Only 36 patients (39%) were in need of the second stage. LSG is a good initial option in those severely comorbid patients
11.	Vidal et al (2007) (Effect of LSG on DM)	35	-	DM resolved in 51.3%, 4 months after LSG
12.	Silecchia et al. (2006)	41 super obese ≥ 2 major comorbidities	One leakage, one bleeding, one transient renal failure	After 12 months, 57.8% of the patients were comorbidity-free
13.	DePaula et al. (2008)	39	Two leakage, two renal failure	50% resolution of DM after 7 months
14.	Madhala et al. (2007)	25	-	-
15.	Till et al. (2008) (LSG in morbid obese children)	4 (≤14.5 years)	-	Comorbidities improved significantly
	Total	**707**	**11 gastric leaks, 1 DEATH, 4 RF, 1 stenosis = 17; 2.4%**	

(BMI: body mass index; DM: diabetes mellitus; GERD: gastroesophageal reflux disease; LSG: laparoscopic sleeve gastrectomy; RF: renal failure)

Laparoscopic Sleeve Gastrectomy in Morbidly Obese Children

Till et al. carried-out LSG in four morbidly obese pediatric patients with multiple comorbidities. Marked improvements in their comorbidities and 23% weight loss had been achieved after 12 months follow-up.

GASTRIC PLICATION

The field of bariatric surgery is evolving continuously. Surgical procedures have now been used to induce weight loss, and many different operations have been tested and dumped owing to the unsatisfactory long-term weight loss or metabolic or mechanical complications.

In sleeve gastrectomy a long staple line is created which can lead to complications, such as bleeding and leaks, and that the operation is irreversible has been a discouragement for few surgeons and patients. So a new operation came into design called laparoscopic gastric plication which is similar in some aspects to sleeve gastrectomy but with reduced risk. It started with the concept of plicating the greater curvature to itself to reduce the lumen of the stomach. Then the procedure was modified by division of the short gastric vessels and inverting and placating the greater curvature without any need for stapling or resection.

Surgical Technique

Two different techniques can be used to achieve laparoscopic gastric volume reduction **(Figs. 12A and B)**.

- In the first group [anterior plication (AP)], the anterior gastric wall was folded inward from the fundus to the antrum using two rows of 2-0 polypropylene running suture. The greater and lesser curvatures were approximated on the anterior surface of the stomach to create an intraluminal fold.
- In the second group [(greater curvature plication (GCP)], the short gastric vessels were divided starting 4 cm from the pylorus and continuing up to the left crus of the diaphragm, similar to the dissection performed for sleeve gastrectomy. After the fundus and body were completely mobilized, the greater curvature was folded inward with two suture lines of 2-0 polypropylene suture to create a large intraluminal gastric fold **(Figs. 13A to D)**. The fold was started just below the angle of His and continued distally to within 4 cm of the pylorus. In both procedure groups, full-thickness suture bites were used to secure the plications **(Fig. 14)**. This was confirmed by intraoperative endoscopy.

Complications

- Gastric obstruction due to fold prolapse or edema
- Adhesions or accumulation of fluid within the gastric fold
- Leak
- Fistula
- Nausea, vomiting, and sialorrhea
- Dysphagia or obstruction

Compared with LSG, laparoscopic gastric plication appears to have worse long-term outcomes (e.g., weight loss and diabetes resolution), more complications, and similar operating time and length of hospital stay. Thus, it is doubtful at this point that the laparoscopic gastric plication will become a meaningful operation for obesity and metabolic control.

MINI GASTRIC BYPASS

The mini gastric bypass (MGB) is a short, simple, successful, reversible laparoscopic gastric bypass weight loss surgery. It has been recently renamed as one anastomosis gastric bypass **(Fig. 15)**. The operation usually takes shorter time with lesser or similar hospital stay as regular bypass. Mini gastric bypass is a feasible and safe bariatric surgical procedure.

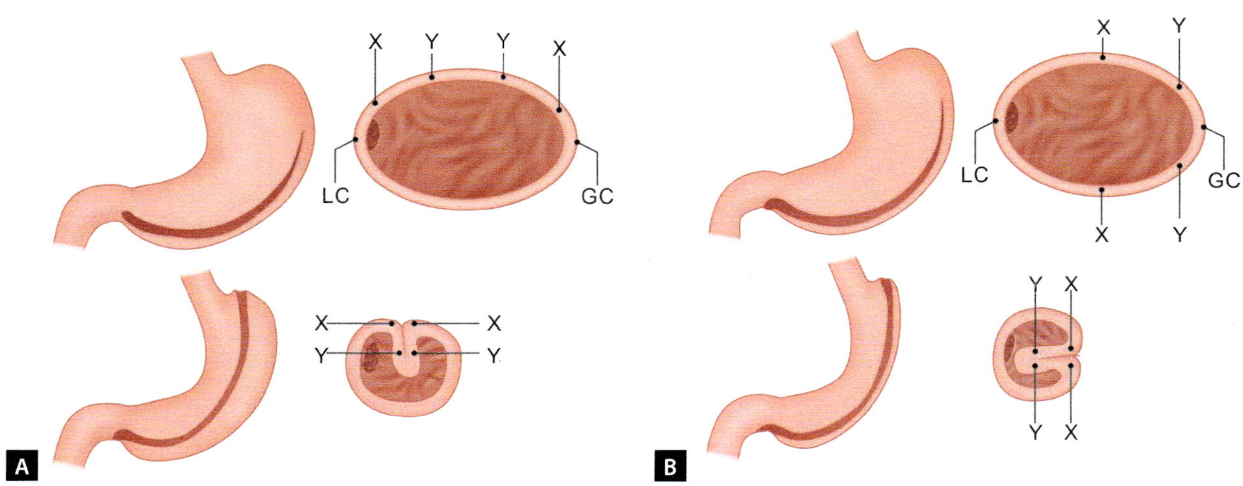

Figs. 12A and B: Different techniques to achieve laparoscopic gastric volume reduction.

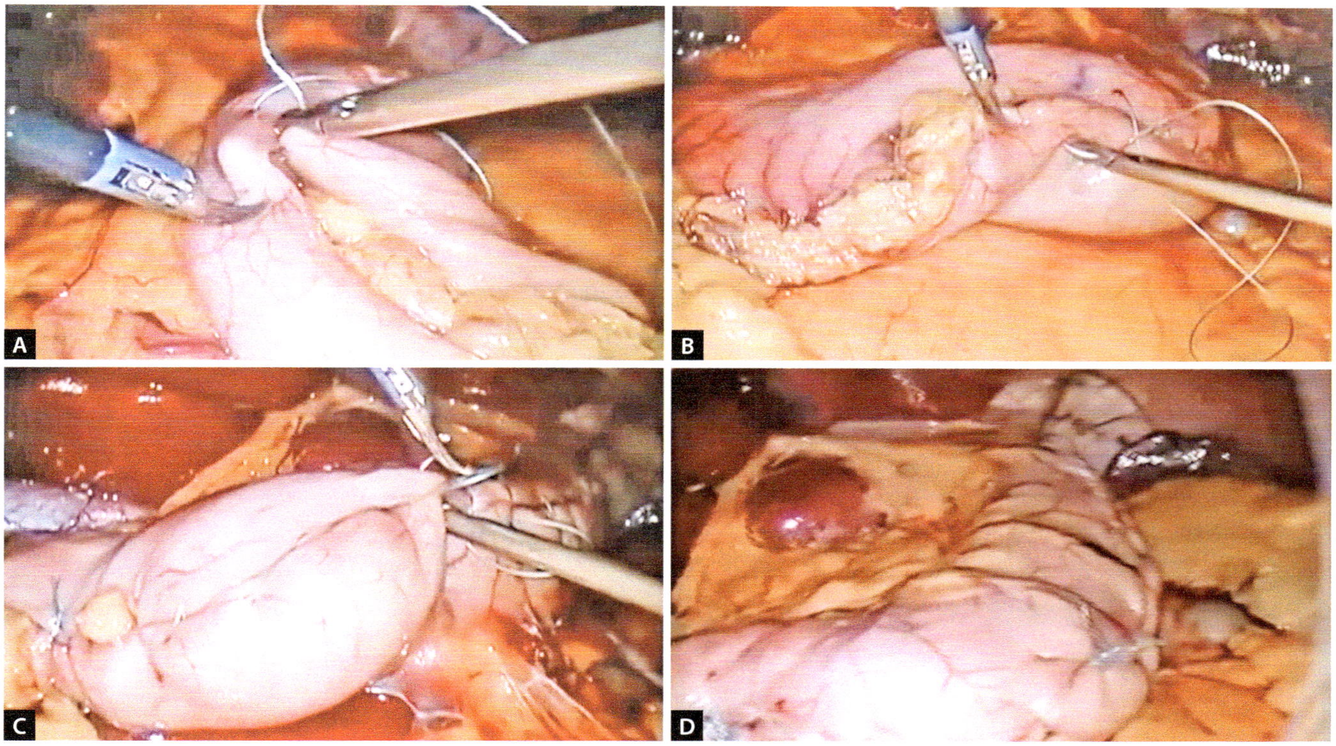

Figs. 13A to D: Steps of gastric plication.

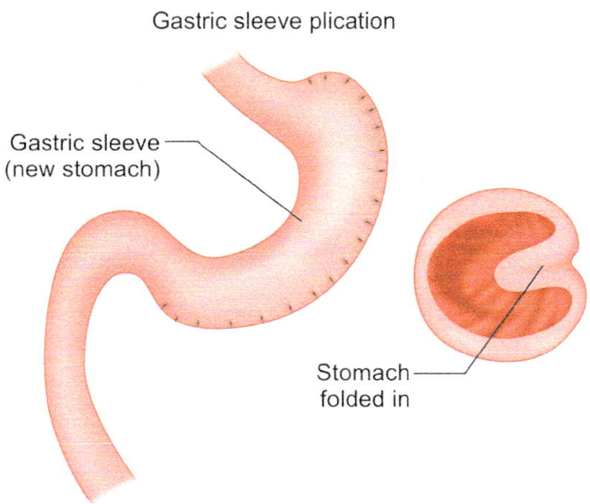

Fig. 14: Folded stomach in gastric plication.

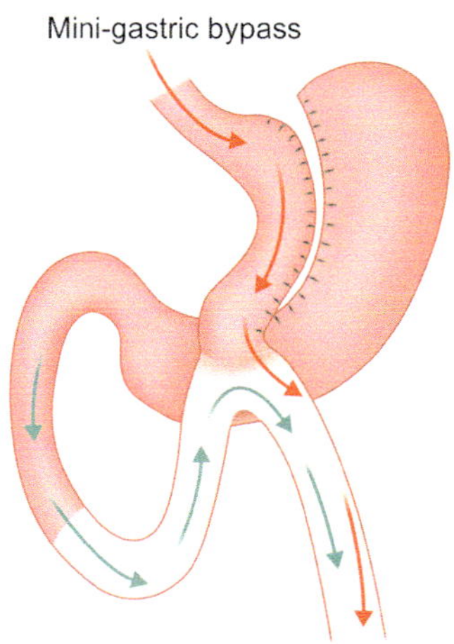

Fig. 15: Mini-gastric bypass.

Indications

It is indicated for people with a BMI of 40 kg/m^2 or more, and also in those whose BMI is 35–39 kg/m^2 that are suffering from obesity associated health conditions such as:

- Type 2 diabetes
- Heart disease
- High blood pressure
- High cholesterol
- Sleep apnea
- Nonalcoholic fatty liver disease
- Cancer

Position of Patient and the Surgical Team

The operation is performed with the patient in the supine position with legs open and with steeply inclined reverse Trendelenburg position. The surgeon stands between the legs with the first assistant, who handles the camera on the right. Antibiotic prophylaxis is routinely administered. The prevention of thrombotic events is made with use of graduated compression stockings and intermittent pneumatic cuffs. A NGT (32-Fr) should be placed. The pneumoperitoneum is performed by means of a direct puncture with a Veress needle in the left upper quadrant, near the costal margin at the level of the midclavicular line (Palmer's point) or some surgeon prefer supraumbilical port. The initial pressure is set at 20 mm Hg, 10 mm permanent trocars for introduction of 30° camera placed at the level of mesogastrium between 12–15 cm below the xiphoid process and 3 cm to the left of the midline. The next trocar of 5 mm is placed near the xiphoid process for the use of liver retractor which is a probe held by the assistant. The next trocar of 12 mm, to be used by the surgeon's left hand, is placed on the right side of the patient in an intermediate position between the previous two, 3–5 cm lateral to the midline. The next trocar of 5 mm is placed along the left costal margin in the anterior axillary line near to the assistant. The last trocar of 12 mm is placed adjacent to the left costal margin in the midclavicular line for surgeon's right hand manipulation.

Surgical Technique (Figs. 16A to E)

The operation begins with the dissection of the angle of His and the opening of the left gastrophrenic ligament with a

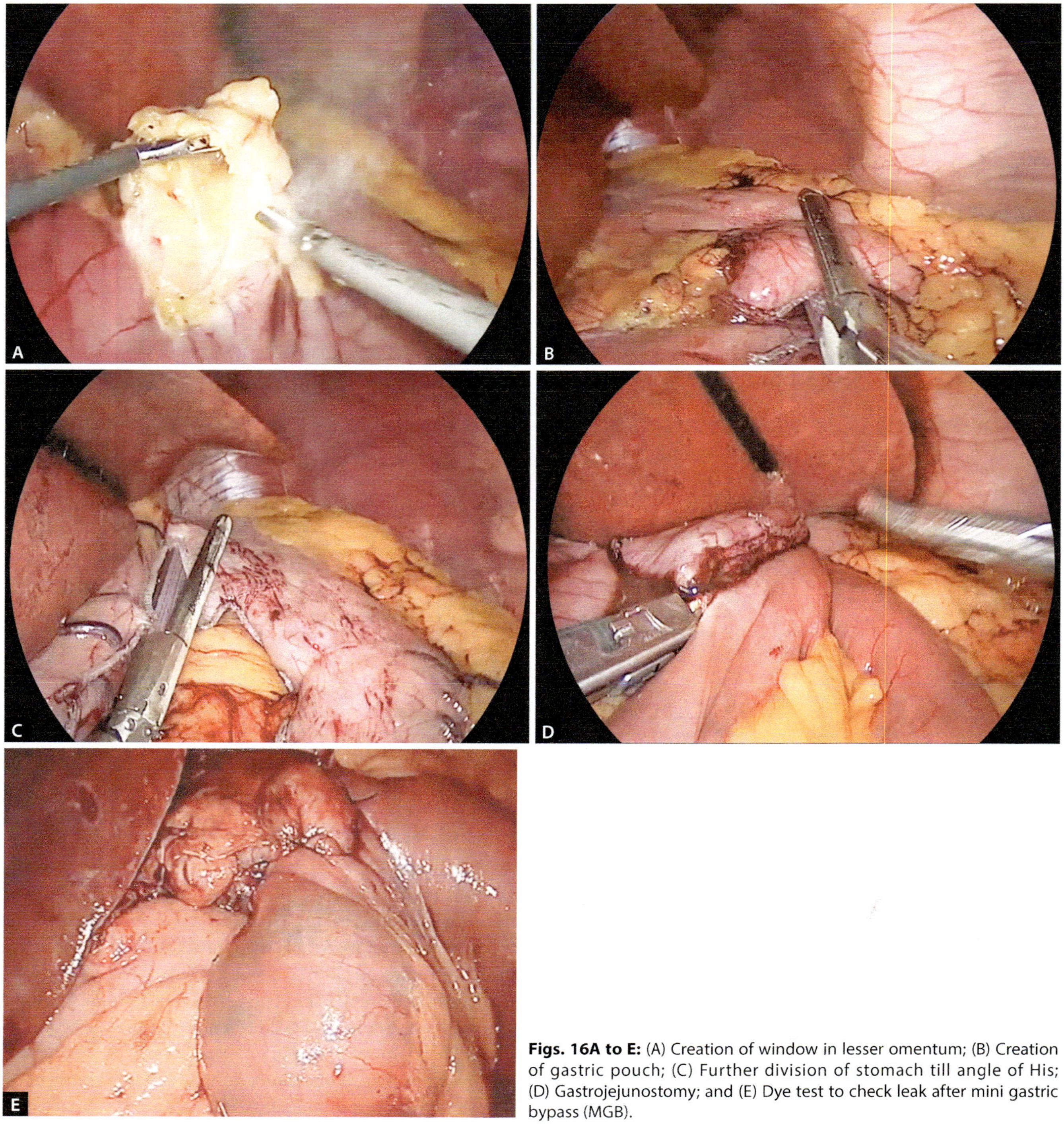

Figs. 16A to E: (A) Creation of window in lesser omentum; (B) Creation of gastric pouch; (C) Further division of stomach till angle of His; (D) Gastrojejunostomy; and (E) Dye test to check leak after mini gastric bypass (MGB).

harmonic scalpel, so as to expose the lateral aspect of the left diaphragmatic crus. Then, the resection of the fat pad of the esophagogastric junction, also known as Belsey's fat, is performed. The surgeon then proceeds to the ligation of the distal lesser sac, next to the insertion of the Latarjet nerve, until the exposure of the posterior gastric wall. The gastric pouch must be lengthy and narrow, measuring around 15–18 cm with a 50–150 mL reservoir capacity. The pouch is created using 45-mm blue cartridges to perform the horizontal section and 2–3 units to perform the vertical section. The stapling lines of the pouch and excluded stomach are then reinforced with a 3-0 polydioxanone continuous suture. The Treitz ligament is then identified and the small bowel is counted until 150–200 cm from the Treitz angle, so that part of the stomach, duodenum, and proximal jejunum gets excluded from the food pathway. This segment is then attached to the pouch and a vertical or slightly oblique omega-loop, isoperistaltic, antecolic, and side-to-side 25-mm gastrojejunostomy is performed using a 45-mm white cartridge; the orifice for the cartridge insertion is then closed by a continuous suture with 3-0 polydioxanone reinforced with separate stitches of 3-0 polyester. The Petersen's defect is closed by means of a continuous suture with 3-0 silk.

Complications

- Breakage
- Dumping syndrome
- Gallstones (risk increases with rapid or substantial weight loss)
- Hernia
- Internal bleeding or profuse bleeding of the surgical wound
- Leakage
- Perforation of stomach or intestines
- Pouch/anastomotic obstruction or bowel obstruction
- Protein or calorie malnutrition
- Pulmonary and/or cardiac problems
- Skin separation
- Spleen or other organ injury
- Stomach or intestine ulceration
- Stricture
- Vitamin or iron deficiency

Mini gastric bypass led to both early morbidity and mortality less than those observed after RYGB. Furthermore, due to its simplified design and the necessity to perform a single anastomosis, it is simpler and potentially more cost-effective since less stapler cartridges are necessary.

LAPAROSCOPIC ROUX-EN-Y GASTRIC BYPASS

Laparoscopic Roux-en-Y gastric bypass (LRYGB) remains the gold standard against which other bariatric procedures are

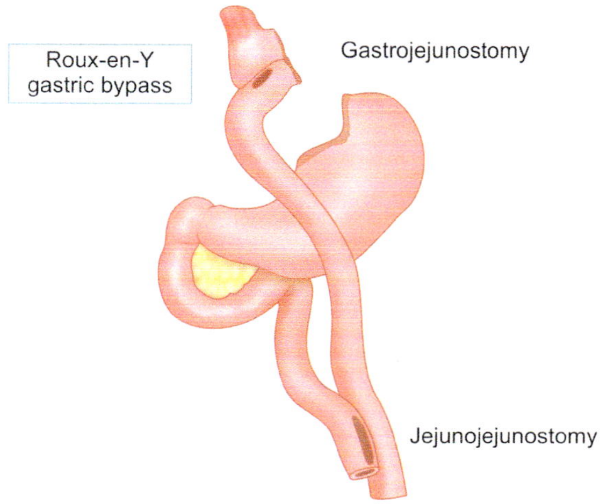

Fig. 17: Roux-en-Y gastric bypass.

measured **(Fig. 17)**. LRYGB induces more weight loss than AGB and more durable weight loss than sleeve gastrectomy. LRYGB, as a bariatric procedure, was first described by Alan Wittgrove in 1994. Over the ensuing decades, the technique of LRYGB as well as perioperative care of patients have been gradually improved and refined. Consequently, the mortality rate associated with the RYGB has decreased from 2.6% at the turn of the century to 0.12%.

Indications

The indications for LRYGB are the same as for all accepted bariatric procedures.

- Body mass index of >40 kg/m^2
- Body mass index of >35 kg/m^2 with one or more obesity-related comorbidities.
- Body mass index of >30 kg/m^2 with uncontrolled type 2 diabetes mellitus or metabolic syndrome.

Because LRYGB treats insulin resistance better than most other bariatric procedures, it may be preferred in patients with uncontrolled type 2 diabetes, nonalcoholic fatty liver disease, metabolic syndrome, or polycystic ovarian syndrome. These conditions are attributable to insulin resistance. Additionally, while sleeve gastrectomy and RYGB are equally effective in improving diabetes in the short term, LRYGB is associated with better long-term control of diabetes and lower rates of relapse.

Surgical Technique of Roux-en-Y Gastric Bypass (Figs. 18A to H)

The patient is placed in a moderate to steep reverse Trendelenburg position. The LRYGB operation is initiated by placing a total of six trocars, of which four are 10 mm and two are 5 mm **(Fig. 19)**. A part of the gastrophrenic ligaments is dissected down at the angle of His. A small gastric pouch is demarcated by creating a window in the lesser sac. After entering the retrogastric space, the surgeon should fully mobilize the angle of His by dividing the cardia's attachments to the overlying diaphragm. Complete mobilization of the fundus, especially a large one, will ensure that the gastric pouch is not created too large. The gastric vascular pedicle is also visualized, and blood supply to the gastric pouch should be preserved. A stapler is used to transect and staple the stomach first horizontally and then vertically to the angle of His. An endoscopic Maloney dilator is used to guide in creating the pouch. A 30-mL pouch has a dimension of approximately 3 × 3 × 3 cm. This can be measured using laparoscopic instruments, rulers placed in the abdomen, or a 30-mL balloon deployed in the proximal stomach as a guide.

When creating the pouch, some surgeons spare the perigastric neurovascular bundle containing vagal fibers, while others divide it routinely. In theory, sparing the vagal nerve fibers may allow better peristalsis and normal emptying

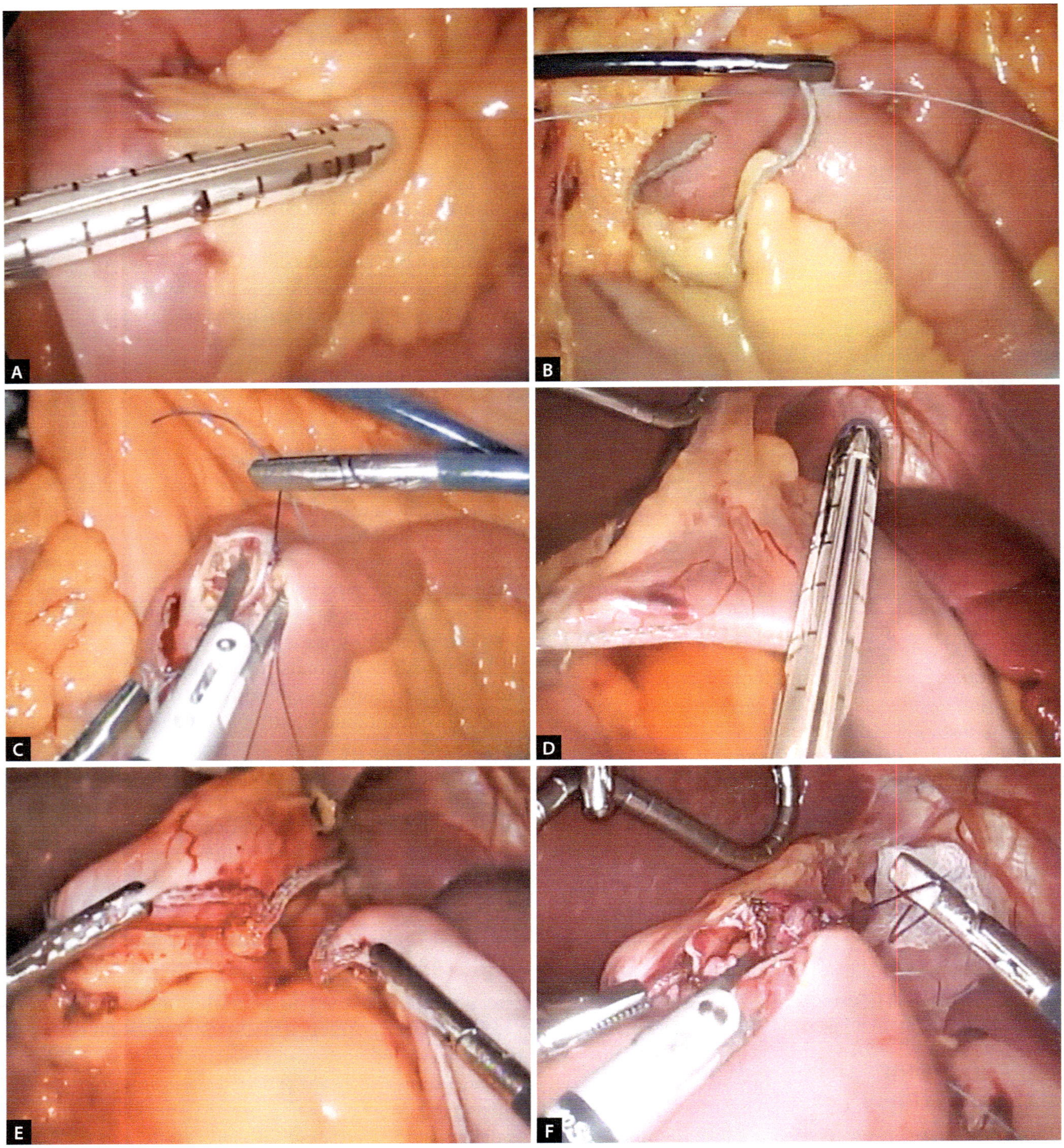

Figs. 18A to F: (A) Division of jejunum at 150 cm; (B) Transected jejunum; (C) Jejunojejunostomy; (D) Stomach pouch; (E) Complete pouch created; (F) Gastrojejunostomy started.

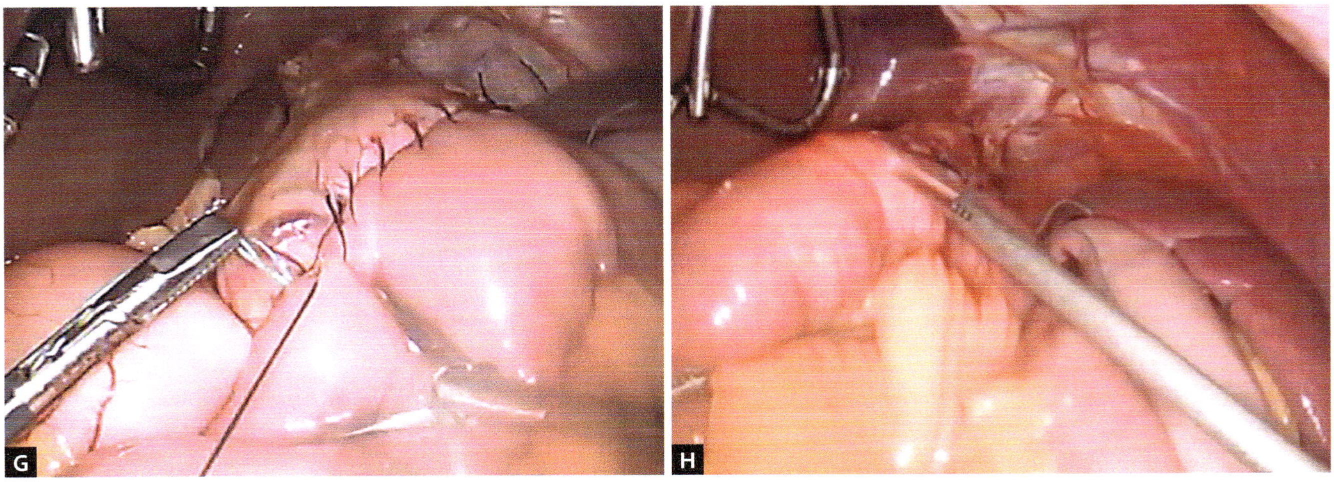

Figs. 18G and H: (G) Gastrojejunostomy near completion; and (H) Dye leak test.

of both the gastric remnant and the gallbladder. Normal gallbladder emptying may help prevent gallstone formation.

After entering the retrogastric space, the surgeon should fully mobilize the angle of His by dividing the cardia's attachments to the overlying diaphragm. The omentum and the transverse colon are retracted cranially, and the ligament of Treitz is thereby exposed. The small bowel is measured 50 cm distal to the ligament of Treitz and is stapled and transected along with mesentery creating a Roux limb. A jejunojejunal anastomosis is performed around 150 cm distally. The common enterotomy of the jejunojejunal anastomosis can be stapled or sewn by hand in a double-layered fashion. The mesenteric defect is then closed to prevent internal hernias.

The Roux limb is brought out in an antecolic and antegastric manner. A gastrojejunal anastomosis between the pouch and the Roux limb is performed in a double-layered fashion as well. A gastrotomy and an enterotomy are created anastomosed using a stapler. The gastrojejunal anastomosis is tested for air leak by submerging the anastomosis with irrigation fluid and inflating the orogastric tube with air. The anastomosis (gastrojejunal or jejunojejunal) can be either stapled or hand sewn. The basic tenets of LRYGB is to create a 30-mL gastric pouch from the proximal stomach, anastomose it to a Roux limb that is 75–150 cm in length, and connect the Roux limb to the biliopancreatic limb to create a common channel. It is generally accepted that the common channel (from the jejunojejunal anastomosis to the cecum) must be >200 cm to permit sufficient absorption of nutrients to prevent malnutrition.

Banded Gastric Bypass

Some laparoscopic surgeons have advocated placing a band (silastic ring) around the gastric pouch during the initial RYGB procedure. Although there have been no randomized trials comparing banded RYGB with standard RYGB, several prospective comparative studies have associated banded RYGB with less weight recidivism and more weight loss,

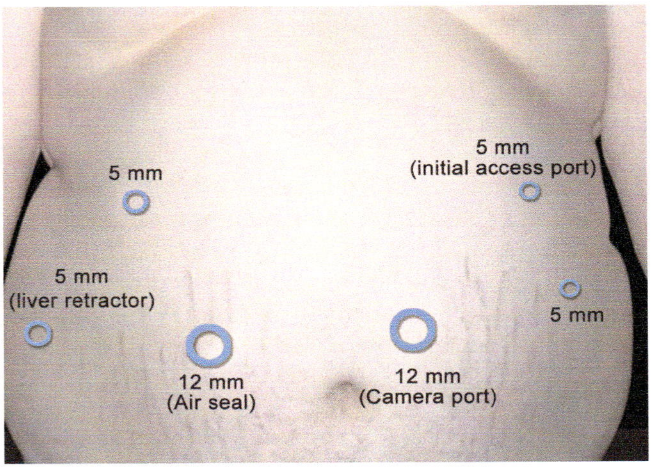

Fig. 19: Port position for Roux-en-Y gastric bypass (RYGB).

especially after the first year following bariatric surgery. Banded RYGB, however, was also associated with more mild complications such as dysphagia as well as vomiting and severe complications such as band eroding through the stomach wall. Thus, banded RYGB has not gained universal acceptance among bariatric surgeons.

Once bypass is successfully performed the pneumoperitoneum is evacuated actively. Trocar incisions that are >10 mm are closed at the fascia level. Because of the large amount of subcutaneous tissue in obese patients, a transfascial suturing device can be used. At this point and under laparoscopic guidance, long-acting local anesthesia is given to assist with postoperative pain control. A drain is only placed in revision operations and when there is concern about the integrity of the gastrojejunostomy anastomosis. The drain can potentially identify a leak and/or potentially help control a small leak.

Prophylaxis against venous thromboembolic events (VTEs) should continue after surgery. Specifically, patients should ambulate on the night of surgery, sequential compression devices (SCDs) should be worn, and chemoprophylaxis should be continued starting from the night after surgery. If a post-RYGB leak test is routine, it is typically performed on the first postoperative day before oral intake is started. If the test is negative for a leak or stenosis, oral intake is started with <30 mL of water every hour. If water is tolerated, the patient can be advanced to a clear liquid diet at breakfast on postoperative day 2 with the rate increased to 30 mL every 15 minutes. If the clear liquid diet is tolerated, the patient is advanced to a full liquid diet for lunch on postoperative day 2. A full liquid diet contains necessary protein supplements that will enable the patient to take in 60 g of protein daily.

Complications

Laparoscopic Roux-en-Y gastric bypass is a major elective surgical procedure. Risks include the following:

- Mortality may occur due to pulmonary embolism or gastrointestinal leak
- Wound infections
- Gastrojejunal stomal stricture
- Marginal ulcers (possibly more common with an antecolic approach than with a retrocolic approach)
- Internal hernia
- Roux limb ischemia
- Blowout of the stomach remnant
- Long-term deficiencies of micronutrients (e.g., vitamin B_{12}, folate, and iron)
- Bleeding from the staple line can become a serious problem. It gets controlled by means of clipping or monopolar cauterization.

CONCLUSION

As the prevalence of morbid obesity continues to escalate, the incidence of progressively complicated patients will rise. Clearly, a valid and effective strategy, beyond the current comprehensive evaluation measures, is needed for the optimal management of these patients.

Bariatric surgery is the most effective treatment for severe obesity, producing durable weight loss, improvement of comorbid conditions, and longer life. Patient selection algorithms should favor individual risk benefit considerations over traditional anthropometric and demographic limits. Bariatric care should be delivered within credentialed multidisciplinary systems. RYGB, AGB, and BPDDS are validated procedures that may be performed laparoscopically. Laparoscopic sleeve gastrectomy is also a promising procedure. Comparative data find that procedures with more dramatic clinical benefits carry greater risks, and those offering greater safety and flexibility are associated with less reliable efficacy.

Sleeve gastrectomy has been introduced and well accepted recently into the armamentarium of bariatric procedures. It was initially intended as a first step for poor-risk patients deemed too ill to undergo BPDDS or RYGB. Some of the patients lost significant weight and declined the proposed second stage, making the first stage with sleeve gastrectomy as a sole procedure. Sleeve gastrectomy has gained popularity with both bariatric surgeons and patients, mainly because of its relative operative simplicity and lower risk profile.

BIBLIOGRAPHY

1. Ahmed AR, Rickards G, Husain S, Johnson J, Boss T, O'Malley W. Trends in internal hernia incidence after laparoscopic Roux-en-Y gastric bypass. Obes Surg. 2007;17:1563-6.
2. Aggarwal S, Kini SU, Herron D. Laparoscopic sleeve gastrectomy for morbid obesity: a review. Surg Obes Relat Dis. 2007;3:189-94.
3. Alfredo G, Roberta M, Massimiliano C, Michele L, Nicola B, Adriano R. Long-term multiple intragastric balloon treatment—a new strategy to treat morbid obese patients refusing surgery: prospective 6-year follow-up study. Surg Obes Relat Dis. 2014;10:307-11.
4. Al Harakeh AB, Kallies KJ, Borgert AJ, Kothari SN. Bowel obstruction rates in antecolic/antegastric versus retrocolic/retrogastric Roux limb gastric bypass: a meta-analysis. Surg Obes Relat Dis. 2016;12:194-8.
5. Al-Mansour MR, Mundy R, Canoy JM, Dulaimy K, Kuhn JN, Romanelli J. Internal Hernia After Laparoscopic Antecolic Roux-en-Y Gastric Bypass. Obes Surg. 2015;25:2106-11.
6. Almogy G, Crookes PF, Anthone GJ. Longitudinal gastrectomy as a treatment for the high risk super-obese patients. Obes Surg. 2004;14:492-7.
7. American Society of Metabolic and Bariatric Surgery. (2018). Estimate of bariatric surgery numbers. [online] Available from http://asmbs.org/resources/estimate-of-bariatric-surgery-numbers (Last accessed August, 2020].
8. American Society for Metabolic and Bariatric Surgery. (2018). Low BMI. [online] Available from https://asmbs.org/resources/bariatric-surgery-in-class-i-obesity [Last accessed August, 2020].
9. Aminian A, Andalib A, Ver MR, Corcelles R, Schauer PR, Brethauer SA. Outcomes of Bariatric Surgery in Patients with Inflammatory Bowel Disease. Obes Surg. 2016;26:1186-90.
10. Aminian A, Brethauer SA, Andalib A, Punchai S, Mackey J, Rodriguez J, et al. Can Sleeve Gastrectomy "Cure" Diabetes? Long-term Metabolic Effects of Sleeve Gastrectomy in Patients With Type 2 Diabetes. Ann Surg. 2016;264:674-81.
11. Angrisani L, Lorenzo M, Borrelli V, Giuffré M, Fonderico C, Capece G. Is bariatric surgery necessary after intragastric balloon treatment? Obes Surg. 2006;16:1135-7.
12. Baltasar A, Serra C, Perez N, Bou R, Bengochea M. Re-sleeve gastrectomy. Obes Surg. 2006;16:1535-8.
13. Birkmeyer NJ, Finks JF, Carlin AM, Chengelis DL, Krause KR, Hawasli AA, et al. Comparative effectiveness of unfractionated and low-molecular-weight heparin for prevention of venous thromboembolism following bariatric surgery. Arch Surg. 2012;147:994-8.
14. Birkmeyer NJ, Finks JF, English WJ, Carlin AM, Hawasli AA, Genaw JA, et al. Risks and benefits of prophylactic inferior vena cava filters in patients undergoing bariatric surgery. J Hosp Med. 2013;8:173-7.
15. Bruzzi M, Rau C, Voron T, Guenzi M, Berger A, Chevallier JM. Single anastomosis or mini-gastric bypass: long-term results and quality of life after a 5-year follow-up. Surg Obes Relat Dis. 2015;11:321-6.
16. Buchwald M, Williams SE. Obesity surgery worldwide. Obes Surg. 2004;14:1157-64.
17. Busetto L, Segato G, De Luca M, Bortolozzi E, MacCari T, Magon A, et al. Preoperative weight loss by intragastric balloon in super-obese patients treated with laparoscopic gastric banding: a case-control study. Obes Surg. 2004;14:671-6.
18. Cottam D, Qureshi FG, Mattar SG, Sharma S, Holover S, Bonanomi G, et al. Laparoscopic sleeve gastrectomy as an initial weight-loss procedure for high-risk patients with morbid obesity. Surg Endosc. 2006;20:859-63.
19. Dapri G, Vaz C, Cadière GB, Himpens J. A prospective randomized study comparing two different techniques for laparoscopic sleeve gastrectomy. Obes Surg. 2007;17:1435-41.
20. DeMaria EJ, Pate V, Warthen M, Winegar DA. Baseline data from American Society for Metabolic and Bariatric Surgery-designated Bariatric Surgery Centers of Excellence using the

Bariatric Outcomes Longitudinal Database. Surg Obes Relat Dis. 2010;6:347-55.
21. Edholm D, Kullberg J, Karlsson FA, Haenni A, Ahlström H, Sundbom M. Changes in liver volume and body composition during 4 weeks of low calorie diet before laparoscopic gastric bypass. Surg Obes Relat Dis. 2015;11:602-6.
22. Eisendrath P, Cremer M, Himpens J, Cadiere GB, Le Moine O, Deviere J. Endotherapy including temporary stenting of fistulas of the upper gastrointestinal tract after laparoscopic bariatric surgery. Endoscopy. 2007;39:625-30.
23. Eynden FV, Urbain P. Small intestine gastric balloon impact on treated by laparoscopic surgery. Obes Surg. 2001;11:646-8.
24. Flum DR, Salem L, Elrod JA, Dellinger EP, Cheadle A, Chan L. Early mortality among Medicare beneficiaries undergoing bariatric surgical procedures. JAMA. 2005;294:1903-8.
25. Frezza EE. Laparoscopic vertical sleeve gastrectomy for morbid obesity. The future procedure of choice? Surg Today. 2007;37:275-81.
26. Genco A, Bruni T, Doldi SB, Forestieri P, Marino M, Busetto L, et al. BioEnterics Intragastric Balloon: the Italian experience with 2,515 patients. Obes Surg. 2005;15:1161-4.
27. Genco A, Cipriano M, Bacci V, Cuzzolaro M, Materia A, Raparelli L, et al. Bioenterics Intragastric Balloon (BIB): a short-term, double blind, randomised, controlled, crossover study on weight reduction in morbidly obese patients. Int J Obes (Lond). 2006;30:129-33.
28. Gumbs A, Gagner M, Dakin G, Pomp A. Sleeve gastrectomy for morbid obesity. Obes Surg. 2007;17:962-9.
29. Hamoui N, Anthone GJ, Kaufman HS, Crookes PF. Sleeve gastrectomy in the high-risk patients. Obes Surg. 2006;16:1445-9.
30. Heshmati K, Lo T, Tavakkoli A, Sheu E. Short-Term Outcomes of Inflammatory Bowel Disease after Roux-en-Y Gastric Bypass vs Sleeve Gastrectomy. J Am Coll Surg. 2019;228:893-901.e1.
31. Kueper MA, Kramer KM, Kirschniak A, Königsrainer A, Pointner R, Granderath FA. Laparoscopic sleeve gastrectomy: standardized technique of a potential stand-alone bariatric procedure in morbidly obese patients. World J Surg. 2008;32:1462-5.
32. Langer FB, Bohdjalin A, Felberbauer FX, Fleischmann E, Reza Hoda MA, Ludvik B, et al. Does gastric dilatation limit the success of sleeve gastrectomy as a sole operation for morbid obesity? Obes Surg. 2006;16:166-71.
33. Lee CM, Cirangle PT, Jossart GH. Vertical gastrectomy for morbid obesity in 216 patients: report of two-year results. Surg Endosc. 2007;21:1810-6.
34. Lehman Center Weight Loss Surgery Expert Panel. Commonwealth of Massachusetts Betsy Lehman Center for Patient Safety and Medical Error Reduction Expert Panel on Weight Loss Surgery: executive report. Obes Res. 2005;13:205-26.
35. le Roux CW, Welbourn R, Werling M, Osborne A, Kokkinos A, Laurenius A, et al. Gut hormones as mediators of appetite and weight loss after Roux-en-Y gastric bypass. Ann Surg. 2007;246:780-5.
36. Maciejewski ML, Arterburn DE, Van Scoyoc L, Smith VA, Yancy WS Jr, Weidenbacher HJ, et al. Bariatric Surgery and Long-term Durability of Weight Loss. JAMA Surg. 2016;151:1046-55.
37. Madhala, Spector R, Wasserberg N, Beglaibter N, Lustigman H, Stein M, et al. Technical aspects of laparoscopic sleeve gastre-ctomy in 25 morbidly obese patients. Obes Surg. 2007;17(6):722-7.
38. Marceau P, Biron S, Bourque RA, Potvin M, Hould FS, Simard S. Biliopancreatic diversion with a new type of gastrectomy. Obes Surg. 1993;3:29-35.
39. Melissas J, Kuokouraki S, Askoxylakis J, Stathaki M, Daskalakis M, Perisinakis K, et al. Sleeve gastrectomy: a restrictive procedure? Obes Surg. 2007;17:57-62.
40. Milone L, Strong V, Gagner M. Laparoscopic sleeve gastrectomy is superior to endoscopic intragastric balloon as a first stage procedure for superobese patients. Obes Surg. 2005;15:612-7.
41. Mognol P, Chosidow D, Marmuse JP. Laparoscopic sleeve gastrectomy as an initial bariatric operation for high-risk patients: initial results in 10 patients. Obes Surg. 2005;15:1030-3.
42. Morino M, Toppino M, Forestieri P, Angrisani L, Allaix ME, Scopinaro N. Mortality after bariatric surgery: analysis of 13,871 morbidly obese patients from a national registry. Ann Surg. 2007;246:1002-7; discussion 1007-9.
43. Nelson DW, Blair KS, Martin MJ. Analysis of obesity-related outcomes and bariatric failure rates with the duodenal switch vs gastric bypass for morbid obesity. Arch Surg. 2012;147:847-54.
44. Nielsen HK. Pathophysiology of venous thromboembolism. Semin Thromb Hemost. 1991;17(Suppl 3):250-3.
45. O'Brien PE, McPhail T, Chaston TB, Dixon JB. Systematic review of medium-term weight loss after bariatric operations. Obes Surg. 2006;16:1032-40.
46. Owens M, Barry M, Janjua AZ, Winter DC. A systematic review of laparoscopic port site hernias in gastrointestinal surgery. Surgeon. 2011;9:218-24.
47. Quesada BM, Roff HE, Kohan G, Salvador Oría A, Chiappetta Porras LT. Laparoscopic sleeve gastrectomy as an alternative to gastric bypass in patients with multiple intra-abdominal adhesions. Obes Surg. 2008;18:566-8.
48. Regan JP, Inabnet WB, Gagner M. Early experience with two stage laparoscopic Roux-en-Y gastric bypass as an alternative in the super-super obese patient. Obes Surg. 2003;13:861-4.
49. Roa PE, Kaidar-Person O, Pinto D, Cho M, Szomstein S, Rosenthal RJ. Laparoscopic sleeve gastrectomy as treatment for morbid obesity: technique ad short-term outcome. Obes Surg. 2006;16:1323-6.
50. Roberts K, Duffy A, Kaufman J, Burrell M, Dziura J, Bell R. Size matters: gastric pouch size correlates with weight loss after laparoscopic Roux-en-Y gastric bypass. Surg Endosc. 2007;21:1397-1402.
51. Rubin M, Yehoshua RT, Stein M, Lederfein D, Fichman S, Bernstine H, et al. Laparoscopic sleeve gastrectomy with minimal morbidity. Early results in 120 morbidly obese patients. Obes Surg. 2008;18:1567-70.
52. Sallet JA, Marchesini JB, Paiva DS, Komoto K, Pizani CE, Ribeiro ML, et al. Brazilian multicenter study on the intragastric balloon. Obes Surg. 2004;14:991-8.
53. Sarr MG, Billington CJ, Brancatisano R, Brancatisano A, Toouli J, Kow L, et al. The EMPOWER study: randomized, prospective, double-blind, multicenter trial of vagal blockade to induce weight loss in morbid obesity. Obes Surg. 2012;22:1771-82.
54. Schigt A, Coblijn U, Lagarde S, Kuiken S, Scholten P, van Wagensveld B. Is esophagogastroduodenoscopy before Roux-en-Y gastric bypass or sleeve gastrectomy mandatory? Surg Obes Relat Dis. 2014;10:411-7.
55. Silecchia G, Boru C, Pecchia A, Rizzello M, Casella G, Leonetti F, et al. Effectiveness of laparoscopic sleeve gastrectomy (first-stage of biliopancreatic diversion with duodenal switch) on co-morbidities in superobese high-risk patients. Obes Surg. 2006;16:1138-44.
56. Skrekas G, Lapatsanis D, Stafyla V, Papalambros A. One year after laparoscopic "tight". sleeve gastrectomy: technique and outcome. Obes Surg. 2008;18:810-3.
57. Till H, Blüher S, Hirsch W, Kiess W. Efficacy of laparoscopic sleeve gastrectomy (LSG) as a stand-alone technique for children with morbid obesity. Obes Surg. 2008;18(8):1047-9.
58. van Wezenbeek MR, van Oudheusden TR, Smulders JF, Nienhuijs SW, Luyer MD. Transection versus preservation of the neurovascular bundle of the lesser omentum in primary Roux-en-Y gastric bypass surgery. Surg Obes Relat Dis. 2016;12:283-9.
59. Weiner RA, Weiner S, Pomhoff I, Jacobi C, Makarewicz W, Weigand G. Laparoscopic sleeve gastrectomy: influence of sleeve size and resected gastric volume. Obes Surg. 2007;17(10):1297-305.
60. Wittgrove AC, Clark GW, Tremblay LJ. Laparoscopic Gastric Bypass, Roux-en-Y: Preliminary Report of Five Cases. Obes Surg. 1994;4:353-7.
61. Yoong W, Saxena S, Mittal M, Stavroulis A, Ogbodo E, Damodaram M. The pressure profile test is more sensitive and specific than Palmer's test in predicting correct placement of the Veress needle. Eur J Obstet Gynecol Reprod Biol. 2010;152:210-3.

CHAPTER 22

Laparoscopic Splenectomy

INTRODUCTION

The first laparoscopic splenectomy was performed by Delaitre and Maignen in 1991. In 1992, Carrol, Philips, Semal, Fellas and Morgenstern of Cedars-Sinai medical center reported three cases of successful laparoscopic splenectomy. The first laparoscopic splenectomy in children was performed in 1993 by Tulman. Laparoscopic splenectomy first started in early 90s, but due to very high conversion rate it was not accepted by most of the laparoscopic surgeons. Now due to increased proficiency in the performance of laparoscopic procedures, conversion rate is now inexistent even with large spleens. To date, this procedure continues to be associated with a steep learning curve but remains very rewarding, elegant procedure. The indications for this procedure have broadened and are now the same as with open procedures. They range from idiopathic thrombocytopenic purpura, unresponsive hemolytic anemia to staging procedures and to primary splenic cysts.

Laparoscopic splenectomy can be safely performed to treat certain conditions such as hereditary hemolytic anemias, autoimmune cytopenias, or symptomatic splenomegaly. One of the most common uses of elective splenectomy is for treatment of idiopathic thrombocytopenic purpura with severe thrombocytopenia that does not respond to a course of glucocorticoids.

Only contraindication of laparoscopic splenectomy is excessively large spleens with weight over 1,000 g. We personally believe that the maneuvers used to remove such large spleens do not warrant these procedures. One should always remember that by laparoscopic approach, the spleen cannot be removed in its integral anatomical form and is usually shredded. If there is any need to preserve splenic integrity, then laparoscopic approach is not indicated.

ANATOMY OF SPLENIC VASCULATURE (FIG. 1A)

For successful laparoscopic splenectomy, the surgeon should be familiar with the three-dimensional relations of the spleen and be conversant with the variations of the blood supply. The important anatomical aspects of the spleen are its vascularization and its great number of relationships with adjacent organs. The spleen being a reticuloendothelial organ is soft, friable and deserves careful handling by the surgeon as well as the assistants. Despite the fragility of the splenic parenchyma, its capsule is solid and can be manipulated without rupture if handled with care. Capsular tears can lead to bleeding, splenosis, and conversion into open.

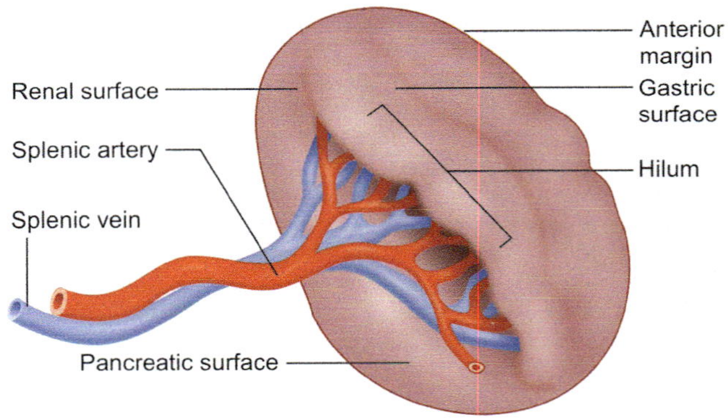

Fig. 1A: Splenic anatomy.

Two types of splenic blood supply exist around spleen are magistral and distributed. Transverse anastomosis exists between the splenic artery branches. The gastrosplenic ligament contains short gastric and gastroepiploic vessels. The lienorenal ligament contains the hilar vessels and the tail of the pancreas. Other suspensory ligaments are avascular, except in portal hypertension and myeloid metaplasia. The tail of the pancreas lies within 1 cm of the inner surface of the spleen in 73% of patients. The tail of the pancreas is in direct contact with the spleen in 30% of patients. The size of the spleen does not determine the number of entering arteries.

The spleen has in essence a double blood supply: short gastric vessels and a main hilar vascular trunk. Although highly variable, splenic artery anatomy has been classified more simply into two patterns: (1) magistral and (2) distributed. The more common distributed type found in around 70% of the dissections and the magistral type found in the rest. By definition, in the distributed type, the trunk is short and many long branches enter over three-fourths the medial surface of the spleen. The branches originate 3–13 cm from the hilum. There are also accessory polar vessels and anastomoses with gastroepiploic vessels. These anatomic details require that the surgeon be completely familiar with variable and anomalous extrasplenic vascular anatomy. The more the number of notches on the spleen, the more is a segmental distributed pattern of blood supply likely. Accessory spleens are more likely with this pattern of blood supply.

ADVANTAGES OF LAPAROSCOPIC SPLENECTOMY

Reasons to prefer laparoscopic splenectomy include the following:

- *Lower surgical mortality*: In a systematic review that included over 6,000 splenectomies for immune thrombocytopenia, laparoscopic splenectomy was associated with a mortality of 0.2% (3 of 1,301 patients) whereas laparotomy with an open procedure was associated with a mortality of 1% (48 of 4,955 individuals).
- *Shorter hospitalization and faster recovery*: One of the reviews from the National Surgical Quality Improvement Program (NSQIP) also evaluated length of hospital stay and found that this was approximately 2 days shorter with the laparoscopic procedures.
- *Reduced complications*: Long-term complications such as infection and venous thromboembolism (VTE) appear similar with open and laparoscopic splenectomy. In the perioperative period, individuals undergoing laparoscopic rather than open splenectomy have been reported to receive fewer transfusions. In a report from a high-volume center, the median blood loss was only 50 mL (interquartile range, 20–150 mL).

DISADVANTAGES OF LAPAROSCOPIC APPROACH

Settings in which an open procedure may be preferred include the following:

- Massive splenomegaly with concern about the ability to remove the spleen via a laparoscopic procedure.
- Local expertise favoring an open procedure or lack of support or equipment for laparoscopy.
- Ability to search more thoroughly for an accessory spleen.
- Cancer surgery or adhesion of the spleen to adjacent organs requiring laparotomy.

In some cases, laparoscopic splenectomy may need to be converted to an open procedure. The likelihood of this happening has been estimated to be in the range of 3–10%. Reasons for conversion included excess bleeding, technical problems, splenic size, and other abnormalities such as friability or infiltration of surrounding structures.

VACCINATION

Patients undergoing laparoscopic splenectomy should receive vaccinations against encapsulated organisms (*Haemophilus influenzae*, *Pneumococcus*, *Meningococcus* species) in order to prevent overwhelming postsplenectomy infection (OPSI). Optimally, vaccinations should be administered 2 weeks prior to surgery. However, in emergent cases, vaccinations can be postponed until 1–2 weeks postoperatively.

OPERATING ROOM SETUP AND PATIENT POSITION

Patient is placed in supine and semi-right lateral position on the table although laparoscopic splenectomy can be performed either in the supine or right semi-lateral decubitus position. Surgeon stands to the right of patient **(Fig. 1B)**. Operating table is flexed at approximately 30 degrees to increase space between the costal margin and iliac crest, and the patient is placed in semi-lateral position.

Semilateral position allows the spleen to hang by its diaphragmatic attachments, thus acting as a natural counter traction while gravity retracts the stomach, transverse colon, and greater omentum inferiorly, and places the hilum of the spleen under tension. Bean bag is used to secure patient position and all pressure points are padded. Camera operator stands to right side of the patient next to the surgeon toward right hand side of surgeon. Monitor is placed left to the patient and Mayo's stand is placed near the feet of the patient **(Figs. 2A and B)**. Various steps of splenectomy shown in **(Fig. 3)**.

Port Position

Port position should be decided according to baseball diamond concept depending on the size of spleen.

Operative Procedure

Laparoscopic splenectomy can be described in five steps:

Step 1: Dissection of the inferior aspect of the spleen.

Step 2: Dissection of the lateral and retroperitoneal attachments.

Step 3: Transection of the splenic hilum.

A 10-mm fan retractor is inserted and will lift the inferior aspect spleen superiorly. The tail of the pancreas should be identified. The splenorenal and colosplenic ligaments are divided with sharp dissection. The splenorenal ligament should be divided without Gerota's fascia. The gastrosplenic ligament containing the short gastric vessels are divided with an energy device. The dissection is continued superior and lateral to mobilize the entire spleen **(Figs. 4 and 5)**. Search for accessory spleens is traditionally performed at the onset of the procedure. Common locations include the splenic hilum, gastrosplenic ligament, splenorenal ligament, and greater omentum. Accessory spleens can also be embedded in the pancreas.

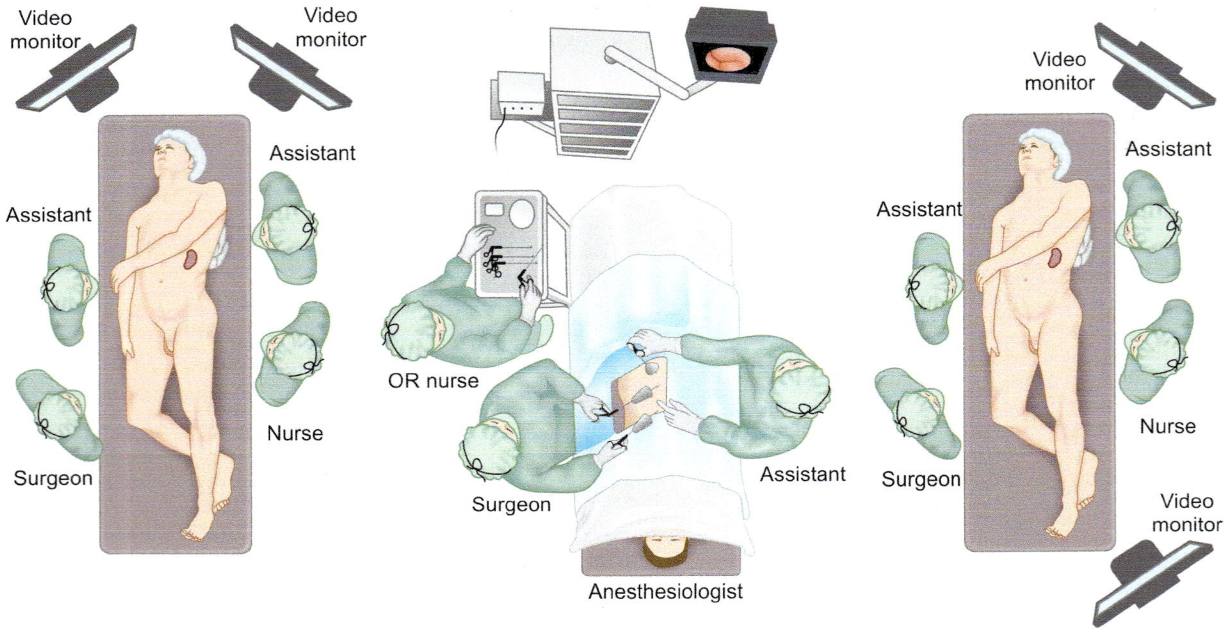

Fig. 1B: Position of surgical team.

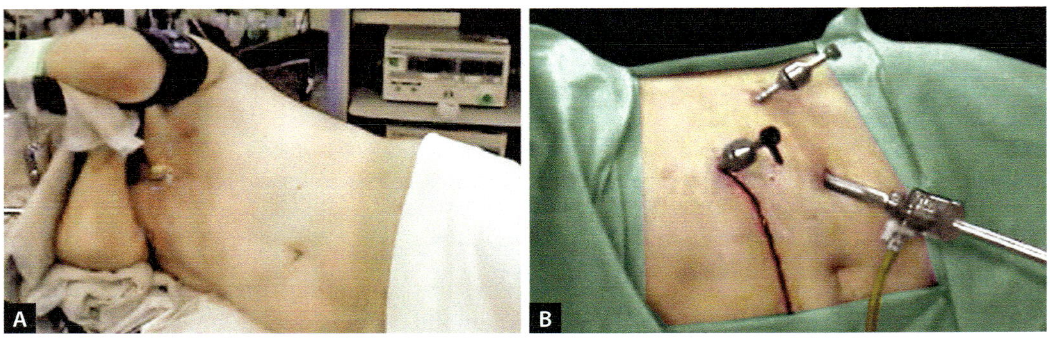

Figs. 2A and B: Position of patient in laparoscopic splenectomy.

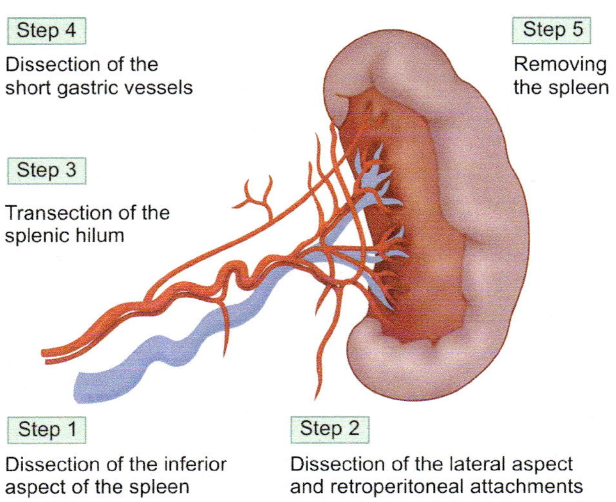

Fig. 3: Various steps of splenectomy.

It is essential to continue our dissection posterior and inferior to the spleen as far as possible. Its purpose is to sufficiently expose the posterior aspect of the splenic hilum **(Fig. 6)**. The entire anterior aspect of the hilum should also be well-visualized **(Figs. 7A to D)**.

Occasionally, the short gastric vessels will have to be first transected to gain additional exposure. While the assistant elevates and retracts the spleen, the hilum should be distinguished from the tail of the pancreas and an endoscopic linear stapler with vascular load should be used to divide the vessels.

Stapler is inserted and each jaw should be positioned anterior and posterior to the splenic vessels **(Figs. 8A to F)**. Advances in linear stapling devices have enhanced laparoscopic splenectomy. In general, 2.5-mm vascular loads are sufficient for hemostasis, but 2.0-mm staple loads are used for thin pedicles and skeletonized vessels. A large spleen dictates an approach to the hilum through less than optimal port placement. The tail of the pancreas should be well visualized to avoid inadvertent injury at the time of firing stapler.

Step 4: Dissection of the short gastric vessels.

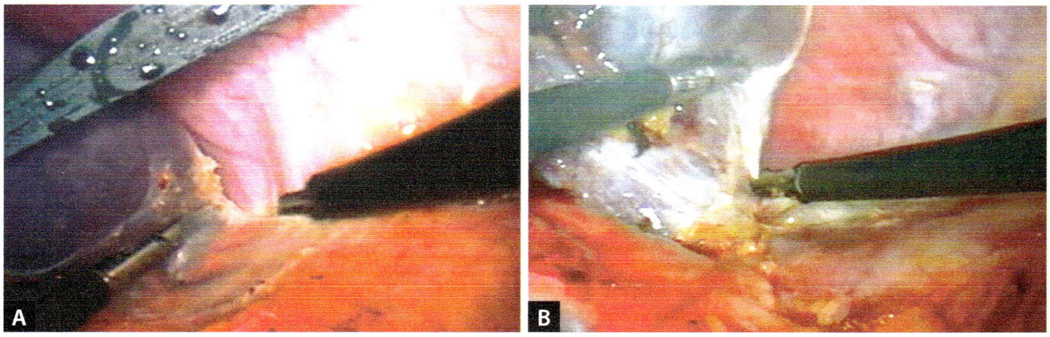

Figs. 4A and B: Dissection of the inferior aspect of the spleen.

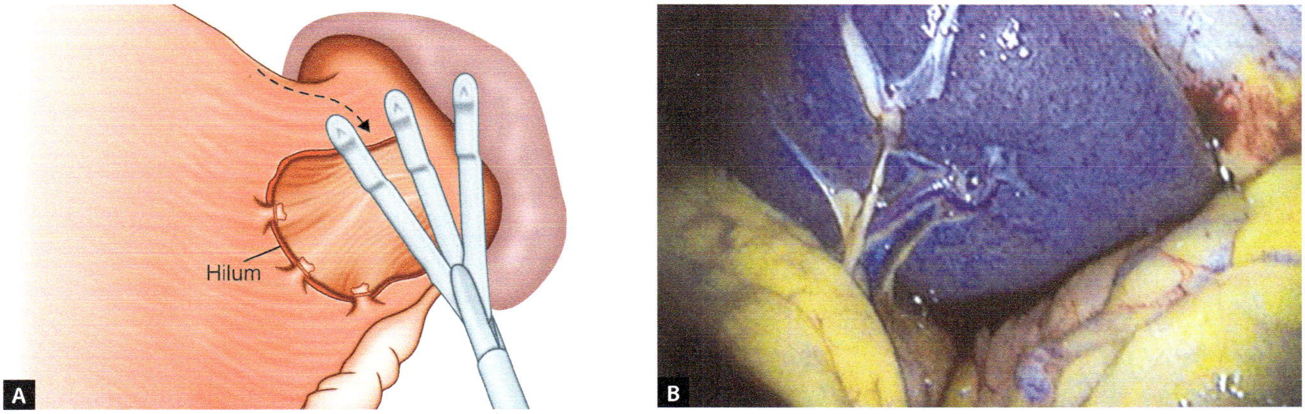

Figs. 5A and B: Retractor is necessary to expose the hilum of spleen.

The short gastric vessels are best divided using energy such as either LigaSure™, harmonic or simple bipolar or tripolar. The clip or stapler may be used also for short gastric vessels. Each time the spleen is moved superiorly, inferiorly or medially and all the attachments should be carefully dissected. With slow and careful separation of ligaments, the spleen should be entirely detached.

Hemorrhage is the most common cause for conversion during laparoscopic splenectomy. A judiciously placed grasper can control the hemorrhage, allowing deliberate suctioning and dissection, rather than blind placing of clips that may cause more bleeding or jam subsequent stapler function. An additional port can also make the difference between continuing laparoscopically and converting to laparotomy. Back bleeding from the spleen can be difficult to identify because of vessel retraction into the spleen and additional parenchymal damage from clips placed to control bleeding. In situations such as this, it is best to progress steadily and expeditiously through the division of the remaining hilum, focusing on control of any bleeding from the proximal side.

Step 5: Removing the spleen.

The most lateral 12-mm trocar is removed; its site is enlarged and replaced by 15-mm trocar. An endobag is introduced and deployed in the intra-abdominal cavity. The spleen is placed in the specimen retrieval bag. The specimen retrieval bag is closed and brought against the anterior abdominal wall. It is open via the enlarged trocar site. The spleen is then sectioned in smaller pieces in the specimen retrieval bag and removed with a large clamp **(Figs. 9A and B)**.

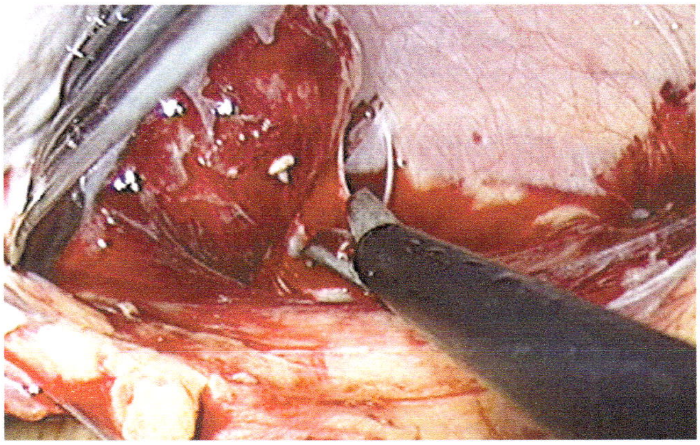

Fig. 6: Transection of the splenic hilum.

A drain is left in the intra-abdominal cavity. The final evaluation of abdominal cavity is done and the instruments are removed. Port is closed according to need.

Simultaneous Cholecystectomy

In some individuals, it may be reasonable to perform cholecystectomy at the same time as splenectomy. This is especially true for those with a history of pigment gallstones,

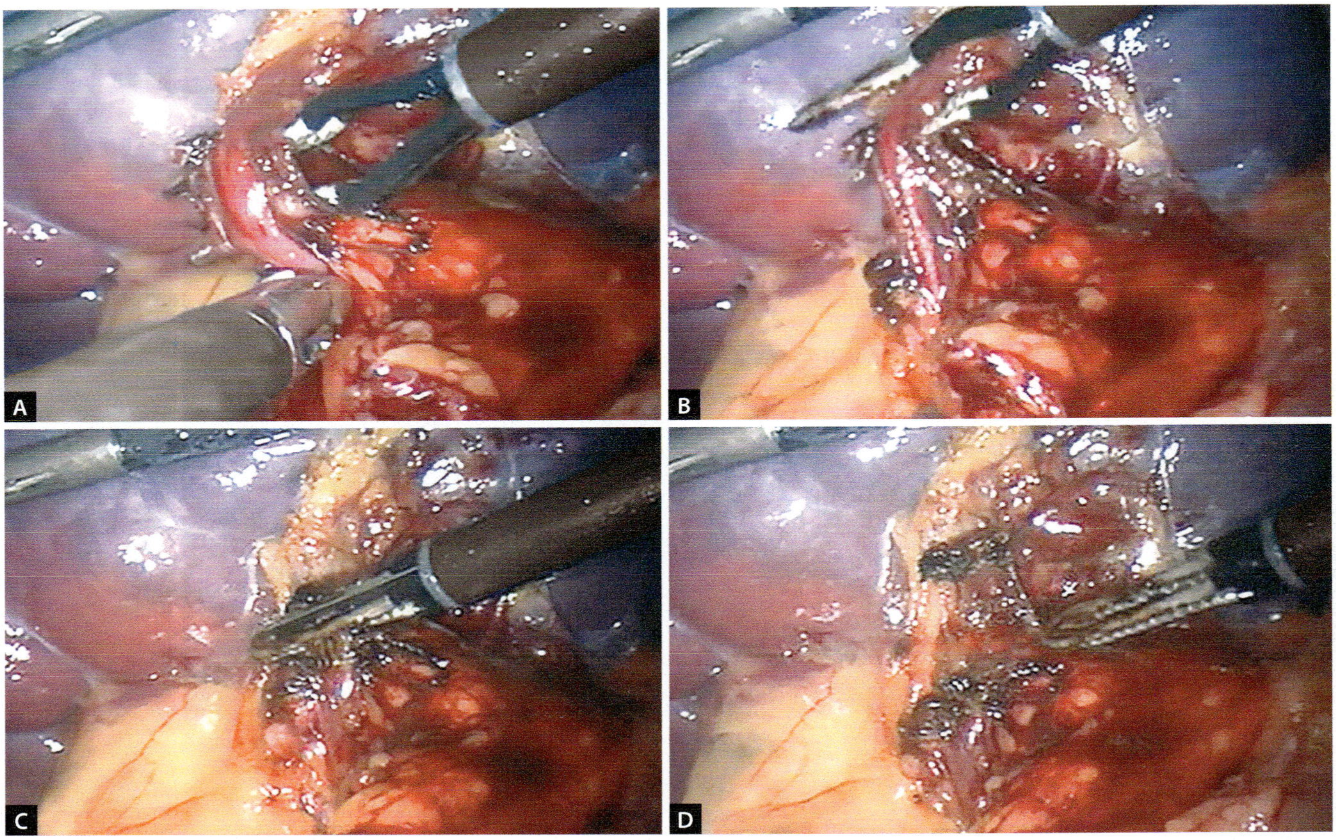

Figs. 7A to D: Dissection of splenic hilum.

which can develop as a complication of chronic hemolysis, such as with an inherited hemolytic anemia.

COMPLICATIONS OF LAPAROSCOPIC SPLENECTOMY

Surgical complications of laparoscopic splenectomy are similar to those for the open splenectomy.

Early complications include:

- Bleeding
- Pneumonia
- Left pleural effusions
- Atelectasis
- Injury to colon, small bowel, stomach, liver, and pancreas

Late complications include:

- Subphrenic abscess
- Splenic or portal vein thrombosis (or both)
- Failure of the procedure to control the primary disease
- Recurrent disease as a result of accessory spleens
- Overwhelming postsplenectomy infection

Independent of any complications inherent to laparoscopic surgery (LS) in general (e.g., related to pneumoperitoneum injuries from trocars), LS is associated with several potential perioperative complications that the surgeon should be aware of and be able to treat. The greatest potential problem is hemorrhage. Hemorrhage from a larger vessel may be an indication for immediate conversion to laparotomy. The best means for its prevention is delicate dissection of the artery and vein to prevent rupture of smaller splenic and pancreatic blood vessels. The dissected artery and vein should then be clipped prior to any movement of the spleen. Injury to these vessels can occur simply due to the rigidity of the clamping instruments. Hemorrhage originating in the parenchyma is less dangerous and can be managed by clamping the artery or by applying slight pressure with gauze, as well as by the use of electrocoagulation.

Another potential complication of LS is injury to the tail of the pancreas. Proper dissection and placement of the endostapler can avoid this problem. A further possible complication of LS is perforation of the diaphragm during dissection of the superior pole of the spleen. A small puncture may be quickly amplified by the presence of pneumoperitoneum, causing a pneumothorax. This can be controlled laparoscopically and by the use of a pleural drain. Other complications reported with LS include deep vein thrombosis, pulmonary embolus, and wound.

Rapid advances in minimal access surgery technology and improvement in noninvasive imaging tests, laparoscopic splenectomy is now being advocated for most of the patient. It has shorter operative time and recovery period and excellent cosmetic results as compared to the open splenectomy. Laparoscopic splenectomy though has a

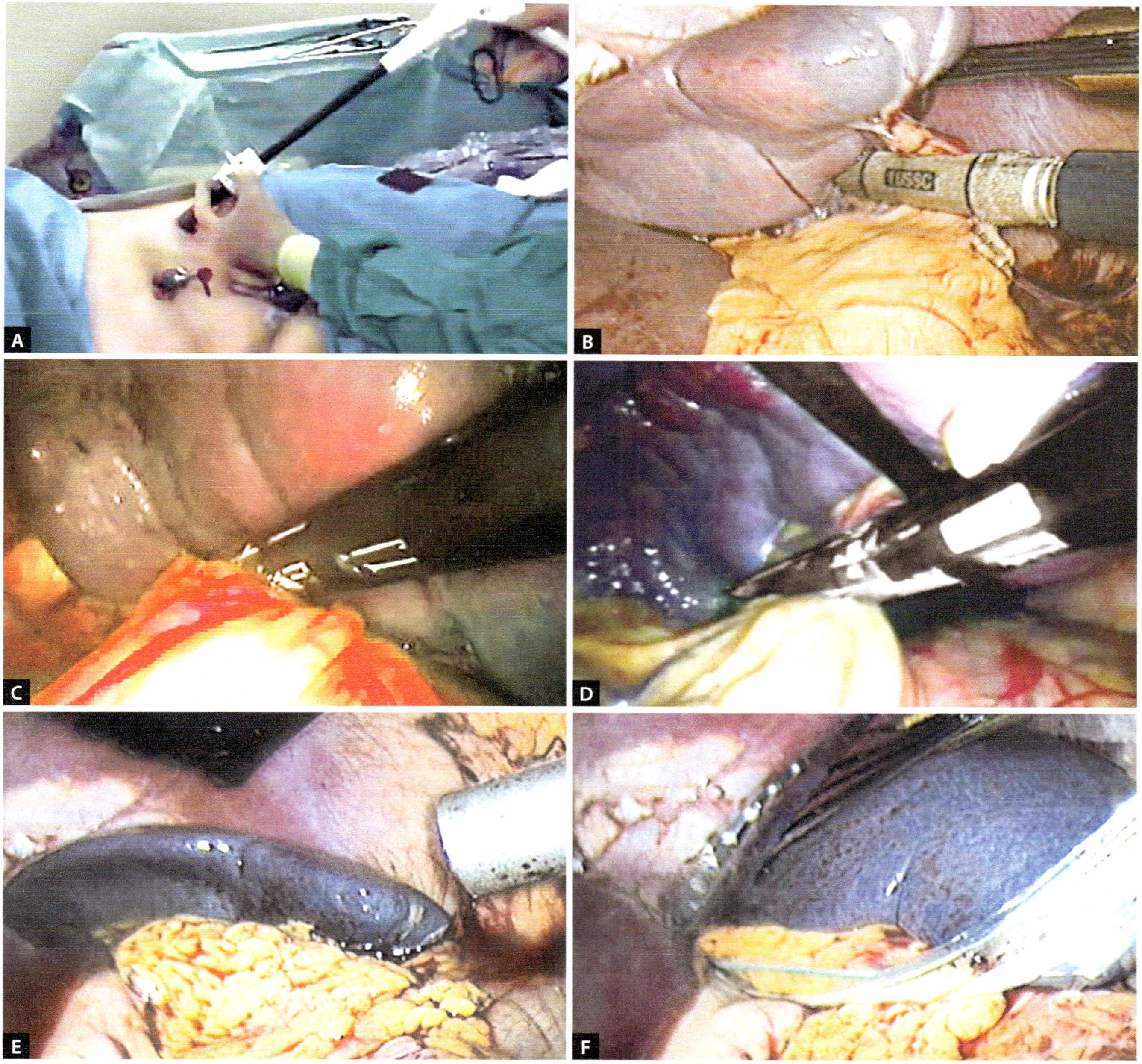

Figs. 8A to F: Use of endo-gastrointestinal (GI) linear stapler or vascular stapler can make the laparoscopic splenectomy easy but many surgeon use extracorporeal knot as their main skill to secure splenic umenti.

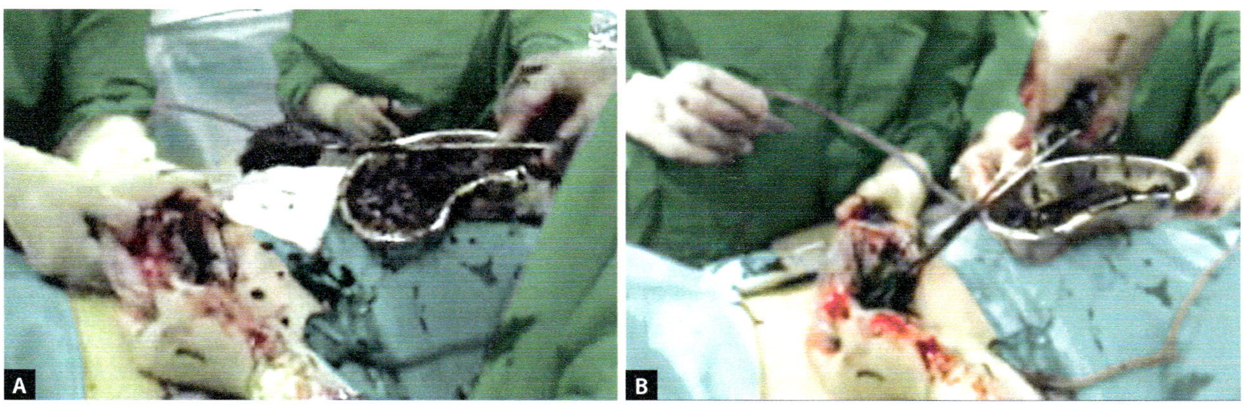

Figs. 9A and B: Manual morcellation of the spleen inside endobag.

definite learning curve is not difficult if one has experience in open splenectomy. Advanced laparoscopic instruments such as harmonic scalpel, endoscopic vascular stapler, LigaSure™, and good quality endobag aid the surgeons in removing spleen.

BIBLIOGRAPHY

1. Baccarani U, Carroll BJ, Hiatt JR, Donini A, Terrosu G, Robert Decker, et al. Comparison of laparoscopic and open staging in Hodgkin disease. Arch Surg. 1998;133:517-22.
2. Baccarani U, Terrosu G, Donini A, Zaja F, Bresadola F, Baccarani M. Splenectomy in hematology: current practice and new perspectives. Haematologica. 1999;84:431-6.
3. Bell RL, Reinhardt KE, Cho E, Flowers JL. A ten-year, single institution experience with laparoscopic splenectomy. JSLS. 2005;9:163-8.
4. Berends FJ, Schep N, Cuesta MA, Bonjer HJ, Kappers-Klunne MC, Huijgens P, et al. Hematological long-term results of laparoscopic splenectomy for patients with idiopathic thrombocytopenic purpura: a case-control study. Surg Endosc. 2004;18:766-70.
5. Brunt LM, Langer JC, Quasebarth MA, Whitman ED. Comparative analysis of laparoscopic versus open splenectomy. Am J Surg. 1996;172:596-9; discussion 599-601.
6. Casaccia M, Torelli P, Squarcia S, Sormani MP, Savelli A, Troilo B, et al. Laparoscopic splenectomy for hematologic diseases: a preliminary analysis performed on the Italian Registry of Laparoscopic Surgery of the Spleen (IRLSS). Surg Endosc. 2006;20:1214-20.
7. Casaccia M, Torelli P, Squarcia S, Sormani MP, Savelli A, Troilo BM, et al. The Italian Registry of Laparoscopic Surgery of the Spleen (IRLSS): a retrospective review of 379 patients undergoing laparoscopic splenectomy. Chir Ital. 2006;58:697-707.
8. Cordera F, Long KH, Nagorney DM, McMurtry EK, Schleck C, Ilstrup D, et al. Open versus laparoscopic splenectomy for idiopathic thrombocytopenic purpura: clinical and economic analysis. Surgery. 2003;134:45-52.
9. Curran TJ, Foley MI, Swanstrom LL, Campbell TJ. Laparoscopy improves outcomes for pediatric splenectomy. J Pediatr Surg. 1998;33:1498-500.
10. Dagash H, Chowdhury M, Pierro A. When can I be proficient in laparoscopic surgery? A systematic review of the evidence. J Pediatr Surg. 2003;38:720-4.
11. Delaitre B, Blezel E, Samama G, Barrat C, Gossot D, Bresler L, et al. Laparoscopic splenectomy for idiopathic thrombocytopenic purpura. Surg Laparosc Endosc Percutan Tech. 2002;12:412-9.
12. Delaitre B, Maignien B. [Splenectomy by the laparoscopic approach: report of a case] Presse Med. 1991;20:2263.
13. Delaitre B, Pitre J. Laparoscopic splenectomy versus open splenectomy: a comparative study. Hepato-gastroenterology. 1997;44:45-9.
14. Diaz J, Eisenstat M, Chung R. A case-controlled study of laparoscopic splenectomy. Am J Surg. 1997;173:348-50.
15. Donini A, Baccarani U, Terrosu G, Corno V, Ermacora A, Pasqualucci A, Bresadola F. Laparoscopic vs open splenectomy in the management of hematologic diseases. Surg Endosc. 1999;13:1220-5.
16. Eden OB, Lilleyman JS. Guidelines for management of idiopathic thrombocytopenic purpura. The British Paediatric Haematology Group. Arch Dis Child. 1992;67:1056-8.
17. Esposito C, Corcione F, Garipoli V, Ascione G. Pediatric laparoscopic splenectomy: are there real advantages in comparison with the traditional open approach? Pediatr Surg Int. 1997;12:509-10.
18. Franciosi C, Caprotti R, Romano F, Porta G, Real G, Colombo G, et al. Laparoscopic versus open splenectomy: a comparative study. Surg Laparosc Endosc Percutan Tech. 2000;10:291-5.
19. Gadenstatter M, Lamprecht B, Klingler A, Wetscher GJ, Greil R, Schmid T. Splenectomy versus medical treatment for idiopathic thrombocytopenic purpura. Am J Surg. 2002;184:606-10.
20. Gadner H. Management of immune thrombocytopenic purpura in children. Rev Clin Exp Hematol. 2001;5:201-22.
21. George JN, Woolf SH, Raskob GE, Wasser JS, Aledort LM, Ballem PJ, et al. Idiopathic thrombocytopenic purpura: a practice guideline developed by explicit methods for the American Society of Hematology. Blood. 1996;88:3-40.
22. Glasgow RE, Mulvihill SJ. Laparoscopic splenectomy. World J Surg. 1999;23:384-8.
23. Joshi M, Kurhade S, Peethambaram MS. Single-incision laparoscopic splenectomy. JAMS. 2011;7:65-7.
24. Jugenburg M, Haddock G, Freedman MH, Ford-Jones L, Ein SH. The morbidity and mortality of pediatric splenectomy: does prophylaxis make a difference? J Pediatr Surg. 1999;34:1064-7.
25. Katkhouda N, Grant SW, Mavor E, Friedlander MH, Lord RV, Achanta K, et al. Predictors of response after laparoscopic splenectomy for immune thrombocytopenic purpura. Surg Endosc. 2001;15:484-8.
26. Katkhouda N, Hurwitz MB, Rivera RT, Chandra M, Waldrep DJ, Gugenheim J, et al. Laparoscopic splenectomy: outcome and efficacy in 103 consecutive patients. Ann Surg. 1998;228:568-78.
27. Khan LR, Nixon SJ. Laparoscopic splenectomy is a better treatment for adult ITP than steroids—it should be used earlier in patient management: conclusions of a ten-year follow-up study. Surgeon. 2007;5:3-4, 6-8.
28. Knauer EM, Ailawadi G, Yahanda A, Obermeyer RJ, Millie MP, Ojeda H, et al. 101 laparoscopic splenectomies for the treatment of benign and malignant hematologic disorders. Am J Surg. 2003;186:500-4.
29. Kojouri K, Vesely SK, Terrell DR, George JN. Splenectomy for adult patients with idiopathic thrombocytopenic purpura: a systematic review to assess long-term platelet count responses, prediction of response, and surgical complications. Blood. 2004;104:2623-34.
30. Konstadoulakis MM, Lagoudianakis E, Antonakis PT, Albanopoulos K, Gomatos I, Stamou KM, et al. Laparoscopic versus open splenectomy in patients with beta thalassemia major. J Laparoendosc Adv Surg Tech A. 2006;16:5-8.
31. Kucuk C, Sozuer E, Ok E, Altuntas F, Yilmaz Z. Laparoscopic versus open splenectomy in the management of benign and malign hematologic diseases: a ten-year single-center experience. J Laparoendosc Adv Surg Tech A. 2005;15:135-9.
32. Kwon HC, Moon CH, Cho YR, Kim MC, Kim KH, Han JY, et al. Prognostic factors of response to laparoscopic, splenectomy in patients with idiopathic thrombocytopenic purpura. J Korean Med Sci. 2005;20:417-20.
33. Lozano-Salazar RR, Herrera MF, Vargas-Vorackova F, Lopez-Karpovitch X. Laparoscopic versus open splenectomy for immune thrombocytopenic purpura. Am J Surg. 1998;176:366-9.
34. Mantadakis E, Buchanan GR. Elective splenectomy in children with idiopathic thrombocytopenic purpura. J Pediatr Hematol Oncol. 2000;22:148-53.
35. Napoli A, Catalano C, Silecchia G, Fabiano P, Fraioli F, Pediconi F, et al. Laparoscopic splenectomy: multidetector row CT for preoperative evaluation. Radiology. 2004;232:361-7.
36. Owera A, Hamade AM, Bani Hani OI, Ammori BJ. Laparoscopic versus open splenectomy for massive splenomegaly: a comparative study. J Laparoendosc Adv Surg Tech A. 2006;16:241-6.
37. Pace DE, Chiasson PM, Schlachta CM, Mamazza J, Poulin EC. Laparoscopic splenectomy: does the training of minimally invasive surgical fellows affect outcomes? Surg Endosc. 2002;16:954-6.

38. Park A, Marcaccio M, Sternbach M, Witzke D, Fitzgerald P. Laparoscopic vs open splenectomy. Arch Surg. 1999;134:1263-9.
39. Peters MB Jr, Camacho D, Ojeda H, Reichenbach DJ, Knauer EM, Yahanda AM, et al. Defining the learning curve for laparoscopic splenectomy for immune thrombocytopenia purpura. Am J Surg. 2004;188:522-5.
40. Pędziwiatr M, Matłok M, Major P, Kuliś D, Budzyński A. Laparoscopic surgery of the spleen through single umbilical incision. Videosurg Miniinv. 2013;1:8-12.
41. Phillips EH, Carroll BJ, Fallas MJ. Laparoscopic splenectomy. Surg Endosc. 1994;8:931-3.
42. Rattner DW, Apelgren KN, Eubanks WS. The need for training opportunities in advanced laparoscopic surgery. Surg Endosc. 2001;15:1066-70.
43. Rege RV, Joehl RJ. A learning curve for laparoscopic splenectomy at an academic institution. J Surg Res. 1999;81:27-32.
44. Rescorla FJ. Laparoscopic splenectomy. Semin Pediatr Surg. 2002;11:226-32.
45. Rhodes M, Rudd M, O'Rourke N, Nathanson L, Fielding G. Laparoscopic splenectomy and lymph node biopsy for hematologic disorders. Ann Surg. 1995;222:43-6.
46. Romano F, Caprotti R, Franciosi C, Finna SD, Colombo G, Uggeri F. Laparoscopic splenectomy using LigaSure. Preliminary experience. Surg Endosc. 2002;16:1608-11.
47. Rothenberg SS. Laparoscopic splenectomy in children. Semin Laparosc Surg. 1998;5:19-24.
48. Sampath S, Meneghetti AT, MacFarlane JK, Nguyen NH, Benny WB, Panton ON. An 18-year review of open and laparoscopic splenectomy for idiopathic thrombocytopenic purpura. Am J Surg. 2007;193:580-4.
49. Sapucahy MV, Faintuch J, Bresciani CJ, Bertevello PL, Habr-Gama A, Gama-Rodrigues JJ. Laparoscopic versus open splenectomy in the management of hemotologic diseases. Rev Hosp Clin Fac Med Sao Paulo. 2003;58:243-9.
50. Sauerland S, Agresta F, Bergamaschi R, Borzellino G, Budzynski A, Champault G, et al. Laparoscopy for abdominal emergencies: evidence-based guidelines of the European Association for Endoscopic Surgery. Surg Endosc. 2006;20:14-29,
51. Schlinkert RT, Mann D. Laparoscopic splenectomy offers advantages in selected patients with immune thrombocytopenic purpura. Am J Surg. 1995;170:624-7.
52. Shimomatsuya T, Horiuchi T. Laparoscopic splenectomy for treatment of patients with idiopathic thrombocytopenic purpura: comparison with open splenectomy. Surg Endosc. 1999;13:563-6.
53. Silecchia G, Boru CE, Fantini A, Raparelli L, Greco F, Rizzello M, et al. Laparoscopic splenectomy in the management of benign and malignant hematologic diseases. JSLS. 2006;10:199-205.
54. Smith CD, Meyer TA, Goretsky MJ, Hyams D, Luchette FA, Fegelman EJ, et al. Laparoscopic splenectomy by the lateral approach: a safe and effective alternative to open splenectomy for hematologic diseases. Surgery. 1996;120:789-94.
55. Tanoue K, Okita K, Akahoshi T, Konishi K, Gotoh N, Tsutsumi N, et al. Laparoscopic splenectomy for hematologic diseases. Surgery. 2002;131:S318-23.
56. Targarona EM, Espert JJ, Balague C, Piulachs J, Artigas V, Trias M. Splenomegaly should not be considered a contraindication for laparoscopic splenectomy. Ann Surg. 1998;228:35-9.
57. Trias M, Targarona EM, Espert JJ, Cerdan G, Bombuy E, Vidal O, et al. Impact of hematological diagnosis on early and late outcome after laparoscopic splenectomy: an analysis of 111 cases. Surg Endosc. 2000;14:556-60.
58. Ucmak H, Buyukbese SS, Buyukbese MA, Kus S. Laparoscopic splenectomy and infection. J Microbiol Infect Dis. 2013;3:1-2.
59. Vecchio R, Cacciola E, Lipari G, Privitera V, Polino C, Cacciola R. Laparoscopic splenectomy reduces the need for platelet transfusion in patients with idiopathic thrombocytopenic purpura. JSLS. 2005;9:415-8.
60. Velanovich V. Laparoscopic vs open surgery: a preliminary comparison of quality-of-life outcomes. Surg Endosc. 2000;14:16-21.
61. Waldhausen JH, Tapper D. Is pediatric laparoscopic splenectomy safe and cost effective? Arch Surg. 1997;132:822-4.
62. Walsh RM, Heniford BT, Brody F, Ponsky J. The ascendance of laparoscopic splenectomy. Am Surg. 2001;67:48-53.
63. Watanabe Y, Horiuchi A, Yoshida M, Yamamoto Y, Sugishita H, Kumagi T, et al. Significance of laparoscopic splenectomy in patients with hypersplenism. World J Surg. 2007;31:549-55.
64. Wu Z, Zhou J, Wang X, Li YB. Laparoscopic splenectomy for treatment of splenic marginal zone lymphoma. World J Gastroenterol. 2013;19:3584-660.
65. Yee LF, Carvajal SH, de Lorimier AA, Mulvihill SJ. Laparoscopic splenectomy: the initial experience at University of California, San Francisco. Arch Surg. 1995;130:874-9.
66. Yuan RH, Chen SB, Lee WJ, Yu SC. Advantages of laparoscopic splenectomy for splenomegaly due to hematologic diseases. J Formos Med Assoc. 1998;97:485-9.

CHAPTER 23

Laparoscopic Management of Hepaticopancreatic Diseases

INTRODUCTION

The indications and preparation for laparoscopic liver surgery remain the same as in open hepatic surgery. Visualization is excellent with the laparoscope, and the addition of laparoscopic ultrasound has been shown to help intraoperative plans in 66% of cases when compared to laparoscopic exploration alone. The ability of visual inspection laparoscopy to assess resectability as opposed to inoperability remains relatively low. It can be improved by extended laparoscopy combined with laparoscopic contact ultrasonography. The technique of extended laparoscopy consists of full inspection of the peritoneal cavity, liver with contact laparoscopic ultrasound scanning, entry and inspection of lesser sac, examination of porta hepatis, duodenum, transverse mesocolon, and celiac and portal vessels. This procedure thus entails extensive dissection and is used to assess operability in patients with pancreatic cancer, hepatic neoplasms and gastroesophageal cancers where it often entails lymph node sampling. Laparoscopic hepatic surgery, while technically difficult, still can be performed safely with good results with careful patient selection. Attention to the etiology of the lesion and its location is essential. Ideal candidates have a large solitary cyst or a symptomatic benign mass located superficially, laterally, or far enough from the pedicle to allow direct clamping of the liver or access to the hilum to perform a Pringle maneuver should bleeding occur. Contraindications to this technique include patients with cirrhosis, hepatocellular carcinoma (HCC), or posterior or centrally located lesions. While we have utilized this approach for solitary small metastatic disease, hydatid disease, hepatic abscess, and polycystic liver disease (PCLD), these should be viewed with a great deal of circumspection. Problems can arise to varying degrees should any of these lesions be spilled. Port site recurrences remain a concern when using laparoscopy in any patient with cancer. This is of special concern when considering pairing this approach with cryoablation. With echinococcal cysts, the risk of spillage is also obvious, although less problematic with calcified cysts. If one does use a laparoscopic approach for hydatid disease, we recommend a cholangiogram to rule out a connection with the biliary system. While fenestration of PCLD has been described both by open and laparoscopic approaches, transcystic fenestration of deeper cysts makes the control of bleeding difficult.

Laparoscopic liver surgery provides advantages over open surgery for the liver since the Chevron incision is completely avoided and the surgery is performed through tiny incisions. As a consequence the duration of stay in hospital, the amount and duration of postoperative discomfort, and the length of recovery are much shorter after the laparoscopic procedure as compared to open surgery. To safely perform liver surgery laparoscopically, the surgeon must be both, an accomplished laparoscopist and hepatic surgeon. Few surgeons, however, are as comfortable with open hepatic surgery as they are with the gallbladder, hernia, appendix, or stomach. Furthermore, only a limited number of lesions, depending upon their location and etiology, can be approached by laparoscopy. The most commonly performed procedures are symptomatic solitary hepatic cyst, symptomatic PCLD, hydatid cyst, focal nodular hyperplasia, adenoma, abscess, metastatic breast cancer, and calcified gallbladder.

TECHNIQUE OF LAPAROSCOPIC MANAGEMENT OF HYDATID CYSTIC LIVER

This procedure is performed with the patient under general anesthesia with oro- or nasogastric decompression and a pneumoperitoneum of 12–14 mm Hg **(Fig. 1)**.

The patients can be placed in the "French" position, a modified lithotomy with minimal flexion of the hips, and the primary surgeon positioned between the legs. The first assistant stands on the patient's left side and the scrub nurse between them. For fenestrations, a four-trocar configuration is used. A 10 mm port at the umbilicus houses the 30° telescope. A 5 mm trocar needs to be placed just below the xiphoid process to the right or the left of the falciform ligament, depending on the location of the cyst. This port is used to expose the liver, often using an irrigation aspiration probe. Two other 5 mm or 10 mm ports, in the right and left flank, allows the surgeon to puncture the cyst dome, aspirate its contents, and excise the cyst wall in a careful sequential fashion to facilitate hemostasis. For more extensive procedures, a strong light source (300 W xenon) and

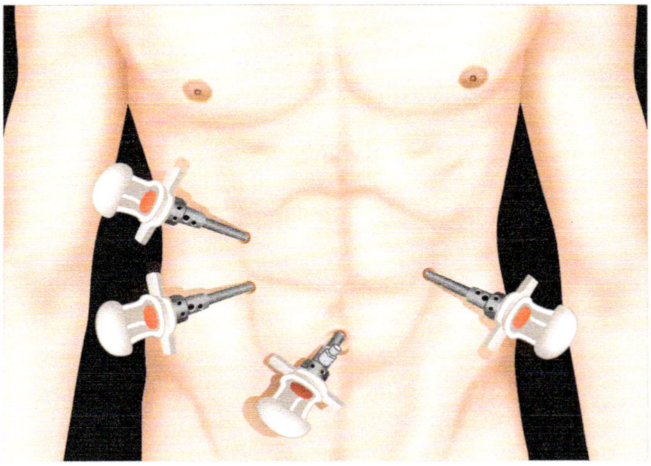

Fig. 1: Port position of the hydatid cyst of left lobe.

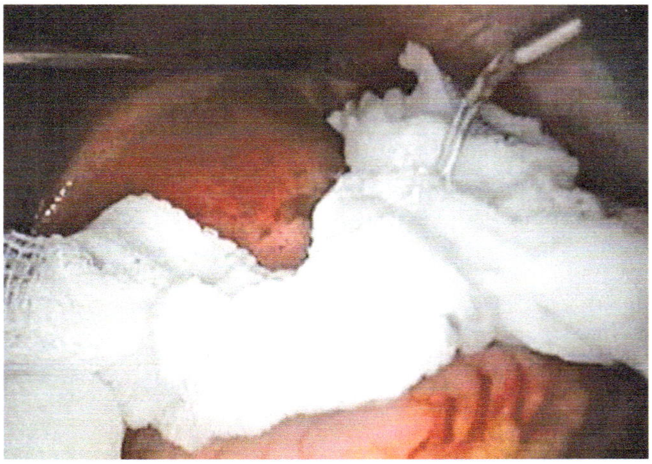

Fig. 2: Gauge piece introduced soaked with 3% saline.

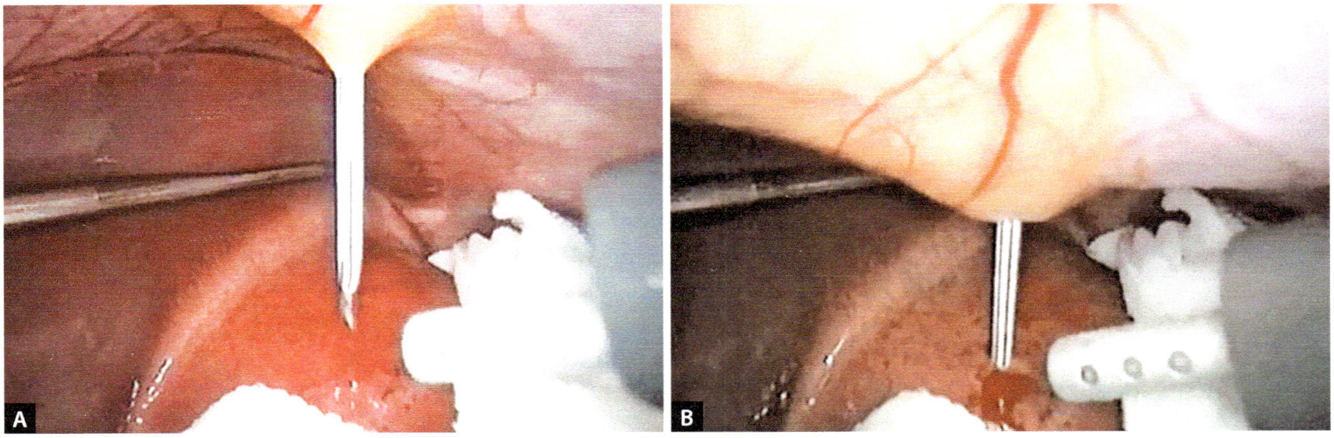

Figs. 3A and B: Instillation of hypertonic saline inside the cyst though percutaneous spinal needle.

high-quality 30° scopes are required. To perform resections safely with a minimum of wasted motion, the four-hand technique is used by many surgeons. This uses 4–6 trocars and allows for the primary surgeon to expose and dissect the liver while second surgeon obtains control and transects the blood vessels and bile ducts. The procedure entails the same components as in open hepatic surgery. First, the patient is explored, both visually and ultrasonographically. Mobilization of the liver and hilar dissection is performed as necessary to obtain vascular control. Division and ligation of the round ligament followed by freeing of the falciform and the right or left triangular ligaments allow access to perform thorough exploration, dissection, and hemostasis. A gauge soaked with 3% saline is kept around the cyst to prevent contamination by spillage **(Fig. 2)**. Spinal needle is used to administer 10% saline inside the cyst **(Figs. 3A and B)**. Dissection is begun by scoring Glisson's capsule with the high frequency electrosurgery **(Fig. 4)**.

Parenchymal dissection can be performed using the ultrasonic dissector. After extraction, the germinal layer is placed in an impermeable specimen bag for removal

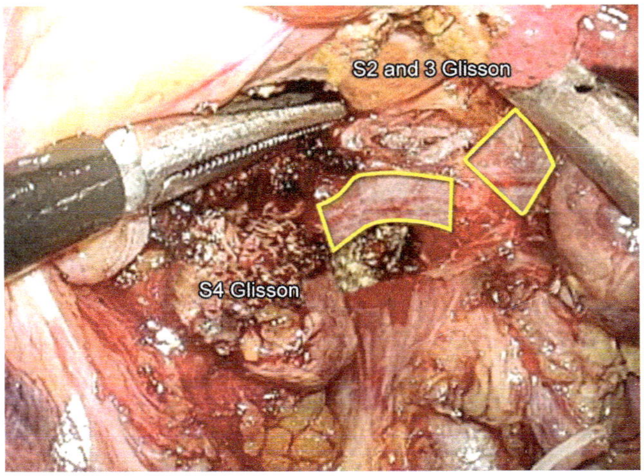

Fig. 4: Glisson's capsule keeps all the lobules together and imparts the liver, some protection from trauma.

(Figs. 5A to D). Cholangiography is very useful to detect possible bile leaks. The raw surface of the liver is then inspected, coagulated and covered with fibrin glue. The specimen is extracted either by partial morcellation, dilatation at the umbilicus, enlarging another port site, or by a small McBurney or subcostal incision **(Figs. 6A and B)**.

LAPAROSCOPIC LIVER RESECTION

The most common indication for laparoscopic liver resection is a solitary liver metastasis from a colorectal cancer, but it may also be used for HCC and for benign liver tumors or cysts.

Laparoscopic liver resections, offer advantages over the conventional open approach in two important respects:

1. Reduced operative blood loss.
2. Lower major postoperative morbidity.

Although laparoscopic staging for intra-abdominal cancer including primary and secondary hepatic tumors has been in established practice for many years, laparoscopic liver resections are still in the early clinical evaluation stage. Nonetheless, the results to date have been uniformly favorable

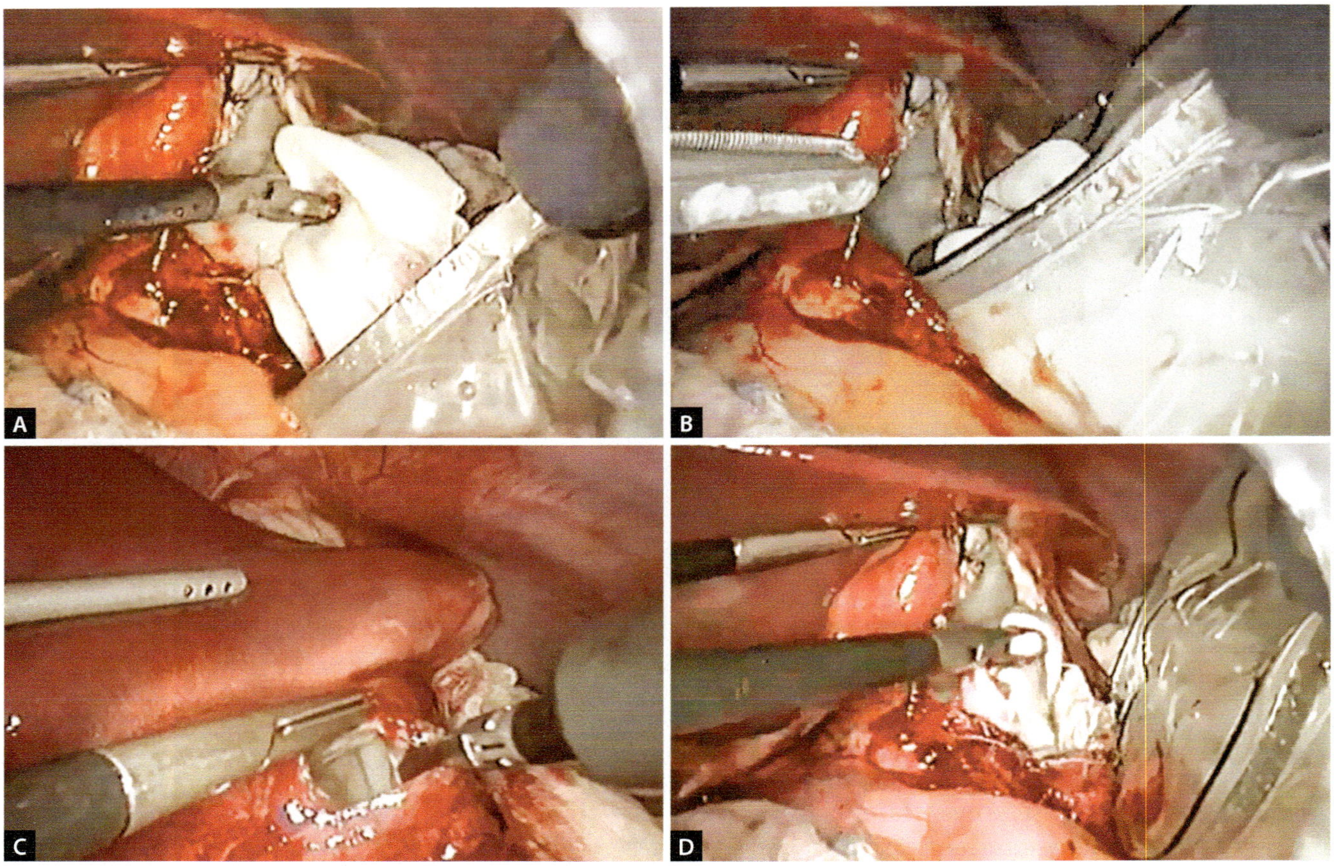

Figs. 5A to D: Opening of the cystic wall and extraction of germinal layer.

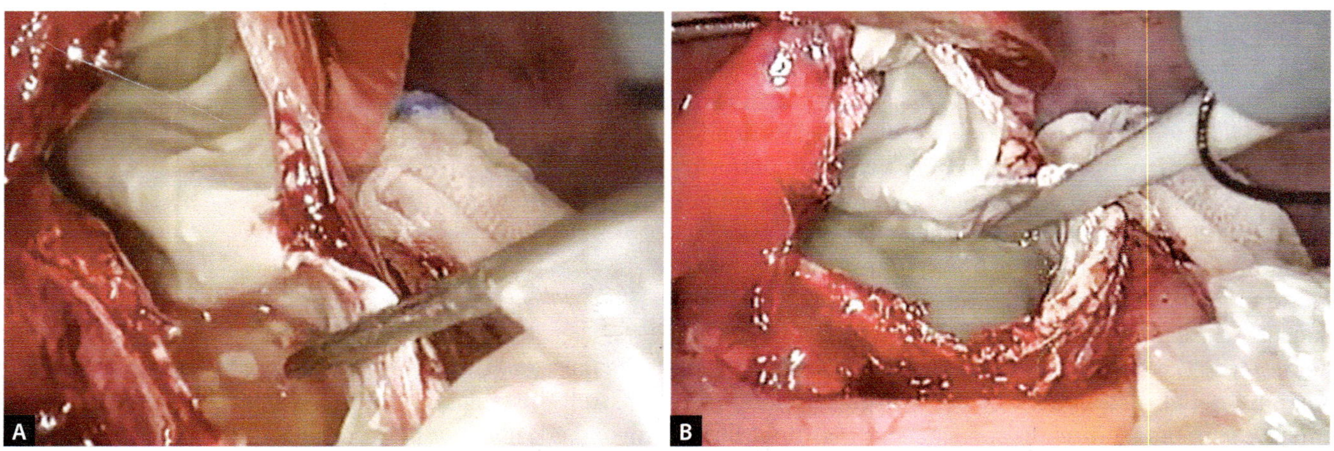

Figs. 6A and B: Removal of cyst with the help of endobag.

especially for left lobectomy and pluri-segmentectomies although right hepatectomy has been performed by the laparoscopically assisted or the hand-assisted laparoscopic surgical (HALS) approach.

The HALS approach, by facilitating these dissections and greatly increasing the safety, makes quite a big difference to the uptake among hepatobiliary and general surgeons with an interest in liver surgery. The procedures, which are in established practice by the laparoscopic and HALS approach, are:

- Extended laparoscopic staging
- Hepatic resections
- Laparoscopic in situ thermal ablation
- Laparoscopic cryosurgery
- Radical de-roofing of simple hepatic cysts
- Hepatic surgery for parasitic cysts.

Laparoscopic Staging of Tumors

Laparoscopy can nicely detect seedling metastases and small hepatic deposits missed by preoperative thin slice multidetector CT or magnetic resonance imaging (MRI). Some surgeons add lavage cytology to diagnostic laparoscopic visual inspection. This detects exfoliated tumors cells in gastrointestinal, pancreatic and ovarian cancers.

HEPATIC RESECTIONS

Approaches

Both the laparoscopic and the HALS approach can be used for hepatic resection **(Fig. 7A)**. The hand-assisted approach expedites the operation and provides an effective safeguard against major hemorrhage that may be encountered during the operation. A 7.0 cm incision is necessary for the insertion of the hand access device, such as the Omniport. This may be introduced through midline for operations on the left lobe or right transverse for resections on the right liver. It is important that the optical port is placed such that it is well clear of the internal hand.

Component Tasks in Laparoscopic Hepatic Resections

These component tasks cover all the surgical technical aspects of the various hepatic resections: hepatectomy, pluri-segmentectomies and segmentectomies.

Contact Ultrasound Localization and Mapping of the Intended Resection

Contact ultrasound is indispensable for hepatic resections **(Fig. 7B)**. The precise localization and extent of the lesion especially when this is intrahepatic can only be determined by contact ultrasound scanning, the findings of which determine the extent of resection segments required. In contrast, the mapping of the outlines of the resection is best carried out by the argon plasma spray coagulation.

Division of Falciform Ligament

Division of falciform ligament is needed for major right and left resections **(Figs. 8A and B)**. The division of the falciform ligament close to the liver substance is best carried out with a combination of scissors and electrocoagulation and is greatly facilitated by the use of curved coaxial instruments. The round ligament (ligamentum teres) can be left undivided except in patients undergoing skeletonization for right extended hepatectomy.

Exposure of Suprahepatic Inferior Vena Cava and Main Hepatic Veins

Exposure of suprahepatic inferior vena cava and main hepatic veins are only required for major hepatectomies. The two leaves of the falciform ligament separate posteriorly to envelop the suprahepatic inferior vena cava and the three main hepatic veins. The right leaf becomes the upper leaf of the right coronary ligament of the liver and the left becomes the upper layer of the left triangular ligament. These both leaves are divided after soft coagulation with the curved coaxial scissors. Ultrasonic shears may be used for this purpose, but this is more difficult as this energized device is straight.

The peritoneal division is extended in both directions to open up the retrohepatic caval space, which consists of relatively avascular loose fibroareolar tissue. The upper end of the caval canal is dissected further with a combination of blunt and sharp scissor dissection to divide fibrous bands. As the dissection precedes, about 1.5 cm of the inferior vena cava, the origin of the right hepatic vein are exposed. Further exposure of the right and middle hepatic veins is achieved beneath the liver and from the right side, required for a right hepatectomy. The left hepatic vein is very easily exposed from the left side above the liver.

Exposure of Infrahepatic Inferior Vena Cava and Division of the Posterior Minor Hepatic Veins

Exposure of infrahepatic inferior vena cava and division of the posterior minor hepatic vein is necessary for the skeletonization of the right liver necessary for a right hepatectomy **(Fig. 9)**. It is performed by retraction of the inferior surface of the right lobe of the liver with an atraumatic flexible ring or fan retractor to put the peritoneum sweeping up from the right kidney to the liver, on the stretch. This peritoneum is divided with the curved coaxial scissors and soft electrocoagulation over a wide front and close to the liver edge. There is usually little fat found underneath the peritoneum except in very obese individuals.

Once the peritoneum is divided, the retractor is replaced which gently lifts the inferoposterior aspect of the liver upward to expose the areolar tissue plane covering the vena cava and the minor retrohepatic veins which vary in number from 3 to 5. The inferoposterior aspect of the liver is lifted

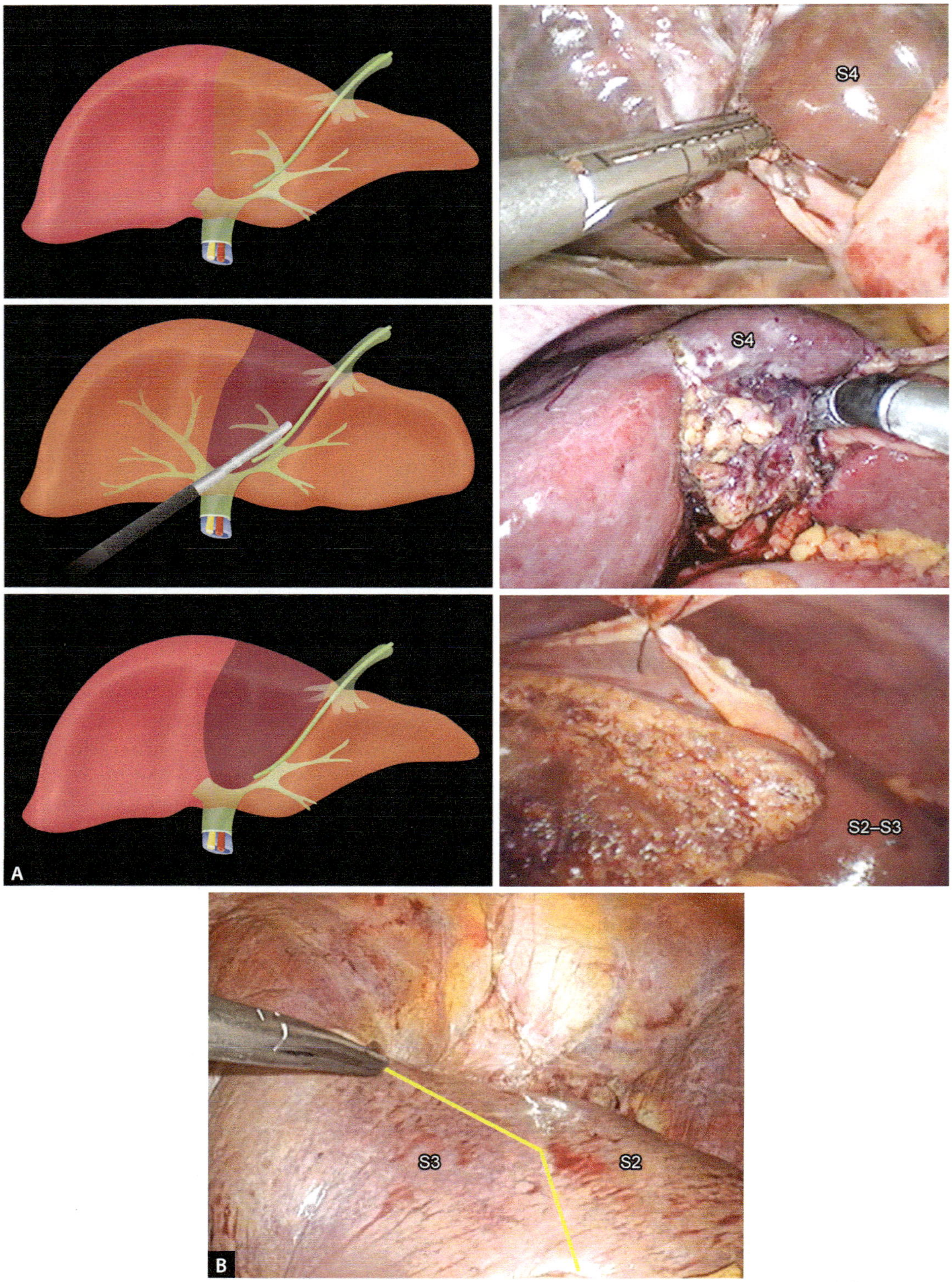

Figs. 7A and B: (A) Laparoscopic liver resection; (B) Mapping of the intended resection.

gently but progressively to expose the vena cava behind the liver. As minor hepatic veins are encountered draining into the inferior vena cava, they are skeletonized by the curved coaxial scissors and then clipped before they are divided. The mobilization continues upward until the right and middle hepatic vein is reached.

Opening the Cave of Retzius

Opening the cave of Retzius is common to both right and left resections. The cave of Retzius refers to the umbilical fissure bridged by variable amount of hepatic tissue anteriorly, which overlies the ligamentum teres containing the obliterated umbilical vein on its way to join the left branch of the portal

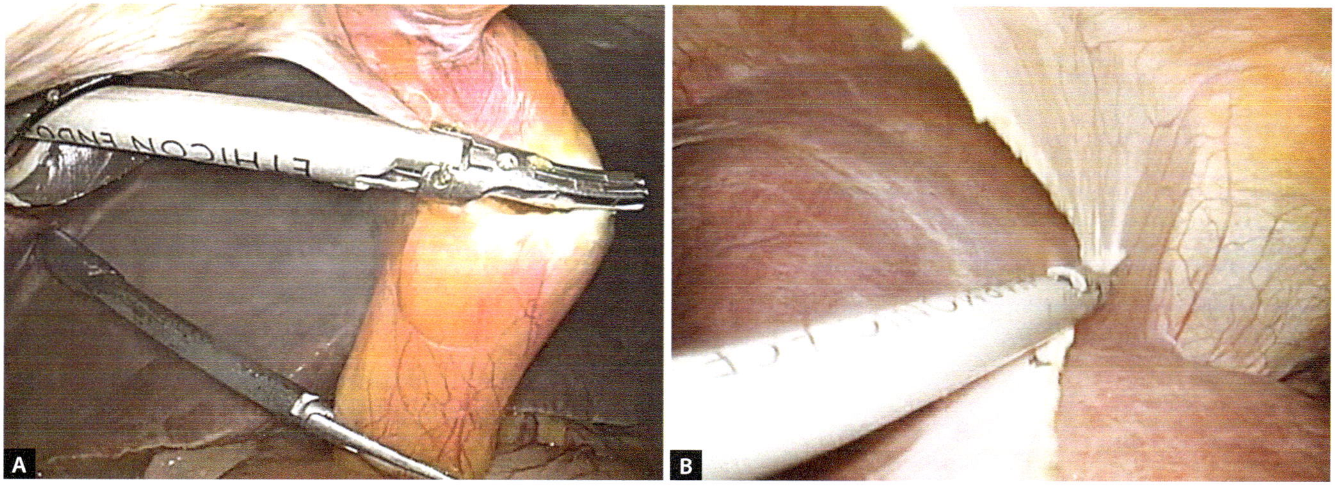

Figs. 8A and B: Division of falciform ligament.

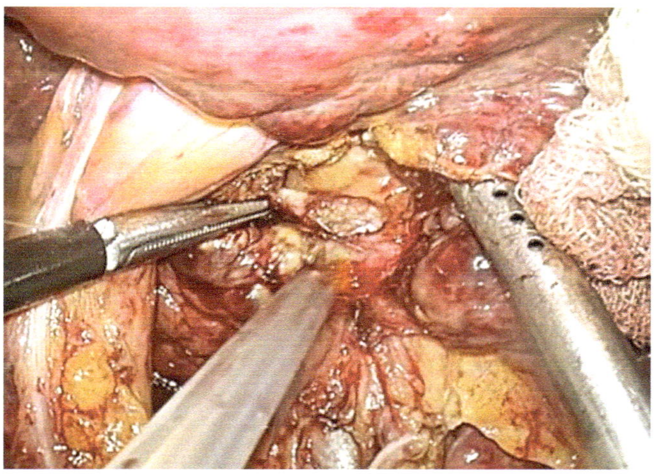

Fig. 9: Exposure of infrahepatic inferior vena cava and division of the posterior minor hepatic veins.

vein at the bottom of the pit. The bridge of liver tissue is crushed and coagulated by an insulated grasping forceps, after which it is divided which will separate segment III on the left side from the quadrate lobe opening up the cave of Retzius, and exposing the terminal segment of the round ligament.

Hilar Dissection

The dissection of the hilum commences by division of the peritoneum along the margin of the hepatic hilum to expose the common hepatic duct and its bifurcation, and the right and left branches of the common hepatic artery. Further dissection is needed to bring down the hilar plate and to skeletonize the right and left hepatic ducts, the two branches of the common hepatic artery and, more posteriorly, the two branches of the portal vein for right and left hepatectomy.

Removal of the Gallbladder

Removal of the gallbladder en bloc with the hepatic substance constitutes an integral part of right hepatectomy and segmentectomy involving segments IVa and V. The dissection of the cystic duct and artery is followed by ligature or clipping of the medial end of the cystic duct and clipping of its lateral end before it is divided.

Inflow Occlusion Prior to Hepatic Resection

Temporary inflow occlusion of the vascular supply to the liver is necessary for major hepatic resections and also to reduce the "heat-sink effect" of the substantial blood flow through the liver during in situ ablation by cryotherapy or radiofrequency thermal ablation. Several types of clamps are available for this purpose but the most suitable are the parallel occlusion clamps, which are introduced through 5.5 mm ports by means of an applicator, which is used to engage and disengage the clamps. Thus, when the clamp is in use it does not occupy a port, which can thus be used for dissection. The application of these parallel occlusion clamps is very easy particularly with the hand-assisted approach and minimal dissection is required. The surgeon just makes a small window through an avascular area of lesser omentum just proximal to the hepatoduodenal ligament enveloping the bile duct, hepatic arteries, and portal vein.

The parallel occlusion clamp is introduced from the right by means of its applicator. The jaws are opened as the hepatoduodenal ligament is reached and applied across the full width of the hepatoduodenal ligament and then released to occlude the bile duct, portal vein, and hepatic arteries. It is extremely important that the period of inflow vascular occlusion to the liver does not exceed 30 minutes at any one-time period.

For removal of the clamp, the introducer is inserted through the port and used to engage the clamp, which then is opened and removed through the same port by the introducer.

Transection of the Hepatic Parenchyma

The transection of the hepatic parenchyma for all the major resections should be carried in the absence of a

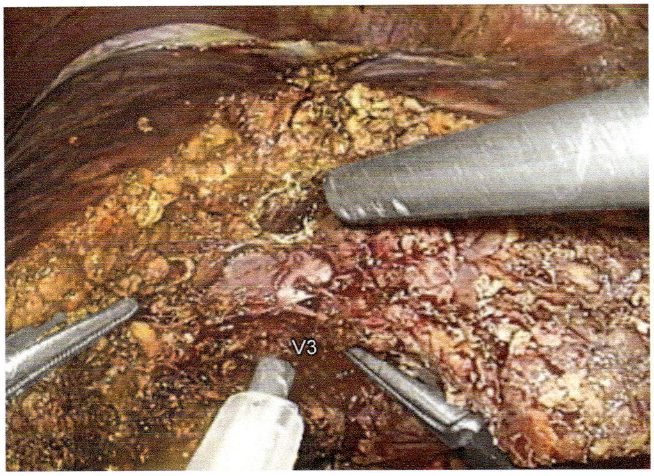

Fig. 10: Transection of the hepatic parenchyma.

positive-pressure pneumoperitoneum **(Fig. 10)**. In hand-assisted laparoscopic surgery, this translates to replacement of the hand access device with a disposable retractor that also acts as a wound protector preventing its contamination by malignant cells during the hepatic resection and removal of the specimen.

The hepatic resection must also be carried out with a low patient central venous pressure (CVP), produced by a head-up tilt and appropriate vasodilator medication by the anesthetist.

The hepatic artery to the resection area is best secured by clips or ligatures in the liver substance rather than extrahepatically. The vascular stapling or ligature and division of the main hepatic veins draining the liver during hepatectomy are carried out at the end of the parenchymal transection.

The actual technique of liver resection varies from simple finger or forceps fracture with individual clipping or ligature of bile ductules to use of energized systems such as ultrasonic dissection or LigaSure™. The liver parenchymal surface is first coagulated and then crushed using a long-jawed crushing laparoscopic forceps to fracture the liver parenchyma exposing sizeable vessels and ducts.

All sizeable blood vessels and bile ducts are clipped before being cut. As the cleft deepens, bands of liver tissue, which are not severed, are presumed to contain large vessels which may be obscured by adherent layer of liver parenchyma. In this situation, palpation of the bridge between the index finger and thumb of the assisting hand will identify the nature of the structure.

All sizeable veins can be transected using an endolinear cutting stapler mounted with 35 mm vascular cartridge introduced through the minilaparotomy wound.

In the case of plurisegmentectomy, after the segment has been separated on three sides, it often remains attached to the liver by bridge of liver tissue. If this connection is no thicker than 1.0 cm, it is simply staple transected by the application of the endolinear cutting stapler to detach completely the area from the liver.

After resection, the specimen is removed through the open minilaparotomy wound. The final stage consists in securing complete hemostasis.

Hemostasis of the Cut Liver Surface

Only minor oozing happens from the cut liver substance if the technique of hepatic transection has been performed correctly and in the presence of a low CVP of patient. Complete hemostasis is achieved by argon plasma coagulation. Application of fibrin glue or other synthetic sealants are very helpful in achieving hemostasis.

Insertion of Drains

Once the resection is complete before the retractor is removed and the wound closed using mass closure with monofilament polydioxanone, a silicon drain should be introduced. It is advisable to insert even two large silicon drains one above and the other below the liver. These must be sutured to the abdominal wall to prevent accidental dislodgment after the operation. Effective drainage is crucial to prevent postoperative biloma.

Postoperative Management

It is important to stress that these patients should be nursed postoperatively in a hepatobiliary unit with immediate access to high dependency and intensive care if needed. The management remains the same as after any other laparoscopic surgery with daily monitoring of the liver function tests, hematology and blood urea nitrogen and serum electrolytes. Opiate medication and sedation are avoided in patients with compromised liver function. Repeated ultrasound scans should be carried out in all patients after hepatic resection. This is necessary to identify early fluid collections most usually bile, which if found are monitored by serial ultrasound studies and aspirated or drained percutaneously under radiological control if persistent.

Using right technique, necessary expertise and appropriate technology, laparoscopic and especially hand-assisted hepatic resections can be carried out safely. The data from the published reports to date indicate benefits over the open approach and these include reduced blood loss and lower postoperative morbidity.

LAPAROSCOPIC PANCREATIC SURGERY

The laparoscopic management of pancreatic disease is one of the most challenging in laparoscopic surgery. This is especially true when considering the procedure of pancreatic resection. Well-trained laparoscopic surgeons have found that operating on the pancreas, such as virtually all intra-abdominal procedures, is technically feasible. Laparoscopic principles suggest that the patient will probably benefit from less postoperative pain, improved wound cosmetics, quicker return to routine activities, and shorter hospital stay. Ultimately the acceptance of many laparoscopic operations is determined by their degree of difficulty, the operating time, the cost (both hospital and societal), and patient outcomes.

In comparison with the literature available on other laparoscopic operations, the information available on pancreatic resection is too scant to draw firm conclusions. However, leaders in the field have demonstrated that pancreatic resection is feasible, and are carefully examining their outcomes to further elucidate the role of this technically demanding procedure.

Laparoscopic procedures for the pancreas fall into four main categories:

1. Laparoscopic staging of pancreatic malignancy.
2. Bilioenteric or gastroenteric bypass.
3. Pancreatic resection.
4. Management of pancreatic pseudocysts.

Anatomic Considerations

The majority of the pancreas lies in a retroperitoneal position, transversely oriented from the second and third portions of the duodenum to the hilum of the spleen. Anterior access to the gland (body and tail) is readily obtained by division of the gastrocolic omentum. This division may be performed by electrocautery, multiple individual clip applications or vascular stapling devices, or ultrasonic dissection.

Access may be obtained through the gastrohepatic ligament, although the exposure is usually less adequate. The patient is positioned in slight head-up position to allow gravity retraction of the viscera. An oblique angle (30° or 45°) telescope is necessary for adequate visualization. Laparoscopic ultrasound is proving to be an essential tool for many aspects of pancreatic surgery.

Laparoscopic Staging of Pancreatic Malignancy

Patients with pancreatic malignancy generally present at later stages of disease. Frequently the disease is unresectable due to tumor size or tumor metastases by the time symptoms occur. Surgical resection for pancreatic cancer still offers the only reasonable chance at a cure. Historically, many patients underwent unnecessary laparotomy in an effort to assess resectability. CT scans have helped many patients avoid the morbidity of a nontherapeutic laparotomy. However, even with this modality, unresectability rates at laparotomy can approach 60%. This is most often due to the presence of unrecognized peritoneal metastases (<1 cm) and tumor invasion not appreciated on CT scan. Spiral CT and MRI are more reliable for predicting unresectability, but are still not adequate in our opinion. Megibow and coworkers reported a sensitivity of 77%, a specificity of 50%, and an overall accuracy of 73% for dynamic CT scanning. Also in their study, they found no additional benefit from MRI.

Diagnostic laparoscopy further narrows patient selection for therapeutic laparotomy. Warshaw and coworkers found that an additional 35% of patients could avoid laparotomy with the use of diagnostic laparoscopy. Despite improving noninvasive imaging methods since Warshaw and coworker's early reports, more recent studies confirm Warshaw and coworker's initial findings that a significantly number of patients (22–35%) can avoid laparotomy with the use of staging laparoscopy.

Further, the sensitivity for evaluation of unresectable disease appears further enhanced with the addition of the laparoscopic ultrasound to the laparoscopic staging procedure. Callery and coworkers use a multifrequency laparoscopic ultrasound probe to search for occult metastases and assess posterior invasion into vascular structures such as the portal vein. Tumors other than pancreatic were also included. Fifty patients were referred for staging laparoscopy after interpretation of conventional noninvasive imaging modalities had determined the tumor to be resectable. Laparoscopic ultrasound established unresectability in 11 patients (22%) in whom staging laparoscopy alone was negative. In another study by John and coworkers involving 40 consecutive patients with pancreatic cancer presenting for diagnostic laparoscopy, laparoscopic ultrasound found an additional 25% (10 patients) whose disease was unresectable when compared with laparoscopy alone. They found the use of ultrasound significantly improved specificity and accuracy as compared with laparoscopy alone (88 and 81% vs. 50 and 60%, respectively).

Staging Laparoscopy Technique

Patients generally undergo staging laparoscopy on the same day they are scheduled for resection. Patients are placed in the supine position on an electrically equipped bed (preferably). A 10 mm trocar is placed in the infraumbilical position to serve as the camera port. The abdomen is insufflated to 15 mm Hg. A 30° laparoscope is used. A second port of 5 mm is placed in the right midclavicular line several centimeters from the subcostal margin. A four-quadrant exploration is then carried out. Grasping devices, biopsy forceps, or electrocautery instruments may be alternatively introduced through the 5 mm port. Important peritoneal surfaces to visualize for areas of metastases include the undersurface of abdomen including falciform, diaphragm, and liver. The omentum must be examined thoroughly and when possible retracted superiorly to evaluate the base of the transverse colon, its mesentery, and the ligament of Treitz (this may require an additional port).

If there is evidence of unresectability, the procedure is terminated. Otherwise laparoscopic ultrasound is carried out. A second 10 mm port is placed in the right midclavicular line at the level of the umbilicus. Laparoscopic ultrasound is then performed using a 9 mm in diameter linear array 7.5 MHz contact ultrasound probe with Doppler flow capability. The liver is systematically scanned (anterior, lateral, inferior) at penetration depths of 7 cm for evidence of metastatic spread or extent of primary tumor invasion. Frequently, biliary and pancreatic metastases to the liver have a characteristic bulls-eye appearance with an echoic rim encircling a mixed-echo tumor center. If found, biopsy for such lesions may be attempted percutaneously, under laparoscopic ultrasound guidance.

Attention is then turned to ultrasonic evaluation of the porta hepatic, peripancreatic, para-aortic, and celiac axis for evidence of nodal disease. Lymph nodes greater than 10 mm may be biopsied. Laparoscopic ultrasound with Doppler flow capability is then used to help locate and assess the potential for tumor extension to surrounding peripancreatic vascular structures (primarily portal vein, but also superior mesenteric vein and artery, and celiac axis).

Bilioenteric or Gastroenteric Anastomosis for Pancreatic Malignancy

Unresectable patients might be candidates for biliary or enteric bypass. The risk and benefits of bypass must be weighed against existing palliative options, the patient's condition, existing or impending obstruction, and expected length of survival based on tumor burden. For most patients with unresectable disease, life expectancy can be expected to be <1 year. Proper management tailored to the individual patient's needs is important so as to offer as much quality of life free from hospitalization as possible.

Commonly, patients will present with some degree of biliary obstruction or will suffer from it during the course of the disease. Most patients with obstructive jaundice are best treated by placing an endoscopic or percutaneous stent. The success rate is high (85%), with a low associated mortality (1–2%). Studies comparing open bypass with those stented endoscopically for obstructive jaundice found no advantage to the surgical approach. Morbidity from stent placement includes potentially frequent admission to hospital (occlusion, infection) and significant cost for endoscopic retrograde cholangiopancreatography (ERCP) and stent. However, repeat placement has become less necessary with the use of improved techniques and stent design. Patients may present or develop distorted duodenal anatomy that makes initial or subsequent stent placement impossible. This finding may be coupled with gastric outlet obstruction. In these patients, bypass procedures may be offered after evaluation of surgical risk or life expectancy.

The morbidity of open surgical bypass is substantial (19%). Laparoscopic biliary (cholecystojejunostomy) or gastric bypass (gastrojejunostomy) is feasible. There is potential for shorter recovery, shorter return to activity; and low morbidity, as evident in several small studies. Nathanson suggests that the bypass should be reserved for a later date from the diagnostic laparoscopy at such time when duodenal obstruction precludes repeat stent or there is stent failure (blockage, recurrent sepsis). For the stomach, failure would include when symptoms of gastric outlet arise. Conditions at initial laparoscopy that might argue for immediate bypass include inability to stent the biliary system in the preoperative setting, endoscopic or radiologic evidence of impending duodenal obstruction, or laparoscopic impression of large locally advanced mass with minimal to no evidence of metastatic spread.

Biliary and Gastric Bypass

Cholecystojejunostomy may be carried out if the gallbladder is present and suitable for anastomosis, and the cystic duct is patent and its junction to the common bile duct (CBD) is far from the tumor. Frequently this information is available by preoperative imaging studies (ERCP or percutaneous transluminal cholangiography). If not, patency of cystic duct and its relation to primary tumor location may be obtained by performing a cholangiogram after cannulation of the gallbladder. Similarly, laparoscopic ultrasound may be used for such an assessment.

For either anastomosis, patients are positioned supine and the port placement is the same. A 10 mm trocar is placed at the inferior umbilical region and a 30° telescope is used. Additional ports and operating room personnel are positioned.

The omentum and transverse colon are elevated with instruments introduced through the epigastric and either 12 mm port. The small bowel is traced back to the ligament of Treitz. A loop of small bowel is then chosen that will comfortably reach stomach and gallbladder without tension (note that this is true once the transverse colon and omentum are allowed to return to normal position). For the biliary bypass, a cholecystotomy is performed with electrocautery on the gallbladder fundus. The biliary contents are then aspirated. An enterotomy is performed on the antimesenteric surface of the chosen small bowel loop. A 30 mm endoscopic stapler is introduced through the right 12 mm port. The jaws of the stapler are opened and one arm of the stapler is inserted into the enterotomy. The jaws of the stapler are then closed to function as a large grasper. The stapler and small bowel contained within are then maneuvered adjacent to the cholecystotomy. The jaws of the stapler are opened again and the free arm of the stapler maneuvered into the cholecystotomy. Assistance is provided by a blunt grasping instrument inserted through the additional ports (epigastric). After proper alignment is assured, the stapler is fired to complete the anastomosis. The original sites may be closed with additional firings of the stapler. At this point the endoscopic stapler will be introduced through the left

12 mm port. Care must be taken not to narrow the anastomosis or the lumen of the small bowel significantly.

To fashion the gastric bypass, a dependent site is chosen along the greater curvature. The gastrocolic omentum is divided close to the greater curve within the gastroepiploic arcade for a distance of approximately 3–4 cm with the ultrasonic scalpel or by electrocautery. A gastrotomy is made on the greater curvature. The anastomosis will be formed along the greater curve but will extend into the posterior wall of the stomach. Typically, the stapled anastomosis will be created by introducing the stapler through the right 12 mm port. The anastomosis should consist of two firings of the 30 mm endoscopic linear cutter.

Ideally, the stapled anastomosis should be aligned to cross the greater curvature to the posterior surface (i.e., through the area of divided gastrocolic omentum). If fashioned in this way, the original puncture sites will be easier to close and the anastomosis more dependent.

Laparoscopic Pancreatic Resection (Figs. 11A to E)

Indications for complete or partial pancreatic resection include:

- Adenocarcinoma
- Insulinoma (neuroendocrine)
- Chronic pancreatitis.

Improved technique and postoperative care have rendered morbidity and mortality for pancreatic resection, including Whipple's procedure, to <5%. Laparoscopic techniques could potentially lower this rate even more or at least accord less pain and a more rapid recovery **(Figs. 11A to E)**.

Laparoscopic Whipple's procedure was first carried out by Gagner in a small series of three patients with various diseases (pancreatitis, ampullary cancer, adenocarcinoma). He subsequently has reported on a pylorus-preserving technique performed in one patient with pancreatitis. The initial experience indicates that it is technically feasible, but because of its operative time, complexity, and as yet no demonstrated improvement in outcome, this procedure must be considered investigational. Hand-assisted laparoscopic surgery may make pancreatic resection more practical.

Laparoscopic pancreatic procedures involving distal pancreatectomy appear to hold more promise at present. Soper and coworkers reported success with his technique in the pig model. Gagner and coworkers successfully performed distal pancreatectomy for a variety of disease processes including islet cell tumors, cystadenocarcinoma, and pseudocyst. The spleen was preserved in all cases and operating times ranged from 2.5 to 5 hours. Cases were managed with the patient in the left lateral position, with pancreatic division carried out with a 60 mm linear cutter. Others are reporting initial success with distal resection.

Laparoscopic Management of Pancreatic Pseudocyst

Pancreatic pseudocysts may be defined as a collection of pancreatic secretions, serous fluid, or necrotic debris surrounded by a nonepithelialized wall made up of

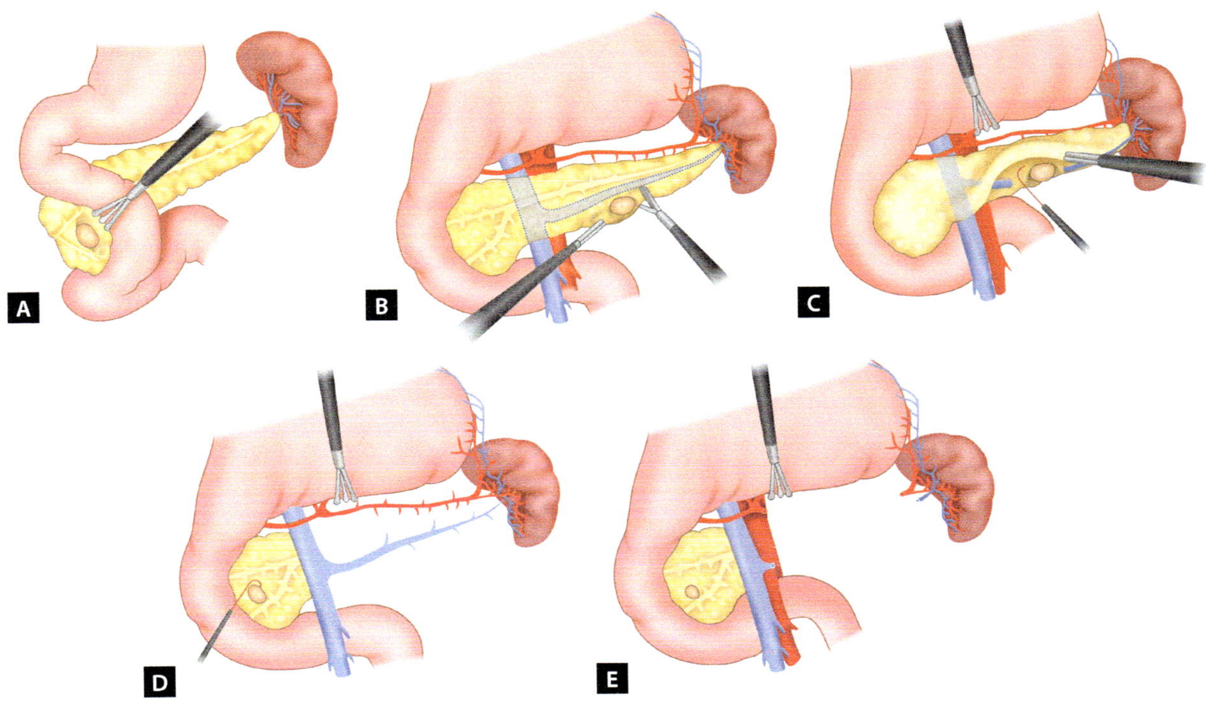

Figs. 11A to E: Laparoscopic pancreatic resection.

granulation tissue and variable degree of fibrous tissue. Pancreatic pseudocysts must be distinguished from true cysts of the pancreas, which are characterized histologically by the presence of an epithelial lining. Pseudocyst formation is the result of a postinflammatory process arising from patients with acute or chronic pancreatitis. An understanding of the natural history of pancreatic pseudocyst is important when deciding on invasive therapy versus expectant management. Studies like those by Bradley and coworkers had a great influence in the management of pseudocystic disease. Bradley and coworkers suggested the likelihood of regression diminished and the likelihood of complications rose dramatically after a 6-weeks period. More recent data suggest that this patient population may be watched safely for longer periods. Yeo and coworkers followed asymptomatic patients with pseudocysts by CT scanning for 1 year (48% were successfully observed with only a 2.7% complication rate). The only predictor for intervention was size >7.4 ± 0.6 cm.

General asymptomatic patients with pancreatic pseudocyst may be followed up for extended periods of time. This conservative approach is more likely to be successful in patients with small 6 cm pseudocysts. Other options are available for drainage procedures (e.g., percutaneous transgastric, ERCP).

LAPAROSCOPIC PSEUDOCYST DRAINAGE

Preoperative decision making and subsequent laparoscopic operative approach should mimic that of open operative planning. The selection of procedure will depend on the anatomic location of the pseudocyst, pseudocyst size, and associated pancreatic duct or distal CBD abnormalities **(Fig. 12)**.

Reports by Newell and coworkers document that pseudocyst-gastrostomy is technically easier than pseudocyst-jejunostomy, while remaining equally efficacious. Laparoscopic pseudocyst-gastrostomy is technically easier, but cyst-jejunostomy is also technically feasible for the cyst not amenable to gastric drainage by standard surgical principles.

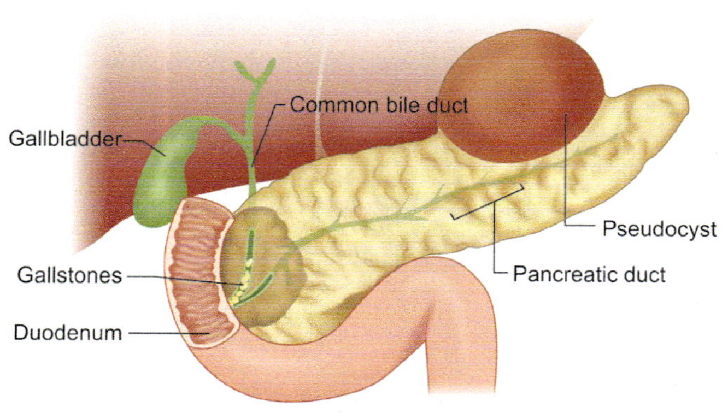

Fig. 12: Pancreatic pseudocyst.

Laparoscopic pseudocyst-gastrostomy was first performed by Petelin in 1991. Principles of operative drainage include biopsy of cyst wall to rule out neoplasm, dependent drainage, and precise hemostatic technique to avoid hemorrhage.

The patient position and port placement are the same as described for the bypass procedure. The pseudocyst may often be seen pushing the stomach forward. A small gastrotomy is established with cautery over the most prominent portion of the pseudocyst. Ultrasound may be helpful in locating the pseudocyst and the site of the initial gastrotomy. The gastrotomy is then extended for several centimeters with electrocautery.

A small window is developed through the posterior wall of the stomach with electrocautery. One must remember that the posterior wall of stomach and cyst capsule will be fused and that this requires a deeper dissection with cautery than felt comfortable by the surgeon. Ultrasound may be helpful to plan dissection where the stomach wall or cyst is thinnest. The window is made large enough to accommodate the endoscopic stapler. A biopsy of the wall may be carried out at this time. Two firings of the stapler are used to create a substantial anastomosis (stapler insertion through the more comfortable 12 mm port, usually the right). Hemostasis at the staple line should be assured. The gastrotomy is closed with either sutures or staples.

CONCLUSION

The laparoscopic approach to hepatic and pancreatic surgery has rapidly been shown to be of considerable value. The laparoscopic approach to the pancreas has value with respect to staging, bypass procedures, and pseudocyst drainage. Pancreatic resection is feasible, but must still be considered investigational.

BIBLIOGRAPHY

1. Adamson GD, Cuschieri A. Multimedia article: laparoscopic infracolic necrosectomy for infected pancreatic necrosis. Surg Endosc. 2003;17:1675.
2. American Joint Commission on Cancer. Exocrine pancreas. In: Greene FL, Page DL, Fleming ID (Eds). AJCC Cancer Staging Manual, 5th edition. New York: Springer-Verlag; 2002. pp. 157-64.
3. Andren-Sandberg A, Lindberg CG, Lundstedt C, Ihse I. Computed tomography and laparoscopy in the assessment of the patient with pancreatic cancer. J Am Coll Surg. 1998;186:35-40.
4. Ashley SW, Perez A, Pierce EA, Brooks DC, Moore FD Jr, Whang EE, et al. Necrotizing pancreatitis: contemporary analysis of 99 consecutive cases. Ann Surg. 2001;234:572-80.
5. Baril NB, Ralls PW, Wren SM, Selby RR, Radin R, Parekh D, et al. Does an infected peripancreatic fluid collection or abscess mandate operation? Ann Surg. 2000;231:361-7.
6. Beger HG, Rau B, Isenmann R. Prevention of severe change in acute pancreatitis: prediction and prevention. J Hepatobiliary Pancreat Surg. 2001;8:140-7.
7. Birkmeyer JD, Stukel TA, Siewers AE, Goodney PP, Wennberg DE, Lucas FL. Surgeon volume and operative mortality in the United States. N Engl J Med. 2003;349:2117-27.

8. Birkmeyer JD, Warshaw AL, Finlayson SR, Grove MR, Tosteson AN. Relationship between hospital volume and late survival after pancreaticoduodenectomy. Surgery. 1999;126:178-83.
9. Buchler MW, Gloor B, Muller CA, Friess H, Seiler CA, Uhl W. Acute necrotizing pancreatitis: treatment strategy according to the status of infection. Ann Surg. 2000;232:619-26.
10. Carter R. Management of infected necrosis secondary to acute pancreatitis: a balanced role for minimal access techniques. Pancreatology. 2003;3:133-8.
11. Castellanos G, Serrano A, Piñero A, Bru M, Párraga M, Marín P, et al. Retroperitoneoscopy in the management of drained infected pancreatic necrosis. Gastrointest Endosc. 2001;53:514-5.
12. Clancy TE, Ashley SW. Current management of necrotizing pancreatitis. Adv Surg. 2002;36:103-21.
13. Conlon KC, Dougherty E, Klimstra DS, Coit DG, Turnbull AD, Brennan MF. The value of minimal access surgery in the staging of patients with potentially resectable peripancreatic malignancy. Ann Surg. 1996;223:134-40.
14. Connor S, Alexakis N, Raraty MG, Ghaneh P, Evans J, Hughes M, et al. Early and late complications after pancreatic necrosectomy. Surgery. 2005;137:499-505.
15. Connor S, Ghaneh P, Raraty M, Sutton R, Rosso E, Garvey CJ, et al. Minimally invasive retroperitoneal pancreatic necrosectomy. Dig Surg. 2003;20:270-7.
16. Connor S, Neoptolemos JP. Surgery for pancreatic necrosis: "whom, when and what." World J Gastroenterol. 2004;10:1697-8.
17. Connor S, Raraty MG, Howes N, Evans J, Ghaneh P, Sutton R, et al. Surgery in the treatment of acute pancreatitis—minimal access pancreatic necrosectomy. Scand J Surg. 2005;94:135-42.
18. Cuschieri A. Laparoscopic hand-assisted surgery for hepatic and pancreatic disease. Surg Endosc. 2000;14:991-6.
19. Cuschieri A. Pancreatic necrosis: pathogenesis and endoscopic management. Semin Laparosc Surg. 2002;9:54-63.
20. Cuschieri A, Hall AW, Clark J. Value of laparoscopy in the diagnosis and management of pancreatic carcinoma. Gut. 1978;19:672-7.
21. Dugernier TL, Laterre PF, Wittebole X, Roeseler J, Latinne D, Reynaert MS, et al. Compartmentalization of the inflammatory response during acute pancreatitis: correlation with local and systemic complications. Am J Respir Crit Care Med. 2003;168:148-57.
22. Fernandez-del Castillo C, Rattner DW, Makary MA, Mostafavi A, McGrath D, Warshaw AL. Debridement and closed packing for the treatment of necrotizing pancreatitis. Ann Surg. 1998;228:676-84.
23. Finlayson EV, Goodney PP, Birkmeyer JD. Hospital volume and operative mortality in cancer surgery: a national study. Arch Surg. 2003;138:721-6.
24. Gupta A, Watson DI. Effect of laparoscopy on immune function. Br J Surg. 2001;88:1296-306.
25. HALS Study Group. Hand-assisted laparoscopic surgery vs standard laparoscopic surgery for colorectal disease: a prospective randomized trial. Surg Endosc. 2000;14:896-901.
26. Hamad GG, Broderick TJ. Laparoscopic pancreatic necrosectomy. J Laparoendosc Adv Surg Tech A. 2000;10:115-8.
27. Horvath KD, Kao LS, Ali A, Wherry KL, Pellegrini CA, Sinanan MN. Laparoscopic assisted percutaneous drainage of infected pancreatic necrosis. Surg Endosc. 2001;15:677-82.
28. Horvath KD, Kao LS, Wherry KL, Pellegrini CA, Sinanan MN. A technique for laparoscopic-assisted percutaneous drainage of infected pancreatic necrosis and pancreatic abscess. Surg Endosc. 2001;15:1221-5.
29. Jimenez RE, Warshaw AL, Rattner DW, Willett CG, McGrath D, Fernandez-del Castillo C. Impact of laparoscopic staging in the treatment of pancreatic cancer. Arch Surg. 2000;135:409-14.
30. Kamei H, Yoshida S, Yamasaki K, Tajiri T, Shirouzu K. Carbon dioxide pneumoperitoneum reduces levels of TNF-a mRNA in the brain, liver, and peritoneum in mice. Surg Endosc. 2001;15:609-13.
31. Kim WW, Jeon HM, Park SC, Lee SK, Chun SW, Kim EK. Comparison of immune preservation between CO_2 pneumoperitoneum and gasless abdominal lift laparoscopy. JSLS. 2002;6:11-5.
32. Lau ST, Simchuk EJ, Kozarek RA, Traverso LW. A pancreatic ductal leak should be sought to direct treatment in patients with acute pancreatitis. Am J Surg. 2001;1:411-5.
33. Laveda R, Martinez J, Munoz C, Penalva JC, Saez J, Belda G, et al. Different profile of cytokine synthesis according to the severity of acute pancreatitis. World J Gastroenterol. 2005;11:5309-13.
34. Lempinen M, Puolakkainen P, Kemppainen E. Clinical value of severity markers in acute pancreatitis. Scand J Surg. 2005;94:118-23.
35. Liu R, Traverso LW. Laparoscopic staging of unresectable pancreatic cancer. Surg Endosc. 2004;18:S256.
36. Louvet C, André T, Lledo G, Hammel P, Bleiberg H, Bouleuc C, et al. Gemcitabine combined with oxaloplatin in advanced pancreatic adenocarcinoma: Final results of a GERCOR multicenter phase II study. J Clin Oncol. 2002;20:1512-8.
37. Papachristou GI, Whitcomb DC. Predictors of severity and necrosis in acute pancreatitis. Gastroenterol Clin North Am. 2004;33:871-90.
38. Pooran N, Indaram A, Singh P, Bank S. Cytokines (IL-6, IL-8, TNF): early and reliable predictors of severe acute pancreatitis. J Clin Gastroenterol. 2003;37:263-6.
39. Ramudo L, Manso MA, De Dios I. Biliary pancreatitis associated ascitic fluid activates the production of tumor necrosis factor-alpha in acinar cells. Crit Care Med. 2005;33:143-8.
40. Raraty MG, Neoptolemos JP. Compartments that cause the real damage in severe acute pancreatitis. Am J Respir Crit Care Med. 2003;168:141-2.
41. Targarona EM, Gracia E, Garriga J, Martínez-Bru C, Cortés M, Boluda R, et al. Prospective randomized trial comparing conventional laparoscopic colectomy with hand-assisted laparoscopic colectomy: applicability, immediate clinical outcome, inflammatory response, and cost. Surg Endosc. 2002;16:234-9.
42. Targarona EM, Gracia E, Rodriguez M, Cerdán G, Balagué C, Garriga J, et al. Hand-assisted laparoscopic surgery. Arch Surg. 2003;138:133-41.
43. Traverso LW, Kozarek RA. Pancreatic necrosectomy: definitions and technique. J Gastrointest Surg. 2005;9:436-9.
44. Tzovaras G, Parks RW, Diamond T, Rowlands BJ. Early and long-term results of surgery for severe necrotising pancreatitis. Dig Surg. 2004;21:41-7.
45. Warshaw AL. Pancreatic necrosis: to debride or not to debride, that is the question. Ann Surg. 2000;232:627-9.
46. West MA, Baker J, Bellingham J. Kinetics of decreased LPS-stimulated cytokine release by macrophages exposed to CO_2. J Surg Res. 1996;63:269-74.
47. Wu FP, Sietses C, von Blomberg BM, van Leeuwen PA, Meijer S, Cuesta MA. Systemic and peritoneal inflammatory response after laparoscopic or conventional colon resection in cancer patients: a prospective, randomized trial. Dis Colon Rectum. 2003;46:147-55.
48. Zengin K, Taskin M, Sakoglu N, Salihoglu Z, Demiroluk S, Uzun H. Systemic inflammatory response after laparoscopic and open application of adjustable banding for morbidly obese patients. Obes Surg. 2002;12:276-9.

CHAPTER 24 Diagnostic Laparoscopy

INTRODUCTION

Diagnostic laparoscopy is a minimally invasive surgical procedure that allows the visual examination of intra-abdominal organs in order to detect any pathology. This procedure allows the direct visual examination of intra-abdominal organs including large surface areas of the liver, gallbladder, spleen, peritoneum, pelvic organs, and retroperitoneum. Biopsies, aspiration, and cultures can be obtained, and laparoscopic ultrasound (US) may be used.

Diagnostic laparoscopy is safe and well tolerated and can be performed in an outpatient or inpatient setting under general anesthesia **(Fig. 1A)**. There may also be unique circumstances where office based diagnostic laparoscopy may be considered under local anesthesia. These circumstances should include only procedures where complications and the need for therapeutic procedures through the same access are extremely unlikely. Manipulation and biopsy of the viscera is possible through additional ports. Diagnostic laparoscopy is the most commonly performed gynecological procedure today. Its greatest advantage is that it has replaced exploratory laparotomy.

Diagnostic laparoscopy was first introduced in 1901, when Kelling, performed a peritoneoscopy in a dog and was called "celioscopy". A Swedish internist named Jacobaeus is credited with performing the first diagnostic laparoscopy on human in 1910. He described its application in patients with ascites and for the early diagnosis of malignant lesions.

In last 10 years, laparoscopy has made a great difference to the diagnosis of abdominal acute and chronic pain. It has evolved as an informative and important method of diagnosing a wide spectrum of both benign and malignant diseases. Exploratory laparoscopy also allows tissue biopsy, culture acquisition, and a variety of therapeutic interventions. Elective diagnostic laparoscopy refers to the use of the procedure in chronic intra-abdominal disorders. Emergency diagnostic laparoscopy is performed in patients presenting with acute abdomen.

INDICATIONS

The indications for diagnostic laparoscopy can be divided into two main groups.

Nontraumatic and Nongynecological Acute Abdomen Like

- Appendicitis
- Diverticulitis
- Duodenal perforation
- Mesenteric adenitis
- Intestinal adhesion
- Omental necrosis
- Intestinal infarction
- Complicated Meckel's diverticulum
- Bedside laparoscopy in the intensive care unit (ICU)
- Torsion of intra-abdominal testis

Gynecological Abdominal Emergencies Like

- Ovarian cysts
- Pelvic inflammatory diseases
- Acute salpingitis
- Ectopic pregnancy
- Endometriosis
- Perforated uterus due to criminal abortion
- Salpingitis

One of the important uses for diagnostic laparoscopy is the investigation of female infertility. Tubal causes of infertility are found in almost 15% of couples. In these patients, laparoscopy not only allows tubal patency to be assessed but also enables other features in the pelvis to be examined. Most important findings related to infertility are kinking of the tube, fimbrial damage or ovarian adhesions. The presence of corpus luteum is considered as good evidence of current ovulation.

If tubal recanalization surgery is planned, it is a good idea to perform a preliminary laparoscopy to assess the prospect of successful anastomosis. If the length of remaining tube is less than 2 cm, the recanalization surgery should not be attempted and in vitro fertilization (IVF) should be recommended.

Ovarian biopsy can also be taken at the time of diagnostic laparoscopy to diagnose the cause of amenorrhea and infertility. Although the functional test of ovarian stimulation by gonadotropin-releasing hormone is more in use, but it can be still of help if the presence of primordial follicles is in doubt in primary amenorrhea or premature ovarian failure.

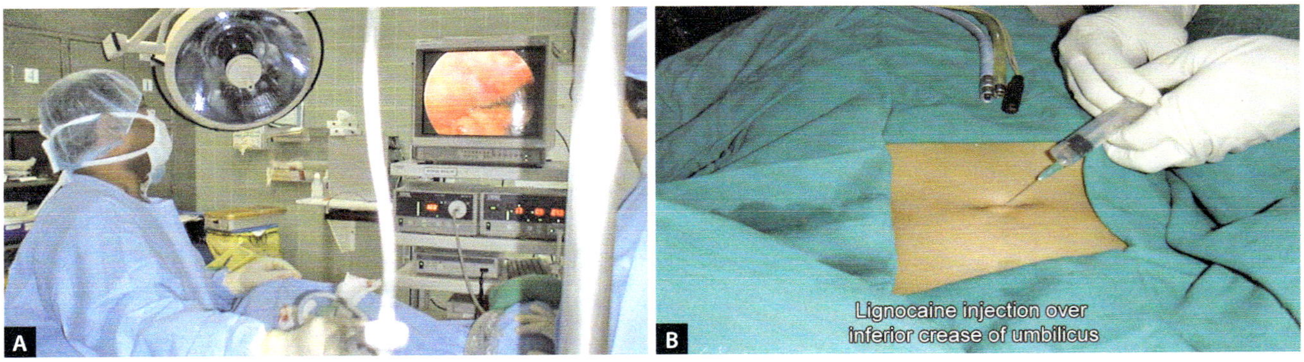

Figs. 1A and B: (A) Diagnostic laparoscopy; (B) Local anesthesia can be used for diagnostic laparoscopy.

RELATIVE CONTRAINDICATIONS

Contraindications may include:

- Hemodynamic instability
- Mechanical or paralytic ileus
- Uncorrected coagulopathy
- Generalized peritonitis
- Severe cardiopulmonary disease
- Abdominal wall infection
- Multiple previous abdominal procedures
- Late pregnancy

However, the final decision is determined not only by the clinical condition of patients, but also by the surgeon's judgment.

Choice of Anesthesia

Diagnostic laparoscopy can be performed under local anesthesia. Sedation with diazepam and pethidine can be used to make patient unaware of procedure because unpleasant sensation of stretching of peritoneum due to pneumoperitoneum cannot be abolished by local anesthesia.

Local anesthetic 4% Xylocaine can be injected subcutaneously over inferior crease of umbilicus **(Fig. 1B)**.

Epidural anesthesia is not preferred by many anesthetists because to anesthetize the entire peritoneum, a high block is necessary which would interfere with intercostal nerves and respiration will be affected. General anesthesia with good muscle relaxation is ideal in laparoscopic surgery.

LAPAROSCOPIC ANATOMY

Diagnostic laparoscopy may be helpful for many undiagnosed surgical problems and therefore knowledge of laparoscopic anatomy of the whole abdomen is necessary. However, most common indications of diagnostic laparoscopy are gynecological and especially related to infertility.

From anterior to posterior, following important tubular structures are found crossing the brim of true pelvis: The round ligament of the uterus, the infundibulopelvic ligament, which contains the gonadal vessels, and the ureter. The ovaries and fallopian tube are found between the round ligament and the infundibulopelvic ligament **(Figs. 2A and B)**.

The fallopian tubes arise from the superior portion of the uterus just above the attachment points of the round ligament. Laparoscopically, the round ligaments overhang the fallopian tube because of uterine manipulation and can be easily mistaken for them. The fallopian tubes towards their lateral end encircle the ovaries partially with their fimbriated ends.

If the uterus is deviated to the contralateral side with the help of uterine manipulator infundibulopelvic ligament is spread out and a pelvic side wall triangle is created. The base of this triangle is the round ligament, the medial side is the infundibulopelvic ligament, and the lateral side is the external iliac artery. The apex of this triangle is the point at which the infundibulopelvic ligament crosses the external iliac artery **(Fig. 3A)**.

Patient Position

The anesthetized patient is placed on the operating table with the legs straight or lithotomy position if patient is female. The lithotomy position will allow the gynecologists and assistant to work simultaneously and uterine manipulation is simultaneously possible. The thighs must not be flexed onto the abdominal wall and should be as they generally are in the full lithotomy position used for other open surgical gynecological procedures. The operating table is tilted head-up or head-down by approximately 15° depending on the main area of examination. Compression bandage may be used on leg during the operation to prevent thromboembolism, especially if patient is in lithotomy position.

Position of the Surgical Team

Before starting diagnostic laparoscopy a best guess is made about the quadrant in which pathology is likely to be found. The surgeon should stand opposite to this quadrant to allow direct view into this quadrant. If the pathology is more likely in pelvic cavity the surgeon stands on left side of the patient **(Fig. 3B)**. The first assistant, whose main task is to position the video camera, is also on the patient's left side.

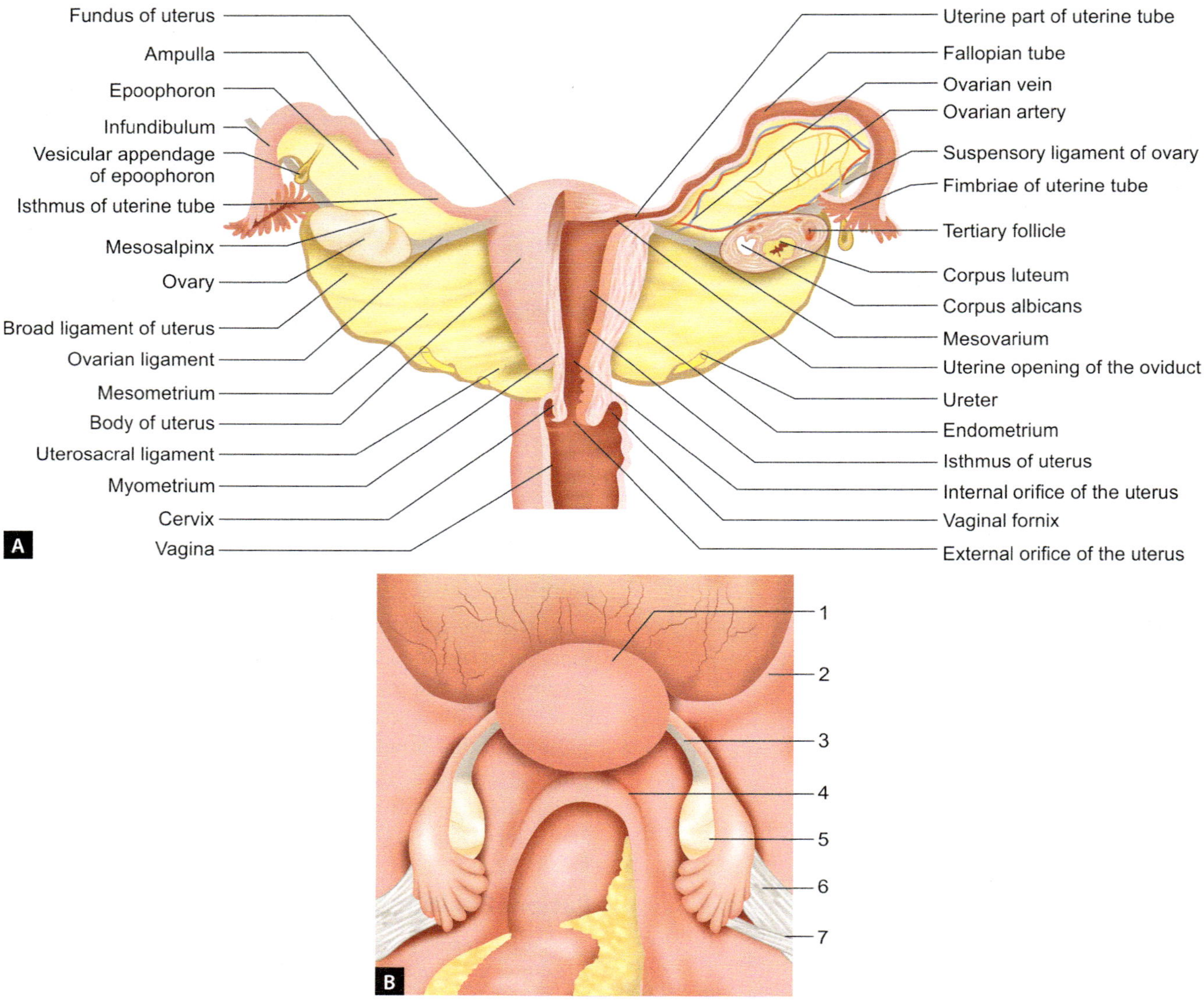

Figs. 2A and B: (A) Anatomy of normal female pelvis; (B) Laparoscopic anatomy of normal female pelvis: (1) Uterus; (2) Round ligament; (3) Utero-ovarian ligament (proper ovarian ligament); (4) Uterosacral ligament; (5) Ovary; (6) Suspensory ligament of the ovary; (7) Ureter.

The instrument trolley is placed on the patient's left, allowing the scrub nurse to assist with placing the appropriate instruments in the operating ports. Television monitors are positioned on either side of the top end of the operating table at a suitable height for surgeon, anesthetists, as well as assistant to see the procedure.

Port Position

Generally one optical port in umbilicus and one 5 mm port in left iliac fossa are required **(Fig. 4A)**. Some gynecologists prefer to put their second port in suprapubic region in midline **(Fig. 4B)**. In our opinion, left iliac fossa port is better because it gives elevation angle of 30° and manipulation angle of 60°, which is ergonomically better. With suprapubic port elevation angle of instrument and tubal structure is 90° and hence lifting up of ovary and tube may be difficult without grasping it.

During diagnostic laparoscopy it is advisable that both telescope and probing instrument is held by surgeon himself as he knows better what he wants to see and where he wants to concentrate more and also which structure he wants to see in magnified close-up view. At the time of diagnostic laparoscopy surgeon should try to be very gentle with the tubal structures and bowel so that adhesions will not form and stricture of tube shall not occur.

Viewing of lateral pelvic organs is helped by the manipulation of mobile structure with a second port introduced through the left iliac fossa port. Many gynecologists introduce the second port in suprapubic region but the elevation angle of the instrument is 90° and the mobilization of organs is difficult.

A three-port approach should be used if there is any difficulty in manipulation with two ports, especially in case of extensive adhesions.

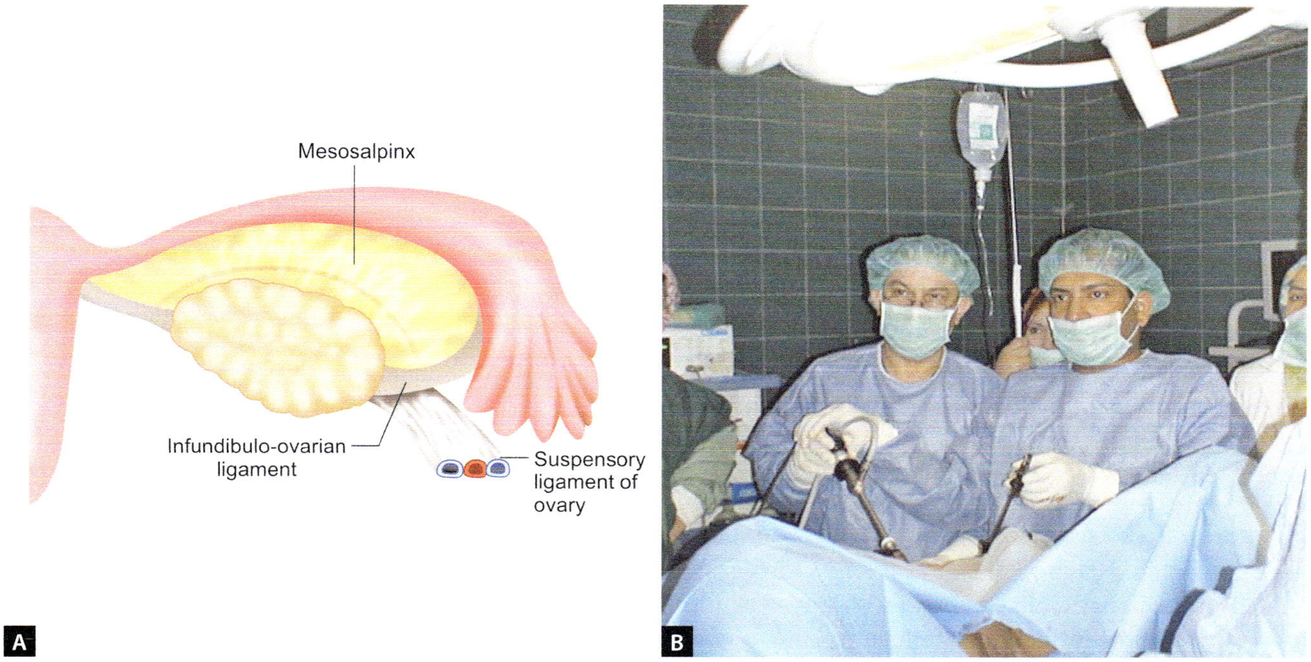

Figs. 3A and B: (A) Anatomy of adnexa; (B) Position of surgical team for diagnostic laparoscopy in female.

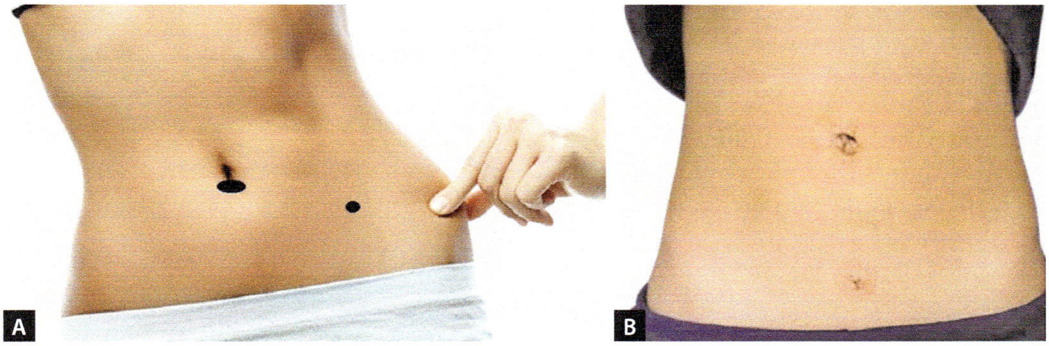

Figs. 4A and B: Port position for diagnostic laparoscopy.

- 10 mm umbilical (optical)
- 5 mm suprapubic
- 5 mm right hypochondrium

A 30° telescope is employed in most instances, as this facilitates easier inspection of the deeper peritoneal cavity and abdominal organs. The secondary ports are inserted under laparoscopic vision. The selected site on the abdominal wall is identified by finger indentation of the parietal peritoneum.

The optimum incision for optical port is in the subumbilical region. The open technique for trocar insertion is recommended if patient presents with severe abdominal distension. Nitrous oxide is preferably used if diagnostic laparoscopy is performed in local anesthesia because nitrous oxide has its own analgesic effect. Carbon dioxide (CO_2) is the preferred gas if diagnostic laparoscopy is performed under general anesthesia. Insufflation should be very slow and with care taken not to exceed 12.0 mm Hg.

Operative Procedure

The first step in diagnostic laparoscopy is thorough exploration, just as during exploratory laparotomy. A systematic approach to exploration is essential to ensure that nothing is missed.

Systemic Plan of Inspection in Mid Abdomen

Positioning is the primary means of displacing the bowel and exposing peritoneal surfaces. In women with a deep pelvis, the bowel should be displaced gently into the upper abdomen, using a blunt probe or closed blunt grasping instrument to avoid laceration of the bowel or mesentery. An additional port with a blunt tipped instrument may be used, if required. Occasionally, fan retractor can be used to retract full sigmoid colon. This instrument can be inserted through a 5 mm trocar cannula and fanned out in the abdomen to retract the bowel. Some common findings are shown in **Figures 5 to 11**.

Inspection of Pelvis

Patient should be again positioned in steep Trendelenburg's position.

After assessing the genital organs, the gynecologist may wish to view areas outside the pelvis. This should be done by tilting the table head up or laterally to examine the paracolic or subdiaphragmatic spaces. Systematic plan of inspection of pelvis is shown in **(Figs. 9A to C)**.

ROLE OF LAPAROSCOPY IN ASCITES

Although the determination of the etiology of ascites is usually straight forward by history, physical examination, and analysis of ascitic fluid, the diagnosis of tuberculous or carcinomatous ascites may be elusive. In such cases, laparoscopy with biopsy is highly accurate. Peritoneal mesothelioma is frequently missed on ascitic fluid by cytology and by blind biopsy. This entity is readily diagnosed by laparoscopy with peritoneal biopsy. Laparoscopy may be useful in the evaluation of hepatic malignancy (both primary or metastatic). About 80–90% of these lesions are present on the hepatic surface and up to two-thirds of the liver surface may be inspected by laparoscopy. When surgical resection is a therapeutic option, laparoscopy may reveal small (1 cm or less) metastatic lesions, peritoneal metastases, or cirrhosis, which represent contraindications to this plan of resection and are frequently missed on computed tomography (CT), magnetic resonance (MRI), and US. The use of laparoscopic US allows detection of deeper lesions and vascular infiltration.

In a study on the role of laparoscopy in the diagnosis and differential diagnosis of ascites, it was found that out of 2,500 patients who underwent laparoscopy, 30.89% had ascites; of which, liver cirrhosis underlays it in 57.78%, peritoneal carcinosis in 26.29%, primary and metastatic carcinoma in 12.95%, and tuberculous peritonitis in 1.42%, more rarely other diseases. Liver cirrhosis, malignant tumors, and the other hepatic affections with concomitant ascites in their course can certainly be diagnosed laparoscopically. Laparoscopy with oriented biopsy of peritoneum and liver is of decisive importance in differentiating peritoneal carcinosis from tuberculosis. In peritoneal carcinosis the diagnosis (as based in clinical and laboratory findings) coincided perfectly with the laparoscopic and histologic one in 24.5%, and partially in 45.5%. In 30% there was no congruence at all. Laparoscopy and the test methods associated with it contributed to the accurate diagnosis of peritoneal carcinosis in 75.5% of the patients. Ovarian carcinoma (20.9%) and cancer of the stomach (16.3%) underlay peritoneal carcinosis most frequently, other diseases were by far more seldom.

Diagnostic peritoneoscopies were performed in 226 patients with ascites. Satisfactory examination was possible in 220 patients. Clinical diagnosis was confirmed at peritoneoscopy in 82.7% of patients. Peritoneoscopic examination corrected the clinical diagnosis in 13.7%, was inconclusive in 2.6% and was incorrect in 0.8% of cases.

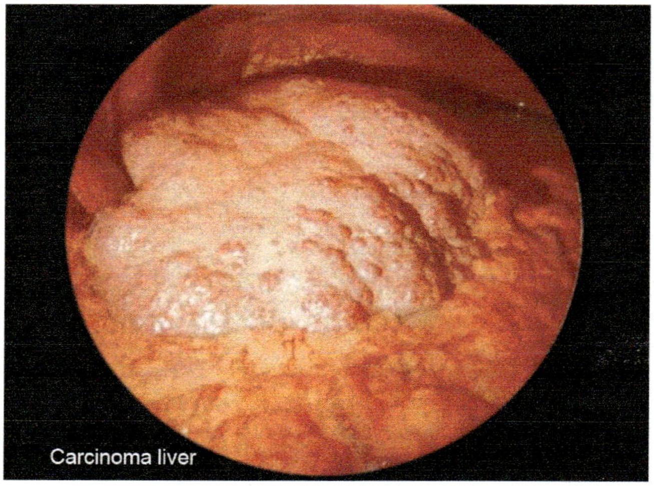

Fig. 5: Hepatic carcinoma.

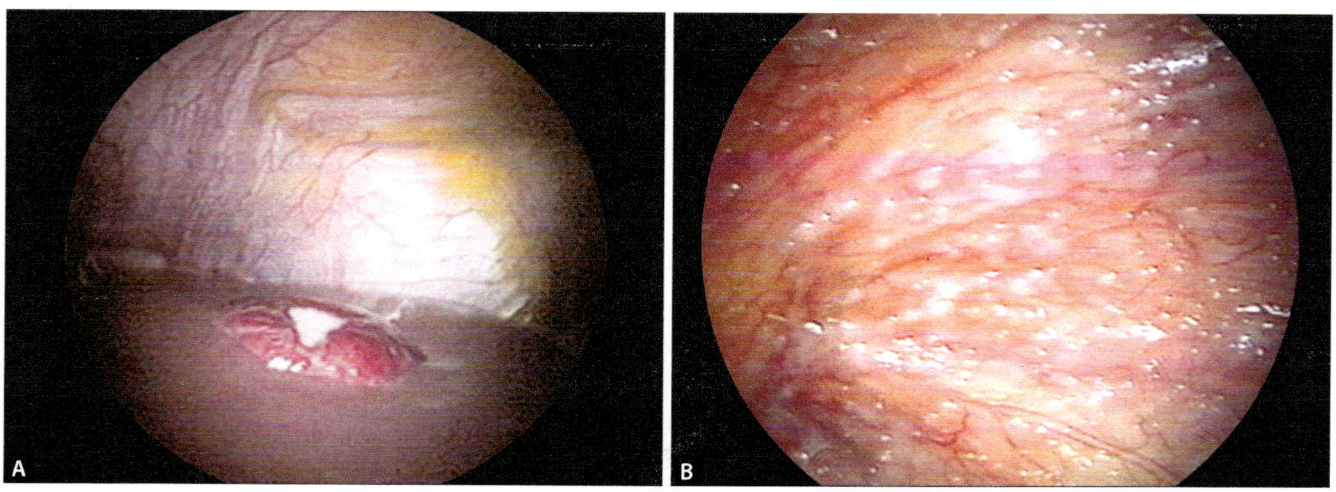

Figs. 6A and B: (A) Hemangioma; (B) Carcinomatosis.

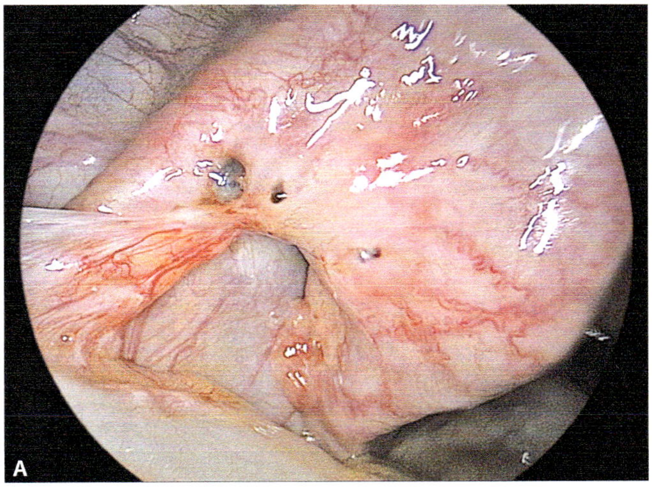

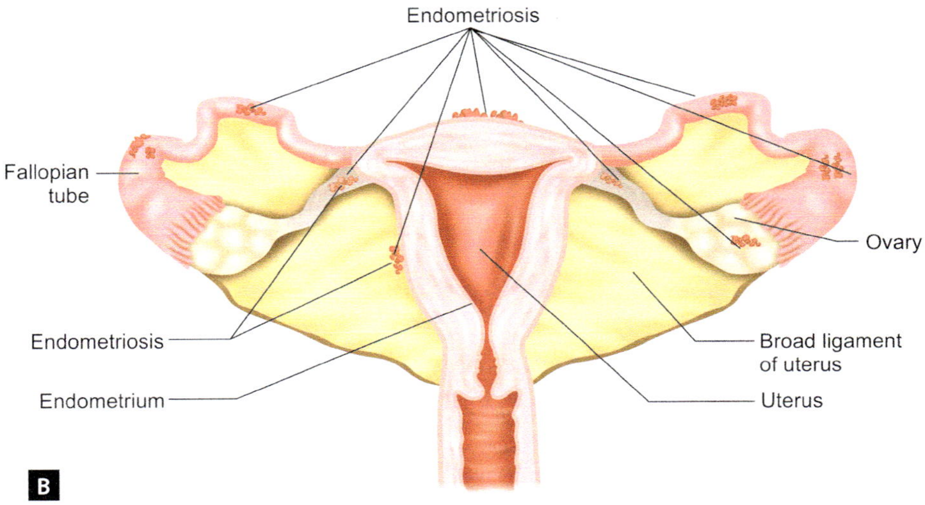

Figs. 7A and B: Endometriosis.

It was 100% diagnostic in malignant peritonitis and 89.5% in patients with tuberculous peritonitis. Pseudomyxoma peritonei and mesothelioma were suspected in one patient each at peritoneoscopy and was confirmed histologically. The utility of routine ascitic fluid examination was reviewed in all patients. The ascitic fluid was transudative in 81.9%, exudative in 8.6% and indeterminate in 9.5% of patients with cirrhosis of liver. Patients with tuberculous peritonitis had exudative, transudative and indeterminate ascites in 71.8%, 3.2%, and 25%, respectively. The ascites in patients with malignant peritonitis was either exudative (80%) or indeterminate (20%). There was considerable overlap in the nature of ascites present in the three groups of patients. We therefore conclude that peritoneoscopy is the most valuable investigation in the diagnosis of ascites, particularly in exudative and indeterminate types.

The Value of Laparoscopic Diagnosis of Tuberculosis

The laparoscopic and pathological diagnosis of 43 patients who underwent abdominal laparoscopy for various indications are presented here. Major indications for the laparoscopy included hepatomegaly in 32 patients, ascites in 28, and pyrexia of unknown origin (PUO) in 18 patients. A combination of two or more of these indications was a more common feature. The most frequently encountered laparoscopic diagnoses were tuberculosis and chronic liver disease (16 patients each), followed by cancer (9 patients). However, on pathological examination of peritoneal or liver biopsy tissue and on follow-up, tuberculosis was confirmed in 12 patients, chronic liver disease in 14 patients, and hepatocellular carcinoma in 11 patients. No complications were encountered during the laparoscopy. Our findings indicate that abdominal laparoscopy is a safe, quick, and inexpensive diagnostic tool, particularly when appropriate and adequate tissue is taken for pathological examination. In such instances, laparoscopy would save an unnecessary laparotomy, especially where tuberculosis and cancer are considered in the differential diagnosis.

Due to its high accuracy, some suggest polymerase chain reaction (PCR) before laparoscopy. In the light of our accumulated experience, we would suggest that PCR of

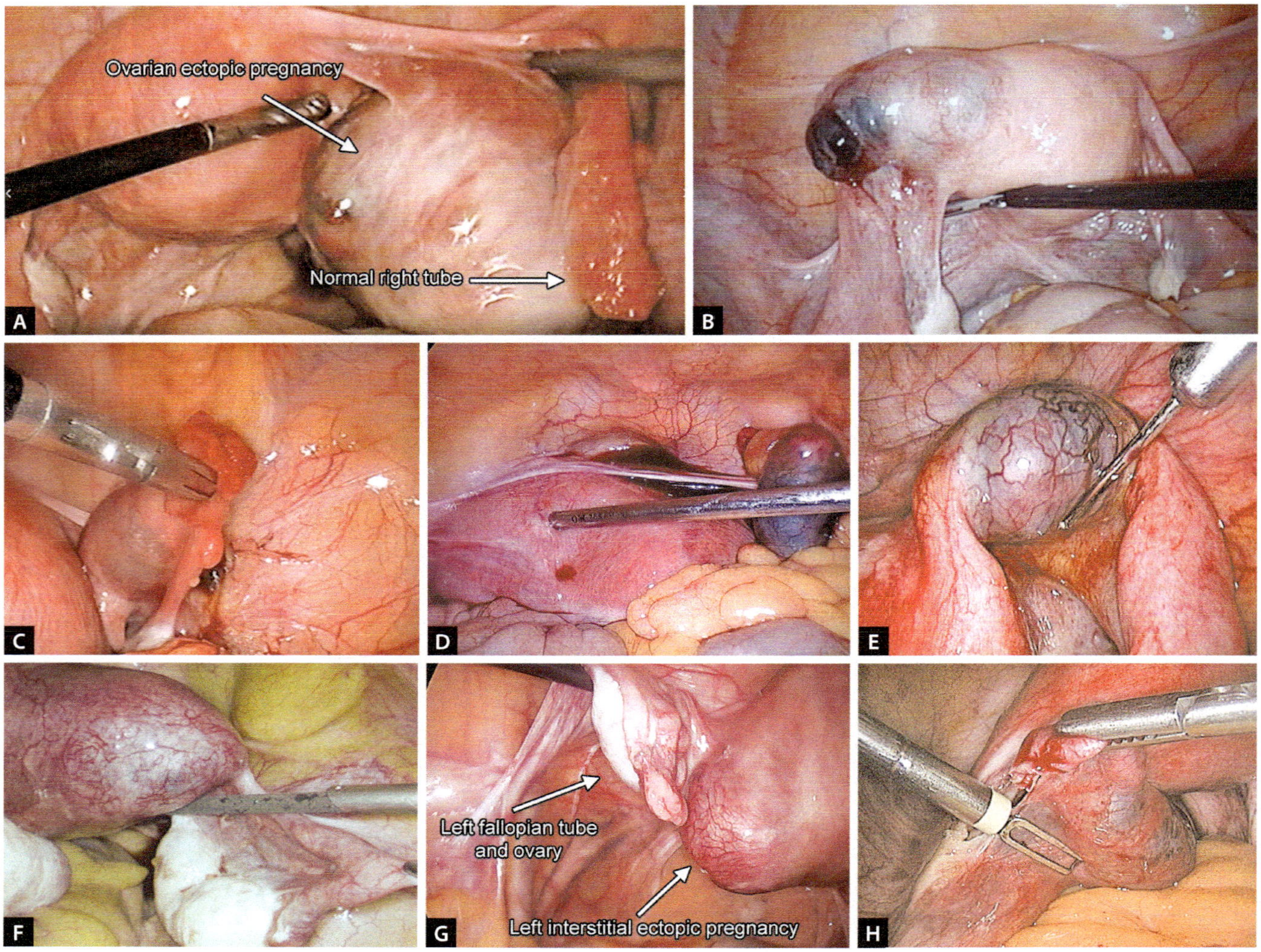

Figs. 8A to H: Ectopic pregnancy.

ascetic fluid obtained by US-guided fine-needle aspiration is now the investigation of choice for patients with the described clinical and radiological presentations and should at least be attempted before surgical intervention. If the result is negative, diagnostic laparoscopy or, if this is not feasible, laparotomy needs to be performed.

Role of Laparoscopy in Carcinoma Assessment

A pretherapeutic staging system to design operative or neoadjuvant treatments in gastric cancer is needed. Laparoscopy can be done even under local anesthesia as it is a sensitive predictor of peritoneal recurrence.

Staging laparoscopy with peritoneal lavage cytology is a safe, effective tool in patients with locally advanced gastric cancer, especially in patients receiving neoadjuvant chemotherapy. The ability of minimally invasive surgeons and endoscopists to diagnose and palliate unresectable pancreatic cancer is likely to continue to improve and these techniques will play an increasingly important role in the care of patients with pancreatic cancer. Likewise, the accuracy of radiological imaging techniques to detect unresectable disease will also continue to advance and further decrease the incidence of nontherapeutic laparotomies. It is valuable and has many therapeutic uses as in staging of tumor, catheter placement in nephrogenic ascites.

Dialysis Catheter and Laparoscopy

Regarding complications of dialysis catheter insertion, Tiong reported many surgical, early and late complications of dialysis catheter of open Tenckhoff catheter insertion under local anesthesia in a single institution. A review was carried out on 164 insertions in 139 patients over a 3-year period. Tenckhoff catheter insertion for continuous ambulatory peritoneal dialysis (CAPD) is a procedure associated with significant surgical morbidity. Patients with diabetes mellitus, glomerulonephritis, and ongoing sepsis are at greater risk of early complications, and hence, must have their conditions stabilized or treated before surgery. In addition, prolonged surgical time and patients with previous abdominal surgery are at increased risk. The rate of complications may be improved by early consideration of patients with poor tolerance of local anesthetic for surgery or

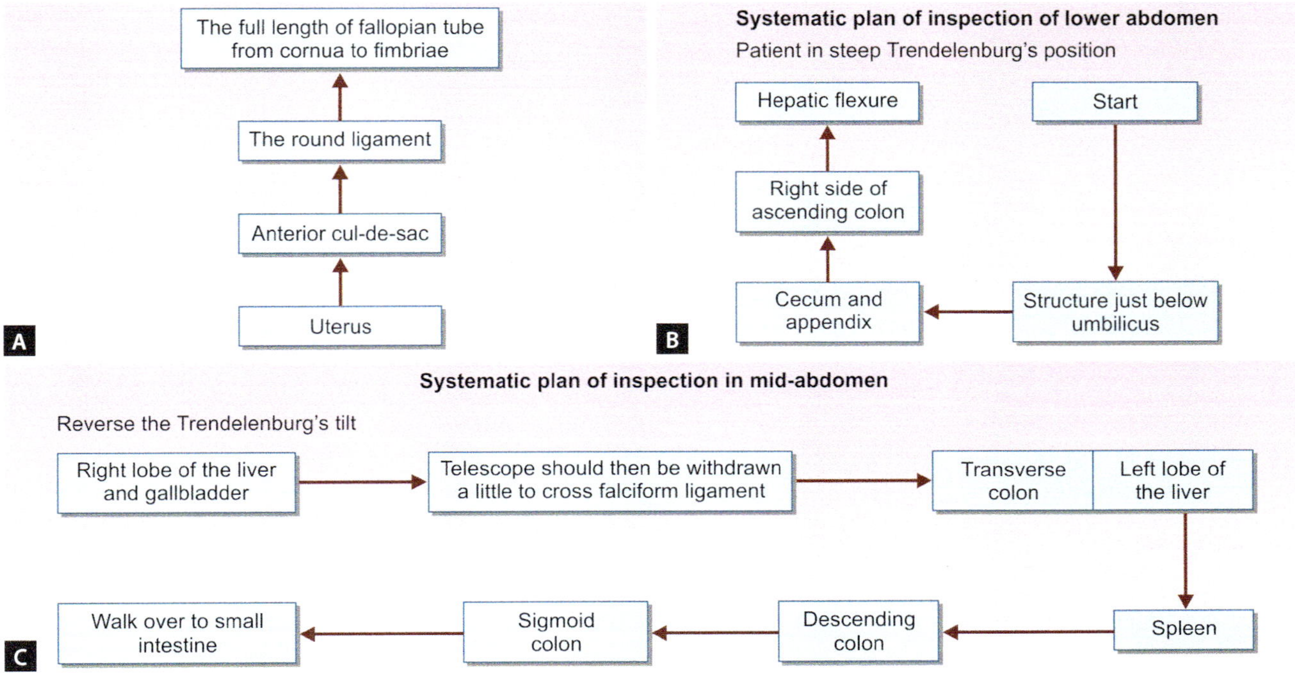

Figs. 9A to C: Systematic plan of inspection of pelvis.

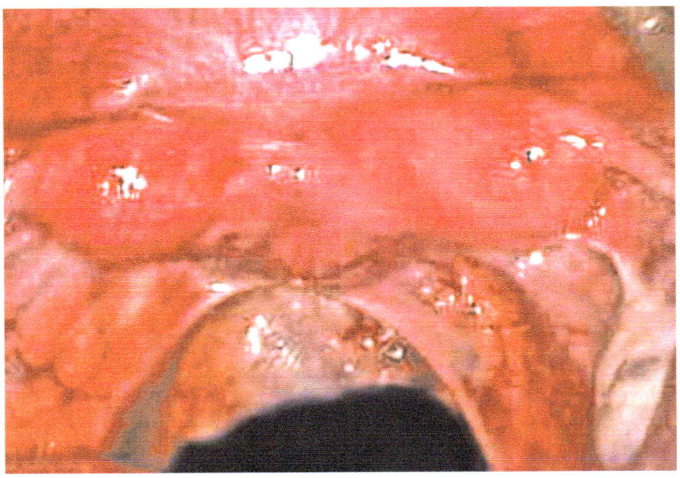

Fig. 10: Bicornuate uterus.

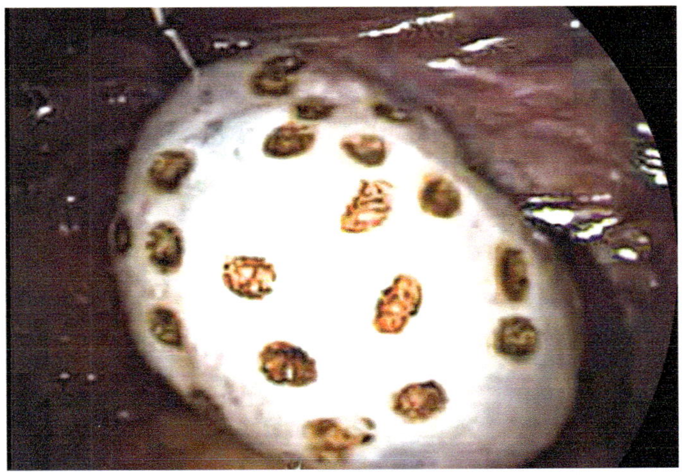

Fig. 11: Polycystic ovary.

with previous abdominal surgery for laparoscopic insertion under general anesthesia. To prevent late complications dominated by CAPD peritonitis, patient's nutritional status and care of the catheter should both be optimized.

Open insertion of peritoneal dialysis (PD) catheters is the standard surgical technique, but it is associated with a relatively high incidence of catheter outflow obstruction and dialysis leak. Omental wrapping is the most common cause of mechanical problem; laparoscopic omental fixation technique is of higher value, in addition laparoscopic surgery also enabled diagnosis of intra-abdominal pathologies and treatment of the accompanying surgical problems during the same operation.

Port-site Metastasis

The risk of port-site metastases in those undergoing laparoscopy for gynecologic malignancy was highest in those with ascites in a study of 82 patients. The study participants underwent 87 procedures that involved 330 trocar sites. The overall risk of port-site metastases per procedure was 2.3%, and per port site was 2.4%, Dr Nimesh Nagarsheth, at an international congress sponsored by the Society of Laparoendoscopic Surgeons reported 39 patients with endometrial cancer, 29 with ovarian cancer, and 14 with cervical cancer. About 20 of those were treated for recurrent cancer, and 10 of them had ascites. They were followed for an average of 361 days. Port-site metastases occurred in two patients. The first developed metastases at five sites, and was diagnosed 13 days after second-look laparoscopy for stage IIIB ovarian cancer. The second had metastases at three sites, and was diagnosed 46 days after second-look laparoscopy for stage IIIC primary peritoneal cancer. Both patients had ascites.

Laparoscopy and Ascites

Laparoscopy in ascites is a safe and cost-effective diagnostic modality and its rules extended the diagnostic procedure often providing definitive diagnosis in unexplained cause of ascites.

In such instances, laparoscopy would save an unnecessary laparotomy; especially where tuberculosis and cancer are considered in the differential diagnosis.

DISCUSSION

The usual site of insertion of the trocar/cannula for diagnostic laparoscopy is below or to the side of the umbilicus. This position may require to be altered in the presence of abdominal scars. The use of a 30° forward oblique telescope is preferable for viewing the surface architecture of organs. By rotation of the telescope, different angles of inspection can be achieved.

The first important step after access to the abdomen has been gained, is to check for damage caused by trocar insertion. A second 5 mm port is then inserted under vision in an appropriate quadrant to take in a palpating rod.

A systematic examination of the abdomen must be performed just as in laparotomy. We begin at the left lobe of the liver but any scheme can be used as long as it is consistent. Next, check around the falciform ligament to the right lobe of liver, gallbladder, and hiatus. After checking the stomach, move onto the cecum and appendix and check the terminal ileum. Follow the colon round to the sigmoid colon, and then check the pelvis. Surgeon should be conversant with sampling and biopsy techniques, and the use of position and manipulation to aid vision.

At the time of diagnostic laparoscopy all the abdominal organs are inspected for any gross anatomical abnormalities. Abdominal cavity is inspected for excess of fluids. Samples are taken if free fluid is present for laboratory tests (chemistry, cytology or bacteriology). Peritoneal lavage and adhesiolysis may need to be performed to improve visualization of organs. At the time of peritoneal lavage, when fluid is sucked from the cul-de-sac, it is important to keep all the holes of the suction-irrigator beneath the level of the fluid to avoid removing pneumoperitoneum. If the suction-irrigator is positioned improperly, the CO_2 gas will be removed undesirably. However, with high-flow insufflators, pneumoperitoneum is rarely lost and quickly restored.

When performing a diagnostic laparoscopy to confirm appendicitis, a-5 mm port is placed in the left iliac fossa to facilitate manipulation. The patient is placed head down and rotated to the left to displace the small bowel from the pelvis and allow the uterus and ovaries to be checked. This, however, should be limited to avoid contamination of subphrenic spaces, if this is not already present.

Ending of the Operation

During diagnostic laparoscopy, surgeon can perform therapeutic laparoscopy if indicated when having a prior consent or can be obtained from patient's relative.

At the end of surgery, abdomen should be re-examined for any possible bowel injury or hemorrhage. The entire accessory instrument and then port is removed. The telescope should be removed leaving gas valve of umbilical port open to let out all the gas. Once the complete gas is out, for removing primary cannula, telescope or any blunt instrument should be introduced again and cannula should be pulled over that instrument to prevent pulling of omentum or bowel. Wound should be closed with suture. Vicryl should be used for rectus and unabsorbable intradermal or stapler for skin. Only 10 mm port wound is necessary to repair. Adhesive sterile dressing over the wound should be applied.

Patient may be discharged on the same day after operation if everything goes well. The patient may have slight pain initially but usually resolves. Diagnostic laparoscopy is a useful method for reducing hospital stay, complications, and return to normal activity if carried on in proper manner.

Laparoscopy for Abdominal Trauma

Trauma is the leading cause of death between 1 and 44 years. In all age groups, it is surpassed only by cancer and atherosclerosis in mortality. The evaluation and treatment of abdominal injuries are critical components in the management of severely injured trauma patients. Because missed intra-abdominal injuries are a frequent cause of preventable trauma deaths, a high index of suspicion is warranted. Multiple factors, including the mechanism of injury, the body region injured, the patient's hemodynamic and neurological status, associated injuries, and institutional resources influence the diagnostic approach and the outcome of abdominal injuries.

Laparoscopy was first used for a trauma patient in 1956 by Lamy, who observed two cases of splenic injury. Since then, Gazzaniga noted that laparoscopy is useful for determining the need for laparotomy. In 1991, Berci reported that he had reduced the number of nontherapeutic laparotomies performed for hemoperitoneum by 25% through the use of laparoscopy in 150 patients with blunt abdominal trauma.

Data show that laparoscopy is a useful modality for evaluating and managing hemodynamically stable trauma patients with penetrating injuries. Increased use of laparoscopy in select patients with penetrating abdominal trauma will decrease the rate of negative and nontherapeutic laparotomies, thus lowering morbidity, decreasing length of hospitalization, and provide for more efficient utilization of available resources. As technology and expertise among surgeons continues to improve, more standard therapeutic interventions may be done laparoscopically in the future. Mandatory surgical exploration for gunshot wounds to the abdomen has been a surgical dictum for the greater part of this century. Although nonoperative management of blunt solid organ injuries and low-energy penetrating injuries such as stab wounds is well established, the same is not true for gunshot wounds. The vast majority of patients who sustain a gunshot injury to the abdomen require immediate laparotomy to control bleeding and contain contamination. Nonoperative treatment of patients with a gunshot injury is gaining acceptance in only a highly selected subset of hemodynamically stable adult patients without peritonitis. Although the physical examination remains the cornerstone in the evaluation of patients with gunshot injury, other techniques such as CT, diagnostic peritoneal lavage (DPL), and diagnostic laparoscopy allows accurate diagnosis of an intra-abdominal injury. The ability to exclude internal organ injury nonoperatively avoids the potential complications of unnecessary laparotomy. Clinical data to support selective nonoperative management of certain gunshot injuries to the abdomen are accumulating, but the approach has risks and requires careful collaborative management by emergency physicians and surgeons experienced in the care of penetrating injury. Sosa reported 121 consecutive abdominal gunshot wounds managed with laparoscopy. About 79 (65%) had negative laparoscopy, and these patients were managed without laparotomy. Another 7.2% avoided nontherapeutic laparotomy.

It is very important to determine the presence, location, and severity of intra-abdominal injury to decide the surgical intervention; and to thoroughly evaluate intra-abdominal organs for associated injuries in the trauma patient. For stab wounds, serial physical examination is supplemented by local wound exploration, DPL, abdominal US, abdominal CT, MRI, and in some cases, angiography to maximize the value of surgical intervention and to reduce negative and nontherapeutic laparotomy. Despite having many positive qualities, these diagnostic methods have some drawbacks. DPL is an invasive but sensitive procedure; it may result in nontherapeutic laparotomy with its attendant morbidity. The use of CT is limited to the hemodynamically stable patient. There has been increasing interest in the use of abdominal US because it is portable, noninvasive, rapid, and easily repeatable. However, it is less accurate for diagnosis of diaphragmatic and hollow viscera injury. With experience in laparoscopic cholecystectomy and the advent of improved and readily accessible laparoscopic equipment and devices, laparoscopic surgery became widespread for intra-abdominal operations, setting the stage for renewed interest in its applications for the diagnosis of traumatic abdominal injuries and examination of their therapeutic potential.

In the evaluation and management of the abdominal injury, current diagnostic methods have a defined sensitivity, specificity, and accuracy, but none of these represents a gold standard. Thus, abdominal exploration by laparotomy should not be discarded as a worthy diagnostic and therapeutic procedure for patients with equivocal and unreliable findings. It is associated with complication rates as high as 40% including a 10–40% negative laparotomy rate, a 20% morbidity rate, a 0–5% mortality rate, and a 3% long-term risk of bowel obstruction secondary to adhesions.

Laparoscopy has been reported infrequently as a therapeutic tool in selected trauma patients. Examples of therapeutic laparoscopy include repair of diaphragmatic lacerations with sutures, staples, or prosthetic mesh; suturing of gastrointestinal perforations; hemostasis of low-grade liver and splenic lacerations; resection of small bowel and colon; cholecystectomy; splenectomy; and distal pancreatectomy. Autotransfusion of collected blood from the hemoperitoneum is another potential application. Fabian in a large study of 182 trauma patients reported one suture repair of diaphragmatic injury. Successful laparoscopic repair of small bowel, colon, and rectal injuries, and laparoscopic repair of a small gastric stab wound using hernia stapler have been reported recently. For the repair of solid visceral injuries, there are three methods that merit investigation: (1) The totally laparoscopic procedure, (2) the laparoscopically assisted procedure, and (3) hand-assisted laparoscopic surgery (HALS). The argon beam coagulator, fibrin glue, topical hemostatic agent, and absorbable mesh may be beneficial for hepatic and splenic lacerations. Laparoscopic repair of bowel injuries can be performed using suture or staples. Primary suture repair of a small bowel injury would be amenable by a totally laparoscopic procedure. Using a porcine model, Pietrafitta and Soperet described a technique for an intraperitoneal functional end-to-end anastomosis of the small intestine. Milsom and Bohm modified these techniques and reported that their technique for intracorporeal intestinal anastomosis has been proven safe in dozens of animal and human procedures, but that it had some drawbacks. It requires a long operating time and needs two or three 30 mm endogastrointestinal anastomosis (GIAs) and a skin incision for specimen retrieval. Recently, animal research has assessed the potential for hand-assisted laparoscopic exploration to detect traumatic injuries. Asbun reported that hand-assisted laparoscopic exploration is more accurate than laparoscopic exploration alone in detecting injuries (63% vs. 38%), but that it still resulted in an unacceptable rate of missed injuries.

Hand-assisted laparoscopic surgery allows for the application of minimally invasive surgical techniques to complex intra-abdominal operations, particularly when specimen removal is required. The rationale for this approach is that the hand offers the surgeon some advantage in terms of tactile feedback, exposure, retraction, and orientation, enabling the surgeon to perform with greater safety and efficiency. Most trauma surgeons consider omental herniation through an anterior abdominal stab wound an indication for laparotomy because frequently there are significant intra-abdominal injuries. As an alternative to laparotomy, the herniated omentum was evaluated and managed, with laparoscopy performed through the abdominal stab wound or using it for accessory trocar. If there are no significant injuries, the wound can be managed without further treatment. Depending on the surgeon's preference, therapeutic laparoscopy can be continued.

The complications of laparoscopy for trauma include not only the usual complications of anesthesia and laparoscopy, but also some that are unique to the trauma patient. Fabian independently reported the development of tension pneumothorax in patients with diaphragmatic injury from positive-pressure pneumoperitoneum. If suspected, induction of pneumoperitoneum is stopped and an immediate needle thoracocentesis is performed, followed by a tube thoracostomy, if needed. However, routine prophylactic tube thoracostomy is not indicated. The risks of gas embolism in patients with intra-abdominal venous injuries, especially liver lacerations, are another problem. Among 133 laparoscopic examinations of trauma, Smith did encounter this complication in two patients with injuries of the inferior vena cava tamponaded by clot.

This potential problem of laparoscopy has stimulated interest in "gasless" laparoscopy based on expansion of the peritoneal cavity by mechanical retractors. In addition to averting the risks of tension pneumothorax and gas embolism, it facilitates the use of conventional instruments such as hemostats, needles, sutures, and electrocautery, resulting in significant cost savings. The major disadvantage of gasless laparoscopy, however, is the excessive cost of the powered mechanical arm and the poor exposure in the lateral gutters. Less expensive apparatus to lift the abdominal wall is expected in times to come. The transperitoneal absorption of CO_2 may cause metabolic and hemodynamic changes such as acidosis, cardiac suppression, atelectasis, subcutaneous emphysema, and increased intracranial pressure, resulting in more profound consequences for the trauma patient. Joseph demonstrated that CO_2 pneumoperitoneum causes significantly increased intracranial pressure in a porcine model of head injury.

The results of this study led them to recommend the avoidance of CO_2 pneumoperitoneum for the evaluation of patients with head injuries. Undoubtedly, gasless laparoscopy could replace CO_2 pneumoperitoneum in these cases. Missed intra-abdominal injuries are among the most frequent causes of potentially preventable trauma deaths. The evaluation and management of abdominal trauma is dependent on multiple factors, including mechanism of injury, location of injury, hemodynamic status of the patient, neurological status of the patient, associated injuries, and institutional resources. Therefore careful selection, high index of suspicion, and a low threshold for laparotomy will provide the patient the benefits of minimal invasive surgery and reducing the rates and morbidity of unnecessary laparotomy.

The diagnostic laparoscopy of various organs is shown in **Figures 12 to 17**.

Complications

Complications may occur during access, trocar insertion, or the diagnostic manipulation of viscera. These complications include, cardiac arrhythmias, hemodynamic instability due to decreased venous return, bleeding, bile leak, perforation of a hollow viscus, laceration of a solid organ, vascular injury, gas embolism, and subcutaneous or extraperitoneal dissection due to the insufflation gas. If proper sterilization

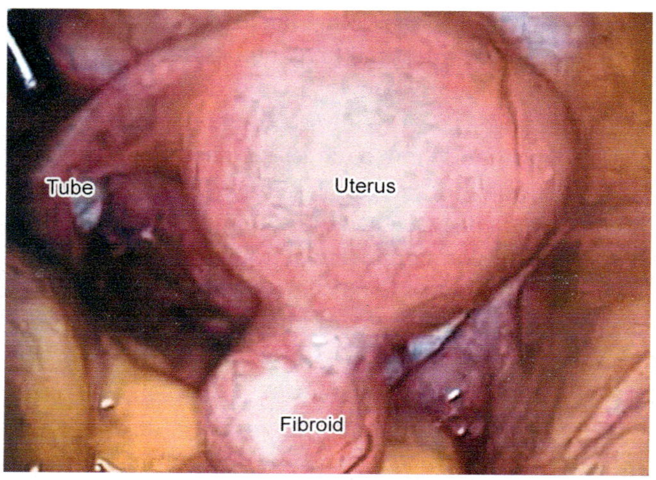

Fig. 12: Fibroid.

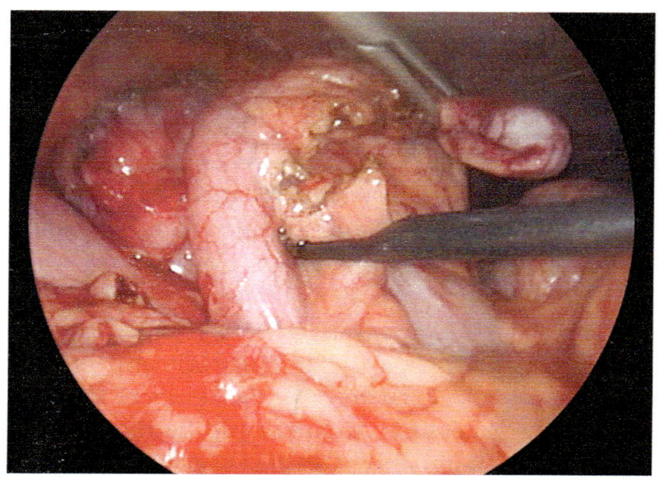

Fig. 13: Adhesion of appendix.

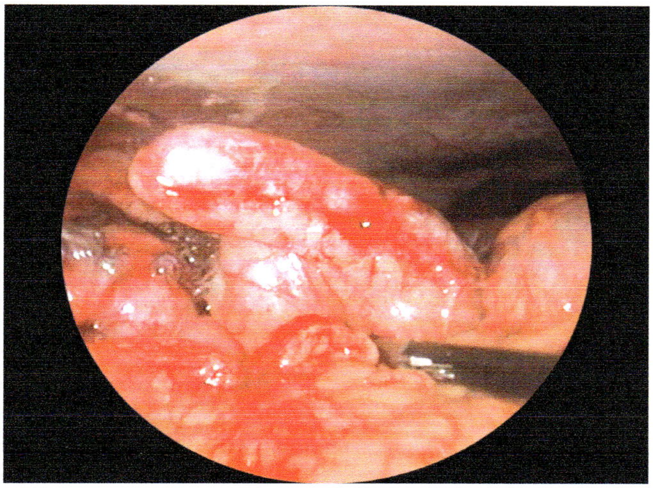

Fig. 14: Acute appendicitis.

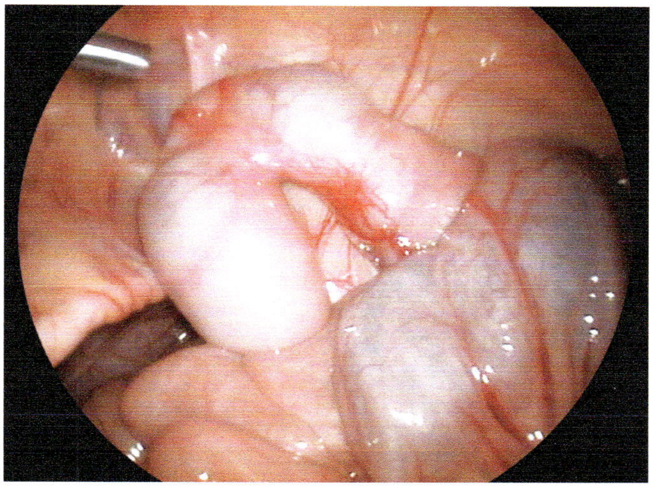

Fig. 15: Diverticulum.

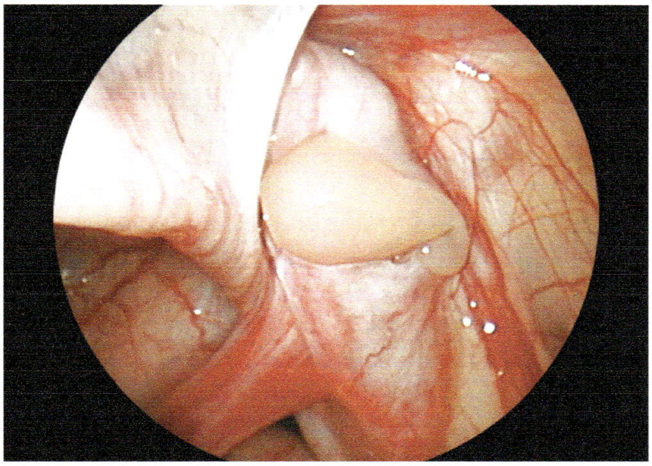

Fig. 16: Impalpable testes.

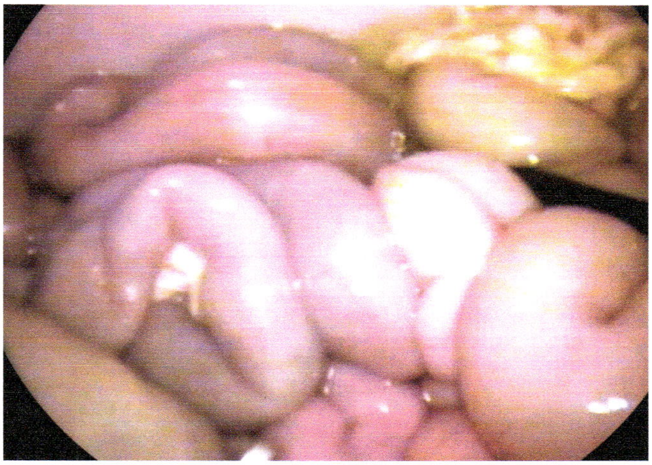

Fig. 17: Perforation of small bowel.

of instrument is not done then wound infection or leakage of ascites may occur postoperatively. Failure to accurately diagnose the extent of intra-abdominal pathology is another potential complication for which patient may have to go for resurgery.

CONCLUSION

Diagnostic laparoscopy is one of the very important methods of investigation for patients in whom the diagnosis or extent of the disease is unclear or the abdominal findings are equivocal. It can be performed safely in an inpatient or outpatient setting, potentially expediting diagnosis, and treatment. This laparoscopic procedure helps to achieve the final diagnosis without any significant complication and less operative time, it can be safely concluded that diagnostic laparoscopy is a safe, quick, and effective adjunct to nonsurgical diagnostic modalities, for establishing a conclusive diagnosis, but whether it will replace imaging studies as a primary modality for diagnosis needs more evidence.

CHAPTER 25

Laparoscopic Small Bowel Surgery

INTRODUCTION

Since the first reports of laparoscopic surgery for inflammatory bowel disease from Peters in 1992, several literatures have subsequently shown the potential advantage of minimal access surgery for small bowel pathologies. The increased use of laparoscopy in the management of gastrointestinal problems continues to expand. Procedures such as jejunostomies, diagnosis of intestinal obstruction or ischemia, resection of the small bowel, and lysis of adhesions can be managed with this technique.

LAPAROSCOPIC RESECTION OF SMALL BOWEL

The role of laparoscopy in resection of the small bowel has increased rapidly in the last 5 years. Laparoscopic small bowel resection can be performed safely in the setting of benign as well as malignant disease and imparts many of the benefits of minimally invasive surgery. The affected small bowel and mesentery can be thoroughly inspected and resected laparoscopically and bowel continuity restored through an entirely intracorporeal technique or laparoscopic-assisted technique.

Indications

A small bowel resection is the surgical removal of one or more segments of the small intestine. Laparoscopic small bowel resection with primary anastomosis is most frequently indicated for benign diseases.

The most common indications are:

- Isolated Crohn's disease
- Gastrointestinal stromal tumors
- Benign strictures, and
- Vascular malformations

Malignant conditions represent relative contra-indications in that they are rare, and if diagnosed or suspected, laparoscopic management should not be considered as the method of choice. The conduct of the laparoscopic operation should be in a manner very similar to that of a conventional small bowel resection.

SURGICAL ANATOMY

The bowel wall is comprised of four layers: (1) the mucosa, (2) submucosa, (3) muscularis propria, and (4) serosa. The submucosa is the "strength" layer of the anastomosis and must be included in every suture pass.

The vascular supply to the bowel is via the mesentery. The superior mesenteric artery gives rise to the arcuate system that supplies the vasa recta of the small intestine. If an anastomosis is constructed off to one side of the bowel, there will be a shorter distance for the blood supply to reach the mesenteric aspect of the anastomosis. However, the blood supply to the antimesenteric aspect of the anastomosis must travel a considerably longer distance over the antimesenteric border of the bowel. That puts the antimesenteric aspect of the anastomosis at a much higher risk of ischemia. For this reason, we suggest centering side-to-side and side-to-end anastomoses on the antimesenteric border of the bowel, rather than off to one side, whenever possible, to minimize ischemia.

Staplers

There are three standard types of surgical staplers used for bowel resection and reconstruction:

1. Transverse anastomosis (TA) staplers are typically noncutting straight staplers that lay down several rows of staples. After stapling with a TA stapler, the specimen needs to be transected with scissors or a scalpel.
2. Linear staplers, most commonly referred to as gastro-intestinal anastomosis (GIA) staplers, are similar to the TA staplers but have an additional cutting mechanism for transection. Three rows of staples are placed on either side of the cut. This type of stapler is ideal for laparoscopic bowel resection.
3. End-to-end anastomosis (EEA) staplers are circular cutting staplers that place several rows of staples on both cut ends as well.

While the individual staples are almost always made of titanium, staplers come in a variety of configurations and lengths for open and laparoscopic procedures. Staplers can also accommodate different cartridges to handle different tissue thickness. Cartridges are preloaded with staples and color coded by the manufacturer to indicate the height of the staples. Typical staple heights range from 2 mm for thin, vascular tissue (e.g., mesentery) to 4.1 mm for thick tissue (e.g., inflamed bowel/colon). The typical staple height used for the majority of bowel resection/anastomosis procedures is 3.5 mm.

Linear Stapled Anastomosis

Side-to-side stapled reconstructions start with sharply removing a portion of the staple line near the antimesenteric border if a stapler has been used to transect the bowel. This also allows bowel viability to be assessed; brisk bleeding from the cut edge implies adequate perfusion for the reconstruction.

The GIA stapler is then introduced into each end of the bowel. Cartridge length is left to the surgeon's discretion, but typically utilizes is a 60-mm load when performing a stapled anastomosis. Using one hand, the bowel is manipulated so that the antimesenteric borders of the bowel are included in the jaws of the stapler as they close. This helps ensure that the anastomosis is perfectly centered on the antimesenteric border of the bowel, which maximizes perfusion.

The stapler is closed, and bowel inspected to ensure that no other intra-abdominal contents have been inadvertently caught by the stapler. Once this is confirmed, a reinforcing silk "crotch" stich may be placed at the distal end of the anastomosis as this area is subject to the most tension. The stapler is then fired. It is then removed and the newly created common channel is inspected for hemostasis with a ring forceps. Interrupted sutures can be used to control larger bleeders from the staple line, though most oozing will be self-limited.

Nowadays, the braided absorbable suture is used to close the common enterotomy in an interrupted fashion. Full-thickness bites are used, taking care to invert the mucosa. The staple lines should be offset to minimize the potential ischemic area.

Patient Positioning and Operating Room Setup

The patient is placed supine in a modified lithotomy position using Dan Allen stirrups. Surgery is begun in the Trendelenburg position (20° head-down tilt) and, after cannula insertion, the patient is tilted left side down for ileal surgery or the right side down for jejunal surgery **(Fig. 1)**.

After insertion of the port, the surgeon stands between the legs. The scrub nurse should stand on the right side of the patient near the knee. The assistant stands on the right side of the surgeon, one monitor is placed close to the patient's right shoulder, and the second monitor is situated near the left shoulder, the best location for viewing by the nurse.

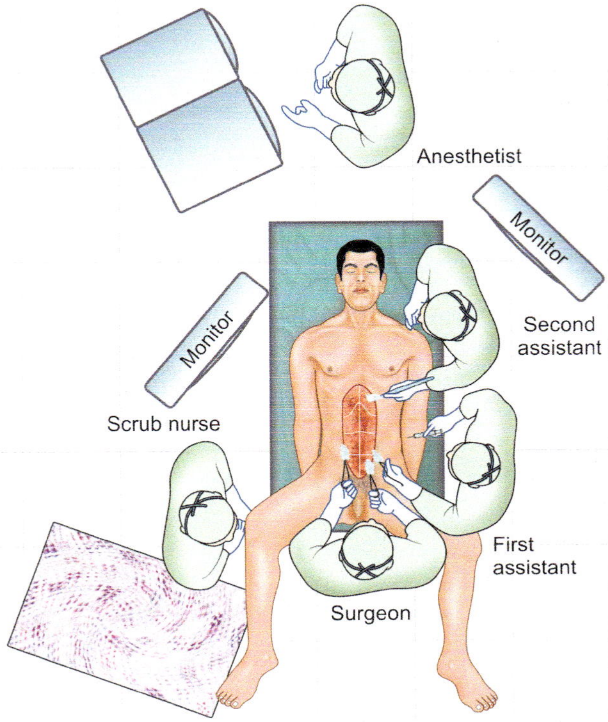

Fig. 1: Position of the surgical team for ileal resection.

Port Position

Port should be positioned according to the baseball diamond concept and should be opposite to the site of pathology.

For jejunal surgery, the left- and right-sided cannulae may suffice. For ileal surgery, it may be preferable to use the suprapubic cannula **(Fig. 2)**.

Operative Technique

Once the preoperative diagnosis is confirmed and the surgeon is confident that laparoscopic procedure appears feasible, the pathology is located by walk over the entire length of the small intestine and placing a suture just upstream of the pathology.

Walk over the small bowel is accomplished from proximal to distal by placing the patient on the left side up, in slight reverse Trendelenburg position until the mid-small bowel is reached, then adjusting the patient to the right side up with Trendelenburg position to run the distal half of the small intestine.

The surgeon should start the "walk over" from between the legs then switch to the left side of the patient for the distal half. The technique of inspection should be "hand-over-hand" or "hand-to-hand" **(Figs. 3A to D)** based on the degree of freedom present within the abdominal cavity.

If it is advantageous to divide the mesenteric vessels before delivery of the specimen through the abdominal incision, this should ideally be done using LigaSure **(Fig. 4)**.

The main vessel supplying the affected segment can also be ligated, leaving the other vessels of the mesentery to be divided through the incision. This may be especially helpful in a patient with a thick abdominal wall. Once the specimen is fully mobilized, a port site is enlarged to 3–5 cm. For small incisions, a transverse incision is preferred. The anterior rectus sheath is transversely incised, the rectus muscles retracted, and the posterior sheath also transversely incised. If the incision has to be larger because of a bulky tumor, a midline longitudinal incision in the midline is accomplished above and below the umbilicus.

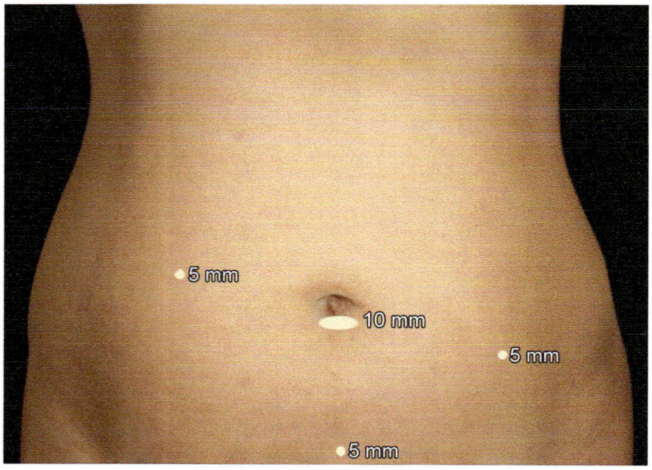

Fig. 2: Position of the cannulae for ileal resection.

The wound is protected using a plastic sheath, and the loop of intestine to be resected is drawn out through the enlarged incision **(Figs. 5A and B)**. Wound protection is important to reduce any contamination by tumor cells or intestine, and it may also facilitate the specimen extraction. The resection and anastomosis are then made in a standard manner extracorporeally, either by a hand-sewn or stapled method. The mesenteric defect is usually closed with a running absorbable suture through the incision **(Figs. 6A and B)**.

After performing the anastomosis, the abdomen is copiously irrigated with warm sterile saline solution through the incision. The fluid is removed by placing the patient in the head-up position and passing a sump suction cannula into the pelvis. After the irrigation of the peritoneal cavity, the abdominal wall is closed with a running suture or a single series suture.

The most important steps of laparoscopically-assisted small bowel surgery are to localize and mobilize the diseased segment and deliver it through a small incision of hand port. The laparoscopic technique has become the procedure of choice for isolated benign small diseases. The intracorporeal

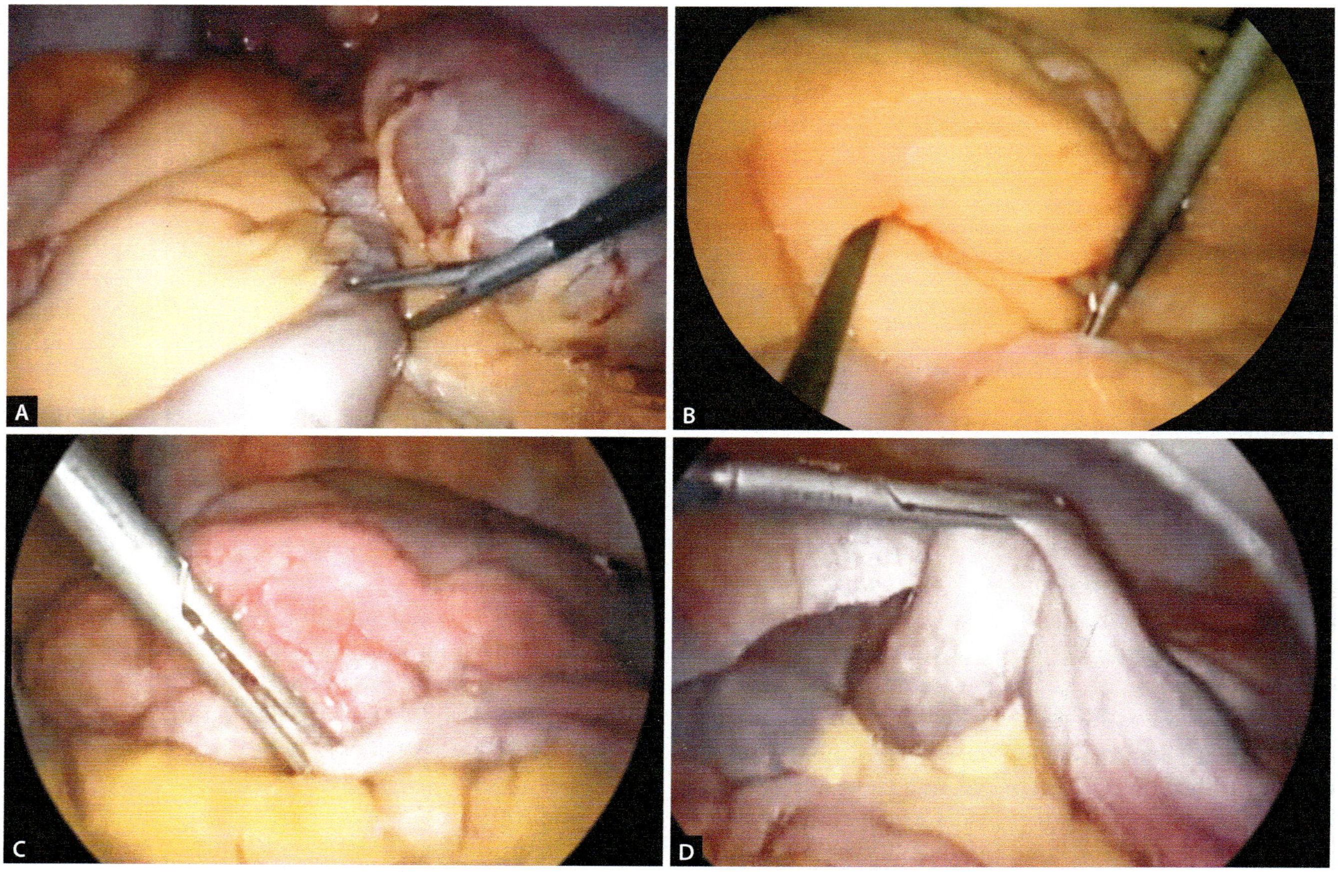

Figs. 3A to D: Walk over to small intestine in order to detect pathology.

anastomosis can also be attempted but extracorporeal anastomosis is more popular at this time because most of the dissection and anastomosis can safely be performed using conventional techniques through a small incision used to remove the specimen.

The role of this approach in cancer surgery is limited. If there is the diffuse spread of the disease, then it may be reasonable to consider a laparoscopic localization of the tumor in order to minimize the incision, or to consider only biopsy and no resection. Because these are rare tumors, and there is no proof yet of the efficacy of a laparoscopic approach.

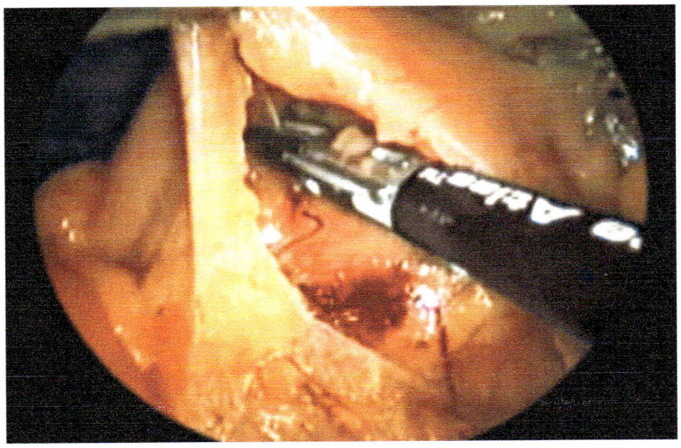

Fig. 4: Dissection mesentery by the help of LigaSure.

ILEOCOLECTOMY

Indications

An ileocolectomy is most frequently indicated in patients with benign disease, i.e., Crohn's disease, cecal diverticulitis, intestinal tuberculosis, enteric Behçet's disease, submucosal tumors (lipoma, gastrointestinal stromal tumor, lymphoma, carcinoid, etc.), giant villous adenoma and polyps, located in the ileocecal regions. Indications for performing a limited ileocecal resection for malignancies of the terminal ileum, the appendix, or the cecum are rare. This may be the procedure of choice in palliative resection for cecal cancer. Before the surgery for Crohn's disease, patients should have a computed tomography scan, small bowel series, and a full colonoscopy to assess the localization and dimension of any phlegmon or abscess or the presence of small bowel stricture or fistula, respectively. The preoperative computed tomography scan

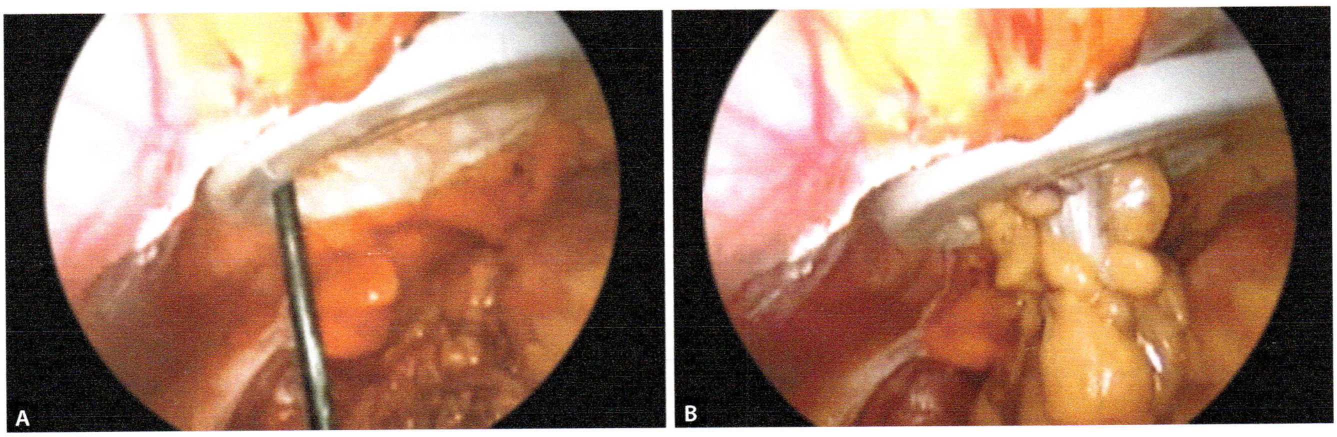

Figs. 5A and B: Loop of intestine to be resected is drawn out through wound protector.

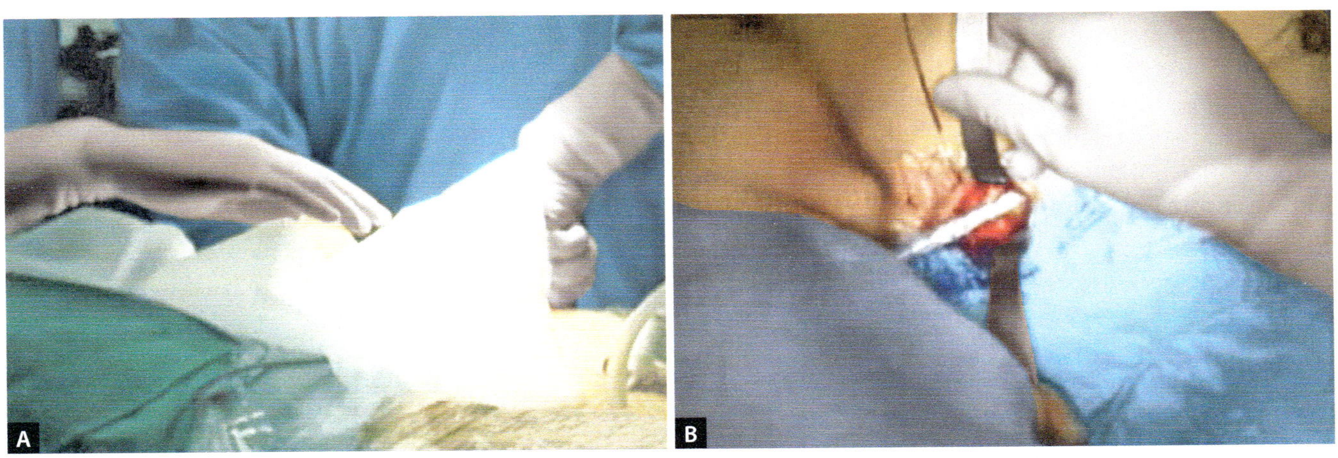

Figs. 6A and B: Resection and anastomosis in a standard manner extracorporeally.

is also useful to evaluate periureteral inflammation and to aid in the decision to use intraoperative ureteric catheters. Preoperative enteral or parenteral nutritional support should be considered in selected patients.

Most surgeons would agree that the laparoscopic approach is contraindicated in patients with nonlocalized intra-abdominal abscesses, multiple previous bowel operations with possible dense adhesions, fixed mass with multiple fistulas, acute intestinal obstruction, and perforation. Although the entire operation can be performed laparoscopically, most surgeons prefer a laparoscopic-assisted procedure by laparoscopic mobilization and extracorporeal resection and anastomosis.

Operative Technique

The patient is placed in the Trendelenburg position, and three or four ports are inserted according to baseball diamond concept. For establishment of pneumoperitoneum, CO_2 is channeled through the infraumbilical trocar until the intra-abdominal pressure reaches 12 mm Hg. Both the operating surgeon and camera holder stand on the patient's left side. After abdominal exploration, the operation table is rotated left side down so the small intestine falls toward the left upper quadrant.

The ascending colon is thoroughly mobilized from the base of the appendix up to the hepatic flexure by cutting the retroperitoneal attachments with electrosurgical scissors and laparoscopic coagulating shears, and bluntly dissecting the retroperitoneal fusion fascia and loose connective tissue. With this procedure, the duodenum, Gerota's fascia, and sometimes more inferiorly the right ureter and the gonadal vessels become visible beneath the retroperitoneal fusion fascia. During dissection, the direct grasping and handling of diseased bowel loops should be avoided, to prevent incidental myotomies and enterotomies.

In patients of Crohn's disease with ileovesical, ileorectal, and gastrocolic fistulas, division with an intracorporeal stapling device by one or two firings of the 45 or 60 mm stapler can be done. After mobilization of the entire ascending colon, meticulous hemostasis is ensured. Then, the patient is placed in a reversed Trendelenburg position temporarily and the abdomen is irrigated with warm sterile saline. Finally patient is placed in a flat supine position, and pneumoperitoneum is released.

To exteriorize the bowel loop a small laparotomy is performed through a 5 cm long skin incision made at the umbilical trocar site or through a Pfannenstiel incision. A wound protector is inserted and the segments of the colon are delivered through this incision. Mesenteric division, ileocolic resection, and anastomosis by Gambee's procedure using 4-0 absorbable sutures, or functional EEA using linear staplers are performed extracorporeally. After closure of the mesenteric defect, the entire residual small bowel is examined through the incision, and drain tube is left in cul-de-sac through the right lateral trocar site if necessary, and every trocar site incision is closed with skin staplers.

Laparoscopic-assisted approach, with an extracorporeal anastomosis, rather than an entirely laparoscopic approach with an intracorporeal anastomosis is more popular. Laparoscopic-assisted approach provides the benefits of laparoscopic surgery while maintaining the advantages of open bowel division and anastomosis, i.e., speed and low risk of intra-abdominal stool spillage. Laparoscopic small bowel surgery for benign conditions continues to evolve. When performed by surgeons with adequate experience, laparoscopic surgery seems to demonstrate advantages over conventional operations. We believe at this time that laparoscopic ileocolectomy should be considered the first-line surgical option for most primary resections for Crohn's disease localized to the ileocolic region.

BIBLIOGRAPHY

1. Altman DG. Practical Statistics for Medical Research. London, England: Chapman and Hall; 1991.
2. American Thoracic Society. Standardization of spirometry: 1987 update. Am Rev Respir Dis. 1987;136:1285-98.
3. Azagra JS, Goergen M, Gilbart E, Jacobs D, Lejeune P, Carlier E. Anterior resection: The total laparoscopic approach. In: Monson JRT, Darzi A (Eds). Laparoscopic Colorectal Surgery. Oxford, England: Isis Medical Media; 1995. pp. 38-55.
4. Bartlett RH, Brennan ML, Gazzaniga AL, Hanson EL. Studies on the pathogenesis and prevention of postoperative pulmonary complications. Surg Gynecol Obstet. 1973;137:925-33.
5. Beecher HK. The measured effect of laparotomy on the respiration. J Clin Invest. 1933;12:639-50.
6. Benhamou D, Simonneau G, Poynard T, Goldman M, Chaput JC, Duroux P. Diaphragm function is not impaired by pneumoperitoneum after laparoscopy. Arch Surg. 1993;128:430-2.
7. Berstein MA, Dawson JW, Reissman P, Weiss EG, Nogueras JJ, Wexner SD. Is complete laparoscopic colectomy superior to laparoscopic assisted colectomy? Am Surg. 1996;62:507-11.
8. Böhm B, Nouchirvani K, Hucke HP, Stock W. Morbidity and mortality after elective resections of colorectal cancers [in German]. Langenbecks Arch Chir. 1991;376:93-101.
9. Bonnet F, Blery C, Zatan M, Simonet O, Brage D, Gaudy J. Effect of epidural morphine on post-operative pulmonary dysfunction. Acta Anaesthesiol Scand. 1984;28:147-51.
10. Chen HH, Wexner SD, Weiss EG, Nogueras JJ, Alabaz O, Iroatulam AJ, et al. Laparoscopic colectomy for benign colorectal disease is associated with a significant reduction in disability as compared with laparotomy. Surg Endosc. 1998;12:1397-400.
11. Christensen EF, Schultz P, Jensen OV. Postoperative pulmonary complications and lung function in high-risk patients: a comparison of three physiotherapy regimens after upper abdominal surgery in general anesthesia. Acta Anaesthesiol Scand. 1991;35:97-104.
12. Craig DB. Postoperative recovery of pulmonary function. Anesth Analg. 1981;60:46-52.
13. Dean PA, Beart RW, Nelson H, Elftmann TD, Schlinkert RT. Laparoscopic assisted segmental colectomy: early Mayo Clinic experience. Mayo Clin Proc. 1994;69:834-40.
14. Duepree HJ, Senagore AJ, Delaney CP, Brady KM, Fazio VW. Advantages of laparoscopic resection for ileocecal Crohn's disease. Dis Colon Rectum. 2002;45:605-10.

15. Dureuil B, Cantineau JP, Desmonts JM. Effects of upper or lower abdominal surgery on diaphragmatic function. Br J Anaesthiol. 1987;59:1230-5.
16. Dureuil B, Viires N, Cantineau JP, Aubier M, Desmonts JM. Diaphragmatic contractility after upper abdominal surgery. J Appl Physiol. 1986;61:1775-80.
17. Erice F, Fox GS, Salib YM, Romano E, Meakins JL, Magder SA. Diaphragmatic function before and after laparoscopic cholecystectomy. Anesthesiology. 1993;79:966-75.
18. Ford GT, Whitelaw WA, Rosenal TW, Cruse PJ, Guenter CA. Diaphragm function after upper abdominal surgery in humans. Am Rev Respir Dis. 1983;127:431-6.
19. Franklin ME, Rosenthal D, Norem RF. Prospective evaluation of laparoscopic colon resection versus open colon resection for adenocarcinoma. Surg Endosc. 1995;9:811-6.
20. Frazee RC, Roberts JW, Okeson GC, Symmonds RE, Snyder SK, Hendricks JC, et al. Open versus laparoscopic cholecystectomy: a comparison of postoperative pulmonary function. Ann Surg. 1991;213:651-4.
21. Gunnarsson L, Tokics L, Gustavsson H, Hedenstierna G. Influence of age on atelectasis formation and gas exchange impairment during general anaesthesia. Br J Anaesth. 1991;66:423-32.
22. Hansen G, Drablos PA, Steinert R. Pulmonary complications, ventilation and blood gases after upper abdominal surgery. Acta Anaesthesiol Scand. 1977;21:211-5.
23. Hansen O, Schwenk W, Hucke HP, Stock W. Colorectal stapled anastomoses: experiences and results. Dis Colon Rectum. 1996;39:30-6.
24. Hedenstierna G. Mechanisms of postoperative pulmonary dysfunction. Acta Chir Scand Suppl. 1989;550:152-8.
25. Hendolin H, Lahtinen J, Lansimies E, Tuppurainen T, Partanen K. The effect of thoracic epidural analgesia on respiratory function after cholecystectomy. Acta Anaesthesiol Scand. 1987;31:645-51.
26. Kanellos I, Zarogilidis K, Ziogas E, Dadoukis I. Prospektiv-vergleichende Studie der Lungenfunktion nach laparoskopischer, Mini-Lap oder konventioneller Cholezystektomie. Minim Invasive Chir. 1995;4:169-71.
27. Kum CK, Eypasch E, Aljaziri A, Troidl H. Randomized comparison of pulmonary function after the "French" and "American" techniques of laparoscopic cholecystectomy. Br J Surg. 1996;83:938-41.
28. Latimer RG, Dickmann M, Day EC. Ventilatory pattern and pulmonary complications after upper abdominal surgery determined by preoperative and postoperative computerized spirometry and blood gas analysis. Am J Surg. 1971;122: 622-32.
29. Lindberg P, Gunnarsson L, Tokics L, et al. Atelectasis and lung function in the postoperative period. Acta Anaesthesiol Scand. 1992;36:546-53.
30. Ludwig KA, Milson JW, Church JM, Fazio VW. Preliminary experience with laparoscopic intestinal surgery for Crohn's disease. Am J Surg. 1996;171:52-6.
31. Marshall BE, Wyche MQ Jr. Hypoxemia during and after anesthesia. Anesthesiology. 1972;37:178-209.
32. McMahon AJ, Baxter JN, Kenney G, O'Dwyer PJ. Ventilatory and blood gas changes during laparoscopic and open cholecystectomy. Br J Surg. 1993;80:1252-4.
33. Milsom JW, Bohm B. Laparoscopic Colorectal Surgery. New York, NY: Springer-Verlag NY Inc; 1996.
34. Milsom JW, Hammerhofer KA, Bohm B, Marcello P, Elson P, Fazio VW. Prospective, randomized trial comparing laparoscopic vs conventional surgery for refractory ileocolic Crohn's disease. Dis Colon Rectum. 2001;44:1-9.
35. Milson JW, Lavery IC, Bohm B, Fazio VW. Laparoscopically assisted ileocolectomy in Crohn's disease. Surg Laparosc Endosc. 1993;3:77-80.
36. Msika S, Iannelli A, Deroide G, Jouët P, Soulé JC, Kianmanesh R, et al. Can laparoscopy reduce hospital stay in the treatment of Crohn's disease? Dis Colon Rectum. 2001;44:326-31.
37. Peters WR. Laparoscopic total proctocolectomy with creation of ileostomy for ulcerative colitis: report of two cases. J Laparoendosc Surg. 1992;2:175-81.
38. Rademaker BM, Ringers J, Odoom JA, de Wit LT, Kalkman CJ, Oosting J. Pulmonary function and stress response after laparoscopic cholecystectomy: comparison with subcostal incision and influence of thoracic epidural analgesia. Anesth Analg. 1992;75:381-5.
39. Rinnert-Gongora S, Tartter PI. Multivariate analysis of recurrence after anterior resection for colorectal carcinoma. Am J Surg. 1989;157:573-6.
40. Sardinha TC, Wexner SD. Laparoscopy for inflammatory bowel disease: pros and cons. World J Surg. 1998;22:370-4.
41. Schauer PR, Luna J, Ghiatas AA, Glen ME, Warren JM, Sirinek KR. Pulmonary function after laparoscopic cholecystectomy. Surgery. 1993;114:389-99.
42. Schoetz DJ, Bockler M, Rosenblatt MS, Malhotra S, Roberts PL, Murray JJ, et al. "Ideal" length of stay after colectomy: whose ideal? Dis Colon Rectum. 1997;40:806-10.
43. Senagore AJ, Lutchfeled MA, Mackeigan JM, Maizer WP. Open colectomy versus laparoscopic colectomy: Are there differences? Am Surg. 1993;59:549-53.
44. Simonneau G, Vivien A, Sartene R, Kunstlinger F, Samii K, Noviant Y, et al. Diaphragm dysfunction induced by upper abdominal surgery: role of postoperative pain. Am Rev Respir Dis. 1983;128:899-903.
45. Sprung J, Cheng EY, Nimphius N, Hubmayr RD, Rodarte JR, Kampine JP. Diaphragm dysfunction and respiratory insufficiency after upper abdominal surgery. Plucne Bolesti. 1991;43:5-12.
46. Stage JG, Schulze S, Møller P, Overgaard H, Andersen M, Rebsdorf-Pedersen VB, et al. Prospective randomized study of laparoscopic versus open colonic resection for adenocarcinoma. Br J Surg. 1997;84:391-6.
47. Stocchi L, Nelson H, Young-Fadok TM, Larson DR, Ilstrup DM. Safety and advantages of laparoscopic vs open colectomy in the elderly. Dis Colon Rectum. 2000;43:326-32.
48. Tabet J, Hong D, Kim CW, Wong J, Goodrace R, Anvari M. Laparoscopic versus open bowel resection for Crohn's disease. Can J Gastroenterol. 2001;15:237-42.
49. UICC International Union Against Cancer. TNM Classification of Malignant Tumours. Berlin, Germany: Springer Publishing Co; 1987.
50. Wahba RWM. Perioperative functional residual capacity. Can J Anaesth. 1991;38:384-400.
51. Williams CD, Brenowitz JB. Ventilatory patterns after vertical and transverse upper abdominal incisions. Am J Surg. 1975;130:725-28.
52. Wu JS, Birbaum EH, Kodner IJ, Read TE, Fleshman JW. Laparoscopic-assisted ileocolic resections in patients with Crohn's disease: are abscess, phlegmons, or recurrent disease contraindications? Surgery. 1997;122:682-9.

CHAPTER 26

Laparoscopic Colorectal Surgery

INTRODUCTION

Laparoscopic colon resections are being performed with increasing frequency all over the world. However, the use of minimal access surgery in colorectal surgery has lagged behind its application in other surgical fields. Since the first laparoscopic colectomy was described in 1991, a great deal of controversy has surrounded its use, particularly in the management of colorectal cancer. After the successful introduction of laparoscopic colectomy by Jacobs, laparoscopic surgery for the treatment of colorectal cancer, especially laparoscopic rectal surgery, has been developed considerably. Several new important studies have demonstrated the benefits and safety of laparoscopic colorectal surgery, making it now the preferred approach in the surgical management of many colorectal diseases.

The technique of laparoscopic colectomy has a long learning curve because of the advanced laparoscopic skills it entails. Unlike other laparoscopic procedures, such as the Nissen fundoplication or cholecystectomy, colorectal procedures involve dissection and mobilization of intra-abdominal organs in multiple quadrants. *Tilting of the operating-room table in various positions during an operation uses gravity to allow intra-abdominal organs to fall away from the area of dissection*, providing necessary exposure that would normally be achieved through the use of retractors. Intestinal resection requires laparoscopic ligation of large vessels, mobilization and removal of a long floppy segment of the colon, and restoration of intestinal continuity. Once the colon segment has been thoroughly mobilized and its blood supply divided, a small skin incision is made to exteriorize the colon, then resection and anastomosis are performed extracorporeally, and the rejoined colon is placed back into the abdomen.

The laparoscopic approach continues to gain popularity and has evolved to include not just "pure" laparoscopic techniques but also hand-assist devices. Hand-assisted surgery can be used as a bridge for surgeons who are not completely familiar or facile with laparoscopic techniques, and even for the most experienced laparoscopic surgeons, it is often the preferred technique for surgery involving left-sided pathology **(Figs. 1A and B)**. The use of a hand-assist device provides tactile feedback for the surgeon and shortens operating-room time while still preserving many of the advantages of laparoscopic surgery. By combining laparoscopic surgery with the tactile feedback of a hand-assisted device, surgeons can reduce operating-room time and have a lower procedure conversion rate. The technique involves making an incision the width of a hand and placing a hand-assist device to facilitate laparoscopic dissection. New handport devices make this technique possible without loss of pneumoperitoneum, which is essential for performing laparoscopic procedures. Because an incision

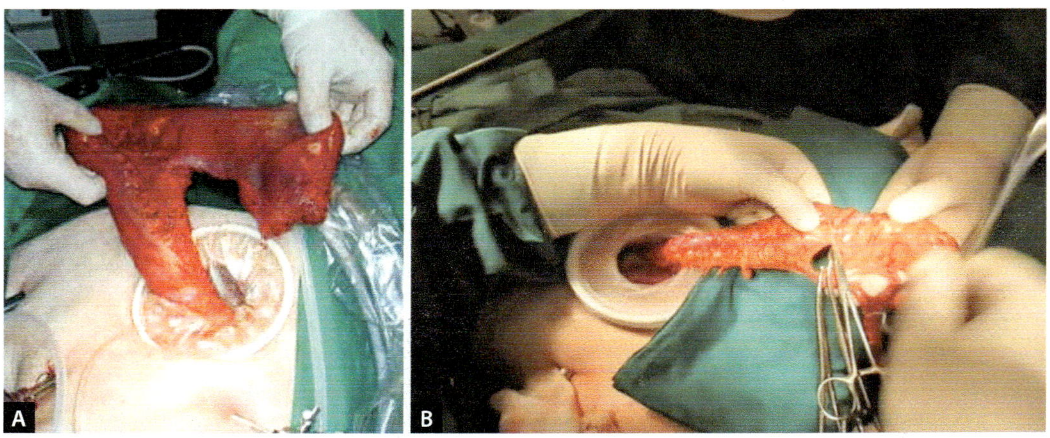

Figs. 1A and B: Hand-assisted colorectal surgery.

(4–5 cm) is necessary to remove the colon specimen at the end of a laparoscopic operation, the difference between a pure laparoscopic procedure and a hand-assisted operation is generally a few additional centimeters (3–4 cm) of incision length. Several clinical trials have demonstrated that there is no difference in patient recovery or discharge for laparoscopic versus hand-assisted techniques. Larger incisions are often needed, and because of the increased risk of wound infections and pulmonary complications, this technique has particular advantages with overweight or obese patients.

Most patients are candidates for a laparoscopic approach. When the surgeon is experienced, even patients with a history of abdominal surgery can form possible candidates. Though there are clear benefits, they have not been as compelling when compared to the clear advantages associated with other laparoscopic procedures. The main reason is that a colectomy, whether open or laparoscopic, results in a delayed return of bowel function. Though recovery of bowel function is quicker after laparoscopic surgery, the difference is on the order of 1 or 2 days, resulting in a similar reduction in length of hospital stay. Also, the laparoscopic approach is associated with longer operating-room times. Even if long-term benefits are equivalent between open and laparoscopic techniques, the short-term benefits are real advantages for patients. In practical terms, the laparoscopic approach is associated with less pain, a faster recovery, earlier return of bowel function, a shorter hospital stay, possible immune benefits, and smaller scars, making it the preferred method for intestinal resection.

The lack of tactile feedback during laparoscopic surgery can make tumor localization difficult, especially if the lesion location has not been tattooed on the colon wall before surgery. It is imperative that the exact location of the tumor is known prior to proceed with colectomy. Even when the lesion location has been tattooed onto the colon, often the mark can be challenging to see, or there may be confusion regarding the location of the tattoo in relation to the tumor (proximal or distal), which can affect surgical margins. Intraoperative colonoscopy is a way of definitively localizing a lesion and should be available during all laparoscopic colectomies. A traditional colonoscopy uses room air as the insufflating gas, which leads to significant bowel distension and requires clamping of the proximal colon to minimize this effect. Clamping the bowel can lead to injury, and even when it is successfully performed, the degree of distension often makes simultaneous laparoscopic visualization difficult. These problems can be circumvented with the use of CO_2, rather than room air, as the insufflating gas. Because CO_2 is absorbed much more rapidly than room air, bowel distension is minimized and dissipates quickly, making proximal clamping unnecessary. The use of CO_2 allows for laparoscopic and endoscopic procedures to be performed simultaneously, and this technique has been shown to be safe and clinically useful. Besides tumor localization, CO_2 colonoscopy may have other potential applications.

PORT-SITE METASTASIS

In the early experience of laparoscopic colectomy for cancer, a few reports described immediate tumor recurrence at the laparoscopic incision sites, referred to as port site recurrences **(Figs. 2A and B)**. It was hypothesized that such early cancer recurrence happened after laparoscopy due to tumor shedding and/or accelerated tumor growth, secondary to the presence of gas in the peritoneal cavity. However, multiple reviews have indicated that this is not the case. In one such study, which included over 2,600 cases, the rate of port-site recurrence was approximately 1%, which is similar to that noted in open colorectal surgery. It is not currently believed that laparoscopic colectomy is associated with early wound recurrences.

Port-site implantation was a concern in the early period, but it has been shown now that it can be prevented by:

- Proper protection of port site while delivering the specimen. (Endobags® and pouches).
- Avoid squeezing of the specimen by taking a liberal incision.

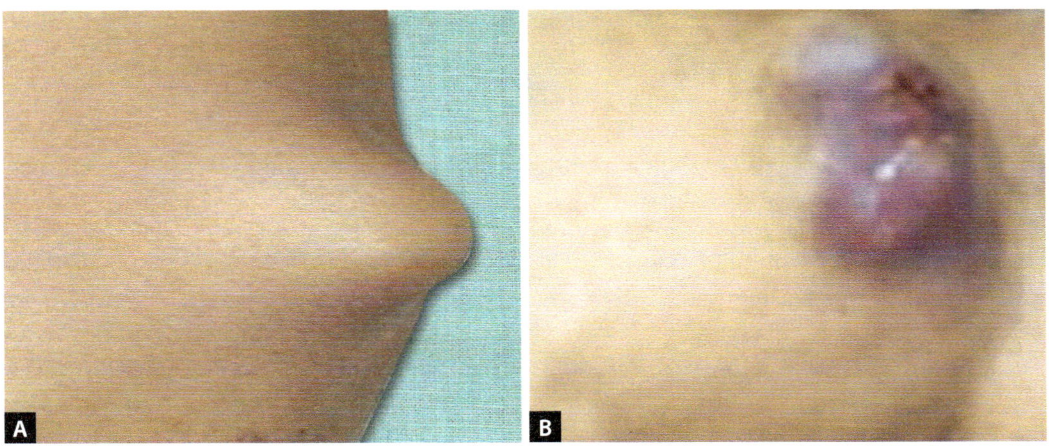

Figs. 2A and B: Port-site metastasis after laparoscopic surgery.

- Thorough wash to the wound, 5FU solution irrigation of all ports
- Slow-release of pneumoperitoneum
- Lap-lift technique

The cost can be brought down by either doing a hand-sewn anastomosis through the specimen delivery site or use of conventional stapler for extracorporeal stapled anastomosis. Minimal use of disposable ports and instruments can further cut down the cost. The use of ultrasonic energy sources in the form of harmonic shears (Ethicon® and USSC®) has added to some of the cost of lap surgery.

The two burning issues are port-site metastasis in malignancies and cost factor due to the use of endo staplers. As mentioned earlier, for a benign condition such as rectal prolapse, adenomas, rectal polyposis, and inflammatory condition such as tuberculosis, ulcerative colitis, and simple diverticulitis, laparoscopic surgery offers a patient-friendly technique. Crohn's disease, though not very common in India, laparoscopy can be offered for the diagnosis, lymph node sampling, and curative resection. Ileocecal tuberculosis is commonly seen in our country, and it is an excellent option to provide the benefits of laparoscopy to these patients whenever surgery is indicated. Incidental colonic resection is unlikely to help the laparoscopic surgeon team in mastering the techniques. The reduction of OT time due to better coordination and cost-benefit to patients can only be offered by repetitive performances. A dedicated team effort will surely bring this specialty under the umbrella of minimal access surgery as has happened in the western world.

BOWEL PREPARATION IN COLORECTAL SURGERY

Though widely accepted as sensible and logical, it has never been subjected to any stringent scrutiny. The ideal method of mechanical preparation should be simple, inexpensive, without distress, and side effects to the patient. However, such an ideal method does not exist. It must be chosen with respect to patient acceptability, efficiency and influence on fluid and electrolyte imbalance and fecal microflora. The conventional method involves a 3-day regimen consisting of low residue and clear liquid diet combined with purgation using laxatives and enemas. Although satisfactory in bowel cleansing in about 70% of patients, it is rather exhausting due to reduced calorie intake. It is time-consuming and may result in dehydration if the patient drinks an inadequate amount of fluids. These disadvantages stimulated the development of more reliable, efficient, and quicker methods, which are given in the following text.

Elemental Diets

Low residue liquid or elemental diets were used with the intention that nutrients could be absorbed in the small intestine. Although, these results in low fecal bulk, satisfactory cleansing is obtained in only 17% of the patients. Nausea and vomiting can occur, and the evidence does not favor elemental diets as a sole means of bowel preparation.

Whole-gut Irrigation

Saline: Normal saline is instilled through a nasogastric tube at a constant rate of 50–70 mL/min in 4 hours, requiring a total of 10–14 L of fluid. Cleansing effect is achieved in 90% of the patients; however, the concentration of colonic bacteria is not reduced unless antibiotics are added. Many patients complain of abdominal distension, nausea, and vomiting. Other drawbacks of this method include the large volume of irrigants, need of nasogastric tube, risk of electrolyte disturbance and water retention, and nursing care required to assist the patient. It is contradicted in patients with gastrointestinal obstruction, perforation, and toxic colitis and has to be used with caution in patients with cardiac problems.

Castor oil: It (30–60 mL) orally achieves good cleansing but requires a large volume of magnesium citrate purgative to achieve the desired results and requires to be given 2 days before surgery followed by anal washouts a day prior which entails preoperative admissions for 3–4 days. Unpalatabilty is another drawback.

Mannitol: Mannitol is a nonabsorbable oligosaccharide which acts as an osmotic agent by pulling fluid into the bowel and producing a purgative effect by irritating the colon. Being a sugar, it is quite palatable and can be flavored by mixing it with fruit juice. Usually, 4 L of 5% solution is consumed over 4 hours, which can be difficult and can result in abdominal discomfort and nausea. To avoid these side effects, hypertonic solutions (10–20%) can be used but these predispose to dehydration and electrolyte losses. Overall, good cleansing is produced in about 80% of the patients, but leads to a high wound infection rate probably by acting as a bacterial nutrient and production of explosive gases as a result of fermentation into methane and hydrogen by anaerobic bacteria is seen. The same can be overcome by using of an antibiotic.

Polyethylene glycol (PEG): To overcome the drawbacks of mannitol, PEG (PEGLEC) in a balanced electrolyte solution was introduced which also acts as an osmotic purgative **(Fig. 3)**.

To achieve satisfactory cleansing in >90% of the patients, an average of 2–4 L of PEGLEC solution must be ingested with tea and lemon. Studies using PEG have shown a significantly lower incidence of fluid retention and lesser aerobic and anaerobic fecal bacterial counts compared to other agents. It is nowadays used as an agent of choice for preparations of the bowel before endoscopy and colonic surgery in a nonobstructed patient.

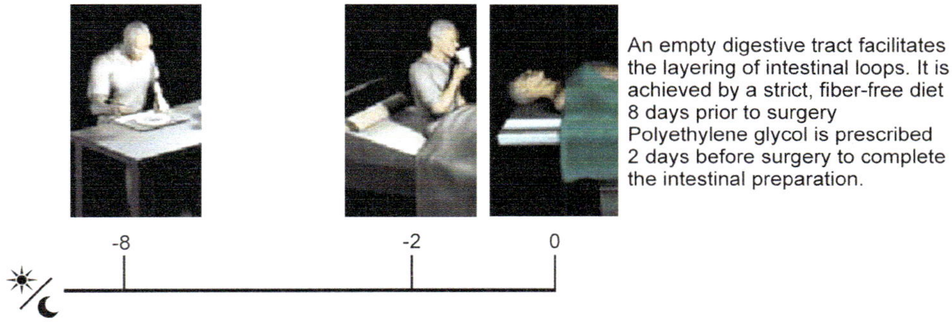

Fig. 3: Bowel preparation in colorectal surgery.

Picolax: It (sodium picosulfate and magnesium citrate) is a stimulant purgative that acts mainly on the left colon after activation by colonic bacteria and on osmotic laxative that cleanses the proximal colon. Two sachets in 2 L of water are administered with dietary restrictions to improve effectiveness. Although acceptable cleansing is achieved in 85% of patients undergoing barium enema and colonoscopy, its efficacy for elective colorectal operations is poorly documented. Picolax is well tolerated but does produces fluid and electrolyte losses.

ANTIBIOTIC BOWEL PREPARATIONS

Mechanical cleansing alone has failed to achieve a significant reduction in the total bacterial load of the colon and, therefore, the associated septic complications. Addition of antibiotics, oral as well as parenteral, to mechanical cleaning has resulted in a significant reduction of the infection rate from 30 to 60% in an uncovered patient to as low as 2–10% in otherwise patients covered with broad-spectrum antibiotics.

Oral Antibiotics

Because the aerobic *Escherichia coli* and the anaerobic *Bacteroides fragilis* are frequently involved organisms in septic complications following colorectal operations; oral antibiotics active against both types of bacteria must be given. Oral administration of erythromycin, neomycin, and metronidazole are popular. Several studies have documented the efficacy of oral antibiotics; however, an antimicrobial used alone without mechanical cleansing has little impact on the postoperative infection rate.

Parenteral Antibiotics

Since parenteral antibiotics are valid only when adequate tissue levels are present at the time of contamination, systemic administration should start immediately before the surgery. A second- or third-generation cephalosporin with metronidazole is the most commonly preferred agent. Studies had shown conflicting results when parenteral antibiotics were compared with oral or both. Whether antibiotics bowel preparation should be oral, systemic, or both are still a controversial issue. The majority of the surgeons would prefer parenteral antibiotics or with concomitant administration of oral antimicrobials together with oral PEGLEC electrolyte solution as the method of choice of preoperative bowel preparation.

Though observational data suggest that mechanical bowel preparation before colorectal surgery reduces fecal mass and bacterial count in the lumen, but the practice has been questioned because the bowel preparation liquefies feces, which could increase the risk for intraoperative spillage, and may be associated with bacterial translocation and electrolyte disturbance. Though commonly practiced without the benefit of evidence from randomized trials, and two of three meta-analyses suggest a higher rate of anastomotic leakage with mechanical bowel preparation thus calling for an end to the practice of mechanical bowel preparation in view of the possible disadvantages of this practice, patient discomfort, and the absence of clinical value. There are others who accept that though routine preoperative bowel cleansing is no longer justified prior to colorectal surgery in general, they call for further evaluation in cases such as total mesorectal resection with low anastomosis where it may still have a role and therefore to consider each case carefully, otherwise the chance of making an inappropriate decision exists with significant consequences for patients.

The majority of surgeons believe that patients should have a standard bowel preparation 48 hours before the operation and should receive a single-dose antibiotic dose immediately preoperatively. For the bowel preparation, patients follow a strictly fiber-free diet eight days before surgery and take a sodium phosphate oral solution the day before surgery. This method is very useful because it ensures an empty digestive tract and a flat small bowel, which facilitates the layering of intestinal loops, a crucial point for achieving adequate exposure. Alternatively, the PEG can be used. In this case, administration 2 days before surgery is preferable to avoid distension of small bowel loops that may be difficult to handle during the surgery.

RIGHT COLECTOMY

A right colectomy or ileocolic resection is the removal of all or part of the right colon and part of the ileum **(Fig. 4)**.

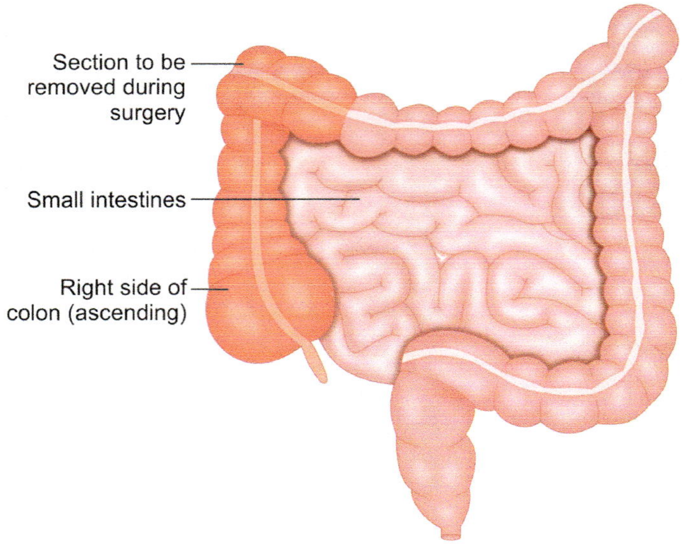

Fig. 4: Section to be removed in right colectomy.

These operations are performed for the removal of cancers, certain non-cancerous growths as well as severe Crohn's disease. If performed by an expert laparoscopic surgeon, laparoscopic right colectomy and ileocolic resection are as safe as "open" surgery in carefully selected cases.

Indications

The advanced laparoscopic skills required for laparoscopic resection of the colon and rectum have precluded wide dissemination of this procedure. By applying certain key principles, laparoscopic right hemicolectomy can be made simple, reproducible, easy to teach, easy to learn, and cost-effective. Although benign tumors not resectable by a colonoscopic procedure and structuring inflammatory bowel disease may be good indications for laparoscopy, they are not so common. The most common disease for right colectomy is right-sided colon cancer. Colon cancer seems to be a good indication for laparoscopic surgery if performed using proper oncologic methods, i.e., early proximal ligation of the major mesenteric vessels and wide mesenteric and intestinal resection with complete lymphadenectomy. For right colectomy, either laparoscopic mobilization of the bowel and/or mesenteric resection, both are performed as for open colectomy, and bowel division and creation of the anastomosis can be performed extracorporeally.

Contraindications

- Patients with complete obstruction caused by the cancer
- Cancer extensively invading adjacent organs
- Bulky cancer >10 cm in size should be excluded.

According to these concepts, a proper oncologic approach using laparoscopy for right colon cancer is described in this chapter.

Equipment and Instruments

One can use the same basic equipment, such as light source, insufflator, 30° angled laparoscope, and 5-mm graspers. To this basic equipment, can be added reusable instruments such as Babcock and alligator clamps, which should be at least 38–40 cm in length to reach from the depths of the pelvis to the upper abdomen using limited port sites. In developing countries, these reusables can be used if necessary but trying to keep disposable equipment to a minimum. Three 10 or 12 mm trocars with stability threads, plus reducers for 5-mm instruments should be used. Cannulas should allow instruments to move through smoothly while maintaining a good seal after multiple instrument passages. An energy source device of one's choice can also be added, such as bipolar, LigaSure™, or harmonic scalpel. Additional disposable equipment is kept readily available in the operating room and used only as needed. These include a clip applier, linear vascular stapler, suction irrigator, and fan retractor.

Patient Positioning and Operating Room Setup

The patient is placed supine, and straps are used to secure the patient during steep table position changes. The patient is fixed in a moldable "bean bag" form with both arms tucked in, and placed in a modified lithotomy position using levitator stirrups **(Figs. 5 and 6)**. A urinary catheter is placed in the bladder, and the stomach is decompressed with a nasogastric tube. Identical operating room personnel is used for the laparoscopic case as for an open right hemicolectomy.

The nurse is on the patient's right. This is also where the assistant stands, with the surgeon on the patient's left side facing the right colon. Hasson (open) technique is preferred to safely insert the first port through the umbilicus. After establishing pneumoperitoneum, the surgeon tries to expose the right mesocolon and to mark the lower border of the ileocolic vessels.

After initial exploration ensures no prohibitive adhesions, two additional 10–12 mm ports are placed under direct visualization, one in the left upper quadrant (in or lateral to the rectus, avoiding the epigastric vessels, approximately a handbreadth from the supraumbilical port) and one in the suprapubic midline. Once all the trocars are in place, the assistant moves to the patient's left side to direct the camera. To start the initial dissection, the surgeon moves between the patient's legs, the assistants position themselves on the patient's left side, and the nurse stands near the patient's right knee. The primary monitor is placed near the patient's right shoulder to give the surgeon and the assistant's optimal viewing **(Fig. 7)**.

The second monitor is placed on the left side close to the head, a location that gives the best view for the nurse.

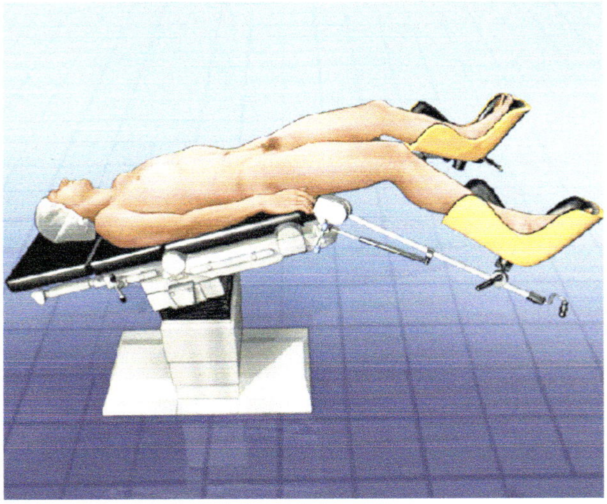

It is essential that the patient be appropriately positioned to avoid complications (nerve and vein compression, injuries to the brachial plexus) and to facilitate the procedure and anesthetic monitoring.
- Trendelenburg position with a 15° to 25° tilt and a 5° to 10° right tilt
- Lithotomy position
- Buttocks placed at the distal edge of the table
- Thighs and legs stretched apart with a slight flexure
- Right arm alongside the body
- Left arm at a right angle or alongside the body (surgeon's preference)
- Gastric tube and urinary catheter
- Heating device

Fig. 5: Position of patient for colorectal surgery.

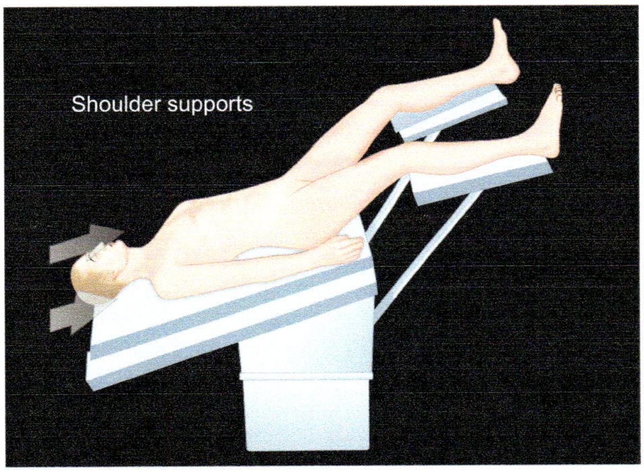

To prevent the patient from sliding, shoulder supports or straps around the thorax may be used.
In our current practice, we rarely use such measures, despite a 20° to 30° Trendelenburg position and a right tilt.

Fig. 6: Shoulder support to prevent sliding during colorectal surgery.

After completing the proximal vessel ligation with lymphadenectomy and mobilization of the terminal ileum and the cecum, the surgeon moves back to the patient's left side, and the first assistant stands between the patient's legs for take-down of right flexure and whole mobilization of the right colon **(Fig. 8)**.

Operative Technique

Right colectomy can be broadly divided in the following steps:
- Ligation of ileocolic vessels
- Identification of right ureter
- Dissection along the superior mesenteric vein
- Division of omentum
- Division of right branch of middle colic vessels
- Transection of the transverse colon
- Mobilization of the right colon
- Transection of the terminal ileum
- Ileocolic anastomosis
- Delivery of specimen

The patient is positioned in Trendelenburg with the right side inclined upward. This allows the small bowel and omentum to fall toward the left upper quadrant, exposing the cecum and assisting in retraction. The omentum and transverse colon are moved toward the upper abdomen, the ventral side of the right mesocolon is well visualized, and the optimal operative field can be achieved. The small bowel is mobilized out of the pelvis by grasping the peritoneum, not bowel wall, near the base of the cecum and pulling cephalad and to the left. The appropriate plane along the base of the small bowel mesentery and around the cecum can be seen and the peritoneum overlying it carefully opened, exposing the correct retroperitoneal plane.

The ureter is identified either before opening the peritoneum in a thin patient or after, being visualized as it courses over the right iliac vessels. Dissection is then continued around the base of the cecum. Moving cephalad and laterally, the white line of Toldt is incised as the right colon is retracted medially and cephalad by grasping the cut edge of the peritoneum, not the bowel.

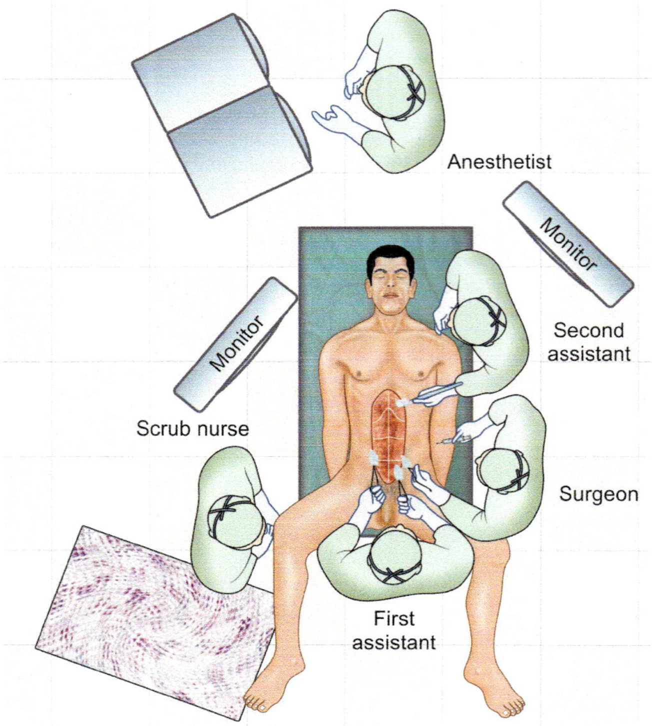

Fig. 7: Position of surgical team during colorectal surgery.

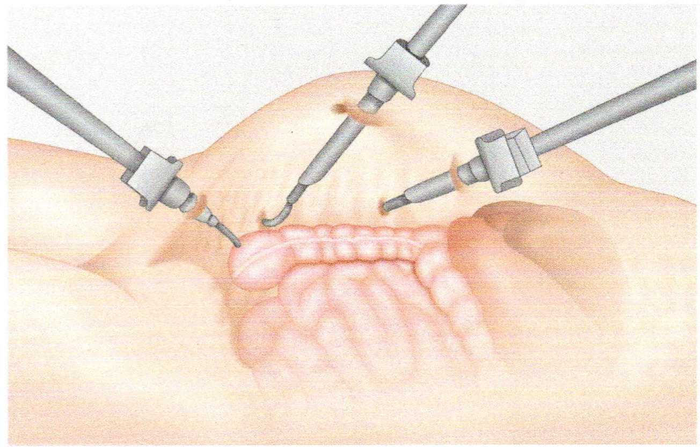

Fig. 8: Mobilization of cecum and right colon.

Before starting the dissection, the ileocolic pedicle must be definitively identified by retracting the right mesocolon. Various approaches, such as lateral-to-medial (lateral approach), medial-to-lateral (medial approach), and retroperitoneal approach, have been documented. The medial approach is quite effective for complete lymphadenectomy with early proximal ligation, minimal manipulation of the tumor-bearing segment, and ideal entry to proper retroperitoneal plane.

Various approaches to the right colon mobilization have been described.

- Lateral to medial ("classic" open approach)
- Medial to lateral approach
- Retroperitoneal approach

It is believed that the medial approach is optimal in order to maintain conventional oncologic principles. First, the mesocolon near the ileocecal junction is lifted to confirm the ileocolic pedicle. The root of the ileocolic pedicle is usually located at the lower border of the duodenum. The independent right colic vessels, if present, are located at the upper border at the duodenum. However, the majority of patients do not have the independent right colic vessels (vessels originating directly from the superior mesenteric artery and vein **(Figs. 9A and B)**. The surgeon should initially stand on the patient's left side to confidently know the ileocolic pedicle from the superior mesenteric vessels, and to mark the lower border of the ileocolic pedicle.

Once the ileocolic pedicle is identified, the surgeon moves between the patient's legs and the scope is inserted through the suprapubic port. The medial side of the right mesocolon is first incised, starting from the previously marked region below the ileocolic pedicle, followed by the incision of the peritoneum over to the superior mesenteric vessels. This is done before mobilization of the right colon. With adequate traction of mesocolon toward the right upper quadrant, the ileocolic vessels are easily mobilized from the subperitoneal fascia leading onto the duodenum. Their origins are identified from the superior mesenteric vessels at the lower border of the duodenum and divided.

The surgeon's first step in the dissection is to mark the inferior border of the ileocolic pedicle. From between the legs, the surgeon dissects the peritoneum overlying the ileocolic vascular pedicle over to the superior mesenteric vessels.

After mobilization of the ileocolic pedicle from the duodenum, the dissection of the ventral side of the superior mesenteric vein (SMV) leads to the dissection of the origin of the ileocolic artery. In type B, the ileocolic artery is running behind the superior mesenteric vein. After mobilization and division of the ileocolic pedicle from the duodenum, the dissection of the ventral side of the SMV leads to a complete dissection of the root of the middle colic artery and vein.

Careful dissection onto the duodenum and the caudad portion of the pancreas must be exercised in the exposure of the middle colic vessels. Dissection around Henle's trunk (the truck of mesenteric veins consisting of the gastroepiploic vein fusing with the right branch of the middle colic vein or the main middle colic vein) may lead to the exposure of an accessory right colic vein. Accessory right colic vein and right branches of middle colic vessels are clipped and divided. However, if an accessory right colic vein is difficult to confirm in this situation, this vein may be easily detected later at the take-down of the right flexure.

After securing the vessels, the operating table is tilted into the steep Trendelenburg position with the right side down to move the small intestine toward the right upper quadrant. After confirming the right ureter and gonadal vessels

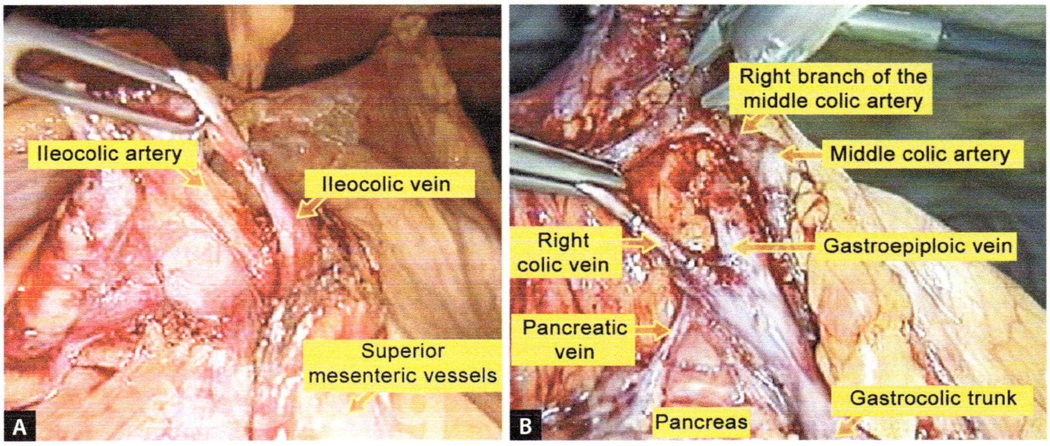

Figs. 9A and B: (A) Position of major blood vessels at the time of surgery; (B) Important vessels supplying right side of colon.

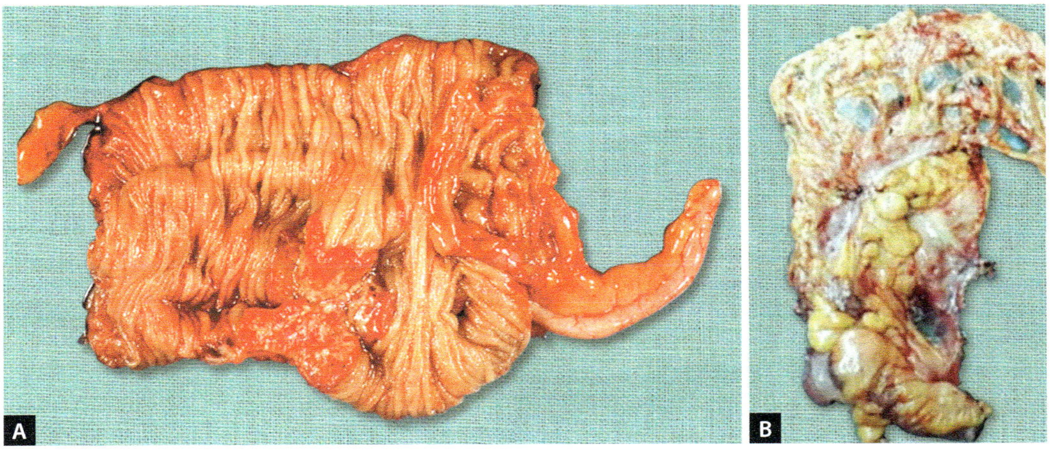

Figs. 10A and B: Specimen of right side of colon after right colectomy.

through the subperitoneal fascia at the right pelvic brim, the peritoneum is incised along the base of the ileal mesentery upward to the duodenum, and the ileocecal region is mobilized medially to lateral. After this mobilization, the surgeon moves back to the patient's left side, and the scope is inserted through the umbilical port. The right mesocolon is mobilized from medial to lateral. Again, this approach allows dissection into the proper retroperitoneal plane. The right gonadal vessels and ureter are safe from injury in this plane, so exposing them is not necessary. This approach also allows the surgeon to work in a straight path from medial to lateral, without tissue to obstruct the vision that can occur while working from lateral to medial. This plane connects the previous dissection plane from the caudad side.

The anatomy around the right flexure is essential to avoid inadvertent bleeding, especially from around Henle's (gastrocolic) trunk. However, if the previous mesenteric dissection is fully performed from the caudad side and the accessory right colic vein is divided, the right flexure is easily taken down only by dividing the hepatotoxic ligament. If the accessory right colic vein is difficult to detect at the previous dissection, it can be easily confirmed from Henle's trunk at this situation and should be divided before extracting the right colon to avoid its injury. Up to this point, the primary tumor has been minimally manipulated using medial to lateral approach. Finally, the right flexure and right colon, including the tumor-bearing segment, are detached laterally, which completes the mobilization of the entire right colon **(Figs. 10A and B)**.

Once the entire right colon is freed, it is withdrawn through an enlargement of the port site at the umbilicus. The wound must be covered with a wound protector to prevent contamination or metastasis. The resection of ileum and transverse colon, and the anastomosis are accomplished extracorporeally by the functional end-to-end anastomotic method using conventional staplers or by a hand-sewn method **(Figs. 11A and B)**. The anastomotic site is returned to the peritoneal cavity. Wounds and peritoneal cavity are copiously irrigated. All wounds are closed, and operation is completed.

The identification of a small tumor in the colon may be difficult even in conventional open surgery. In laparoscopic surgery, where there is no tactile sensation, pre- or intraoperative marking of the tumor is frequently needed.

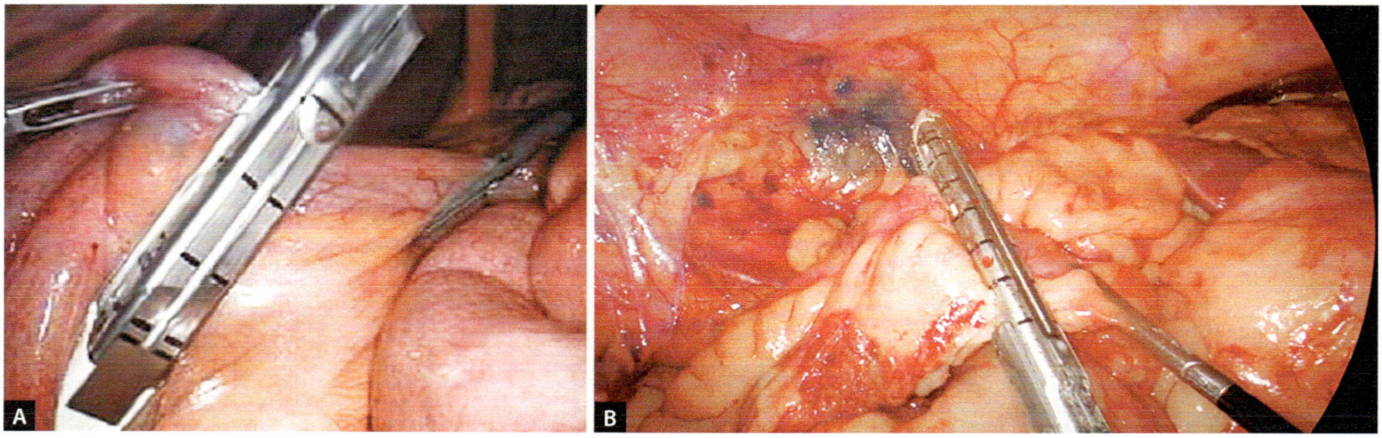

Figs. 11A and B: Transaction of ileum by the stapler.

Various kinds of marking methods are available, e.g., dye injection and mucosal clip placement by preoperative colonoscopy, which has been reported for the tumor localization. Several reports demonstrated the usefulness of tattooing the colonic wall adjacent to the tumor with India ink in four quadrants using preoperative colonoscopy.

However, effective injection in all four points of the bowel is sometimes challenging to achieve. In some cases, surgeons failed to achieve serosal staining visible at laparoscopy, which forced them to use intraoperative colonoscopy. This complicated the laparoscopic colonic resection because of the distended bowel related to air insufflation during colonoscopy.

Conclusion

Right-sided colon cancer can be adequately treated by proper laparoscopic procedures adherent to the oncologic principles. Port-site metastasis after laparoscopic colon cancer surgery is unlikely to be a major risk factor when the procedure is performed according to oncologic principles. It is believed that laparoscopic right colectomy for cancer performed by expert surgeons is accepted as less invasive surgery without sacrificing the survival benefit compared with conventional open right colectomy.

SIGMOIDECTOMY

Laparoscopic sigmoid colon resection is indicated for both benign (diverticulitis, segmental Crohn's disease, polyp unresectable by colonoscopy) and malignant (primary colon cancer) etiologies, and is one of the most common operations done by laparoscopic methods. In chronic diverticular disease, the indications for laparoscopic sigmoid resection are the same as for open surgery. Sigmoid colectomy for diverticulitis can be technically challenging because of severe inflammation in the left lower quadrant and pelvis.

Patient Positioning and Operating Room Setup

A proper patient position is key to both facilitating operative maneuvers and preventing complications such as nerve and vein compression and traction injuries to the brachial plexus. The patient is placed supine, in the modified lithotomy position, with legs abducted and slightly flexed at the knees. The patient's right arm is alongside the body, whereas the left arm is usually placed at a 90° angle. Adequate padding is used to avoid compression on bone prominences.

A nasogastric or orogastric tube and a urinary catheter are placed. Adequate thromboembolism prophylaxis should be used, as preferred by the surgeon, and intermittent leg compression stockings can be used as well. The procedure is usually performed with two assistants and a scrub nurse **(Fig. 12)**. The surgeon is on the right side of the patient, and the second assistant is also on the right side. The first assistant stands between the patient's legs and the scrub nurse at the lower right side of the table. The team remains in the same position throughout the entire procedure. It is advisable to use a table that can be easily tilted laterally and placed into steep Trendelenburg and reverse Trendelenburg position in order to facilitate exposure of the pelvic space and of the splenic flexure. The laparoscopic unit with the main monitor is located on the left side of the table. It is useful to use a second monitor placed above the patient's head.

Cannula Positioning

Standardize cannula placements are five or six cannulae for left-sided colectomies. This allows us to achieve excellent exposure, which may be particularly valuable at the beginning of a surgeon's learning curve. Using six cannulae allows the use of more instruments in the abdominal cavity for retraction of bowel and structures, especially in the presence of abundant intra-abdominal fat or the dilated small bowel, as well as during mobilization of the splenic flexure.

Cannula fixation to the abdominal wall is essential, to avoid CO_2 leakage, and in cases of malignancy, to minimize the passage of tumor cells and help reduce the incidence of port-site metastases. This is mainly achieved by fitting the size of the incision to the cannula size or by fixing the

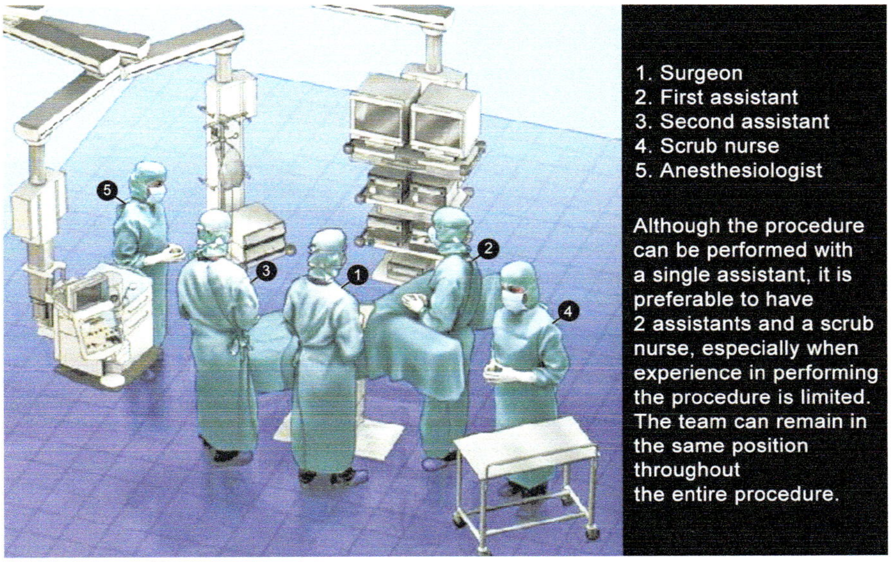

Fig. 12: Position of surgical team in colorectal surgery.

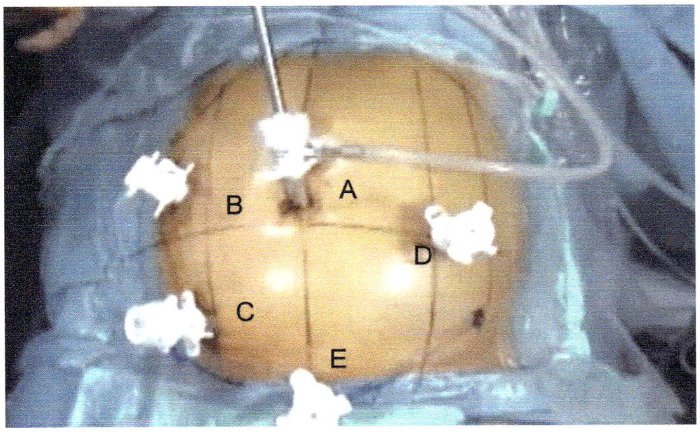

Fig. 13: Port position for sigmoidectomy for benign disease.

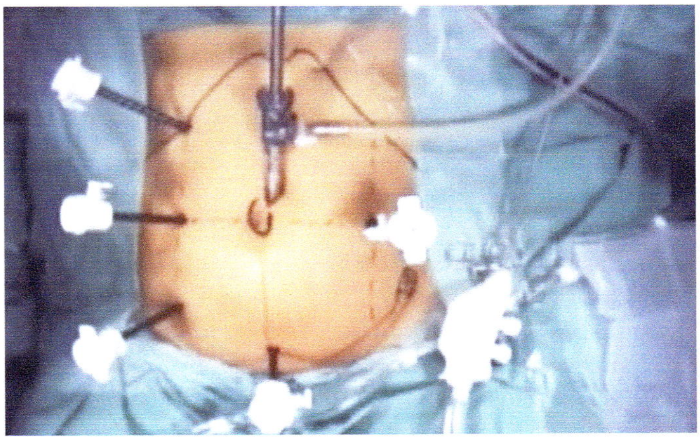

Fig. 14: Alternating port position for sigmoidectomy for malignant disease.

cannula to the abdomen with a suture placed around the stopcock of the cannula. Use of screw-like cannulae has drawbacks that it increases the parietal trauma. Generally, it is better to perform an "open" technique for the insertion of the first cannula, which is placed at the midline, above the umbilicus, to reduce the risk of injury of abdominal organs. With some experience, the task becomes easy and very rapid. However, in the case of previous abdominal surgery, we usually inflate the abdominal cavity using the Veress needle in the left subcostal area, in order to insert the first cannula as far lateral as possible, in the right hypochondrium, to avoid potential areas of adhesions.

The first cannula (12 mm), which is used for the optical device, is positioned on the midline 3–4 cm above the umbilicus. The two operating cannulae are introduced, one at the junction between the umbilical line and the right midclavicular line, and the other 8–10 cm inferiorly, on the same line. The latter is a 12 mm operating cannula to allow the introduction of a linear stapler at the time of bowel resection. This cannula accommodates the following: scissors (monopolar, high-frequency hemostasis device, clip, staplers), a monopolar hook, surgical loops, a suction-irrigation device, and an atraumatic grasper. A fourth cannula is placed on the left midclavicular line at the level of the umbilicus. This is a 5-mm cannula, which accommodates an atraumatic grasper used for retraction and exposure during the medial approach for the dissection of the left mesocolon. When performing mobilization of the splenic flexure, this cannula becomes an operating cannula. A fifth 5-mm cannula is placed 8–10 cm above the pubic bone, on the midline, and is used for retraction **(Figs. 13 and 14)**.

For most of the procedure, it accommodates a grasper used to expose the sigmoid and descending mesocolon. At the end of the procedure, the incision at this cannula's site is lengthened to allow extraction of the specimen. Some surgeons sometimes use an additional cannula, which is a

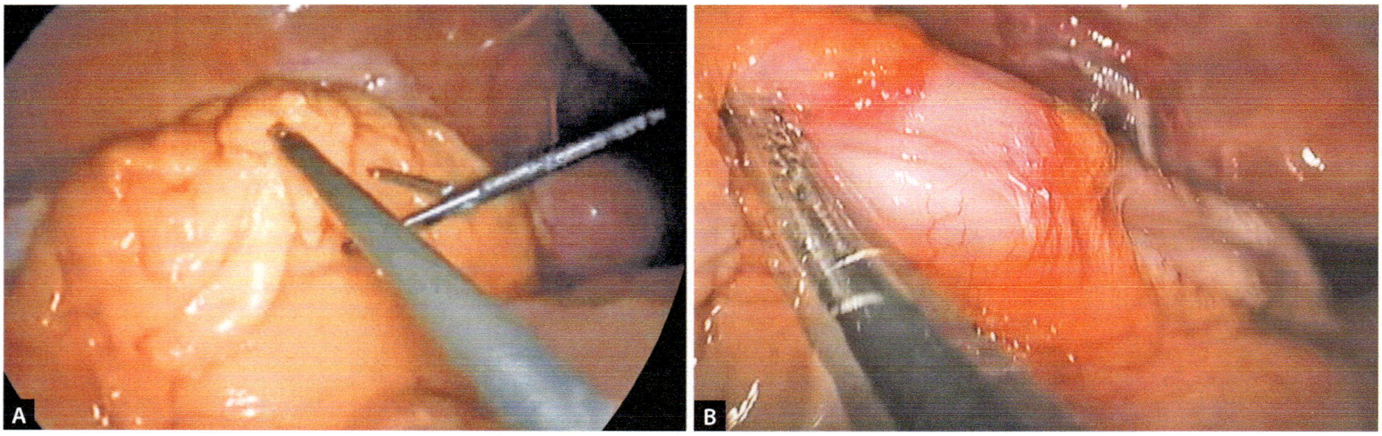

Figs. 15A and B: Exposure of sigmoid colon after shifting the omentum upward.

5 mm cannula situated on the right midclavicular line in the subcostal area and accommodates an atraumatic grasper used to retract the terminal portion of the small intestine laterally at the beginning of the dissection and to retract the transverse colon during the mobilization of the splenic flexure.

Operative Technique

Exposure

To complete exposure of the operative field, active positioning of the bowel is usually necessary in addition to the passive action of gravity, especially in the presence of obesity or bowel dilatation. The greater omentum and the transverse colon are placed in the left subphrenic region and maintained in this position by the Trendelenburg tilt. An atraumatic retractor, introduced through the cannula on the left side, may also be used. Subsequently, the proximal small bowel loops are placed in the right upper quadrant using gentle grasping **(Figs. 15A and B)**.

The distal small bowel loops are placed in the right lower quadrant with the cecum and maintained there with gravity. If gravity is not sufficient, as occurs mainly in the presence of abundant intra-abdominal fat or dilated bowel, an additional maneuver is used. An instrument passed through the right subcostal cannula is passed at the root of the mesentery and grasps the parietal peritoneum of the right iliac fossa; the shaft of the grasper thus provides an autostatic retraction of the bowel loops, keeping them away from the midline and the pelvic space. This technique of exposure offers an excellent view of the sacral promontory and the aortoiliac axis. This particular view on the operative field is essential for the medial-to-lateral vascular approach.

The uterus may be an obstacle to adequate exposure in the pelvis. In postmenopausal women, the uterus can be suspended to the abdominal wall by a suture **(Fig. 16)**. This suture is introduced halfway between the umbilicus and the pubis and opens the rectovaginal space. In younger women, the uterus can be retracted using a similar suspension by a suture around the round ligaments or using a 5-mm

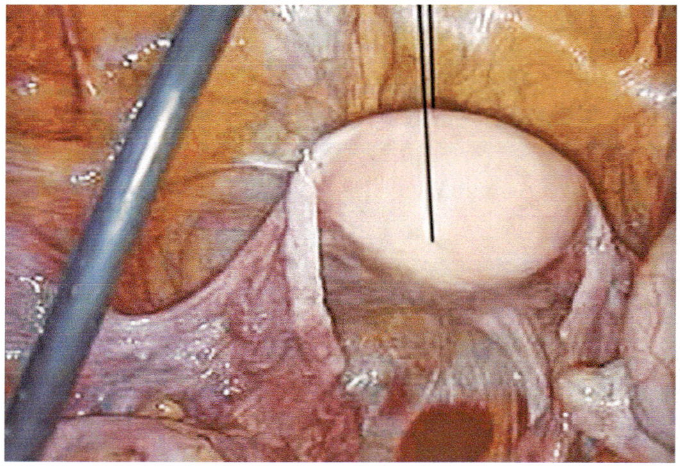

Fig. 16: Securing the uterus by suture for proper exposure of rectum.

retractor passed through the suprapubic cannula. Very often, conversion to open surgery is caused by difficulty in exposure, not only at the beginning but also throughout the procedure.

To perform a medial approach, time is dedicated to the perfect achievement of this exposure, which will serve not only for the initial vascular approach, but also for about half of the remaining operative time. After adequate exposure has been achieved, the following steps of the technique include the vascular approach, the medial posterior mobilization of the sigmoid, the extraction of the specimen, and the anastomosis. Additional steps include the mobilization of the splenic flexure, performed when further lengthening of the bowel is needed to perform a tension-free anastomosis.

This step of the exposure is preliminary, and it is done in a similar manner, regardless of the type of disease. The remainder of the procedure is different if the indication for surgery is cancer or benign disease.

Sigmoid Colon Resection for Cancer

In laparoscopic colorectal sigmoidectomy for cancer or for benign disease, the vascular approach is the first step of the dissection. It is believed that it allows us to avoid unnecessary manipulation of the colon and tumor, which may cause tumor cell exfoliation, and to perform a good lymphadenectomy following the vascular anatomy. The vessels are gradually exposed once the peritoneum at the base of the sigmoid mesocolon is incised **(Figs. 17A and B)**. The medial-to-lateral view allows us to see the sympathetic nerve plexus trunks, the left ureter, and gonadal vessels, avoiding ureteral injuries and possibly preserving genital function.

Primary Vascular Approach (Medial Approach)

Peritoneal Incision

The sigmoid mesocolon is retracted anteriorly, using a grasper introduced through the suprapubic cannula: This exposes the base of the sigmoid mesocolon. The visceral peritoneum is incised at the level of the sacral promontory **(Figs. 18A to D)**. The incision is continued upward along the right anterior border of the aorta up to the ligament of

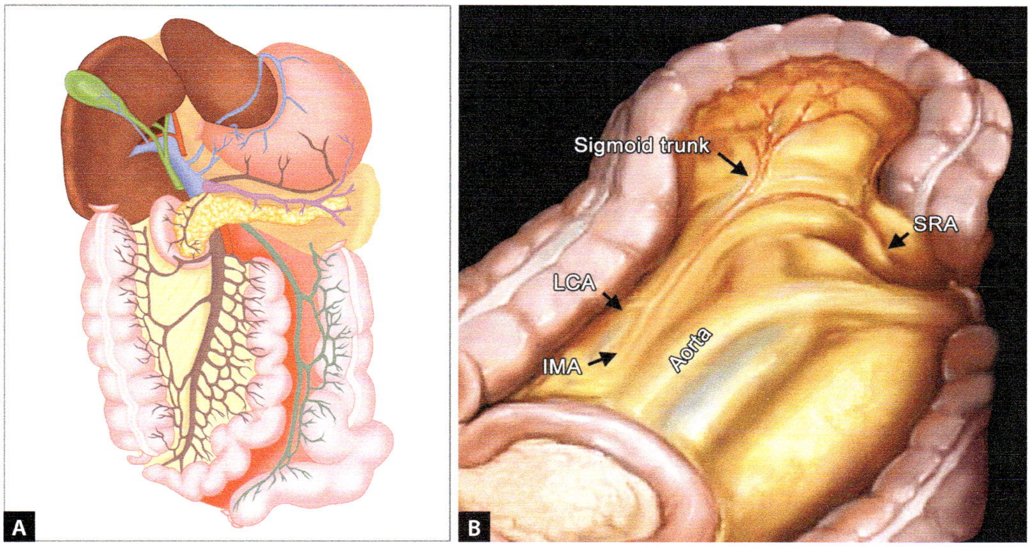

Figs. 17A and B: Vascular supply of left side of colon.
(SRA: superior rectal artery; LCA: left colic artery; IMA: inferior mesenteric artery)

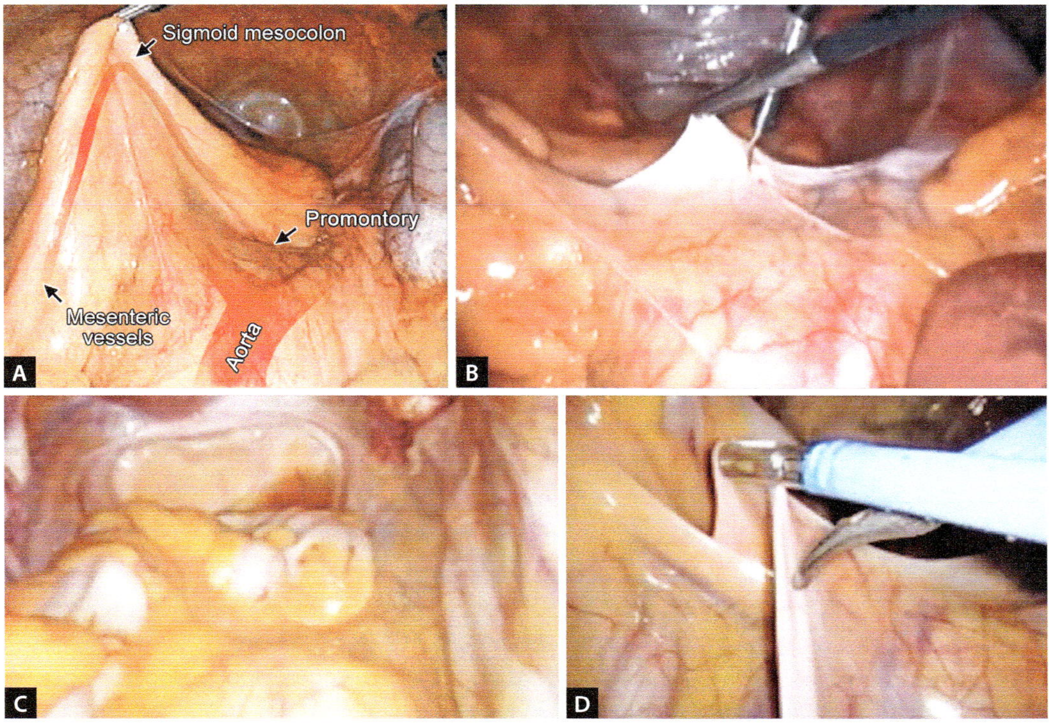

Figs. 18A to D: Incision of peritoneum over sacral promontory.

Treitz. The pressure of the pneumoperitoneum facilitates the dissection, as the diffusion of CO_2 opens the avascular planes.

Identification of the Inferior Mesenteric Artery

The dissection of the cellular adipose tissue is continued upward by gradually dividing the sigmoid branches of the right sympathetic trunk. The dissection behind the inferior mesenteric artery (IMA) involves preservation of the main hypogastric nerve trunks but also division of the small branches traveling to the colon to expose the origin of the IMA (**Figs. 19A and B**). To ensure an adequate lymphadenectomy, the first 2 cm of the IMA are dissected free, and the artery is skeletonized before it is divided.

This dissection at the origin of the IMA involves a risk of injury to the left sympathetic trunk situated on the left border of the inferior mesenteric artery. A meticulous dissection of the artery (skeletonization) helps to avoid this risk, because only the vessel will be divided, and not the surrounding tissues. Dissection performed close to the artery also minimizes the risk of ureteral injury during the ligation of the inferior mesenteric artery. The IMA can then be divided between clips, or by using a linear stapler (vascular 2.5 or 2.0-mm cartridges. The artery is divided at 1–2 cm distal to its origin from the aorta ideally after the take-off of the left colic artery **(Figs. 20A to H)**.

Identification of the Inferior Mesenteric Vein

The inferior mesenteric vein (IMV) terminates when reaching the splenic vein, which goes on to form the portal vein with the SMV. Anatomical variations include the IMV draining into the confluence of the SMV and splenic vein and the IMV draining in the SMV.

The IMV is identified to the left of the IMA or in case of difficulty, higher, just to the left of the ligament of Treitz junction **(Fig. 21)**. The vein is divided below the inferior border of the pancreas or above the left colic vein. Once again, clips are sure options to ligate and divide this vessel **(Figs. 22A to D)**.

Mobilization of the Sigmoid and Descending Colon

The mobilization of the sigmoid colon follows the division of the vessels. This step includes the freeing of posterior and lateral attachments of the sigmoid colon and mesocolon and the division of the rectal and sigmoid mesenteries. The approach is either medial or lateral. It is wise to routinely perform this medial-to-lateral laparoscopic dissection for all indications. The medial approach is well adapted for laparoscopy because it preserves the working space and demands the least handling of the sigmoid colon. In a randomized trial comparing the medial-to-lateral laparoscopic dissection with the classical lateral-to-medial approach for resection of rectosigmoid cancer, Liang et al. showed that the medial approach reduces operative time and the postoperative proinflammatory response. Besides the potential oncologic advantages of early vessel division and "no-touch" dissection, it is believed that he longer the lateral abdominal wall attachments of the colon are preserved, the easier are the exposure and dissection.

Posterior Detachment

The sigmoid mesocolon is retracted anteriorly using the suprapubic cannula to expose the posterior space. The plane between Toldt's fascia and the sigmoid mesocolon can then be identified. This plane is avascular and easily divided.

The dissection continues posteriorly to the sigmoid mesocolon going laterally toward Toldt's line. The sigmoid colon is then completely free, and the lateral attachments can then be divided using a lateral approach.

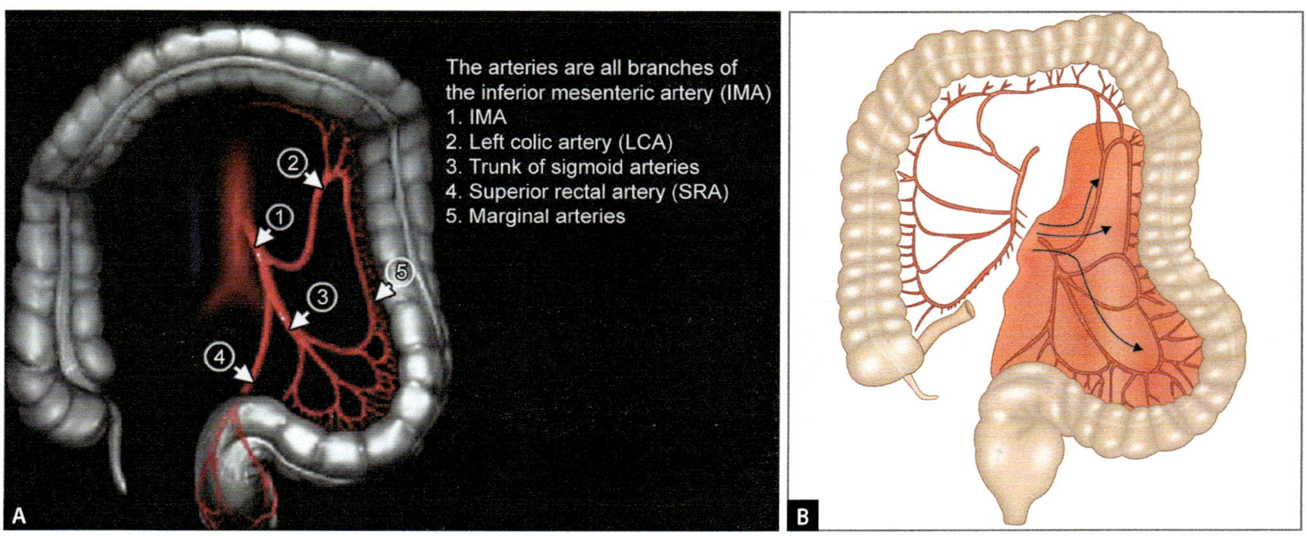

Figs. 19A and B: Arterial supply of sigmoid colon.

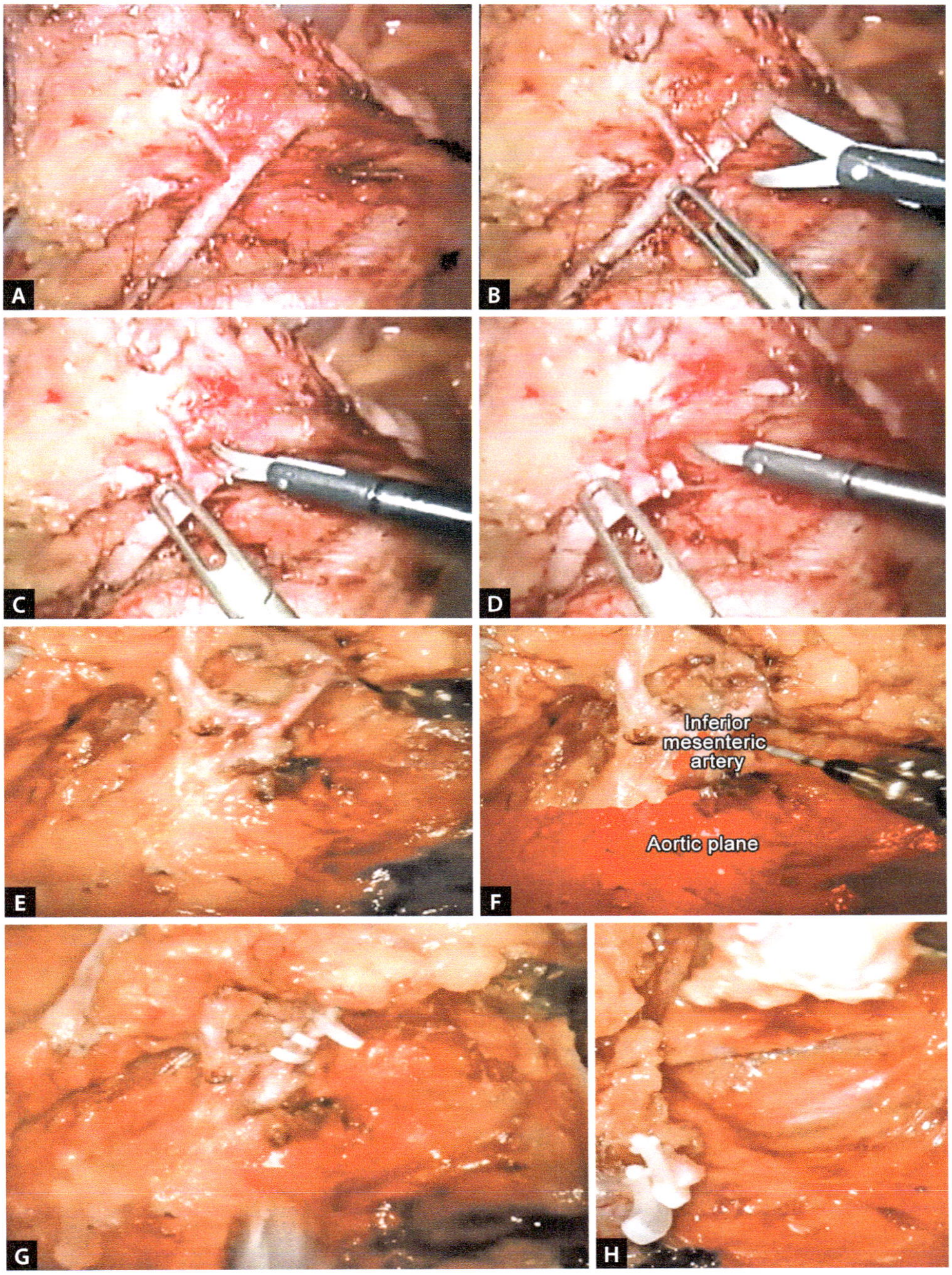

Figs. 20A to H: Dissection of inferior mesenteric artery

Lateral Mobilization

The extent of the dissection is superiorly formed by the inferior border of the pancreas, laterally following Gerota's fascia and inferiorly the psoas muscle where the ureter crosses the iliac vessels. The sigmoid loop is pulled toward the right upper quadrant (grasper in right subcostal cannula) to exert traction on the line of Toldt **(Fig. 23)**. The peritoneal fold is opened cephalad and caudad, and the dissection joins the one previously performed medially. During this step, care must be taken to avoid the gonadal vessels and the left ureter because they can be attracted by the traction exerted on the

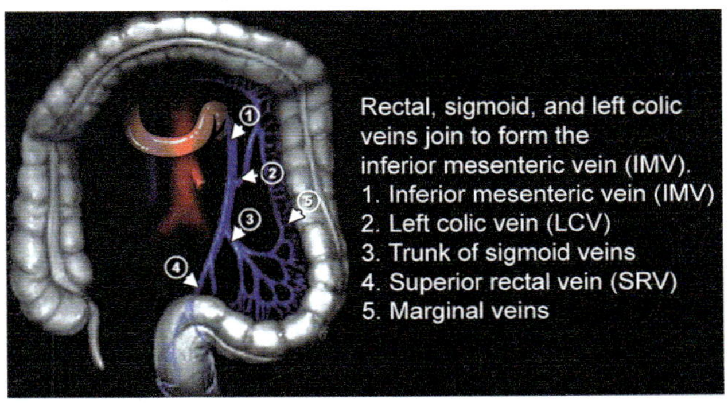

Fig. 21: Venous supply of sigmoid colon.

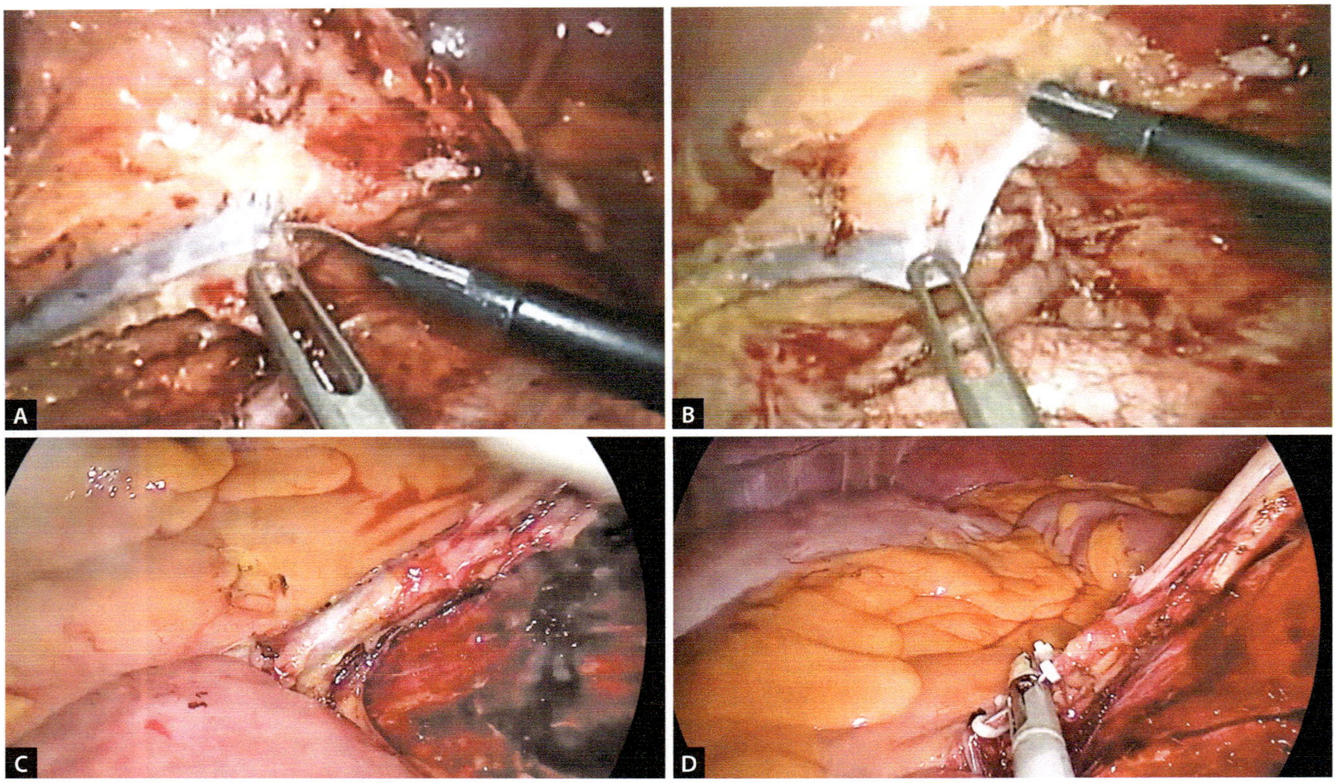

Figs. 22A to D: Dissection of inferior mesenteric vein.

mesentery. Ureteral stenting (infrared stents) can be useful in cases in which inflammation, tumoral tissue, or adhesions and endometriosis make planes difficult to recognize.

Dissection of the Upper Mesorectum

This area of dissection should be approached with caution, especially on the left side: The mesorectum there is closely attached to the parietal fascia where the superior hypogastric nerve and the left ureter are situated. The upper portion of the rectum is mobilized posteriorly following the avascular plane described before, then laterally, until a sufficient distal margin is achieved **(Figs. 24A to D)**.

Resection of the Specimen

Division of the Rectum

Once the upper rectum is freed, the area of distal resection is chosen, allowing a distal margin of at least 5 cm. The fat surrounding this area is cleared, using monopolar cautery, ultrasonic dissection, or the LigaSure™ device. Doing so, the superior hemorrhoidal arteries are divided in the posterior upper mesorectum. The distal division is performed using a linear stapler.

The stapler is introduced through the right lower quadrant cannula. It is wise to use stapler loads 3.5 mm, 45 mm blue cartridges, which are applied perpendicular to the bowel **(Figs. 25A to F)**. Articulated staplers can also be useful, although they are usually unnecessary at the level of the upper rectum **(Figs. 26A and B)**.

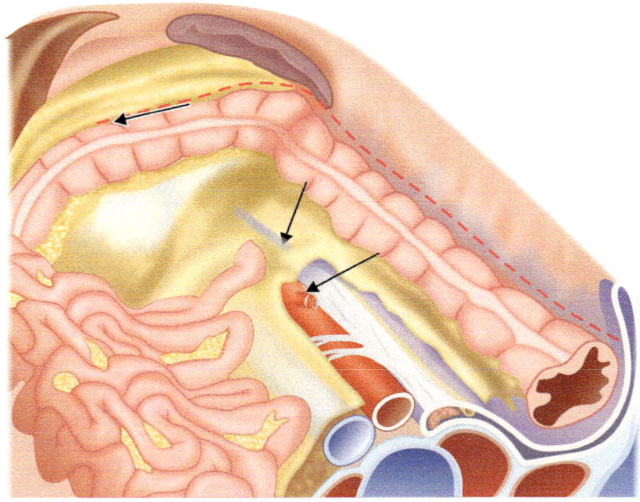

Fig. 23: Lateral approach.

Proximal Division

The proximal division site should be located at least 10 cm proximal to the tumor. It is performed by first dividing the mesocolon and, subsequently, the bowel **(Fig. 27)**.

The division of the mesocolon is more easily performed with the harmonic scalpel, or the LigaSure™, although linear staplers can also be used. The distal portion of the divided

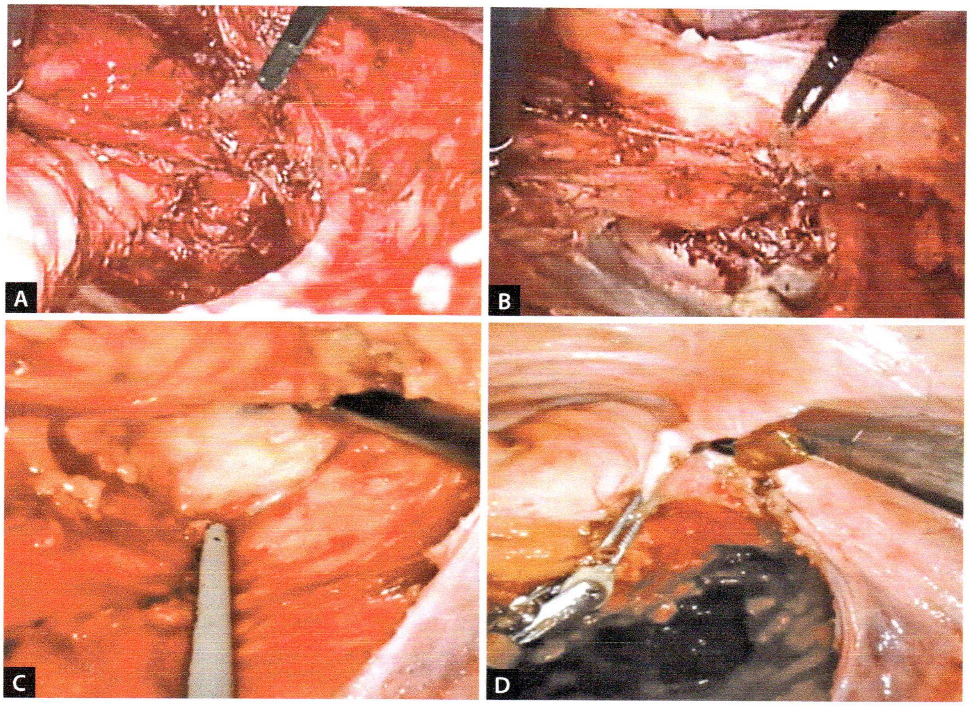

Figs. 24A to D: Dissection of upper mesorectum.

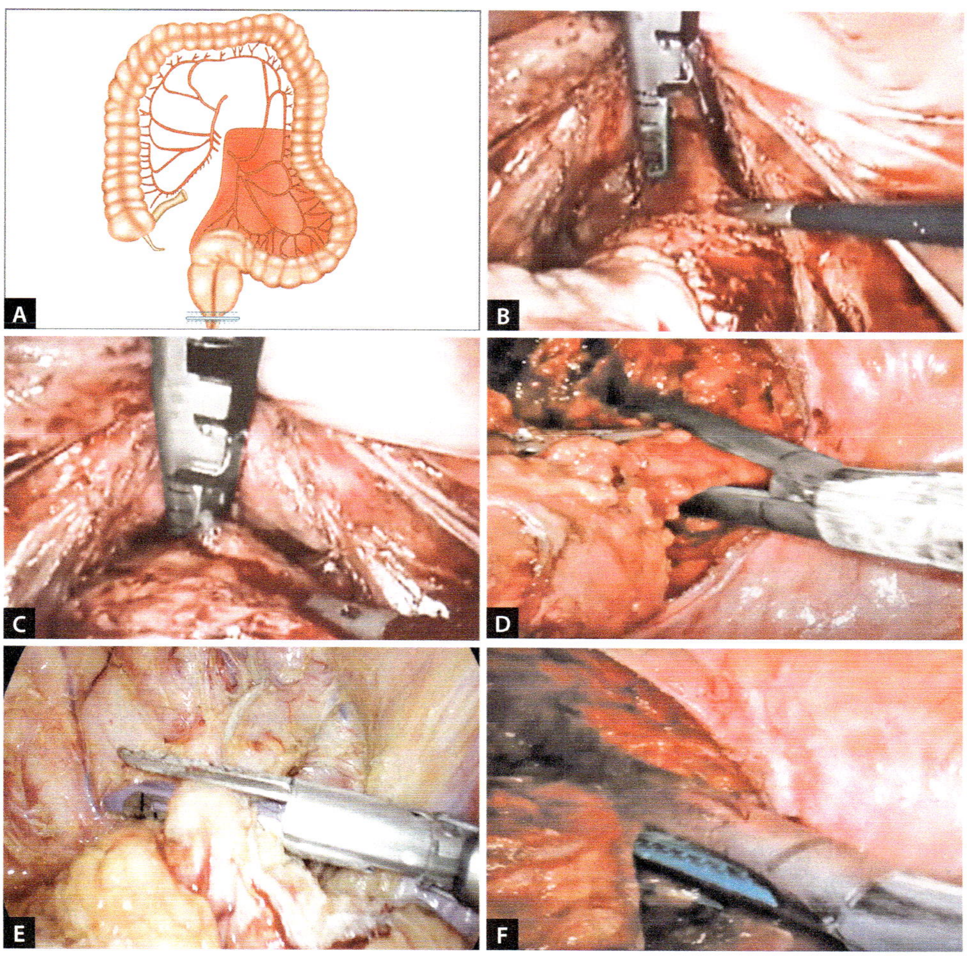

Figs. 25A to F: Division of rectum using stapler.

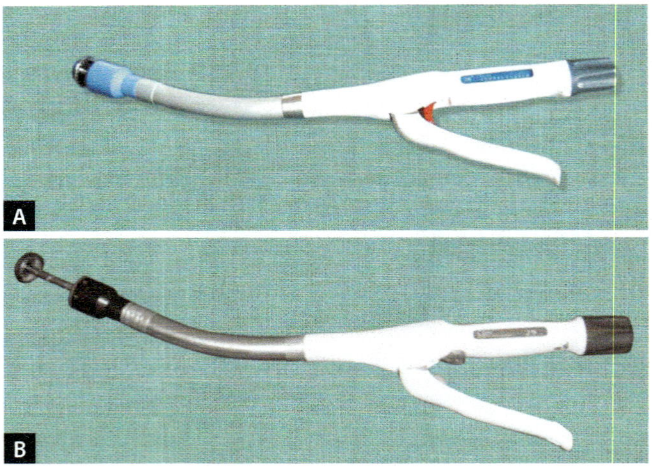

Figs. 26A and B: Disposable circular staplers used in colorectal surgery.

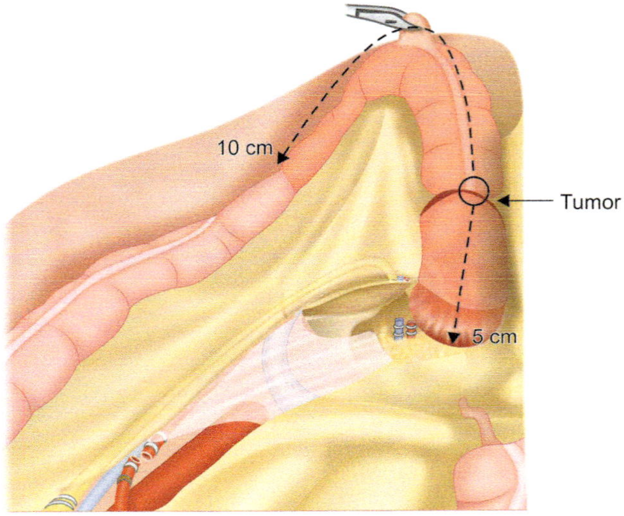

Fig. 27: Division 10 cm proximal and 5 cm distal to tumor.

IMA is identified, and the division of the mesocolon starts right at this level and continues toward the chosen proximal section site at a 90° angle. A linear stapler is then fired across the bowel. The stapler (blue load) is introduced through the right lower quadrant cannula. The specimen is placed in a plastic retrieval sac introduced through the same cannula. This permits the continuation of the procedure without manipulation of the bowel and tumor. If the resected specimen is large and obscures the operative fields, the extraction can be done before completing the mobilization of the left colon.

Mobilization of the Splenic Flexure

In the frequent event that a long segment of the sigmoid colon has been resected, mobilization of the splenic flexure is required. This can be achieved in different ways. It is important for the surgeon to be familiar with all approaches in order to select the most suitable approach. Sufficient mobilization of the splenic flexure may be achieved by simply freeing the posterior and lateral attachments of the descending colon. This is begun by a medial approach to free the posterior attachments of the descending and distal transverse colon, followed by the dissection of the lateral attachments, or by doing the same task in the reverse order. Lateral mobilization is sometimes sufficient in cases of sigmoid cancer, where the posterior mobilization can be omitted.

Lateral Mobilization of the Splenic Flexure

This approach is often used in open surgery and can also be used in simple laparoscopic colectomies. The first step is the section of the lateral attachments of the descending colon. An ascending incision is made along the line of Toldt using scissors introduced via the left-sided cannula. The phrenicocolic ligament is then divided using scissors introduced through this cannula. Retraction of the descending colon and the splenic flexure toward the right lower quadrant using graspers introduced through the right lower and suprapubic cannulae helps to expose the correct plane **(Figs. 28A and B)**. The attachments between the transverse colon and the omentum are divided close to the colon until the lesser sac is opened. The division of these attachments is continued as needed to facilitate the mobilization of the colon into the pelvis.

Medial Mobilization

This approach dissects the posterior attachments of the transverse and descending colon first. The dissection plane naturally follows the plane of the previous sigmoid colon mobilization, cephalad, and anterior to Toldt's fascia. The transverse colon is retracted anteriorly to expose the inferior border of the pancreas, and the root of the transverse mesocolon is divided anterior to the pancreas and at a distance from it, to enter the lesser sac. The dissection then follows toward the base of the descending colon and distal transverse colon, dividing the posterior attachments of these structures. The division of the lateral attachments, as described above, then follows the full mobilization of the splenic flexure. If the mobilized colon reaches the pelvis easily, it may be safely assumed the anastomosis will be tension free as well.

Extraction of Colon

The extraction of the specimen is performed using double protection: A wound protector as well as a retrieval sac **(Figs. 29 and 30)**. The wound protector is also helpful to ensure that there is no CO_2 leak during the intracorporeal colorectal anastomosis, which follows the extraction. This allows a reduction of the size of the incision and potentially minimizes the risk of tumor cell seeding.

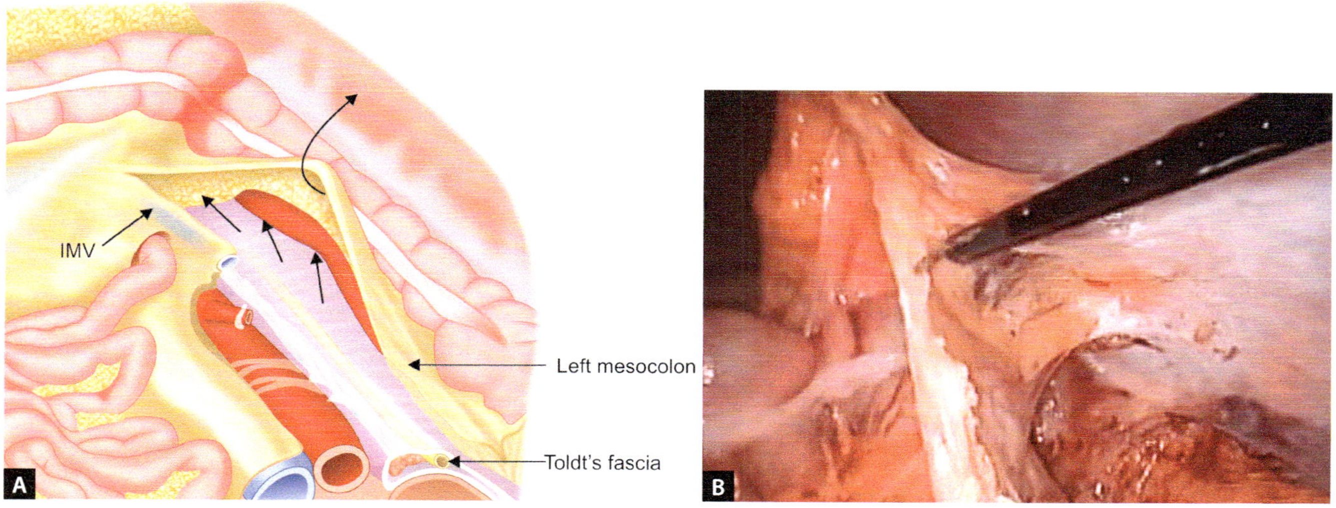

Figs. 28A and B: Mobilization of the splenic flexure of the colon. (IMV: inferior mesenteric vein)

The Incision to Extract the Specimen

The size of the incision, its location, and the extraction technique take into account the volume of the specimen, the patient's body habitus, cosmetic concerns, and the type of disease. The incision is generally performed in the suprapubic region. The proximal division is performed intracorporeally, as described above, and the specimen placed into a thick plastic bag before being extracted through the incision at the suprapubic area.

Anastomosis

For anastomosis, a mechanical circular stapling device passed transanally to perform the anastomosis is used. Performing the anastomosis includes an extra-abdominal preparatory step, and an intra-abdominal step performed laparoscopically.

The extra-abdominal step takes place after the extraction of the specimen. The instrument holding the proximal bowel presents it at the incision where it can easily be grasped with a Babcock clamp and pulled out. If necessary, the colon is divided again in a healthy and well-vascularized zone **(Figs. 31A and B)**.

The anvil (at least 28 mm in diameter) is then introduced into the bowel lumen and closed with a purse-string; then, the colon is reintroduced into the abdominal cavity **(Fig. 32)**. The abdominal incision is closed to re-establish the pneumoperitoneum. For an air-tight closure, it is sufficient to twist the wound protector at the level of the incision using a large clamp **(Figs. 33A and B)**. The circular stapler is introduced into the rectum through the gently dilated anus. The rectal stump is then transfixed with the tip of the head of the circular stapler. In women, the posterior vaginal wall should be retracted anteriorly by the assistant passing the stapler **(Fig. 34)**. Once the center rod and anvil are clicked into the distal part of the circular stapler, twisting of the colon and the mesentery should be checked. The stapler is then fired after ensuring that the neighboring organs are away from the stapling line. The stapler is then twisted open and withdrawn. The anastomosis is checked for leaks by verifying the integrity of the proximal and distal rings, as well as performing an air test **(Figs. 35 and 36)**.

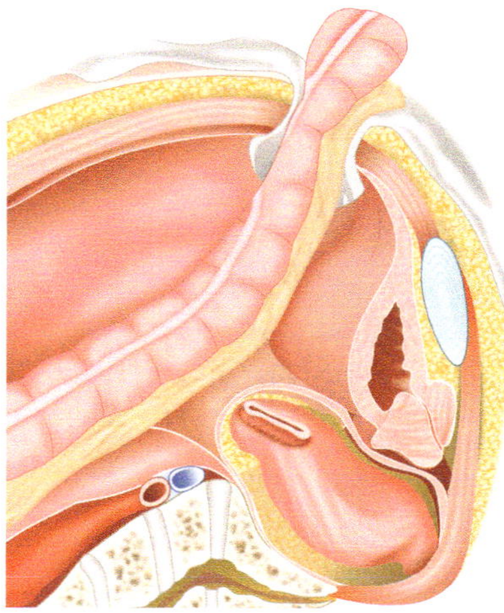

Fig. 29: Extraction of colon.

Wound Closure

The cannula sites are checked internally for possible hemorrhage. To do so, a grasper is passed through the cannula, and the cannula is removed, leaving the grasper in the abdomen. Because of the smaller diameter of the grasper compared with the cannula, if the bleeding was so far concealed by the tamponade effect of the cannula, it would be revealed promptly. The cannula is then reintroduced to allow maintenance of the pneumoperitoneum while performing the same check at all cannula sites.

When the check is completed, the CO_2 is desufflated through the cannulae, and cannulae are removed. No routine

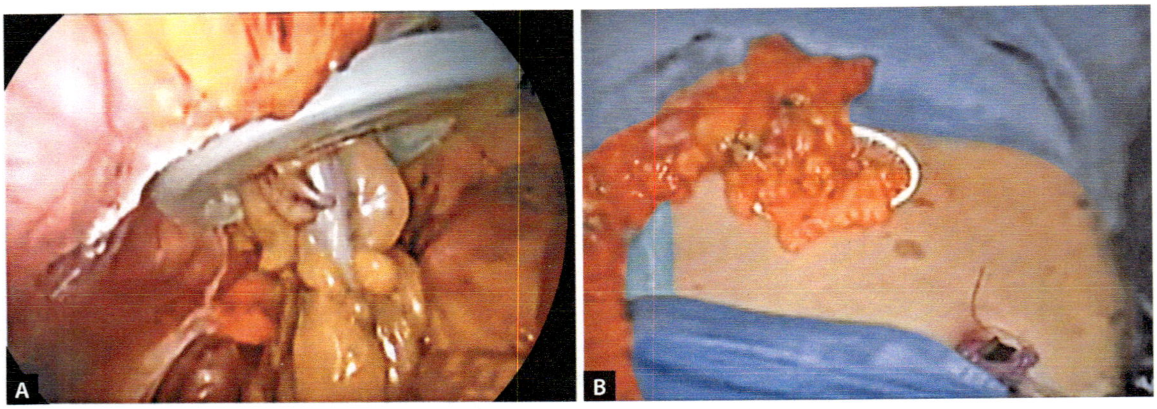

Figs. 30A and B: Extraction of specimen through wound protector.

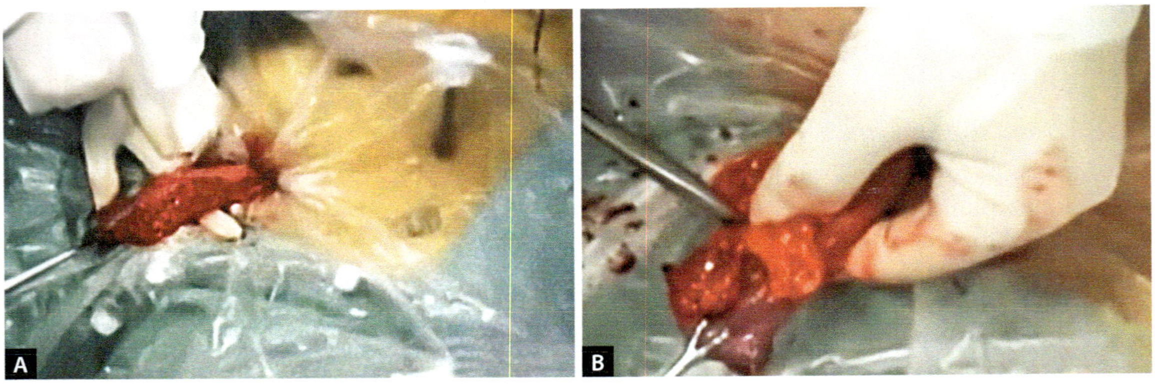

Figs. 31A and B: Preparation of the proximal loop of the colon for anastomosis.

drainage of the anastomotic area is performed. The suprapubic incision is closed in layers using running absorbable sutures, and all fascial defects of 10 mm and more are closed. The skin is closed with a subcuticular absorbable suture.

Sigmoidectomy for Diverticular Disease

The outcomes after laparoscopic sigmoidectomy for diverticulitis are similar or even better to those seen in the open method, with faster recovery and decreased postoperative pain. Hand-assisted laparoscopic sigmoid resection for diverticulitis is also an attractive alternative to a "pure" laparoscopic method in complicated cases.

The vascular approach for patients with benign diseases of the sigmoid colon is performed with the following steps.

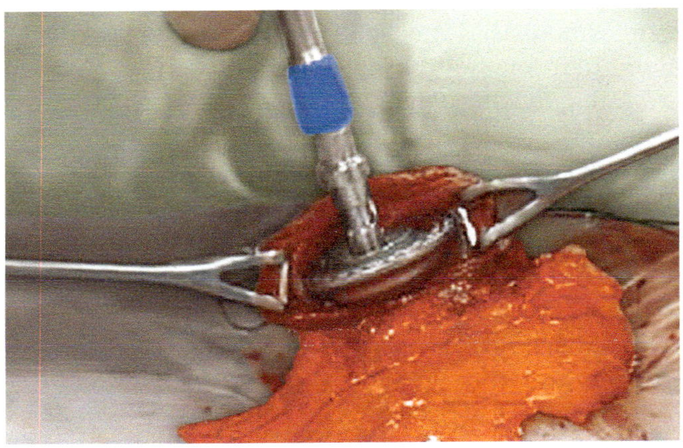

Fig. 32: Fixing the anvil on the proximal loop of colon.

Peritoneal Incision

The peritoneal incision can be similar to the cancer technique, particularly in difficult cases (obesity, inflammatory mesocolon). In most cases, the surgeon should try to preserve the vascularization of the rectum and the left colic vessels. The opening of the peritoneum can be limited to the mesosigmoid parallel to the colon at mid-distance between the colon and the root of the mesosigmoid. An initial lateral mobilization of the sigmoid can be useful in this approach. The branches of the sigmoid arterial trunk can be divided separately anteriorly to inferior mesenteric vessels or together after creating windows in the mesentery to divide the various branches. A linear stapler or, better, the LigaSure™ Atlas 10-mm device can be used for this task.

Resection of the Specimen

In diverticular disease, one should perform the distal resection of the bowel below the rectosigmoid junction.

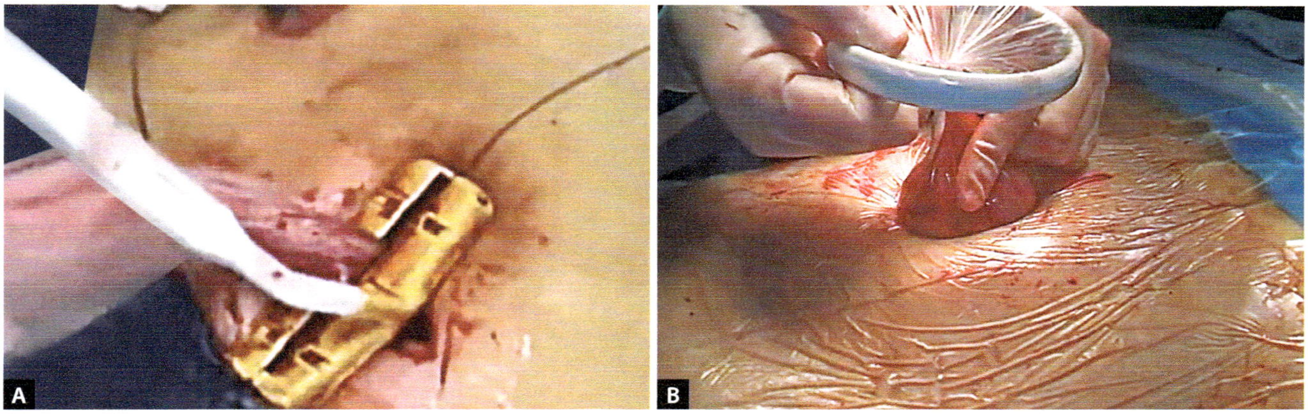

Figs. 33A and B: Clamping and twisting of wound protector to prevent gas leak.

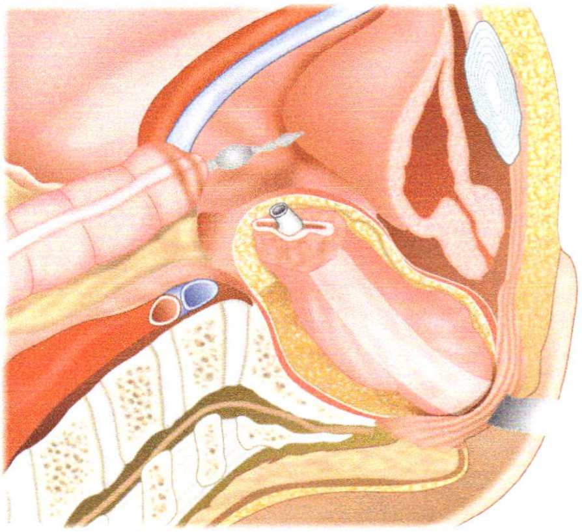

Fig. 34: Anvil and stapler ready for anastomosis.

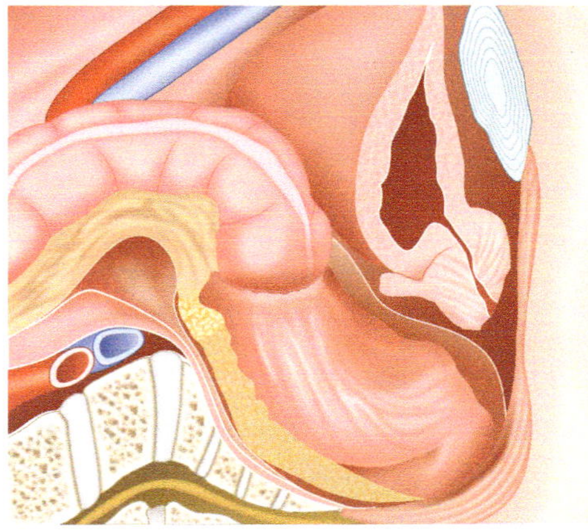

Fig. 35: End-to-end anastomosis done with the help of circular stapler.

The rectosigmoid junction is located just above the peritoneal reflection at the pouch of Douglas **(Fig. 37)**. It is preferred to perform the mobilization of the splenic flexure at this moment, before resection at the proximal limit, using the same principles as described above.

Extraction of the Specimen

Before extracting the colon, it is important to divide the mesocolon at the level of the proximal side of the division. After adequate mobilization is achieved, the colon is extracted through a suprapubic incision, protected by the plastic drape described above, and proximal division performed externally on a compliant and well-vascularized part of the colon. The anastomosis is performed as described above for cancer.

Special Considerations

Ureteral injuries are one of the most important complications, which can be avoided by a perfect exposure and the respect of the correct plane of dissection. Indeed, a dissection properly performed above the Toldt's fascia does not expose the ureter to accidental injury. Difficult cases, such as important inflammatory reaction, cancer invasion or adhesions, and, sometimes, endometriosis, may alter the anatomy of the region and render the identification of the ureter troublesome. In these special cases, prevention of ureteral injury may be facilitated by the use of infrared wires inserted in ureteral stents. The infrared light is cold and safe for use in close contact with the ureteral tissue, and, on the other side, makes it easy to recognize the structure under the light of an adequate laparoscope.

LOW ANTERIOR RESECTION

Two surgical procedures with curative intent are available to patients with rectal cancer:

1. Lower anterior resection
2. Abdominoperineal resection

Lower anterior resection may improve quality of life and functional status. Lower anterior resection, formally known as anterior resection of the rectum and anterior excision of the rectum or simply anterior resection, is a common surgery for rectal cancer. It is commonly abbreviated as LAR. LAR is generally the preferred treatment for rectal cancer insofar as this is surgically feasible. Laparoscopic low anterior resection for rectal cancer has gained full acceptance among general surgeons. Hand-assisted laparoscopic surgery (HALS) LAR also has equal recognition, mainly due to the technical difficulties encountered during pelvic dissection.

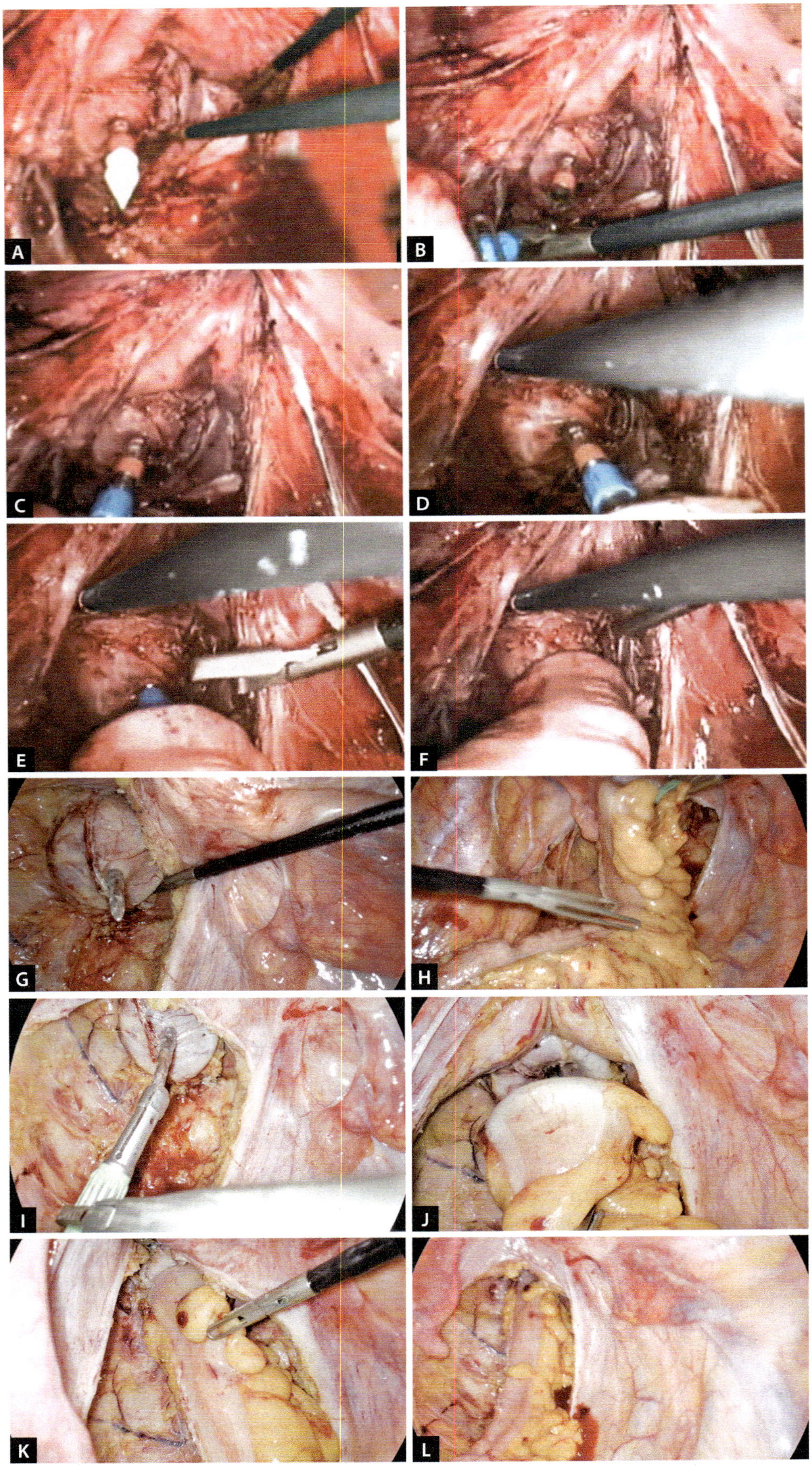

Figs. 36A to L: Anastomosis by the help of a circular stapler.

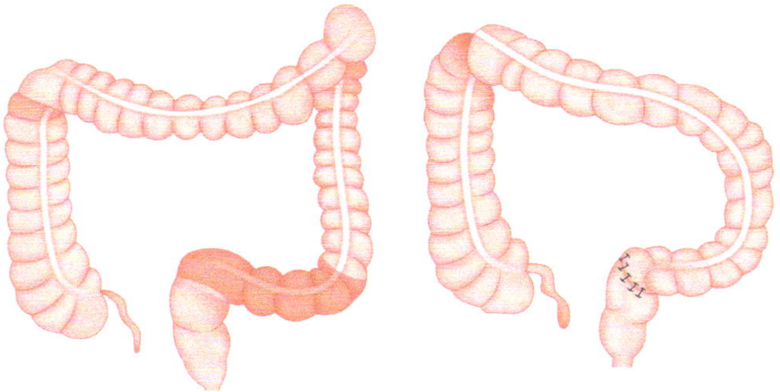

Fig. 37: Before and after sigmoidectomy.

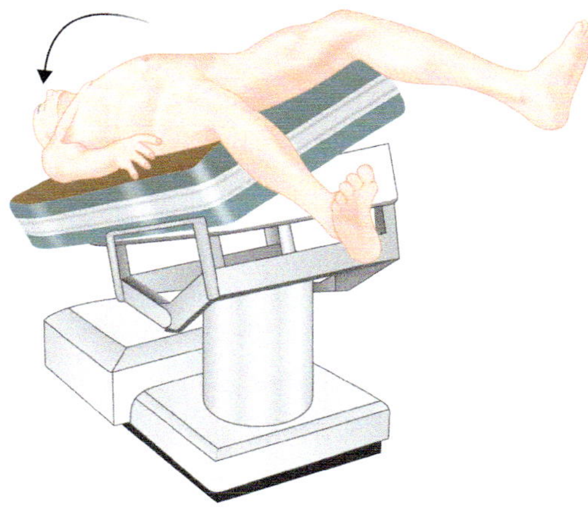

Fig. 38: Patient position for low anterior resection.

Patient Positioning

The patient is placed supine on the operating table **(Fig. 38)**. After induction of general anesthesia and insertion of an orogastric tube and Foley catheter, the legs are placed in stirrups. The arms are tucked at the patient's side, and the beanbag is aspirated. The abdomen is prepared with an antiseptic solution and draped routinely.

Position of Surgical Team

The primary monitor is placed on the left side of the patient at approximately the level of the hip. The operating nurse is placed between the patient's legs. There should be sufficient space to allow the surgeon to move from either side of the patient to between the patient's legs, if necessary. The primary operating surgeon stands on the right side of the patient with the assistant standing on the patient's left and moving to the right side, caudad to the surgeon, once ports have been inserted **(Fig. 39)**. A 30-degree telescope is used.

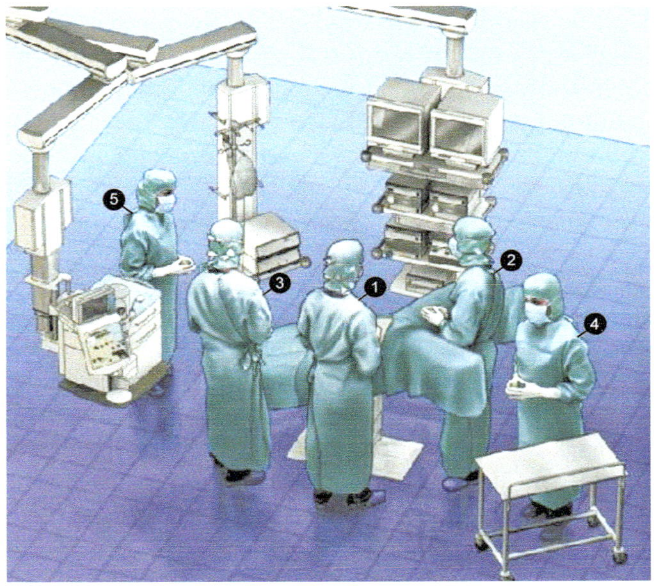

Fig. 39: Position of the surgical team for LAR.
(LAR: low anterior resection)

Port Position

The primary optical port is introduced subumbilical using a modified Hasson approach. Having confirmed entry into the peritoneal cavity, a purse-string suture is placed around the subumbilical fascial defect, the abdomen to be insufflated with CO_2 to a pressure of 12 mm Hg.

The telescope is inserted into the abdomen and an initial diagnostic laparoscopy is performed, carefully evaluating the liver, small bowel, and peritoneal surfaces. A 12-mm port is inserted in the right lower quadrant approximately 2–3 cm medial and superior to the anterior superior iliac spine. It is carefully inserted lateral to the inferior epigastric vessels, paying attention to keep track of the port going as perpendicular as possible through the abdominal wall. A 5-mm port is then inserted in the right upper quadrant at least a hand's breadth superior to the lower quadrant port. A left lower quadrant 5-mm port is inserted. A 5-mm left upper quadrant port is also inserted to aid splenic flexure mobilization. Again, all of these remaining ports are kept lateral to the epigastric vessels. This may be ensured by diligence to anatomic port site selection and using the laparoscope to transilluminate the abdominal wall before making the port-site incision to identify any obvious superficial vessels.

The assistant now moves to the patient's left side, standing caudad to the surgeon. The patient is rotated with the left side up and right side down, to approximately 15–20° tilt, and often as far as the table can go. This helps to move the small bowel over to the right side of the abdomen. The patient is then placed in the Trendelenburg position. This again helps gravitational migration of the small bowel away from the operative field. The surgeon then inserts two atraumatic bowel clamps through the two right-sided abdominal ports. The greater omentum is reflected over the transverse colon so that it comes to lie on the stomach. If there is no space in the upper part of the abdomen, one must confirm that the orogastric tube is adequately decompressing the stomach. The small bowel is moved to the patient's right side, allowing visualization of the medial aspect of the rectosigmoid mesentery. This may necessitate the use of the assistant's 5-mm atraumatic bowel clamp through the left lower quadrant to tent the sigmoid mesentery cephalad.

Defining and Dividing the Inferior Mesenteric Pedicle

An atraumatic bowel clamp is placed on the rectosigmoid mesentery at the level of the sacral promontory, approximately halfway between the bowel wall and the promontory itself. This area is then stretched up toward the left lower quadrant port, stretching the inferior mesenteric vessels away from the retroperitoneum. In most cases, this demonstrates a groove between the right or medial side of the inferior mesenteric pedicle and the retroperitoneum. Electrosurgery or harmonic is used to open the peritoneum along this line, opening the plane cranially up to the origin of the inferior mesenteric artery, and caudally up to the sacral promontory. Blunt dissection is then used to lift the vessels away from the retroperitoneum and presacral autonomic nerves. The ureter is then looked for under the inferior mesenteric artery. If the ureter cannot be seen, and the dissection is in the correct plane, the ureter should be just deep to the parietal peritoneum, and just medial to the gonadal vessels. Care must be taken not to dissect too deep and injure the iliac vessels.

If the ureter cannot be found, it has usually been elevated on the back of the inferior mesenteric pedicle, and one needs to stay very close to the vessel not only to find the ureter but also to protect the autonomic nerves. If the ureter still cannot be found, the dissection needs to come in a cranial direction, which is usually into clean tissue allowing it to be found. If this fails, a lateral approach can be performed. This usually gives a fresh perspective to the tissues, and the ureter can often be found quite easily. In very rare cases, the ureter still may not be found. The ureteric stent should be used, and it helps in easy identification of ureter and prevents it from getting injured. It is good not to proceed if the ureter cannot be defined. The dissection is continued up to the origin of the inferior mesenteric artery, which is carefully defined and divided using a high ligation, above the left colic artery. A clamp is placed on the origin of the vessel to control it if clips or other energy sources do not adequately control the vessel. Endo Gia stapler can also be used for easy division of the vessel.

Having divided the vessels at the origin of the artery, the plane between the descending colon mesentery and the retroperitoneum is developed laterally, out toward the lateral attachment of the colon, and superiorly, dissecting the bowel off the anterior surface of the Gerota's fascia up toward the splenic flexure. This makes the inferior vein quite obvious, and this vessel can also be divided just inferior to the pancreas. This allows increased reach for a coloanal anastomosis with or without neorectal reservoir.

Mobilization of the Lateral Attachments of the Rectosigmoid and Descending Colon

The surgeon now grasps the rectosigmoid junction with his left-hand instrument and draws it to the patient's right side. This allows the lateral attachments of the sigmoid colon to be seen and divided using electrosurgery or harmonic.

Bruising from the prior retroperitoneal mobilization of the colon can usually be seen in this area. Once this layer of peritoneum has been opened, one immediately enters into the space opened by the retroperitoneal dissection. Dissection now continues up along the white line of Toldt, toward the splenic flexure. As the dissection continues, the surgeon's left-hand instrument needs to be gradually moved up along the descending colon to keep the lateral attachments under tension. In this way, the lateral and any remaining posterior attachments are freed, making the left colon and sigmoid a midline structure. Elevating the descending colon and drawing it medially is useful, as this keeps small bowel loops out of the way of the dissecting instrument and facilitates the dissection. In some patients, particularly very obese or otherwise large patients, it is difficult to reach high enough through the right lower quadrant port. For this reason, the surgeon's right-hand instrument is moved to the left lower quadrant port site. This permits greater reach along the descending colon.

Mobilization of the Splenic Flexure

Complete lateral mobilization of the left colon up to the splenic flexure is performed as an initial step. The descending colon is pulled medially using an atraumatic bowel clamp in the right lower quadrant port, and the scissors are placed in the left iliac fossa port. A 5-mm left upper quadrant port may be necessary, particularly in those with a very high splenic flexure, or in very tall or obese individuals. The lateral attachments of the left colon are divided, and the colon is dissected off the Gerota's fascia over the left kidney.

Once the lateral attachments of the colon have been freed, it is necessary to move medially and enter the lesser sac. Some surgeons prefer to perform this as an initial step before lateral mobilization. To enter the lesser sac, the patient is tilted to a slight reverse Trendelenburg position. An atraumatic bowel clamp is inserted through the right upper quadrant port. If the left upper quadrant port is available, this can also be used. The assistant holds up the greater omentum, toward its left side, like a cape. The surgeon grasps the transverse colon toward the left side using a grasper in the right lower quadrant port to aid the identification of the avascular plane between the greater omentum and the transverse mesocolon. Harmonic scalpel or monopolar scissors can be used through the left lower quadrant port to dissect this plane and enter the lesser sac. The surgeon usually moves to stand between the patient's legs for this part of the procedure. This dissection is continued toward the splenic flexure.

Following separation of the omentum off the left side of the transverse colon, connection to the lateral dissection allows the splenic flexure to be fully mobilized. The colon at the flexure is retracted caudally and medially, and any remaining restraining attachments are divided.

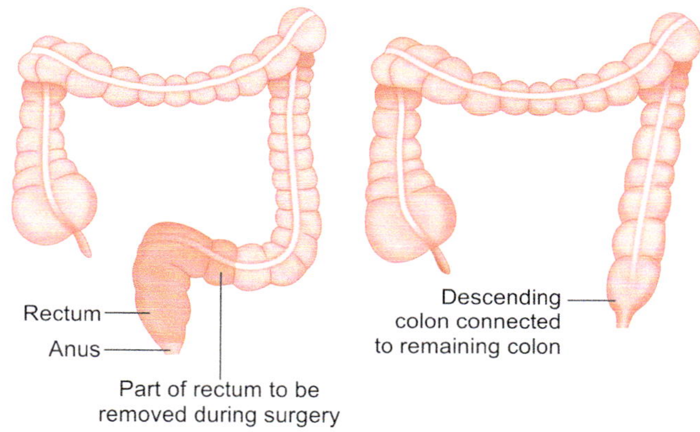

Fig. 40: Low anterior resection.

Rectal Mobilization

The patient is returned to the Trendelenburg position, and the small bowel is reflected cranially. Atraumatic bowel clamps inserted through the left-sided ports are used to elevate the rectosigmoid colon out of the pelvis and away from the retroperitoneum and sacral promontory, to enable entry into the presacral space. The posterior aspect of the mesorectum can be identified and the mesorectal plane dissected with diathermy, preserving the hypogastric nerves as they pass down into the pelvis, anterior to the sacrum. Dissection continues down the presacral space in this avascular plane toward the pelvic floor.

Attention is now switched to the peritoneum on the right side of the rectum. This is divided into the level of the seminal vesicles or rectovaginal septum. This is repeated on the peritoneum on the left side of the rectum. This facilitates further posterior dissection along the back of the mesorectum to the pelvic floor, to a level inferior to the lower edge of the mesorectum, just posterior to the anal canal. For an LAR, it is necessary to perform a total mesorectal excision and hence the rectum must be dissected down to the muscle tube of the rectum below the inferior extent of the mesorectum. In many cases, particularly in those who are obese or men with a narrow pelvis, some or all of the anterior and lateral dissection must be completed to get adequate visualization, to complete the posterior dissection.

An atraumatic bowel clamp through the left iliac fossa port is used to retract the peritoneum anterior to the rectum forward. The peritoneal dissection is continued from the free edge of the lateral peritoneal dissection, anteriorly. Lateral dissection is continued on both sides of the rectum and is extended anterior to the rectum, posterior to Denonvilliers' fascia, separating the posterior vaginal wall from the anterior wall of the rectum or down to the level of the prostate in men. The difficulty of dissection will vary depending on the body habitus of the patient, the diameter of the pelvis, and the size of the tumor. Occasionally, rectal mobilization can be very difficult to perform laparoscopically. In some cases, it may need to be completed in an open manner through a small Pfannenstiel incision.

Division of Rectum

The lower rectum may be divided with a stapler either laparoscopically or by open surgery, depending on the ease of access related to the size of the pelvis **(Fig. 40)**. A rotaculator laparoscopic stapler may be used to divide the muscle tube of the rectum below the level of the mesorectum. The stapler is inserted through the right lower quadrant incision, and two firings of the stapler are usually required to divide the rectum. There is no residual mesorectum to divide at this level. A digital examination is performed to confirm the location of the distal staple line. If there is any doubt about the adequacy of the distal margin, a rigid proctoscopy is performed.

It is sometimes impossible to divide the rectum laparoscopically as the angulation of the endovascular stapler is limited to 45°, necessitating the open division of the rectum. In some patients, getting an assistant to push up on the perineum with their hand may lift the pelvic floor enough to get the first cartridge of the stapler low enough. In some cases, placing a suprapubic port allows easier access with the stapler to allow the division of the rectum.

Some patients are either too obese or have a very narrow pelvis or a long anal canal, and the stapler cannot be passed low enough. Two options exist. One is to perform a transanal intersphincteric dissection, remove the specimen, and then perform a handsewn coloanal anastomosis. The second is to perform a short Pfannenstiel incision, which allows a linear 30-mm stapler to be positioned and the rectum divided.

Extraction and Anastomosis

The specimen can be extracted either through a Pfannenstiel incision or a left iliac fossa incision; in both incisions, a wound protector is used in cases with a polyp or cancer to reduce the risk of tumor implantation in the wound. The left colon mesentery is divided with cautery. The left colon is divided, and the specimen is removed. Pulsatile mesenteric bleeding is confirmed and the vessels ligated with 0 polyglycolate suture ties. Depending on the preference of the operating surgeon, a colonic pouch or coloplasty may

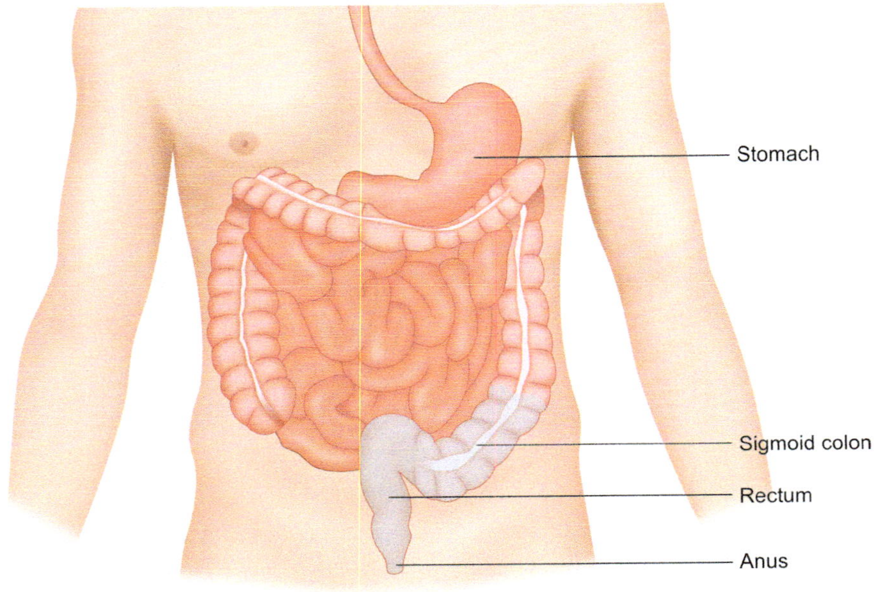

Fig. 41: Anus, rectum, and sigmoid colon removed in APR.
(APR: abdominoperineal resection)

be performed. A 2/0 Prolene purse-string suture is inserted into the distal end of the left colon or pouch, the anvil of a circular stapling gun inserted, and the purse-string suture is tied tightly. If a Pfannenstiel incision has been made, the coloanal anastomosis can be performed under direct vision and open manipulation following the insertion of a circular stapling gun into the rectal stump. If a left iliac fossa incision has been used, the colon is returned to the abdomen, and the incision closed, the pneumoperitoneum recreated, and the anastomosis is formed laparoscopically. The anastomosis can be leak-tested by filling the pelvis with saline and inflating the neorectum using a proctoscope or bulb syringe.

ABDOMINOPERINEAL RESECTION

Laparoscopic abdominoperineal resection is an operation in which the anus, rectum, and sigmoid colon are removed **(Fig. 41)**. It is used to treat cancer located very low in the rectum or in the anus, close to the sphincter muscles. Laparoscopic surgery for anorectal carcinoma is steadily gaining acceptance. The advantage offered by laparoscopy has always centered on improved vision. This advantage seems to be put to best use in the case of rectal cancer surgery, where logistic impediments, viz., narrow pelvis and impaired visibility as the dissection proceeds caudad, have proved to be obstacles to colorectal surgeons during open surgery. Recent studies have shown that the size of the tumor does not hamper the feasibility of performing laparoscopic abdominoperineal resection. We need to consider the possibility of an increased circumferential margin rate for large-size tumors. This may be addressed by preoperative radiotherapy and chemotherapy before undertaking surgery on these large tumors. It is important to note, though, that the oncological safety is not only dependant on the abdominal procedure but also the adequacy of the perineal part of the operation. Besides, should tumor injury be detected intraoperatively, it is advisable to convert to open surgery to control the amount of contamination and complete the rest of the procedure.

Patient Position

The patient is placed supine on the operating table on a beanbag. After induction of general anesthesia and insertion of an orogastric tube and Foley catheter, the legs are placed stirrups. The arms are tucked at the patient's side. The abdomen is prepared with an antiseptic solution and draped routinely.

Position of Surgical Team

The primary monitor is placed on the left side of the patient up toward the patient's feet. The secondary monitor is placed on the right side of the patient at the same level and is primarily for the assistant during the early phase of the surgery and port insertion. The operating nurse's instrument table is placed between the patient's legs. There should be sufficient space to allow the surgeon to move from either side of the patient to between the patient's legs, if necessary. The primary operating surgeon stands on the right side of the patient with the assistant standing on the patient's left and moving to the right side, caudad to the surgeon, once ports have been inserted.

Port Position

This is performed using a Hasson approach. A 10-mm smiling subumbilical incision is made. This is deepened down to the linea alba, which is then grasped on each side of the midline using Kocher clamps. A scalpel (No. 15 blades) is used to open the fascia between the Kocher clamps, and a Kelly forceps is used to open the peritoneum bluntly. Having confirmed entry into the peritoneal cavity, a purse-string suture of 0 polyglycolic acids is placed around the subumbilical fascial defect. A 10-mm reusable port is inserted through this port wound, allowing the abdomen to be insufflated with CO_2 to a pressure of 12 mm Hg. The laparoscope is inserted into the abdomen and an initial laparoscopy is performed, carefully evaluating the liver, small bowel, and peritoneal surfaces. A 12-mm port is inserted in the right lower quadrant approximately 2–3 cm medial and superior to the anterior superior iliac spine. This is carefully inserted lateral to the inferior epigastric vessels, paying attention to keep track of the port going as perpendicular as possible through the abdominal wall. A 5-mm port is then inserted in the right upper quadrant at least a hand's breadth superior to the lower quadrant port. A left lower quadrant 5-mm port is also inserted.

Exposure and Dissection of Retroperitoneum

The assistant now moves to the patient's left side, standing caudad to the surgeon. The patient is rotated with the left side up and right side down, to approximately 15–20° tilt, and often as far as the table can go. This helps to move the small bowel over to the right side of the abdomen. The patient is then placed in the Trendelenburg position. This again helps gravitational migration of the small bowel away from the operative field. The surgeon then inserts two atraumatic bowel clamps through the two right-sided abdominal ports. The greater omentum is reflected over the transverse colon so that it comes to lie on the stomach. If there is no space in the upper part of the abdomen, one must confirm that the orogastric tube is adequately decompressing the stomach. The small bowel is moved to the patient's right side, allowing visualization of the medial aspect of the rectosigmoid mesentery pedicle. This may necessitate the use of the assistant's 5-mm atraumatic bowel clamp through the left lower quadrant to tent the sigmoid mesentery cephalad. Complete mobilization of the left colon is not required. Adequate mobilization must allow the formation of a left iliac fossa colostomy without tension. Following the division of the inferior mesenteric artery, the left mesocolon is separated from the retroperitoneum in a medial-to-lateral direction using a spreading movement. An atraumatic bowel clamp inserted through a right-sided port is placed under the left colonic mesentery, which is elevated away from the retroperitoneum, and using a scissors inserted through the other right-sided port, the attachments to the retroperitoneum are swept down, until the lateral abdominal wall is reached.

Division of the Left Colon

The mesentery of the left colon is divided from the free edge, cranial to the previously divided inferior mesenteric artery, toward the left sigmoid colon. The mesentery can be divided with diathermy, and the marginal artery can be clipped and then divided. Alternatively, an energy source such as a LigaSure™ may be used to divide the mesentery up to the edge of the bowel. This may be done before freeing the lateral attachments of the sigmoid and left colon as it aids in retraction.

After the division of the mesentery, the lateral attachments of the sigmoid to the abdominal wall are divided along the white line. Care is taken to avoid damage to the retroperitoneal structures. The colon is then divided using a linear endoscopic stapler at the site where the colonic mesentery has been divided.

Rectal Mobilization

In women, the uterus may be hitched out of the area of dissection with a suture. Atraumatic bowel clamps that are inserted through the left-sided ports are used to elevate the rectosigmoid colon out of the pelvis and away from the retroperitoneum and sacral promontory, to enable entry into the presacral space. The posterior aspect of the mesorectum can be identified and the mesorectal plane dissected with diathermy, preserving the hypogastric nerves passing down into the pelvis anterior to the sacrum. Dissection continues down the presacral space in this avascular plane toward the pelvic floor. Attention is now switched to the peritoneum on the right side of the rectum. This is divided to the level of the seminal vesicles or rectovaginal septum. This is repeated on the peritoneum on the left side of the rectum. This facilitates further posterior dissection along the back of the mesorectum to the pelvic floor, to a level inferior to the lower edge of the mesorectum. Usually, when the approach is low on the posterior surface of the mesorectum, it becomes necessary to perform a lateral and anterior dissection.

A bowel grasper inserted through the left iliac fossa port is used to retract the peritoneum anterior to the rectum forward. The peritoneal dissection is continued from the free edge of the lateral peritoneal dissection, anteriorly. Lateral dissection is continued on both sides of the rectum. It is extended anteriorly to the rectum in front of Denonvilliers' fascia, separating the posterior vaginal wall from the anterior wall of the rectum or down past the level of the prostate in men. The most inferior rectal dissection can be completed from the perineal approach. For anterior tumors, the dissection may be performed anterior to Denonvilliers' fascia, or by taking one side of the fascia to protect the anterolateral nerve bundle.

It is necessary to perform a total mesorectal excision and hence the rectum must be dissected down close to the muscle tube of the rectum below the level of the mesorectum.

The levators may then be divided from above, staying well wide of any potential tumor, or the division may be performed from below after making the perineal incision.

Formation of Trephine Left Iliac Fossa Colostomy

The divided distal end of the left sigmoid colon is grasped with atraumatic bowel clamps, which are locked. A trephine colostomy is made in the left iliac fossa at a site that has been marked by an enterostomal therapist before surgery. A skin disk is excised, and a longitudinal incision is made in the anterior rectus sheath, and the left rectus muscle is split. The peritoneum is held with two hemostats and incised. The stapled colon is delivered to the trephine and grasped with Babcock forceps and delivered through the trephine.

The staple line is excised, and the end colostomy is matured using 3/0 chromic catgut sutures.

Perineal Dissection

The perineal dissection is performed with a conventional open approach **(Figs. 42A and B)**. The anus is sutured closed with 0 nylon, and an elliptical skin incision is made. The incision is deepened using diathermy, and the ischiorectal fossae are entered on either side, well lateral to the external sphincter muscle. The dissection continues laterally and posteriorly to expose the levator ani muscles **(Fig. 43)**. The tip of the coccyx is used as the posterior landmark, and the pelvic cavity is entered by dividing the levator ani muscle just anterior to the tip of the coccyx. A finger can be placed into the pelvis onto the upper border of the levator ani, which is divided with diathermy onto the underlying finger. Care is taken anteriorly to divide the remaining levator ani while protecting the posterior surface of the vagina or prostate/urethra. The specimen may then be delivered out of the pelvis, which facilitates the division of the remaining anterior attachments of the rectum, reducing the risk of damage to the prostate or posterior wall of the vagina. The specimen is removed, the pelvic cavity irrigated of blood or debris, and the perineal tissue closed in layers using polydioxanone sutures.

HARTMANN REVERSAL

The Hartmann procedure is a standard life-saving operation for acute left colonic complications. It is usually performed

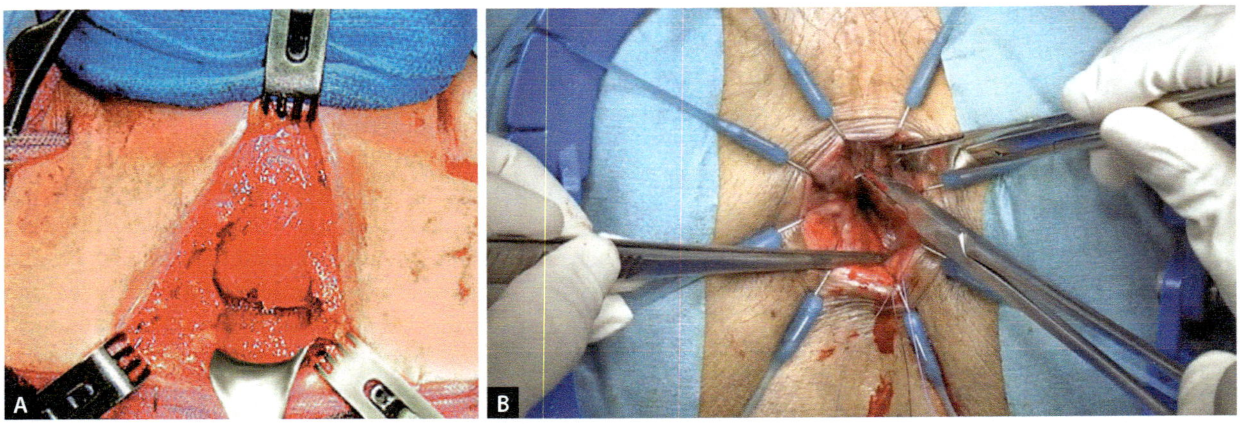

Figs. 42A and B: Perineal dissection.

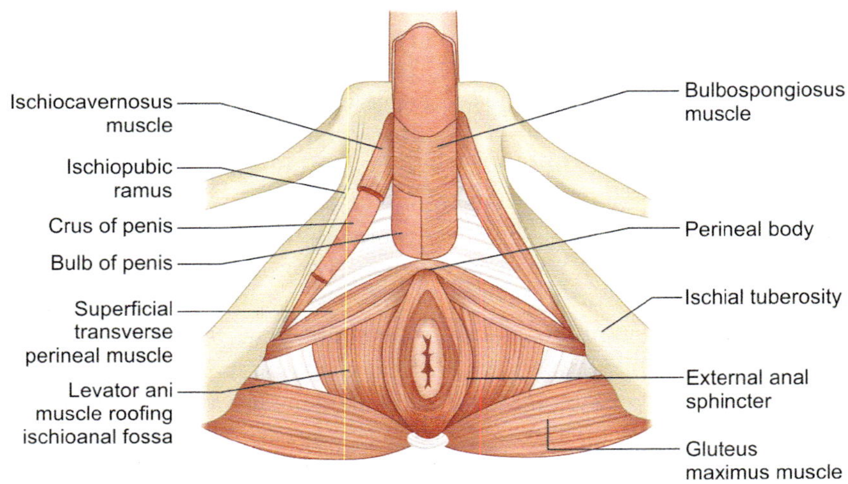

Fig. 43: Perineal anatomy.

as a temporary procedure with the intent to reverse it later on. This reversal is associated with considerable morbidity and mortality by the open method. The laparoscopic reestablishment of intestinal continuity after Hartmann procedure has shown better results in terms of a decrease in morbidity and mortality.

There are several laparoscopic techniques of the reversal of the Hartmann procedure. The principle common to all techniques is a tension-free intracorporeal stapler anastomosis. The introduction of a circular stapler in the rectal stump helps in the identification and mobilization of the rectal stump. Others have mobilized the colostomy first and have used the colostomy site as a first port or used a standard umbilical port.

It is technically challenging and requires an experienced laparoscopic surgeon but offers clear advantages to patients. Main reasons reported for conversion to open were dense abdominal–pelvic adhesions secondary to diffuse peritonitis at the primary operation, the short delay before the reconstruction, difficulty in finding the rectal stump, and rectal scarring. Leaving long, nonabsorbable suture ends at the rectal stump or suturing it to the anterior abdominal wall helps in its localization. Other relative limitation factors could be a large incisional hernia from the previous laparotomy and contraindications to general anesthesia and laparoscopy.

Patient Position

The patient is placed supine on the operating table, on a beanbag. After induction of general anesthesia and insertion of an orogastric tube and Foley catheter, the legs are placed in a lithotomy stirrup position. The arms are tucked at the patient's side, and the beanbag is aspirated.

The abdomen is prepared with an antiseptic solution and draped routinely.

Position of Surgical Team

The primary monitor is placed on the left side of the patient at approximately the level of the hip. The secondary monitor is placed on the right side of the patient at the same level and is primarily for the assistant during the early phase of the surgery and port insertion. The operating nurse's instrument table is placed between the patient's legs. There should be sufficient space to allow the surgeon to move from either side of the patient to between the patient's legs, if necessary. The primary operating surgeon stands on the right side of the patient with the assistant standing on the patient's left and moving to the right side, caudad to the surgeon once ports have been inserted. A 30-degree camera lens is better to be used.

The colostomy is mobilized and all adhesions dissected through the fascial opening until an adequate segment of bowel has been freed from the surrounding tissues. The bowel is trimmed as necessary, and a purse-string suture is positioned before insertion of the anvil of a curved EEA stapling device. The bowel is returned to the abdomen, the fascia is closed with a monofilament suture, but before tying the suture a 12-mm port is inserted at this site, and the abdomen is insufflated.

The laparoscope is inserted into the abdomen through the stoma port to assess adhesions and allow direct visualization for subsequent port insertion, and an initial laparoscopy is performed, carefully evaluating the liver, small bowel, and peritoneal surfaces. A 10-mm port is inserted in the umbilicus for camera location. A 5-mm right lower quadrant trocar is placed approximately 2–3 cm medial to the anterior superior iliac spine. This is carefully inserted lateral to the inferior epigastric vessels, paying attention to keep track of the port going as perpendicular as possible through the abdominal wall. A 5-mm port is then inserted in the right upper quadrant at least a hand's breadth superior to the lower quadrant port. A left upper quadrant 5-mm port is inserted. Again all of these remaining ports are kept lateral to the epigastric vessels. This may be ensured by diligence to anatomic port site selection and using the laparoscope to transilluminate the abdominal wall before making the port-site incision to identify any obvious superficial vessels.

The assistant now moves to the patient's right side, standing caudad to the surgeon. The patient is rotated with the left side up and right side down, to approximately 15–20° degrees tilt, and often as far as the table can go. This helps to move the small bowel over to the right side of the abdomen. The patient is then placed in the Trendelenburg position. This again helps gravitational migration of the small bowel away from the operative field. The surgeon then inserts two atraumatic bowel clamps through the two right-sided abdominal ports. The greater omentum is reflected over the transverse colon so that it comes to lie on the stomach. If there is no space in the upper part of the abdomen, one must confirm that the orogastric tube is adequately decompressing the stomach. The small bowel is moved to the patient's right side, allowing visualization of the proximal rectum. Variable degrees of adhesiolysis may be required. This may necessitate the use of the assistant's 5-mm atraumatic bowel clamp through the stoma trocar or left upper quadrant.

Left Colon Mobilization

An atraumatic bowel clamp is placed on the descending colon to take down the inflammatory and native attachments to free it laterally. The omentum is dissected off the transverse colon, and the lesser sac is entered. The splenic flexure is released to allow a tension-free reach to the proximal rectum. The colonic mesentery should be mobilized off the Gerota's fascia. The left ureter is identified at the pelvic brim and freed from the proximal rectum to avoid injury. The ureter should be just deep to the parietal peritoneum, and just medial and posterior to the gonadal vessels. Care must be taken not to dissect too deep or caudad, leading to injury of the iliac vessels.

Mobilization of Rectum

An atraumatic bowel clamp inserted through the left lower quadrant port is used to elevate the proximal rectum out of the pelvis and away from the retroperitoneum and sacral promontory, to enable entry into the presacral space. The posterior aspect of the mesorectum can be identified and the mesorectal plane dissected with diathermy, preserving the hypogastric nerves as they pass down into the pelvis anterior to the sacrum. Dissection needs to progress only to allow the advancement of the circular stapler to the end of the rectum and assure that all the sigmoid has been resected. If residual sigmoid is present, the linear endoscopic stapler should be used to divide the bowel at the level of the proximal rectum. A site for rectal division should be chosen in proximal, peritonealized rectum, which assures that the anastomosis will be distal to the sacral promontory. The rectum is divided laparoscopically with a linear endoscopic stapler through the right lower quadrant trocar. One or two firings of the stapler may be required to divide the rectum. The mesorectum is divided using monopolar and bipolar cautery at this level.

Specimen Extraction and Anastomosis

If residual sigmoid is required, the specimen is extracted through the stoma site port. Pneumoperitoneum is recreated, and the circular stapled anastomosis is formed under laparoscopic guidance. The anastomosis can be leak-tested by filling the pelvis with saline and inflating the neorectum using a proctoscope or bulb syringe, and the orientation and lack of tension confirmed. The fascia of all the 10 mm or above port is closed, and the usual manner is followed for skin dressing.

Conclusion

The reversal of the Hartmann procedure can be difficult due tendency of the Hartmann segment to become densely adherent deep in the pelvis. The laparoscopic reversal has made this major operation easier, safe, and practical. As a majority of these patients is in the elderly age group, it has the advantage of early mobilization, less pain, short hospital stay, and returns to normal life.

RESECTION RECTOPEXY

Total rectal prolapse with chronic constipation and anal incontinence is a devastating disorder. It is more common in the elderly, especially women, although why it happens is unclear. Rectal prolapse can cause complications (such as pain, ulcers, and bleeding), and cause fecal incontinence **(Figs. 44A to C)**. Surgery is commonly used to repair the prolapse. Rectopexy with or without bowel resection is the most frequent surgical procedure, with 0–9% recurrence rates in many years. Laparoscopic resection rectopexy is safely feasible as a minimally invasive treatment option for rectal prolapse.

Patient Position

The patient is placed supine on the operating table, on a beanbag. After induction of general anesthesia and insertion of an orogastric tube and Foley catheter, the legs are placed in Dan Allen stirrups. The arms are tucked at the patient's side. The abdomen is prepared with an antiseptic solution and draped routinely.

Position of Surgical Team

The primary monitor is placed on the left side of the patient at approximately the level of the hip. The secondary monitor is placed on the right side of the patient at the same level and is primarily for the assistant during the early phase of the surgery and port insertion. The operating nurse's instrument table is placed between the patient's legs. There should be sufficient space to allow the surgeon to move from either side of the patient to between the patient's legs, if necessary. The primary operating surgeon stands on the right side of the patient with the assistant standing on the patient's left and moving to the right side, caudad to the surgeon once ports have been inserted. A 0-degree camera lens is used.

Port Position

This is performed using a Hasson approach. A smiling 10-mm subumbilical incision is made. This is deepened down to the linea alba, which is then grasped on each side of the midline using Kocher clamps. A scalpel (No. 15 blades) is used to open the fascia between the Kocher clamps, and a Kelly forceps is used to open the peritoneum bluntly. The telescope is inserted into the abdomen, and an initial laparoscopy is performed, carefully evaluating the liver, small bowel, and peritoneal surfaces. A 12-mm port is inserted in the right lower quadrant approximately 2–3 cm medial and superior to the anterior superior iliac spine. This is carefully inserted lateral to the inferior epigastric vessels, paying attention to keep track of the port going as perpendicular as possible through the abdominal wall. A 5-mm port is then inserted in the right upper quadrant at least a hand's breadth superior to the lower quadrant port. A left lower quadrant 5-mm port is inserted. All the ports are more or less obeying the baseball diamond concept.

Dissection

The patient is rotated with the left side up and right side down, to approximately 15–20° tilt, and often as far as the table can go. This helps to move the small bowel over to

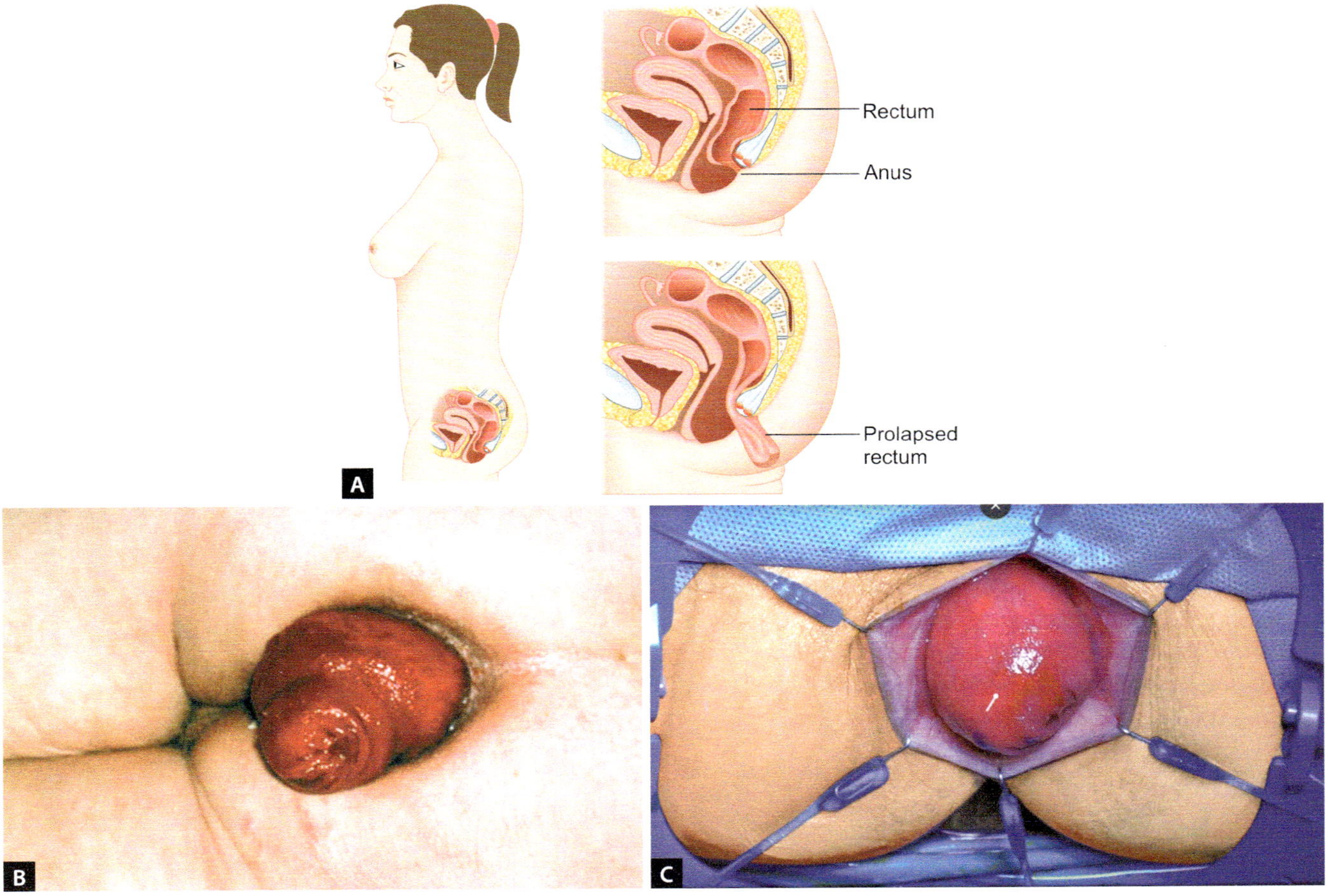

Figs. 44A to C: Rectal prolapse

the right side of the abdomen. The patient is then placed in the Trendelenburg position. This again helps gravitational migration of the small bowel away from the operative field. The surgeon then inserts two atraumatic bowel clamps through the two right-sided abdominal ports. The greater omentum is reflected over the transverse colon so that it comes to lie on the stomach. If there is no space in the upper part of the abdomen, one must confirm that the orogastric tube is adequately decompressing the stomach. The small bowel is moved to the patient's right side, allowing visualization of the medial aspect of the rectosigmoid mesentery. This may necessitate the use of the assistant's 5-mm atraumatic bowel clamp through the left lower quadrant to tent the sigmoid mesentery cephalad.

Division of Inferior Mesenteric Vessel

An atraumatic bowel clamp is placed on the rectosigmoid mesentery at the level of the sacral promontory, approximately halfway between the bowel wall and the promontory itself. This area is then stretched up toward the left lower quadrant port, stretching the inferior mesenteric vessels away from the retroperitoneum. In most cases, this demonstrates a groove between the right or medial side of the inferior mesenteric pedicle and the retroperitoneum. Cautery is used to open the peritoneum along this line, opening the plane cranially up to the origin of the inferior mesenteric artery, and caudally past the sacral promontory. Blunt dissection is then used to lift the vessels away from the retroperitoneum and presacral autonomic nerves. The ureter is then looked for under the inferior mesenteric artery. If the ureter cannot be seen, and the dissection is in the correct plane, the ureter should be just deep to the parietal peritoneum, and just medial to the gonadal vessels. Care must be taken not to dissect too deep or caudad, leading to injury of the iliac vessels.

If the ureter cannot be found, it has usually been elevated on the back of the inferior mesenteric pedicle, and one needs to stay very close to the vessel not only to find the ureter but also to protect the autonomic nerves. If the ureter still cannot be found, the dissection needs to come in as a cranial dissection, which is usually into clean tissue allowing it to be found. If this fails, a lateral approach can be performed. This usually gives a fresh perspective to the tissues, and the ureter can often be found quite easily. In very rare cases, the ureter still may not be found.

The dissection should allow sufficient mobilization of the IMA so that the origin of the left colic artery is seen. The vessel is carefully defined and divided just distal to the left colic artery. A clamp is placed on the origin of the vessel to control it if clips or other energy sources do not adequately control the vessel. In general, a cartridge of the endoscopic linear stapler is used to divide the vessel. Having divided the pedicle, the plane between the sigmoid colon mesentery and the retroperitoneum is developed laterally, out toward the lateral attachment of the colon. Limited mobilization of the mesentery of the anterior surface of Gerota's fascia and of the left colon should be performed to enhance the fixation of the rectum.

Mobilization of the Lateral Attachments of the Rectosigmoid

The surgeon now grasps the rectosigmoid junction with his left-hand instrument and draws it to the patient's right side. This allows the lateral attachments of the sigmoid colon to be seen and divided using cautery. Bruising from the prior retroperitoneal mobilization of the colon can usually be seen in this area. Once this layer of peritoneum has been opened, one immediately enters into the space opened by the retroperitoneal dissection. No dissection should be performed more proximally along the white line of Toldt, toward the splenic flexure.

Mobilization of Rectum

An atraumatic bowel clamp inserted through the left lower quadrant port is used to elevate the rectosigmoid colon out of the pelvis and away from the retroperitoneum and sacral promontory, to enable entry into the presacral space. The posterior aspect of the mesorectum can be identified, and the mesorectal plane dissected with diathermy, preserving the hypogastric nerves as they pass down into the pelvis anterior to the sacrum. Dissection continues down the presacral space in this avascular plane toward the pelvic floor. Only the posterior 60% of the rectum needs to be mobilized; however, dissection should be continued all the way to the levator ani muscles. A transanal examining finger should be used to confirm the distal extent of the dissection. The lateral stalks should be preserved. The peritoneum on either side of the rectum should be incised to the level of the lateral stalks. The lateral stalks should generally be preserved, the exception being when further dissection must completely reduce a very distal prolapsing segment.

Rectal Division

The fully mobilized rectum should be elevated out of the pelvis and a site selected for optimal rectal tension to maintain a full reduction of the prolapse. A site for rectal division should be chosen in proximal, peritonealized rectum, which assures that the anastomosis will be rostral to the sacral promontory. The rectum is divided laparoscopically with a linear endoscopic stapler through the right lower quadrant trocar. One or two firings of the stapler may be required to divide

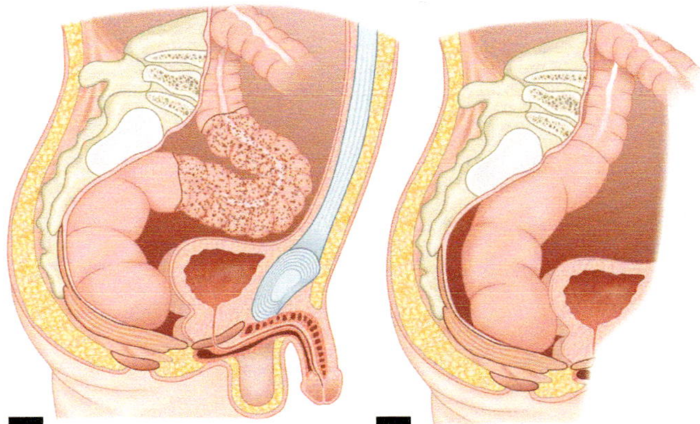

A **B**

Figs. 45A and B: Resection rectopexy.

the rectum. The mesorectum is divided using monopolar and bipolar cautery at this level.

Specimen Extraction and Anastomosis

The specimen is extracted through a left iliac fossa incision. Before making the incision, the proximal colonic transaction point should be grasped with a locking atraumatic bowel grasper. This site should allow a colorectal anastomosis that will provide a safe amount of tension on the rectum to maintain prolapse reduction. After extracorporeal bowel transaction, adequate vascularity of the colon should be assured. A 2/0 Prolene purse-string suture is inserted into the distal end of the left colon; the anvil of a circular stapling gun is inserted, and the purse-string suture is tied tightly. The colon is returned to the abdomen, and the left iliac fossa incision is closed in layers with 0 polyglycolic acid suture. Pneumoperitoneum is recreated, and the circular stapled anastomosis is formed under laparoscopic guidance. The anastomosis can be leak-tested by filling the pelvis with saline and inflating the neorectum using a proctoscope or bulb syringe.

Rectopexy (Figs. 45A and B)

The rectum is retracted rostrally to the desired tension to allow complete reduction of the prolapse. The rectopexy is then performed from the right side using the two remaining ports. Two or three nonabsorbable sutures are used to attach the mesorectum distal to the anastomosis to the sacral promontory. Alternatively, nitinol or titanium tackers may be employed using one of the mechanical fixation devices used for mesh hernia repairs.

WELLS OR MARLEX RECTOPEXY

Rectal prolapse is a distressing condition, especially when associated with fecal incontinence and constipation. It usually occurs in children or the elderly. Presently laparoscopic approach is favored as it has better results, especially in terms of less postoperative pain, shorter hospital stay, and lower cost. The pelvic sympathetic and parasympathetic nerves run along with the rectum; if dissection is not carried out in the proper plane, injury can occur, leading to bladder dysfunction, impotence, and retrograde ejaculation. This is an important consideration when trying to decide which procedure to perform, especially in men, although the risk of injury should be <1–2%. Perineal procedures and anterior resection have a low risk of outlet obstruction. Abdominal procedures of rectopexy that tack the rectum to the sacrum can cause outlet obstruction if the rectum is wrapped circumferentially, often requiring the release of the fixation to treat the problem.

In a Marlex rectopexy (Ripstein procedure), the entire rectum is mobilized down to the coccyx posteriorly, the lateral ligaments laterally, and the anterior cul-de-sac anteriorly. A nonabsorbable material, such as Marlex mesh or an Ivalon sponge, is then fixed to the presacral fascia. The rectum is then placed on tension, and the material is partially wrapped around the rectum to keep it in position. The anterior wall of the rectum is not covered with the sponge or mesh in order to prevent a circumferential obstruction. The peritoneal reflections are then closed to cover the foreign body. The Marlex mesh or sponge causes an inflammatory reaction that scars and fixes the rectum into place.

The Wells procedure was followed by rectal dysfunction accompanied by increased constipation and evacuation problems. The Ripstein procedure, preserving the lateral ligaments, appears not to affect such symptoms adversely. Modified mesh rectopexy aligns the rectum, avoids excessive mobilization and division of lateral ligaments, thus preventing constipation and preserving potency. We recommend this technique for patients with complete rectal prolapse with up to grades 1, 2, and 3 incontinence based on Browning and Parks classification.

During wells rectopexy, the dissection should allow sufficient mobilization of the IMA so that the origin of the left colic artery is seen. The pedicle is not divided.

The plane between the sigmoid colon mesentery and the retroperitoneum is developed laterally, out toward the lateral attachment of the colon. Limited mobilization of the mesentery of the anterior surface of Gerota's fascia and of the left colon should be performed to enhance the fixation of the rectum.

Ripstein operation often improved anal continence in patients with rectal prolapse and rectal intussusception. This improvement was accompanied by increased maximum resting pressure (MRP) in patients with rectal prolapse, indicating recovery of internal anal sphincter function. In one of the studies at the Department of Surgery, Karolinska Institute at Danderyd Hospital, Stockholm, Sweden, MRP (52+/- 23 mm Hg) was found in patients with rectal prolapse who underwent Ripstein operation than in patients with rectal intussusception. No postoperative increase in MRP was found in patients with rectal intussusception. This suggests an alternate mechanism of improvement in patients with rectal intussusception.

Mobilization of the Lateral Attachments of the Rectosigmoid

For rectal prolapse surgery lateral mobilization, the surgeon grasps the rectosigmoid junction with his left-hand instrument and draws it to the patient's right side. This allows the lateral attachments of the sigmoid colon to be seen and divided using cautery. Bruising from the prior retroperitoneal mobilization of the colon can usually be seen in this area. Once this layer of peritoneum has been opened, one immediately enters into the space opened by the retroperitoneal dissection. No dissection should be performed more proximally along the white line of Toldt, toward the splenic flexure.

Rectal Mobilization

An atraumatic bowel clamp inserted through the left lower quadrant port is used to elevate the rectosigmoid colon out of the pelvis and away from the retroperitoneum and sacral promontory, to enable entry into the presacral space. The posterior aspect of the mesorectum can be identified, and the mesorectal plane dissected with diathermy, preserving the hypogastric nerves as they pass down into the pelvis anterior to the sacrum. Dissection continues down the presacral space in this avascular plane toward the pelvic floor. Only the posterior 60% of the rectum needs to be mobilized; however, dissection should be continued all the way to the levator ani muscles. A transanal examining finger should be used to confirm the distal extent of the dissection. The peritoneum on either side of the rectum should be incised to the level of the lateral stalks. The lateral stalks should generally be preserved, the exception being when further dissection must completely reduce a very distal prolapsing segment. The rectum is not divided in the case of Wells rectopexy.

Rectopexy

A 2–4 cm portion of polypropylene mesh is rolled and inserted through the umbilical trocar. The camera is reinserted, and the mesh is positioned at the sacral promontory. A mechanical device used for hernia mesh fixation is used to fix the mesh to the promontory. This may be inserted through the right lower quadrant port, but if adequate access cannot be obtained, a 5-mm suprapubic port may be inserted. Great care must be taken not to tear or strip off the presacral fascia when stapling the mesh in place.

The rectum is retracted rostrally to the desired tension to allow complete reduction of the prolapse, which is confirmed by digital rectal examination. The rectopexy is then performed from the right side using the two right-sided trocars. Two or three nonabsorbable sutures are used to attach the distal mesorectum to the mesh at the promontory, sufficient to maintain adequate tension. Alternatively, the mechanical fixation device used for mesh fixation may be employed.

The Complications of Colorectal Surgery

The exact frequency and severity of complications are difficult to determine due to heterogeneous definitions, patient populations, procedures, comorbidities, and intensity of follow-up. One perspective of the incidence of complications can be gleaned from four recent randomized controlled trials comparing laparoscopic to open colon resections for cancer **(Table 1)**.

The risk factors related to colorectal surgery include:

- Perioperative blood transfusion
- American Society of Anesthesiology (ASA) score grade 2 or 3
- Male gender
- Surgeons
- Types of operation
- Creation of an ostomy
- Contaminated wound
- Use of a drain
- Obesity
- Long duration of operation

Wound Infection

Superficial wound infections are the most common complication of colorectal surgery. The previously held belief that preoperative cathartic and oral antibiotic bowel preparation was mandatory to prevent postoperative infections has recently been debunked by multiple randomized controlled trials. Superficial wound infections are recognized by any combination of erythema, induration, tenderness, or drainage at the wound site. Systemic signs of fever and tachycardia may also be present. The infection may manifest as an abscess, cellulitis, or a combination of the two. When suspected, the wound should be carefully inspected, and when a collection is detected, it is drained by reopening the wound. Gram stain can assist in the management and antibiotic selection.

Anastomotic Leak

During laparoscopic colorectal surgery, the anastomotic leak is a common, potentially life-threatening complication associated with significant morbidity, increased risk of local recurrence of cancer, decreased functional outcomes, increased length of stay, high risk of (permanent) ostomy, and death. Leaks are variably defined in the literature, but in general, regarded as perianastomotic stool, gas, or abscess, peritonitis, or a fecal fistula. The incidence of an anastomotic leak following colectomy is generally reported between 2 and 6%. Anastomotic leaks present in one of three ways:

1. Asymptomatic leak
2. Subtle, insidious leak
3. Dramatic early leak

After surgery, the asymptomatic leak is incidentally found during endoscopic or radiographic studies. The incidence of radiographically detected leaks is 4–6 times higher than clinically detected leaks. These leaks, which often present weeks or months later, are typically walled off sinuses, and are, as a general rule, harmless. Treatment is rarely necessary. The subtle, insidious leak can present perioperatively with nonspecific signs and symptoms common in the postoperative period. Such signs include low-grade fevers, mild leukocytosis, protracted ileus, and failure to thrive and occur 5–14 days following surgery. Management of the stable patient without signs of peritonitis usually begins with imaging to identify and localize the process. Traditionally, water-soluble contrast enema has been the primary study to identify leaks. Drawbacks include lower sensitivity for right-sided anastomosis as the contrast dilutes out before reaching the proximal bowel. It also provides little information on extracolonic conditions such as ileus and collections.

TABLE 1: Complication rates following laparoscopic and open colon resections.

	Barcelona trial	*Cost trial*	*Classic trial*	*Color trial*
Wound infection	11.9%	2.5	8.7	3.3%
Persistent ileus	5.5%	2.8		
Evisceration	0.9%			0.8%
Bleeding	0.5%	1.2%	4.8%	1.9%
Anastomotic leak	0.9%		6.0%	2.3%
Pneumonia	0%		6.5%	1.9%
UTI	0.5%	1.2%		2.3%
ARF	1.4%			
DVT			1%	
Cardiac		2.6%		1.2%

(ARF: acute renal failure; DVT: deep venous thrombosis; URI: urinary tract infection)

Abdominopelvic CT scan with triple contrast (oral, intravenous, and rectal) has become the imaging modality of choice to evaluate suspected postoperative intra-abdominal infection. Specificity during the first 5 days postoperative, however, is reduced. During this period, infectious processes may be challenging to differentiate from acute postoperative inflammation and fluid collections. Sensitivity is much improved beyond 5–7 days. CT scan and contrast enema can also be used as complementary studies.

If there are large collections, it can often be amenable to percutaneous, transgluteal, or transanal image-guided catheter drainage. The images should be reviewed with an interventional radiologist to identify a safe window of access that avoids vascular structures and other organs. Abscesses <3–4 cm are too small for most pigtail catheters and will often resolve with a course of antibiotics. In the era of modern CT scanning and interventional radiology, the routine practice of repeat laparotomy, abdominal washouts, large sump drains, and open abdominal wound management is rarely necessary and can be reserved for patients who fail to respond to, deteriorate following, or are not candidates for percutaneous drainage.

Sometimes the management of the patient with progressive generalized peritonitis with or without septic shock requires resuscitation in ICU with broad spectrum antibiotics and urgent laparotomy. Laparoscopic management may be considered if the surgeon has sufficient laparoscopic skills and operative experience. At the time of surgery, the anastomosis should be scrutinized for signs, which led to its failure. This can guide the appropriate method of repair.

After laparoscopic colorectal surgery, if the findings at operation show ischemia and necrosis of greater than one third of the anastomosis, the anastomosis should be resected with the creation of a stoma. If the mucous fistula can be brought up to the skin, it should ideally be fashioned through the same site as the proximal ostomy. When performed in this fashion, subsequent ostomy reversal can be done via a circumstomal incision, obviating the need for formal laparotomy and its associated morbidity. If the findings at operation identify a smaller leak with healthy bowel, the anastomosis can usually be salvaged with suture repair, proximal diversion, and washout of the distal segment. Our preferred diversion is a loop ileostomy.

Early Postoperative Small Bowel Obstruction

After colorectal laparoscopic surgery, early postoperative bowel obstruction is rare, occurring in 1% of patients. This time period accounts for 5–29% of all small bowel obstructions. Most obstructions are caused by adhesions which form within 72 hours of surgery and then become very dense and vascular after 2–3 weeks. Obstructions are more common following colorectal and gynecological procedures than following appendectomy or procedures located above the transverse colon. Signs and symptoms of early postoperative small bowel obstruction are similar to and hard to differentiate from the more common paralytic ileus. Patients typically develop abdominal distention, nausea, and vomiting, but cannot tolerate nasogastric tube clamping or removal. Most patients have a slow, smoldering course, with emergencies being the exception.

The surgeon should try to manage obstruction conservatively initially. There is a fine balance between waiting for the obstruction to resolve and rushing a patient to the operating room. In the first week following surgery, obstruction is hard to differentiate from ileus. Between 2 weeks and 2 months, postoperative adhesions become thick, vascular, and obliterate natural planes, making surgery much more difficult and prone to complications. The decision to operate should, therefore, occur between 7 and 14 days.

If the patient has symptoms of obstruction, plain films readily diagnose most small bowel obstructions. Oral administration of water-soluble contrast followed by a plain abdominal film or CT scan 4 hours later is a good predictor of the resolution of a small bowel obstruction. The contrast in the colon indicates the obstruction is likely to resolve with nonoperative means. CT scan may be useful in identifying signs of ischemia, other intra-abdominal processes and in localizing the site of obstruction for operative planning.

Initial management of the stable patient involves fluid and electrolyte replacement, bowel rest, nasogastric tube drainage, and nutritional evaluation. Total parenteral nutrition should be started as soon as the detected leak. Operation is advised for high-grade or complete bowel obstruction, concern for strangulated bowel, or unresolved small bowel obstruction despite prolonged NGT decompression.

If proper care is ensured, most patients resolve with nonoperative management. If surgery becomes necessary, it should occur prior to the 2 weeks mark, after which the acute adhesions become dense, vascular, and problematic. Surgery involves careful re-exploration and lysis of adhesions. Operative findings usually reveal either a single adhesive band or multiple matted adhesions, each occurring with similar frequency.

After colorectal surgery, if obstruction develops, laparoscopic exploration and adhesiolysis is being increasingly utilized for small bowel obstructions. Advanced laparoscopic skills and experience are a prerequisite because access is difficult in these patients. Poor candidates for laparoscopic management include patients with signs of peritonitis, multiple previous operations for small bowel obstruction, small bowel diameter >4 cm, or other medical contraindication to laparoscopy. Pneumoperitoneum should be established with an open technique at a site remote from the previous incision. Atraumatic graspers are used to explore the bowel in a retrograde fashion beginning with decompressed bowel at the ileocecal valve. Distended bowel is fragile and should not be grasped: grasping the adjacent mesentery reduces the risk of inadvertent bowel perforation. Adhesiolysis is best performed with scissors or bipolar cautery devices to reduce the risk of adjacent bowel injury. Conversion rates range from 7 to 43%. Proactive reasons to convert include poor visualization, nonviable intestine, multiple dense adhesions, deep pelvic adhesions, and failure to progress in a reasonable time.

Sexual Dysfunction

Sexual dysfunction following rectal surgery is related to the extent of pelvic nerve dissection and occurs in both men and women. In men, damage to the sympathetic nerves during high ligation of the IMA or posterior dissection at the sacral promontory can lead to retrograde ejaculation. In addition, damage to the parasympathetic plexus (nerve erigentes) during lateral and anterior dissection can lead to erectile dysfunction. The pathophysiology of sexual dysfunction in women is likely multifactorial and includes damage to the parasympathetic nerves during deep pelvic dissection as well as postoperative mechanical changes in the pelvis, which contribute to loss of sexual desire, vaginal dryness, altered orgasm, and dyspareunia. Sexual dysfunction is more difficult to diagnose in women, in part because the presence of incontinence often discourages women from engaging in sexual activity.

TIPS AND TRICKS

To avoid intraoperative complications:

- Create adequate exposure.
- Use proper traction and counter traction.
- Develop the right planes.
- Standardize the assistant's role.
- Beware of the variations of vasculature and anatomy.
- Should visualization be compromised during the procedure?, it is easy to switch to a 30° laparoscope for a more topographical view. Applying the angled 30° laparoscope can also be helpful to manage external arm collisions during tight set-up situations, as the camera arm angle changes depending on the endoscopy used. Additionally, with an angled 30° laparoscope, the surgeon has the ability to rotate the viewing angle of the scope (out of the horizontal image plane) and minimize collisions as well.
- Leave 1–1.5 cm on either side of the transacted IMA and IMV so that if any bleeding occurs, grasping of the vessel is still possible to allow the application of the hemostatic technique (clips, LigaSure™ or suture).
- Distance the ports as much as possible from each other during initial port placement (minimum of 7.5 cm). Placing the patient in a steeper Trendelenburg position can increase the vertical spacing between the arms and potentially eliminate or minimize arising collisions.
- Before dividing any tissues, identify the ureter and gonadal vessels one more time.
- During all procedure steps, clear communication with the patient-side assistant is essential.

CONCLUSION

The laparoscopic technique reduces parietal aggression and achieves the same results as traditional surgery. Patients recover faster and experience less pain, with fewer wound infections, postoperative hernias, less time in the hospital, and reduced costs. But laparoscopic colonic surgery requires extensive and highly specialized training, with few surgeons qualified to perform these procedures. The recent conclusion of the oncologic debate, together with the rapid development of technological means and the increase in public awareness, will probably result in a substantial increase in the number of surgeons performing laparoscopic colorectal surgery. The laparoscopic technique is an excellent approach, though not yet the gold standard. Smooth performance of this technique depends on the quality of the equipment, perfect knowledge of the operative steps, exposure of operative field, and the experience of the surgical team. Operative times are somewhat longer than open procedures but become shorter along the learning curve. Right colectomies are shorter and easier to perform than left-sided and rectal resections and should be employed for teaching residents. The conversion rate would not necessarily drop after the first 50 cases and should reflect good surgical judgment rather than a surgical failure.

BIBLIOGRAPHY

1. Anderson J, Luchtefeld M, Dujovny N, Hoedema R, Kim D, Butcher J. A comparison of laparoscopic, hand-assist and open sigmoid resection in the treatment of diverticular disease. Am J Surg. 2007;193(3):400-3.
2. Bartels SA, D'Hoore A, Cuesta MA, Bensdorp AJ, Lucas C, Bemelman WA . Significantly increased pregnancy rates after laparoscopic restorative proctocolectomy: a cross-sectional study. Ann Surg. 2012;256:1045.
3. Belizon A, Balik E, Feingold DL, Bessler M, Arnell TD, Forde KA, et al. Major abdominal surgery increases plasma levels of vascular endothelial growth factor: open more so than minimally invasive methods. Ann Surg. 2006;244(5):792-8.
4. Bender JS, Magnuson TH, Zenilman ME, Smith-Meek MM, Ratner LE, Jones CE, et al. Outcome following colon surgery in the octogenarian. Am Surg. 1996;62(4):276-9.
5. Berends FJ, Kazemier G, Bonjer HJ, Lange JF. Subcutaneous metastases after laparoscopic colectomy. Lancet. 1994; 344(8914):58.
6. Chang YJ, Marcello PW, Rusin C, Roberts PL, Schoetz DJ. Hand-assisted laparoscopic sigmoid colectomy: helping hand or hindrance? Surg Endosc. 2005;19(5):656-61.
7. Dean PA, Beart RWJr, Nelson H, Elftmann TD, Schlinkert RT. Laparoscopic-assisted segmental colectomy: early Mayo Clinic experience. Mayo Clin Proc. 1994;69(9):834-40.
8. Djokovic JL, Hedley-Whyte J. Prediction of outcome of surgery and anaesthesia in patients over 80. JAMA. 1979; 242(21):2301-6.
9. Döbrönte Z, Wittmann T, Karácsony G. Rapid development of malignant metastases in the abdominal wall after laparoscopy. Endoscopy. 1978;10(2):127-30.

10. Falk PM, Beart RW Jr, Wexner SD, et al. Laparoscopic colectomy: a critical appraisal. Dis Colon Rectum. 1993;36(1):28-34.
11. Fallahzadeh H, Mays ET. Preexisting disease as a predictor of the outcome of colectomy. Am J Surg. 1991;162(5):497-8.
12. Fleshman JW, Fry RD, Birnbaum EH, Kodner IJ. Laparoscopic-assisted and minilaparotomy approaches to colorectal diseases are similar in early outcome. Dis Colon Rectum. 1996;39(1):15-22.
13. Franklin ME, Rosenthal D, Abrego-Medina D, Dorman JP, Glass JL, Norem R, et al. Prospective comparison of open vs laparoscopic colon surgery for carcinoma. Five-year results. Dis Colon Rectum. 1996;39(10 Suppl):S35-46.
14. Frazee RC, Roberts JW, Okeson GC, Symmonds RE, Snyder SK, Hendricks JC, et al. Open versus laparoscopic cholecystectomy. A comparison of postoperative pulmonary function. Ann Surg. 1991;213(6):651-3.
15. Gellman L, Salky B, Edye M. Laparoscopic assisted colectomy. Surg Endosc. 1996;10:1041-4.
16. Goh YC, Eu KW, Seow-Choen F. Early postoperative results of a prospective series of laparoscopic vs. open anterior resections for rectosigmoid cancers. Dis Colon Rectum. 1997;40:776-80.
17. Hasegawa H, Kabeshima Y, Watanabe M, Yamamoto S, Kitajima M. Randomized controlled trial of laparoscopic versus open colectomy for advanced colorectal cancer. Surg Endosc. 2003;17(4):636-40.
18. Hoffman GC, Baker JW, Fitchett CW, Vansant JH. Laparoscopic-assisted colectomy. Initial experience. Ann Surg. 1994;219:732-40.
19. Hughes ESR, McDermott FT, Polglase AL, Johnson WR. Tumor recurrence in the abdominal wall scar after large-bowel cancer surgery. Dis Colon Rectum. 1983;26(9):571-2.
20. Keats AS. The ASA classification of physical status-a recapitulation. Anesthesiology. 1978;49:233-6.
21. Khalili TM, Fleshner PR, Hiatt JR, Sokol TP, Manookian C, Tsushima G, et al. Colorectal cancer: comparison of laparoscopic with open approaches. Dis Colon Rectum. 1998;41(7):832-8.
22. Kirman I, Cekic V, Poltoratskaia N, Sylla P, Jain S, Forde KA, et al. Open surgery induces a dramatic decrease in circulating intact IGFBP-3 in patients with colorectal cancer not seen with laparoscopic surgery. Surg Endosc. 2005;19(1):55-9.
23. Kranczer S. Banner year for US longevity. Star Bull Metrop Insur Co. 1998;79:8-14.
24. Lacy AM, García-Valdecasas JC, Delgado S, Castells A, Taurá P, Piqué JM, et al. Laparoscopy-assisted colectomy versus open colectomy for treatment of non-metastatic colon cancer: a randomised trial. Lancet. 2002;359(9325):2224-9.
25. Lacy AM, Garcia-Valdecasas JC, Pique JM, Delgado S, Campo E, Bordas JM, et al. Short-term outcome analysis of a randomized study comparing laparoscopic vs open colectomy for colon cancer. Surg Endosc. 1995;9(10):1101-5.
26. Lange MM, Marijnen CA, Maas CP, Putter H, Rutten HJ, Stiggelbout AM, et al. Risk factors for sexual dysfunction after rectal cancer treatment. Eur J Cancer 2009; 45:1578.
27. Lechaux D, Trebuchet G, Le Calve JL. Five-year results of 206 laparoscopic left colectomies for cancer. Surg Endosc. 2002;16(10):1409-12.
28. Liberman MA, Phillips EH, Carroll BJ, Fallas M, Rosenthal R. Laparoscopic colectomy vs traditional colectomy for diverticulitis. Outcome and costs. Surg Endosc. 1996;10:15-8.
29. Lord SA, Larach SW, Ferrara A, Williamson PR, Lago CP, Lube MW. Laparoscopic resections for colorectal carcinoma: a three-year experience. Dis Colon Rectum. 1996;39:148-54.
30. Loungnarath R, Fleshman JW. Hand-assisted laparoscopic colectomy techniques. Semin Laparosc Surg. 2003;10(4): 219-30.
31. Lumley JW, Fielding GA, Rhodes M, Nathanson LK, Siu S, Stitz RW. Laparoscopic-assisted colorectal surgery: lessons learned from 240 consecutive patients. Dis Colon Rectum. 1996;39:155-9.
32. Masui H, Ike H, Yamaguchi S, et al. Male sexual function after autonomic nerve-preserving operation for rectal cancer. Dis Colon Rectum. 1996;39(10):1140-5.
33. MilsomJW, Bohm B, Hammerhofer KA, Fazio V, Steiger E, Elson P. A prospective, randomized trial comparing laparoscopic versus conventional techniques in colorectal cancer surgery: a preliminary report. J Am Coil Surg. 1998;187:46-54.
34. Nakajima K, Lee SW, Sonoda T, Milsom JW. Intraoperative carbon dioxide colonoscopy: a safe insufflation alternative for locating colonic lesions during laparoscopic surgery. Surg Endosc. 2005;19(3):321-5.
35. Ng CSH, Whelan RL, Lacy AM, Yim AP. Is minimal access surgery for cancer associated with immunologic benefits? World J Surg. 2005;29(8):975-81.
36. Olsen KO, Joelsson M, Laurberg S, Oresland T. Fertility after ileal pouch-anal anastomosis in women with ulcerative colitis. Br J Surg. 1999;86:493.
37. Ørding Olsen K, Juul S, Berndtsson I, Tom Oresland, Søren Laurberg. Ulcerative colitis: female fecundity before diagnosis, during disease, and after surgery compared with a population sample. Gastroenterology. 2002;122:15.
38. Ortega AE, Beart RW Jr, Steele GD Jr, Winchester DP, Greene FL. Laparoscopic bowel surgery registry: preliminary results. Dis Colon Rectum. 1995;38:681-5.
39. Peters WR, Barrels TL. Minimally invasive colectomy: are the potential benefits realized? Dis Colon Rectum. 1993;36: 751-6.
40. Peters WR, Fleshman JW. Minimally invasive colectomy in elderly patients. Surg Laparosc Endosc. 1995;5:477-9.
41. Reilly WT, Nelson H, Schroeder G, et al. Wound recurrence following conventional treatment of colorectal cancer. Dis Colon Rectum. 1996;39(2):200-7.
42. Reissman P, Agachan F, Wexner SD. Outcome of laparoscopic colorectal surgery in older patients. Am Surg. 1996;62:1060-3.
43. Senagore AJ, Luchtefeld MA, Mackeigan JM, Mazier WP. Open colectomy versus laparoscopic colectomy: are there differences? Am Surg. 1993;59:549-53.
44. Spivak H, Maele DV, Friedman I, Nussbaum M. Colorectal surgery in octogenarians. J Am Coil Surg. 1996;183:46-50.
45. Stocchi L, Nelson H. Laparoscopic colectomy for colon cancer: trial update. J Surg Oncol. 1998;68:255-67.
46. Veldkamp R, Kuhry E, Hop WC; Colon cancer Laparoscopic or Open Resection Study Group (COLOR). Laparoscopic surgery versus open surgery for colon cancer: short-term outcomes of a randomized trial. Lancet Oncol. 2005;6(7):477-84.
47. Vukasin P, Ortega AE, Greene FL, Steele GD, Simons AJ, Anthone GJ, et al. Wound recurrence following laparoscopic colon cancer resection. Results of the American Society of Colon and Rectal Surgeons Laparoscopic Registry. Dis Colon Rectum. 1996;39(10 Suppl):S20-3.
48. Waljee A, Waljee J, Morris AM, Higgins PD. Threefold increased risk of infertility: a meta-analysis of infertility after ileal pouch anal anastomosis in ulcerative colitis. Gut. 2006;55:1575.
49. Walsh TH. Audit of outcome of major surgery in the elderly. Br J Surg. 1996;83:92-7.
50. Weeks JC, Nelson H, Gelber S; Clinical Outcomes of Surgical Therapy (COST) Study Group. Short-term quality of life outcomes following laparoscopic-assisted colectomy vs open colectomy for colon cancer: a randomized trial. JAMA. 2002;287(3):321-8.
51. Whittle J, Steinberg EP, Anderson GF, Herbert R. Results of colectomy in elderly patients with colon cancer, based on Medicare claims data. Am J Surg. 1992;163:57245.
52. Wise WE Jr, Padmanabhan A, Meesig DM, Arnold MW, Aguilar PS, Stewart WR. Abdominal colon and rectal operations in the elderly. Dis Colon Rectum. 1991;34:959-63.
53. Young-Fadok T, Radice E, Nelson H. Benefits of laparoscopic-assisted colectomy for colon polyps: a casematched series. [meeting abstract] Dis Colon Rectum. 1998;41:A47.

CHAPTER 27

Laparoscopic Adhesiolysis

INTRODUCTION

Peritoneal adhesions are a common cause of bowel obstruction, pelvic pain, and infertility. More often than not, these adhesions need to be released surgically for the management of these complications. Proper technique of adhesiolysis is very important, and operating surgeons should have a clear concept of the mechanism of adhesion formation.

The adhesions that form in the abdomen following abdominal or pelvic surgery are a normal response to injury of the peritoneal surfaces during surgery. Although adhesions have some beneficial effects, they also cause significant morbidity, including adhesive small bowel obstruction, female infertility, chronic abdominal pain, and increased difficulty with subsequent surgery.

Normal fibrinolytic activity prevents fibrinous attachments for 72–96 hours after surgery and mesothelial repair occurs within 5 days of trauma. Within these 5 days a single cell layer of new peritoneum covers the injured raw area, replacing the fibrinous exudates. However, if the fibrinolytic activity of the peritoneum is suppressed, fibroblasts will migrate, proliferate, and form fibrous adhesions. Collagen is deposited, and neovascular formation starts.

The most important factors which suppress fibrinolytic activity and promote adhesion formation are:

- Port wound just above the target of dissection
- Tissue ischemia
- Drying of serosal surfaces
- Excessive suturing of omental patches
- Traction of peritoneum
- Blood clots, stones or dead tissue retained inside
- Prolonged operation
- Visceral injury
- Infection
- Delayed postoperative mobilization of the patient
- Postoperative pain due to inadequate analgesia

Laparoscopic adhesiolysis was first described by a gynecologist for the treatment of chronic pelvic pain and infertility. In the early days of laparoscopy, previous abdominal surgery was a relative contraindication for most laparoscopic procedures. Laparoscopic surgery to relieve bowel obstructions was not routinely performed. However, in 1991, Bastug et al. reported the successful use of laparoscopic adhesiolysis for small bowel obstruction in one patient with a single adhesive band.

Since then, many case series have documented this technique. Advanced technology with high-definition imaging, smaller cameras, and better instrumentation have allowed for an increasing number of adhesiolysis to be performed laparoscopically with good outcomes.

Compared with the open approach to adhesiolysis, the laparoscopic approach offers the following:

- Less postoperative pain
- Decreased incidence of ventral hernia
- Reduced recovery time with the earlier return of bowel function
- Shorter hospital stay

INDICATIONS

Patient selection is important in the success of the procedure. Laparoscopic adhesiolysis has a number of potential advantages, but these advantages are realized only if the procedure is performed in patients best suited for it.

Laparoscopic adhesiolysis is indicated in the following patients:

- Patients with a complete small bowel obstruction or partial small bowel obstruction not resolving with nonoperative therapy, but without signs of peritonitis or bowel perforation or ischemia.
- Patients with resolved bowel obstruction but with a history of recurrent and chronic small bowel obstruction demonstrated by a contrast study.

Controversy exists regarding whether patients with chronic pelvic pain benefit from laparoscopic adhesiolysis or whether any seeming benefit is a placebo effect. This controversy notwithstanding, the procedure should be offered to patients with chronic pelvic pain if no other etiology of pain is found in the previous workup.

CONTRAINDICATIONS OF LAPAROSCOPIC ADHESIOLYSIS

- Hemodynamic instability
- Uncorrected coagulopathy

- Severe cardiopulmonary disease
- Abdominal wall infection
- Multiple previous upper abdominal procedures
- Late pregnancy

Patient Position

The anesthetized patient is placed on the operating table with the legs straight or in a lithotomy position if female. The lithotomy position will allow the gynecologists and assistant to work simultaneously, and uterine manipulation would be possible in case it is required. The thighs must not be flexed onto the abdominal wall as they would be in the full lithotomy position used for other open surgical, gynecological procedures. The operating table is tilted head up or down by approximately 15° depending on the main area of examination. Compression bandage may be used on legs during the operation to prevent thromboembolism, especially if the patient is in the lithotomy position.

Position of the Surgical Team

Before starting diagnostic laparoscopy, the best guess is made about the quadrant in which adhesions are more likely to be found. The surgeon should stand opposite to this quadrant to allow a direct view into this quadrant. If the pathology is more likely in the pelvic cavity the surgeon stands on left side of the patient. The first assistant, whose main task is to position the video camera, is also on the patient's left side. The instrument trolley is placed on the patient's left, allowing the scrub nurse to assist with placing the appropriate instruments in the operating ports. Television monitors are positioned on either side of the bottom end of the operating table at a suitable height for surgeon, anesthetists, as well as assistant to see the procedure. For adhesions involving other quadrants of the abdomen, the surgeon, assistants, and monitors are placed accordingly.

Port Position

For the adhesiolysis of gynecological purposes, generally, one optical port in umbilicus and two 5 mm port in left and right iliac fossa should be introduced according to the baseball diamond concept after visualizing the target of dissection. Port should be in a position to provide an elevation angle of 30° and a manipulation angle of 60°, which is a standard and considered ergonomically better. Some gynecologists prefer suprapubic port, but with a suprapubic port, the elevation angle of the instrument and tubal structure is 90°, and hence lifting of ovary and tube may be difficult without grasping it.

A three or four ports approach should be used if there is any difficulty in manipulation with two ports, especially in case of extensive adhesions **(Figs. 1A and B)**.

For adhesiolysis in right lower quadrant, the preferred port positions should be:

- 10 mm umbilical (optical)
- 5 mm suprapubic
- 5 mm right hypochondrium

A 30° telescope is employed in most instances, as this facilitates easier inspection of the deeper peritoneal cavity and abdominal organs. The secondary ports are inserted under laparoscopic vision. The selected site on the abdominal wall is identified by finger indentation of the parietal peritoneum.

The open technique for trocar insertion is recommended if extensive adhesion is suspected. At the time of laparoscopic adhesiolysis, surgeon should try to be very gentle with the tubal structure and bowel so that readhesions are prevented and stricture of tube may not occur.

Viewing of lateral pelvic organs is helped by the manipulation of mobile structures with a second port introduced through the left iliac fossa.

PATHOGENESIS

At the molecular level, adhesion formation involves a complex interaction of cytokines, growth factors, cell adhesion molecules, neuropeptides, and numerous other factors secreted by cells in or near the area of trauma. The early balance between fibrin deposition and degradation (i.e., fibrinolysis) appears to be a critical factor in the pathogenesis of adhesions.

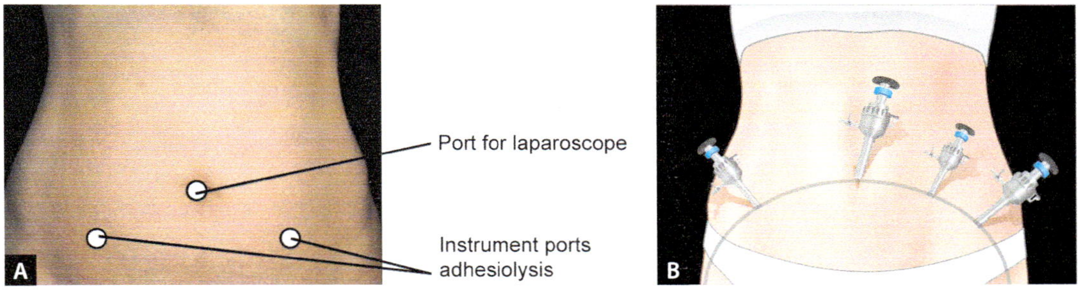

Figs. 1A and B: Ports for pelvic adhesiolysis.

LAPAROSCOPIC ADHESIOLYSIS TECHNIQUE

Animal studies have proved that laparoscopy leads to less adhesion formation compared to open surgery. The low adhesion forming tendency after laparoscopic surgery is because very less retraction is used, packing of the abdominal cavity is not required that can damage peritoneum. In laparoscopic surgery, there are fewer chances of drying of tissues because the inside environment is cutoff from outside. Also, the excellent visualization and magnification result in less likelihood of tissue injury and adhesions. In laparoscopy, port wound and wound at the target of dissection is far away from each other, so the chances of adhesions are less likely to the peritoneum because, for adhesions to form, both the raw layers which tends to adhere should be in contact. At least three ports should be used to perform laparoscopic adhesiolysis. After access and introduction of telescope, two other ports should be introduced according to the baseball diamond concept, keeping in mind the center of adhesions as a target of dissection.

If the adhesions are thin and avascular, it is easily lysed, and the chances of recurrence are not much. In contrast, if adhesions are thick and highly vascular, then it is difficult to separate. These adhesions usually require the use of energy sources (ultrasonic dissector, unipolar, or bipolar). Regular achieving of hemostasis and meticulous sharp dissection with scissors is necessary **(Figs. 2A and B)**.

Adhesiolysis can be safely performed if dissection is done carefully through avascular planes. The laparoscopic approach precludes feeling through these adhesions. Accordingly, a general rule that can be followed in this setting is, if you can see through it, you can cut it.

An atraumatic grasper is introduced to hold the adhesions or involved organs. It should be stretched gently, and boundaries of adhesion are identified. The avascular area is chosen with the close-up magnified view of the telescope. The opposite trocar on the side of the surgeon is used for scissors and adhesions should be cut close to the affected organ. Vascular adhesions should be coagulated using an electrosurgical instrument, preferably, bipolar. Scissors should be used only if flimsy avascular adhesions are found **(Figs. 3A and B)**. Thick vascular adhesions should be first tried with blunt dissection, or otherwise must be coagulated before being cut. A suction irrigation instrument is good if blunt dissection is the main line of action.

Try to get a sense of the tissue. Some patients have tissue that will tear easily, whereas others have tissue that readily

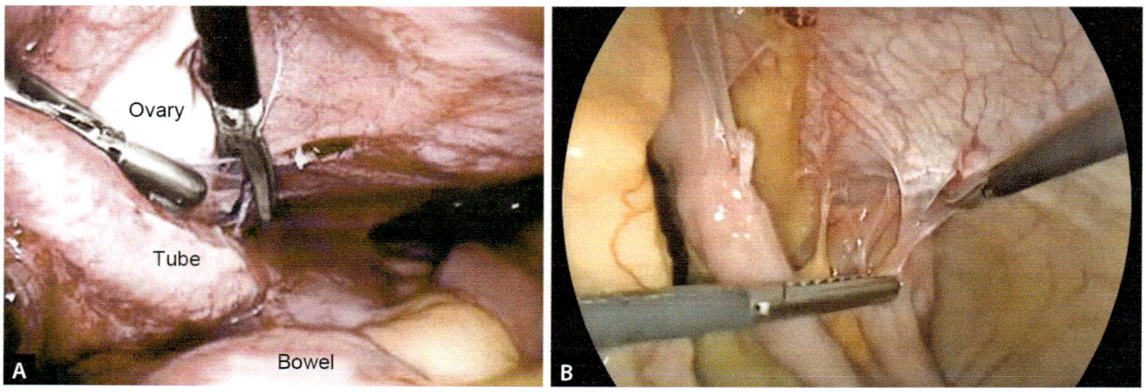

Figs. 2A and B: Sharp dissection with scissors for bowel is involved.

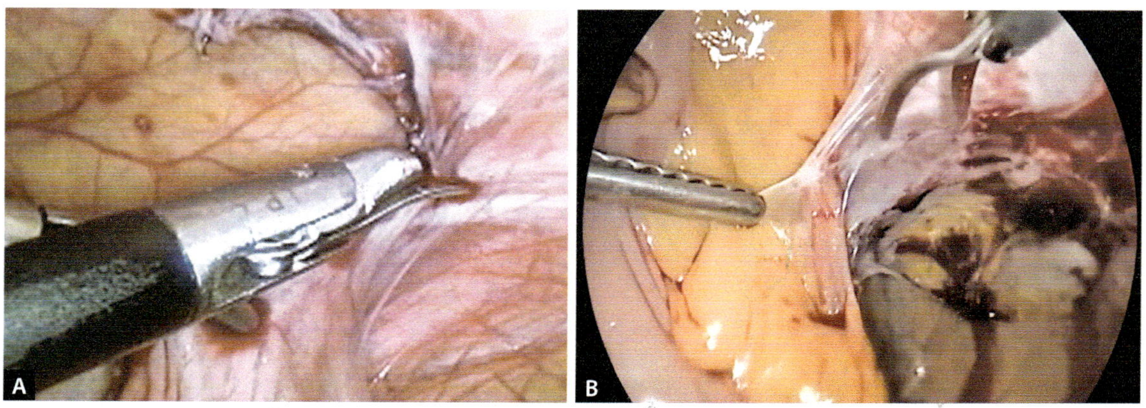

Figs. 3A and B: Sharp dissection with scissors if the bowel is involved.

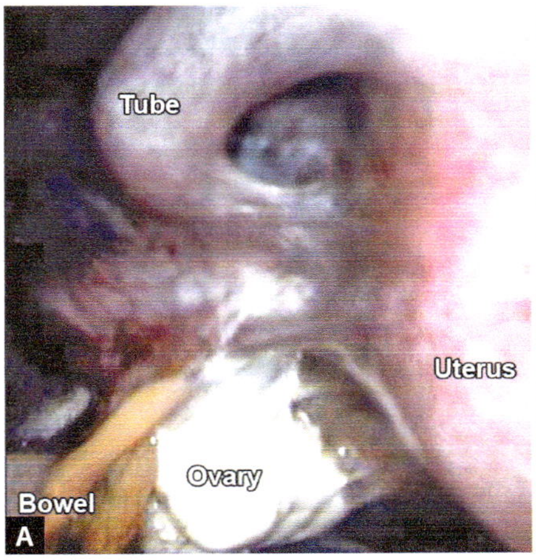

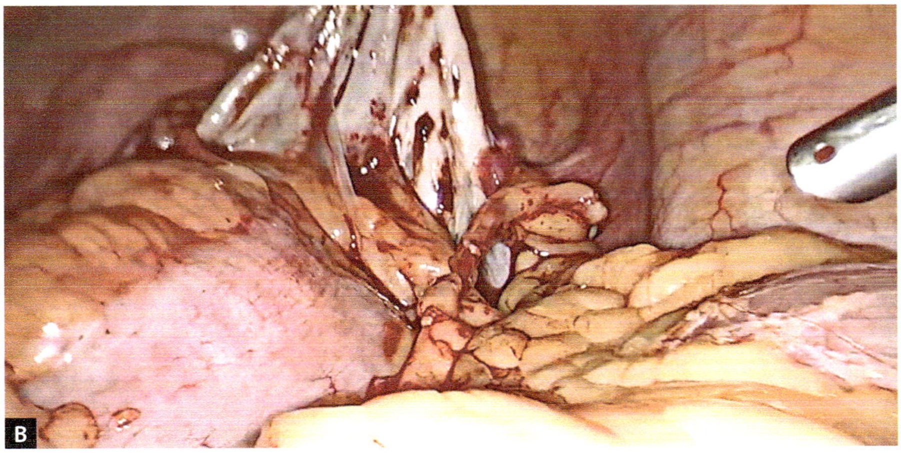

Figs. 4A and B: Tubo-ovarian mass with bowel involvement.

permits blunt dissection. An individualized approach to each patient's tissues is important.

Bowel injury is not very uncommon during enterolysis and patients who have a history of the previous laparotomy should undergo a preoperative bowel preparation **(Figs. 4A and B)**. If an inadvertent injury occurs, then enterorrhaphy can be accomplished with one layer closure using Vicryl.

After adhesiolysis, some fluid can be left inside to which may help prevent a recurrence. Steroids and antihistamines have been tried, but are now used infrequently because of the adverse effect of delayed wound healing and high risk of dehiscence.

High-molecular weight dextran has also been tested to prevent readhesions because it is absorbed over a period of 7–10 days. Its osmotic effect draws the fluid into the peritoneal cavity, and so the mobile peritoneal organ floats, reducing adherence between intraperitoneal organs. Although the study in animals has demonstrated reduced postoperative adhesion, its efficacy is not fully confirmed.

Adhesion barrier membranes have also been tried. These absorbable membranes separate the peritoneal lining from potentially likely to adhere to organs and thus prevent fibrous bands from different binding structures. Two such materials are Interceed and Gore-Tex. Interceed is an absorbable fabric of oxidized regenerated cellulose, and Gore-Tex is a nonabsorbable and nonreactive surgical membrane. Animal studies have demonstrated good results using these membranes.

MEASURES FOR PREVENTING PERITONEAL ADHESIONS

Fundamentals

Methods for preventing adhesions are directed at the mechanisms of adhesion formation.

- Minimize injury
- Introduce a barrier between injured surfaces
- Prevent coagulation of the serous exudate
- Remove or dissolve the deposited fibrin
- Inhibit the fibroblastic response to the tissue injury
- Involve recombinant tissue plasminogen activator and novel fibrinolytic

Methods for preventing adhesions can be classified broadly as technical measures; physical barriers, which may be solid or liquid; and pharmacologic therapies.

Gentle Tissue Handling

A good surgical technique is the first defense against adhesion formation. Meticulous hemostasis and gentle, minimal tissue handling are important for limiting the extent of the initial peritoneal injury. Damage to the serosa can be prevented by minimizing trauma, bleeding, and ischemia and by keeping the surgical field moist with frequent irrigation to prevent tissues from drying out. Laparoscopy offers certain advantages over open abdominal surgery concerning adhesion formation. The abdominal incisions are small and there is less handling of tissue and exposure to foreign bodies, all of which may help to decrease tissue trauma, compared with laparotomy, and thus to reduce the risk for adhesion formation, especially to the abdominal wall.

Physical Barriers

Physical barriers include solid materials (absorbable sheets and nonabsorbable prosthetic materials) and viscous fluids introduced into the abdomen. All are aimed at keeping damaged peritoneal surfaces separated during the first 5–7 days after surgery until after reepithelialization has occurred. Although barriers do appear to limit the extent of adhesion formation, whether they improve clinically important outcomes by reducing the risks for intestinal obstruction, infertility, and chronic abdominal or pelvic pain is less.

Solid Barriers (Sheets)

Two absorbable membrane sheets are commercially available. One is a sodium hyaluronate-based carboxymethylcellulose sheet (Seprafilm) **(Figs. 5A and B)**,

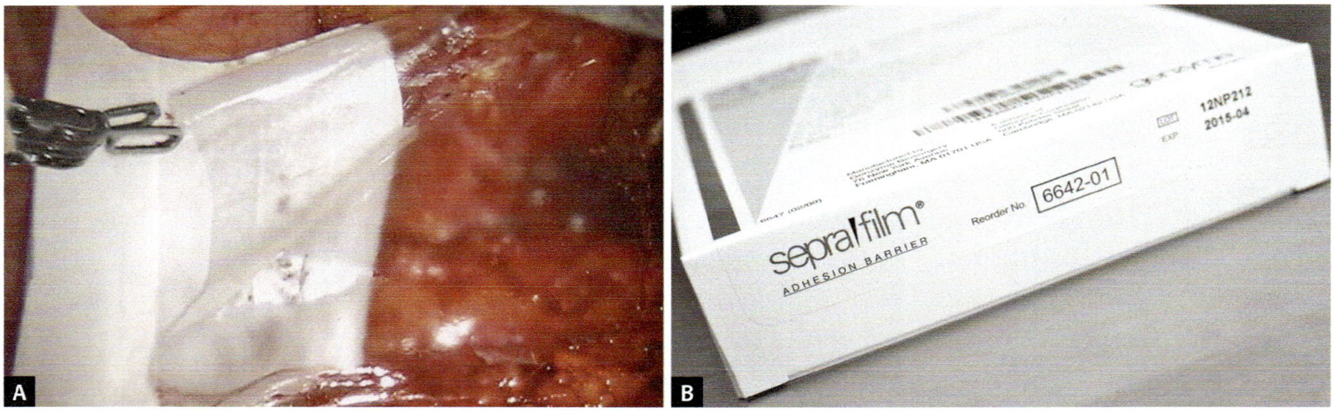

Figs. 5A and B: Seprafilm an adhesive barrier.

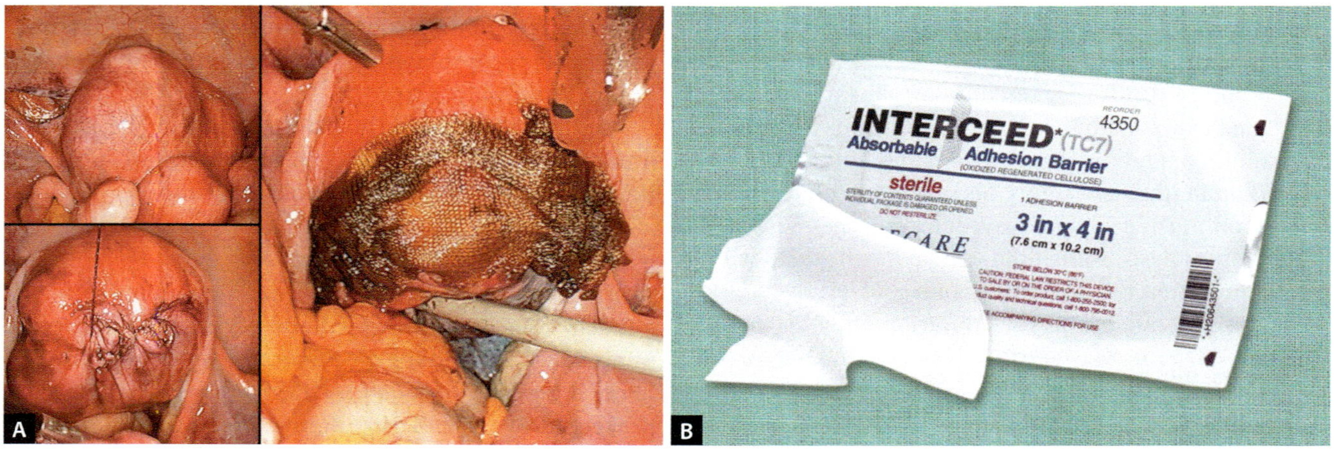

Figs. 6A and B: Interceed an adhesive barrier.

and the second is an oxidized regenerated cellulose sheet (Interceed) **(Figs. 6A and B)**. Both appear safe and effective for preventing adhesions between surfaces to which they are applied but are somewhat tricky to handle and do not avert adhesion formation at other sites within the abdomen. In addition, there is one nonabsorbable solid barrier [expanded polytetrafluoroethylene (ePTFE)] that has been found to prevent adhesions in clinical studies.

Expanded Polytetrafluoroethylene

Expanded polytetrafluoroethylene is a nonabsorbable, flexible prosthetic material used for a variety of surgical reconstructions. The ePTFE is trimmed to overlap the denuded area by 1 cm and sutured into place with nonabsorbable sutures, usually a 7-0 or 8-0 nylon or polypropylene.

A small trial of patients having open myomectomy randomly assigned 28 subjects to the application of ePTFE suture over the uterine incision or to no barrier. At second-look laparoscopy, more patients receiving ePTFE were adhesion free compared with untreated controls (55% vs. 7%).

Liquid Barriers (Instillates)

Polyethylene Glycol

Polyethylene glycol (PEG) adhesion barrier (SprayGel and SprayShield) is a synthetic hydrogel that forms within seconds after simultaneous spray of two solutions of PEG-based liquids onto targeted tissue. Crosslinking between the solutions forms an absorbable, flexible, and adherent gel barrier that remains intact for 5–7 days before degrading into its components, which are then resorbed and excreted through the kidneys. SprayGel is available in Europe but is not yet approved for use in the United States.

Icodextrin Solution

A 4% isosmolar solution of icodextrin (Adept) is an alpha-1,4 glucose polymer with the prolonged peritoneal residence. It is used as an irrigant during surgery (minimum 100 mL/30 min) and is the most promising intraoperative instillate for adhesion prevention. It can be used following laparoscopic adhesiolysis and is the only agent approved in the United States for preventing peritoneal adhesions in gynecologic laparoscopy.

Hyaluronic Acid Solution, Gel, and Powder

Hyaluronic acid is an anionic, nonsulfated glycosaminoglycan distributed in connective tissue. A systematic review identified four trials comparing hyaluronic acid-containing solutions with placebo and found no difference in overall mean adhesions scores, but also found that the solutions significantly reduced the proportion of women with adhesions or the extent of adhesions at time of second-look laparoscopy.

Promotion of Bowel Motility

As an adjunct to the physical separation of healing surfaces, maintenance of relative motion between healing surfaces, mimicking normal peristalsis and mobility, has been proposed to prevent or limit adhesion formation. In humans, impaired postoperative intestinal motility may cause a postoperative ileus, further exacerbated by postoperative pain management with opiates. The small intestine has impaired motility for 1-2 days postoperatively, whereas the colon has impaired motility for 2-3 days on average.

A number of other agents have been applied in attempts to prevent postoperative peritoneal adhesions but are considered generally ineffective and possibly harmful. Crystalloid solutions should not be expected to prevent adhesion formation because of their short intraperitoneal time of residence, and this prediction is consistent with clinical observations installation of nonbarrier fluid into the peritoneal cavity after surgery is associated with numerous theoretical and practical concerns. Fluid overload may potentially lead to pulmonary edema and may cause abdominal pain and dyspnea. Fluid may potentially leak through laparoscopic incisions, which may cause distress to the patient and require frequent bandage replacement. Extravasation to the vulvar region has been reported in up to 2% of patients receiving dextran 70. Excess intraperitoneal fluid also may reduce opsonization of foreign cells, impair host cell phagocytosis, and lead to infectious complications. In one animal study, dextran significantly reduced adhesion formation but resulted in peritonitis rather than in abscesses as was observed with the instillation of saline.

Other solutions instilled into the peritoneum to reduce adhesion formation have been evaluated and are ineffective. A systematic review found no significant benefit from the use of intraoperative irrigation or infusion of various drugs and liquids, including intraperitoneal steroids, dextran, or heparin. Antibiotic solutions also are ineffective for preventing adhesions, and, in rats, irrigation of the abdominal cavity with cefazolin and tetracycline resulted in increased formation of peritoneal adhesions.

BIBLIOGRAPHY

1. De Wilde RL. Goodbye to late bowel obstruction after appendicectomy. Lancet. 1991;338:1012.
2. Diamond MP, Daniell JF, Feste J, Surrey MW, McLaughlin DS, Friedman S, et al. Adhesion reformation and de novo adhesion formation after reproductive pelvic surgery. Fertil Steril. 1987;47(5):864-6.
3. Easter DW, Cushieri A, Nathanson LK, Lavelle-Jones M. The utility of diagnostic laparoscopy for abdominal disorders. Audit of 120 patients. Arch Surg. 1992;127(4):379-83.
4. Eypasch E, Spangenberger W, Williams JI, Ure B, Neugebauer W, Wood-Dauphinee S, et al. Frfihe postoperative Verbesserung der Lebensqualitfit nach laparoskopischer Cholecystektomie. In: Hfiring R (Ed). Diagnostik und Therapie des Gallensteinleidens im Wandel der Zeit. Berlin: Blackwell; 1992. pp. 481-91.
5. Fervers C. Die Laparoskopie mit dem Cystoskop. Ein Beitrag zur Vereinfachung der Technik und zur endoskopischen Strangdurchtrennung in der Bauchhohle. Med Klin Chir. 1933;178:288.
6. Fuchs KH, Freys SM, Heimbucher J, Thiede A. Laparoskopische Cholecystektomie—lohnt sich die laparoskopische Technik in "schwierigen" Ffillen? Chirurg. 1992;63:296-304.
7. Klaiber C, Metzger A. Manual der laparoskopischen Chirurgie. Bern: Verlag Hans Huber; 1992. pp. 185-206.
8. Kolmorgen K, Schulz AM. Results of laparoscopic lysis of adhesions in patients with chronic pelvic pain. Zentralbl Gynakol. 1991;113(6):291-5.
9. Kresch AJ, Seifer DB, Sachs LB, Banner I. Laparoscopy in 100 women with chronic pelvic pain. Obstet Gynecol. 1984;64(5):672-4.
10. Luciano AA, Maier DB, Koch EI, Nulsen JC, Whitman GF. A comparative study of postoperative adhesions following laser surgery by laparoscopy versus laparotomy in the rabbit model. Obstet Gynecol. 1989;74(2):220-4.
11. Mecke H, Semm K, Lehmann-Willenbrock E. Pelviscopic adhesiolysis. Successes in the treatment of chronic abdominal pain caused by adhesions in the lower and middle abdomen. Geburtshilfe Frauenheilkd. 1988;48(3):55-9.
12. Meiser G, Waclawiczek HW, Heinerman M, Boeckl O. Der intermittierende inkomplette Dtinndarmileus—sonographische Diagnostik und Trendbeobachtung. Chirurg. 1990;61:651-6.
13. Nezhat CR, Nezhat FR, Metzger DA, Luicano A. Adhesion reformation after reproductive surgery by videolaseroscopy. Fertil Steril. 1990;53(6):1008-11.
14. Peters AA, Trimbos-Kemper GC, Admiraal C, Trimbos JB, Hermans J. A randomized clinical trial on the benefit of adhesiolysis in patients with intraperitoneal adhesions and chronic pelvic pain. Br J Obstet Gynaecol. 1992;99(1):59-62.
15. Raf LE. Causes of abdominal adhesions in cases of intestinal obstruction. Acta Chir Scand. 1969;135:73-6.
16. Rapkin AJ. Adhesions and pelvic pain: a retrospective study. Obstet Gynecol. 1986;68(1):13-5.
17. Riedel HH, Haag GM. Late sequelae of appendectomy with special reference to adhesions in the lower abdomen, chronic abdominal pain and sterility. Zentralbl Gynakol. 1989;111(16):1101-12.
18. Riedel HH, Lehmann-Willenbrock E, Mecke H, Serum K. The frequency distribution of various pelviscopic (laparoscopic) operations, including complications rates—statistics of the Federal Republic of Germany in the years 1983-1985. Zentralbl Gynakol. 1989;111:78-91.
19. Serum K. Operationslehre ftir endoskopische Abdominalchirurgie. Stuttgart: Schattauer; 1984.
20. Serum K. Sichtkontrollierte Peritoneumperforation zur operativen Pelviskopie. Geburtshilfe Frauenheilkd. 1988;48: 436-9.
21. Tavmergen EN, Mecke H, Serum K. Hfiufigkeit intra-abdomineller Adhfisionen nach Pelviskopie und Laparotomie. Zentralb Gynakol. 1990;112:1163-9.
22. Troidl H, Spangenberger W, Dietrich A, Neugebauer F. Laparoskopische Cholecystektomie. Erste Erfahrungen und Ergebnisse bei 300 Operationen: eine prospektive Beobachtungsstudie. Chirurg. 1991;62:257-65.

SECTION 3

Laparoscopic Gynecological Procedures

CHAPTER 28

Laparoscopic Sterilization

INTRODUCTION

Laparoscopic sterilization was the first popular minimal access surgical procedure ever performed. Laparoscopic sterilization is very straightforward procedure. Worldwide laparoscopic sterilization is now the most commonly applied method for family planning **(Figs. 1A and B)**.

Laparoscopic tubal ligation is considered as a surgical sterilization procedure in which a woman's fallopian tubes are either clamped and blocked or severed and sealed. Both methods prevent eggs from being fertilized. Tubal ligation is a permanent method of sterilization. Laparoscopic sterilization has been evolved by Palmer and Steptoe in USA by monopolar technique. Rioux and Kleppinger developed the bipolar technique for sterilization because of more cases of bowel injury were being reported with the use of monopolar. Later silastic band and spring clips were invented for occlusive method of sterilization.

LAPAROSCOPIC ANATOMY

From anterior to posterior, following important tubular structures are found crossing the brim of true pelvis: the round ligament of the uterus, the infundibulopelvic ligament, which contains the gonadal vessels, and the ureter. The ovaries and fallopian tube is found between the round ligament and the infundibulopelvic ligament.

The main problem that can arise in laparoscopic sterilization surgery is mistaking the round ligament for fallopian tube. This mistake was more common when single puncture sterilization was used with laparocator. In laparocator, the image of the target organ and instrument were in the same axis and this was the cause of more incidence of failure. The next most common mistake is injury of the ureter during dissection of the infundibulopelvic ligament. If the uterus is deviated to the contralateral side with the help of uterine manipulator infundibulopelvic ligament is spread out and a pelvic side wall triangle is created. The base of this triangle is the round ligament, the medial side is the infundibulopelvic ligament, and the lateral side is the external iliac artery. The apex of this triangle is the point at which the infundibulopelvic ligament crosses the external iliac artery.

INDICATIONS

- Desire for permanent sterilization
- Completed childbearing

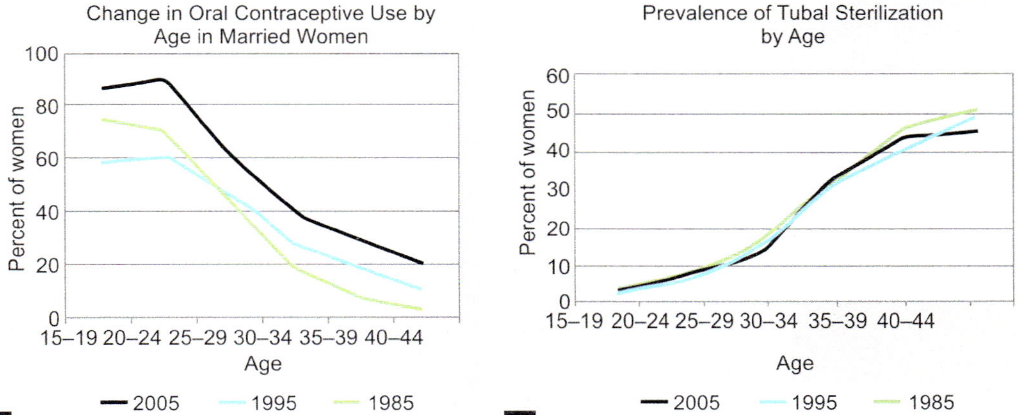

A B

Figs. 1A and B: Trend of family planning.

CONTRAINDICATIONS

- Hemodynamic instability
- Uncorrected coagulopathy
- Severe cardiopulmonary disease
- Abdominal wall infection
- Multiple previous upper abdominal procedures
- Late pregnancy

Patient Position

Patient should be in steep Trendelenburg's and lithotomy position. One assistant should remain between the legs of patient to do uterine manipulation, whenever required.

Port Position

Generally, laparoscopic sterilization is possible with two ports only. Many gynecologists like to perform tube ligation with one port in umbilicus and other in suprapubic region. In our practice, we like to put port in left iliac fossa. The left iliac fossa port will allow elevation angle of instrument at 30° and this angle is better for manipulation of fallopian tube and good ergonomics **(Fig. 2)**.

Operative Procedure

Methods of Tubal Sterilization (Fig. 3)

- *Destructive*:
  - Unipolar
  - Bipolar
  - Coagulation using thermal cautery
  - Ligation and cutting by scissors (Pomeroy technique)
- *Occlusive* ***(Figs. 4 and 5)***:
  - Filshie clip
  - Falope ring
  - Hulka clip

Laparoscopic sterilization by occlusive method is most popular method of interval sterilization in USA. Use of laparoscopic sterilization in immediate postpartum period is not wise and usually planned 4–6 weeks after delivery. During the time of postpartum laparoscopic tubal sterilization, the chances of some complications if performed laparoscopically. Also in the period of immediate postpartum, the uterus is approximately 20 weeks in size and fills the entire pelvis, rendering insertion of the Veress needle and laparoscopic trocar difficult. Making the subumbilical minilaparotomy incision is fast and easy; often it can be performed under regional anesthesia. There seems no advantage to performing postpartum tubal sterilization laparoscopically.

Laparoscopic sterilization can be planned together with first trimester medical termination of pregnancy (MTP), but in second trimester again an interval of 6 weeks is essential. The main risk of laparoscopic sterilization just after delivery or after second trimester MTP is because uterus is large and may be injured by trocar.

The occlusion of tube in the luteal phase may lead to pregnancy just after sterilization. This may create a medicolegal problem for gynecologist. To avoid this problem, a urine pregnancy test should be obtained on the morning of surgery and patient should be advised to return for MTP, if sign of intrauterine or ectopic pregnancy develops.

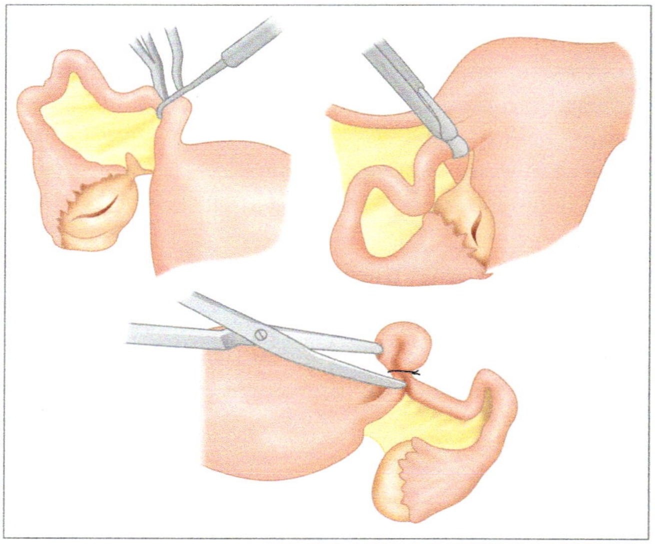

Fig. 3: Methods of sterilization.

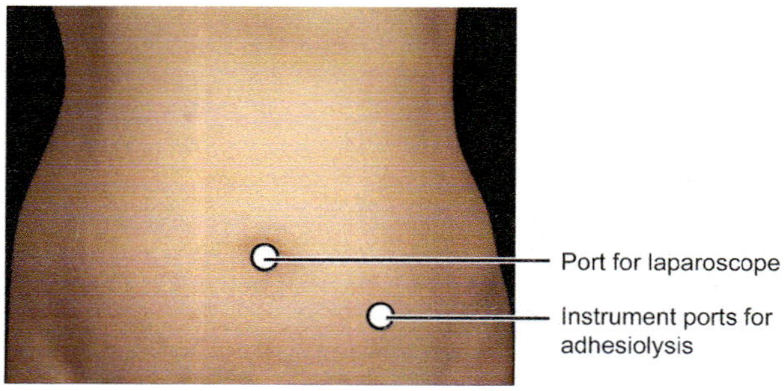

Fig. 2: Port position for tubal sterilization.

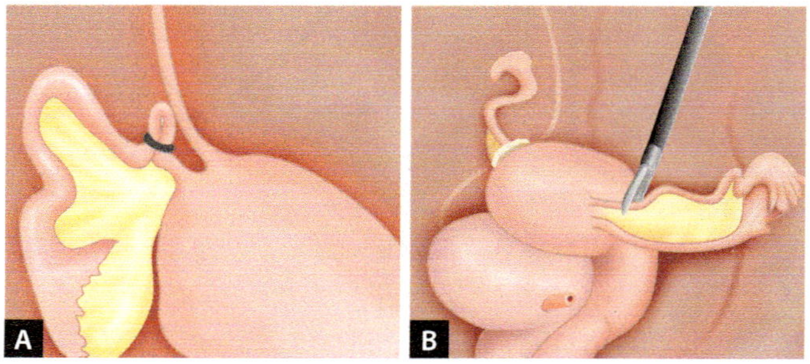

Figs. 4A and B: Falope ring and Filshie clip.

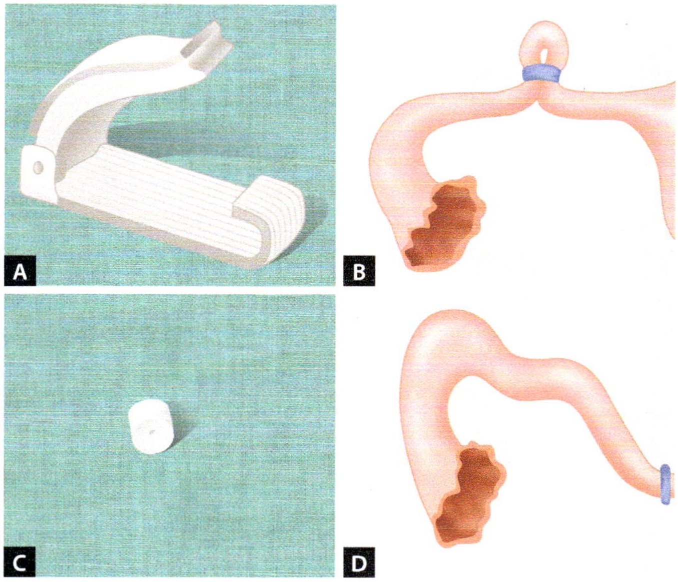

Figs. 5A to D: Various occlusive devices for sterilization.

BIPOLAR COAGULATION

Two port techniques are used for sterilization by electrosurgery. One in umbilicus and one in left iliac fossa. Gynecologist stands left to the patient and camera assistant right to the gynecologist. Uterine manipulator is helpful to bring both the tube under vision.

Fallopian tube is grasped 2 cm lateral to the uterine end and bipolar is activated. If tube is coagulated very close to uterus, there is chance of development of uteroperitoneal fistula containing endometrial tissue due to continuous contractility of uterus. Activation of bipolar should be intermittent and after each activation jaw of bipolar should be slightly opened to avoid sticking of jaw of bipolar with tube. The procedure should be repeated at three adjacent areas.

If the jaw of bipolar gets adhered with tube forceps should be gently twisted clockwise and counterclockwise and at the same time the pressure from the handle of grasper is decreased.

Some gynecologists prefer coagulation and division of tube between coagulated area, but study has shown that coagulation of 2–3 cm of tube without division is better because division lead to significant incidence of bleeding from underlying vessels. Bipolar should be applied always at three places. If only "one place bipolar coagulation" per tube is performed, there is always a risk of spontaneous recanalization in about 3 months.

It is worth noting that, in a study done, the risk of ectopic pregnancy was also highest among the bipolar coagulation group (65% of pregnancies were ectopic), Falope ring group (29%), and spring clip group (15%). The high bipolar cauterization ectopic rate is thought to result from inadequate cauterization. These cases were done prior to the routine use of a power meter to monitor tissue desiccation. The Filshie clip was not included in this study.

FALOPE RING APPLICATION

Yoon in 1974 described silastic band technique for occlusive tubal sterilization. The Falope ring is applied with the help of Falope ring applicator **(Figs. 6A to D)**.

Operative Technique

Sterilization using Falope ring application gained popularity in the 1970s. Initially, failure rate was high with single-puncture technique using laparocator **(Fig. 7)**.

These days double-puncture technique is preferred and has less failure rate compared to single-puncture technique. Pneumoperitoneum is created in usual manner. First of all diagnostic laparoscopy should be performed to exclude any other abnormality. The Filshie clip or Falope ring is loaded into the receiving edge of the applicator **(Figs. 8A to C)**. The clip or ring should be applied across the narrow ischemic area about 2 cm from the cornua **(Figs. 9A to D)**. This area is very mobile and easy to see. In case of desired reanastomosis, this area is easier to anastomose.

Once the fallopian tube is found, the atraumatic grasping forceps is used to pick up one of the tubes, around 2 cm lateral to the corneal end of uterus. The jaw of Falope ring applicator is pushed out and tube is then drawn into the inner cylinder of Falope ring applicator **(Figs. 6A to D)**. Once the Falope ring applicator is fully fired either one or two silicon rubber bands are applied to the grasped segment of the fallopian tube. After application of Falope ring the grasping forceps is moved forward out of the inner cylinder to release the occluded segment of tube **(Figs. 10A to D)**. In the similar manner, the contralateral tube is grasped and the ring is applied. After both the tubes are occluded, some gynecologists inject indigo carmine dye through uterus to confirm tubal lumen occlusion. The blanching of the tube after clip application can also be seen after successful application of ring. Blanch is due to ischemia and this means that the sterilization is perfect.

If everything goes well, then patient can be discharged on the same day. The snapshot pictures and video recording of all the procedure is good practice for future references.

Filshie and Hulka clip is also applied with same manner, only difference is that clips does not form loop. Hence, the chances of successful reversal of sterilization are better compared to Falope rings **(Figs. 11 and 12)**.

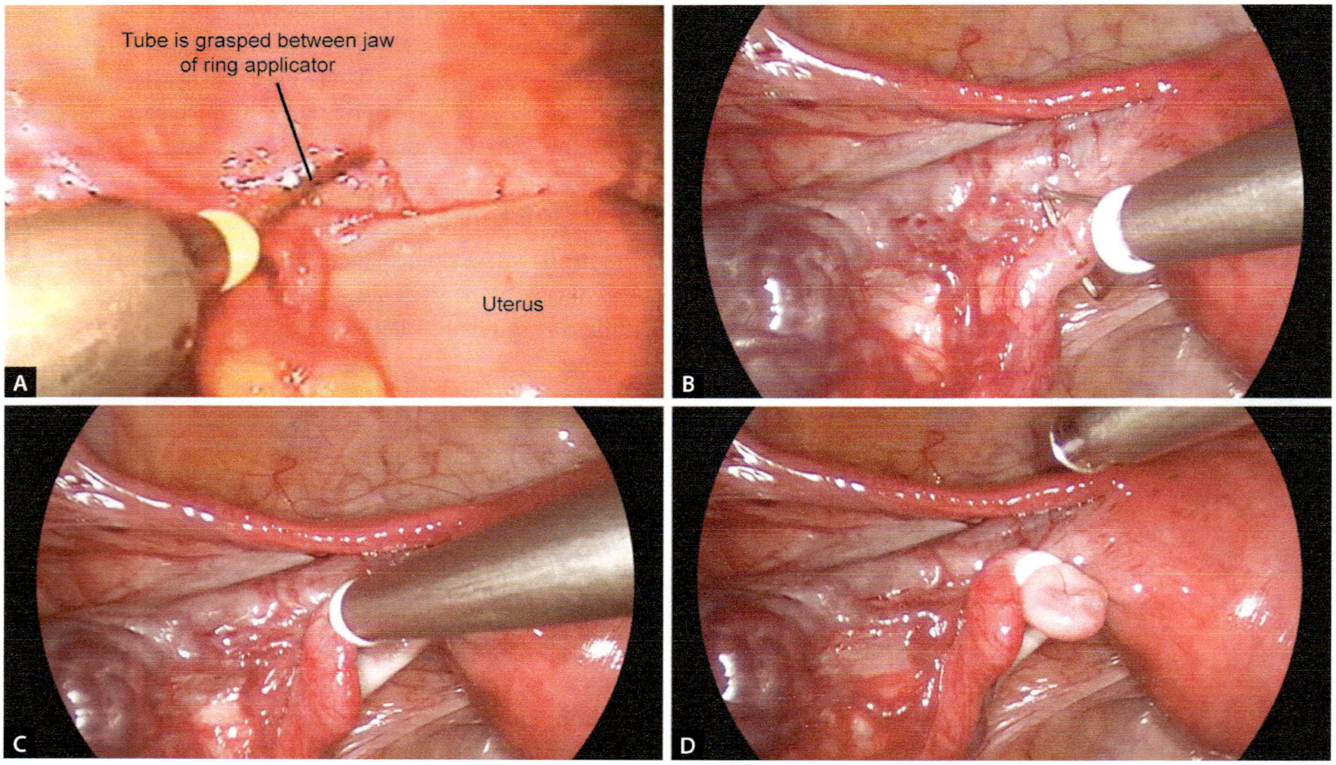

Figs. 6A to D: Tubal sterilization by Falope ring applicator.

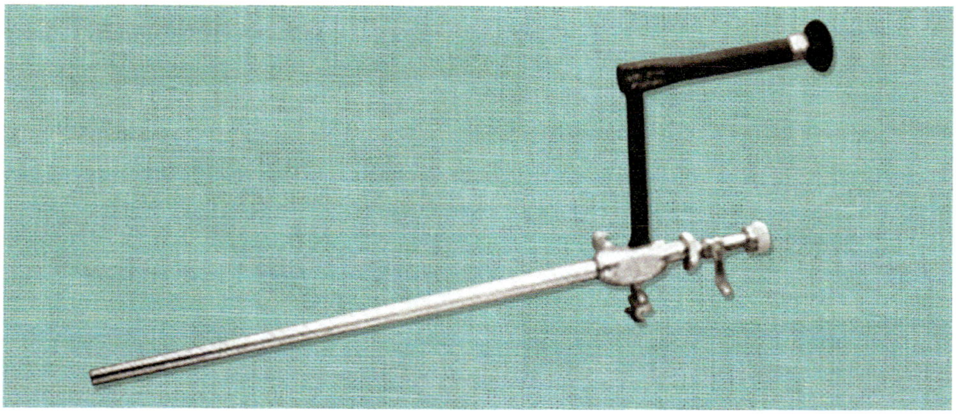

Fig. 7: Laparocator for single puncture tubal ligation.

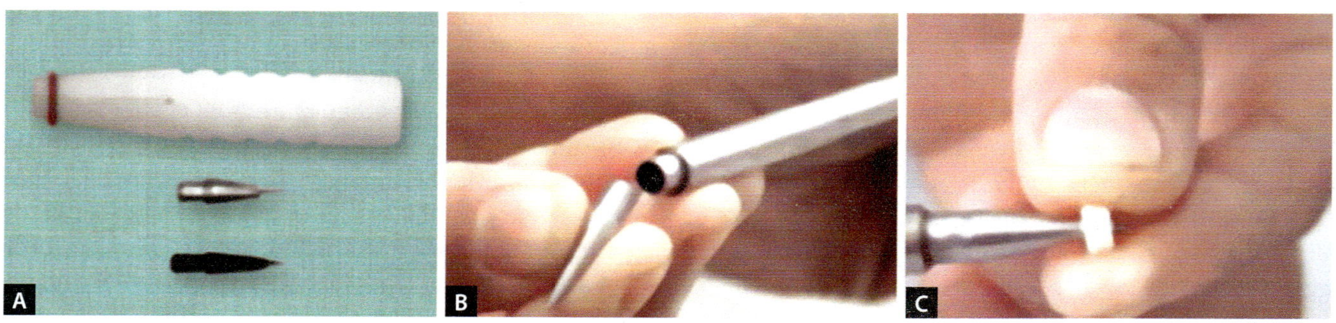

Figs. 8A to C: Ring loading.

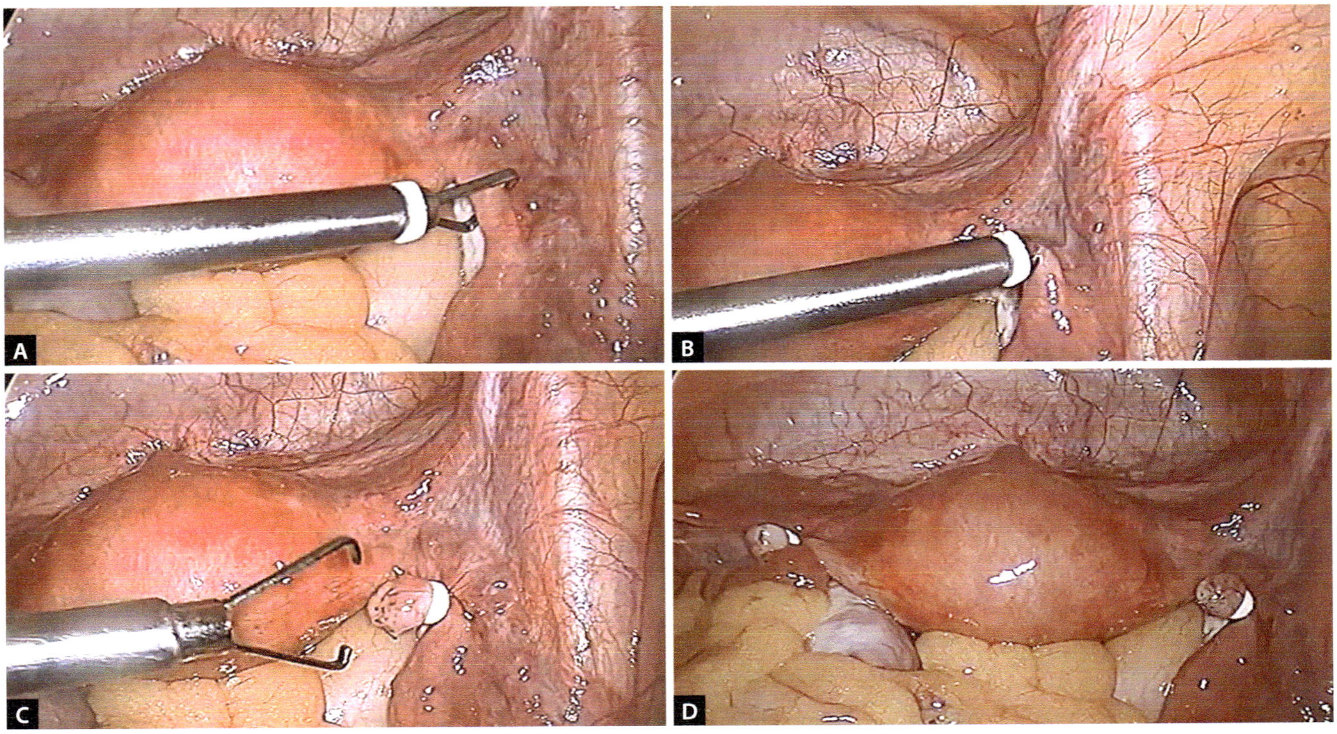

Figs. 9A to D: Methods of sterilization in isthmus.

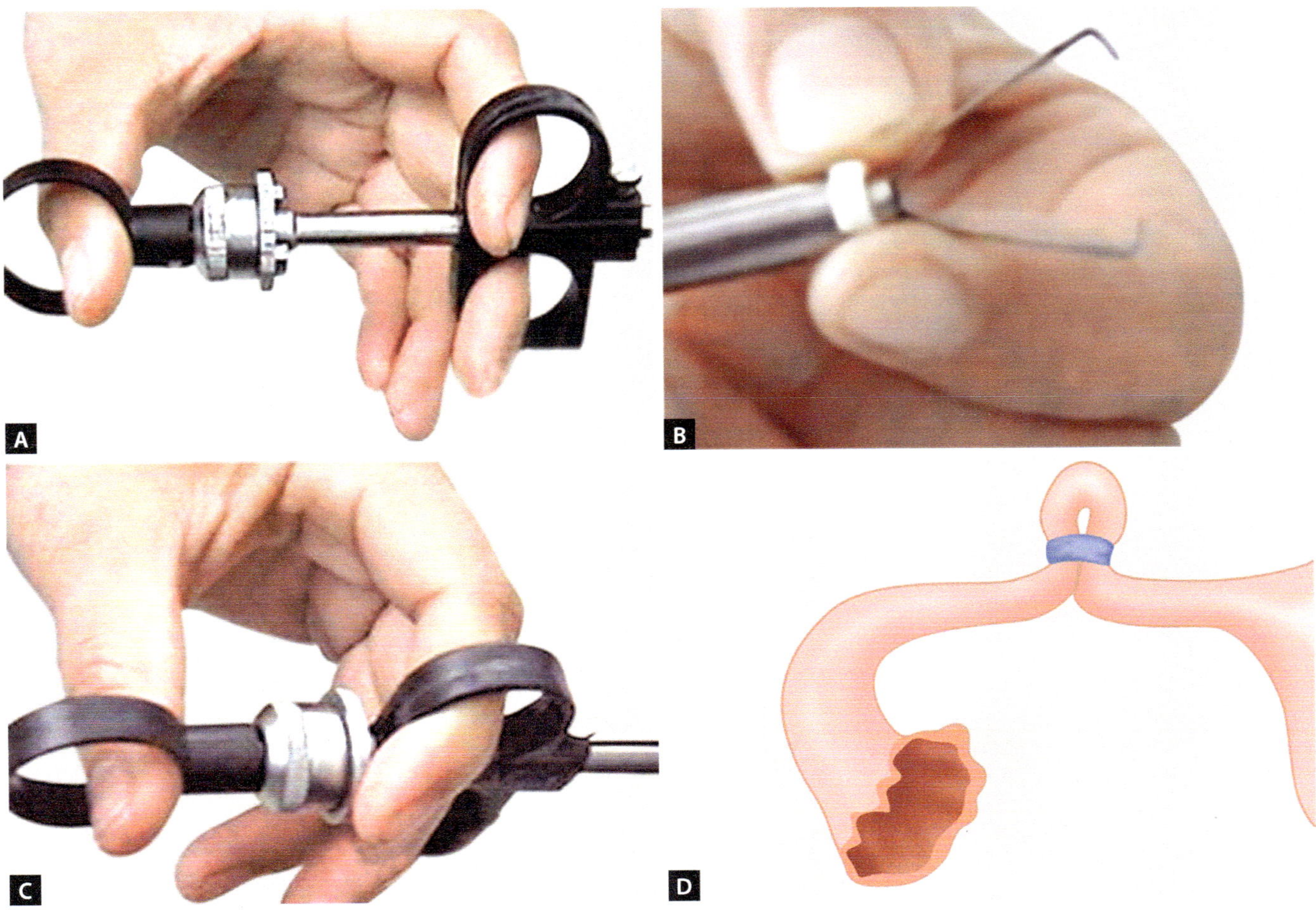

Figs. 10A to D: Loading of Falope ring.

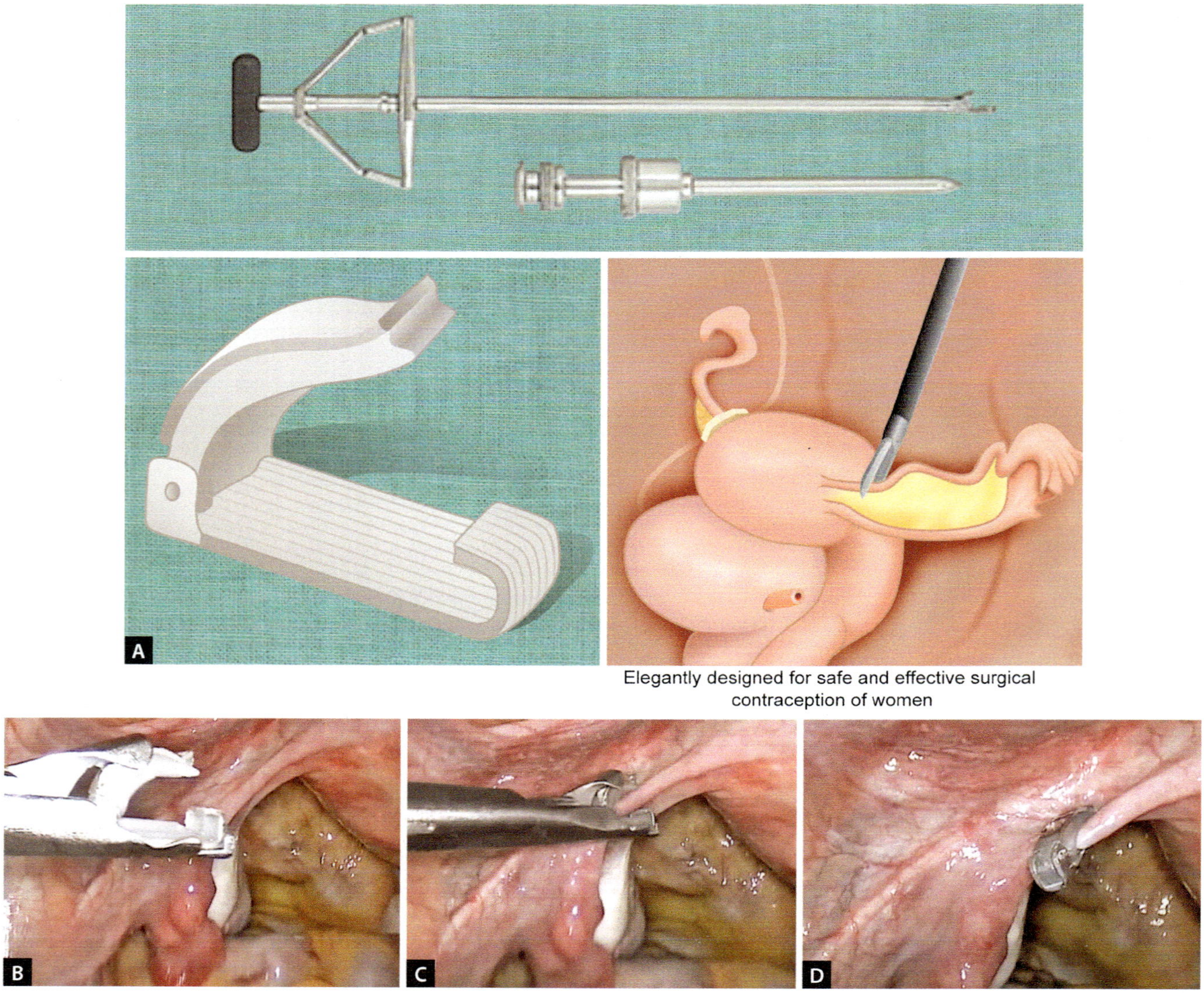

Figs. 11A to D: Filshie clip.

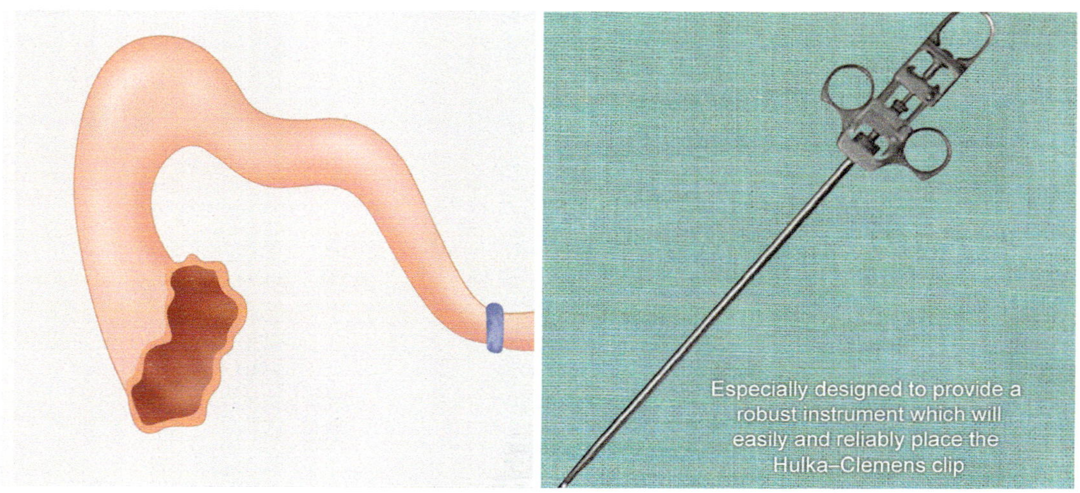

Fig. 12: Hulka clip.

BIBLIOGRAPHY

1. Benhamou D, Narchi P, Mazoit JX, Fernandez H. Postoperative pain after local anesthetics for laparoscopic sterilization. Obstet Gynecol. 1994;84:877-80.
2. Bordahl PE, Raeder JC, Nordentoft J, Kirste U, Refsdal A. Laparoscopic sterilization under local or general anesthesia? A randomized study. Obstet Gynecol. 1993;81:137-41.
3. Cooper JM. Hysteroscopic sterilization. Clin Obstet Gynecol. 1992;35:282-98.
4. Davis A, Millar JM. Postoperative pain: a comparison of laparoscopic sterilisation and diagnostic laparoscopy. Anaesthesia. 1988;43:796-7.
5. De Wilde RL. Goodbye to late bowel obstruction after appendicectomy. Lancet. 1991;338:1012.
6. Diamond MP, Daniell JF, Feste J, Surrey MW, McLaughlin DS, Friedman S, et al. Adhesion reformation and de novo adhesion formation after reproductive pelvic surgery. Fertil Steril. 1987;47(5):864-6.
7. Easter DW, Cushieri A, Nathanson LK, Lavelle-Jones M. The utility of diagnostic laparoscopy for abdominal disorders. Audit of 120 patients. Arch Surg. 1992;127(4):379-83.
8. Fraser RA, Hotz SB, Hurtig JB, Hodges SN, Moher D. The prevalence and impact of pain after day-care tubal ligation surgery. Pain. 1989;39:189-201.
9. JF Kerin, Cooper JM, Price T, Herendael BJ, Cayuela-Font E, Cher D, et al. Hysteroscopic sterilization using a micro-insert device: results of a multicentre Phase II study. Hum Reprod. 2003;18:1223-30.
10. Kerin JF, Carignan CS, Cher D. The safety and effectiveness of a new hysteroscopic method for permanent birth control: results of the first Essure PBC clinical study. Aust NZJ Obstet Gynecol. 2001;41:364-70.
11. Kerin JF, Williams DB, San Roman GA, Pearlstone AC, Grundfest WS, Surrey ES. Falloposcopic classification and treatment of fallopian tube lumen disease. Fertil Steril. 1992;57:731-41.
12. Kerin JF. New methods for transcervical cannulation of the fallopian tube. Int J Gynaecol Obstet. 1995;51:S29-39.
13. Klaiber C, Metzger A. Manual der laparoskopischen Chirurgie. Bern: Verlag Hans Huber; 1992. pp. 185-206.
14. Kolmorgen K, Schulz AM. Results of laparoscopic lysis of adhesions in patients with chronic pelvic pain. Zentralbl Gynakol. 1991;113(6):291-5.
15. Kresch AJ, Seifer DB, Sachs LB, Banner I. Laparoscopy in 100 women with chronic pelvic pain. Obstet Gynecol. 1984;64(5):672-4.
16. Ligt-Veneman NG, Tinga DJ Kragt H, Brandsma G, van der Leij G. The efficacy of intratubal silicone in the Ovabloc hysteroscopic method of sterilization. Acta Obstet Gynecol Scand. 1999;78: 824-5.
17. Lindblom B, Norstrom A. The smooth-muscle architecture of the human fallopian tube. In: Siegler AM, Ansari AH (Eds). The Fallopian Tube. Mount Kisco, New York, USA: Futura Publishing Company, Inc; 1986. pp. 13-20.
18. Luciano AA, Maier DB, Koch EI, Nulsen JC, Whitman GF. A comparative study of postoperative adhesions following laser surgery by laparoscopy versus laparotomy in the rabbit model. Obstet Gynecol. 1989;74(2):220-4.
19. MacKay AP, Kieke BA Jr, Koonin LM, Beattie K. Tubal sterilization in the United States, 1994-1996. Fam Plann Perspect. 2001;33:161-5.
20. Mecke H, Semm K. Pelviscopic adhesiolysis. Successes in the treatment of chronic abdominal pain caused by adhesions in the lower and middle abdomen. Geburtshilfe Frauenheilkd. 1988;48(3):155-9.
21. Nezhat CR, Nezhat FR, Metzger DA, Luicano A. Adhesion reformation after reproductive surgery by video-laseroscopy. Fertil Steril. 1990;53(6):1008-11.
22. Peters AA, Trimbos-Kemper GC, Admiraal C, Trimbos JB, Hermans J. A randomized clinical trial on the benefit of adhesiolysis in patients with intraperitoneal adhesions and chronic pelvic pain. Br J Obstet Gynaecol. 1992;99:59-62.
23. Peterson HB, Xia Z, Hughes JM, Wilcox LS, Tylor LR, Trussell J. The risk of pregnancy after tubal sterilization: findings from the US Collaborative Review of Sterilization. Am J Obstet Gynecol. 1996;174:1161-70.
24. Räf LE. Causes of abdominal adhesions in cases of intestinal obstruction. Acta Chir Scand. 1969;135:73-6.
25. Rapkin AJ. Adhesions and pelvic pain: a retrospective study. Obstet Gynecol. 1986;68:13-5.
26. Riedel HH, Haag GM. Late sequelae of appendectomy with special reference to adhesions in the lower abdomen, chronic abdominal pain and sterility. Zentralbl Gynakol. 1989;111(16):1101-12.
27. Ryder RM, Vaughan MC. Laparoscopic tubal sterilization: Methods, effectiveness, and sequelae. Obstet Gynecol Clin North Am. 1999;26:83-97.
28. Sciarra JJ, Keith L. Hysteroscopic sterilization. Obstet Gynecol Clin North Am. 1995;22:581-9.
29. Tool AL, Kammerer-Doak DN, Nguyen CM, Cousin MO, Charsley M. Postoperative pain relief following laparoscopic tubal sterilization with silastic bands. Obstet Gynecol. 1997;90:731-4.
30. Valle RF, Carignan CS, Wright TC. Tissue response to the STOP microcoil transcervical permanent contraceptive device: results from a prehysterectomy study. Fertil Steril. 2001;76:974-80.

CHAPTER 29

Laparoscopic Ovarian Surgery

INTRODUCTION

Most ovarian abnormalities can be managed laparoscopically. Ovarian pathology can occur at any time from fetal life to menopause. First laparoscopic salpingo-oophorectomy was performed by Semm in 1984. He reported his experience with a laparoscopic approach to oophorectomy and salpingo-oophorectomy.

Laparoscopy management may be an alternative in those cases where hysterectomy is being planned and a more conservative management of pain caused by adnexal disease can be performed. If necessary, even oophorectomy can be performed laparoscopically with a short hospital stay and recovery period at a later date.

LAPAROSCOPIC OVARIAN ANATOMY

The ovaries are seen clearly by laparoscope because of their whiteness and knobby texture **(Fig. 1)**. They may be seen more clearly if uterine manipulator is used and uterus is pushed towards anterior abdominal wall. Ovaries hang down in the laparoscopic field. A normal ovary is almond shaped and approximately 3 cm in diameter **(Fig. 2)**.

The ovarian ligaments run from the ovaries to the lateral border of the uterus. Ovary is attached to the pelvic sidewall with infundibulopelvic ligament, which carries ovarian artery **(Fig. 3)**. One of the common mistakes that a surgeon can land into is injury of the ureter during dissection of the infundibulopelvic ligament. If the uterus is deviated to the contralateral side with the help of uterine manipulator, infundibulopelvic ligament is spread out and a pelvic side wall triangle is created. The base of this triangle is the round ligament, the medial side

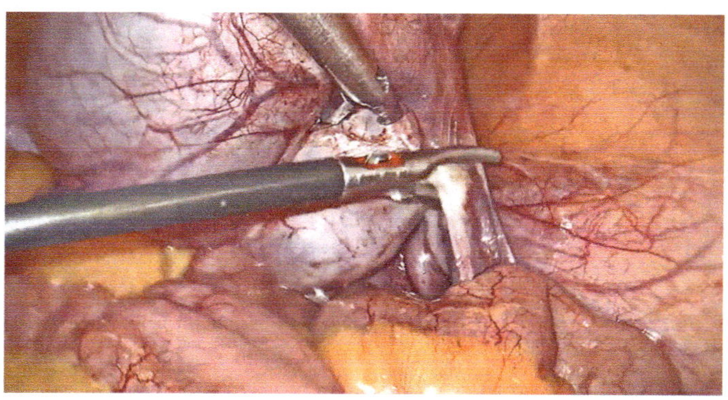

Fig. 1: Laparoscopic oophorectomy using bipolar.

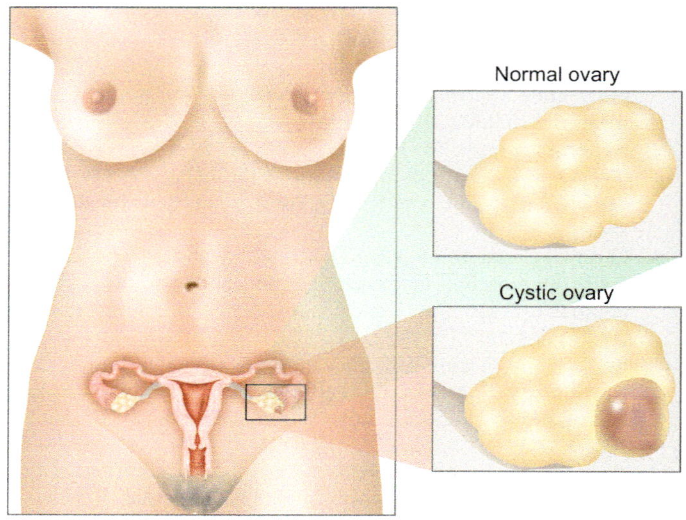

Fig. 2: Anatomy of ovary.

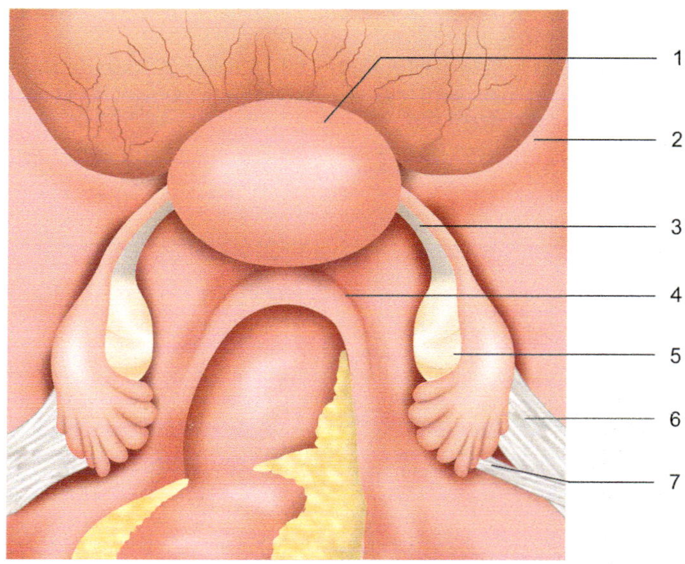

Fig. 3: Position of ovary: (1) Uterus; (2) Round ligament; (3) Utero-ovarian ligament (proper ovarian ligament); (4) Uterosacral ligament; (5) Ovary; (6) Suspensory ligament of the ovary; (7) Ureter.

is the infundibulopelvic ligament, and the lateral side is the external iliac artery. The apex of this triangle is the point at which the infundibulopelvic ligament crosses the external iliac artery.

The ovarian arteries arise from the aorta to descend lateral to the ureter and genitofemoral nerve. The artery and accompanying vein cross over the external and internal iliac vessels to enter the pelvis. The left ovarian vein joins the left renal vein and right ovarian vein joins the inferior vena cava.

LAPAROSCOPIC MANAGEMENT OF OVARIAN CYST

Ovarian cysts are sacs filled with fluid or a semisolid material that develops on or within the ovary. Surgery is indicated if the growth is larger than 4 inch (10 cm), complex, growing, persistent, solid and irregularly shaped, on both ovaries, or causes pain or other symptoms.

Laparoscopic management of ovarian cyst depends on the patient's age, pelvic examination, sonographic images, and serum markers. When surgery is indicated for benign ovarian disease, preservation of ovarian tissue via cystectomy or enucleation of a solid tumor from the ovary is generally preferable to complete oophorectomy. When the ovary cannot be salvaged or insufficient viable tissue remains after attempts at conservation, oophorectomy is usually performed. A large, solid, fixed, or irregular adnexal mass accompanied by ascites is suspicious for malignancy. Cul-de-sac nodularity, ascites, cystic adnexal structures, and fixed adnexae occur with endometriosis and sometimes ovarian malignancy. Before selecting any case for laparoscopy, CA-125, which is an ovarian cancer marker, should be estimated, that may help to identify cancerous cysts in older women. Although ovarian neoplasms can occur at any age, the risk of malignancy is highest during prepuberty and menopause. Malignancy is not the only concern in managing an ovarian cyst. Patients who wish to preserve their reproductive organs should have the least aggressive therapy. In a postmenopausal patient whose family has a history of ovarian cancer, CA-125 levels may help to detect it in the early stages. However, surgeon should keep in mind that many benign gynecologic disorders are also associated with elevated CA-125 levels, including fibroid uterus, endometriosis, and salpingitis that could lead to unnecessary concern and intervention.

Because the risk of malignancy is relatively low in young women, preoperative evaluation should include a history and physical examination. Pelvic ultrasound should be performed to evaluate both ovaries to rule out bilateral endometriomas or teratoma. Removing cysts in a specimen bag reduces both operating time and spillage. Controlled intraperitoneal spillage of benign cyst contents (e.g., cystic teratoma) does not increase postoperative morbidity as long as the spillage is aspirated, and the peritoneal cavity is lavaged. A solid adnexal mass that is small enough to be removed intact via colpotomy or via a laparoscopic bag can be managed with laparoscopy. Solid masses can also be mobilized via laparoscopic technique and then removed through a minilaparotomy incision or morcellated inside a specimen bag.

Hormone levels [such as luteinizing hormone (LH), follicle-stimulating hormone (FSH), estradiol, and testosterone] may be checked to evaluate for associated hormonal conditions. The persistent ovarian cysts must be treated surgically, and evolving laparoscopic technology has enabled endoscopic management of most of them. Although most are benign, the possibility of malignancy usually requires a laparotomy using a midline incision.

Oral contraceptives have been prescribed for some small cystic adnexal masses in reproductive-aged women on the assumption that decreasing gonadotropin stimulation to a functional cyst will hasten its resolution. Either danazol (800 mg/day) or oral contraceptive pills with 50 pg estrogen are advised for any cyst suspected of being functional.

Crossing the true brim of pelvis the following important tubular structures are found. The round ligament of the uterus, the infundibulopelvic ligament which contains the gonadal vessels and the ureter. The ovaries and fallopian tube are found between the round ligament and the infundibulopelvic ligament.

Patient Position

Patient should be in steep Trendelenburg's and lithotomy position. One assistant should remain between the legs of patient to do uterine manipulation whenever required.

Port Position

Port position should be in accordance with baseball diamond concept. If the cyst is of right side, one port should be in left iliac fossa and another in right hypochondrium **(Fig. 4)**.

Operative Procedure

After access, the pelvis and upper abdomen are examined, and the cyst contents should be aspirated. Once the capsule is opened, the interior of the capsule is examined and

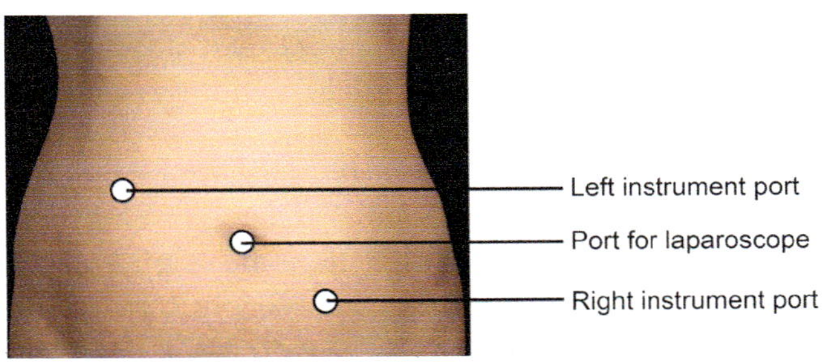

Fig. 4: Port position for right-sided ovarian surgery.

suspicious areas should be sent for biopsy. The entire cyst capsule must be removed to search for an early carcinoma. Whether to perform oophorectomy or cystectomy depends on the patient's age and characteristics of the mass.

Ovarian Cystectomy

Medical management of endometriomas has proven ineffective, and nowadays either laparotomy or operative laparoscopy is necessary. Laparoscopic ovarian cystectomy removes the cyst with minimal trauma to the residual ovarian tissue. Laparotomy for ovarian cystectomy is not a good procedure because of increased risk of ovarian adhesion formation. Three methods to manage such cysts are drainage, excision, and thermal coagulation. By excising the unruptured cyst, histopathologic examination is more complete and the risk of recurrence is minimized, but laparoscopic removal of intact cyst is very difficult and aspiration is recommended for functional cysts, which are diagnosed laparoscopically. Many cysts get ruptured during their manipulation despite a delicate technique.

Thermal ablation does not destroy the entire cyst wall, and the underlying ovarian cortex can be damaged by the heat. Therefore, excision of entire cyst wall with the help of blunt stripping and sharp dissection by scissors are recommended.

The removal of small cyst is possible without aspirating it. A careful dissection should be performed to strip out ovarian cortex with inner cystic layer and it can be extracted safely transferring in the endobag **(Figs. 5A to F)**.

The removal of a cyst 10 cm or larger is difficult laparoscopically. Aspiration before removal of large cysts is practical and can be accomplished using an 18 gauge needle passed through the separate puncture of abdominal wall while stabilizing the cyst. The suction irrigation instrument can also be used to aspirate the content of the cyst **(Fig. 5G)**.

If gross characteristics of ovary look suspicious for malignancy, some gynecologists recommend peritoneal washing before puncturing an ovarian cyst, because any cyst may turn out to be malignant. The peritoneal fluid or washings should be sent for cytological examination.

After aspiration capsule of cyst is stripped from the ovarian stroma using two grasping forceps and the suction-irrigator probe for traction and counter traction **(Fig. 6)**. The electrosurgery can be used at low power to seal blood vessels at the base of the capsule and at higher powers to vaporize small remnants of capsule. Bipolar forceps can also be used to control bleeding. The open jaw of bipolar can be touched to the oozing area and hemostasis can be achieved. Sometimes it is difficult to remove the capsule from the ovarian cortex so that injecting dilute vasopressin between the capsule and cortex facilitates the stripping procedure **(Fig. 7)**. If the cyst wall cannot be identified clearly, the edge of the ovarian incision can be "freshened" with scissors and the resulting clean edge reveals the two layers, outer layer will be ovarian and inner cystic. If this does not free the capsule, the base of the cyst is grasped and traction applied to the cyst with counter traction to the ovary. Sometime the complete cyst or portions of the wall may be densely adherent to the ovary, requiring sharp or electrosurgical dissection to completely free the cyst wall. Generally, when the cyst capsule is removed from the ovary, the contraction of the ovarian capsule provides significant hemostasis. Bleeding can occur at the base, particularly if the cyst was close to the hilum. Under these circumstances, a needle electrode or a fine bipolar forceps can be used to minimize thermal damage. Large cysts sometime need partial oophorectomy, to remove the distorted portion of the ovary, and the remaining cyst wall can be stripped from the ovarian stroma.

Teratoma often can be excised intact, but often the cyst ruptures. After extraction, if the ovarian edges overlap itself, the defect is left to heal without suturing because adhesions are more likely following the use of suture. In rare instances one or two fine, absorbable monofilament sutures may be needed to approximate the ovarian edges. The sutures are placed inside the ovary to decrease formation of adhesions.

Endometriomas

Ovarian endometriosis causes the adhesions between the ovarian surface and the broad ligament. As the ovary enlarges, endometriomas form. Sometime surface endometrial implants penetrate more deeply into the cyst wall, making excision more difficult. The degree of endometrial invasion of the cyst wall forms the basis for differentiating between these two subtypes and is characterized by the progressive difficulty in removing the cyst wall.

The least invasive and the technically simplest approach to endometriomas involve laparoscopic fenestration and removal of "chocolate" fluid without cystectomy or ablation of the cyst wall. However, fenestration and irrigation are associated with a 50% recurrence rate compared to 8% in the group with the capsule removed. Postoperatively, either danazol 800 mg/day or a gonadotropin-releasing hormone (GnRH) analog is used for 6–8 weeks. Large hematomas are associated with periovarian adhesions attaching them to the pelvic sidewall and the back of the uterus, and tend to rupture during separation. After mobilizing the ovary, the contents of the cyst are removed with the suction-irrigator probe and the cavity is irrigated. The inside of the cyst is evaluated and the portion of ovarian cortex involved with endometriosis is removed. Using the grasping forceps and the suction-irrigator probe, the cyst wall is grasped and separated from the ovarian stroma by traction and counter traction. Small blood vessels from the ovarian bed and bleeding from the ovarian hilum can be controlled with bipolar electrocoagulation.

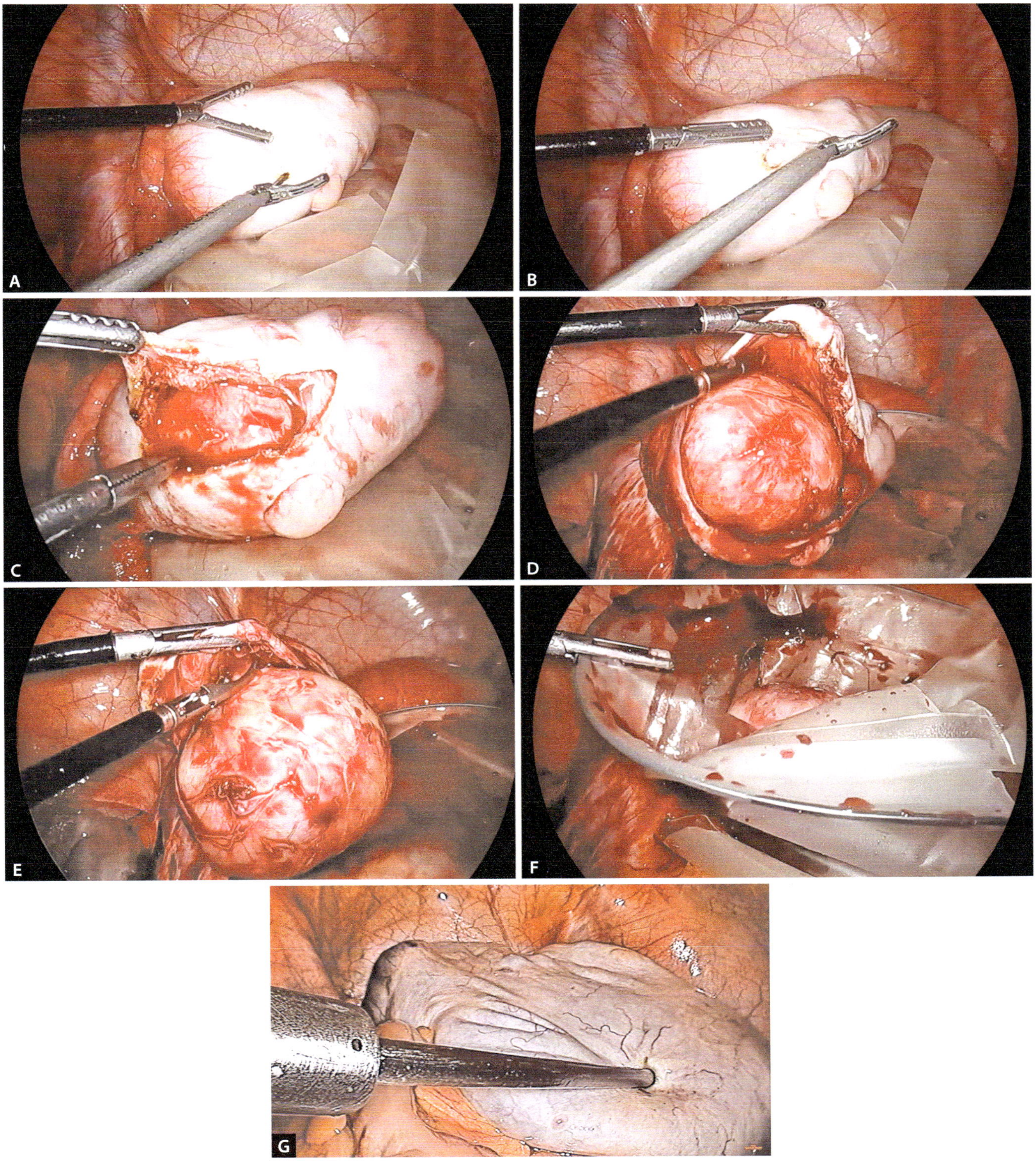

Figs. 5A to G: (A to F) Ovarian cystectomy without aspirating the cyst and taking it in the endobag; (G) Ovarian cyst is aspirated for ovarian cystectomy.

The remaining ovarian tissue is approximated with low-power laser or electrosurgery to avoid adhesions. Low-power, continuous laser or bipolar coagulation applied to the inside wall of the redundant ovarian capsule causes it to invert, but excessive coagulation of the adjacent ovarian stroma must be avoided. Sutures, if needed, are placed inside the capsule and 4-0 polydioxanone sutures are preferred. Fewer sutures result in fewer adhesions.

The ability to diagnose and treat endometriosis at earlier stages may prevent its progression and invasion, reducing its adverse impact on health, quality of life, and fertility potential.

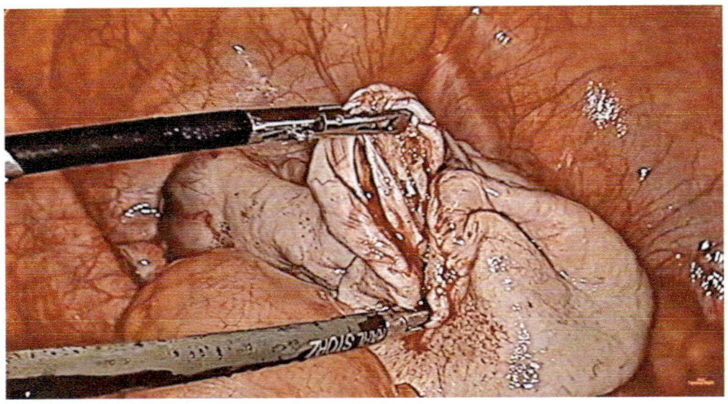

Fig. 6: Cystic wall is stripped out from ovarian cortex.

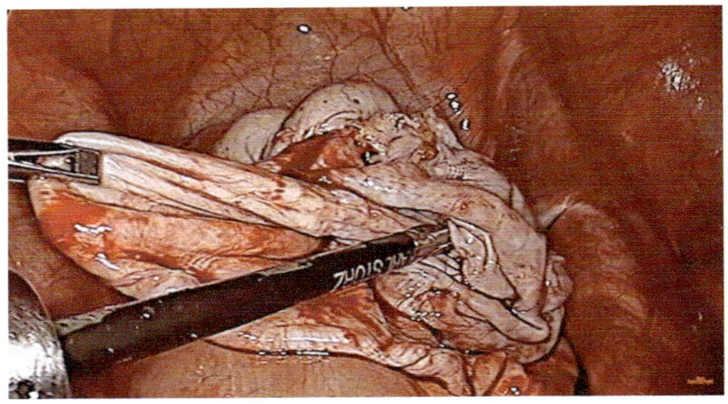

Fig. 7: Cyst is being separated from ovary.

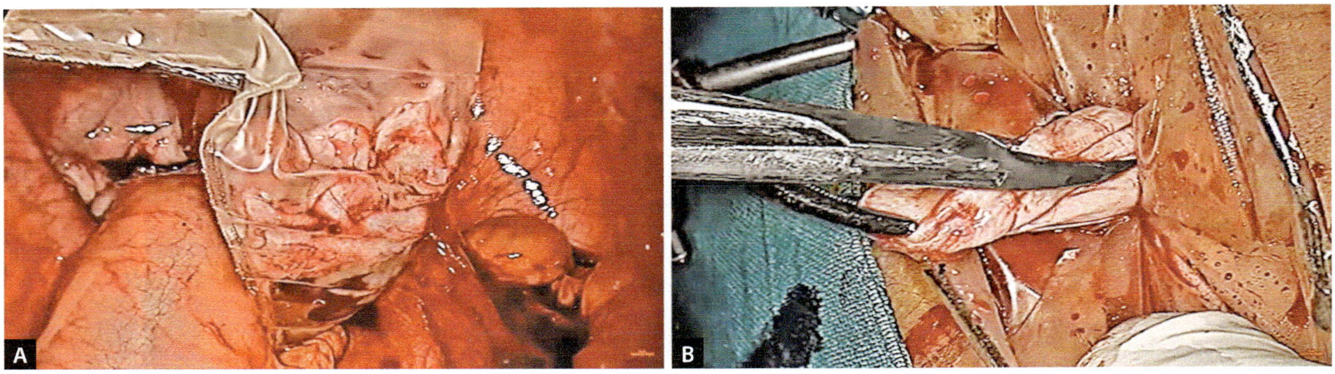

Figs. 8A and B: Extraction of ovary.

Benign Cystic Teratoma

These germ cell tumors occur predominantly in young women. A cystic teratoma contains sebaceous material that is irritating to peritoneal surfaces and can cause chemical peritonitis and possible adhesions. The surgeon should avoid rupturing the cyst. If the cyst does get ruptured during excision, it is important to clean the body cavity of all sebaceous material and hair. If it ruptures at the time of excision, without spending much time, the suction-irrigator is placed in the cyst, the contents aspirated, and the cavity copiously irrigated. The interior of the cyst is inspected and its lining is grasped and removed from the ovary. The lining is removed from the pelvis through a 10 mm port. In case of intact cyst an endobag may be necessary **(Figs. 8A and B)**. A colpotomy can be made through which the cyst is pulled into it and then incised and drained and its capsule removed. These same procedures can be performed through a mini-laparotomy incision. The cyst wall is punctured and the contents rapidly aspirated. The wall is removed, placed in an endobag, and removed through the cul-de-sac or through one of the port wound. Following removal, it is critical to irrigate the pelvis copiously with 5–10 L of warm Ringer's lactate. The sebaceous material is less dense than water and shall float, facilitating removal. Occasionally, when the cyst is mainly solid, it should be removed intact without rupturing. The cyst wall should be sent for histopathological examination. The pelvis is irrigated with lactated Ringer's solution until all evidence of sebaceous material is removed because incomplete removal of this material can cause peritonitis. During irrigation, the ovarian stroma is inspected to verify hemostasis. If bleeding is present, bleeder points are controlled with a monopolar fulguration or bipolar forceps.

If the teratomas are greater than 8 cm, the ovary can be placed in the cul-de-sac adjacent to a colpotomy incision. Cyst is removed transvaginally which minimizes the risk of contamination of upper abdomen and port wound and maintains a minimally invasive approach. The vagina should be cleaned thoroughly and prepared with betadine before colpotomy. In elderly women or for those patients in whom the ovary and tube cannot be conserved, salpingo-oophorectomy should be considered. When the cyst wall is benign and the tissue is fragmented, it can be removed through a 10 mm suprapubic port. No tissue should be left in the pelvic cavity or on the abdominal wall. Contamination of the anterior abdominal wall should be avoided and if this happens, all tissue must be removed and the incision copiously irrigated and washed. Abdominal wall metastasis has been reported following contamination of the wall during laparoscopy for ovarian cancer.

LAPAROSCOPIC OOPHORECTOMY

Indications

The most common indications for oophorectomy are:

- Persistent localized pain despite previous lysis of adhesions or ablation of endometriosis
- Residual ovary syndrome
- Dysgenetic gonads
- Ovarian cysts greater than 5 cm
- Tubo-ovarian abscess
- Prophylactic therapy for advanced breast cancer
- Early ovarian cancer in young women

Contraindications

- Hemodynamic instability
- Uncorrected coagulopathy
- Severe cardiopulmonary disease
- Abdominal wall infection
- Multiple previous upper abdominal procedures
- Late pregnancy

Operative Procedure

The port position is shown in **Figure 9**. Properly placed uterine manipulator is important to get a good exposure of ovary and tube. It is sometime difficult to immobilize the ovary because of its smooth surface and finer texture. In case of difficulty in immobilizing the ovary, the uterine-ovarian ligament can be grasped by one of the atraumatic grasper to lift and isolate the ovary or the ovary can be wedged against the pelvic sidewall using the flattened edges of the opened or closed forceps. It is important to remember that overly aggressive manipulation can cause lacerations in the capsule, follicles, or cysts and result in bleeding. Before starting the procedure, it is important to observe the course of the ureter as it crosses the external iliac artery near the bifurcation of the common iliac artery at the pelvic brim. The left ureter can be more difficult to find because it is often covered by the base of the sigmoid mesocolon. If the ureter is difficult to identify transperitoneally it must be identified by retroperitoneal approach. If previous hysterectomy is done it is better to insert a vaginal probe or sponge stick through the vagina so that the surgeon can maintain orientation, particularly with procedures involving extensive adhesions. Many time anatomic landmarks are distorted by adhesions, endometriosis, or prior surgical extirpation. In those cases dissection should be started from the most normal area and then it should proceed toward the more distorted parts of the operative field. Attention should be given that complete ovary must be removed to prevent ovarian remnant syndrome or tumor development in a dysgenetic gonad. At the end of the procedure, the operative field is inspected and any clots are removed with a suction-irrigator or grasping forceps. Pedicles are inspected under water and with decreased pneumoperitoneum and any bleeding if present can be controlled with bipolar electrocoagulation.

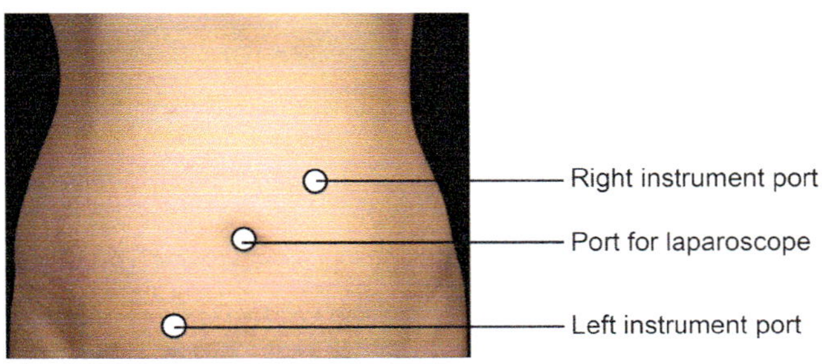

Fig. 9: Port position for laparoscopic left oophorectomy.

Dissection of the Infundibulopelvic Ligament

Three techniques have been described for managing the infundibulopelvic ligament:

1. Bipolar electrodesiccation
2. Suture ligation with pretied loop
3. Stapling

Patient cost for the linear stapler is approximately ₹ 4,500 and ₹ 250 for each pretied ligature. Considering these expenses bipolar electrosurgery is most economical way of dissection and it is preferable for hemostasis of the infundibulopelvic ligament.

Endoloop cannot be applied in the presence of adhesions and distorted anatomy. Sometime it is difficult to place endoloop sutures on large bunch of pedicles such as the mesovarium and infundibulopelvic ligament. If extracorporeal slip knot is applied over wide pedicle, the slipknot can loosen under the tension of the large pedicle. It may increase the risk of intraoperative hemorrhage. If the stump is large a piece of the ovary may get left in the pedicle, predisposing the patient to ovarian remnant syndrome.

Aside from cost, the linear stapling device has several other drawbacks. It needs to be introduced though a 12 mm trocar. Insertion of bigger trocar can lead to injury of the inferior epigastric artery and predispose the patient to a postoperative hernia. The linear stapler instrument is bulky and the operator must be careful to its proximity to the ureter, bowel, and bladder. If correct size staple is not selected the staples may dislodge and bleeding may start.

Salpingo-oophorectomy

If complete salpingo-oophorectomy is planned, the ovary and tube can be approached either from the infundibulopelvic or utero-ovarian ligament. Filmy adhesion limiting the mobilization of ovary should be dissected first. If ovarian cyst is found it should be aspirated and deflated, making removal of the ovary easier. The preferred approach is that dissection should begin with the infundibulo-ligament because it

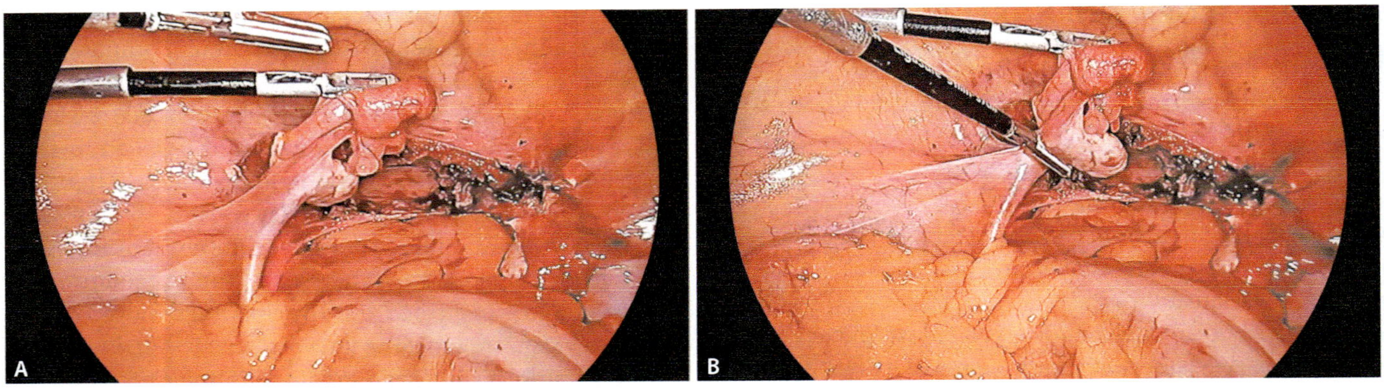

Figs. 10A and B: Dissection at the level of infundibulopelvic ligament.

is easier and this approach becomes essential if prior hysterectomy has been performed. The lateral approach is also essential if the hemostasis from ovarian vessel is of primary consideration. The ovary is held with a grasping forceps and infundibulopelvic ligament is put under traction by pulling it up and medially **(Figs. 10A and B)**.

The infundibulopelvic ligament is desiccated with bipolar forceps and cut with scissors from lateral to medial.

It is important to use appropriate traction away from lateral pelvic wall to prevent excessive coagulation and damage to the lateral pelvic structures like ureter or vessels in triangle of doom.

Laparoscopic linear stapling and cutting device can also be used for salpingo-oophorectomy in selected cases. Laparoscopic extracorporeal Roeder's or Meltzer's knot can also be applied. Pretied loop are easy to use, but pedicle should not be wide. In cases of wide pedicel window can be created in midpoint of infundibulopelvic ligament and extracorporeal knot for continuous structure should be applied.

Dysgenic Gonads

Sometime dysgenic gonads can be found at the time of laparoscopy and require gonadectomy to prevent gonadoblastoma. The laparoscopic removal technique of dysgenic gonad is same as removing an ovary with adhesion to lateral pelvic wall. In these difficult cases hydrodissection is of utmost importance.

Ovarian Wedge Resection and Ovarian Drilling

Drilling of polycystic ovary is a common procedure performed laparoscopically. Polycystic disease of ovary has various manifestations, but its hallmark is chronic anovulation. Ovarian wedge resection is advocated for these enlarged ovaries. However, chances of returning to previous inoculators state are quite high after several months. There is also an increased risk of adhesion formation after laparoscopic ovarian wedge resection. Availability of ovulation inducing medicines like clomiphene citrate (CC) around 1970s has offered a nonsurgical management of this disease. Initially wedge resection of polycystic ovary was tried, but later laparoscopic ovarian drilling evolved to be simpler and associated with comparable rates of ovulation and conception.

Theoretically wedge resection of ovary and ovarian drilling work by reducing androgen production by ovarian stroma. Ideal patient of ovarian wedge resection or ovarian drilling are those women who fail to ovulate after 3–4 months treatment with CC.

The laparoscopic technique uses a 5 mm or 10 mm umbilical port for telescope and 5 mm port in left iliac fossa or suprapubic region. With the help of one atraumatic grasper one ovary is kept held by utero-ovarian ligament. At laparoscopy, multiple symmetrically placed holes are made over subcapsular follicular cystic stroma. Polycystic drilling generally does not bleed like physiological follicular cyst following incision. Each ovary is treated symmetrically and cysts are vaporized. The ovaries are irrigated and hemostasis is obtained by the help of bipolar forceps. If aspiration needle is used for monopolar drilling 30–40 watt current is used in a cutting mode. The power is activated just before touching the ovary and it should be penetrated at four to eight sites at a depth of 4 mm.

Ovarian Torsion

Adnexal torsion is a surgical emergency and if diagnosed early, the adnexae can be unwound and saved. It occurs most frequently if there is an adnexal lesion. It occurs generally in young women in whom preservation of ovary may be necessary. If diagnosis is delayed the adnexae may become gangrenous **(Fig. 11A)**.

If conservative treatment is planned the torted structure is straightened to assess the viability and even ovary that appears infarcted at laparotomy might regain normal color after untwisting. Causes of ovarian torsion include

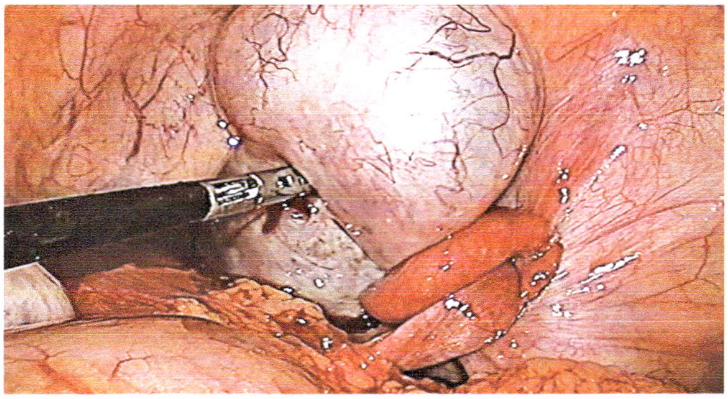

Fig. 11A: Torsion of ovary.

paraovarian cyst, functional and pathologic ovarian cyst, ovarian hyperstimulation, ectopic pregnancy, adhesions, and congenital malformations.

Ischemic structure is straightened gently with the atraumatic forceps to avoid additional adnexal damage. In women with ovarian hyperstimulation, the functional cyst should be drained before untwisting. The abnormalities contributing to torsion should be treated. It may be necessary to shorten the utero-ovarian ligament, if its length has contributed to ovarian torsion. A running suture of monofilament material is placed along the utero-ovarian ligament and tied to shorten it, limiting ovarian mobility.

After ovarian torsion if the ovary cannot be salvaged or insufficient viable tissue remains after attempts at conservation, oophorectomy is usually performed. Traditionally, less effort was made to preserve ovarian function in postmenopausal patients because of the thought that the ovary no longer functioned. In toted ovarian cyst if oophorectomy is required extracorporeal Mishra's knot also can be used **(Figs. 11B to I)**.

Ovarian Remnant Syndrome

In premenopausal women who had undergone bilateral oophorectomy, small piece of functional ovarian tissue can respond to hormonal stimulation with growth, cystic degeneration or hemorrhage and produce pain. Ovarian remnant remains because of dense adhesion and distorted anatomic relationship, which invariably worsen with subsequent operation. It is not unusual for these patients to have had previous attempt to excise an ovarian remnant. Complete removal of the ovarian tissue is preferred. Diagnosis is based on history and localization of pelvic pain. Although some patients have cystic adnexal structure or ill-defined fixed masses, others have normal pelvic findings. Vaginal ultrasound helps to locate the ovarian remnants. Low or borderline FSH levels in patients with documented bilateral oophorectomy are consistent with the presence of active ovarian tissue. Hormonal suppression, with oral contraceptives or GnRH agonist provides no relief in most patients. CC or human menopausal gonadotropin (hMG) may be used to increase the ovarian remnant size to confirm the diagnosis preoperatively or to aid in locating the tissue intraoperatively.

The anatomy of the retroperitoneal space should be identified when the ovarian remnant is adherent to the lateral pelvic wall. Space beneath the peritoneum is injected with Ringer's lactate solution and the peritoneum is opened close to the infundibulopelvic ligament or its remnant. Adhesions are lysed until the course of the major pelvic blood vessels and ureter can be traced and if necessary dissected. The ovarian blood supply is desiccated with bipolar forceps and ovarian tissue is excised and submitted for histological examination.

Paraovarian Cysts

These cysts are most commonly found over the serosa surrounding the tubal fimbriae. Usually puncture with fine electrode is sufficient for these patients. Only 40–50 watt of cutting current is required for a fraction of second and cyst will burst. Sometime if these paraovarian cysts are large and intermingled with the serosa surrounding the fimbriae may be attached with lateral pelvic wall. In these cases, opening of peritoneum is necessary for hydrodissection. Once the cyst will leave the pelvic wall; using scissors, laser or electrode, it can be dissected nicely.

Ovarian Drilling for Polycystic Ovarian Disease

Although ovarian drilling is a controversial surgery it is performed some times when medical management of polycystic ovarian disease (PCOD) fails. Ovarian drilling, also known as multiperforation or laparoscopic ovarian diathermy, is a surgical technique of puncturing the membranes surrounding the ovary with a laser beam or a surgical needle using minimally invasive laparoscopic procedures. Women with polycystic ovarian syndrome (PCOS) usually have ovaries with a thick outer layer. The ovaries make more testosterone. High testosterone levels can lead to irregular menstrual periods, acne, and extra body hair.

Ovarian drilling works by breaking through the thick outer surface and lowering the amount of testosterone made by the ovaries. This can help the ovaries release an egg each month and start regular monthly menstrual cycles. This may make it easier to get pregnant **(Figs. 12A to E)**.

In some of the studies, the long-term follow-up for ovarian drilling, which usually takes up to 36 months, showed a successful pregnancy rate of 60.4% and an increased pregnancy rate of 75%; however, some women got pregnant within only 12 months. PCOS is a frequent disorder, affecting approximately 5–10% of infertile women. It can represent more than 80% of cases of infertility due to anovulation. The main goal of treatment is the induction of mono-ovulatory cycles.

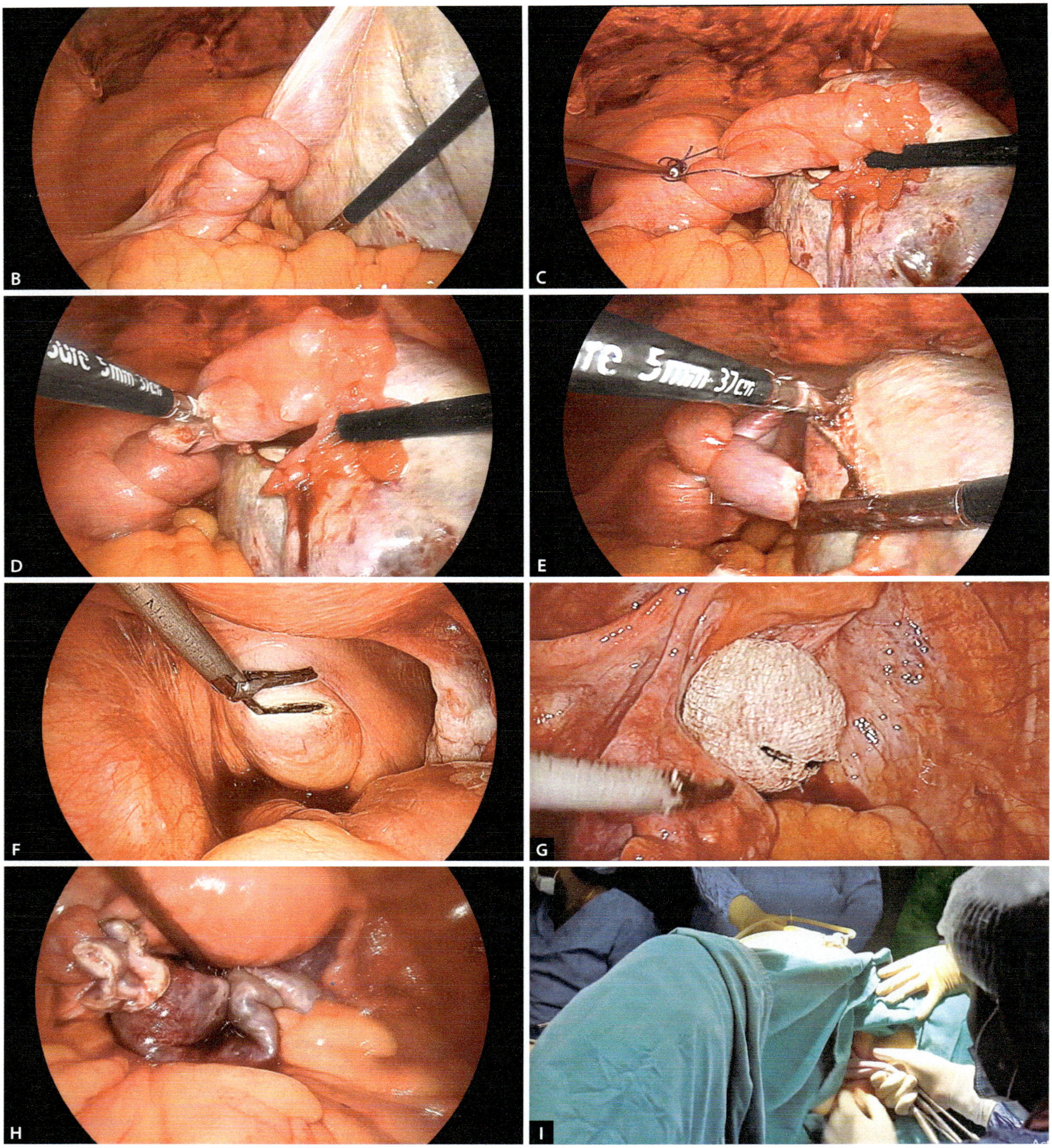

Figs. 11B to I: Oophorectomy and removal through colpotomy.

A pragmatic management of infertility in PCOS will allow most patients to conceive. Weight loss and clomiphene citrate are the first-line components of patients treatment before gonadotropins are used. However, during gonadotropin administration, there is a high risk of ovarian hyperstimulation and multiple pregnancies. So, surgery with laparoscopic ovarian drilling is often used before gonadotropins in order to obtain normal ovulatory cycles. The main benefits of ovarian drilling are shorter time to pregnancy and less need to ovulation induction drugs. The other advantages of this technique are more comfort, cost-effectiveness, and possibility to be performed ambulatory day care surgery.

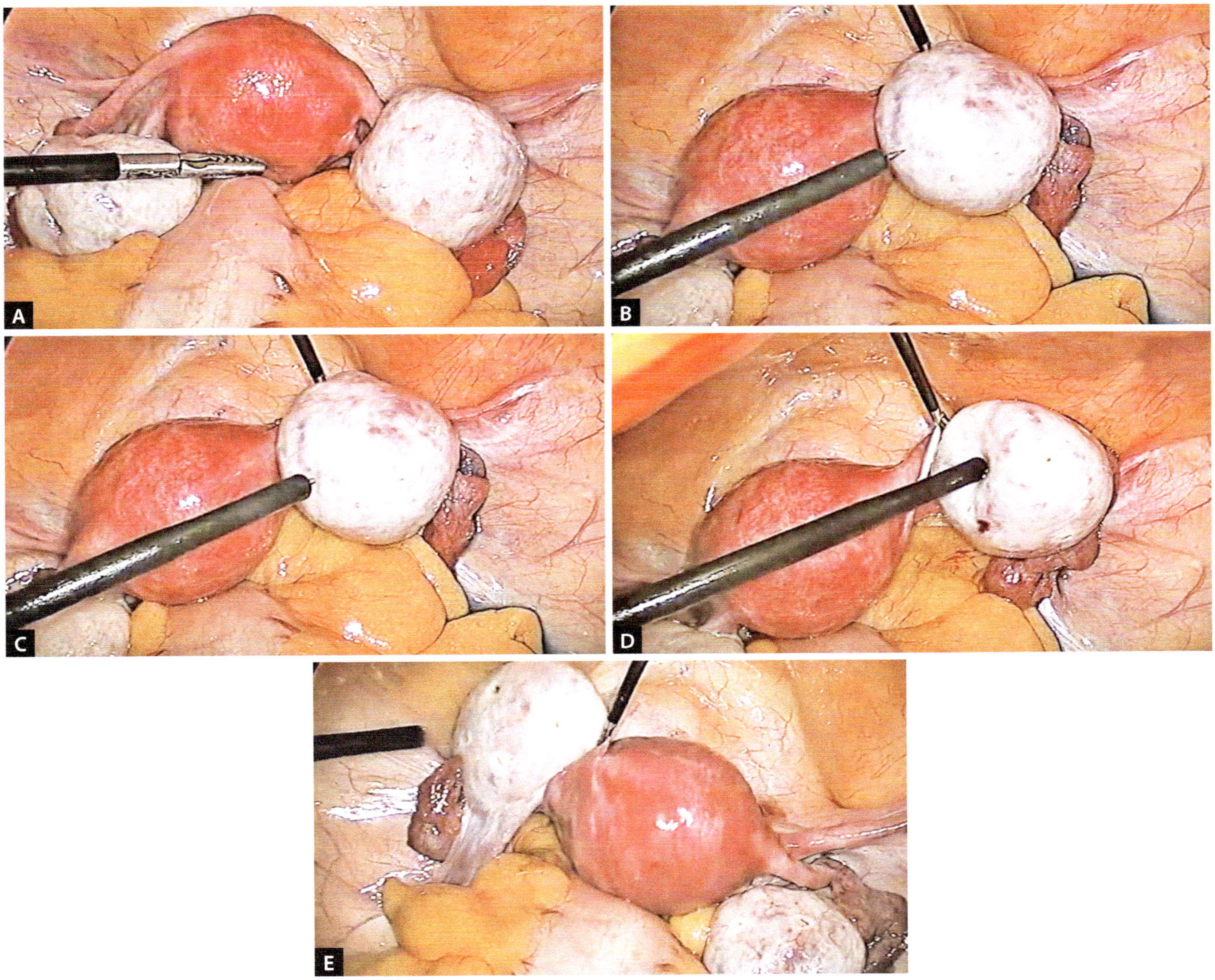

Figs. 12A to E: Polycystic ovary syndrome.

BIBLIOGRAPHY

1. Acs G. Serous and mucinous borderline (low malignant potential) tumors of the ovary. Am J Clin Pathol. 2005;123:S13-57.
2. Barnhill DR, Kurman RJ, Brady MF, Omura GA, Yordan E, Given FT, et al. Preliminary analysis of the behavior of stage I ovarian serous tumors of low malignant potential: a Gynecologic Oncology Group study. J Clin Oncol. 1995;13:2752-6.
3. Blanc B, D'Ercole C, Nicoloso E, Boubli L. Laparoscopic management of malignant ovarian cysts: a 78-case national survey. Part 2: Follow-up and final treatment. Eur J Obstet Gynecol Reprod Biol. 1995;61:147-50.
4. Boran N, Cil AP, Tulunay G, Ozturkoglu E, Koc S, Bulbul D, et al. Fertility and recurrence results of conservative surgery for borderline ovarian tumors. Gynecol Oncol. 2005;97:845-51.
5. Bostwick DG, Tazelaar HD, Ballon SC, Hendrickson MR, Kempson RL. Ovarian epithelial tumors of borderline malignancy. A clinical and pathologic study of 109 cases. Cancer. 1986;58:2052-65.
6. Camatte S, Morice P, Atallah D, Thoury A, Pautier P, Lhomme C, et al. Clinical outcome after laparoscopic pure management of borderline ovarian tumors: results of a series of 34 patients. Ann Oncol. 2004;15:605-9.
7. Camatte S, Morice P, Pautier P, Atallah D, Duvillard P, Castaigne D. Fertility results after conservative treatment of advanced stage serous borderline tumour of the ovary. BJOG. 2002;109:376-80.
8. Candiani M, Vasile C, Sgherzi MR, Nozza A, Maggi F, Maggi R. Borderline ovarian tumors: laparoscopic treatment. Clin Exp Obstet Gynecol. 1999;26:39-43.
9. Chan JK, Lin YG, Loizzi V, Ghobriel M, DiSaia PJ, Berman ML. Borderline ovarian tumors in reproductive-age women. Fertility-sparing surgery and outcome. J Reprod Med. 2003;48:756-60.
10. Crispens MA. Borderline ovarian tumours: a review of the recent literature. Curr Opin Obstet Gynecol. 2003;15:39-43.
11. Darai E, Teboul J, Fauconnier A, Scoazec JY, Benifla JL, Madelenat P. Management and outcome of borderline ovarian tumors incidentally discovered at or after laparoscopy. Acta Obstet Gynecol Scand. 1998;77:451-7.
12. Darai E, Teboul J, Walker F. Epithelial ovarian carcinoma of low malignant potential. Eur J Obstet Gynecol Reprod Biol. 1996;66:141-5.
13. Deffieux X, Morice P, Camatte S, Fourchotte V, Duvillard P, Castaigne D. Results after laparoscopic management of serous borderline tumor of the ovary with peritoneal implants. Gynecol Oncol. 2005;97:84-9.

14. Desfeux P, Camatte S, Chatellier G, Blanc B, Querleu D, Lecuru F. Impact of surgical approach on the management of macroscopic early ovarian borderline tumors. Gynecol Oncol. 2005;98:390-5.
15. Donnez J, Bassil S. Indications for cryopreservation of ovarian tissue. Hum Reprod Update. 1998;4:248-59.
16. Donnez J, Munschke A, Berliere M, Pirard C, Jadoul P, Smets M, et al. Safety of conservative management and fertility outcome in women with borderline tumors of the ovary. Fertil Steril. 2003;79:1216-21.
17. Fauvet R, Boccara J, Dufournet C, David-Montefiore E, Poncelet C, Darai E. Restaging surgery for women with borderline ovarian tumors: results of a French multicenter study. Cancer. 2004;100:1145-51.
18. Fauvet R, Poncelet C, Boccara J, Descamps P, Fondrinier E, Darai E. Fertility after conservative management for borderline ovarian tumors: a French multicenter study. Fertil Steril. 2005;83:284-90.
19. Gershenson DM. Contemporary treatment of borderline ovarian tumors. Cancer Invest. 1999;17:206-10.
20. Gotlieb WH, Flikker S, Davidson B, Korach Y, Kopolovic J, Ben-Baruch G. Borderline tumors of the ovary: fertility treatment, conservative management, and pregnancy outcome. Cancer. 1998;82:141-6.
21. Havrilesky LJ, Peterson BL, Dryden DK, Soper JT, Clarke-Pearson DL, Berchuck A. Predictors of clinical outcomes in the laparoscopic management of adnexal masses. Obstet Gynecol. 2003;102:243-51.
22. International Federation of Gynecology and Obstetrics. Annual report and results of treatment in gynaecologic cancer. Int J Gynaecol Obstet. 1989;28:189-90.
23. International Federation of Gynecology and Obstetrics. Changes in definitions of clinical staging for carcinoma of the cervix and ovary. Am J Obstet Gynecol. 1987;156:263-4.
24. International Federation of Gynecology and Obstetrics. Classification and staging of malignant tumors in the female pelvis. Acta Obstet Gynecol Scand. 1971;50:1-7.
25. Kaern J, Trope CG, Abeler VM. A retrospective study of 370 borderline tumors of the ovary treated at the Norwegian Radium Hospital from 1970 to 1982. A review of clinicopathologic features and treatment modalities. Cancer. 1993;71:1810-20.
26. Lim-Tan SK, Cajigas HE, Scully RE. Ovarian cystectomy for serous borderline tumors: a follow-up study of 35 cases. Obstet Gynecol. 1988;72:775-81.
27. Lin PS, Gershenson DM, Bevers MW, Lucas KR, Burke TW, Silva EG. The current status of surgical staging of surgical staging of ovarian serous borderline tumors. Cancer. 1999;85:905-11.
28. Maneo A, Vignali M, Chiari S, Colombo A, Mangioni C, Landoni F. Are borderline tumors of the ovary safely treated by laparoscopy? Gynecol Oncol. 2004;94:387-92.
29. Morice P, Camatte S, El Hassan J, Pautier P, Duvillard P, Castaigne D. Clinical outcomes and fertility after conservative treatment of ovarian borderline tumors. Fertil Steril. 2001;75:92-6.
30. Morice P, Camatte S, Wicart-Poque F, Atallah D, Rouzier R, Pautier P, et al. Results of conservative management of epithelial malignant and borderline ovarian tumours. Hum Reprod Update. 2003;9:185-92.
31. Nezhat F, Nezhat C, Welander CE, Benigno B. Four ovarian cancers diagnosed during laparoscopic management of 1011 women with adnexal masses. Am J Obstet Gynecol. 1992;167:790-6.
32. Pejovic T, Nezhat F. Laparoscopic management of adnexal masses the opportunities and the risks. Ann N Y Acad Sci. 2001; 943:255-68.
33. Querleu D, Papageorgiou T, Lambaudie E, Sonoda Y, Narducci F, LeBlanc E. Laparoscopic restaging of borderline ovarian tumours: results of 30 cases initially presumed as stage IA borderline ovarian tumours. BJOG. 2003;110:201-4.
34. Rao GG, Skinner EN, Gehrig PA, Duska LR, Miller DS, Schorge J. Fertility-sparing surgery for ovarian low malignant potential tumors. Gynecol Oncol. 2005;98:263-6.
35. Romagnolo C, Gadducci A, Sartori E, Zola P, Maggino T. Management of borderline ovarian tumors: Results of an Italian multicenter study. Gynecol Oncol. 2006;101(2):255-60.
36. Rota SM, Zanetta G, Iedà N, Rossi R, Chiari S, Perego P, et al. Clinical relevance of retroperitoneal involvement from epithelial ovarian tumors of borderline malignancy. Int J Gynecol Cancer. 1999;9:477-80.
37. Salomon LJ, Lhommé C, Pautier P, Duvillard P, Morice P. Safety of simple cystectomy in patients with unilateral mucinous borderline tumors. Fertil Steril. 2006;85:1510.e1-4.
38. Scully RE. World Health Organization classification and nomenclature of ovarian cancer. Natl Cancer Inst Monogr. 1975;42:5-7.
39. Seidman JD, Kurman RJ. Ovarian serous borderline tumors: a critical review of the literature with emphasis on prognostic indicators. Hum Pathol. 2000;31:539-57.
40. Seracchioli R, Venturoli S, Colombo FM, Govoni F, Missiroli S, Bagnoli A. Fertility and tumor recurrence rate after conservative laparoscopic management of young women with early-stage borderline ovarian tumors. Fertil Steril. 2001;76:999-1004.
41. Steinberg M. Cox regression examples. SPSS Advanced Models 9.0. Chicago: SPSS Inc; 1999. p. 258.
42. Tazelaar HD, Bostwick DG, Ballon SC, Hendrickson MR, Kempson RL. Conservative treatment of borderline ovarian tumors. Obstet Gynecol. 1985;66:417-22.
43. Tinelli R, Tinelli A, Tinelli FG, Cicinelli E, Malvasi A. Conservative surgery for borderline ovarian tumours: a review. Gynecol Oncol. 2006;100:185-91.
44. Trimble EL, Trimble LC. Epithelial ovarian tumors of low malignant potential. In: Markman M, Hoskins WJ (Eds). Cancer of the Ovary. New York: Raven Press; 1993. pp. 415-29.
45. Trope CG, Kristensen G, Makar A. Surgery for borderline tumor of the ovary. Semin Surg Oncol. 2000;19:69-75.
46. Vergote I, De Brabanter J, Fyles A, Bertelsen K, Einhorn N, Sevelda P, et al. Prognostic importance of degree of differentiation and cyst rupture in stage I invasive epithelial ovarian carcinoma. Lancet. 2001;357:176-82.
47. Winter WE III, Kucera PR, Rodgers W, McBroom JW, Olsen C, Maxwell GL. Surgical staging in patients with ovarian tumors of low malignant potential. Obstet Gynecol. 2002;100:671-6.
48. Zanetta G, Chiari S, Rota S, Bratina G, Maneo A, Torri V, et al. Conservative surgery for stage I ovarian carcinoma in women of childbearing age. BJOG. 1997;104:1030-35.
49. Zanetta G, Rota S, Chiari S, Bonazzi C, Bratina G, Mangioni C. Behavior of borderline tumors with particular interest to persistence, recurrence, and progression to invasive carcinoma: a prospective study. J Clin Oncol. 2001;19:2658-64.

CHAPTER 30

Laparoscopic Tubal Surgery

INTRODUCTION

Tubal diseases are one of the frequent causes of infertility. The most common predisposing factor is pelvic inflammatory disease (PID). Distal tubal obstruction has been managed previously by open surgery using microsurgical technique. The pregnancy rate after reconstructive surgery is 20–30% 2 years postoperatively. Laparoscopy for tubal infertility has been a significant factor in reducing—costs, hospitalization, and recuperation. Recently, in women with severe tubal damage, in vitro fertilization (IVF) offers a better chance for term pregnancy (72.3%) compared to reconstructive surgery (27.3%). Fimbrioplasty and lysis of peritubal and periovarian adhesions have been associated with good pregnancy rates. In these patients, IVF is appropriate when pregnancy is not achieved postoperatively after a few years.

LAPAROSCOPIC TUBAL ANATOMY

The fallopian tubes arise from the superior portion of the uterus just above the attachment points of the round ligament. Laparoscopically, the round ligaments overhang the fallopian tube because of uterine manipulation and can be easily mistaken for them. The fallopian tubes toward its lateral end encircle the ovaries partially with their fimbriated ends **(Fig. 1)**.

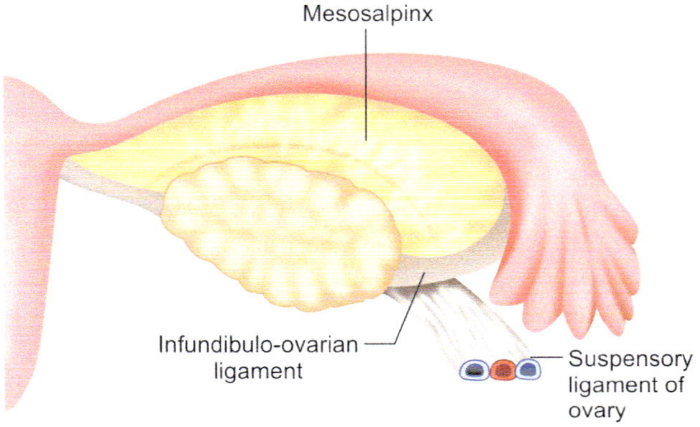

Fig. 1: Tubal anatomy.

From anterior to posterior, following important tubular structures are found crossing the brim of true pelvis; the round ligament of the uterus, the infundibulopelvic ligament, which contains the gonadal vessels and the ureter. The ovaries and fallopian tube is found between the round ligament and the infundibulopelvic ligament.

The ovarian ligaments run from the ovaries to the lateral border of the uterus. Ovary is attached to the pelvic side wall with infundibulopelvic ligament, which carries ovarian artery. One of the common mistakes that a surgeon can land into is injury of the ureter during dissection of the infundibulopelvic ligament. If the uterus is deviated to the contralateral side with the help of uterine manipulator, infundibulopelvic ligament is spread out and a pelvic side wall triangle is created. The base of this triangle is the round ligament, the medial side is the infundibulopelvic ligament, and the lateral side is the external iliac artery. The apex of this triangle is the point at which the infundibulopelvic ligament crosses the external iliac artery.

The ureters enter the pelvis in close proximity to the female pelvic organs and are at risk for injury during laparoscopic surgery of these organs. As the ureter courses medially over the bifurcation of the iliac vessels, they pass obliquely under the ovarian vessels and then run in close proximity to the uterine artery.

Patient Position

Patient should be in steep Trendelenburg's and lithotomy position. One assistant should remain between the legs of patient to do uterine manipulation whenever required.

Port Position

Port position should be in accordance with baseball diamond concept. If the left side of tube has to be operated, one port should be in right iliac fossa and another below left hypochondrium **(Fig. 2)**.

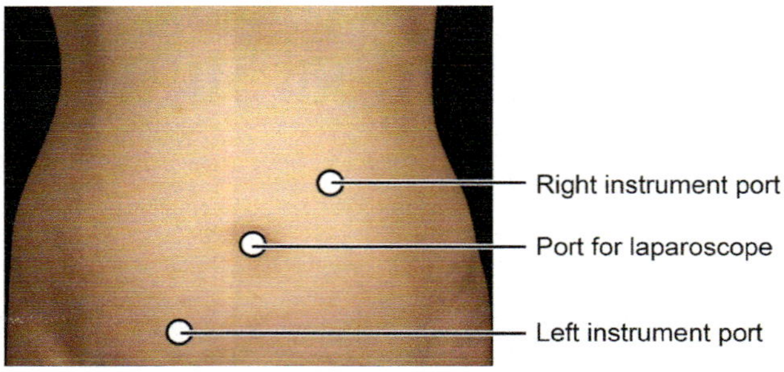

Fig. 2: Port position tubal surgery left side.

OPERATIVE PROCEDURE

Management of Acute Pelvic Inflammatory Disease

Pelvic inflammatory disease usually results from sexually transmitted diseases caused by *Chlamydia* or *Gonococcus* infection, an intrauterine device (IUD), postpartum endometritis, or hysteroscopy at the time of endometrial infection.

Pelvic inflammatory disease has four primary sequelae:

1. Infertility
2. Ectopic pregnancy
3. Chronic pelvic pain
4. Recurrent upper UTI.

One of the worst outcomes of PID is adhesions of reproductive organ leading to infertility and pain. The degree of tubal damage and pelvic adhesions often depends on the severity of the infection, the number of PID episodes, and etiology. Severe peritonitis is associated with a 17% risk of infertility compared to 3% for mild infection. With each successive episode of PID, the risk of infertility doubles. Despite its typically mild presentation, chlamydial PID results in a threefold increase in infertility compared to gonococcal PID. The risk of ectopic pregnancy is 6–10 times higher in women who have had PID. In addition, chronic pelvic pain has been shown to occur in 15–18% of patients after PID, usually because of adhesions. Up to 20–25% of patients will have at least one recurrent infection because damaged fallopian tubes are more susceptible to infection.

Laparoscopy is being used increasingly in patients suspected of having PID to make a precise diagnosis and thereby avoid the potential sequelae. Prompt surgical confirmation of the diagnosis is possible with laparoscopy. A tubo-ovarian abscess (TOA) can be drained, reducing the risk of serious morbidity associated with rupture. The clinical diagnosis of PID is difficult because of the wide variation in symptoms and signs. Many women with PID report subtle, vague, or mild symptoms that are not specific, such as dyspareunia, postcoital spotting, or abnormal uterine bleeding. In these situations, a bimanual examination may demonstrate cervical mobility or adnexal tenderness.

Tubo-ovarian abscess is a severe sequelae and occurs in as many as 34% of patients hospitalized with PID. Symptomatic or subclinical infections can progress rapidly into a TOA. These abscesses can rupture, resulting in severe peritonitis.

At present, surgical intervention is used to treat a tubo-ovarian mass only when medical management is ineffective. The laparoscopic procedure for managing pelvic abscesses has been described by several authors. Once TOA is diagnosed laparoscopically, two 5 mm trocars are placed in both the flanks according to baseball diamond concept through which a suction-irrigator probe and grasping forceps are inserted. The pelvis, upper abdomen, and pelvic gutters should be examined for free or loculated purulent material and the course of both ureters should be identified. Purulent fluid is aspirated from the pelvis, and cultures are taken from the aspirated fluid and the inflammatory exudates. If necessary, the suction-irrigator is used to mobilize the omentum, small bowel, rectosigmoid junction. Tubo-ovarian adhesions should be dissected until the abscess cavity is localized. After the abscess cavity is drained, the suction-irrigator is used to separate the bowel and omentum completely from the reproductive organs. Chromotubation is not indicated in case of PID because edema in the interstitial tissue of the tube occludes the lumen.

At the end of the procedure, whole peritoneal cavity is irrigated with normal saline until the effluent is clear. Between 300 and 400 mL of irrigation fluid are left in the pelvis to distance these organs during the early healing phase.

Adhesiolysis is technically difficult and associated with a high risk of complications. Hydrodissection decreases the potential for intestinal or ureteral injury; the laser and electrosurgery should be used sparingly.

Laparoscopy for Adnexal Torsion

Adnexal torsion is a rare gynecologic emergency of women who are mostly in reproductive ages. So there is an increasing trend toward conservative approach for preservation of fertility in young women. Literature has all come to a point of agreement that, as minimal surgery as possible and sparing of adnexa for these women of reproductive age should be done, since torted adnexa has a benign histopathology in most cases. Operative laparoscopic procedures are being performed increasingly in gynecology in recent years. It delivers some main advantages over laparotomy. Smaller surgical scars which have better healing process than a single big scar, reduced postoperative pain and morbidity; and shorter hospital stays, recovery periods with a lower cost are the major advantages of laparoscopy for a number of gynecologic conditions (ectopic pregnancy, benign ovarian cysts, tuba peritoneal infertility, etc). The results of laparoscopic treatment are comparable with those of laparotomy. For these reasons operative laparoscopy has become the surgical treatment of choice for the conditions listed above. Like all surgeries, operative laparoscopy does bring with it a risk of complications which need to be assessed.

Since mostly the lesions are benign in nature, simply detorsion of the torted adnexa and if necessary the cyst excision is the preferred procedure. But what is very important, is the time period between the diagnosis and treatment of the pathology. Since the torsion of adnexa causes a relative ischemia of the ovarian tissue, it may result in failure and loss of ovarian function.

In older studies, it was advised to remove the necrotic adnexa since they thought that it might lead to pulmonary emboli. But in recent literature, it is not advised to remove the adnexa even if the adnexa looks necrotic because even severely necrotic looking adnexa may save its function after surgery.

Some literature suggest that only simple detorsion procedure may cause retorsion and the rate of retorsion is higher patients with normal looking adnexa and is lower in the patients who have pathological adnexa and some other procedure should also applied along with detorsion. Ovariopexy may be applied additionally, especially if there is a long ovarian pedicle, but more studies are needed to evaluate its value.

In the literature, it is shown in retrospective studies that in the patient selection for laparoscopic surgeries, size of the adnexal cystic pathology is an important criteria that is the mean size of the cyst, which is smaller in laparoscopic surgeries compared to laparotomy.

Risk factors for conversion to laparotomy are studied in some articles and it is found that the most important risk factor for conversion to laparotomy is previous pelvic surgery and especially hysterectomy. In cases where laparoscopic access cannot be performed, minilaparotomy is an alternative method and the results are comparable to laparoscopic surgery.

Adnexal torsion in pregnant patients may occur due to drugs used for ovarian hyperstimulation at infertility therapy that increases the size of ovary or due to persistence of corpus luteum or other pathologies of the adnexa. Laparoscopic detorsion and cyst excision procedures were safely applied in pregnant patients even in third trimester of pregnancy. The maternal and fetal outcomes after procedure were satisfactory and comparable to laparotomy. Open laparoscopy technique is advised in literature as more safe procedure even in advanced pregnancy.

In case of premenarchal and adolescence period, although very rare, adnexal torsion may occur and sometimes an additional congenital malformation may accompany. With the advent of new and smaller instrumentation, laparoscopic surgery has extended to include the neonate as well as the pediatric patient. Laparoscopic detorsion and the sparing of the adnexa is the type of treatment encouraged in the literature in case of benign neoplasm, although the patient's numbers are very limited. Some authors suggest contralateral oophoropexy in case of normal appearing adnexa.

In postmenopausal women due to increase in rate of malignant transformations, preoperative investigations for predicting malignant and benign lesions is very important. Literature supports that in case of good analyses of the patient preoperatively and the criteria for the lesion to be benign are fulfilling, laparoscopic surgery is safe and if the intraoperative histopathological diagnosis is also benign, bilateral salpingo-oophorectomy is the treatment of choice. But in advanced centers with a skilled surgeon at malignant procedures, laparoscopic surgery and laparoscopic staging may be performed in case there is suspicion of malignancy.

Laparoscopic Tubal Reconstruction and Anastomosis

Prior to laparoscopy, most tubal recanalization operations were performed by an operating microscope or with magnifying loupes **(Figs. 3 and 4)**. These reduced tissue trauma and increased the detection of abnormalities. Magnification, which enabled the use of microsurgical instruments and fine, nonreactive sutures, was an

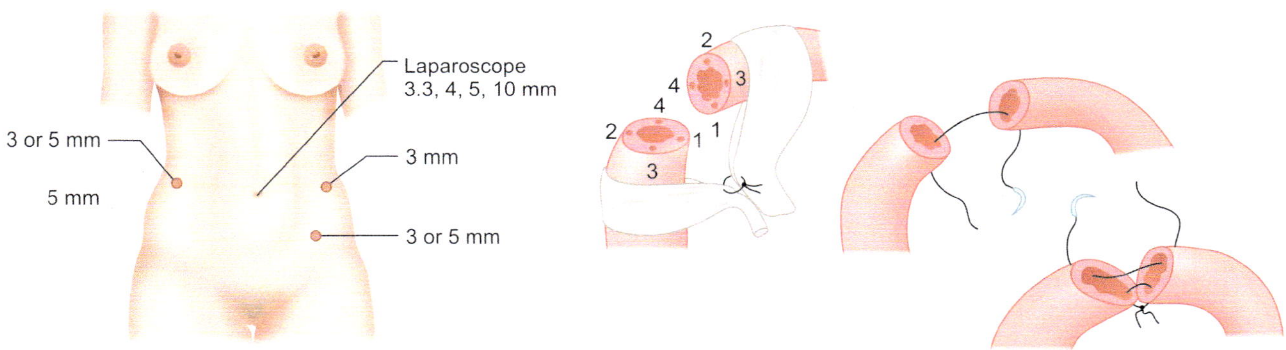

Fig. 3: Tubal recanalization surgery.

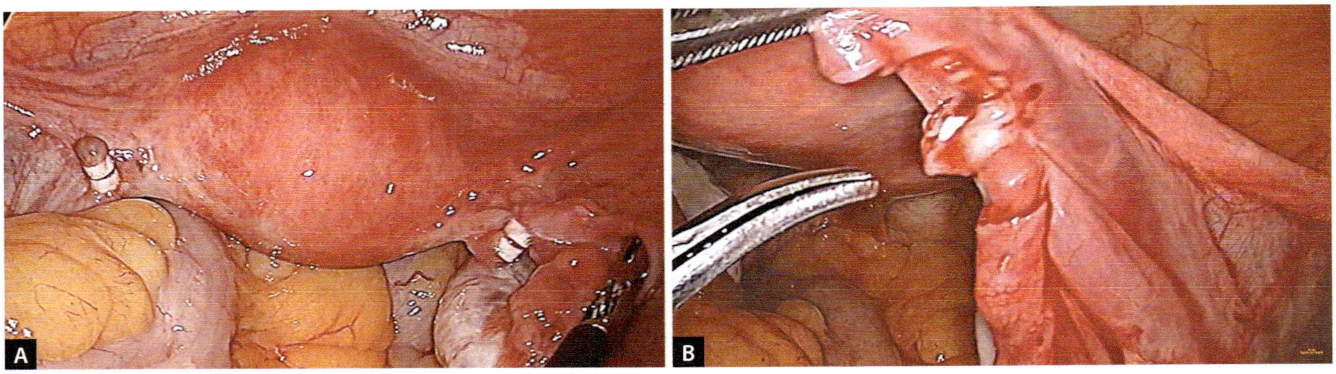

Figs. 4A and B: Tubal recanalization.

improvement over macrosurgical techniques. The combination of the laparoscope and the video monitor make it possible to perform tubal microsurgery using laparoscopic instruments due to the magnification.

The serosa of the fallopian tube is delicate and easily traumatized, especially when graspers are used to apply traction. Although laparoscopic Babcock's clamps allow atraumatic manipulation of the tube, it is still possible to tear the mesosalpinx and lacerate vessels. It is preferable to use a manipulating probe, a closed grasper, or the suction-irrigator to position the tube and apply traction. If really necessary, the tubal serosa should be held behind the fimbria on the antimesenteric aspect using atraumatic grasping forceps.

The fimbria is very vascular and bleeds with little provocation. The bleeding is difficult to localize precisely and frequent attempts to achieve hemostasis may damage tubes. An injection of 3–5 mL of dilute Pitressin in the mesosalpinx can be used to decrease bleeding. The removal of any large clots is vital to prevent adhesion formation.

Outcome of tuboplasty depends on the extent of adnexal disease and the degree of postoperative adhesion formation. The adhesions can be filmy, dense, and vascular and involve the tubes and ovaries. Tubal abnormality and other pelvic disease (i.e., endometriosis, fibroids) also affect the outcome.

Judicious use of suture can improve the operative outcome. A monofilament suture is recommended (i.e., 4-0 PDS or similar type) **(Fig. 3)**.

Desire to perform minimally invasive surgery has resulted in the continued better performance of anastomosis by laparoscopy. However, the reproductive outcome after tubal anastomosis by laparoscopy has been slightly poor than open procedure. Patients who want reversal of sterilization should show the documentation of the sterilization procedure previously. If previous sterilization is performed near fimbria, the reversal is seldom successful and in these patients, IVF is recommended. If the mechanical occlusion was used for previous sterilization, the tube is not much destroyed and reversal is more successful. The ability to perform laparoscopic tubal reversal is limited by the fine suture and needles required for anastomosis **(Figs. 5A to E)**. Gynecologists who want to perform recanalization surgery should have good practice of intracorporeal suturing. However, it is possible to prepare the tubes through the laparoscope and either bring the ends through a minilaparotomy incision or bring the entire uterus out to perform the anastomosis under the operating microscope, using 8-0 polydioxanone suture.

Successful tubal anastomosis depends on precise apposition of tissues to ensure and restore anatomic integrity **(Fig. 6)**.

Fine suture material can minimize tissue reaction and excessive scar formation. Several obstacles have limited the performance of tubal anastomosis at laparoscopy. One of the limiting factors of lesser success rate of laparoscopic anastomosis is inappropriate intracorporeal suturing skill.

In Europe, the availability of fibrin glue has increased the options for joining tissues without suture. Recently performed randomized prospective study has compared microsurgical tubal anastomosis with anastomosis using fibrin glue. Postoperative adhesions and pregnancy rates did not differ between the two groups.

If surgeon does not have sufficient laparoscopic intracorporeal suturing skill, the ends of the tube are exteriorized through a minilaparotomy incision and the lumen is approximated with 8-0 or finer Vicryl. Exteriorization is aided by using traction on the uterine manipulator to properly position the uterus. Patients are discharged the same day or the following morning.

The anastomosis is considered as complete after four 6/0 sutures have been placed. Methylene blue dye injected into the uterine cavity emerges from the end of the tube with no leakage at the joint.

With continuous progress in development of laparoscopic microinstruments, with refinement of video cameras, and with further improvement of endoscopic surgical suturing skills, it is now possible to perform tubal anastomosis entirely by laparoscopy. However, the success of the anastomosis should never be sacrificed for the sake of performing the procedure by laparoscopy and increasing skill on human patients.

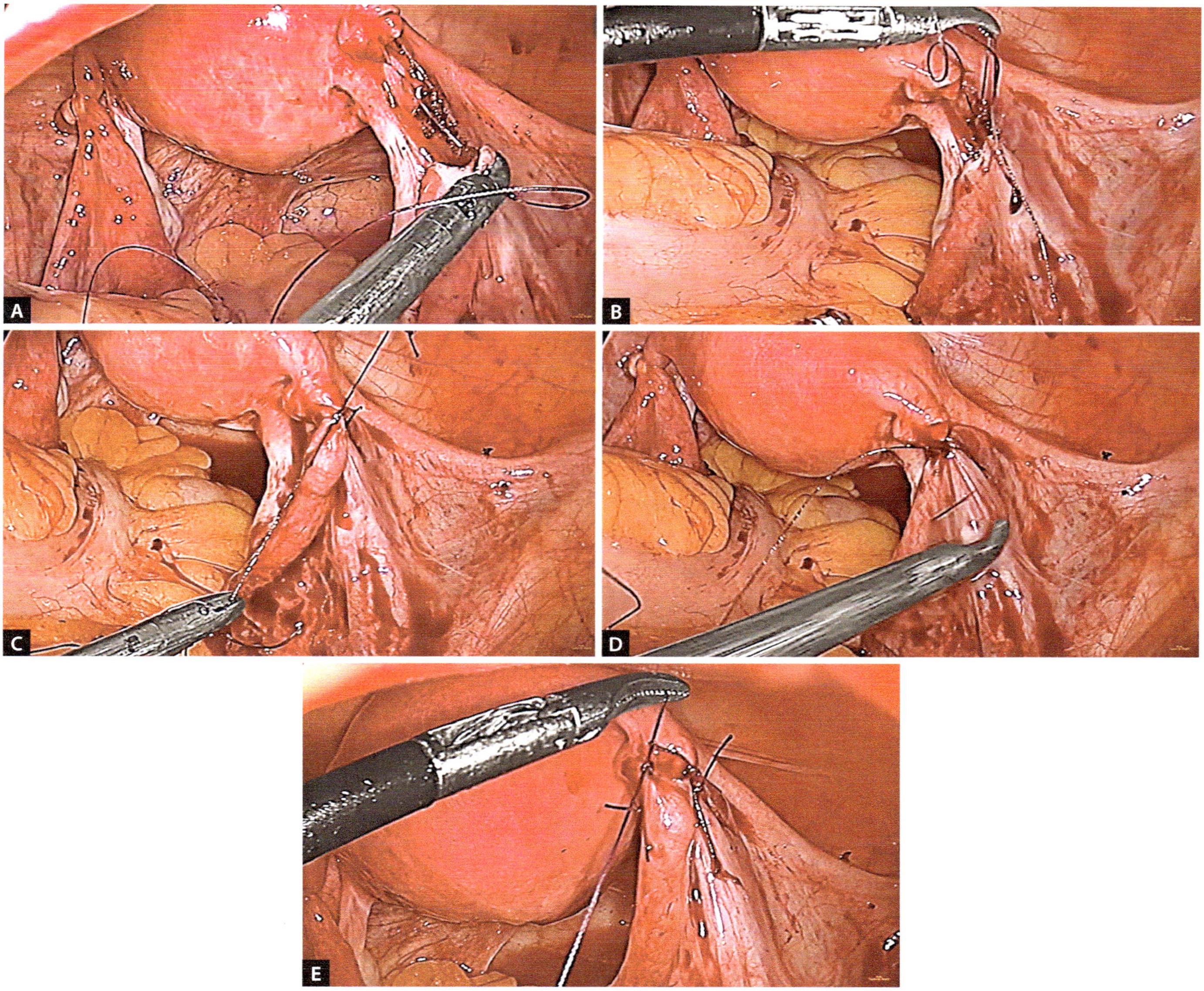

Figs. 5A to E: 6-0 Vicryl is used for tubal recanalization surgery.

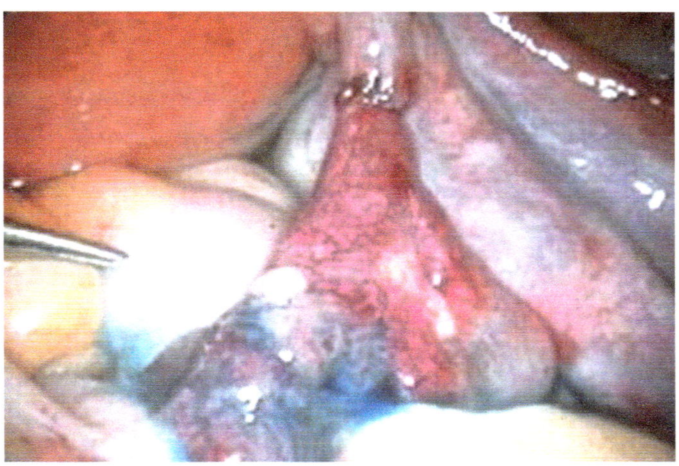

Fig. 6: Chromotubation after recanalization.

Laparoscopic Management of Distal Tubal Occlusion

A hydrosalpinx is caused by distal tubal occlusion and is characterized by a dilated tube filled with clear fluid. It is usually a consequence of infectious salpingitis and is associated with intrinsic tubal disease. Distal tubal obstruction also can be caused by ruptured appendix, adhesions from previous pelvic surgery, or endometriosis, all of which result in extrinsic disease and do not significantly affect the delicate tubal mucosa.

The pregnancy outcome following tuboplasty is related to many variables that reflect the severity of pre-existing disease. Only a small percentage of patients achieve intrauterine pregnancy.

In contrast, pregnancy rates approached zero when there were numerous dense adhesions. No clear pattern was associated with the risk for ectopic pregnancy. Several scoring systems have been proposed to predict the probability of conception.

To free the fimbria, a closed 3-mm forceps is inserted into the fallopian tube through the phimotic opening. The jaws of the forceps are opened within the tube; the open forceps are withdrawn. This procedure is repeated until satisfactory.

Neosalpingostomy

Once the laparoscope is inserted, two more suprapubic trocars are placed; the suction-irrigator and grasping forceps can be introduced. The distal portion of the tube is manipulated into position with the grasper or the uterine fundus. Fluid distention of the tube using chromotubation allows identification of the avascular central point, which is generally the thinnest portion of the tube. A cruciate incision should be given using the scissor.

Neosalpingostomy also can be performed by opening the distended end of the tube and then grasping the endosalpinx with an atraumatic grasping forceps, pulling it out and back over the tube like a sleeve. The defocused laser may be used to further evert the edges. The edges of the tube are sutured to the tubal serosa using 6-0 PDS. Tubal patency is confirmed by injecting diluted indigo carmine through the cannula of the uterine manipulator. The presence of fimbrial adhesions may be assessed on close-up view of the fimbria as the dye is injected. The condition of the tubal mucosa can be evaluated by salpingoscopy.

Salpingoscopy

Until recently, it was not possible to examine the tubal mucosa endoscopically. As previously noted, the degree of tubal mucosa damage is probably the major factor in establishing a prognosis for tubal reconstructive surgery. It has been assumed that tubal patency on hysterosalpingogram (HSG) indicated tubal normality. Thus, the selection of patients who could benefit from tubal reconstructive surgery was based on preoperative HSG and laparoscopic appearance of the tubes. Although the mucosal folds can be outlined by HSG, the correlation between radiological studies and endoscopy in assessing the tubal mucosa is poor.

For salpingoscopy first laparoscopy is performed by introducing the laparoscope through the umbilicus and inserting two other accessory ports in both the iliac fossa. The tube is manipulated gently with atraumatic forceps applied to the antimesenteric serosal surface close to the fimbria. Once the fimbrial end is in the line, a 3-mm telescope is inserted through the ipsilateral accessory port and gently inserted in the tubal lumen. Normal saline is infused through the Cohen cannula, which has been attached to the cervix. The saline infusion is an essential part of the procedure because it creates space and makes the anatomy of the mucosa fold more visible.

The distal end of the tube can be occluded with an atraumatic grasper if distention of the tube is inadequate. The scope is slowly and gently advanced under direct vision into the tubal infundibulum where the major and minor folds can be seen. In a normal tube, the folds are well formed, parallel to each other, and freely move in the distending fluid. The tubal lumen is followed into the ampulla by advancing the scope and carefully negotiating the bends. In the ampulla there are 4–6 major folds, each about 4 mm in height, with accessory folds arising from them. Between the major folds there are several minor folds approximately 1 mm in height. When the junction of ampulla and isthmus is reached, the major folds give way to three or four rounded folds. With experience, it is usually possible to follow the lumen as far as the isthmic-ampullary junction.

Salpingoscopy revealed various lesions such as synechiae and denuded areas that were unsuspected from HSG appearance, for a false-negative rate of 45%. If the tubal mucosa seemed to have an abnormality on HSG, a normal mucosa was discovered at salpingoscopy 21% of the time. These data suggest that salpingoscopy more accurately indicates the condition of the tubal mucosa than HSG and that assessment of tubal status by salpingoscopy allows a better assessment of treatment options.

Currently, more infertility surgery is performed by laparoscopy than by laparotomy.

Laparoscopic salpingoscopy permits detailed examination of the ampullary portion of the tubal mucosa and is particularly useful to:

- Detect unsuspected tubal lesions not previously identified on HSG.
- Evaluate the extent of mucosal damage in a woman who has PID.
- Evaluate the status of tubal mucosa in patients who have known tubal disease with or without a hydrosalpinx.
- Decide on management of the contralateral tube in a woman with an ectopic pregnancy.
- Examine tubes before the granulocyte immunofluorescence test.

Complications from this operation are rare; however, it is possible to damage the fimbriae with the forceps, causing minor bleeding or adhesion formation. The most serious complication, perforation of the tubal mucosa, may occur when the scope is advanced blindly or with unnecessary force. Occasionally, bleeding will occur at the level of the fimbria, but usually ceases spontaneously.

Salpingectomy

There are occasions when a fallopian tube is damaged to such an extent that its removal is indicated **(Figs. 7A and B)**. Circumstances that frequently require salpingectomy

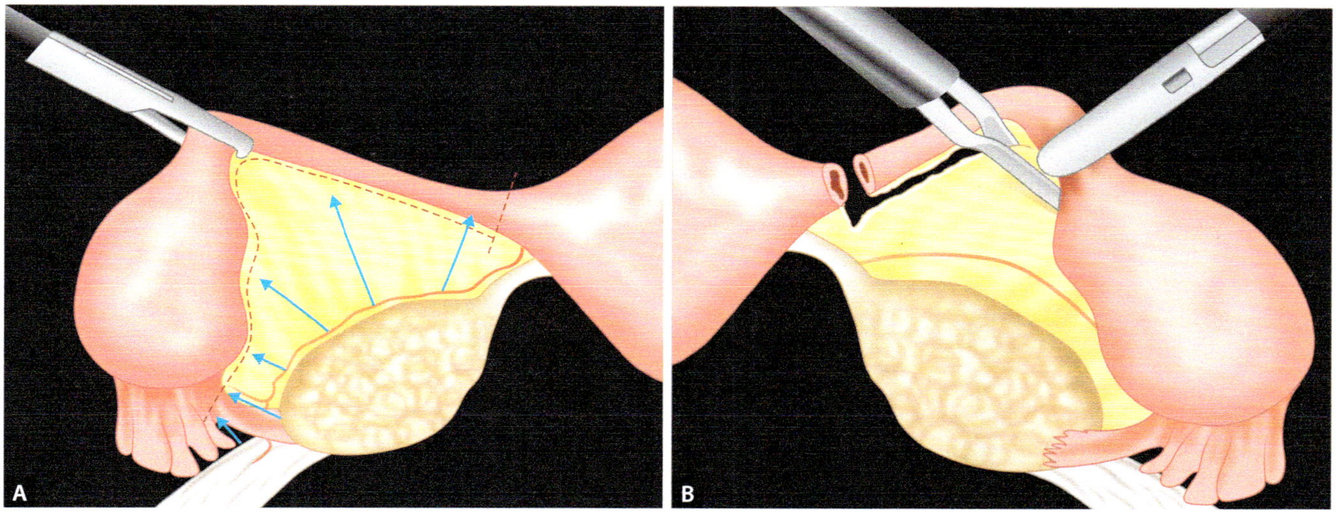

Figs. 7A and B: Laparoscopic salpingectomy.

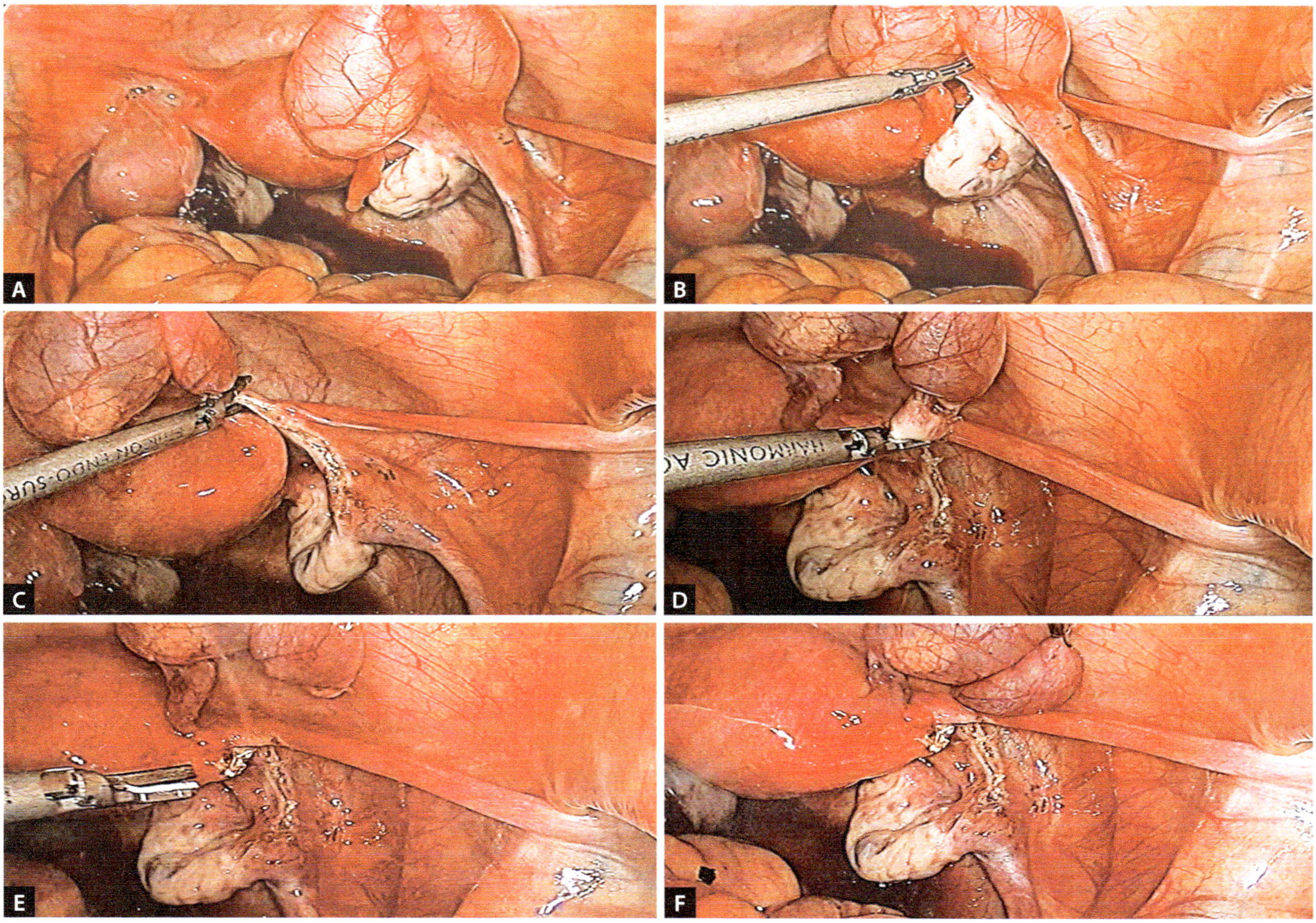

Figs. 8A to F: Salpingectomy by harmonic scalpel.

include pathologic conditions such as ruptured ectopic pregnancy, more than two ectopic pregnancies in the same tube, severe tubal damage, particularly if the contralateral tube is normal, severe pelvic adhesions, pain caused by recurrent hydrosalpinx, and large hydrosalpinx or torsion with nonviability of the tube.

Salpingectomy is a relatively easy procedure, requiring those instruments commonly used to perform tubal electrocoagulation for sterilization. The minimum instruments necessary are bipolar electrocoagulator, grasping forceps, scissors, and laparoscope. Once the patient is anesthetized, the laparoscope and two other ports are placed, through which the graspers and bipolar electrocoagulator are inserted. Adhesions that limit mobility of the fallopian tube are lysed and it is grasped at the isthmic portion. The most proximal portion of the isthmus is coagulated and cut using bipolar. If scissors are used, the bipolar electrocoagulator must be removed and replaced with the scissors through the same secondary trocar, or a third accessory trocar is placed. The harmonic scalpel or LigaSure generally is faster and more precise than the scissors with monopolar **(Figs. 8A to F)**. Cutting is performed in layers so there is less chance to cut beyond the coagulated area. Once the isthmus of the tube is transected, the mesosalpinx is alternatively coagulated and cut at intervals of 1–2 cm in the direction of the tubo-ovarian ligament.

Alternatives to bipolar electrocoagulation of the mesosalpinx are the automated stapling device, and Endoloop suture. The stapling device is introduced through a 12-mm trocar incision. After lysing significant adhesions and mobilizing the tube, it is pulled up and put under traction. The stapler is used from the proximal to the distal end to staple and cut the tube. One to two applications are sufficient for the entire tube. Before using the Endoloop ligature, both the proximal portion of the tube and its distal attachment to the ovary are coagulated and cut. The Endoloop is passed around the tube, and the mesosalpinx is ligated with one Endoloop and removed. The mesosalpinx is cut above the ligature.

Once detached, the fallopian tube is removed from the pelvis through one of the 10-mm cannula or the operating channel of the laparoscope. The removal of a larger tube, ruptured tubal pregnancy or hydrosalpinx, may require an endobag.

BIBLIOGRAPHY

1. American Fertility Society. The American Fertility Society classification of adnexal adhesions, distal tubal occlusion, secondary to tubal ligation, tubal pregnancies, Müllerian anomalies, and intrauterine adhesions. Fertil Steril. 1988;49:944-9.
2. Baumgartel PB, Fleischer AC, Cullinan JA, Bluth RF. Color Doppler sonography of tubal torsion. Ultrasound Obstet Gynecol. 1996;7:367-70.
3. Bernardus RE, Van der Slikke JW, Roex AJ, Dijkhuizen GH, Stolk JG. Torsion of the fallopian tube: some considerations on its etiology. Obstet Gynecol. 1984;64:675-8.
4. Blair CR. Torsion of the fallopian tube. Surg Gynecol Obstet. 1962;114:727-30.
5. Bland-Sutton T. Salpingitis and some of its effects. Lancet. 1890;2:1146.
6. Bruhat MA, Manhes H, Mage G, Pouly JL. Treatment of ectopic pregnancy by means of laparoscopy. Fertil Steril. 1980;33:411-4.
7. Clasen K, Camus M, Tounaye H, Devroy P. Ectopic pregnancy: let's cut! Strict laparoscopic approach to 194 consecutive cases and review of literature on alteratives. Hum Reprod. 1997;12:596-601.
8. Cropp CC, Cowell PD, Rock JA. Failure of tubal closure following laser salpingostomy for ampullary tubal ectopic pregnancy. Fertil Steril. 1987;48:887-8.
9. DeCherney AH, Diamond MP. Laparoscopic salpingostomy for ectopic pregnancy. Obstet Gynecol. 1987;70:948-50.
10. DeCherney AH, Kase N. The conservative surgical management of unruptured ectopic pregnancy. Obstet Gynecol. 1979;54:451-5.
11. DeCherney AH, Romero R, Naftolin F. Surgical management of unruptured ectopic pregnancy. Fertil Steril. 1981;35:21-4.
12. Fernandez H, Yves Vincent SC, Pauthier S, Audibert F, Frydman R. Randomized trial of conservative laparoscopic treatment and methotrexate administration in ectopic pregnancy and subsequent fertility. Hum Reprod. 1998;13:3239-43.
13. Fujishita A, Ishimaru T, Hideaki M, Samejima T, Matsuwaki T, Chavez RO, et al. Local injection of methotrexate dissolved in saline versus methotrexate suspensions for conservative treatment of ectopic pregnancy. Hum Reprod. 1995;10:101-4.
14. Ghosh S, Mann C, Khan K, Gupta JK. Laparoscopic management of ectopic pregnancy. Semin Laparosc Surg. 1999;6:68-72.
15. Gross M, Blumstein SL, Chow LC. Isolated fallopian tube torsion: a rare twist on a common theme. Am J Radiol. 2005;185:1590-2.
16. Hajenius PJ, Mol F, Mol BW, Bossuyt PM, Ankum WM, van der Veen F. Interventions for tubal ectopic pregnancy. Cochrane Database Syst Rev. 2007;2007:CD000324.
17. Hansen OH. Isolated torsion of the fallopian tube. Acta Obstet Gynecol Scand. 1970;49:3-6
18. Kawauchi H, Iino J, Ishii T, Nakai M, Kenmochi M. Laparoscopic salpingotomy for tubal pregnancy. Jpn J Gynecol Obstet Endos. 1994;10:140.
19. Krissi H, Shalev J, Bar-Hava I, Langer R, Herman A, Kaplan B. Fallopian tube torsion: laparoscopic evaluation and treatment of a rare gynecological entity. J Am Board Fam Pract. 2001;14:274-7.
20. Lang PF, Tamusssion K, HoÈnigl W, Ralph G. Treatment of unruptured tubal pregnancy by laparoscopic instillation of hyperosmolar glucose solution. Am J Obstet Gynecol. 1992;154:1216-21.
21. Lavy G, Diamond MP, DeCherney AH. Ectopic pregnancy: its relationship to tubal reconstructive surgery. Fertil Steril. 1987;47:543-56.
22. Lindblom B, Halin M, Lundorff P, Thorbun L. Treatment of tubal pregnancy by laparoscope-guided injection of prostaglandin F2a. Fertil Steril. 1990;54:404-8.
23. Lundorff P, Thorburn J, Lindblom B. Second-look laparoscopy after ectopic pregnancy. Fertil Steril. 1990;53:604-9.
24. Mecke H, Semm K, Lehmann-Willenblock E. Results of operative pelvicoscopy in 202 cases of ectopic pregnancy. Int J Fertil. 1989; 34:93-100.
25. Nelson LM, Margara RA, Winston RM. Primary and secondary closure to ampullary salpingotomy compared in the rabbit. Fertil Steril. 1986;45:292-5.
26. Pouly JL, Mahnes H, Mage G, Canis M, Bruhat MA. Conservative laparoscopic treatment of 321 ectopic pregnancies. Fertil Steril. 1986;46:1093-7.
27. Raziel A, Mordechai E, Friedler S, Schachter M, Pansky M, Ron-El R. Isolated recurrent torsion of the fallopian tube: case report. Hum Reprod. 1999;14:3000-1.
28. Reich H, Freifeld ML, McGlynn F, Reich E. Laparoscopic treatment of tubal pregnancy. Obstet Gynecol. 1987;69:275-9.
29. Semm K. Advances in pelviscopic surgery. Curr Probl Obstet Gynecol. 1982;5:20-5.
30. Tulandi T, Guralnick M. Treatment of ectopic pregnancy by salpingostomy with or without tubal suturing and salpingectomy. Fertil Steril. 1991;55:53-5.
31. Tulandi T, Saleh A. Surgical management of ectopic pregnancy. Clin Obstet Gynecol. 1999;42:31-8.
32. Vermesh M, Presser SC. Reproductive outcome after linear salpingostomy for ectopic gestation: a prospective 3-year follow up. Fertil Steril. 1992;57:682-4.
33. Vermesh M. Conservative management of ectopic gestation. Fertil Steril. 1989;51:559-67.
34. Yao M, Tulandi T. Current status of surgical and nonsurgical management of ectopic pregnancy. Fertil Steril. 1997;67:421-33.

CHAPTER 31

Laparoscopic Management of Ectopic Pregnancy

INTRODUCTION

An ectopic pregnancy is a pregnancy outside of the uterine cavity. The majority of ectopic pregnancies occurs in the fallopian tube, but other possible sites include cervical, interstitial, hysterotomy scar, intramural, ovarian, or abdominal. In addition, in rare cases, a multiple gestation may be heterotopic.

Ectopic pregnancy is a potentially life-threatening condition. While surgical approaches are the gold-standard treatment, advances in early diagnosis in the 1980s facilitated the introduction of medical therapy with methotrexate. With the routine use of early ultrasound, diagnosis of ectopic pregnancy can be established early and medical treatment can be administered in most cases. The overall success rate of medical treatment in properly selected women is nearly 90%. In select cases of early ectopic pregnancy or pregnancy of unknown location, expectant management is an option.

ECTOPIC PREGNANCY

The risk of ectopic pregnancy is higher in white women. It increases three to four times in women between the age of 35 and 44 years compared to those from 15 to 24 years. About 64% of ectopic pregnancies occur in the ampulla where fertilization occurs. The recent increase in incidence of ectopic pregnancy has been attributed to a greater incidence of sexually transmitted disease (STD), delayed childbearing, previous sexual organ surgical interference, and successful clinical detection. Any condition that prevents or retards migration of fertilized ovum to the uterine cavity could predispose a woman to an ectopic gestation **(Fig. 1)**.

Ectopic pregnancy usually occurs in the fallopian tube in 99% of cases **(Fig. 1)**. Its distribution is as follows:

- The ampulla (64%)
- The isthmus (25%)
- The infundibulum (9%)
- The intramural junction (2%)
- Ovarian (0.5%)
- Cervical (0.4%)
- Abdominal (0.1%)
- Intraligamental (0.05%)

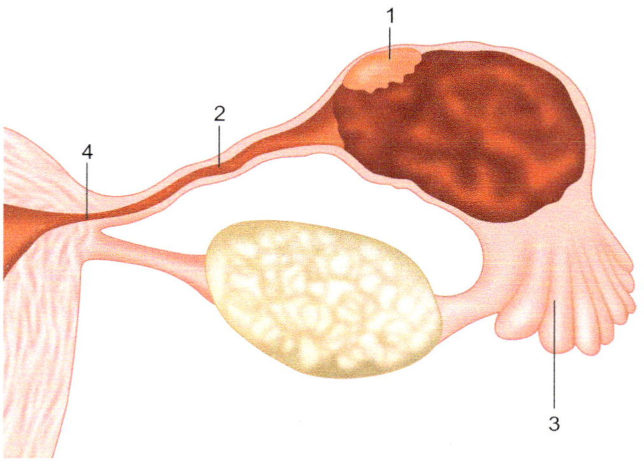

Fig. 1: Tubal pregnancy: (1) the ampulla; (2) the isthmus (3) the infundibulum; and (4) the intramural junctions.

Major contributing factors and associated relative risks for ectopic pregnancy are as follows:

- Current use of intrauterine device (11.5%)
- Use of clomiphene citrate (10%)
- Prior tubal surgery (5.6%)
- Pelvic inflammatory disease (4.0%)
- Infertility (2.9%)
- Induced abortion (2.5%)
- Adhesions (2.4%)
- Abdominal surgery (2.3%)
- T-shaped uterus (2%)
- Myoma (1.7%)
- Progestin only contraceptives (1.6%)

If laparoscopy is planned, the location, the size, and the nature of the tubal pregnancy should be ascertained preoperatively. If the bleeding has ceased or can be arrested adequately, ruptured tubal pregnancies can be treated successfully endoscopically. Once bleeding is controlled, the products of conception and blood clots are removed. If there is >1,500 cc hemoperitoneum, laparoscopic approach is contraindicated. Heparinized saline should be used in cases of large hematoma. Large ruptured ectopic may require extracorporeal knotting.

A 10-mm suction instrument is used to clean the abdominal cavity. Forced irrigation with normal saline should dislodge the clot and trophoblastic tissue from the serosa of the peritoneal organs with minimal injury to these structures **(Figs. 2A to H)**.

For unruptured tubal pregnancy, the involved fallopian tube is identified and mobilized to minimize bleeding, a 5–8 mL of diluted solution containing five unit vasopressin in 20 mL of saline is injected with a 20 G spinal or a laparoscopic needle. It should be injected in the mesosalpinx just below the ectopic and over the antimesenteric surface of the tubal segment containing gestational product. The needle must not be inserted deep within a blood vessel because intravascular injection may precipitate acute arterial hypertension, bradycardia, and sometime, it may even be fatal **(Fig. 3)**.

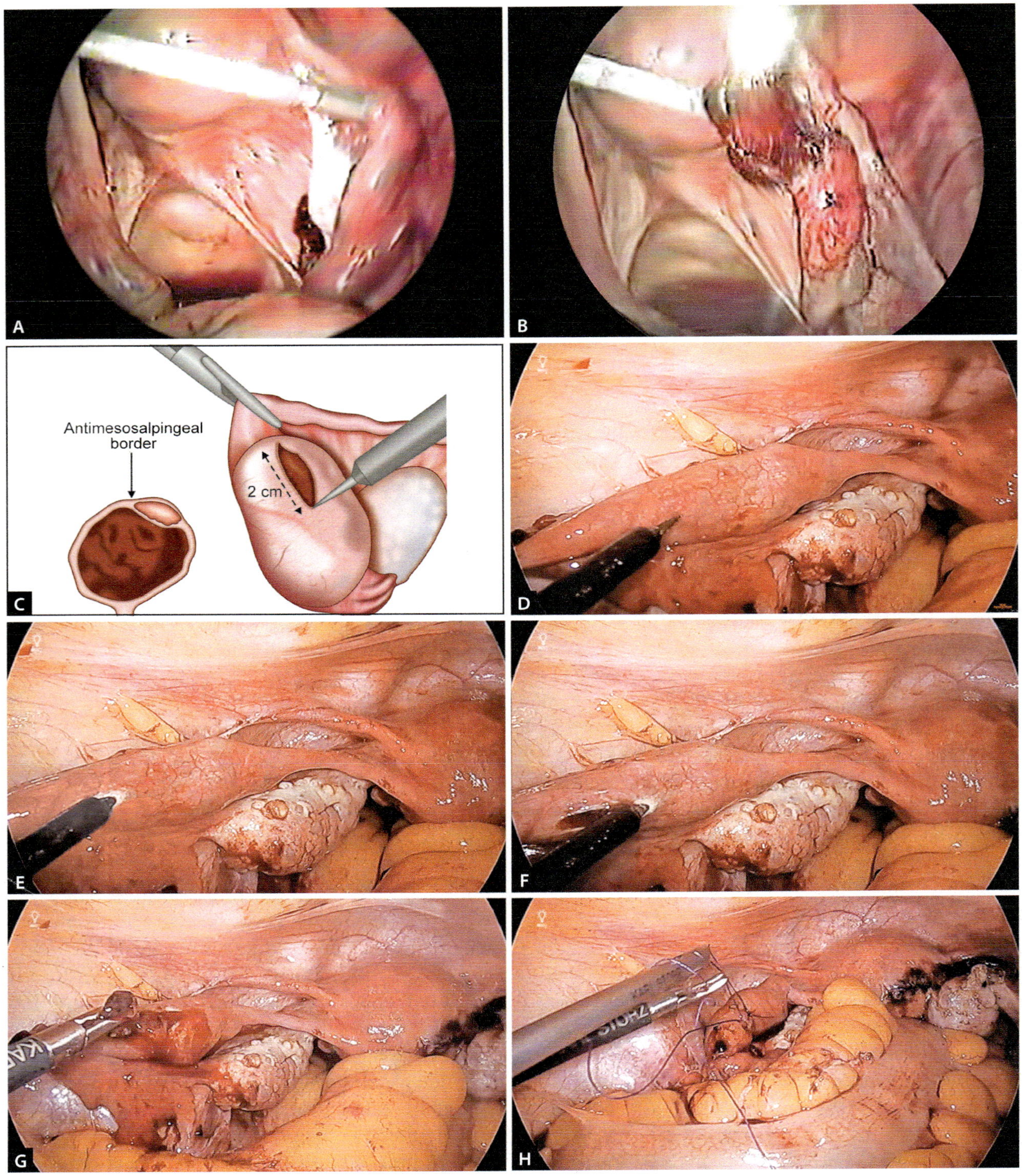

Figs. 2A to H: Salpingotomy for unruptured ectopic pregnancy.

After stabilizing the tube by grasper in one hand and microelectrode in other, a linear incision is made on the antimesenteric surface extending 1–2 cm over the thinnest portion of tube. The fine needle tip should be used in the cutting mode, and should barely touch the tissue surface. With electrosurgery, thermal damage may spread if large tips are used on large surface areas in contact with tissue. It is important to remain aware of the location of underlying or adjacent structures. If the gynecologists are not careful, there may be a chance of adjacent visceral injury. The pregnancy usually should protrude through the incision and slowly slips out of tube. It may be teased gently out using hydrodissection or laparoscopic atraumatic forceps. Sometimes forceful irrigation in the tubal opening can dislodge the gestation from implantation. As pregnancy is pulled out or extrudes from the tube, some of the products of conception can remain adhered to the implantation site by a ligamentous structure containing blood vessels. Using bipolar, this structure should be coagulated before removing the tissue. Depending upon the size of the product of conception, ectopic mass is removed, usually through a 10 mm trocar sleeve.

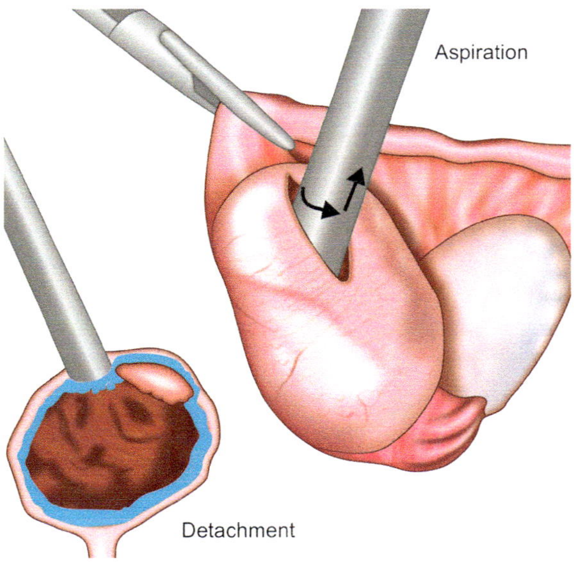

Fig. 3: Suction of trophoblast for unruptured ectopic pregnancy.

Resection of the tubal segment containing the gestation is preferable to salpingostomy for an isthmic pregnancy or a ruptured tube or if hemostasis is difficult to obtain. Segmental tubal resection is performed by the help of bipolar forceps or harmonic scalpel. Automatic stapling or suturing devices can be used for bloodless tubal resection. If the mesosalpinx bleeds, it should be cauterized by using bipolar forceps, particular attention being given to the arcuate anastomosing branches of the ovarian and uterine arteries. Total salpingectomy is performed by progressively coagulating and cutting the mesosalpinx, beginning with the proximal portion to fimbrial end. It is separated from the uterus using bipolar coagulation and scissors **(Figs. 4A and B)**. The isolated segment containing the tubal pregnancy is removed intact or in sectioned part, through the 10 mm trocar sleeve. The products of conception can be placed in a plastic bag and removed. Multefire stapling devices for salpingectomy require a 10 mm trocar. If the tissue is bulky and cannot be accommodated through cannula, an endobag can be used for retrieval of tissue.

Adhesions or other pathologic processes such as endometriosis can be treated simultaneously during the removal of ectopic pregnancy without significantly prolonging the operation. In 1 week, the beta-human chorionic gonadotropin (β-hCG) should return to baseline, i.e., undetectable or very low.

If the pregnancy is interstitial, it may be associated with traumatic rupture, hemorrhagic shock, and there is twofold increase in maternal mortality over other tubal pregnancies. Delayed diagnosis and increased vascularity of this make laparoscopic procedure difficult. Only 2–4% of ectopic are interstitial. The anatomy of ectopic accommodates the growing gestation, accounting for its late recognition. The traditional management is better in these cases, i.e., salpingectomy with or without corneal resection and in some difficult cases, hysterectomy may be necessary. Interstitial pregnancy can be suspected at the time of laparoscopy when large and asymmetrical uterus is seen.

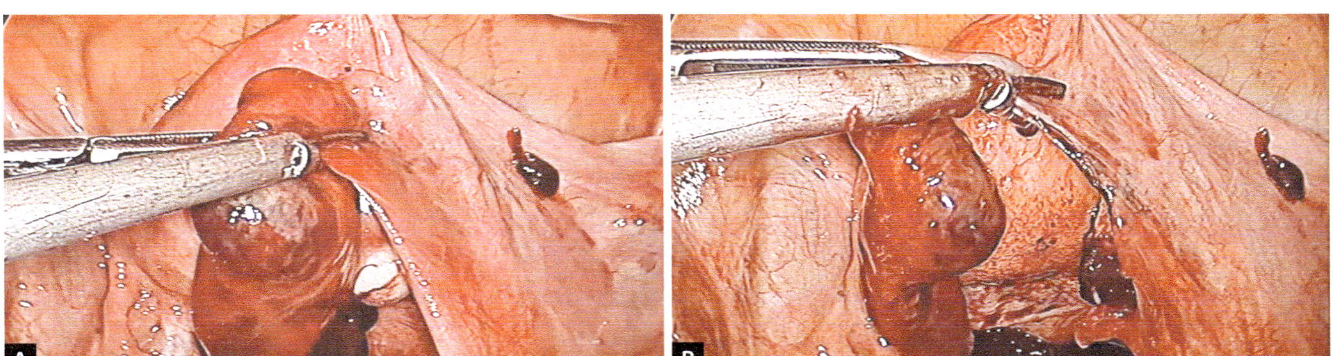

Figs. 4A and B: Salpingectomy for tubal ectopic.

Most patients are discharged within 48 hours. There is a higher fertility rate/intrauterine pregnancy rate in subsequent pregnancies with laparoscopic techniques **(Figs. 4A and B)**.

Laparoscopic surgery is a good option for ruptured ectopic and a rupture does not necessarily warrant a laparotomy for mild hemoperitoneum **(Fig. 5)**. If the patient is hemodynamically stable and initial laparoscopic examination indicates a moderate blood loss, it may be possible to control bleeding laparoscopically and perform any indicated procedures. If the patient is in stage II or stage III shock who has a large hemoperitoneum, laparotomy is the better choice **(Figs. 6A and B)**. Managing ruptured ectopic pregnancies involves examining the pelvis, localizing the ectopic, aspirating blood and clots, localizing and controlling the bleeding points, and performing either salpingectomy or in rare situations, an oophorectomy needs to be performed concurrently.

Controlling bleeding is the most critical part of the procedure, and several methods can be attempted sequentially to achieve hemostasis:

- Identification of the bleeding point followed by careful bipolar electrodesiccation
- Injection of vasopressin into the mesosalpinx
- Electrodesiccation of the mesosalpinx

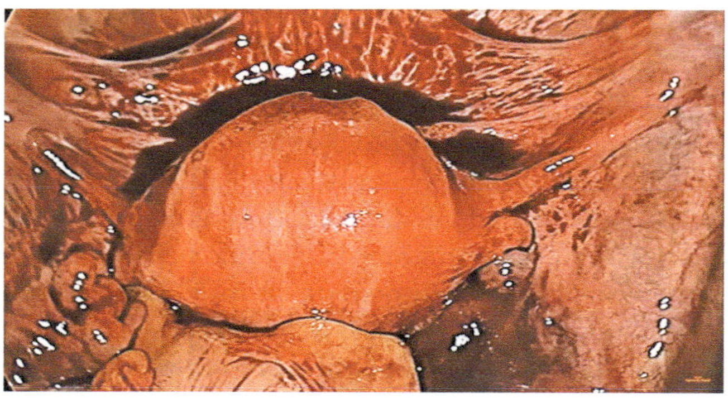

Fig. 5: Mild hemoperitoneum (Laparoscopic appearance).

- If bleeding does not stop by these means, then partial or complete salpingectomy is required, depending on the portion of tube involved and the patient's desire for fertility.

After successfully managing the ectopic pregnancy laparoscopically, the patient can be discharged on the second day. The patient should come again for a serum β-hCG 1 week postoperatively to ascertain resolution of the ectopic gestation. The β-hCG level should be either undetectable or very low after 1 week of surgery. If it is above 20 mIU/ mL, a repeat blood test is ordered 1–2 weeks later when the β-hCG should be undetectable.

DISCUSSION

Ectopic pregnancy was first discovered in the 11th century, and until the middle of the 18th century, it was usually fatal. John Bard reported the first successful surgical intervention to treat an ectopic pregnancy in 1759.

According to Sepilian, the survival rate in the 19th century was dismal; however, in the beginning of the 20th century, improvement in blood transfusion, anesthesia, and antibiotics contributed to the decrease in the maternal mortality. Ectopic pregnancy currently is the leading cause of pregnancy-related deaths in the first trimester. Sepilian stated that ectopic pregnancy is derived from the Greek word "ektopos" meaning out of place, and it refers to the implantation of the fertilized ovum in a location outside of the uterine cavity including the fallopian tubes, cornual or interstitial region of the uterus and fallopian tubes, cervix, ovary, and the abdominal cavity. This abnormally implanted pregnancy grows and draws its blood supply from the site of abnormal implantation, as the gestation enlarges, it creates the potential for organ rupture because only the uterine cavity is designed to expand and accommodate fetal development. The arterial blood supply to the mesosalpinx provided by branches of the ovarian artery that derive directly from the aorta as well as the branches from the uterine artery that derive from the internal iliac artery provides the fallopian

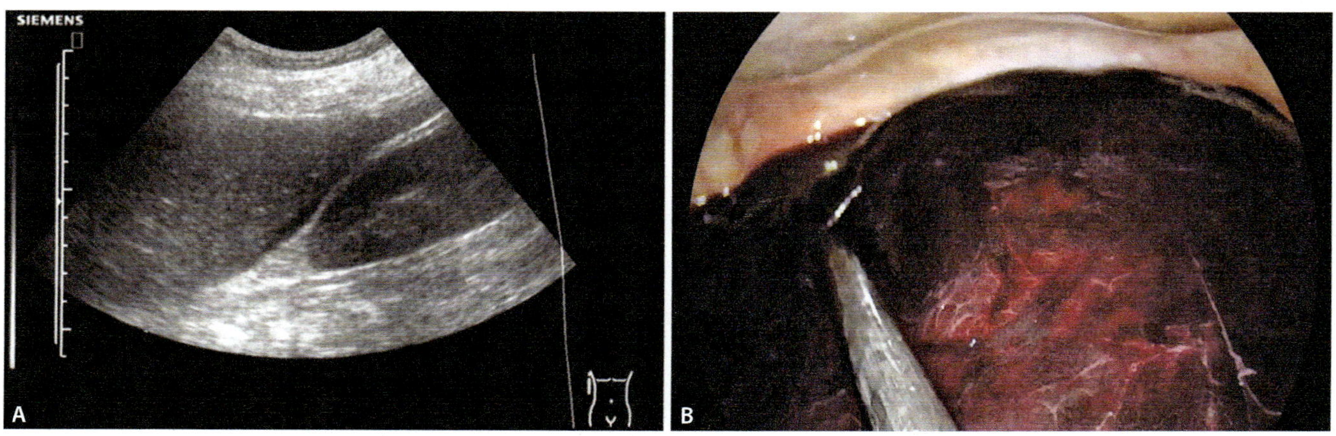

Figs. 6A and B: (A) Ultrasonography (USG); and (B) Massive hemoperitoneum.

tubes with a rich arterial supply that can bleed in the event of a perforated tube, to massive catastrophic hemorrhage and maternal death.

Seeber in 2006 from a study at the University of Pennsylvania reported that the incidence of ectopic pregnancy has increased sixfold since 1970, and is responsible for approximately 9% of all pregnancy related deaths in the United States. The author further reported that a rise in the quantitative beta subunit of hCG of a maximum of 53% over 2 days would be required for a viable pregnancy, and a decline of 21–35% in 48 hours would be mandatory for a diagnosis of spontaneous abortion.

Seeber stated that the absence of an intrauterine pregnancy above an established threshold point of hCG is consistent with an abnormal pregnancy, but does not distinguish a miscarriage from an ectopic pregnancy.

Seeber stated that the symptoms of abdominal pain or pelvic pain and vaginal bleeding are the most common complaints suggestive of ectopic pregnancy. The multiple potential sites of ectopic pregnancies add to the complexity of the diagnosis. Seeber also stated that these symptoms may be erratic and variable, and in some cases, absent. Likewise, such symptoms are nonspecific, and also have been associated with spontaneous abortion, cervical irritation, or trauma, and infection.

Sepilian wrote that the classic triad of amenorrhea, pain, and vaginal bleeding has been strongly associated with the clinical presentation of ectopic pregnancy. However, 50% of patients with ectopic pregnancy present without this triad. They may have symptoms associated with early pregnancy, including nausea, fatigue, lower abdominal pain, painful uterine cramping, recent dyspareunia, and shoulder pain.

Due to increased technology, nowadays most ectopics are diagnosed prior to rupture. Sepilian reported that approximately 20% of ectopic patients are hemodynamically unstable at initial presentation suggesting a ruptured ectopic gestation. There is a 10–25% chances of a recurrent ectopic pregnancy.

Risk factor included progesterone intrauterine device. Increasing maternal age plays important roles in ectopic pregnancy and women aged 35–44 years have a three- to fourfold higher chances as compared to women aged 15–24 years.

Smoking may alter tubal and uterine motility, and is associated with a risk of 1.6–3.5 times more than non-smokers. Other factors associated with an increased risk of ectopic pregnancies include prior abdominal surgery, a ruptured appendix, exposure to diethylstilbestrol, and uterine developmental abnormalities.

Most authors also list prior tubal infection as a cause. Chlamydia may remain asymptomatic and untreated as well as other infectious agents are associated with an increased risk of salpingitis and potential tubal damage. Sepilian stated that within the last two decades, there has been a more conservative surgical approach to unruptured ectopic gestation. Utilizing minimally invasive surgery, laparoscopy has become the recommended approach in most cases. Laparotomy has been usually reserved for cases where the patients are hemodynamically unstable, or when the surgeon is inexperienced in laparoscopy.

Seeber stated that laparoscopic minimally invasive approach has become the preferred surgical approach, and laparotomy is reserved for hemodynamically unstable patients. Other situations in which the open surgical approach may be preferable include extensive pelvic adhesions where adequate visualization of the ectopic is impossible or extratubal, intra-abdominal ectopic gestation, where risk of injury to other pelvic structures is high. Bruhart reported the first laparoscopic surgery for ectopic pregnancy in 1980.

LAPAROSCOPY VERSUS LAPAROTOMY IN TREATMENT OF ECTOPIC PREGNANCIES

El-Tabbakh reported the results of a trial in Kuwait from March 1999 to October 2001, involving 207 patients to compare laparoscopy versus laparotomy for surgical treatment of ectopic pregnancy. A total of 184 patients were treated by laparoscopy and 23 by laparotomy of the 207 patients with a diagnosis of ectopic pregnancy based on clinical symptoms, history, physical examination, positive serum β-hCG, transvaginal ultrasonography, and an ectopic pregnancy conformed at laparoscopy. Following surgery, patients were followed with serial quantitative β-hCG on Days 4 and 7, then weekly until levels <20 IU/L were obtained. Those treated with laparoscopy had an overall success rate of 98.9%. Moreover, the patients treated by laparoscopy had significantly lower blood loss. Blood transfusion was required by 13% in the laparoscopically treated group compared to 23% in the laparotomy group. All patients had the ectopic pregnancy confirmed by laparoscopy and the decision to proceed with operative laparoscopy or laparotomy depended on the minimal invasive surgery experience of the surgeon on call. There were no intraoperative complications and the duration of surgery ranged from 66 to 72 minutes for both groups. The Kuwait study led the author to conclude that laparoscopic treatment offered benefits superior to laparotomy with less blood loss, therefore, a reduced need for transfusion. The patients experienced less need for analgesia, and a shortened postoperative hospitalization.

Yuen's study included 105 patients in Hong Kong, there were no differences in age, parity, gestational age, and pregnancy of previous laparotomy patients between the groups that underwent a diagnostic laparoscopy prior to laparotomy. The laparoscopy group had a lower incidence of hemoperitoneum (45.9% vs. 75%); Yuen's study was performed in Hong Kong. Yuen stated that operative laparoscopy has the advantage of combining diagnostic and therapeutic procedures in a single operation is a better approach than laparotomy for the management of tubal pregnancy.

Xiang's study was conducted in Shanghai. Seventy-two of ectopic pregnancy patients were treated laparoscopically. The author concluded that while it was more expensive than laparotomy, the operating time and postoperative hospitalization were shortened. In the laparoscopic studies, the authors stressed reduced blood loss, shortened hospital stay, and reduced need for postoperative analgesia as recurrent positive findings throughout the various studies.

Seeber commented on the laparoscopic treatment of salpingostomy versus salpingectomy. Seeber noted that if salpingostomy had not resulted in the improvement of subsequent pregnancy rate over salpingectomy, then she would have recommended salpingostomy for all ectopic pregnancy patients. However, she states that the data to support this contention are not clear cut. The approximate 50% subsequent pregnancy rate has been noted with either method. The rate of recurrent ectopic pregnancy appeared higher in the salpingostomy (15–10%). The decision to perform salpingostomy as opposed to salpingectomy is often made intraoperatively. In case of severe damage or tubal rupture, tubal conservation is not indicated. Moreover, if tubal bleeding occurs that requires extensive coagulation, then salpingectomy may be preferred due to tubal damage. The success of *in vitro* fertilization has been beneficial for those patients who have had salpingectomy. The formation of adhesions postoperatively has been more extensive with laparotomy. Seeber noted that ectopic pregnancy occurs most frequently as a result of fallopian tube pathology; therefore, there is a risk of recurrence in both the affected and contralateral tube. Women who underwent salpingectomy will have a risk of subsequent ectopic pregnancy in the remaining tube.

As the surgeons gain more experience and training with laparoscopic surgery for ectopic pregnancy, it has become the preferred choice when skill, equipment, and resources are available.

BIBLIOGRAPHY

1. American College of Obstetricians and Gynecologists. ACOG Practice Bulletin No. 94: Medical management of ectopic pregnancy. Obstet Gynecol. 2008;111(6):1479-85.
2. American Fertility Society. The American Fertility Society classification of adnexal adhesions, distal tubal occlusion, secondary to tubal ligation, tubal pregnancies, Miillerian anomalies, and intrauterine adhesions. Fertil Steril. 1988;49(6):944-9.
3. Barnhart KT, Gosman G, Ashby R, Sammel M. The medical management of ectopic pregnancy: a meta-analysis comparing "single dose" and "multidose" regimens. Obstet Gynecol. 2003;101(4):778-84.
4. Baumgartel PB, Fleischer AC, Cullinan JA, Bluth RF. Color Doppler sonography of tubal torsion. Ultrasound Obstet Gynecol. 1996;7(5):367-70.
5. Bernardus RE, Van der Slikke JW, Roex AJ, Dijkhuizen GH, Stolk JG. Torsion of the fallopian tube: some considerations on its etiology. Obstet Gynecol. 1984;64(5):675-8.
6. Bouyer J, Coste J, Fernandez H, Pouly JL, Job-Spira N. Sites of ectopic pregnancy: a 10 year population-based study of 1800 cases. Hum Reprod. 2002;17(12):3224-30.
7. Farquhar CM. Ectopic pregnancy. Lancet. 2005;366(9485): 583-91.
8. Hajenius PJ, Mol F, Mol BW, Bossuyt PMM, Ankum WM, van der Veen F. Interventions for tubal ectopic pregnancy. Cochrane Database Syst Rev. 2007;2007(1):CD000324.
9. Kelly H, Harvey D, Moll S. A cautionary tale: fatal outcome of methotrexate therapy given for management of ectopic pregnancy. Obstet Gynecol. 2006;107(2 Pt 2):439-41.
10. Lipscomb GH. Medical therapy for ectopic pregnancy. Semin Reprod Med. 2007;25(2):93-8.
11. Mol F, Mol BW, Ankum WM, van der Veen F, Hajenius PJ. Current evidence on surgery, systemic methotrexate and expectant management in the treatment of tubal ectopic pregnancy: a systematic review and meta-analysis. Hum Reprod Update. 2008;14(4):309-19.
12. Morlock RJ, Lafata JE, Eisenstein D. Cost-effectiveness of single-dose methotrexate compared with laparoscopic treatment of ectopic pregnancy. Obstet Gynecol. 2000;95(3):407-12.
13. Practice Committee of American Society for Reproductive Medicine. Medical treatment of ectopic pregnancy: a committee opinion. Fertil Steril. 2013;100(3):638-44.
14. Teal SB. A cautionary tale: fatal outcome of methotrexate therapy given for management of ectopic pregnancy. Obstet Gynecol. 2006;107(6):1420-1.
15. Willner N, Storch S, Tadmor T, Schiff E. Almost a tragedy: severe methotrexate toxicity in a hemodialysis patient treated for ectopic pregnancy. Eur J Clin Pharmacol. 2014;70(3):261-3.

Chapter 32

Laparoscopic Surgery in Pregnancy: Precautions and Complications

INTRODUCTION

Since the advent of laparoscopic surgery in the 1980s, laparoscopic surgery has been popularized by surgeons throughout the world. However, routine laparoscopic surgery has been slow to catch the pregnant patient. Treatment of surgical disease in the gravid patient requires a unique and careful approach where safety of both the mother and the fetus are considered.

During pregnancy, due to the physiological changes that take place in the mother and considering the presence of a living fetus in utero, surgical conditions are handled with a lot of care and cautions. In past, pregnancy was considered to be absolutely contraindicated for laparoscopic intervention, but with better understanding of physiology of pregnancy and improved anesthetic and laparoscopic techniques, emergency laparoscopic procedures such as diagnostic laparoscopy for pain abdomen, appendicectomy, splenectomy, pheochromocytoma, and cholecystectomy are feasible in pregnancy. Lachman et al. have already reported 300 laparoscopic procedures during pregnancy.

The advantages of laparoscopic surgery are similar for pregnant and nonpregnant women; nevertheless, this procedure had been avoided during pregnancy because of concerns that it may be harmful to the fetus. Potential concerns include:

- The rise in intra-abdominal pressure during pneumoperitoneum could decrease uteroplacental blood flow and result in fetal hypoxia.
- Fetal acidosis could develop from absorption of carbon dioxide (CO_2).
- The fetus could be injured directly or indirectly if the uterus is perforated by a trocar or Veress needle.
- Uterine perforation may result in preterm premature rupture of the membranes and preterm delivery.

However, multiple case reports and case series describing the safe performance of laparoscopic procedures in pregnant patients have been published, resulting in a paradigm shift. Appendicitis, gallbladder disease, mesenteric cysts, and adnexal masses/torsion have been successfully managed laparoscopically during pregnancy. More advanced laparoscopic procedures, such as radical nephrectomy, splenectomy, adrenalectomy, retroperitoneal lymphadenectomy, and ventral hernia repair, have also been reported in gravid patients.

The responsibility of caring for two patients during one operation and the concern over potential harm to the unborn fetus due to the pneumoperitoneum and/or instrumentation are factors that have played a role in the delay of adapting laparoscopic surgery to the pregnant patient **(Fig. 1)**. However, recent evidence suggests that not only is laparoscopic surgery safe in the pregnant patient in all three trimesters, but it is also often preferable.

During pregnancy, usually all surgical procedures are avoided to minimize various risks of anesthesia and

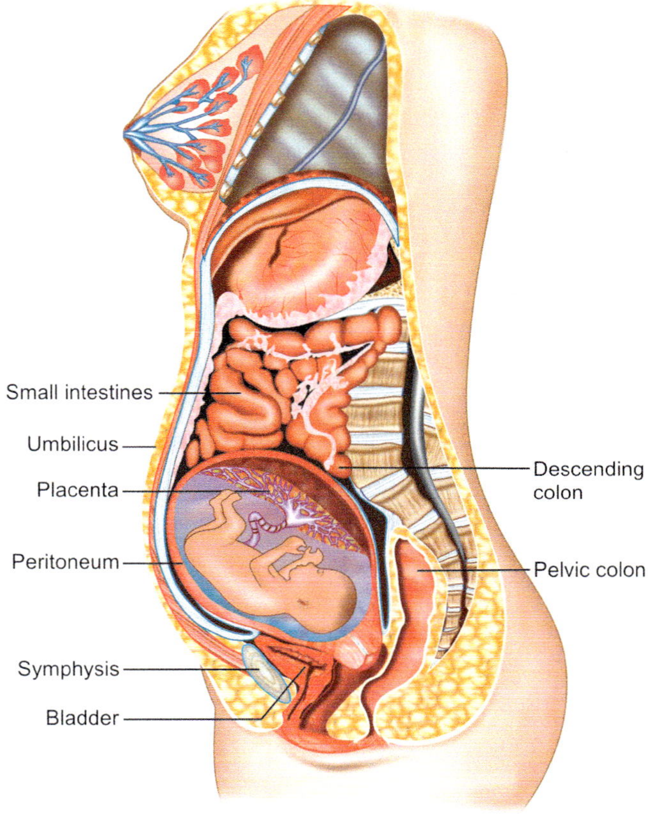

Fig. 1: Anatomical changes inside abdominal cavity during pregnancy.

procedure to mother and fetus. At times, emergency surgical conditions make it absolutely necessary for intervention. With increasing progress in minimal access surgery more and more surgeons have found the skill and interest to perform the emergency procedures laparoscopically. Laparoscopy was first done in pregnancy for diagnosis and evaluation. The first laparoscopic appendicectomy in pregnancy was performed by Scheiber in 1990. The first laparoscopic cholecystectomy in laparoscopy was first done in pregnancy for diagnosis and evaluation of acute abdominal pain in 1980.

However, surgical intervention in pregnant ladies needs special consideration of well-being of both mother and fetus; if intrauterine viable fetus is present, and in cases of ectopic pregnancy or heterotrophic pregnancy, the pathophysiological changes brought about during pregnancy should be considered for the safety of patient **(Fig. 2)**. Furthermore, with advancement of pregnancy laparoscopic diagnosis and procedures become more challengingly difficult as the gravid uterus displaces the organs and becomes completely an abdominal organ.

Up-to-date the data on laparoscopic procedures during pregnancy are still limited, but with growing ability of minimal access surgeons, the recent accumulating data shows that laparoscopic procedures such as diagnostic laparoscopy, adnexal surgery, appendicectomy, splenectomy, cholecystectomy, and management of ectopic and heterotrophic pregnancies are relatively safe and effective during pregnancy, if certain precautions are taken. But of course like all surgical procedures in pregnancy, there is an increased risk of certain complications with laparoscopic intervention in pregnancy.

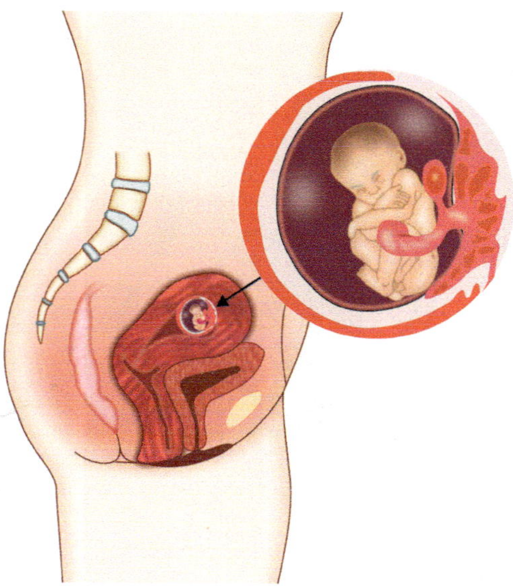

Fig. 2: Proper evaluation of patient is necessary to evaluate pathophysiological changes.

PHYSIOLOGICAL CHANGES IN PREGNANCY

Almost all the organ systems undergo physiological changes in pregnancy. These changes should be considered during operative procedures in pregnancy.

Gastrointestinal System

Due to enlarged gravid uterus, stomach is pushed toward diaphragm and assumes a more horizontal position. The viscera, such as transverse, ascending, and descending colon, are displaced, so location of abdominal pain and tenderness, especially in condition such as appendicitis, is altered. The hormonally-induced decrease lower esophageal sphincter tone causes gastroesophageal regurgitation which places the pregnant lady at higher risk of aspiration, so nasogastric tube suction and careful airway management is necessary for all pregnant patients undergoing laparoscopy.

Cardiovascular and Hematological Changes

Cardiac output and blood volume increase by 30–40%, but as RBC volume does not expand by same ratio, this results in physiological anemia, especially noticed in the second trimester. After 20 weeks' gestation, the gravid uterus compresses the aorta and inferior vena cava and may cause supine hypotension syndrome; so during surgery, the patient should be positioned in lateral recumbent position to avoid vena caval compression. A vasomotor block caused by spinal anesthesia produces more severe hypotension than in nonpregnant individuals. During pregnancy, WBC count increases to 12,000–14,900/mm.

A hypercoagulable state is physiologically developed in pregnancy due to increase in fibrinogen and other coagulation factors such as factor VII, factor VIII, factor IX, and factor X. Thus, the risk of thromboembolism increases in pregnancy.

Respiratory System

Due to enlarging gravid uterus, gradually the chest movements are restricted. There is an increase in minute ventilation and oxygen consumption and decrease in residual volume, also mixed venous oxygen content and functional reserve capacity also decreases so the patient is prone to hypoxemia and hypocapnia. $PaCO_2$ of 28–32 mm Hg, pH of 7.44, and decreased bicarbonate levels are detected due to chronic respiratory alkalosis which has to be maintained during pregnancy. The patient gains more weight during pregnancy and there is more edema in soft tissues of neck, so the anesthetist may face more difficulties in airway management.

Urinary System

Hydroureter, decreased urethral peristalsis, and bladder expansion increase incidence of urinary tract infection. There is an increased retention of water and electrolytes.

Other Changes

In addition to the respiratory changes, there are mild hematologic abnormalities in the pregnant patient. Levels of fibrinogen, factor VII, and factor XII are increased, whereas there are decreased levels of antithrombin III, all of which result in an increased risk of venous thromboembolism. When considering the acute abdomen in a pregnant patient, making the correct diagnosis may often be difficult. Nausea and vomiting, leukocytosis, low-grade fever, mild hypotension, and anorexia are common. The gravid uterus pushes the abdominal contents cephalad, displacing organs and inhibiting the migration of the omentum, causing altered landmarks and often distorting the clinical picture. During the second and third trimesters, the gravid uterus may cause decreased gastric motility and may lead to an increased risk of gastroesophageal reflux disease (GERD) and aspiration as well.

FETAL CONSIDERATION

Fetus is a hidden patient in the womb of the pregnant mother and its health should be considered by surgeon and anesthetist both. It is important to:

- Maintain uteroplacental blood flow and oxygenation. Decreased uteroplacental blood flow may be due to maternal hypotension or increase in uterine artery resistance.
- Maternal hypoxia causes fetal hypoxia and metabolic acidosis and in long-term; it may be fatal to infant, so it should be prevented.
- Avoid teratogenic drugs during anesthesia. Cocaine is known to have teratogenic effect so products containing cocaine should be avoided. Diazepam and nitrous oxide are considered safe during anesthesia as no teratogenicity was detected clinically.
- Avoid preterm labor. Try to manipulate uterus minimum as possible. Although, there is an increased incidence of spontaneous abortion, premature delivery, and low birth weight following anesthesia but in emergency situations operation is unavoidable.

EFFECTS OF PNEUMOPERITONEUM IN PREGNANCY DURING LAPAROSCOPIC PROCEDURE

In pregnant patient, the pneumoperitoneum increases the intra-abdominal pressure and this causes decreased inferior vena caval return to the heart, hence decreased cardiac output. With reverse Trendelenburg position, decreased cardiac output is even worsened, cardiac index decreases, and when this is combined with mothers hypoxia can cause fetal death. Increased intra-abdominal pressure also leads to decreased uterine blood flow and increased intrauterine pressure; these may, in turn cause fetal hypoxia and may lead to fetal death. Pneumoperitoneum decreases the diaphragmatic movement; in pregnant lady, already the movement of diaphragm is decreased due to bulky uterus, this further decreases the movement due to pneumoperitoneum causing increased peak airway pressure, decreased functional reserve capacity, increased ventilation-perfusion mismatch, decreased thoracic cavity compliance, and increased pleural pressure.

The use of CO_2 for causing pneumoperitoneum leads to hypercarbia and further hypoxemia. The CO_2 absorbs across the peritoneum and leads to respiratory acidosis in the patient and her fetus. If pCO_2 increases above 40 mm Hg, decreased removal of CO_2 occurs leading to fetal acidosis. Fetal tachycardia and hypotension may develop as a result of fetal hypocarbia. This can be corrected by maintaining mild maternal respiratory alkalosis, by hyperventilating the mother during surgery. Monitoring maternal arterial blood gases is better than monitoring $PaCO_2$ during laparoscopic procedures.

N_2O as the gas for pneumo-peritonization will not cause fetal respiratory acidosis, but it is highly combustible.

CRITERIA FOR PATIENT SELECTION

A safe laparoscopic procedure can be performed in all the three trimesters of pregnancy from 2 to 31 weeks.

During the first trimester, there is increase risk of abortion up to 12% also risk of teratogenesis increases in first trimester. In the third trimester, there is a 40% risk of preterm labor and 30% risk of premature birth. Also the visualization in laparoscopic procedure is decreased due to enlarged uterus.

Therefore, second trimester is considered as the safest time for laparoscopic surgery in pregnancy. The risk of abortion is not increased, no risk of teratogenesis, and risk of preterm labor is only 5% in second trimester.

ADVANTAGES OF LAPAROSCOPY IN PREGNANCY

- Short hospital stay
- Early return to normal activities
- Small incision, so rapid postoperative recovery and less incision complications such as hernia, postoperative wound infection and pain
- Less uterine manipulation and hence decreased uterine irritability and fetal loss

Risks of Laparoscopy in Pregnancy

- More chance of uterine injury during port entry as uterus becomes an abdominal organ after first trimester **(Fig. 3)**
- Problems associated with pneumo-peritonization as discussed already

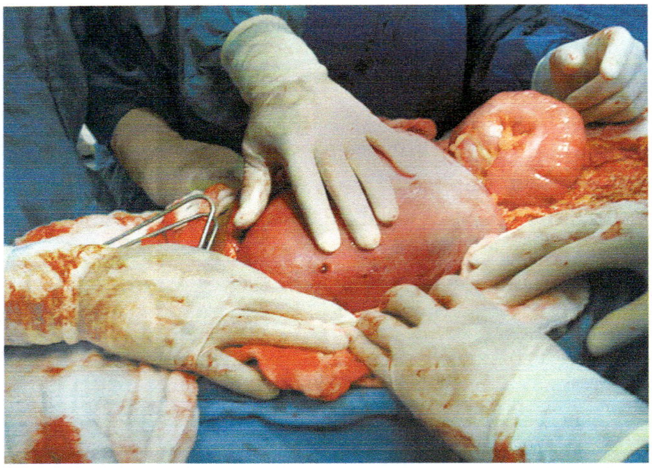

Fig. 3: Injury of pregnant uterus.

- CO_2 absorption causes increased CO_2 pressure and decreased arterial pH
- Risk of exposure to intra-abdominal smoke including carbon monoxide generated by electrosurgery and laser

Strategies for Safe Laparoscopic Surgery in Pregnancy

- Surgery should be done in second trimester.
- If patient presents in late third trimester, surgery should be postponed if possible until after delivery.
- Nasogastric incubation is a must in all cases, as there is a high risk of aspiration into the lungs.
- Patient can be placed in dorsal lithotomy position in the first-half of pregnancy, but in second-half to prevent inferior vena cava compression patient is ideally placed in lateral recumbent position.
- Hypotension should be avoided; proper fluid replacement should be done.
- Ideal method for commencing pneumoperitoneum is open Hasson trocar method. Placement of trocar depends on the size of gravid uterus.
- Tocolysis is indicated if signs of uterine irritability are present.
- Decrease operation time by using adequate number of ports, and using the most experienced surgeons.
- Maternal hyperventilation to maintain end-tidal CO_2 pressure at 32 mm Hg
- Lower CO_2 insufflations pressure of <12 mm Hg should be used to avoid fetal acidosis.
- Electrocautery should be used with care; the smokes containing carbon monoxide should be evacuated promptly to avoid toxic effect to fetus.
- Entry of all instruments must be under direct vision; care should be taken to avoid injury to the gravid uterus.
- All specimens should be removed with endobag to avoid spillage.
- Manipulators should never be fixed to vagina or cervix.

SAGES (Society of American Gastrointestinal Endoscopic Surgery) Recommendations

- Obstetrical consultation should be obtained preoperatively.
- When possible, operative intervention should be deferred until the second trimester, when fetal risk is lowest.
- Pneumoperitoneum enhances lower extremity venous stasis already present in the gravid patient and pregnancy induces a hypercoagulable state. Therefore, pneumatic compression devices should be utilized whenever possible.
- Fetal and uterine status, as maternal end tidal CO_2 and/or arterial blood gases, should be monitored.
- The uterus should be protected with a lead shield if intraoperative cholangiography is a possibility.
- Fluoroscopy should be utilized selectively.
- Given the enlarged gravid uterus, abdominal access should be attained using an open technique.
- Dependent positioning should be utilized to shift the uterus away from the inferior vena cava.
- Pneumoperitoneum pressures should be kept at 10 mm Hg.
- Further studies into methods that increase the safety of laparoscopy in pregnant patient should be done.

DISCUSSION

Advances in laparoscopic surgery have led to development of methods to perform abdominal surgery and reduce morbidity using minimal access surgery techniques. In 1999, Lachman et al. reported on a series of pregnant women undergoing 518 surgical procedures. Cholecystectomy (45%) is the most common procedures performed during pregnancy followed by adnexal surgery (34%) and appendicectomy (15%).

Operative procedures are postponed in pregnant patient until after delivery, but in acute emergency conditions even if the patient is pregnant, operation should be performed.

According to the recent studies done, the second trimester is ideal for laparoscopic intervention.

Most cases reported and small series indicate that laparoscopy can be safely performed during pregnancy. The incidence of prematurity and intrauterine growth restriction was reported to be higher in the open surgical group too.

Two recent studies suggest that there is no difference in fetal outcome for patient with singleton pregnancies undergoing laparoscopy or laparotomy. In one study, the resultant children born after laparoscopic surgery was performed on their mother during their intrauterine life, were monitored and no evidence of developmental or physical abnormality was detected during the study period. Despite the growing clinical experience suggesting that laparoscopy is as safe as laparotomy in pregnancy, more long-term clinical studies are required.

CONCLUSION

A laparoscopic access to pathology in pregnancy has many benefits for the patient, but it is important that the surgeon and anesthetist both have an immense knowledge of maternal fetal physiology. An experienced surgeon can continue to perform laparoscopy safely in all trimesters by without significant increases in either maternal or fetal morbidity or mortality. Further controlled clinical studies are needed to clarify many other unknown issues, and revision may be necessary as new data appear.

BIBLIOGRAPHY

1. Adelstein S. Administered radionuclides in pregnancy. Teratology.1999;59(4):236-9.
2. Affleck DG, Handrahan DL, Egger MJ, Price RR. The laparoscopic management of appendicitis and cholelithiasis during pregnancy. Am J Surg. 1999;178(6):523-9.
3. Akira S, Yamanaka A, Ishihara T, Takeshita T, Araki T. Gasless laparoscopic ovarian cystectomy during pregnancy: comparison with laparotomy. Am J Obstet Gynecol. 1999;180(3 Pt1):554-7.
4. Al-Fozan H, Tulandi T. Safety and risks of laparoscopy in pregnancy. Curr Opin Obstet Gynecol. 2002;14:375-9.
5. Ames Castro M, Shipp TD, Castro EE, Ouzounian J, Rao P. The use of helical computed tomography in pregnancy for the diagnosis of acute appendicitis. Am J Obstet Gynecol. 2001;184:954-7.
6. Amos JD, Schorr SJ, Norman PF, Poole GV, Thomae KR, Mancino AT, et al. Laparoscopic surgery during pregnancy. Am J Surg. 1996;171(4):435-7.
7. Andreoli M, Servakov M, Meyers P, Mann Jr WJ. Laparoscopic surgery during pregnancy. J Am Assoc Gynecol Laparosc. 1999;6(2):229-33.
8. Andriulli A, Loperfido S, Napolitano G, Niro G, a Valvano MR, Spirito F, et al. Incidence rates of post-ERCP complications: a systematic survey of prospective studies. Am J Gastroenterol. 2007;102(8):1781-8.
9. Arvidsson D, Gerdin E. Laparoscopic cholecystectomy during pregnancy. Surg Laparosc Endosc. 1991;1(3):193-4.
10. Barone JE, et al. Outcome study of cholecystectomy during pregnancy. Am J Surg.1999;177(3):232-6.
11. Buser KB. Laparoscopic surgery in the pregnant patient-one surgeon's experience in a small rural hospital. 2002;6(2):121-4.
12. Canis M, Rabischong B, Houlle C, Botchorishvili R, Jardon K, Safi A, et al. Laparoscopic management of adnexal masses: a gold standard? Curr Opin Obstet Gynecol. 2002;14(4):423-8.
13. Clark SL, Cotton DB, Pivarnik JM, Lee W, Hankins GD, Benedetti TJ, et al. Position change and central hemodynamic profile during normal third-trimester pregnancy and post- partum. Am J Obstet Gynecol. 1991;164(3):883-7.
14. Conron RW Jr, Abbruzzi K, Cochrane SO, Sarno AJ, Cochrane PJ. Laparoscopic procedures in pregnancy. Am Surg. 1999;65(3):259-63.
15. Cosenza CA, Saffari B, Jabbour N, Stain SC, Carry D, Parekh D, et al. Surgical management of biliary gallstone disease during pregnancy. Am J Surg. 1999;178:545-8.
16. Costantino GN, Vincent GJ, Mukalian GG, Kliefoth WL Jr. Laparoscopic cholecystectomy in pregnancy. J Laparoendosc Surg. 1994;4(2):161-4.
17. Curet MJ. Special problems in laparoscopic surgery. Previous abdominal surgery, obesity, and pregnancy. Surg Clin North Am. 2000;80(4):1093-110.
18. Curet MJ, Vogt DA, Schob O, Qualls C, Izquierdo LA, Zucker KA. Effects of CO_2 pneumoperitoneum in pregnant ewes. J Surg Res. 1996;63(1):339-44.
19. Curet MJ, Allen D, Josloff RK, Pitcher DE, Curet LB, Miscall BG, et al. Laparoscopy during pregnancy. Arch Surg. 1996;131(5): 546-50; discussion 550-51.
20. Davis A, Katz VL, Cox R. Gallbladder disease in pregnancy. J Reprod Med. 1995;40:759-62.
21. De Wilde JP, Rivers AW, Price DL. A review of the current use of magnetic resonance imaging in pregnancy and safety implications for the fetus. Prog Biophys Mol Biol. 2005;87 (2-3):335-53.
22. Doll R, Wakeford R. Risk of childhood cancer from fetal irradiation. Br J Radiol. 1997;70:130-09.
23. Elkayam UGN. Cardiovascular physiology of pregnancy. Cardiac problems in pregnancy: diagnosis and management of maternal and fetal disease. New York: Alan R Liss; 1982. p. 5.
24. Eyvazzadeh AD, Levine D. Imaging of pelvic pain in the first trimester of pregnancy. Radiol Clin North Am. 2006;44(6): 863-77.
25. Fallon WF Jr, Newman JS, Fallon GL, Malangoni MA. The surgical management of intra-abdominal inflammatory conditions during pregnancy. Surg Clin North Am. 1995;75(1):15-31.
26. Fatum M, Rojansky N. Laparoscopic surgery during pregnancy. Obstet Gynecol Surv. 2001;56:50-9.
27. Forsted DH, Kalbhen CL. CT of pregnant women for urinary tract calculi, pulmonary thromboembolism, and acute appendicitis. Am J Roentgenol. 2002;178(5):1285.
28. Friedman JD, Ramsey PS, Ramin KD, Berry C. Pneumoamnion and pregnancy loss after second-trimester laparoscopic surgery. Obstet Gynecol. 2002;99(3):512-3.
29. Garcia-Bournissen F, Shrim A, Koren G. Safety of gadolinium during pregnancy. Can Fam Physician. 2006;52:309-10.
30. Geisler JP, Rose SL, Mernitz CS, Warner JL, Hiett AK. Non-gynecologic laparoscopy in second and third trimester pregnancy: obstetric implications. JSLS. 1998;2(3):235-8.
31. Glasgow RE, Visser BC, Harris HW, Patti MG, Kilpatrick SJ, Mulvihill SJ. Changing management of gallstone disease during pregnancy. Surg Endosc. 1998;12:241-6.
32. Gordon MC. Maternal physiology in pregnancy. In: Gabbe SG, Niebyl JR, Simpson JL (Eds). Obstetrics: Normal and Problem Pregnancies. Philadelphia: Churchill Livingstone: 2002. pp. 63-91.
33. Graham G, Baxi L, Tharakan T. Laparoscopic cholecystectomy during pregnancy: a case series and review of the literature. Obstet Gynecol Surv. 1998;53:566-74.
34. Guidelines for laparoscopic surgery during pregnancy. Surg Endosc.1998;12(2):189-90.
35. Gurbuz AT, Peetz ME. The acute abdomen in the pregnant patient: is there a role for laparoscopy? Surg Endosc. 1997;11:98-102.
36. Halpern NB. Laparoscopic cholecystectomy in pregnancy: a review of published experiences and clinical considerations. Semin Laparosc Surg. 1998;5(2):129-34.
37. Hiatt JR, Hiatt JC, Williams RA, Klein SR. Biliary disease in pregnancy: strategy for surgical management. Am J Surg. 1986;151:263-5.
38. Hume RF, Killiam AP. Maternal physiology, in obstetrics and gynecology. In: Scott JR, KiSaia J, Hammon DB (Eds). Philadelphia: JB Lippincott; 1990. pp. 93-100.
39. Hunter JG, Swanstrom L, Thornburg K. Carbon dioxide pneumoperitoneum induces fetal acidos is in a pregnant ewe model. Surg Endosc. 1995;9(3):272-7; discussion 277-9.
40. Hurwitz LM, Yoshizumi T, Reiman RE, Goodman PC, Paulson EK, Frush DP, et al. Radiation dose to the fetus from body MDCT during early gestation. Am J Roentgenol. 2005;186(3):871-6.
41. Iafrati MD, Yarnell R, Schwaitzberg SD. Gasless laparoscopic cholecystectomy in pregnancy. J Laparoendosc Surg. 1995;5(2):127-30.
42. Kammerer WS. Nonobstetric surgery during pregnancy. Med Clin North Am. 1979;63:1157-64.

43. Karam PA. Determining and reporting fetal radiation exposure from diagnostic radiation. Health Phys. 2000;79(5):S85-90.
44. Kennedy A. Assessment of acute abdominal pain in the pregnant patient. Semin Ultrasound CT MR. 2000;21(1):64-77.
45. Kort B, Katz VL, Watson WJ. The effect of nonobstetric operation during pregnancy. Surg Gynecol Obstet. 1993;177:371-6.
46. Lachman E, Schienfeld A, Voss E, Gino G, Boldes R, Levine S, et al. Pregnancy and laparoscopic surgery. J Am Assoc Gynecol Laparosc. 1999;6(3):347-51.
47. Lemaire BM, van Erp WF. Laparoscopic surgery during pregnancy. Surg Endosc. 1997;11:15-8.
48. Leyendecker JR, Gorengaut V, Brown JJ. MR imaging of maternal diseases of the abdomen and pelvis during pregnancy and the immediate postpartum period. Radiographics. 2004;24(5):1301-16.
49. Lim HK, Bae SH, Seo GS. Diagnosis of acute appendicitis in pregnant women: value of sonography. Am J Roentgenol. 1992;159:539-42.
50. Lowe SA. Diagnostic radiography in pregnancy: risks and reality. Aust NZ J Obstet Gynaecol. 2004;44(3):191-6.
51. Malangoni MA. Gastrointestinal surgery and pregnancy. Gastroenterol Clin North Am. 2003;32(1):181-200.
52. Matsumoto T, Mutsumasa N, Miyuki Y, Masaharu I. Laparoscopic treatment of uterine prolapse during pregnancy. Obstet Gynecol. 1999;93 (5 pt2):849.
53. McKellar DP, Anderson CT, Boynton CJ, Peoples JB. Cholecystectomy during pregnancy without fetal loss. Surg Gynecol Obstet. 1992;174(6):465-8.
54. McKenna DA, Meeha CP, Alhajeri AN, Regan MC, O'Keeffe DP. The use of MRI to demonstrate small bowel obstruction during pregnancy. Br J Radiol. 2007;80(949):11e-14e.
55. Medical radiation exposure of pregnant and potentially pregnant women (1977). Report No. 054–National Council on Radiation Protection and Measurements. [online] Available from https://ncrponline.org/shop/reports/report-no-054-medical-radiation-exposure-of-pregnant-and-potentially-pregnant-women-1977/# [Last accessed August, 2020].
56. Melgrati L, Damiani A, Franzoni G, Marziali M, Sesti F. Isobaric (gasless) laparoscopic myomectomy during pregnancy. J Minim Invasive Gynecol. 2005;12(4):379-81.
57. Menias CO, Elsayes KM, Peterson CM, Huete A, Gratz BI, Bhalla S. CT of pregnancy-related complications. Emerg Radiol. 2007;13(6):299-306.
58. Moore C, Promes SB. Ultrasound in pregnancy. Emerg Med Clin North Am. 2004;22(3):697-722.
59. Muench J, Albrink M, Serafini F, Rosemurgy A, Carey L, Murr MM. Delay in treatment of biliary disease during pregnancy increases morbidity and can be avoided with safe laparoscopic cholecystectomy. Am Surg. 2001;67(6):539-42; discussion 542-3.
60. Murakami T, Noda T, Okamura C, Terada Y, Morito Y, Okamura K. Cul-de-sac packing with a metreurynter in gasless laparoscopic cystectomy during pregnancy. J Am Assoc Gynecol Laparosc. 2003;10(3):421-3.
61. Nagayama M, Watanabe Y, Okumura A, Amoh Y, Nakashita S, Dodo Y. Fast MR imaging in obstetrics. Radiographics. 2002; 22(3):563-80; discussion 580-2.
62. Nelson MJ, Cavalieri R, Graham D, Sanders RC. Cysts in pregnancy discovered by sonography. J Clin Ultrasound. 1986;14(7):509-12.
63. Nezhat FR, Tazuke S, Nezhat CH, Seidman DS, Phillips DR, Nezhat CR. Laparoscopy during pregnancy: a literature review. JSLS. 1997;1(1):17-27.
64. Oelsner G, Stockheim D, Soriano David, Goldenberg M, Seidman DS, Cohen SB, et al. Pregnancy outcome after laparoscopy or laparotomy in pregnancy. J Am Assoc Gynecol Laparosc. 2003;10(2):200-4.
65. Oguri H, Taniguchi K, Fukaya T. Gasless laparoscopic management of ovarian cysts during pregnancy. Int J Gynaecol Obstet. 2005;91(3):258-9.
66. Osei EK, Faulkner K. Fetal doses from radiological examinations. Br J Radiol. 1999;72(860):773-80.
67. Pucci RO, Seed RW. Case report of laparoscopic cholecystectomy in the third trimester of pregnancy. Am J Obstet Gynecol. 1991;165(2):401-2.
68. Quan WL, Chia CK, Yim HB. Safety of endoscopical procedures during pregnancy. Singapore Med J. 2006;47(6):525-8.
69. Qureshi WA, Rajan E, Adler DG, Davila RE, Hirota WK, Jacobson BC, et al. ASGE guideline: guidelines for endoscopy in pregnant and lactating women. Gastrointest Endosc. 2005;61(3):357-62.
70. Reedy MB, Galan HL, Bean-Lijewski JD, Carnes A, Knight AB, Kuehl TJ. Maternal and fetal effects of laparoscopic insufflation in the gravid baboon. J Am Assoc Gynecol Laparosc. 1995; 2(4):399-406.
71. Reedy MB, Kallen B, Kuehl TJ. Laparoscopy during pregnancy: a study of five fetal outcome parameters with use of the Swedish Health Registry. Am J Obstet Gynecol. 1997;177:673-9.
72. Reedy MB, Galan HL, Richards WE, Preece CK, Wetter PA, Kuehl TJ. Laparoscopy during pregnancy. A survey of laparoendoscopic surgeons. J Reprod Med. 1997;42(1):33-8.
73. Rizzo AG. Laparoscopic surgery in pregnancy: long-term follow-up. J Laparoendosc Adv Surg Tech A. 2003;13(1):11-5.
74. Rollins MD, Chan KJ, Price RR. Laparoscopy for appendicitis and cholelithiasis during pregnancy: a new standard of care. Surg Endosc. 2004;18(2):237-41.
75. Romer T, Bojahr B, Schwesinger G. Treatment of a torqued hematosalpinx in the thirteenth week of pregnancy using gasless laparoscopy. J Am Assoc Gynecol Laparosc. 2002;9(1):89-92.
76. Schmidt T, Nawroth F, Foth D, Rein DT, Römer T, Mallmann P. Gasless laparoscopy as an option for conservative therapy of adnexal pedical torsion with twin pregnancy. J Am Assoc Gynecol Laparosc. 2001;8(4):621-2.
77. Scott LD. Gallstone disease and pancreatitis in pregnancy. Gastroenterol Clin North Am. 1992;21:803-15.
78. Shay DC, Bhavani-Shankar K, Datta S. Laparoscopic surgery during pregnancy. Anesthesiol Clin North Am. 2001;19(1):57-67.
79. Society of American Gastrointestinal Endoscopic Surgeons (SAGES). Guidelines for laparoscopic surgery during pregnancy. Surg Endosc. 1998;12:189-90.
80. Soriano D, Yefet Y, Seidman DS, Goldenberg M, Mashiach S, Oelsner G. Laparoscopy versus laparotomy in the management of adnexal masses during pregnancy. Fertil Steril. 1999; 71(5):955-60.
81. State-specific changes in singleton preterm births among black and white women-United States, 1990 and 1997. Morb Mortal Wkly Rep. 2000;49:837-40.
82. Stepp K, Falcone T. Laparoscopy in the second trimester of pregnancy. Obstet Gynecol Clin North Am. 2004;31(3):485-96.
83. Timins JK. Radiation during pregnancy. N J Med. 2001;98(6): 29-33.
84. Toppenberg KS, Hill DA, Miller DP. Safety of radiographic imaging during pregnancy. Am Fam Physician. 1999;59(7):1813-20.
85. Visser BC, Glasgow RE, Mulvihill KK, Mulvihill SJ. Safety and timing of nonobstetric abdominal surgery in pregnancy. Dig Surg. 2001;18(5):409-17
86. Wang CJ, Yen CF, Lee CL, Soong YK. Mini laparoscopic cystectomy and appendectomy in late second trimester. JSLS. 2002;6(4):373-75.
87. Weber AM, Bloom GP, Allan TR, Curry SL. Laparoscopic cholecystectomy during pregnancy. Obstet Gynecol. 1991; 78(5 Pt2):958-9.
88. Williams JK, Rosemurgy AS, Albrink MH, Parsons MT, Stock S. Laparoscopic cholecystectomy in pregnancy. A case report. J Reprod Med. 1995;40(3):243-5.

CHAPTER 33

Laparoscopic Management of Endometriosis

INTRODUCTION

Endometriosis is a progressive and often debilitating disease, affecting 10–15% of women during their reproductive years. Among gynecologic disorders, endometriosis is surpassed in frequency only by leiomyomas. Endometriosis is defined as endometrial glands and stroma that occur outside the uterine cavity. The endometriotic lesions are typically located in the pelvis but can occur at multiple sites, including the bowel, diaphragm, and pleural cavity. While endometriosis is a common and nonmalignant process, ectopic endometrial tissue and resultant inflammation can cause dysmenorrhea, dyspareunia, chronic pain, and infertility. Symptoms can range from minimal to severely debilitating. Endometriosis is an estrogen-dependent, benign, inflammatory disease that affects women during their premenarcheal, reproductive, and postmenopausal hormonal stages. Laparoscopy and the surgical laser have allowed definitive treatment following diagnosis. The debate continues as to whether laparotomy or operative laparoscopy is more effective for the treatment of endometriosis.

In women with bowel symptoms such as dyschezia, tenesmus, or cyclic rectal bleeding without any other pathology, a sigmoidoscopic examination should be done at the time of menstruation to rule out bowel involvement by an endometrial implant. However, many women do not demonstrate rectal lesions, but at the time of laparoscopy, significant bowel involvement is seen. It should be remembered that a negative sigmoidoscopy does not rule out bowel involvement in patients of endometriosis. In patients who have significant rectovaginal nodularity on physical examination, preoperative bowel preparation is necessary and antibiotics are administered on the day of surgery. Gynecologists should also consult with a general surgeon experienced in laparoscopic bowel resections. A preoperative ultrasound can assess the ovaries for endometriomas. Preoperative hormonal suppressive therapy can be useful in decreasing the inflammation, bleeding, and possible postoperative adhesion formation.

The goals of surgery are to remove all implants, resect adhesions, relieve pain, reduce the risk of recurrence, and to prevent postoperative adhesion formation. It should also restore the involved organ's reasonable anatomical and physiological condition. In the case of infertility, restoration of tubo-ovarian relationship is essential to restore fertility.

Hysterectomy with bilateral salpingo-oophorectomy is a definitive treatment of endometriosis. In advanced disease, the ovary may have adhered to the pelvic sidewall. Ovarian dissection may increase the risk of injury to the ureter and vessels in the triangle of doom. The retroperitoneal approach is helpful in these cases and ensures complete removal of ovarian tissue. It also avoids the ovarian remnant syndrome.

Bilateral oophorectomy must be performed to eliminate the estrogen that sustains and stimulate the ectopic endometrium. Following hysterectomy and bilateral oophorectomy, the patient often requires hormone replacement therapy (HRT). Administering the minimal effective dose of estrogen is sometimes associated with a small risk of recurrence. HRT should begin postoperatively. Patients with residual disease may benefit from receiving progesterone from 2 to 6 months, followed by combined progesterone and estrogen for an additional 9 months. Conservative surgery is indicated for women who desire pregnancy and whose disease is responsible for the symptoms of pain and infertility. Surgery improves the likelihood of pregnancy and offers pain relief. Twenty-five percent of patients undergoing conservative operation may require a subsequent operation. The rate of resurgery directly depends on the extent of disease. Those who achieve pregnancy after surgery, only 10% require another operation. Conservative operations are cytoreductive, and recurrence of symptom most likely is caused by the progression of existing pathology that was missed during laparoscopy.

Complete removal of endometriosis is difficult to achieve because there is variability in appearance and visibility. Powder-burn lesions represent foci of inactive disease containing stroma and gland embedded in hemosiderin deposit. These presentations are more common in older lesions and sometimes without any symptoms. When endometriosis involve uterosacral ligament, they are palpable as tender nodule and may cause dysmenorrhea and dyspareunia. Superficial endometriosis is treated optimally by electrosurgical fulguration or ablation. If large areas of peritoneum are involved with endometriosis or if a woman has recurrent endometriosis in an area previously ablated by electrosurgery or laser, it may be better to excise that entire area of the peritoneum to prevent a recurrence. Especially, areas with scarring or fibrosis should be excised carefully because there may be endometriosis beneath them. One concern in laser ablation or excising large areas of the peritoneum is the chance of adhesion formation. Animal studies indicate that these areas are reperitonealized in 24–48 hours by the migration of surrounding peritoneum and that adhesion formation is low after laparoscopy. However, the surgeon should be cautious, particularly when excising areas of the peritoneum, which are opposed by pelvic organs.

Sometimes atypical lesions are seen as a clear vesicle, pink vascular pattern, white scarred lesion, red lesion, yellow-brown patches, and peritoneal windows, which represent active endometriosis **(Fig. 1A)**. These lesions secrete prostaglandin into the peritoneal fluid. The depth of endometrial implants may be related to the level of disease activity and symptoms. The peritoneum must be examined from all the angles and from different degrees of illumination to see all types of lesions. The peritoneal folds must be stretched and search for small and atypical lesions. Normal appearing ovaries sometime may contain endometriosis under the apparently normal cortex. By inserting the needle in the ovary, small endometriosis can be identified by observing the color of aspirated content.

All the pelvic organs are inspected thoroughly. In 15% of cases, the appendix is involved, and so it should be examined. The endometriosis, which has penetrated retroperitoneally several centimeters, is called an iceberg lesion. It can be detected laparoscopically by palpating areas of the pelvis and bowel with the suction irrigation probe. With the forceps or probe, the endometriotic implant is examined, and their size, depth, and proximity to the normal pelvic structure is evaluated.

The diagnostic laparoscopy can be converted into operative one (if required) if the surgeon has preoperative consent. The operative procedure begins by removing adhesions if present between the bowel and pelvic organs to adequately expose the pelvic cavity. The ovaries and tube may be adhered with cul-de-sac or pelvic sidewall. These organs are freed from adhesions and chromotubated. Endometrial implants and endometriomas are resected or vaporized, and if the patient has significant central pelvic pain, uterosacral nerve ablation or presacral nerve resection is performed.

LYSIS OF BOWEL ADHESIONS

Tubo-ovarian mass with bowel adhesion is a common finding in extensive endometriosis. Bowel adhesions vary in thickness, vascularity, and cohesiveness. Some adhesions are stretched without tearing the tissue and should be excised with electrosurgery at the points of attachment to the pelvic organs. Dense adhesions are excised either with scissors or by the ultrasonic dissector. The adhered structures requiring separation are pulled apart with forcers, and a cleavage plane is formed. Hydrodissection is useful to identify and develop the dissection plane, which is ablated or excised, using dissecting scissors.

PERITONEAL IMPLANTS

At the time of treating peritoneal endometriosis, the implants should be destroyed in the most effective and least traumatic manner to minimize postoperative adhesions and injury to retroperitoneal vessels and nerves. Although different modalities have been used, but hydrodissection and high-power fulguration or CO_2 laser are the best choices for endometriosis treatment **(Fig. 1B)**.

Superficial peritoneal endometriosis may be vaporized with monopolar or bipolar current or excised. Implants less than 2 mm are coagulated, vaporized, or excised. As lesions exceed 3 mm, vaporization or excision is needed. For lesions greater than 5 mm, deep vaporization or excisional techniques are required. If vaporization is chosen, it is important to copiously irrigate and remove the charred areas to confirm complete removal of the lesion and to avoid confusing endometriosis with a carbon deposit.

RESECTION OF OVARIAN ENDOMETRIOSIS

The ovaries are a common site for endometriosis. Endometrioma is formed when ectopic endometrial tissue within the ovary bleeds and results in a hematoma surrounded by duplicated ovarian parenchyma **(Figs. 1C and D)**. Both ovaries are involved in one-third of patients. Endometrial implants or endometriomas less than 2 cm in diameter are coagulated, laser-ablated, or excised using scissors, biopsy forceps, or electrodes. For successful eradication, all visible lesions and scars must be removed from the ovarian surface. Entrapment of oocytes within the luteinized ovarian follicle, as reported in experimental animal models, must be avoided. Endometriomas more than 2 cm diameter must be resected thoroughly to prevent recurrence **(Figs. 2A to D)**. Draining the endometriomas or partial resection of its wall is inadequate because the endometrial tissue lining the cyst is likely to remain functional and can cause the symptoms to recur **(Figs. 3A and B)**. Many gynecologists like to perform ovarian cytology and biopsy of the cyst wall before ablating the cyst. By using a double optic laparoscope, which involves the passage of a smaller operative endoscope through the channel of the main laparoscope, the ovarian cyst may be punctured, drained, the fluid sent for cytology, and the lining of the inner cystic wall is visually inspected. Once it confirmed that the cyst is not malignant, its wall is ablated to a depth of 3–4 mm.

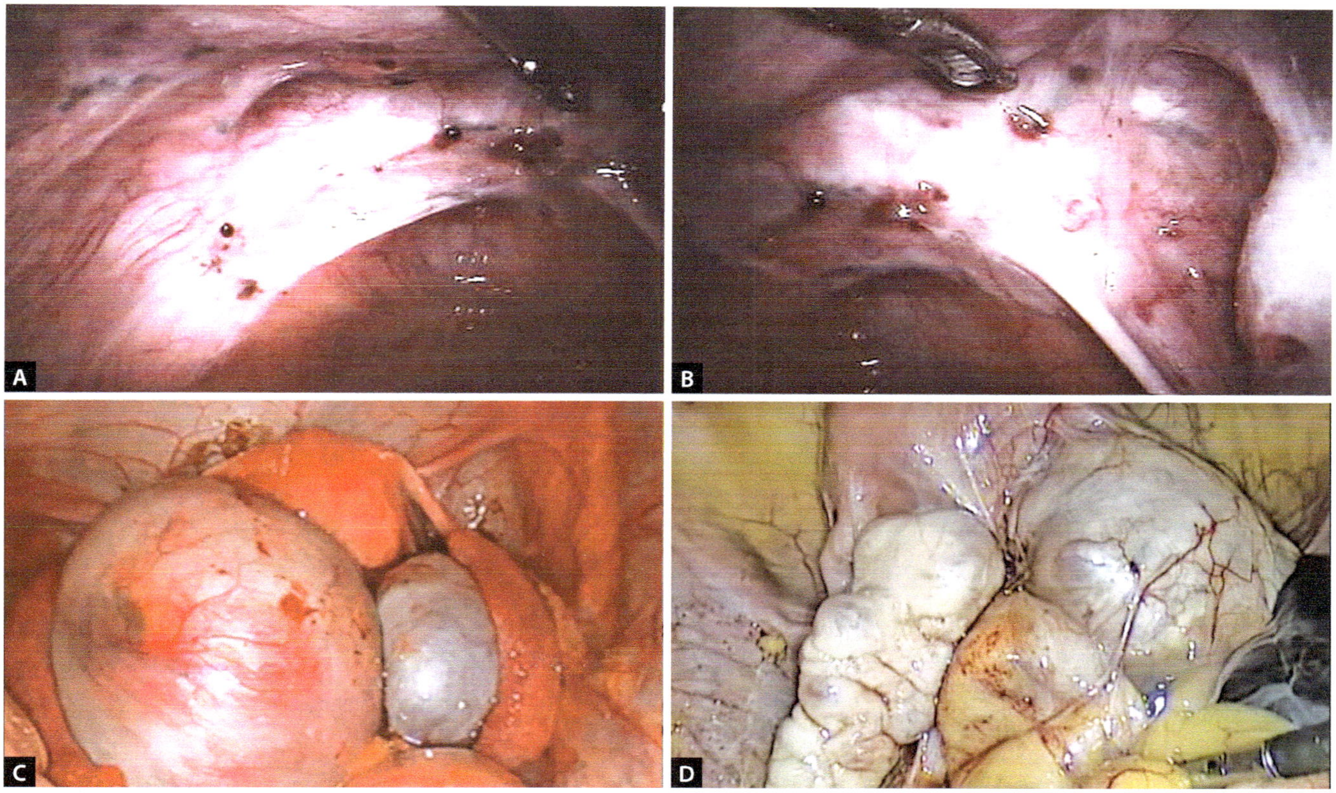

Figs. 1A to D: Endometriosis and endometrioma.

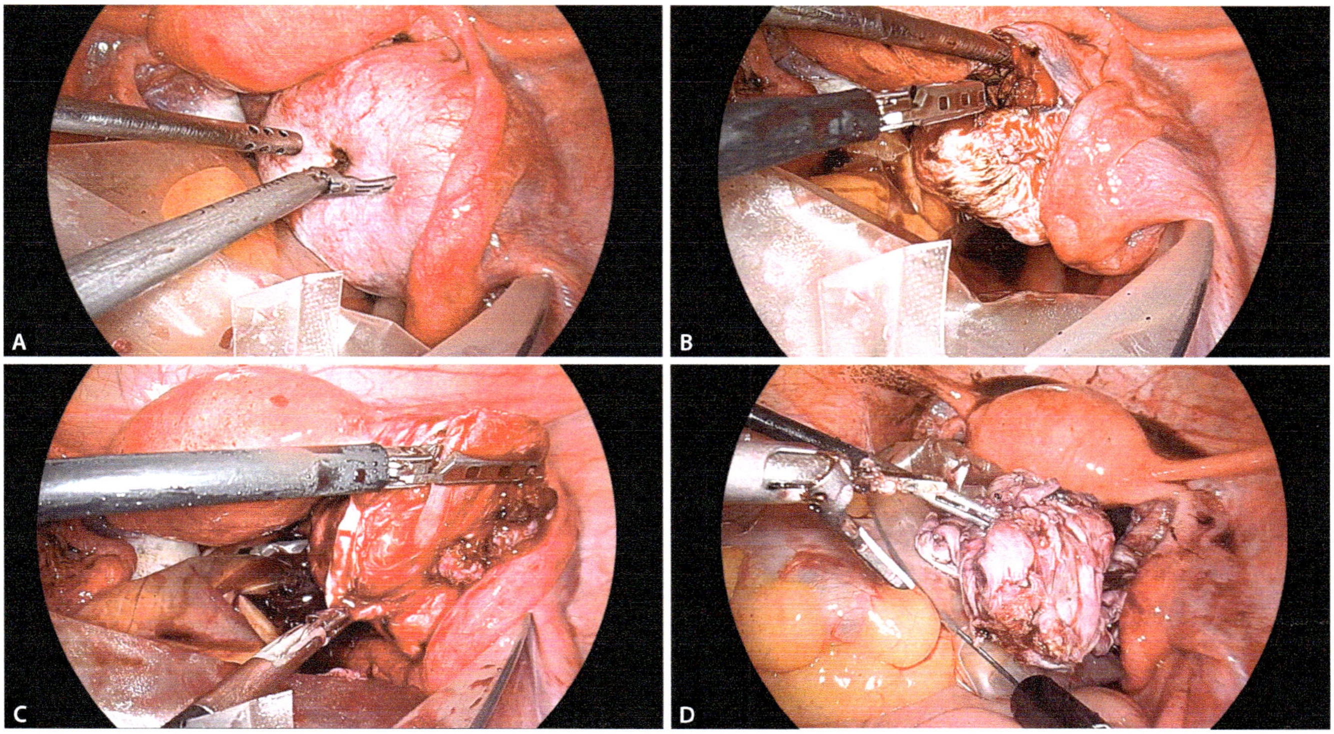

Figs. 2A to D: Endometrioma dissection.

For endometriomas over 2 cm in diameter, the cyst is punctured with aspiration needle and aspirated with the suction-irrigator probe. Deroofing of the cyst wall is performed. The cyst wall should be removed by grasping its base with laparoscopic forceps and peeling it from the ovarian stroma. If the peeling of the remaining wall is not possible, it

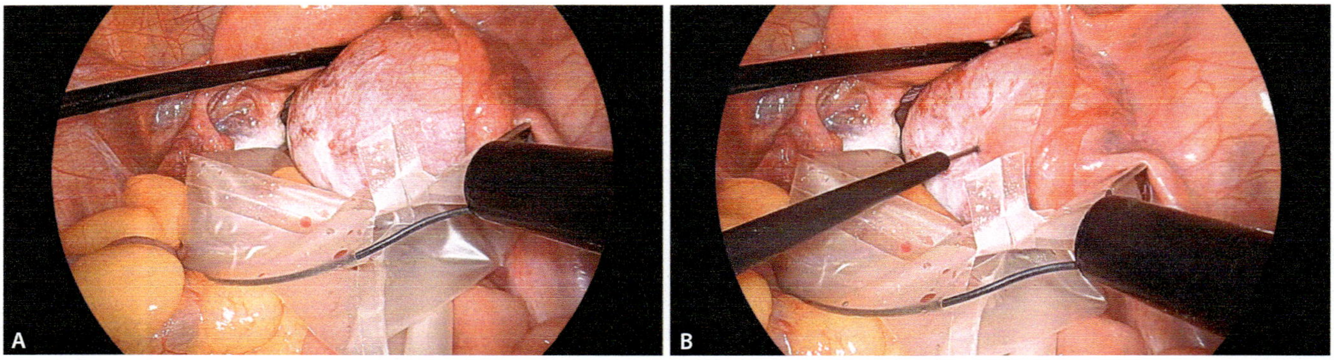

Figs. 3A and B: Chocolate cyst kept inside endobag and aspirated.

should be ablated using electrosurgical fulguration. When the entire cyst wall is ablated, representative biopsies are taken for histological diagnosis.

Cyst wall closure is not necessary, according to animal experiments for large defects that result from resecting endometriomas larger than 5 cm; the edges of the ovarian cortex are approximated with a single suture placed within the ovarian stroma. Fibrin sealant has been described to atraumatically approximate the edges of large ovarian defects, without adhesion formation. Although rare, some patients present with localized symptoms and severe involvement of only one ovary with disease and adhesions while the opposite ovary is normal. These patients are benefited by unilateral salpingo-oophorectomy. By removing the diseased ovary, the risk of disease recurrence is minimized, and the fertility potential is improved by limiting ovulation to the healthy side.

GENITOURINARY ENDOMETRIOSIS

Ureteral involvement has been reported in 1–11% of women diagnosed with endometriosis. Endometriosis of the urinary tract generally tends to be superficial but can be invasive and cause complete ureteral obstruction. The symptom constellation of dysuria, urinary frequency and urgency, bladder infection, and hematuria is suggestive of bladder endometriosis in both women with known endometriosis and those who have not been diagnosed with endometriosis **(Fig. 4)**.

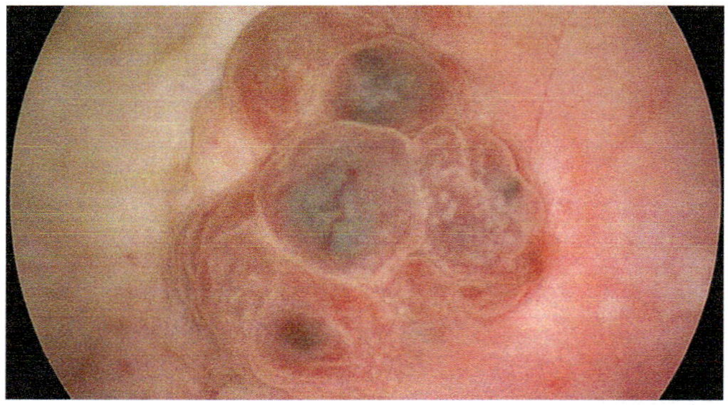

Fig. 4: Bladder endometriosis hysteroscopic view.

Decreased bladder capacity and stability, which is unresponsive to conventional therapy, may result from endometriosis. When bladder symptoms are present, a course of danazol may be tried to see the improvement in bladder instability. Clinicians should consider endometriosis in cases of refractory and unexplained urinary complaints.

If urinary tract endometriosis is suspected, a complete preoperative evaluation is performed, including an intravenous pyelogram, ultrasound of the kidneys, and routine blood and urine workup. In selected cases of recurrent hematuria, cystoscopy is indicated. Superficial implants over the ureter can be treated by a variation of hydrodissection. Approximately 20–30 mL of Ringer's lactate is injected subperitoneally on the lateral pelvic wall; this elevates the peritoneum and backs it with a bed of fluid to prevent injury at the time of fulguration. The peritoneum is held with an atraumatic grasping forceps and peeled away with the help of a suction irrigation probe. Following hydrodissection of the broad ligaments and the pelvic sidewall, many patients develop swelling of the external genitalia, most likely from the penetration of water through the inguinal canal to the labia majora. This swelling resolves in most cases within 1–2 hours without sequelae.

The incidence of ureteral obstruction by endometriosis is low, and conventional therapy previously consisted of laparotomy followed by resection of the obstructed segment of the ureter. Laparoscopic ureteroureterostomy can be performed under direct laparoscopic observation.

The bladder wall is one of the sites least frequently involved with endometriosis. If the lesions are superficial, hydrodissection and vaporization are adequate for removal. Using hydrodissection, the areolar tissue between the serosa and muscularis beneath the implants is dissected. The lesion is circumcised with the laser or monopolar and fluid is injected into the resulting defect. The lesion is grasped with forceps and dissected with the help of either sharp or electrosurgical dissection. Traction allows the small blood vessels supplying the surrounding tissue to be coagulated as the lesion is resected. Frequent irrigation is necessary

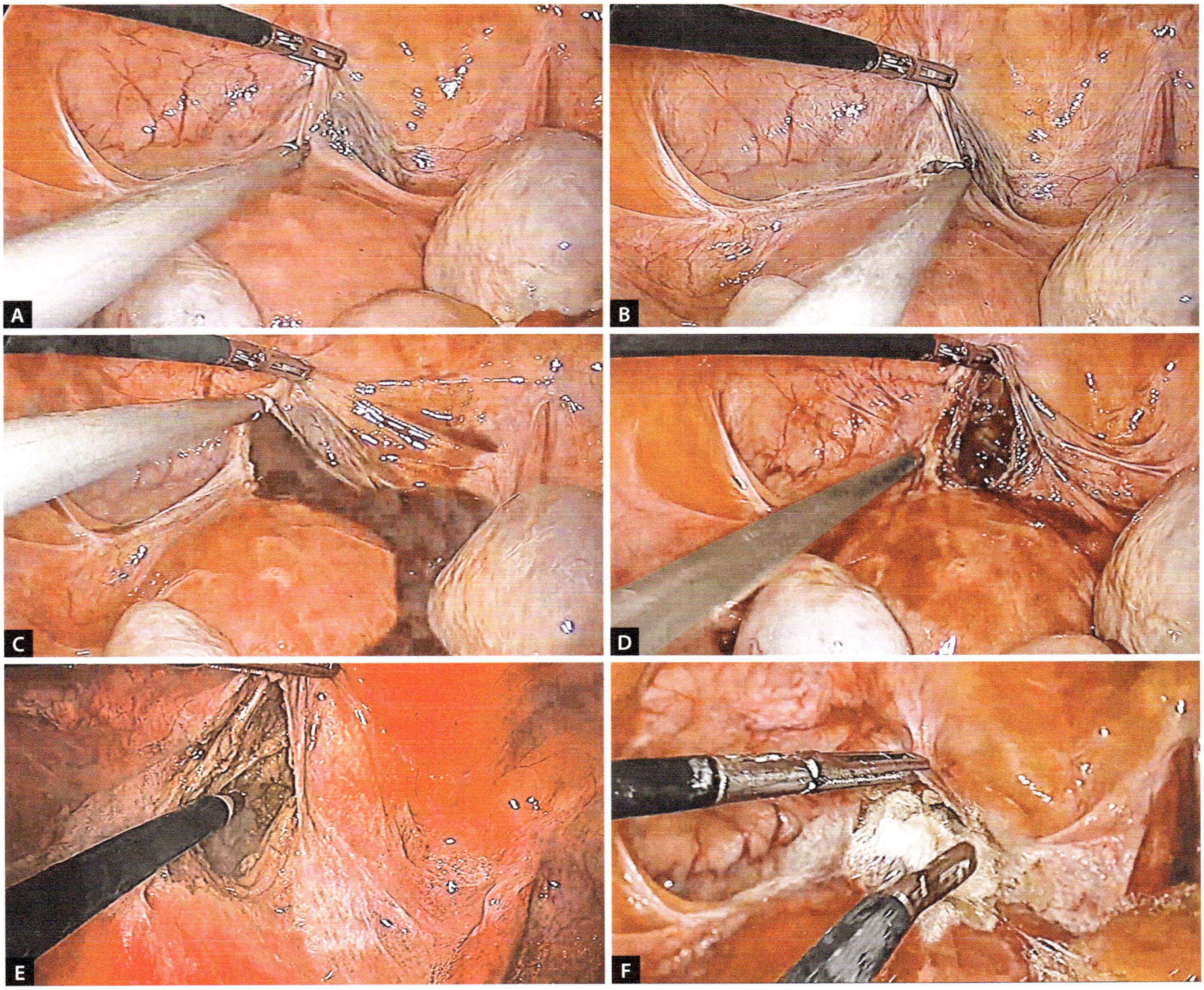

Figs. 5A to F: Dissection of bladder endometriosis, fulguration and packing with surgicel snow.

to remove char, ascertain the depth of vaporization, and ensure that the lesion does not involve the muscularis and the mucosa. After proper fulguration of endometriotic tissue bladder integrity should be checked and surgical snow can be packed in the defect **(Figs. 5A to F)**.

Endometriosis extending to the muscularis but without mucosal involvement can be treated laparoscopically and any residual or deeper lesions may be treated successfully with postoperative hormonal therapy. When endometriosis involves full bladder wall thickness, the lesion is excised and the bladder may be reconstructed laparoscopically.

GASTROINTESTINAL ENDOMETRIOSIS

Gastrointestinal endometriosis is believed to occur in 3–37% of women suffering from endometriosis. Endometriosis can involve rectovaginal septum, rectosigmoid colon, between the small intestines and anal canal. The symptoms are lower abdominal pain, backache, dysmenorrhea, dyspareunia, diarrhea, constipation, and tenesmus. Occasionally rectal bleeding is also noticed. Typically these symptoms occur cyclically at or about the time of menstruation. Surgical intervention is necessary to dissect and resect the infiltrating bowel endometriosis. Intestinal endometriosis involves the rectum and sigmoid colon in 76% of cases, the appendix in 18%, and the cecum in 5%. Appendiceal lesion requires an appendectomy. In cases of severe disease of the bowel wall, resection and anastomosis is done laparoscopically. In cases of cul-de-sac endometriosis, because ureter is lateral to the uterosacral ligament, surgeons should try to dissect in between them. If the dissection is extended lateral to the uterosacral ligament, the ipsilateral ureter should be identified by opening the overlying peritoneum and kept safe and away from the area of the lesion. The ureter, uterine artery, and vein should be identified, and bipolar forceps or titanium clips must be used if bleeding starts.

DIAPHRAGMATIC ENDOMETRIOSIS

Endometriosis sometimes affects diaphragm also. In these cases, pleuritic shoulder or upper abdominal pain is present at the time of menses. Laparoscopy is an excellent modality to diagnose and treat diaphragmatic endometriosis. Follow-up medical treatment is necessary because extensive surgery can damage or even rupture the diaphragm. Bilateral oophorectomy is promising, and further intervention may not be necessary. Three cannulas are required in the upper quadrant according to the site of the lesion on the diaphragm. A liver retractor is used by one port, and lesions are removed using hydrodissection and vaporization or excision. If the injury to diaphragm happens, it should be repaired with a 4-0 PDS. Cardiopulmonary resuscitation may be necessary after surgery.

PROGNOSIS

Complete surgical removal of endometriosis is associated with long-term control of symptoms. In the largest case series of 275 women surgically treated for deeply infiltrating endometriosis, 10% required repeat surgery, all women reported an improvement in pain symptoms, and 77% reported the pain improvement as "excellent" during a mean follow-up of 5 years. The incidence of endometriosis in women with dysmenorrhea is up to 40–60%, whereas in women with subfertility is up to 20–30%. The recurrence of endometriosis varies greatly among different studies. The overall recurrence rates range between 6 and 67% according to the criteria that are taken into consideration. Which of the various reasons is more predictive for recurrence is still unclear and controversial. The main aim of postoperative medical treatment is suppressing ovarian activity leading to atrophy of endometriotic lesions. The success of treatment depends on the resorption of all visible residual lesions and the eradication of microscopic implants. The recurrent lesions might originate from residual lesions or from de novo cells. Determining risk factors for recurrence may allow the identification of subgroups at risk for disease control. Potential biomarkers for recurrence could also maintain targeted therapy. It is difficult to eliminate the risk of endometriosis recurrence. Various risk factors have been suggested for recurrence in the literature, and these are both patient- and surgeon-dependent. According to the risk factor and the follow-up period, the recurrence rates may also alter. Finding an ideal biomarker may clarify the recurrence process so that individualized treatment can be maintained.

BIBLIOGRAPHY

1. Adamson GD, Kennedy S, Hummelshoj L. Creating solutions in endometriosis: global collaboration through the World Endometriosis Research Foundation. J Endometriosis. 2010;2:3-6.
2. Anglesio MS, Papadopoulos N, Ayhan A, Nazeran TM, Noë M, Horlings HM, et al. Cancer-associated mutations in endometriosis without cancer. N Engl J Med. 2017;376:1835.
3. Audebert A, Petousis S, Margioula-Siarkou C, Ravanos K, Prapas N, Prapas Y, et al. Anatomic distribution of endometriosis: a reappraisal based on series of 1101 patients. Eur J Obstet Gynecol Reprod Biol. 2018;230:36-40.
4. Ballard KD, Seaman HE, de Vries CS, Wright JT. Can symptomatology help in the diagnosis of endometriosis? Findings from a national case-control study--Part 1. BJOG. 2008;115:1382.
5. Blanco RG, Parithivel VS, Shah AK, Gumbs MA, Schein M, Gerst PH. Abdominal wall endometriomas. Am J Surg. 2003;185:596.
6. Brosens I, Puttemans P, Benagiano G. Endometriosis: a life cycle approach? Am J Obstet Gynecol. 2013;209:307.
7. Brosens IA, Puttemans PJ, Deprest J. The endoscopic localization of endometrial implants in the ovarian chocolate cyst. Fertil Steril. 1994;61:1034.
8. Burney RO, Giudice LC. Pathogenesis and pathophysiology of endometriosis. Fertil Steril. 2012;98:511.
9. Canlorbe G, Laas E, Cortez A, Daraï E. Spontaneous hymeneal endometriosis: a rare cause of dyspareunia. BMJ Case Rep. 2014;2014.
10. Chatman DL, Ward AB. Endometriosis in adolescents. J Reprod Med. 1982;27:156.
11. Clement PB. The pathology of endometriosis: a survey of the many faces of a common disease emphasizing diagnostic pitfalls and unusual and newly appreciated aspects. Adv Anat Pathol. 2007;14:241.
12. Czernobilsky B, Morris WJ. A histologic study of ovarian endometriosis with emphasis on hyperplastic and atypical changes. Obstet Gynecol. 1979;53:318.
13. De Cicco C, Corona R, Schonman R, Mailova K, Ussia A, Koninckx Pr. Bowel resection for deep endometriosis: a systematic review. BJOG. 2011;118:285.
14. Dovey S, Sanfilippo J. Endometriosis and the adolescent. Clin Obstet Gynecol. 2010;53:420.
15. Du H, Taylor HS. Contribution of bone marrow-derived stem cells to endometrium and endometriosis. Stem Cells. 2007;25:2082.
16. Dwivedi AJ, Agrawal SN, Silva YJ. Abdominal wall endometriomas. Dig Dis Sci. 2002;47:456.
17. Eskenazi B, Warner ML. Epidemiology of endometriosis. Obstet Gynecol Clin North Am. 1997;24:235.
18. Farland LV, Eliassen AH, Tamimi RM, Spiegelman D, Michels KB, Missmer SA. History of breast feeding and risk of incident endometriosis: prospective cohort study. BMJ. 2017;358:j3778.
19. Fukunaga M, Nomura K, Ishikawa E, Ushigome S. Ovarian atypical endometriosis: its close association with malignant epithelial tumours. Histopathology. 1997;30:249.
20. Giudice LC. Clinical practice. Endometriosis. N Engl J Med. 2010;362:2389.
21. Goldstein DP, deCholnoky C, Emans SJ, Leventhal JM. Laparoscopy in the diagnosis and management of pelvic pain in adolescents. J Reprod Med. 1980;24:251.
22. Gruenwald P. Origin of endometriosis from the mesenchyme of the celomic walls. Am J Obstet Gynecol. 1942;44:470.
23. Gustofson RL, Kim N, Liu S, Stratton P. Endometriosis and the appendix: a case series and comprehensive review of the literature. Fertil Steril. 2006;86:298.
24. Halme J, Hammond MG, Hulka JF, Raj SG, Talbert LM. Retrograde menstruation in healthy women and in patients with endometriosis. Obstet Gynecol. 1984;64:151.
25. Harris HR, Wieser F, Vitonis AF, Rich-Edwards J, Boynton-Jarrett R, Bertone-Johnson ER, et al. Early life abuse and risk of endometriosis. Hum Reprod. 2018;33:1657.
26. Hediger ML, Hartnett HJ, Louis GM. Association of endometriosis with body size and figure. Fertil Steril. 2005;84:1366.
27. Hickey M, Ballard K, Farquhar C. Endometriosis. BMJ. 2014; 348:g1752.

28. Horton JD, Dezee KJ, Ahnfeldt EP, Wagner M. Abdominal wall endometriosis: a surgeon's perspective and review of 445 cases. Am J Surg. 2008;196:207.
29. Jaime TJ, Jaime TJ, Ormiga P, Leal F, Nogueira OM, Rodrigues N. Umbilical endometriosis: report of a case and its dermoscopic features. An Bras Dermatol. 2013;88(1):121-4.
30. Jansen RP, Russell P. Nonpigmented endometriosis: clinical, laparoscopic, and pathologic definition. Am J Obstet Gynecol. 1986;155:1154.
31. Javert CT. The spread of benign and malignant endometrium in the lymphatic system with a note on coexisting vascular involvement. Am J Obstet Gynecol. 1952;64:780.
32. Jenkins S, Olive DL, Haney AF. Endometriosis: pathogenetic implications of the anatomic distribution. Obstet Gynecol. 1986;67:335.
33. Kavoussi SK, Odenwald KC, As-Sanie S, Lebovic DI. Incidence of ovarian endometrioma among women with peritoneal endometriosis with and without a history of hormonal contraceptive use. Eur J Obstet Gynecol Reprod Biol. 2017; 215:220.
34. Kirshon B, Poindexter AN 3rd. Contraception: a risk factor for endometriosis. Obstet Gynecol. 1988;71:829.
35. Laufer MR, Goitein L, Bush M, Cramer DW, Emans SJ. Prevalence of endometriosis in adolescent girls with chronic pelvic pain not responding to conventional therapy. J Pediatr Adolesc Gynecol. 1997;10:199-202.
36. Lee HJ, Park YM, Jee BC, Kim YB, Suh CS. Various anatomic locations of surgically proven endometriosis: a single-center experience. Obstet Gynecol Sci. 2015;58:53.
37. Longo LD. Classic pages in obstetrics and gynecology. Aberrant portions of the müllerian duct found in an ovary: William Wood Russell Johns Hopkins Hospital Bulletin, vol. 10, pp. 8--10, 1899. Am J Obstet Gynecol. 1979;134:225.
38. Mahmood TA, Templeton A. Prevalence and genesis of endometriosis. Hum Reprod. 1991;6:544.
39. Marinis A, Vassiliou J, Kannas D, Theodosopoulos TK, Kondi-Pafiti A, Kairi E, et al. Endometriosis mimicking soft tissue tumors: diagnosis and treatment. Eur J Gynaecol Oncol. 2006;27:168.
40. Marsh EE, Laufer MR. Endometriosis in premenarcheal girls who do not have an associated obstructive anomaly. Fertil Steril. 2005;83:758.
41. Minaglia S, Mishell DR Jr, Ballard CA. Incisional endometriomas after cesarean section: a case series. J Reprod Med. 2007;52:630.
42. Missmer SA, Chavarro JE, Malspeis S, Bertone-Johnson ER, Hornstein MD, Spiegelman D, et al. A prospective study of dietary fat consumption and endometriosis risk. Hum Reprod. 2010;25:1528.
43. Missmer SA, Hankinson SE, Spiegelman D, Barbieri RL, Malspeis S, Willett WC, et al. Reproductive history and endometriosis among premenopausal women. Obstet Gynecol. 2004;104: 965-74.
44. Missmer SA, Hankinson SE, Spiegelman D, Barbieri RL, Marshall LM, Hunter DJ. Incidence of laparoscopically confirmed endometriosis by demographic, anthropometric, and lifestyle factors. Am J Epidemiol. 2004;160:784.
45. Missmer SA, Hankinson SE, Spiegelman D, Barbieri RL, Michels KB, Hunter DJ. In utero exposures and the incidence of endometriosis. Fertil Steril. 2004;82:1501.
46. Morales Martínez C, Tejuca Somoano S. Abdominal wall endometriosis. Am J Obstet Gynecol. 2017; 217:701.
47. Mowers EL, Lim CS, Skinner B, Mahnert N, Kamdar N, Morgan DM, et al. Prevalence of endometriosis during abdominal or laparoscopic hysterectomy for chronic pelvic pain. Obstet Gynecol. 2016;127:1045.
48. Muzii L, Bianchi A, Bellati F, Zullo MA, Angioli R, Panici PB, et al. Histologic analysis of endometriomas: what the surgeon needs to know. Fertil Steril. 2007;87:362.
49. Nnoaham KE, Webster P, Kumbang J, Kennedy SH, Zondervan KT. Is early age at menarche a risk factor for endometriosis? A systematic review and meta-analysis of case-control studies. Fertil Steril. 2012;98:702.
50. Ogawa S, Kaku T, Amada S, Kobayashi H, Hirakawa T, Ariyoshi K, et al. Ovarian endometriosis associated with ovarian carcinoma: a clinicopathological and immunohistochemical study. Gynecol Oncol. 2000;77:298.
51. Olive DL, Henderson DY. Endometriosis and mullerian anomalies. Obstet Gynecol. 1987;69:412.
52. Parazzini F, Cipriani S, Bianchi S, Gotsch F, Zanconato G, Fedele L. Risk factors for deep endometriosis: a comparison with pelvic and ovarian endometriosis. Fertil Steril. 2008;90:174.
53. Prefumo F, Todeschini F, Fulcheri E, Venturini PL. Epithelial abnormalities in cystic ovarian endometriosis. Gynecol Oncol. 2002;84:280.
54. Rahmioglu N, Nyholt DR, Morris AP, Missmer SA, Montgo GW. Genetic variants underlying risk of endometriosis: insights from meta-analysis of eight genome-wide association and replication datasets. Hum Reprod Update. 2014;20:702.
55. Redwine DB. Diaphragmatic endometriosis: diagnosis, surgical management, and long-term results of treatment. Fertil Steril. 2002;77:288.
56. Reese KA, Reddy S, Rock JA. Endometriosis in an adolescent population: the Emory experience. J Pediatr Adolesc Gynecol. 1996;9:125.
57. Sampson JA. Peritoneal endometriosis due to the menstrual dissemination of endometrial tissue into the peritoneal cavity. Am J Obstet Gynecol. 1927;14:422.
58. Sangi-Haghpeykar H, Poindexter AN 3rd. Epidemiology of endometriosis among parous women. Obstet Gynecol. 1995;85:983.
59. Seidman JD. Prognostic importance of hyperplasia and atypia in endometriosis. Int J Gynecol Pathol. 1996;15:1.
60. Shafrir AL, Farland LV, Shah DK, Harris HR, Kvaskoff M, Zondervan K, et al. Risk for and consequences of endometriosis: a critical epidemiologic review. Best Pract Res Clin Obstet Gynaecol. 2018;51:1.
61. Sinaii N, Plumb K, Cotton L, Lambert A, Kennedy S, Zondervan K, et al. Differences in characteristics among 1,000 women with endometriosis based on extent of disease. Fertil Steril. 2008;89:538.
62. Soliman AM, Surrey E, Bonafede M, Nelson JK, Castelli-Haley J. Real-world evaluation of direct and indirect economic burden among endometriosis patients in the United States. Adv Ther. 2018;35:408.
63. Strathy JH, Molgaard CA, Coulam CB, Melton LJ 3rd. Endometriosis and infertility: a laparoscopic study of endometriosis among fertile and infertile women. Fertil Steril. 1982;38:667.
64. Treloar SA, Bell TA, Nagle CM, Purdie DM, Green AC. Early menstrual characteristics associated with subsequent diagnosis of endometriosis. Am J Obstet Gynecol. 2010;202:534.e1-6.
65. Vercellini P, Viganò P, Somigliana E, Fedele L. Endometriosis: pathogenesis and treatment. Nat Rev Endocrinol. 2014;10:261.
66. Victory R, Diamond MP, Johns DA. Villar's nodule: a case report and systematic literature review of endometriosis externa of the umbilicus. J Minim Invasive Gynecol. 2007;14:23.
67. Woodward PJ, Sohaey R, Mezzetti TP Jr. Endometriosis: radiologic-pathologic correlation. Radiographics. 2001;21:193.
68. Zhao X, Lang J, Leng J, Liu Z, Sun D, Zhu L, et al. Abdominal wall endometriomas. Int J Gynaecol Obstet. 2005;90:218.

CHAPTER 34 Laparoscopic Hysterectomy

INTRODUCTION

The first laparoscopic hysterectomy (LH) was performed in January 1988 by Harry Reich in Pennsylvania. There has been a great increase in interest following the introduction of LH but most surgeons now perform laparoscopically-assisted vaginal hysterectomy (LAVH) and then total laparoscopic hysterectomy (TLH). This minimal access surgical procedure was designed to be an alternative to abdominal hysterectomy and not vaginal hysterectomy. Benign uterine diseases of uterus are very common and often need hysterectomy and laparotomy.

There are several subtypes of LH, including:

- *Total laparoscopic hysterectomy*: The uterus and cervix are removed. The entire procedure, including suturing of the vaginal vault, is performed laparoscopically. The uterine specimen is typically removed through the vaginal vault, either intact or after morcellation.
- *Laparoscopic subtotal (supracervical) hysterectomy (LSH)*: The uterus is removed; the cervix is conserved. The uterine specimen is extracted via the abdominal ports or incisions.
- *Laparoscopic-assisted vaginal hysterectomy*: The laparoscopic approach is utilized to perform any needed adnexal surgery and control the adnexal blood supply. The remainder of the procedure is performed vaginally, including entry into the peritoneal cavity and ligation of the uterine vessels from below.

LAPAROSCOPIC ANATOMY OF UTERUS

The normal nulliparous uterus is approximately 8 cm in length and angled forward so the fundus lies over the posterior surface of the bladder. Uterus is all around covered with peritoneum except where the bladder touches the lower uterine segment at the anterior cul-de-sac and laterally at the broad ligaments **(Fig. 1)**.

Two important arteries, uterine and ovarian, are of great significance in uterine surgery. The uterine arteries arise from the internal iliac arteries. They pass medially on the levator ani muscle, cross the ureter and ultimately divide into ascending and descending branch. The uterine artery runs in a tortuous course within the broad ligaments. The uterine arteries ascending branch terminates by anatomizing with the ovarian artery.

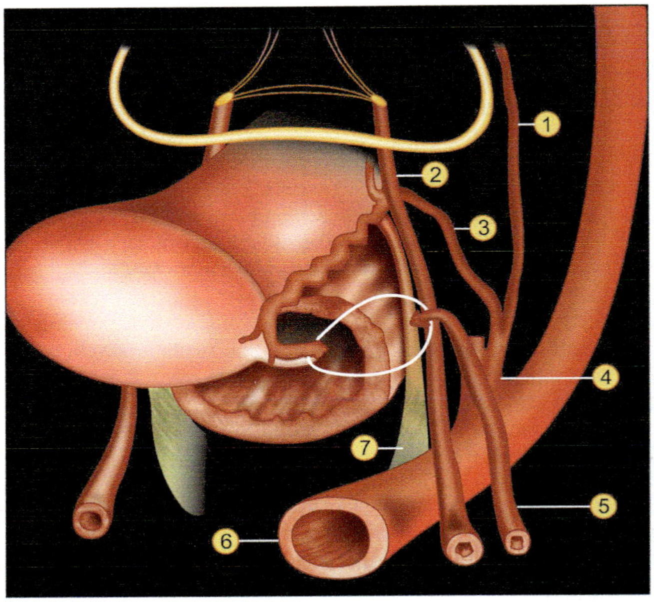

Fig. 1: Anatomy of uterus. (1) Umbilical artery; (2) Ureter; (3) Uterine artery; (4) Internal iliac artery; (5) Ovarian artery; (6) Common iliac artery; (7) Uterosacral ligament.

From anterior to posterior, following important tubular structures are found crossing the brim of true pelvis: the round ligament of the uterus, the infundibulopelvic ligament, which contains the gonadal vessels and the ureter. The ovaries and fallopian tube are found between the round ligament and the infundibulopelvic ligament **(Fig. 2)**.

The ovarian ligaments run from the ovaries to the lateral border of the uterus. Ovary is attached to the pelvic side wall with infundibulopelvic ligament, which carries ovarian artery. One of the common mistakes that may happen is injury of the ureter during dissection of the infundibulopelvic ligament. If the uterus is deviated to the contralateral side with the help of uterine manipulator infundibulopelvic ligament is spread out and a pelvic side wall triangle is created. The base of this triangle is the round ligament, the medial side is the infundibulopelvic ligament, and the lateral side is the external iliac artery. The apex of this triangle is the point at which the infundibulopelvic ligament crosses

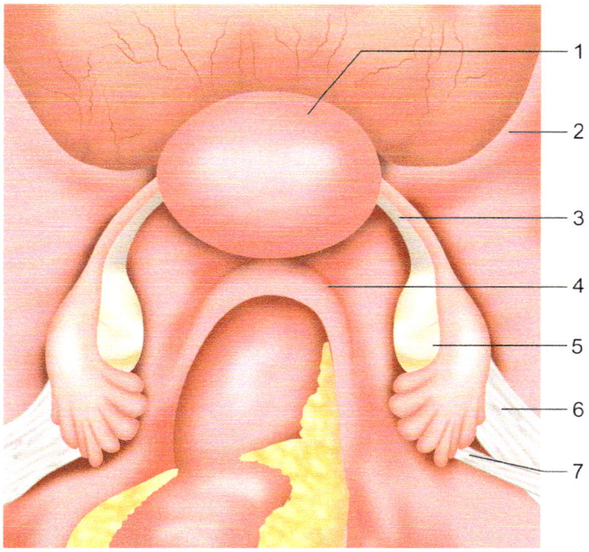

Fig. 2: Position of uterus. (1) Uterus; (2) Round ligament; (3) Utero-ovarian ligament (proper ovarian ligament); (4) Uterosacral ligament; (5) Ovary; (6) Suspensory ligament of the ovary; (7) Ureter.

the external iliac artery. The ureter always enters medial to this triangle into the pelvis. It is visible under the peritoneum overlying the external iliac artery.

The ureters enter the pelvis in close proximity to the female pelvic organ and are at risk for injury during laparoscopic surgery of these organs. As the ureters course medially over the bifurcation of the iliac vessels, they pass obliquely under the ovarian vessels and then run in close proximity to the uterine artery.

Laparoscopy hysterectomy needs careful identification of ureter with some dissection of retroperitoneum. An incision is made in the peritoneum overlying the pelvic side wall triangle between the fallopian tube and iliac vessel.

Pelvic lymph node dissection is also necessary if gynecologist plans to perform radical LH. Node dissection as far distal as Cloquet's node in the femoral triangle may be included and proximally dissection may be necessary up to para-aortic lymph nodes.

If a vaginal hysterectomy can be performed in the first place, there would be no point in adding the costs and complications of laparoscopy. Its greatest benefit is the potential to convert what would have been an abdominal hysterectomy into a vaginal hysterectomy. An abdominal hysterectomy requires both a vaginal incision and a 4–6 inch long incision in the abdomen, which is associated with greater postoperative discomfort and a longer recovery period than for a vaginal procedure. Another advantage of the LH may be the removal of the tubes and ovaries which on occasion may not be easily removed with a vaginal hysterectomy.

The most common medical reasons for performing hysterectomies include uterine fibroids (30%), abnormal uterine bleeding (20%), endometriosis (20%), genital prolapse (15%), and chronic pelvic pain (10%). For most of these conditions, other treatments should first be considered, and hysterectomy should be reserved as a last resort.

TABLE 1: Postoperative pain levels.

Day	*LAVH (n = 19)*	*TAH (n = 19)*	*p*
1	6.6	6.4	NS
3	4.4	4.3	NS
7	2.8	3.6	S
14	1.6	2.4	S
21	1.46	1.8	S
Week 6	1.35	1.4	NS

Wilcoxon's signed-rank test.
Ten-point activity scale: 1 = no pain; 10 = unbearable pain.
S = significant at $p < 0.005$; NS = not significant at $p < 0.01$

TABLE 2: Postoperative activity levels.

Day	*LAVH (n = 19)*	*TAH (n = 19)*	*p*
1	3.4	3.3	NS
3	5.4	4.4	NS
7	7.8	5.8	S
14	9.2	6.4	S
21	9.6	7.9	S
Week 6	9.95	8.5	S

Wilcoxon's signed-rank test.
Ten-point activity scale: 1 = extremely limited activity, 10 = no limits on activity
S = significant at $p < 0.005$; NS = not significant at $p < 0.01$

Laparoscopic hysterectomy results in a significantly shorter hospital stay, and a much more rapid return to normal activities than in total abdominal hysterectomy (TAH). The drug requirement to control pain and the level of pain patients experienced were also significantly less. Blood loss was not different for the two procedures **(Tables 1 and 2)**.

Postoperative recovery times and pain levels were assessed in 37 patients with a primary complaint of pelvic pain and diagnoses of fibroid uterus, adenomyosis, and severe endometriosis who underwent LH. Women reported an activity level of 8.7 on a scale of 1–10 (10 no limits on activity) by postoperative day 14. In another study, those undergoing abdominal hysterectomy had a mean uterine weight of 418 g compared with 150 g for those undergoing LAVH. The mean hospital stay after abdominal hysterectomy was 4.5 days and after LH 2.5 days. An important public policy issue now confronts us. As it is currently performed, LH is more expensive than TAH. The issue is whether the benefits of shorter convalescence and faster return to the work force, shorter hospitalization, and less need for narcotics for postoperative pain outweigh the disadvantage of the higher cost. If total healthcare system costs are evaluated, the short-term disability costs of 2 weeks of recovery after LH should be compared with disability costs of 6–8 weeks of recovery after abdominal hysterectomy.

For LH to be economically viable compared with TAH, savings in disability costs and the increased contribution to the gross domestic product must offset the increased healthcare costs. In the current system, insurance companies and hospitals do not have share in these benefits, only consider the costs. The economic impact of laparoscopic surgery must take into account both the cost to the hospital and insurance payers and these productivity and social issues. Insurance is based on a risk pool whereby the cost of a premium is based on the cost of treatment, not the ability of the subscriber to return to work. An economic and social cost–benefit analysis must be performed before decisions are made to modify or judge a procedure that provides substantial benefits to the patient.

Since its introduction in 1989, no one could have imagined that with continued improvement of techniques will progress so rapidly that LH can be performed on daycare basis for many women, and will result in shorter recovery time. Thus, the increased operating room time of approximately 46 minutes is significantly outweighed by the benefits available with widespread application of this procedure.

CLASSIFICATION

Garry and Reich Classification of Laparoscopic Hysterectomy

- *Type 1*: Diagnostic lap + VH
- *Type 2*: Lap vault suspension after VH
- *Type 3*: LAVH
- *Type 4*: LH (lap ligation of uterine artery)
- *Type 5*: TLH
- *Type 6*: LSH (lap supracervical hysterectomy)
- *Type 7*: LHL (lap hysterectomy with lymphadenectomy)
- *Type 8*: LHL + O (as above + omentectomy)
- *Type 9*: RLH (radical lap hysterectomy)

AAGL Classification of Laparoscopic Hysterectomy

American Association of Gynecologic Laparoscopists (AAGL) classification of laparoscopic hysterectomy is shown in **Table 3**.

TABLE 3: Laparoscopic hysterectomy classification according to American Association of Gynecologic Laparoscopists.

Type 0	Laparoscopic-directed preparation for vaginal hysterectomy	
*Type I**	Dissection up to but not including uterine arteries	
	Type IA	Ovarian artery pedicle(s) only
	Type IB¶	IA + anterior structures
	Type IC	IA + posterior culdotomy
	Type ID¶	IA + anterior structures and posterior culdotomy
*Type II**	Type I + uterine artery occlusion and division, unilateral or bilateral	
	Type IIA	Ovarian artery(ies) and uterine artery(ies) occlusion and division only
	Type IIB¶	IIA + anterior structures
	Type IIC	IIA + posterior culdotomy
	Type IID¶	IIA + anterior structures and posterior culdotomy
*Type III**	Type II + portion of cardinal-uterosacral ligament complex only, unilateral or bilateral	
	Type IIIA	Uterine and ovarian artery pedicles with portion of the cardinal-uterosacral complex only, unilateral or bilateral
	Type IIIB¶	IIIA + anterior structures
	Type IIIC	IIIA + posterior culdotomy
	Type IIID¶	IIIA + anterior structures and posterior culdotomy
*Type IV**	Type II + total cardinal-uterosacral ligament complex, unilateral or bilateral	
	Type IVA	Uterine and ovarian artery pedicles with complete detachment of the total cardinal-uterosacral ligament complex only, unilateral or bilateral
	Type IVB¶	IVA + anterior structures
	Type IVC	IVA + posterior culdotomy
	Type IVD¶	IVA + anterior structures and posterior culdotomy
	Type IVE	Laparoscopically directed removal of entire uterus

(AAGL: American Association of Gynecologic Laparoscopists)
The system describes the portion of the procedure completed laparoscopically.
*A suffix "o" may be added if unilateral or bilateral oophorectomy is performed concomitantly (e.g., type IoA).
¶The B and D subgroups may be further subclassified according to the degree of dissection involving the bladder and whether an anterior culdotomy is created: (1) incision of vesicouterine peritoneum only, (2) dissection of any portion of bladder from cervix, and (3) creation of an anterior culdotomy.

LAPAROSCOPIC-ASSISTED VAGINAL HYSTERECTOMY

Laparoscopically-assisted vaginal hysterectomy is one of the most frequently performed gynecologic operations, and numerous authors have demonstrated its safety and feasibility. A laparoscopic-assisted vaginal hysterectomy is a type 3 Garry and Reich hysterectomy in which the adnexal pedicles of the round ligament, fallopian tube, and ovarian ligament are released abdominally through laparoscopic approach while the uterine artery and vein are secured through the vaginal approach. Further dissection of the broad ligament anteriorly to free the bladder from the uterovesical fold is done laparoscopically. A 2 cm posterior colpotomy in between the uterosacral ligaments at the base of the pouch of Douglas is also done laparoscopically. This dissection allows completion of the surgery vaginally with ease.

Preoperative Measures

Patients are evaluated same way as that of any major surgery. Routine preoperative tests include a complete blood count with differential, serum electrolyte, bleeding time, and urinalysis. More comprehensive blood studies include thrombin time, partial thrombin time, ECG, chest X-ray, and endometrial biopsy. Mechanical and antibiotic bowel preparation is advised. Peglec powder 1 sachet with water a night prior to surgery is advised.

Patient Position

Patient should be in steep Trendelenburg and lithotomy position. One assistant should remain between the legs of patient to do uterine manipulation whenever required **(Figs. 3A and B)**.

Position of Surgical Team (Fig. 4)

Surgeon stand left to the patient, camera assistant should be left to the surgeon. Second assistant should be the opposite side of the body of patient. One more assistant is required between the legs to handle uterine manipulator. The patient should ideally get general anesthesia with endotracheal intubation. A Foley catheter should be inserted to provide bladder drainage throughout the operation.

Port Position

A 10-mm umbilical port for camera should be along the inferior crease. Two 5-mm ports should be placed at 5 cm away from umbilicus on either side. Sometime, accessory port at right or left iliac region may be required according to need. Port position should be in accordance with baseball diamond concept. If the left side of tube has to be operated, one port should be in right iliac fossa and another below left iliac fossa **(Fig. 5)**.

Operative Technique

It is important throughout the procedure to be able to manipulate the uterus for optimal observation.

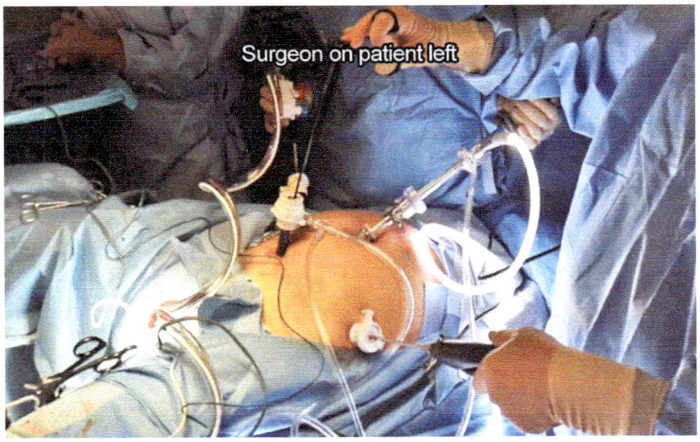

Fig. 4: Surgical team position in laparoscopically-assisted vaginal hysterectomy.

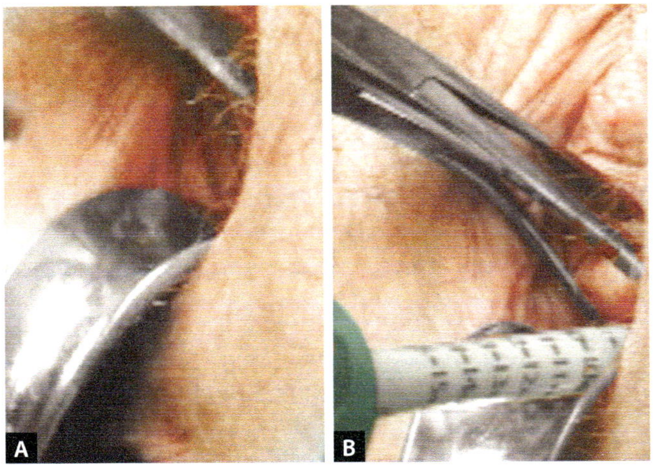

Figs. 3A and B: Pervaginal examination should be routine.

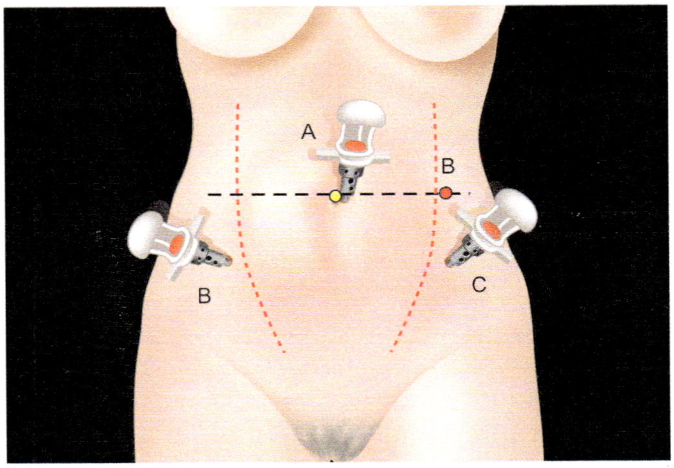

Fig. 5: Port position for laparoscopically-assisted vaginal hysterectomy.

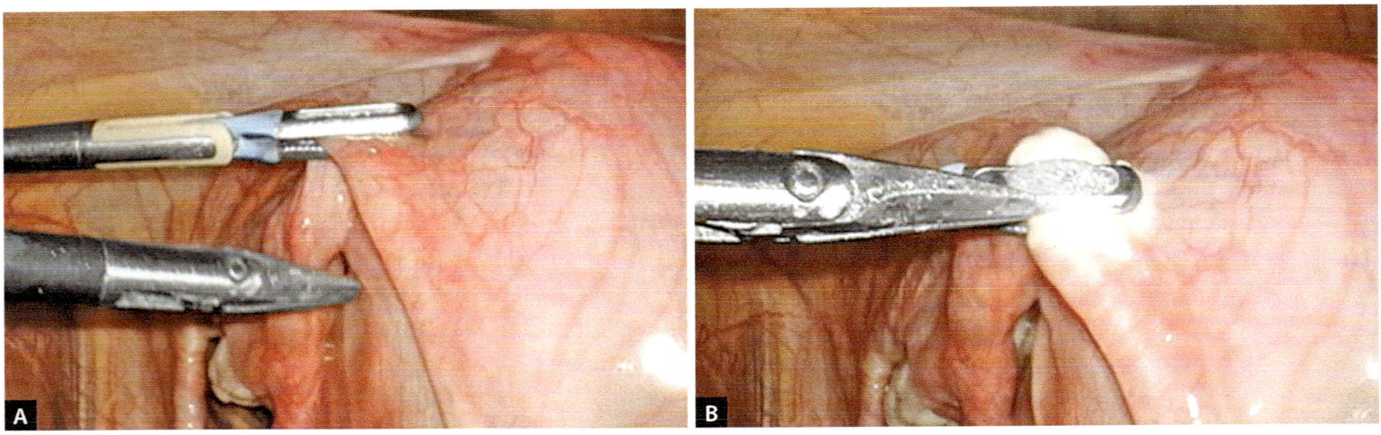

Figs. 6A and B: Laparoscopically-assisted vaginal hysterectomy using bipolar.

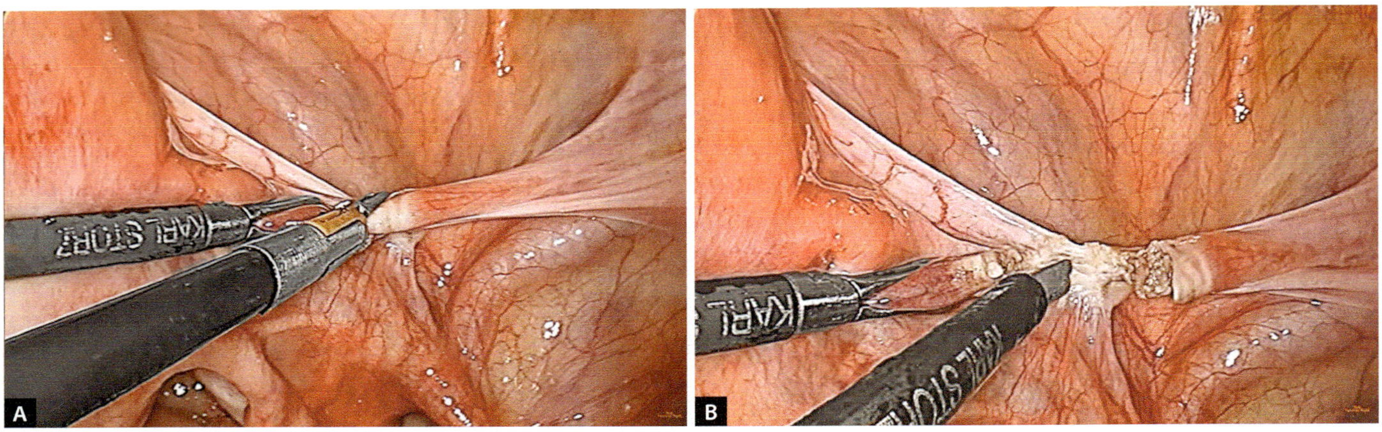

Figs. 7A and B: Successive desiccation and dissection.

Different types of uterine manipulators are available. Depending on the laparoscopic procedure, digital examination, probes, and sponge stick applicators are used in the cul-de-sac for identification of structures during laparoscopy. The direction and location of both ureters should be identified as much as possible **(Figs. 6A and B)**.

With the patient in lithotomy position, after the pneumoperitoneum insufflated to a pressure of 12–14 mm Hg, three ports should be introduced. The 10 mm optical umbilical trocar, 5 mm in lateral border of the right rectus abdominis in right iliac fossa, 5 mm in the same position on the left side for the Ligasure forceps. The ureters were visualized transperitoneally. If adnexectomy is planned, following electrodesiccation and cutting of the round ligaments 2–3 cm from the uterus, then infundibulopelvic ligament is desiccated and cut, taking progressive bites of tissue starting at pelvic brim and moving towards the round ligament. It is important to avoid the coagulation of the round ligament near the uterus because of higher bleeding **(Figs. 6A and B)**. In order to preserve the adnexa, the coagulation and section is performed proximal to the fallopian tubes and the utero-ovarian ligament. The dissection continues posteriorly on the broad ligament, taking care not to cut the uterine pedicle's vessels **(Figs. 7A and B)**.

The anterior leaf of the broad ligament is opened towards the vesicouterine fold and bladder flap is developed. The anterior leaf of the broad ligament is grasped with forceps, elevated and dissected from the anterior lower uterine segment. The utero-ovarian ligament, proximal tube, and mesosalpinx are progressively dissected and cut and posterior leaf of the broad ligament is opened. Similarly, the round ligament, fallopian tube, and utero-ovarian ligament are grasped closed to their insertion into the uterus then secured with the bipolar, Ligasure, or harmonic scalpel and cut. The distal end of the energized instruments must be kept free of the bladder and ureter **(Fig. 8)**.

The uterovesical junction is identified, grasped, and elevated with forceps while being cut with scissors. The bladder pillars are identified desiccated and cut. The bladder can be completely freed from the uterus by pushing downward with the tip of a blunt probe along the vesicocervical plane until the anterior cul-de-sac is exposed completely. In patients with severe anterior cul-de-sac

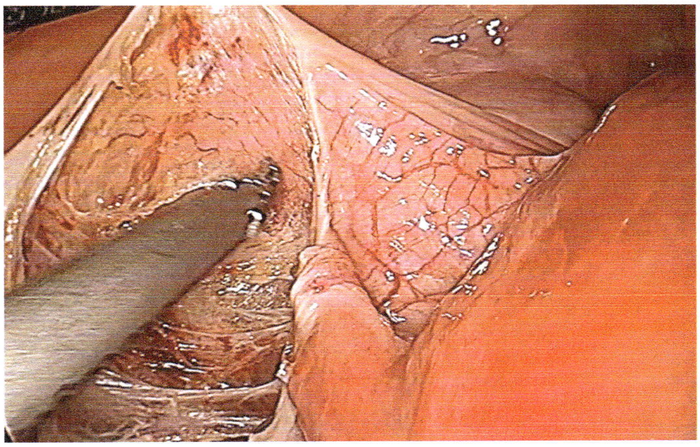

Fig. 8: Dissection of bladder peritoneum.

endometriosis, previous CS or adhesions, sharp dissection can be performed. Injecting 5 mL of indigo carmine in the patient's bladder helps to detect bladder trauma **(Figs. 9 and 10)**.

Colpotomy

A folded gauze in sponge forceps is used to mark the fornix. The vaginal wall is tented and transacted horizontally with hook electrode **(Figs. 11A to C)**. Once the dissection is extended to the lower uterine segment or to the level of cardinal ligament, laparoscopic procedure is temporarily terminated and vaginal part of LAVH started.

VAGINAL PART OF LAPAROSCOPIC-ASSISTED VAGINAL HYSTERECTOMY

The sponge forceps occluding the colpotomy is withdrawn together with the uterine manipulator. Three vaginal specula are used to get proper access for vaginal part of LAVH **(Figs. 12A to D)**. With aid of appropriate-sized speculum and adequate lateral and anterior retraction by the assistant, the anterior and posterior lips of the cervix are held by tenaculum. Using monopolar energy in circumcision of the skin at 2.5 cm above the external os towards the vaginal vault is done. Further dissection with gloved finger or dissecting scissors creates a flap in which the superior Sims speculum or narrow angled retractor is placed to lift the bladder away. Gradual release of the tissues results in entry to the abdominal cavity **(Figs. 13A to H)**.

Using appropriate-sized caucus clamp, the uterosacral pedicles are identified bilaterally clamped, secured, cut, and tied with the tail of the thread left as mark or coagulated with Ligasure, harmonic scalpel, or bipolar instrument specially made for vaginal hysterectomy **(Figs. 12A to D)**. With release of the uterosacral, the uterus descends into the vaginal cavity. Similarly, the cardinal ligaments are bilaterally clamped, secured, cut, and tied with a mark or coagulated and dissected. Further descent of the uterus is gained, and the uterine pedicles are clamped, secured, cut and tied.

The uterus is then delivered vaginally. Once the uterus is removed, the vaginal vault is closed to ensure support of the vault; the vaginal angles are attached to the uterosacral and cardinal ligaments with 2-0 vicryl. Any coexisting cystocele or rectocele is repaired. A very large fibroid uterus should be debulked by morcellation for removal vaginally. It can be combined with laparoscopic adnexal surgery, e.g., ovariectomy or adhesiolysis. Once the vaginal surgery is completed again laparoscopic inspection of the pelvis is done.

Total Laparoscopic Hysterectomy

Preparation and Positioning of Patient

Preoperative check of consent form and patient past medical history should be taken followed by proper preanesthetic checkup (PAC). Patients is placed in a dorsal lithotomy position. The arms are tucked at the sides and a foam mattress is situated directly under the patient to prevent sliding during steep Trendelenburg. Gynecologist should keep the table in a low position and have a monitor directly facing each surgeon to promote an ergonomic working environment **(Fig. 14)**.

Abdominal Entry and Trocar Placement

A 10-mm supraumbilical skin incision is made using a #15 blade and insert a Veress needle is introduced into the peritoneal cavity. Once intraperitoneal pressure has reached 15 mm Hg, insert trocar through the supraumbilical incision, followed by a complete survey of the abdomen to rule out any visceral injury at the time of entry. The lower quadrant trocar sleeves are placed under direct vision. These trocars are placed lateral to the rectus abdominis muscles, 2 cm above and 2 cm medial to the anterior superior iliac spine. These secondary trocar position varies according to the size of uterus. Usually, a 5-mm trocar is placed on the right and a 5-mm trocar on the left. For TLH port position can be ipsilateral or contralateral. Two ports on the left greatly facilitate suturing and help to maintain an ergonomic position for the surgeon throughout the procedure **(Figs. 15A and B)**.

Insertion of a Uterine Manipulator

Different types of uterine manipulators are available. Generally, most of the gynecologists use the RUMI® or Mangeshkar Uterine Manipulator; however, in patients with a very narrow introitus the VCare® Uterine Manipulator is useful because this is easier to insert **(Fig. 16)**.

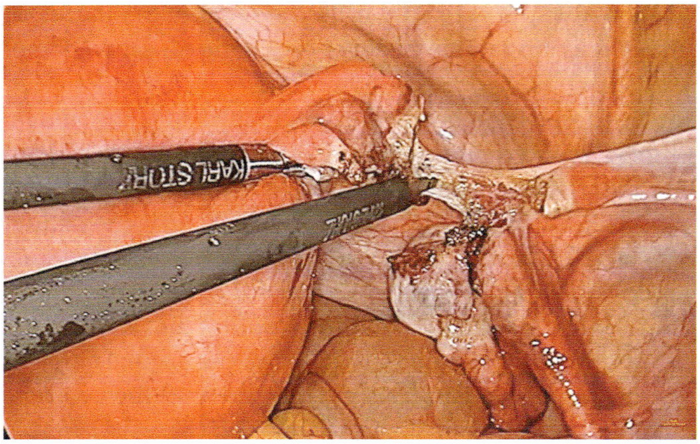

Fig. 9: Opening of anterior and posterior leaf broad ligament.

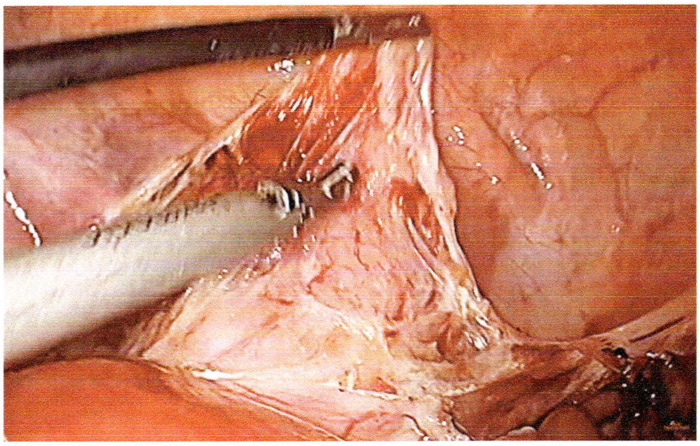

Fig. 10: Separation of bladder.

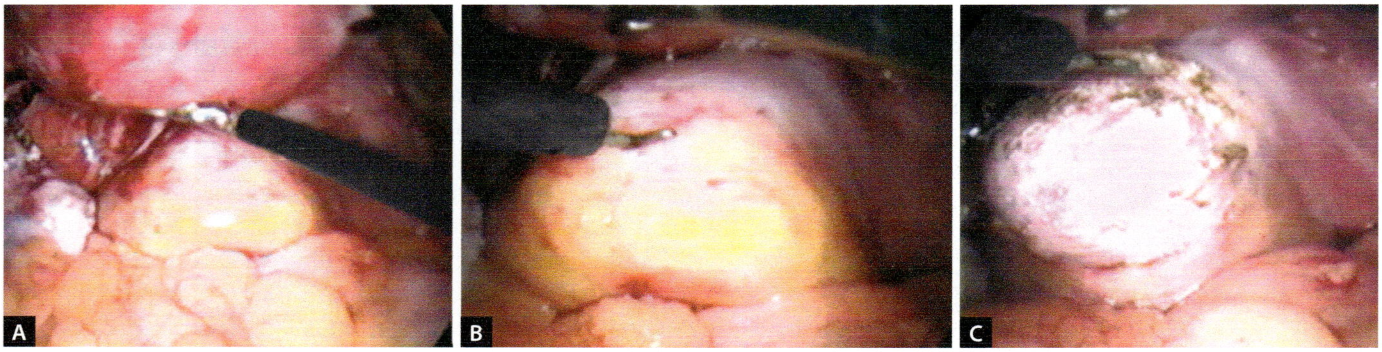

Figs. 11A to C: Steps of colpotomy.

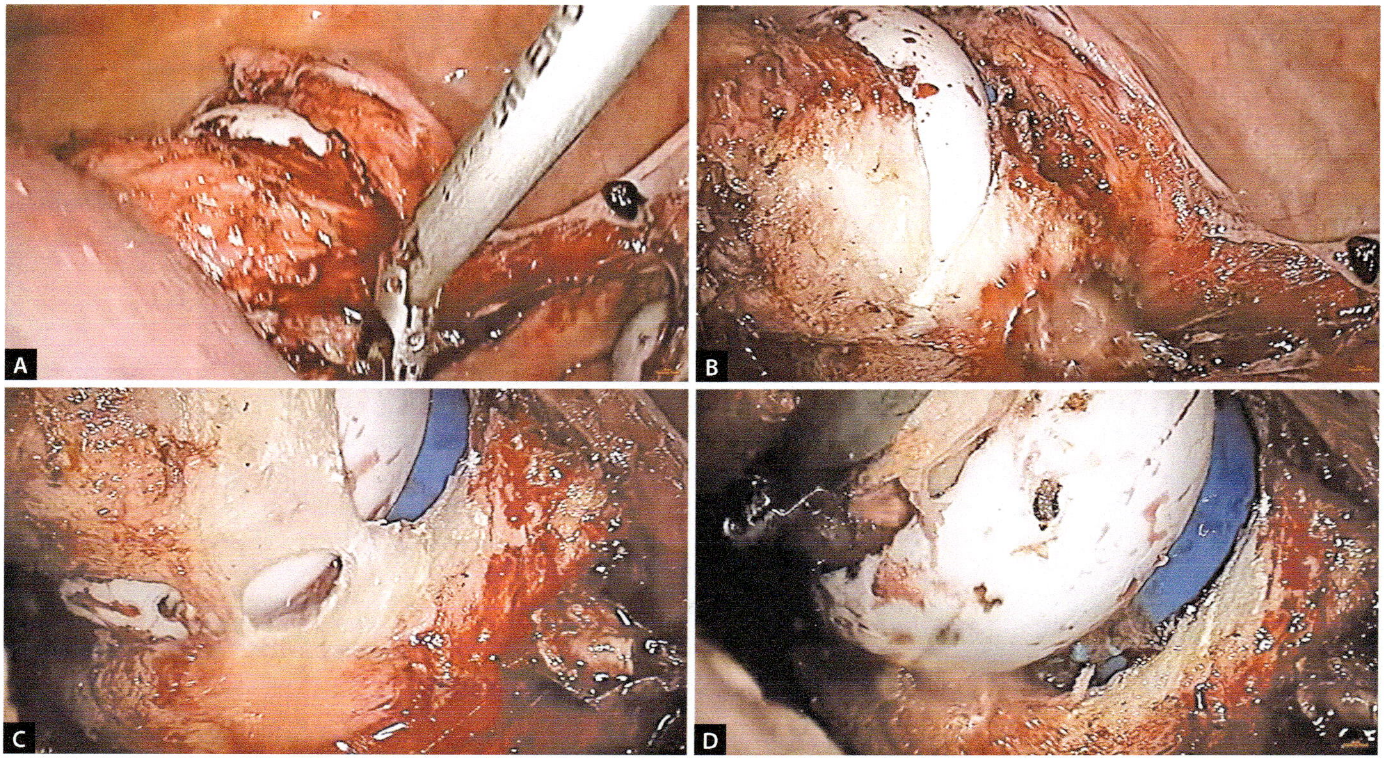

Figs. 12A to D: Anterior and posterior colpotomy.

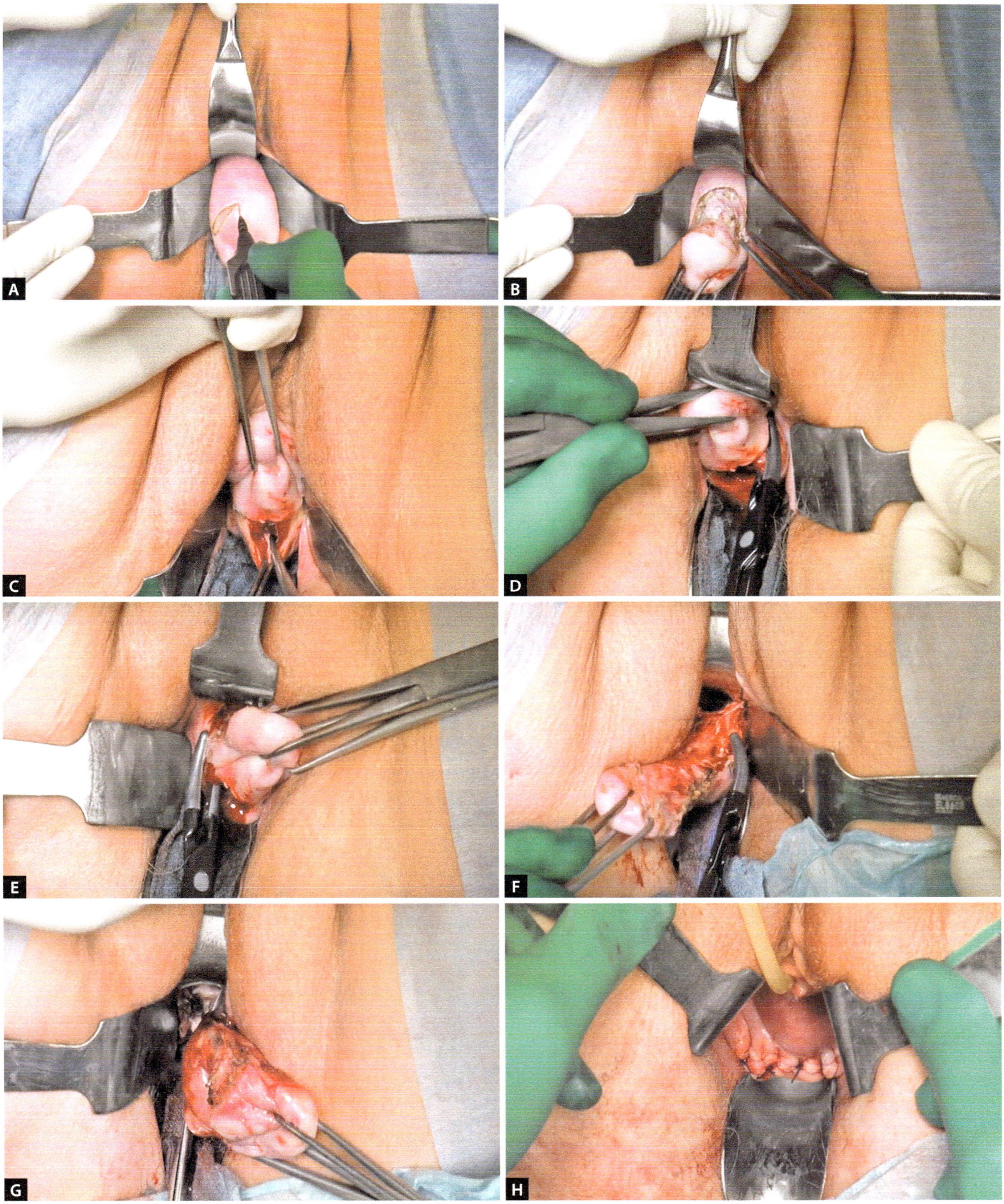

Figs. 13A to H: Successive clamping and desiccation of uterine pedicle through the vaginal route using bipolar.

Dissection of Infundibulopelvic Ligament

The infundibulopelvic (IP) ligament or the utero-ovarian ligament is initially desiccated with a reusable bipolar grasper, Ligasure, or harmonic scalpel. It is important to stay close to the ovary as this helps to avoid the pelvic sidewall during ovarian removal and the ascending uterine vessel during ovarian conservation. The gynecologists should take special care to desiccate the parametrial veins that run between the ovary and the round ligament as these can be quite tortuous and tend to bleed if left unattended. The IP ligament or utero-ovarian ligament is then transacted close to the ovary. During this step of the procedure, the uterine manipulator is being pushed upward and to the contralateral side to provide maximal visualization **(Fig. 17)**.

Mobilization of the Bladder

Transect the round ligament and separate the anterior and posterior leaves of the broad ligament with the harmonic scalpel or monopolar scissors. It is important to find the correct plane; this is where the peritoneum separates easily with gentle manipulation. After peritoneal separation, identify the vesicouterine peritoneal fold and continue the dissection anteriorly, thereby mobilizing the bladder off the lower uterine segment. It is important to stay in the loose areolar tissue if at all possible. In patients who have had a prior cesarean section, this area may be scarred and it is important to stay relatively high on the uterus during the dissection. In case of adhesion a pledget dissection combined with sharp dissection with cold scissors is helpful. A reevaluation of the route of dissection is advised if fat is encountered because the fat belongs to the bladder; this may indicate that the dissection is moving too close to the bladder **(Fig. 18)**.

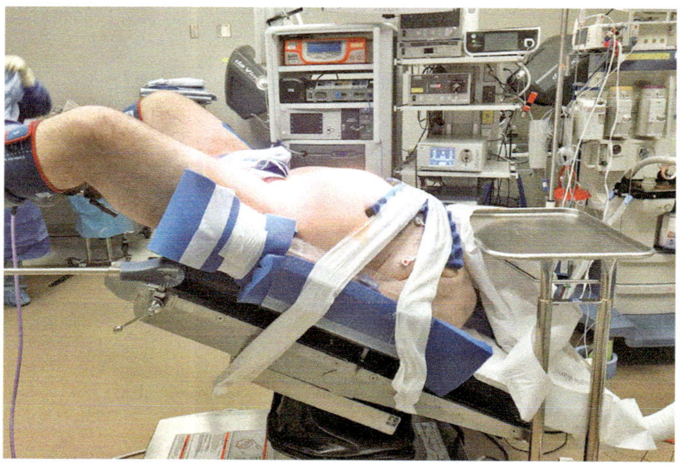

Fig. 14: Position of the patient for total laparoscopic hysterectomy.

Securing the Uterine Vessels

Uterine artery course is diverse and due to a wide variety in anatomy and in the course of the uterine vessels, it is helpful to initially skeletonize them with the harmonic scalpel. Then desiccate the ascending uterine vessels with the bipolar grasper or Ligasure at the level of internal cervical os. Note that pushing cephalad with the uterine manipulator helps to move the uterine vessels away from the ureter. Complete desiccation of the vessels can be assessed visually by observing the bubbles coming and going during this process; when the bubbles stop forming and tissue color turns brown the vessel is desiccated and safe to transect with the harmonic scalpel or Ligasure. It is important to take the uterine vessels high and then dissect medially to the uterine vessels down to the cup of colpotomizer. This averts ureteral injury and provides a healthy vascular pedicle that can be safely desiccated further in the event of bleeding **(Figs. 19A and B)**.

Colpotomy

After dissection of uterine pedicle the next step is to identify the vaginal fornices while pushing cephalad with the uterine manipulator. Gynecologist will either see the indentation of the KOH colpotomizer or be able to palpate it with a laparoscopic instrument. The harmonic scalpel is then used to cut circumferentially around the cup. Take care not to direct the harmonic scalpel directly into the metal because this may result in failure of the device and may even break

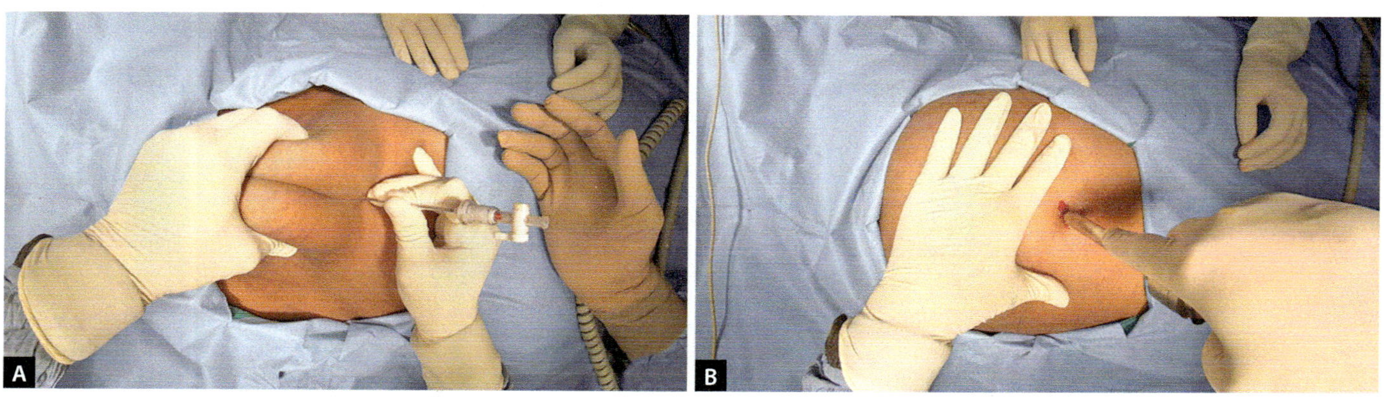

Figs. 15A and B: Abdominal entry and trocar placement.

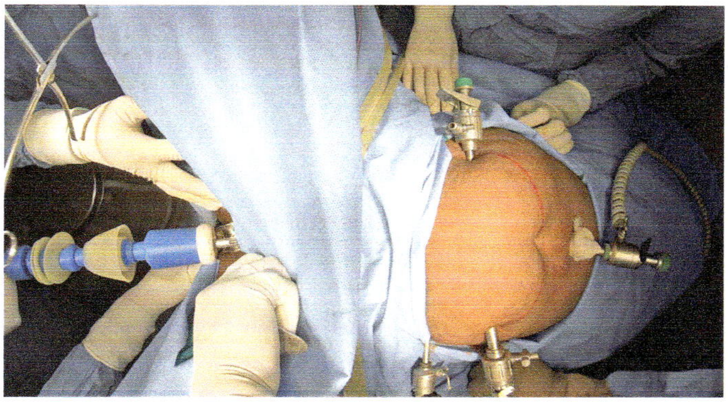

Fig. 16: Insertion of a uterine manipulator.

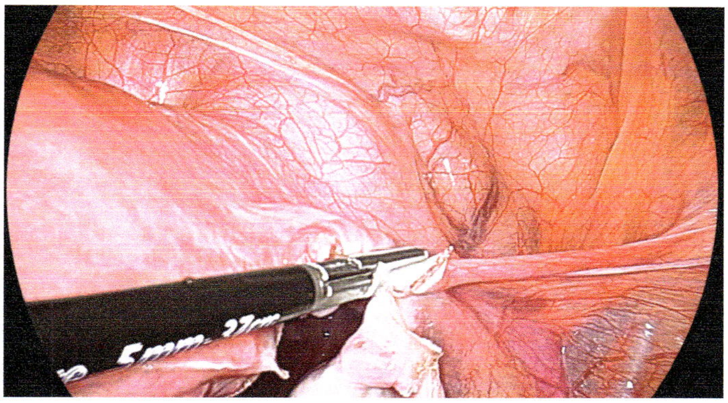

Fig. 17: Dissection of upper pedicle, conserving ovary.

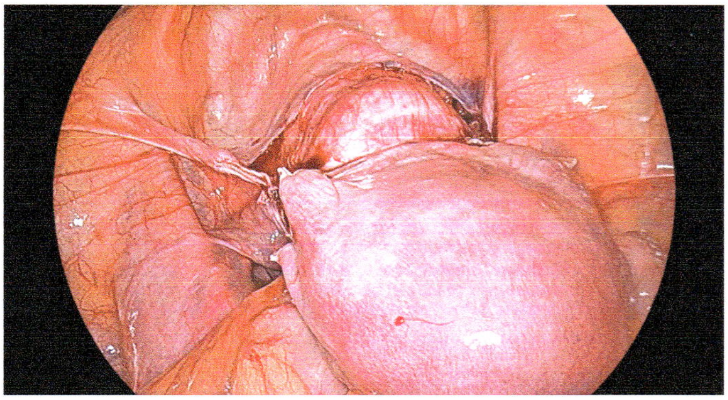

Fig. 18: Mobilization of bladder.

the active blade or harmonic **(Figs. 20A to D)**. For colpotomy hook can also be used if harmonic is not available.

Removal of the Uterus

Once complete separation of uterus with vaginal cuff is achieved pull the uterus into the vagina if it fits **(Figs. 21A and B)**. The uterus can remain there to maintain pneumoperitoneum during suturing. Alternatively, the uterus is removed and a glove with a pair of 4 × 4 sponges is placed into the vagina to maintain pneumoperitoneum. If the uterus is too large to fit through the vagina, it can be carefully morcellated transvaginally by using a 10-blade scalpel and triple hooks for retraction. In patients with limited vaginal access, the uterus can be morcellated laparoscopically using an electronic morcellator. It is important to keep the tip of the morcellator in clear view at all times.

Vaginal Cuff Closure

There are various ways of vaginal cuff closure **(Figs. 22A to D)**. One can use barbed suture, extracorporeal square knot, intracorporeal continuous suture, or interrupted suture. Most commonly used technique of vault closure is intracorporeal continuous suturing. Closure begins at the distal angle of the vaginal cuff and proceeds in a running fashion, making sure to include the vaginal mucosa and the pubocervical and rectovaginal fascia. Many surgeons do not tie a knot at the end of vault if they use barbed suture. Extracorporeal knot with Clark knot pusher is also very good to close the vault especially in deep pelvis. The pelvis can now be irrigated and hemostasis at all sites is assured.

Port Site Closure

The fascia at the 10 mm incision is closed using 0 vicryl sutures with a fascia closure device. The skin is closed with 4-0 monocryl suture in a continuous subcutaneous fashion or skin stapler. The 5-mm incisions are closed with Dermabond. Many gynecologists then inject 20 cc of 0.5% Marcaine at all incision sites to reduce immediate postoperative pain. It is not necessary to perform cystoscopy routinely, but in selected cases cystoscopy is performed after vaginal closure to check ureteral patency and for any signs of bladder injury. The patient is given 5 cc of Indigo carmine intravenously 5 minutes prior to closure. Please note that a normal cystoscopy does not exclude a delayed thermal injury to either the ureters or the bladder.

Subtotal Hysterectomy

Supracervical hysterectomy is performed to preserve libido of patient. The procedure is performed fully laparoscopically. After desiccating and cutting the uterine vessels at the level of cardinal ligaments above the uterosacral ligament, uterus is retracted, and its lower segment is amputated with the scissors and unipolar cutting current. After transecting the uterus from the cervix, uterine manipulator is removed vaginally, the cervical stump is irrigated, and hemostasis is achieved. The endocervical epithelium, lining the cervical canal, is vaporized or coagulated with laser or electrosurgery. The rest of the endocervical canal is ablated vaginally to reduce the risk of intraepithelial cervical neoplasia. The cervical stump is closed with interrupted absorbable sutures and covered with peritoneum, which is stitched transversely with interrupted sutures. The dissected uterus is morcellated and removes through a 10-mm cannula. Mini-laparotomy or posterior colpotomy can also be performed to remove the uterus in case of subtotal hysterectomy. These patients are advised for annual examination for Pap smear.

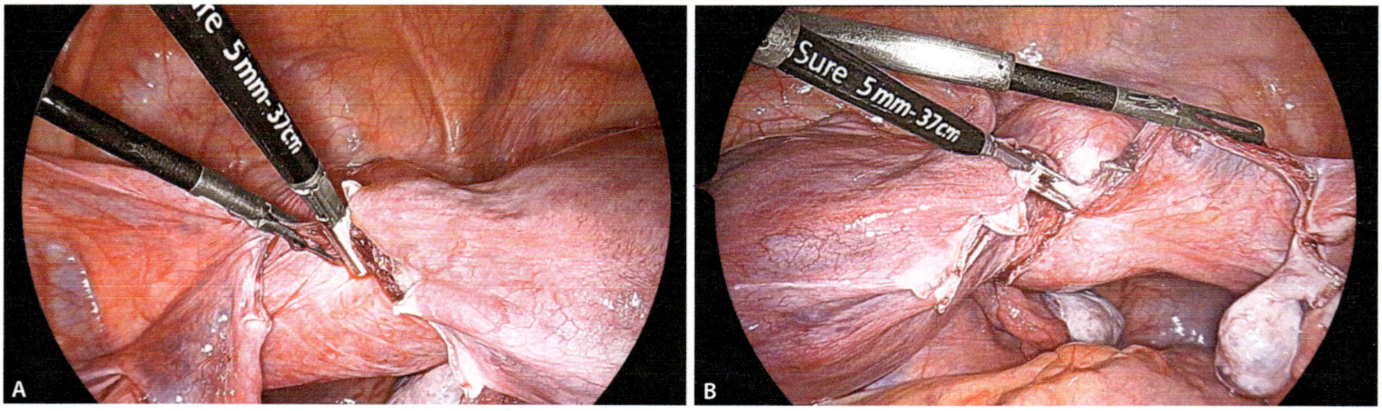

Figs. 19A and B: Securing uterine artery.

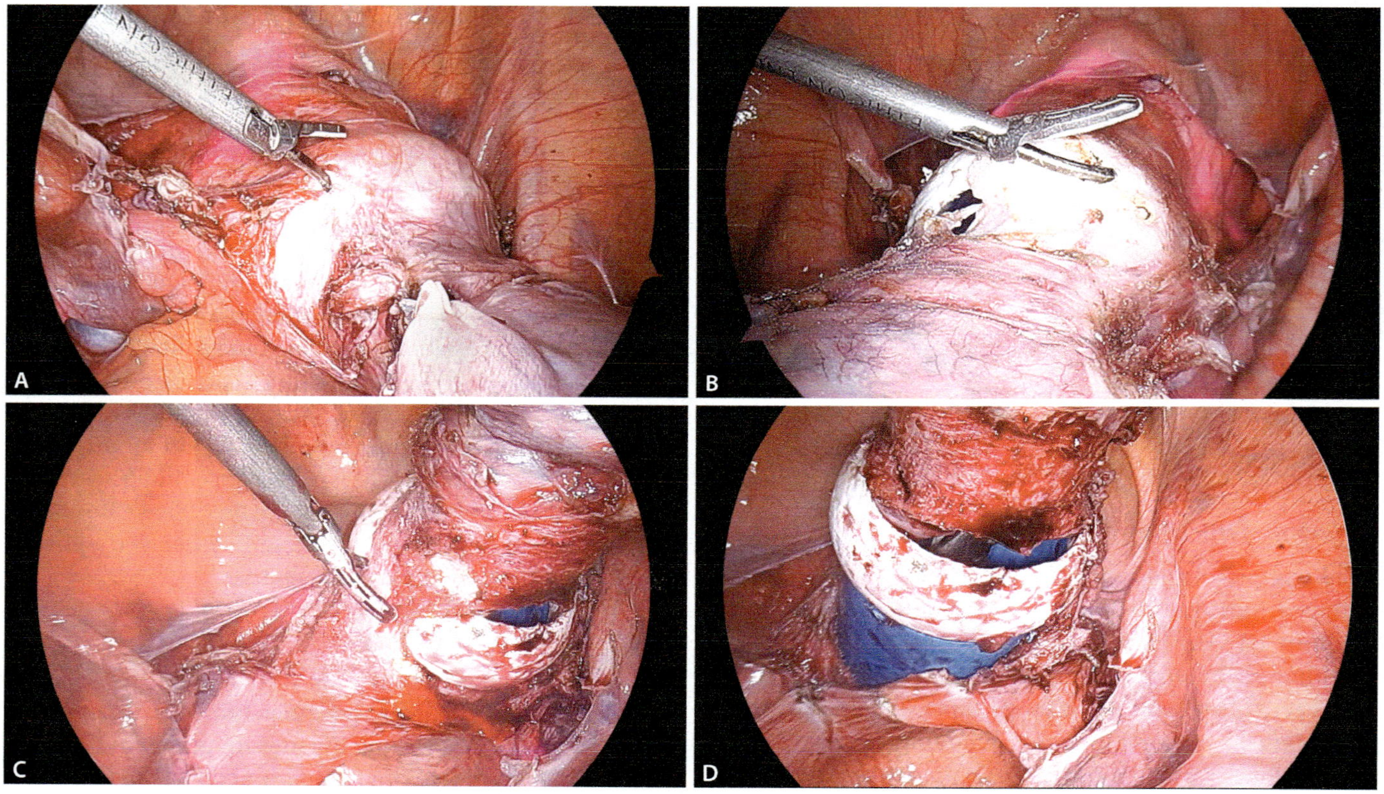

Figs. 20A to D: Colpotomy by harmonic scalpel.

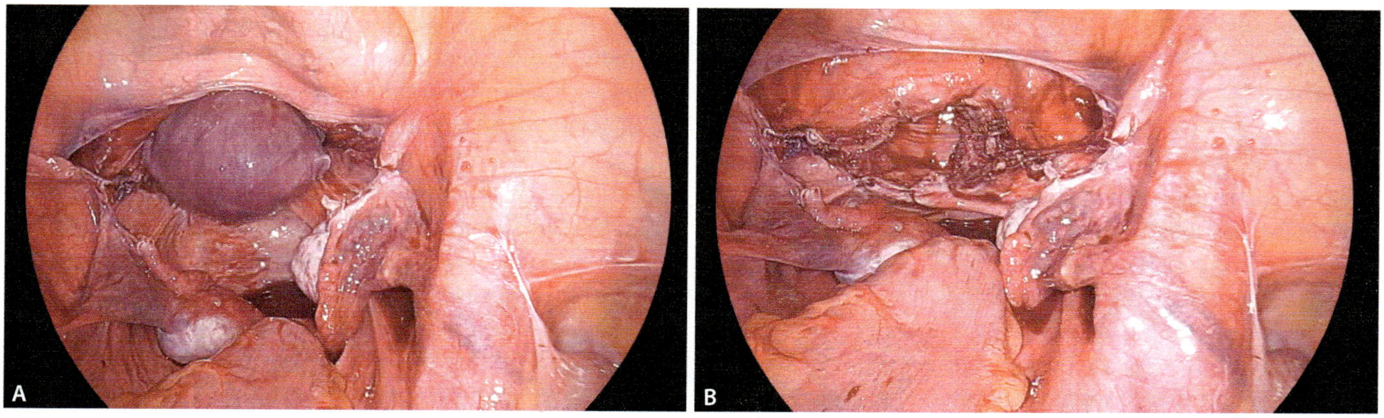

Figs. 21A and B: Removal of uterus through the vaginal route.

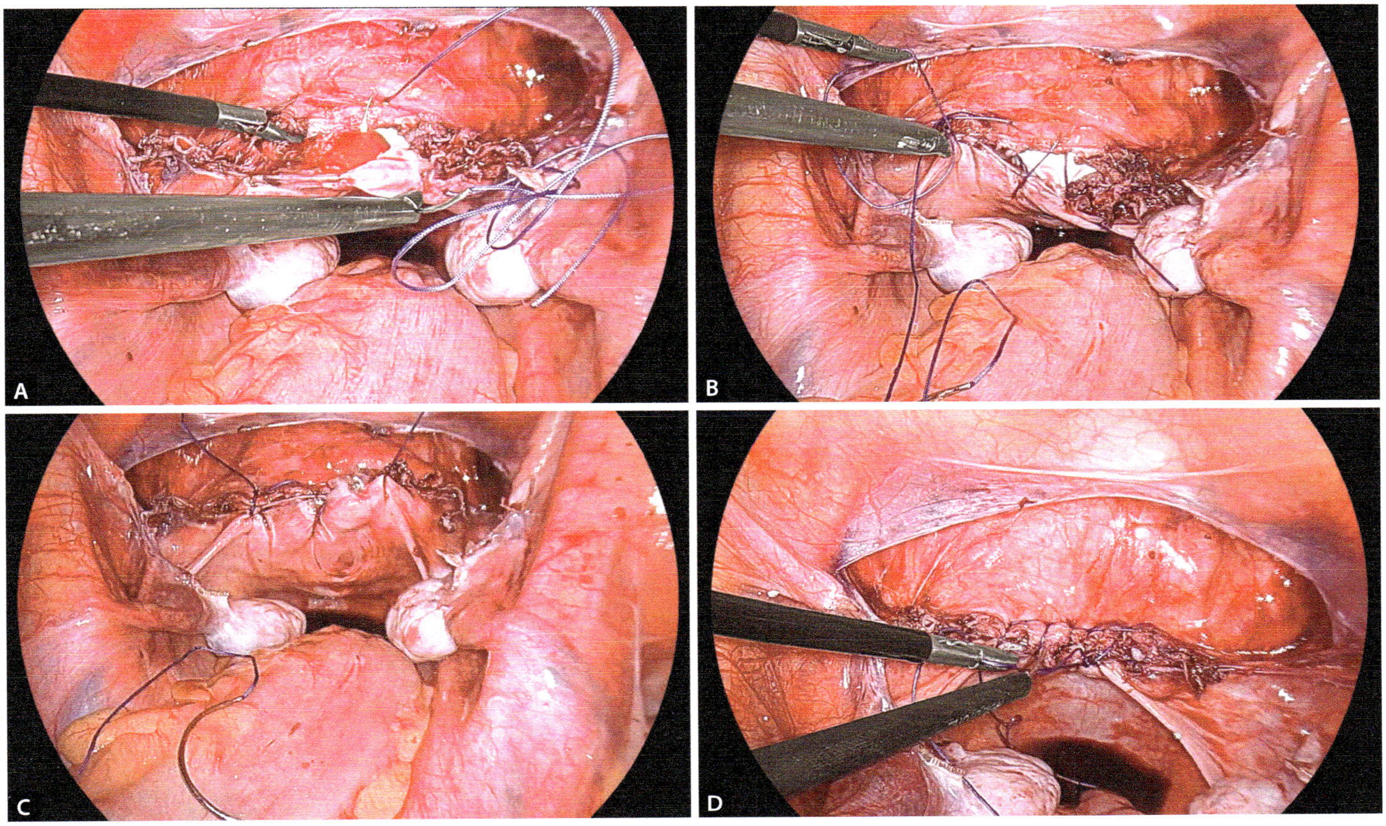

Figs. 22A to D: Vault closure with by continuous suturing.

Ending the Procedure

One of the benefits of LAVH or TLH over nondescent vaginal hysterectomy (NDVH) is inspection of pedicles at the end of surgery. The vaginal cuff can be closed from below or above but after that pneumoperitoneum is again restored to see the pelvic and abdominal cavity. Irrigation and suction should be performed. In case of any residual bleeding it is controlled laparoscopically. At the end pelvis is filled with 300 mL Ringer's lactate and it should be seen for any change in color. Once inspection is satisfactory, the fluid is sucked and instrument and cannula are removed after deflating the abdominal cavity.

It has been demonstrated that TLH and LAVH are associated with a shorter hospital stay and patients require less pain medication compared to TAH. LAVH or TLH can replace most of the abdominal hysterectomy for the benign disease of uterus and with the technology available today, it has definite benefit over nondescended vaginal hysterectomy.

DISCUSSION

Vaginal hysterectomy is a part of repertoire of every trained gynecologist. It is considered as a feasible option to abdominal hysterectomy and many studies have shown that vaginal hysterectomy has fewer complications, short recovery, and smaller hospital stay than laparotomy. LH requires greater surgical expertise and has a steep learning curve. Randomized trials have shown advantages of laparoscopy vs. laparotomy, including reduced postoperative pain, shorter hospitalization, rapid recovery, and substantial financial benefits to society. The objective of performing hysterectomy laparoscopically can be achieved but the question is, does this offer any advantage over vaginal route? Every mode of hysterectomy has advantages and disadvantages but the indications for each remain controversial. Good surgical practice is when the indication for hysterectomy is considered as the primary criterion for selecting the route of hysterectomy and not factors such as surgeon's choice and experience. A major determinant of the route of hysterectomy is not the clinical situation but the attitude of the surgeon. There is no need for extra training and special skills or complicated equipment for vaginal hysterectomy.

Laparoscopic hysterectomy took a long time to perform in all studies. However, with increasing weight of the uterus, there was a linear increase in operating time and blood loss in hysterectomy performed vaginally which was not observed in laparoscopic-assisted vaginal hysterectomy. There is no statistically significant difference in postoperative analgesia requirement, hospital stay, recovery milestones, or complication rates. The biggest drawback of laparoscopic route over vaginal one is its cost due to expensive disposable instruments, prolonged operating and anesthesia time, and the need for a trained senior gynecologist. For laparoscopic-assisted vaginal hysterectomy to be cost effective expensive disposable instruments must be eliminated.

Laparoscopic surgeons argue that subtotal hysterectomy can be performed laparoscopically but most randomized trials have failed to demonstrate any benefit of subtotal hysterectomy over total hysterectomy. In women who wish to retain their cervix vaginal subtotal hysterectomy described by Döderlein-Krönig technique can be performed. The disadvantage of vaginal approach is vault hematomas. The abdominal approach to hysterectomy does ensure good hemostasis under direct vision, while during the vaginal operation, the vault is closed and subsequent bleeding from the vagina between the mucosa and the peritoneum can give rise to problems, especially if a vasoconstrictor has been given that subsequently wears off. Laparoscopic approach can help check hemostasis and reduce the incidence of vault hematomas. However; this aspect needs to be evaluated in studies.

Lack of uterine descent and nulliparity, fibroid uterus, need for oophorectomy, and previous pelvic surgery are no more considered as contraindications to the vaginal route. With adequate vaginal access and technical skill, and good uterine mobility, vaginal hysterectomy can easily be achieved. Multiparity, lax tissues due to poor involution following multiple deliveries and lesser tissue tensile strength afford a lot of comfort to vaginal surgeon even in the presence of significant uterine enlargement. None of the evidence supports the use of LH rather than VH if latter can be performed safely. No outcomes are significantly worse for vaginal hysterectomy as compared to LAVH. There are clinical situations where vaginal surgeries are not appropriate such as dense pelvic adhesions, severe endometriosis, adnexal disease, when vaginal access is reduced wherein LH is indicated as it has advantages over the abdominal approach. Laparoscopic approach may be helpful postoperatively to rule out hemorrhage in some cases. Laparoscopic assistance should not be used to supplant inadequate skills of vaginal hysterectomy.

Lack of training in laparoscopic surgery is not a reason for not removing uteri vaginally. The learning curve of VH is noticeably short as compared to laparoscopic surgery, however, the current scenario in residency programs is not providing a level of surgical competency in performing difficult vaginal hysterectomies. There is a need to improve this training.

In order to compare the complication rates of different types of hysterectomies, considering an incidence of 4–5% of serious complications of hysterectomies, at least 1,460 women would be required in each arm of the study to detect 50% increase in the complication rate. Therefore, larger randomized controlled trials are required to compare different types of hysterectomies.

When the size of the uterus is greater than 16 weeks gestation, there is an increase in the operative time and blood loss in VH compared to LAVH which is statistically significant.

Laparoscopically-assisted vaginal hysterectomy is a useful adjunct to transvaginal hysterectomy for lysis of extensive adhesions and sometimes for certain concomitant adnexal surgery. Besides, LAVH can also secure almost all the main blood supplies to the uterus, i.e., the uterine vessels and the adnexal collaterals. Although, a skilled surgeon can do transvaginal hysterectomy with a larger uterus by employing volume-reducing techniques, Kohler reported that laparoscopic coagulation hemostasis of the uterine vessels was associated with less blood loss. It may take time to achieve these goals, but they may make subsequent extirpation or volume-reducing procedures easier and safer to perform. Therefore, the average operative time and estimated blood loss for LAVH remained almost constant regardless of increasing uterine weight. Generally, the average operative time for LAVH is longer than that for transvaginal hysterectomy. It takes time to secure the uterine blood supply before extirpation and volume-reducing procedures, but it also makes LAVH superior to transvaginal hysterectomy when dealing with a larger uterus. In our opinion, LAVH might be considered for a larger uterus in view of the relatively shorter operative time and less blood loss, whereas transvaginal hysterectomy is preferable for a small uterus, not only for shorter operative time and minimal wound, but also for much lower costs.

BIBLIOGRAPHY

1. Carley ME, McIntire D, Carley JM, Schaffer J. Incidence, risk factors and morbidity of unintended bladder or ureter injury during hysterectomy. Int Urogynecol J Pelvic Floor Dysfunct. 2002;13:18-21.
2. Chapron C, Dubuisson JB, Aubert V. Total laparoscopic hysterectomy: preliminary results. Hum Reprod. 1994;9: 2084-9.
3. Chapron C, Dubuisson JB. Laparoscopic hysterectomy. Lancet. 1995;345:593.
4. Chapron C, Fauconnier A, Goffinet F, Bréart G, Dubuisson JB. Laparoscopic surgery is not inherently dangerous for patients presenting with benign gynaecologic pathology. Results of a meta-analysis. Hum Reprod. 2002;17:1334-42.
5. Chapron C, Laforest L, Ansquer Y, Fauconnier A, Fernandez B, Breart G, et al. Hysterectomy techniques used for benign disorders: results of a French multicentre study. Hum Reprod. 1999;14:2464-70.
6. Chauveaud A, de Tayrac R, Gervaise A, Anquetil C, Fernandez H. Total hysterectomy for a nonprolapsed, benign uterus in women without vaginal deliveries. J Reprod Med. 2002;47:4-8.
7. Cosson M, Querleu D, Crepin G (Eds). Hystérectomies pour pathologies bénignes. Masson: Paris; Williams et Wilkins; 1997. pp. 160.
8. Councell RB, Thorp JM Jr, Sandridge DA, Hill ST. Assessments of laparoscopic-assisted vaginal hysterectomy. J Am Assoc Gynecol Laparosc. 1994;2:49-56.

9. Dandolu V, Mathai E, Chatwani A, Harmanli O, Pontari M, Hernandez E. Accuracy of cystoscopy in the diagnosis of ureteral injury in benign gynecologic surgery. Int Urogynecol J Pelvic Floor Dysfunct. 2003;14:427-31.
10. Daraï E, Soriano D, Kimata P, Laplace C, Lecuru F. Vaginal hysterectomy for enlarged uteri, with or without laparoscopy assistance: randomized study. Obstet Gynecol. 2001;97:712-6.
11. Davies A, Vizza E, Bournas N, O'Connor H, Magos A. How to increase the proportion of hysterectomies performed vaginally. Am J Obstet Gynecol. 1998;179:1008-12.
12. Dicker RC, Greenspan JR, Strauss LT, Cowart MR, Scally MJ, Peterson HB, et al. Complications of abdominal and vaginal hysterectomy among women of reproductive age in the United States. The Collaborative Review of Sterilization. Am J Obstet Gynecol. 1982;144:841-8.
13. Dorairajan G, Rani PR, Habeebullah S, Dorairajan LN. Urological injuries during hysterectomies: a 6-year review. J Obstet Gynaecol Res. 2004;30:430-5.
14. Dorsey JH, Steinberg EP, Holtz PM. Clinical indications for hysterectomy route: patient characteristics or physician preference? Am J Obstet Gynecol. 1995;173:1452-60.
15. Dwyer PL, Carey MP, Rosamilia A. Suture injury to the urinary tract in urethral suspension procedures for stress incontinence. Int Urogynecol J Pelvic Floor Dysfunct. 1999;10:15-21.
16. Farquhar CM, Steiner CA. Hysterectomy rates in the United States 1990–1997. Obstet Gynecol. 2002;99:229-34.
17. Garry R, Fountain J, Brown J, Manca A, Mason S, Sculpher M, et al. Evaluate hysterectomy trial. A multicentre randomised trial comparing abdominal, vaginal and laparoscopy methods of hysterectomy. Health Technol Assess. 2004a;8:1-154.
18. Garry R, Fountain J, Mason S, Hawe J, Napp V, Abbott J, et al. (2004b) The evaluate study: two parallel randomised trials, one comparing laparoscopy with abdominal hysterectomy, the other comparing laparoscopy with vaginal hysterectomy. BMJ. 2004;328:129. Erratum in BMJ. 2004;328:494.
19. Gilmour DT, Das S, Flowerdew G. Rates of urinary tract injury from gynecologic surgery and the role of intraoperative cystoscopy. Obstet Gynecol. 2006;107:1366-72.
20. Gilmour DT, Dwyer PL, Carey MP. Lower urinary tract injury during gynecologic surgery and its detection by intraoperative cystoscopy. Obstet Gynecol. 1999;94:883-9.
21. Gimbel H, Settnes A, Tabor A. Hysterectomy on benign indication in Denmark 1988–1998. Acta Obstet Gynecol Scand. 2001;80:267-72.
22. Härkki-Siren P, Kurpi T, Sjöbery J, Tiitinen A. Safety aspects of laparoscopic hysterectomy. Acta Obstet Gynecol Scand. 2001;80:383-91.
23. Härkki-Siren P, Sjöberg J, Mäkinen J, Heinonen PK, Kaudo M, Tomas E, et al. Finnish national register of laparoscopic hysterectomies: A review and complications of 1165 operations. Am J Obstet Gynecol. 1997;176:118-122.
24. Härkki-Siren P, Sjöberg J, Tiitinen A. Urinary tract injury after hysterectomy. Obstet Gynecol. 1998;92:113-8.
25. Harris MB, Olive DL. Changing hysterectomy patterns after introduction. Gynecol. 1994;171:340-3.
26. Hurd WW, Bude RO, De Lancey JO, Pearl ML. The relationship of the umbilicus to aortic bifurcation: implications for laparoscopic technique. Obstet Gynecol. 1992;80:48-51.
27. Hwang JL, Seow KM, Tsai YL, Huang LW, Hsieh BC, Lee C. Comparative study of vaginal, laparoscopically-assisted vaginal and abdominal hysterectomies for uterine myoma larger than 6 cm in diameter or uterus weighing at least 450 g: a prospective randomized study. Acta Obstet Gynecol Scand. 2002;81:1132-8.
28. Johns DA, Carrera B, Jones J, DeLeon F, Vincent R, Safely C. The medical and economic impact of laparoscopically-assisted vaginal hysterectomy in a large, metropolitan, not-for-profit hospital. Am J Obstet Gynecol. 1995;172:1709-15.
29. Johnson N, Barlow D, Lethaby A, Tavender E, Curr E, Garry R. Surgical approach to hysterectomy for benign gynaecological disease. Cochran Database Syst Rev. 2006;(2):CD003677.
30. Johnson N, Barlow D, Lethaby A, Tavender E, Curr L, Garry R. Methods of hysterectomy: systematic review and meta-analysis of randomised controlled trials. Br Med J. 2005;330:1478.
31. Kadar N. Dissecting the pelvic retroperitoneum and identifying the ureters. A laparoscopic technique. J Reprod Med. 1995;40:116-22.
32. Kreiker G, Bertoldi A, Sad Larcher J, Ruiz Orrico G, Chapron C. Prospective evaluation of the learning curve of total laparoscopic hysterectomy in a university hospital. J Am Assoc Gynecol Laparosc. 2004;11:229-35.
33. Leonard F, Chopin N, Borghese B, Fotso A, Foulot H, Coste J, et al. Total laparoscopic hysterectomy: preoperative risk factors for conversion to laparotomy. J Minim Invasive Gynecol. 2005;12:312-17.
34. Leonard F, Chopin N, Borghese B, Fotso A, Foulot H, Coste J, et al. Total laparoscopy hysterectomy: preoperative risk factor for conversion to laparotomy. J Minim Invasive Gynecol. 2005;12:312-7.
35. Liu CY, Reich H. Complications of total laparoscopic hysterectomy in 518 cases. Gynecol Endoscopy. 1994;3:203-8.
36. Mäkinen J, Johansson J, Tomas C, Tomas E, Heinonen PK, Laatikainen T, et al. Morbidity of 10110 hysterectomy by type approach. Hum Reprod. 2001;16:1473-8.
37. McMaster-Fay RA, Jones RA. Laparoscopic hysterectomy and ureteric injury: a comparison of the initial 275 cases and the last 1,000 cases using staples. Gynecol Surg. 2006;3:118-21.
38. Meikle SF, Nugent EW, Orleans M. Complications and recovery from laparoscopy-assisted vaginal hysterectomy compared with abdominal and vaginal hysterectomy. Obstet Gynecol. 1997;89:304-11.
39. Mteta KA, Mbwambo J, Mvungi M. Iatrogenic ureteric and bladder injuries in obstetric and gynaecologic surgeries. East Afr Med J. 2006;83:79-85.
40. National Centre for Disease Control and Prevention 1997. Hysterectomy surveillance United States 1980–1993. CDC surveillance summaries, August. Mabille de Poncheville L (1998) Coeliochirurgie gynécologique en France, instantanée 1996. Résultats d'une enquête nationale. Thèse de médecine, Tours, France. Moller C, Kehlet H and Ottesen BS. Hospita- lization and convalescence after hysterectomy. Open or laparoscopy surgery? Ugeskr Laeger. 1999;161:4620-4.
41. Nezhat F, Nezhat C, Admon D, Gordon S, Nezhat C. Complications and results of 361 hysterectomies performed at laparoscopy. J Am Coll Surg. 1995;180:307-16.
42. O'Shea RT, Petrucco O, Gordon S, Seman E. Adelaide laparoscopic hysterectomy audit (1991–1998): realistic complications rates. Gynaecol Endoscopy. 2000;9:369-72.
43. Oh BR, Kwon DD, Park KS, Ryu SB, Park YI, Presti JC Jr. Late presentation of ureteral injury after laparoscopic surgery. Obstet Gynecol. 2000;95:337-39.
44. Ou CS, Beadle E, Presthus J, Smith M. A multicenter review of 839 laparoscopic-assisted vaginal hysterectomies. J Am Assoc Gynecol Laparosc. 1994;1:417-22.
45. Paulson JD. Laparoscopically-assisted vaginal hysterectomy. A protocol for reducing urinary tract complications. J Reprod Med. 1996;41:623-8.
46. Phipps JH, Tyrrell NJ. Transilluminating ureteric stents for preventing operative ureteric damage. Br J Obstet Gynaecol. 1992;99:81.
47. Reich H, De Caprio J, McGlynn F. Laparoscopic hysterectomy. J Gynecol Surg. 1989;5:213-6.
48. Ribeiro S, Reich H, Rosenberg J, Guglielminetti E, Vidali A. The value of intraoperative cystoscopy at the time of laparoscopic hysterectomy. Hum Reprod. 1999;14:1727-9.

49. Ribeiro SC, Ribeiro RM, Santos NC, Pinotti JA. A randomized study of total abdominal, vaginal and laparoscopy hysterectomy. Int J Gynaecol Obstet. 2003;83:37-43.
50. Rutkow IM. Obstetric and gynecologic operations in the United States, 1979 to 1984. Obstet Gynecol. 1986;67:755-9.
51. Saidi MH, Sadler RK, Vancaillie TG, Akright BD, Farhart SA, White AJ. Diagnosis and management of serious urinary complications after major operative laparoscopy. Obstet Gynecol. 1996;87:272-6.
52. Shen CC, Wu MP, Kung FT, Huang FJ, Hsieh CH, Lan KC, et al. Major complications associated with laparoscopic-assisted vaginal hysterectomy: ten-year experience. J Am Assoc Gynecol Laparosc. 2003;10:147-53.
53. Soriano D, Goldstein A, Lecuru F, Daraï E. Recovery from vaginal hysterectomy compared with laparoscopy-assisted vaginal hysterectomy: a prospective, randomized, multicenter study. Acta Obstet Gynecol Scand. 2001;80:337-41.
54. University of York (UK) Centre for Health Economics. The management of menorrhagia. Effective Healthcare. 1991;1(9).
55. Vakili B, Chesson RR, Kyle BL, Shobeiri SA, Echols KT, Gist R, et al. The incidence of urinary tract injury during hysterectomy: a prospective analysis based on universal cystoscopy. Am J Obstet Gynecol. 2005;192:1599-1604.
56. Vessey MP, Villard-Mackintosh L, McPherson K, Coulter A, Yeates D. The epidemiology of hysterectomy: findings in a large cohort study. Br J Obstet Gynaecol. 1992;99:402-7.
57. Visco AG, Taber KH, Weidner AC, Barber MD, Myers ER. Cost-effectiveness of universal cystoscopy to identify ureteral injury at hysterectomy. Obstet Gynecol. 2001;97:685-92.
58. Wattiez A, Soriano D, Cohen SB, Nervo P, Canis M, Botchorisvili R, et al. The learning curve of total laparoscopic hysterectomy: comparative analysis of 1647 cases. J Am Assoc Gynecol Laparosc. 2002;9:339-45.
59. Wood EC, Maher P, Pelosi MA. Routine use of ureteric catheters at laparoscopic hysterectomy may cause unnecessary complications. J Am Assoc Gynecol Laparosc. 1996;3:393-7.
60. Wu SM, Chao Yu YM, Yang CF, Che HL. Decision making tree for women considering hysterectomy. J Adv Nurs. 2005;51:361-8.

CHAPTER 35

Laparoscopic Myomectomy

INTRODUCTION

Fibroids or leiomyomas are a very commonly occurring uterine tumor affecting up to 20–25% of women. Fibroid develops from benign transformation of a single smooth muscle cell. The growth of myoma is dependent on many factors. Increased estrogen stimulation alone or together with growth hormone or human placental lactogen appears to be the major growth regulator of fibroid. The severities of symptoms depend on the number of tumors, size, and location. Many a time, they can cause abdominal pressure leading to urinary frequency, abdominal pain, or constipation. One of the common occurrences is dysfunctional uterine bleeding (DUB) due to altered blood flow through the uterus. The fibroids many a time do not affect pregnancy.

Fibroids are clinically diagnosed in 25% of women, although their actual incidence is probably much higher since they are frequently found on routine ultrasound. In women with menorrhagia, the hematocrit is used to assess the degree of anemia. Patients with large broad ligament fibroid may require an intravenous pyelogram to rule out any ureteral obstruction. For anemic patients, preoperative treatment with gonadotropin-releasing hormone (GnRH) may enable restoration of a normal hematocrit and decrease the size of myoma and, thus, reduce the risk of transfusion.

Fibroid types are defined by where they grow in relation to the uterine wall **(Fig. 1)**. There are four types of uterine fibroids:

1. *Submucosal fibroids*: Grow in the submucosa, which means just below the thin layer of tissue found in the uterus. These fibroids can protrude into the uterine cavity. These are the rarest type of fibroid.
2. *Intramural fibroids*: Grown in and are contained within the uterine wall. These are the most common type of fibroid.
3. *Subserosal fibroids*: Grown on the outside of the uterine wall.
4. *Pedunculated fibroids*: Types of fibroids that grow on stalks or stems. These stems are attached to the uterine wall and can grow either outside the uterus or inside the uterine cavity.

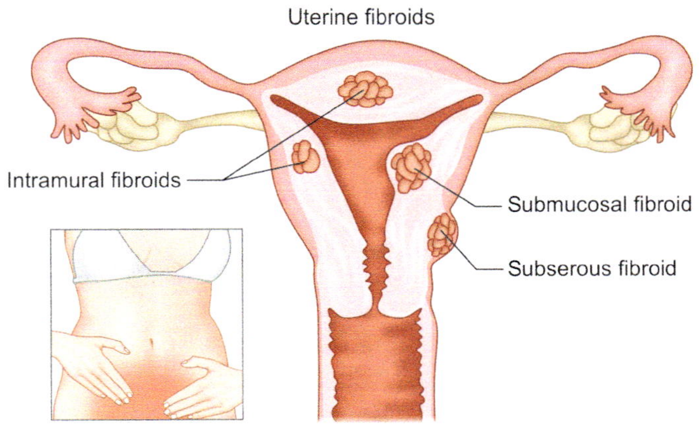

Fig. 1: Different types of fibroid uterus.

Uterine leiomyomas are the most frequent indication for hysterectomy all over the world. Many patients with symptomatic leiomyomas desire to retain the option of future childbearing or simply want to preserve their uterus. For these women, myomectomy, the removal of the myomas with reconstruction and preservation of the uterus, is an important option.

Over the past 10 years, several studies have demonstrated that laparoscopic myomectomy has several advantages over laparotomic and minilaparotomic approaches, including lower operative hemoglobin drop, shorter hospital stays, less postoperative pain, and faster recovery times. On the other hand, laparoscopy itself is a surgical technique that may present significant challenge to the surgeons. The suture of the uterine wall defect is probably the most difficult and time-consuming task for surgeons performing laparoscopic myomectomy.

INDICATIONS

The decision to perform surgery for uterine leiomyoma is complex and varies from patient to patient based on their medical conditions, surgical history, clinical picture, and patient preference. In general, consideration for a hysterectomy is given in patient with:

- *Excessive uterine bleeding*:
  - Profuse bleeding causing lifestyle derangements that is refractory to medical management
  - Uterine bleeding that results in anemia

- *Pelvic discomfort caused by myomas*:
  - Acute and severe
  - Chronic lower abdominal pain or low back or pelvic pressure with evidence of sizeable leiomyoma on imaging studies
- Leiomyomas that are palpable abdominally.

CONTRAINDICATIONS

- Endometrial cancer
- Uterine sarcoma

Intraoperatively use of dilute vasopressin helps to minimize the blood loss. Vertical uterine incisions bleed less than transverse incisions.

Single, vertical, anterior, and midline incisions are least likely to form adhesion. Although sutures predispose to adhesions, they are almost always necessary to close the uterine defect.

If during myomectomy, the endometrial cavity is entered due to large size of myoma, then such a patient when subsequently becomes pregnant should necessarily undergo cesarean delivery.

Preoperative GnRH agonist has been used by some gynecologists to decrease myomas and intraoperative blood loss. The risk of future uterine rupture is a major concern following myomectomy. The difficulty of adequately closing the layers laparoscopically and use of electrocoagulation may contribute to the risk of uterine rupture.

Uteroperitoneal fistulas may follow laparoscopic myomectomy because meticulous laparoscopic approximation of all layers is very difficult. Use of electrosurgery for hemostasis inside the uterine defect may also increase the risk of uteroperitoneal fistula formation.

The chances of postoperative adhesion are also quite high in case of laparoscopic myomectomy. A single uterine incision for removal of multiple leiomyomas and subserosal approximation of the uterine defect should be done.

Laparoscopic-assisted myomectomy (LAM) can reduce the chance of this complication. Here, the suturing is done outside by open method so decreasing the operating time and secure-layered suturing ensures that uterus does not rupture in later pregnancy. Pelvic observation during the laparoscopy allows the diagnosis and treatment of any other disease such as endometriosis or adhesion in the same setting. The criteria for LAM are myoma >5 cm, numerous myomas, requiring vigorous use of morcellator, deep intramural myoma, and removal that require uterine repair with sutures in multiple layers.

PATIENT POSITION

Correct patient positioning is a key component of successful laparoscopic myomectomy **(Fig. 2)**. Table height should be at or below the waistline of the operating surgeon to avoid muscular fatigue from the nonphysiological position of the surgeon's arms during the procedure. The patient's knees should be widely separated in Allen-type stirrups. Padded supports should be applied to the foot and posterior calf. Deep vein thrombosis (DVT) prophylaxis stockings above knee type should be applied before positioning the legs in stirrups. Sequential calf muscle compressors should be in place over DVT stockings. Both upper limbs are tucked on the patient's sides with the IV line in place with extension tubing.

POSITION OF THE SURGICAL TEAM

Surgeon should stand in the left side of the patient during Veress needle insertion and opposite to the side of pathology to start surgery, monitor, target organ, and surgeons visual axis in coaxial line, camera assistant should be in the right side of the surgeon, two assistant surgeons one in the right side opposite to the main surgeon and the second for holding uterine manipulator, and scrubbed nurse should be in the left side of the surgeon. Preparation of parts is done by scrubbing and draping under aseptic techniques **(Fig. 3)**.

PORT PLACEMENT

The insertion of the trocars is a crucial issue to accomplish the operation. In most instances, when small-to-midsize

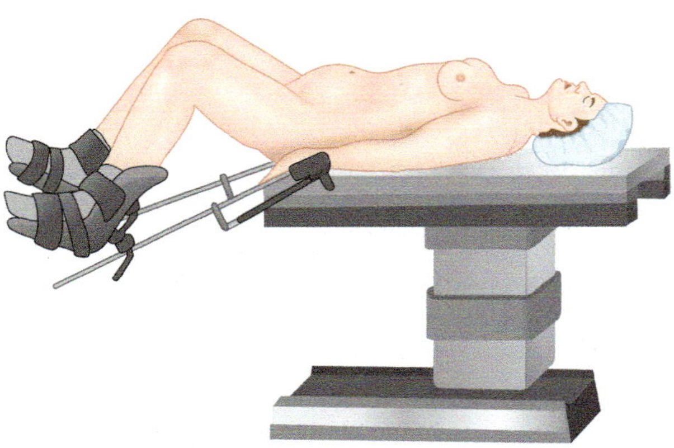

Fig. 2: Patient position in laparoscopic myomectomy.

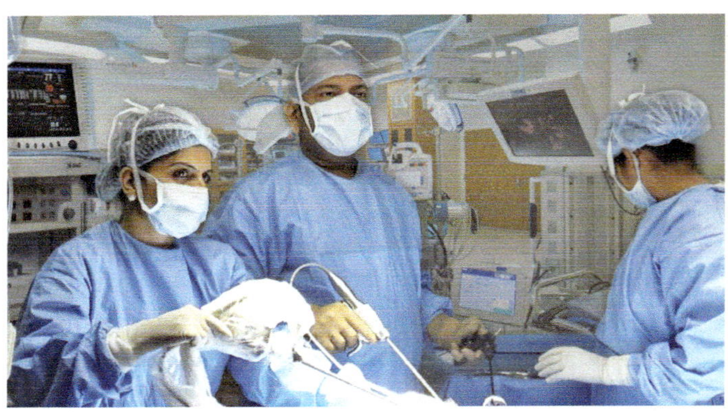

Fig. 3: Position of surgical team during laparoscopic myomectomy.

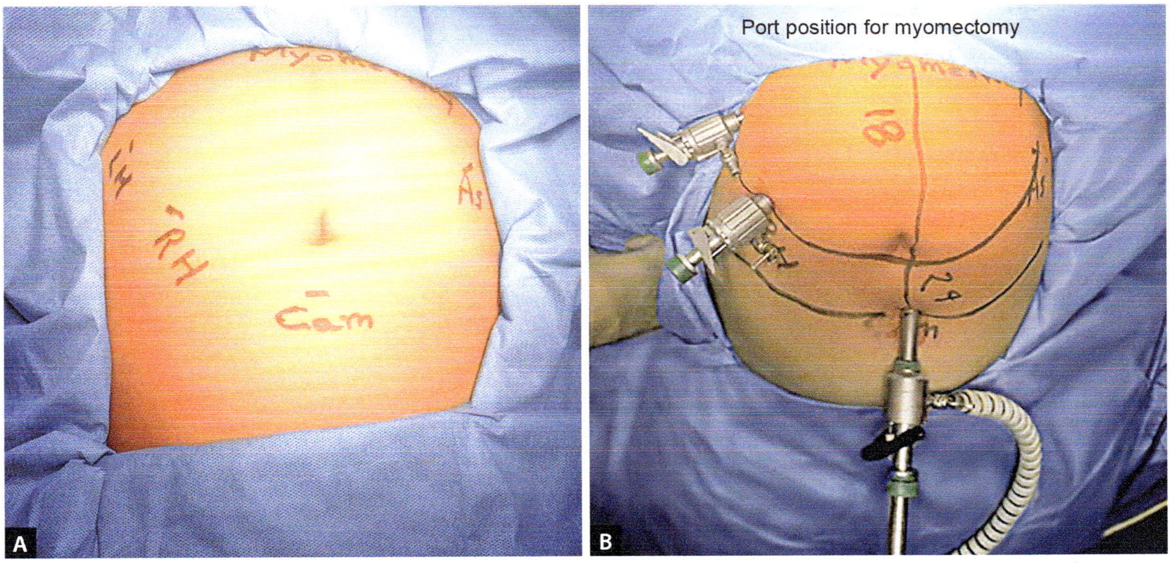

Figs. 4A and B: Port position for laparoscopic myomectomy.

fibroids are concerned, the laparoscope can be placed in standard umbilical position, using the closed- or open-entry technique of choice. However, depending on the size of the uterus, a supraumbilical insertion may be required for large myomas to gain optimal view and room for surgical manipulation. Lee and Wang (2009) suggest placing the laparoscope at the midpoint between the umbilicus and the xiphoid process (Lee–Huang point), if the uterine size is >14 weeks of gestation; the Lee–Huang point could be useful not only to increase the working distance in case of large myomas, but also to prevent injuries in the umbilical area when adhesions are expected, notably in patients with previous abdominal or pelvic surgery **(Fig. 4A)**.

Secondary ports for laparoscopic myomectomy depend on size of uterus. Port position depends on baseball diamond concept **(Fig. 4B)**. Myomectomy usually needs two ipsilateral and one contralateral port position. Base of the myoma should be the target and telescope should be placed 24 cm from the target. This usually comes from supraumbilical port in between umbilicus and xiphisternum. Working ports should be 18 cm from the target and this should be two ipsilateral and one contralateral.

PROCEDURE

Pedunculated myomas are easiest to remove by just coagulating and cutting the stalk. Diluted vasopressin may be injected in the base of stalk. Intramural fibroids require more manipulation, so diluted vasopressin should be injected between the myometrium and the fibroid capsule **(Fig. 5)**. Dilute vasopressin (20 units in 100 mL of normal saline) is injected just beneath the capsule of the fibroid enough to make a bleb. Enough is injected to penetrate the capsule of the fibroid, causing the area injected to appear white or pale. This also facilitates dissection of the fibroid.

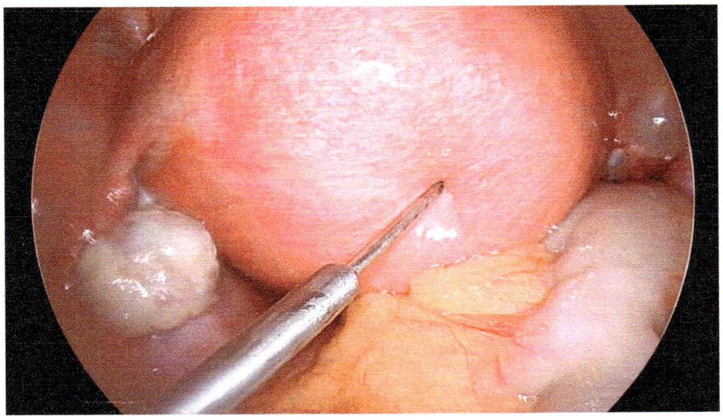

Fig. 5: Injection of vasopressin.

A vertical or horizontal incision depends on port position is made on the serosa overlying the leiomyomas using the monopolar electrode or harmonic scalpel **(Fig. 6)**. The incision is extended until it reaches the capsule. The myometrium retracts as incision is made, exposing the myoma. Two grasping tooth forceps hold the edges of myometrium and the suction irrigator is used as blunt probe to remove the covering of the leiomyomas from its capsule.

The myoma screw should be inserted into the fibroid to apply traction, while the suction irrigation instrument can be used as a blunt dissector **(Fig. 7)**. The harmonic scalpel, monopolar hook, or CO_2 laser can be used to further dissect capsular attachment. Vessels are electrocoagulated before being cut **(Fig. 8)**.

After complete myoma removal, the uterine defect is irrigated; bleeding points are identified and controlled with the open jaw of bipolar. If the fibroid is small and patient does not want baby, the edges of the uterine defects are approximated by coagulating the myometrium. If the deeper defect is formed and cavity is opened, then the edges of defect should be approximated by using 4-0 polydioxanone (PDS).

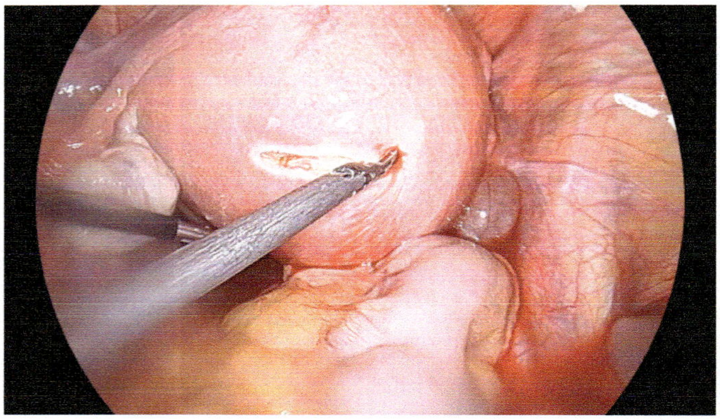

Fig. 6: Incision on seromuscular layer to start laparoscopic myomectomy.

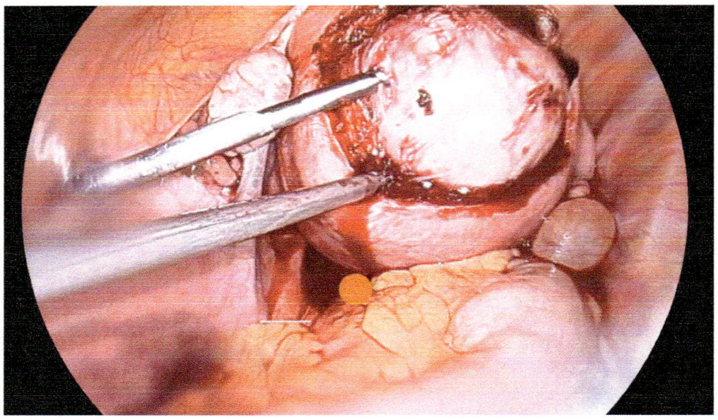

Fig. 7: Use of myoma screw for enucleation of intramural myoma.

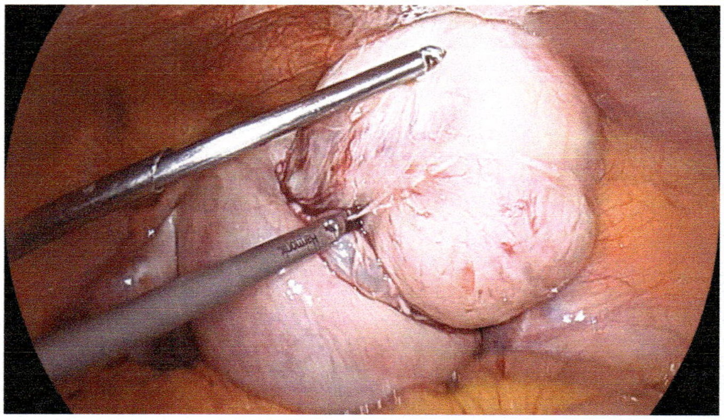

Fig. 8: Traction and countertraction for enucleation of intramural myoma.

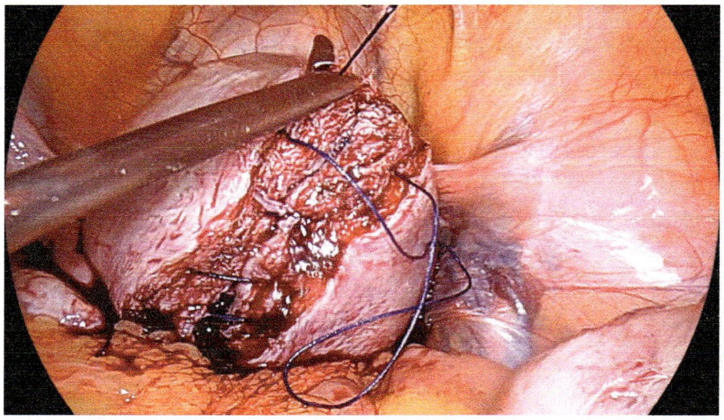

Fig. 9: Suturing of muscle layer of uterus after removal of myoma.

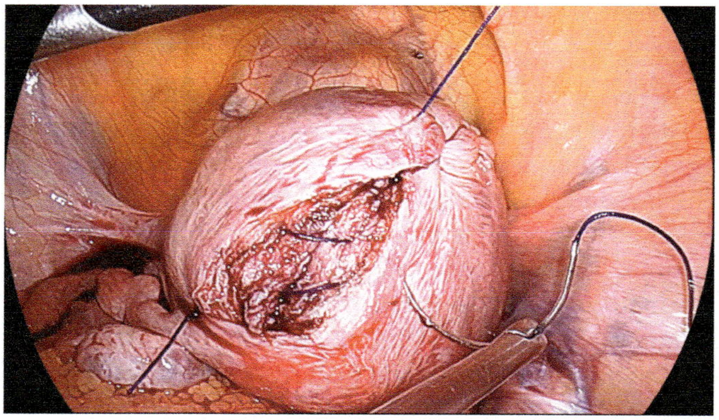

Fig. 10: Suturing of serosal layer after suturing muscle layer of uterus.

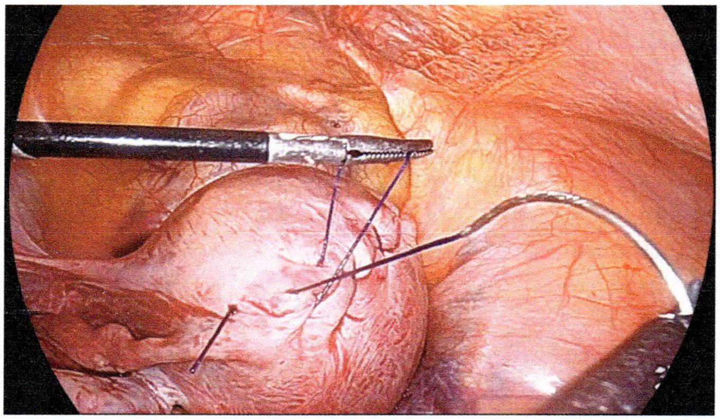

Fig. 11: Continuous suturing of layers of uterus after removal of myoma.

The repair mainly involves suturing of muscle layer and subserosal layer by No. 1 Vicryl or PDS by continuous suture or can be done en masse as one single layer interrupted extracorporeal square knot. Sutures are applied at a distance of 5–10 mm depending on vascularity of myoma in multiple layers according to depth of intramural myoma **(Figs. 9 to 13)**. A new kind of suture, bidirectional barbed thread (Quill™ Self-Retaining System; Angiotech Pharmaceuticals, Inc., Vancouver, British Columbia, Canada), has been recently made available to surgeons; this suture consists of standard material with tiny barbs cut into the length of the thread facing in opposite directions from the midpoint and with a needle at each end.

Common methods of extraction include removal via posterior colpotomy and by electric morcellation **(Figs. 14 and 15)**. The performance of posterior colpotomy is facilitated by an assistant elevating the posterior fornix of the vagina from below with a veil held by a sponge forceps

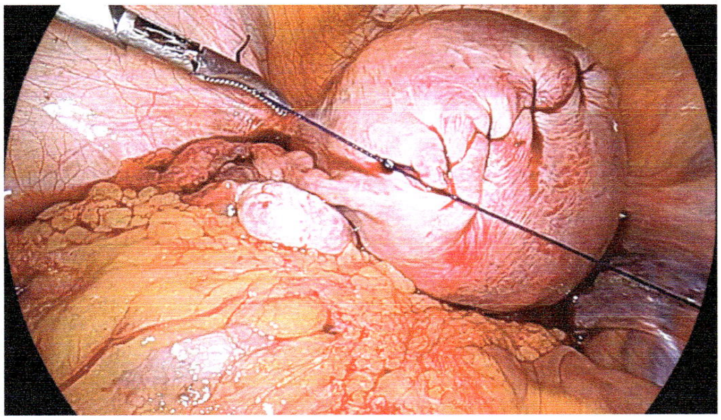

Fig. 12: Suturing knot termination of all the layers of uterus after removal of myoma.

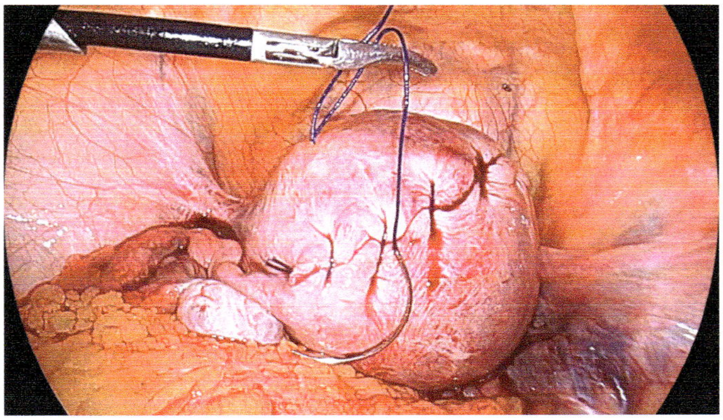

Fig. 13: Completion of suturing of muscle layer and serosal layer after removal of myoma.

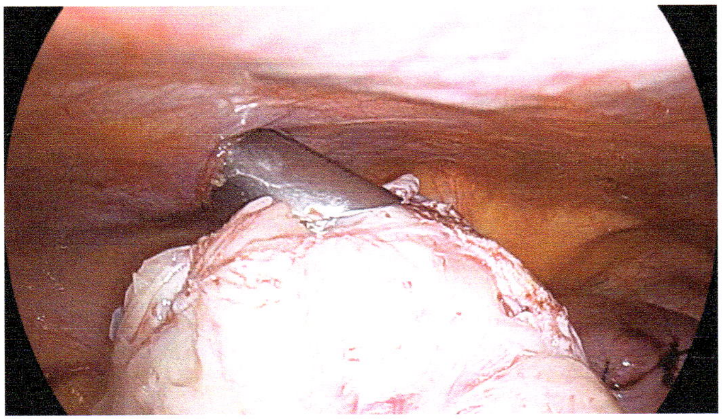

Fig. 14: Careful morcellation of fibroid uterus.

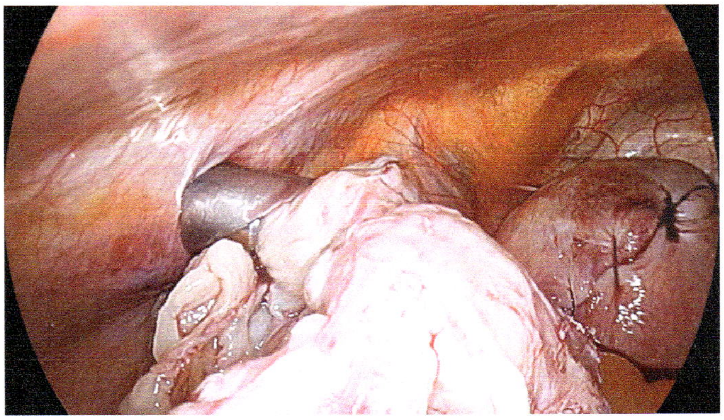

Fig. 15: Morcellation of fibroid uterus should be always under vision.

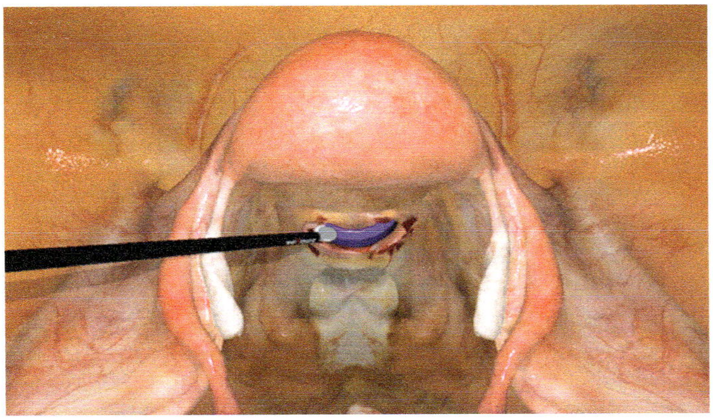

Fig. 16: Posterior colpotomy for removal of myoma with the help of spatula or hook.

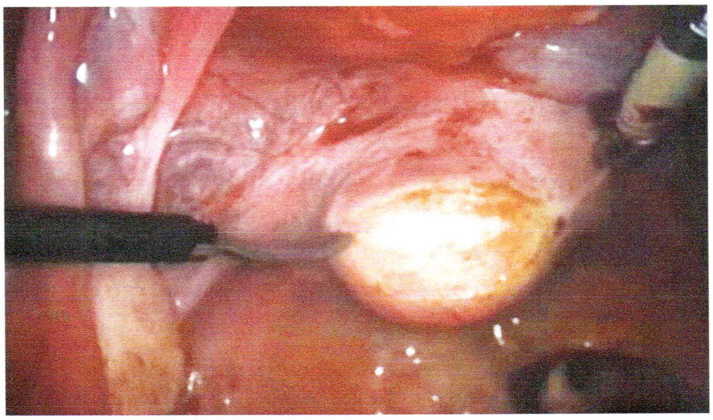

Fig. 17: Posterior colpotomy for removal of myoma with the help of monopolar scissors.

or colpotomizer **(Fig. 16)**. The posterior colpotomy is made about 2 cm above the vaginal attachment of the uterosacral ligaments using monopolar cutting current of spatula, hook, monopolar scissors, or harmonic scalpel **(Fig. 17)**.

A 10-mm forceps with jaws are inserted through the colpotomy under direct vision and this is used to grasp the myoma **(Fig. 18)**. Depending on the size, the myoma may be extracted whole or if large morcellated before extraction through the colpotomy. Alternatively, the 10 mm accessory port may be enlarged to 12–15 mm to allow the introduction of an electric morcellator **(Fig. 19)**. Claw forceps are inserted through the morcellator channel and used to grasp the myoma, which is then progressively cut by the morcellator and extracted piecemeal. The morcellator should be held as if pointing to the abdominal wall in such a way as to avoid the risk of injury to surrounding organs by the morcellator

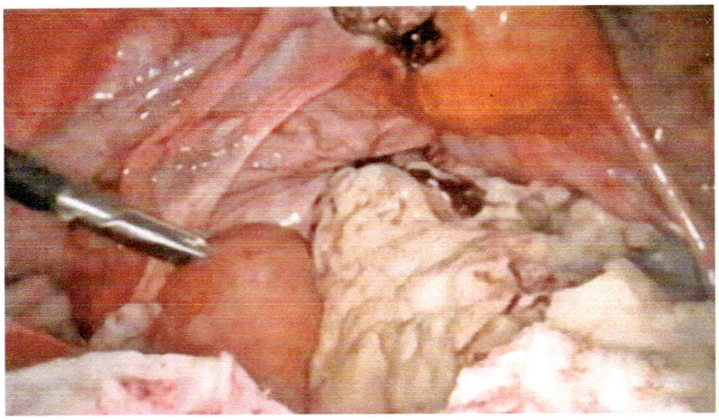

Fig. 18: Extraction of myoma through colpotomy.

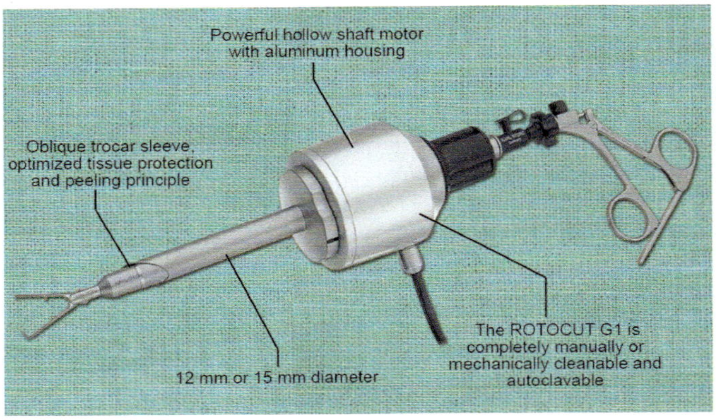

Fig. 19: Morcellator is necessary equipment for myoma tissue retrieval.

blade **(Figs. 14 and 15)**. Following extraction, irrigation is performed as deemed adequate using normal saline. Especially in cases with associated infertility, Interceed may be placed along suture lines as further prophylaxis against adhesions.

After repair, thorough suction and irrigation should be performed. Some gynecologist uses adhesive medical glues over the suture line to prevent adhesion. Even in the hands of an expert, the laparoscopic myomectomy is difficult and challenging. Tumble square knot is advisable, if the edges are in tension. Dundee jamming knot with continuous suturing may be used, if the tension is not too much, followed by Aberdeen termination. Precise suturing of several layers is almost impossible laparoscopically.

Intraligamentous and broad ligament fibroids are difficult to remove due to the risk of injury to ureter and uterine artery at the time of dissection. Following a thorough exposure of ureter and vessels and depending on the location of myoma, an incision is made on the anterior or posterior leaf of the broad ligament and the leiomyomas are slowly shelled as any other subserosal or intramural fibroid.

Throughout the procedure, the location of the ureter is monitored and bleeding points are controlled by bipolar. The broad ligament and peritoneum are not closed in cases of broad ligament myoma. If postoperative oozing is anticipated, a drain should be left.

Upon completion, ports are removed under vision. It is important to ensure that all gas is let out. The 12 mm port is closed using Cobbler needle or Veress needle technique under vision. The port with the telescope is removed last with the telescope in place such that the cannula comes out of the incision before the tip of the telescope. This technique is employed to prevent omentum or bowel entrapment in the incision. The port is closed with sutures previously placed with Cobbler or Veress needle technique. The 5 mm ports do not require closure. The skin incision is closed with staples or Steri-Strip and a dry dressing is applied.

REMOVAL OF MYOMA MORSAFE

The Food and Drug Administration (FDA) looked at studies about the use of power morcellation to find out how often problems occur. They found that anywhere from 1 in 225 to 1 in 580 women treated for fibroids by having their uterus or fibroids removed were later found to have uterine sarcoma. Fibroid removal is one of the difficult and time-consuming procedures. Larger myomas may be removed through a posterior colpotomy. In women with concurrent posterior cul-de-sac pathology, posterior colpotomy is not safe. Medium- and large-sized fibroids are morcellated using a morcellator. The process is ineffective for calcified myomas. For infected tissue and in case of suspected carcinoma, tissue retrieval bag should be used **(Figs. 20 and 21)**. Many sizes of disposable tissue retrieval bags are available and hard rim of these retrieval bags is easy to negotiate inside the abdominal cavity. Morcellation of a malignancy is contraindicated and women should be evaluated preoperatively to identify malignancy. However, leiomyosarcoma cannot be reliably diagnosed preoperatively; thus, there is a risk that a woman with a presumed leiomyoma may have a malignancy that may be spread through morcellation, leading to a potentially worsened prognosis. Although an abdominal hysterectomy or myomectomy may reduce the chance of spreading cancer cells in women with undiagnosed leiomyosarcoma, it is associated with increased morbidity when compared with minimally invasive approaches. The obstetrician–gynecologist and patient should engage in shared decision-making, including informed consent explaining the risks and benefits of each approach to surgery for presumed leiomyomas, the risks and benefits of morcellation, and alternatives to morcellation.

COMPLICATIONS

Laparoscopic myomectomy has all of the usual risks of laparoscopy, predominantly those related to trocar placement. This includes injury to bladder, bowel, ureter,

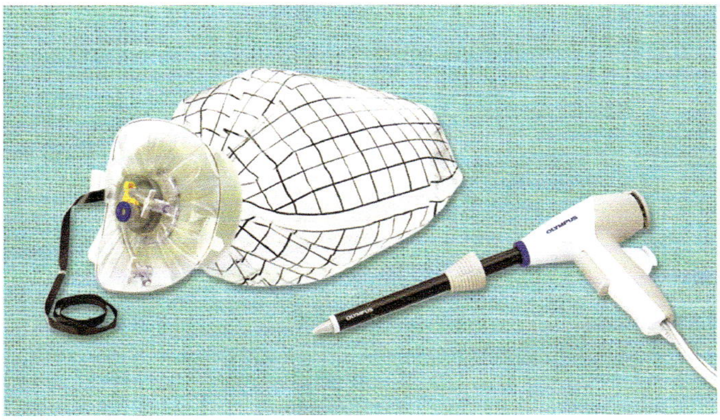

Fig. 20: Morcellation of myoma in Endobag.

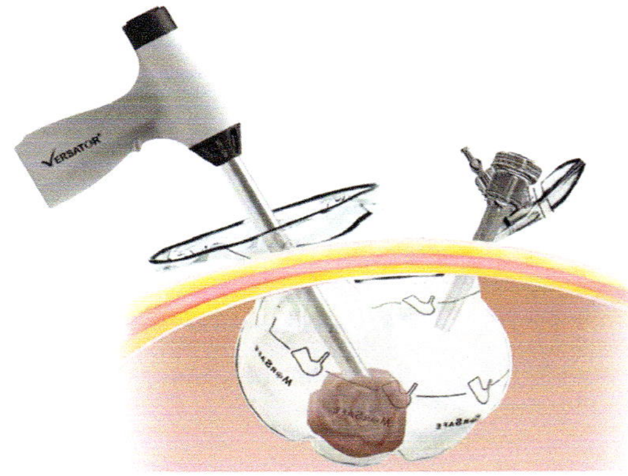

Fig. 21: Morcellation of myoma in Morsafe Endobag.

and blood vessels, and the need to convert to a laparotomy. Rates of conversion vary from very low to 8–10%, largely depending on the complexity of the case.

Suboptimal defect closures are of great concern for uterine rupture in future labor. A number of case reports have been published that describe uterine rupture after laparoscopic myomectomy. Two retrospective analyses evaluating uterine rupture after laparoscopic myomectomy showed no cases of uterine rupture. Another retrospective study showed a rupture rate of 3.7% (2/54 patients). The largest published series of laparoscopic myomectomy reported one uterine rupture per 213 patients. The risk of unexpected leiomyosarcoma is uncertain, but estimates range from 1 in 498 to <1 in 10,000. For women undergoing surgery for presumed leiomyomas, the higher procedural risk of abdominal hysterectomy or myomectomy (to avoid the risk of spreading malignant cells from an unsuspected leiomyosarcoma) must be balanced against the risk of morcellating an unanticipated malignancy and its associated morbidity and mortality. Based on existing data, this balance may favor a minimally invasive approach for younger women. However, because of the increasing prevalence of leiomyosarcoma with advancing age (and interpreting the age cutoff of 50 years used in the decision analyses as a proxy for menopause), for postmenopausal women, this balance may favor procedures that do not involve morcellation.

CONCLUSION

Laparoscopic myomectomy can be regarded as an alternative to open myomectomy in well-selected patients. Most studies failed to document significant differences between the two techniques as to the rate of complications and showed better figures of recovery and hospital stay in the laparoscopy group. Although laparoscopic myomectomy is still an operation that requires high skills, it is possible that the increasing laparoscopic competence of gynecologist, along with the advances in surgical instrumentation and the availability of new suturing materials, will contribute to make it a more widespread procedure.

BIBLIOGRAPHY

1. AAGL Advancing Minimally Invasive Gynecology Worldwide. AAGL practice report: Morcellation during uterine tissue extraction. J Minim Invasive Gynecol. 2014;21:517-30.
2. ACOG Committee Opinion No. 770: Uterine morcellation for presumed leiomyomas. Obstet Gynecol. 2019;133:e238-48.
3. American Cancer Society (ACS). (2021). Survival rates for uterine sarcoma. [online] Available from https://www.cancer.org/cancer/uterine-sarcoma/detection-diagnosis-staging/survival-rates.html. [Last accessed May, 2021].
4. Banas T, Klimek M, Fugiel A, Skotniczny K. Spontaneous uterine rupture at 35 weeks' gestation, 3 years after laparoscopic myomectomy, without signs of fetal distress. J Obstet Gynaecol Res. 2005;31:527-30.
5. Brölmann H, Tanos V, Grimbizis G, Ind T, Philips K, van den Bosch T, et al. Options on fibroid morcellation: a literature review. Gynecol Surg. 2015;12:3-15.
6. Desai VB, Wright JD, Schwartz PE, Gross CP, Xu X. In reply. Obstet Gynecol. 2018;132:519-20.
7. Dubuisson J, Fauconnier A, Deffarges J, Norgaard C, Kreiker G, Chapron C. Pregnancy outcome and deliveries following laparoscopic myomectomy. Hum Reprod. 2000;15:869-73.
8. Dubuisson JB, Fauconnier A, Chapron C, Kreiker G, Norgaard C. Reproductive outcome after laparoscopic myomectomy in infertile women. J Reprod Med. 2000;45:23-30.
9. Einstein MH, Barakat RR, Chi DS, Sonoda Y, Alektiar KM, Hensley ML, et al. Management of uterine malignancy found incidentally after supracervical hysterectomy or uterine morcellation for presumed benign disease. Int J Gynecol Cancer. 2008;18:1065-70.
10. Farmer RM, Kirschbaum T, Potter D, Strong TH, Medearis AL. Uterine rupture during trial of labour after previous cesarean section. Am J Obstet Gynecol. 1991;65:996-1001.
11. Flamm BL, Goings JR, Liu Y, Wolde-Tsadik G. Elective repeat cesarean delivery versus trial of labor: a prospective multicenter study. Obstet Gynecol. 1994;83:927-32.
12. Glaser LM, Friedman J, Tsai S, Chaudhari A, Milad M. Laparoscopic myomectomy and morcellation: a review of techniques, outcomes, and practice guidelines. Best Pract Res Clin Obstet Gynaecol. 2018;46:99-112.
13. Golan D, Aharoni A, Gonen R, Boss Y, Sharf M. Early spontaneous rupture of the post myomectomy gravid uterus. Int J Gynaecol Obstet. 1990;31:167-70.

14. Grande N, Catalano GF, Ferrari S, Marana R. Spontaneous uterine rupture at 27 weeks of pregnancy after laparoscopic myomectomy. J Minim Invasive Gynecol. 2005;12:301.
15. Hensley ML, Leitao MM. (2021). Treatment and prognosis of uterine leiomyosarcoma. [online] Available from https://www.uptodate.com/contents/treatment-and-prognosis-of-uterine-leiomyosarcoma. [Last accessed May, 2021].
16. Hurst BS, Matthews ML, Marshburn PB. Laparoscopic myomectomy for symptomatic uterine myomas. Fertil Steril. 2005;83:1-23.
17. Kumakiri J, Takeuchi H, Kitade M, Kikuchi I, Shimanuki H, Itoh S, et al. Pregnancy and delivery after laparoscopic myomectomy. J Minim Invasive Gynecol. 2005;12:241-6.
18. Landi S, Fiaccavento A, Zaccoletti R, Barbieri F, Syed R, Minelli L. Pregnancy outcomes and deliveries after laparoscopic myomectomy. J Am Assoc Gynecol Laparosc. 2003;10:177-81.
19. Lieng M, Istre O, Langebrekke A. Uterine rupture after laparoscopic myomectomy. J Am Assoc Gynecol Laparosc. 2004;11:92-3.
20. Lynam S, Young L, Morozov V, Rao G, Roque DM. Risk, risk reduction and management of occult malignancy diagnosed after uterine morcellation: a commentary. Womens Health (Lond). 2015;11:929-44.
21. Malin JL, Kahn KL, Adams J, Kwan L, Laouri M, Ganz PA. Validity of cancer registry data for measuring the quality of breast cancer care. J Natl Cancer Inst. 2002;94:835-44.
22. Moore BJ, White S, Washington R, Coenen N, Elixhauser A. Identifying increased risk of readmission and in-hospital mortality using hospital administrative data: The AHRQ Elixhauser Comorbidity Index. Med Care. 2017;55:698-705.
23. Mowers EL, Skinner B, McLean K, Reynolds RK. Effects of morcellation of uterine smooth muscle tumor of uncertain malignant potential and endometrial stromal sarcoma: case series and recommendations for clinical practice. J Minim Invasive Gynecol. 2015;22:601-6.
24. Nielsen TF, Ljungblad U, Hagberg H. Rupture and dehiscence of cesarean section during pregnancy and delivery. Am J Obstet Gynecol. 1989;160:569-73.
25. Nkemayim DC, Hammadeh ME, Hippach M, Mink D, Schmidt W. Uterine rupture in pregnancy subsequent to previous laparoscopic electromyolysis: case report and review of the literature. Arch Gynecol Obstet. 2000;264:154-6.
26. Oduyebo T, Rauh-Hain AJ, Meserve EE, Seidman MA, Hinchcliff E, George S, et al. The value of re-exploration in patients with inadvertently morcellated uterine sarcoma. Gynecol Oncol. 2014;132:360-5.
27. Ozeren M, Ulusov M, Uvanik E. First-trimester spontaneous uterine rupture after traditional myomectomy: case report. Isr J Med Sci. 1997;33:752-3.
28. Pelosi MA, Pelosi MA. Spontaneous uterine rupture at thirty-three weeks subsequent to previous superficial laparoscopic myomectomy. Am J Obstet Gynecol. 1997;177:1547-9.
29. Phelan JP, Clark SL, Diaz F, Paul RH. Vaginal birth after cesarean. Am J Obstet Gynecol. 1987;157:1510-15.
30. Pirracchio R, Resche-Rigon M, Chevret S. Evaluation of the propensity score methods for estimating marginal odds ratios in case of small sample size. BMC Med Res Methodol. 2012;12:70.
31. Pisarska MD, Carson SA. Incidence and risk factors for ectopic pregnancy. Clin Obstet Gynecol. 1999;42:2-8.
32. Raine-Bennett T, Tucker LY, Zaritsky E, Littell RD, Palen T, Neugebauer R, et al. Occult uterine sarcoma and leiomyosarcoma: incidence of and survival associated with morcellation. Obstet Gynecol. 2016;127:29-39.
33. Ramirez PT, Frumovitz M, Pareja R, Lopez A, Vieira M, Ribeiro R, et al. Minimally invasive versus abdominal radical hysterectomy for cervical cancer. N Engl J Med. 2018;379:1895-904.
34. Raspagliesi F, Maltese G, Bogani G, Fucà G, Lepori S, De Iaco P, et al. Morcellation worsens survival outcomes in patients with undiagnosed uterine leiomyosarcomas: a retrospective MITO group study. Gynecol Oncol. 2017;144:90-5.
35. Roopnarinesingh S, Suratsingh J, Roopnarinesingh A. The obstetric outcome of patients with previous myomectomy or hysterotomy. West Indian Med J. 1985;34:59-62.
36. Seagle BLL, Sobecki-Rausch J, Strohl AE, Shilpi A, Grace A, Shahabi S. Prognosis and treatment of uterine leiomyosarcoma: A National Cancer Database study. Gynecol Oncol. 2017;145:61-70.
37. Seinera P, Farina C, Todros T. Laparoscopic myomectomy and subsequent pregnancy: results in 54 patients. Hum Reprod. 2000;15:1993-6.
38. Siedhoff MT, Doll KM, Clarke-Pearson DL, Rutstein SE. Laparoscopic hysterectomy with morcellation vs abdominal hysterectomy for presumed fibroids: an updated decision analysis following the 2014 Food and Drug Administration safety communications. Am J Obstet Gynecol. 2017;216:259.e1-6.
39. Sizzi O, Manganaro L, Rossetti A, Saldari M, Florio G, Loddo A, et al. Assessing the risk of laparoscopic morcellation of occult uterine sarcomas during hysterectomy and myomectomy: Literature review and the ISGE recommendations. Eur J Obstet Gynecol Reprod Biol. 2018;220:30-8.
40. Stewart EA. (2020). Uterine fibroids (leiomyomas): Differentiating fibroids from uterine sarcomas. [online] Available from https://www.uptodate.com/contents/uterine-fibroids-leiomyomas-differentiating-fibroids-from-uterine-sarcomas. [Last accessed May, 2021].
41. Stringer NH, Strassner HT, Lawson L, Oldham L, Estes C, Edwards M, et al. Pregnancy outcomes after laparoscopic myomectomy with ultrasonic energy and laparoscopic suturing of the endometrial cavity. J Am Assoc Gynecol Laparosc. 2001;8:129-36.
42. Tantitamit T, Huang KG, Manopunya M, Yen CF. Outcome and management of uterine leiomyosarcoma treated following surgery for presumed benign disease: review of literature. Gynecol Minim Invasive Ther. 2018;7:47-55.
43. Tissue Extraction Task Force Members. Morcellation during uterine tissue extraction: an update. J Minim Invasive Gynecol. 2018;25:543-50.
44. Tulandi T, Ferenczy A. Biopsy of uterine leiomyomata and frozen sections before laparoscopic morcellation. J Minim Invasive Gynecol. 2014;21:963-6.
45. Wright JD, Cui RR, Wang A, Chen L, Tergas AI, Burke WM, et al. Economic and survival implications of use of electric power morcellation for hysterectomy for presumed benign gynecologic disease. J Natl Cancer Inst. 2015;107:djv251.

CHAPTER 36

Laparoscopic Management of Stress Incontinence

INTRODUCTION

Genuine stress incontinence is the involuntary loss of urine, which occurs when the intravesical pressure exceeds the maximum urethral pressure in the absence of a detrusor contraction. The preferred therapy for genuine stress incontinence is surgery. Urinary incontinence is becoming more prevalent as the population ages. A significant improvement in the psychological status of these patients after the successful surgical cure of stress incontinence has been demonstrated.

PATHOPHYSIOLOGY

In genuine stress incontinence, the proximal urethra is displaced outside the abdominal cavity. Stress incontinence then results from inadequate transmission of increase in intra-abdominal pressure to the proximal urethra. The urethra has, in fact, lost its retropubic position due to attenuated support. As a result, coughing will produce an immediate increase in intravesical pressure but not a concomitant increase in intraurethral pressure and a dribble of urine results **(Fig. 1)**.

More than 160 types of operations are available to correct stress urinary incontinence (SUI), an optimal approach has not yet been developed. On April 16, 2019, the Food and Drug Administration (FDA) ordered all manufacturers of surgical mesh intended for transvaginal repair of SUI. Surgical mesh has been used for urogynecologic procedures, including repair of pelvic organ prolapse (POP) and SUI. It is permanently implanted to reinforce the weakened vaginal wall for POP repair or support the urethra or bladder neck for the repair of SUI. There are three main surgical procedures performed with surgical mesh to treat pelvic floor disorders with surgical mesh:

1. Transvaginal mesh to treat POP
2. Transabdominal mesh to treat POP
3. Mesh sling to treat SUI

Each of these procedures has unique risks and benefits and it is important not to confuse the procedures and their risks and benefits. Since the FDA has not received sufficient evidence to assure that the probable benefits of these devices outweigh their probable risks, the agency has concluded that these products do not have reasonable assurance of safety and effectiveness.

The Burch procedure is considered by many to be the gold standard for surgical treatment of genuine stress incontinence **(Fig. 2)**. The Burch procedure requires the elevation of the anterior wall of the vagina to the level of the origin of the paravaginal fascia by suspension from Cooper's ligaments (iliopectineal ligaments). A properly performed Burch procedure cures in up to 93% of cases.

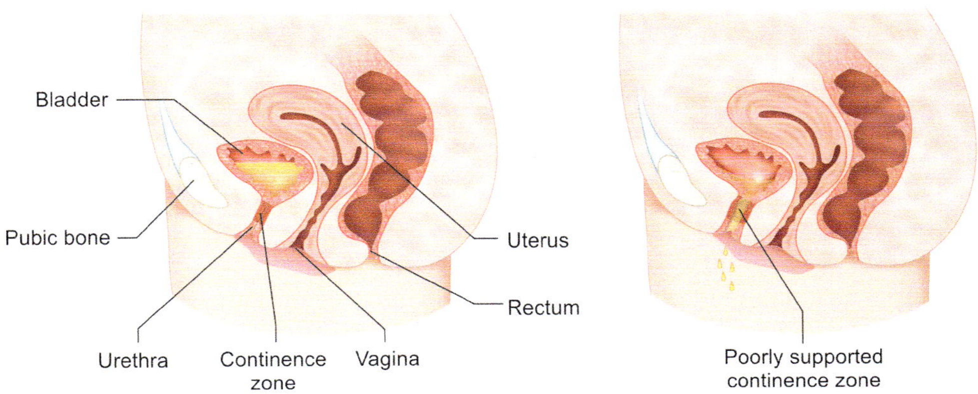

Fig. 1: Pathophysiology of stress urinary incontinence.

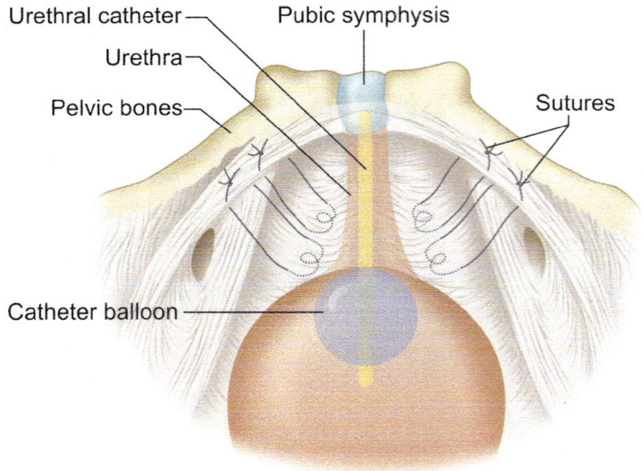

Fig. 2: Laparoscopic Burch suspension.

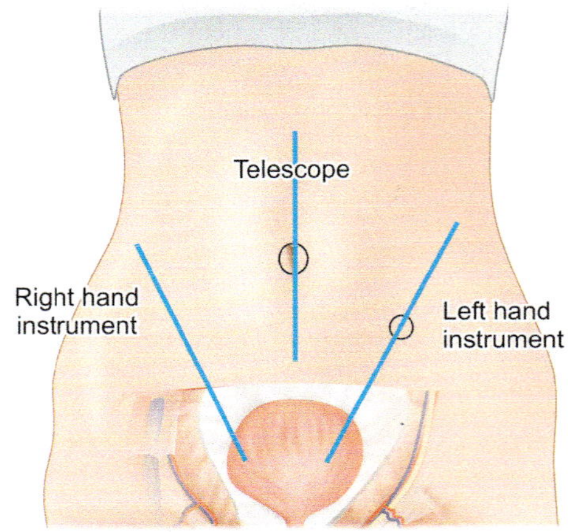

Fig. 3: Port position for Burch suspension surgery.

INDICATIONS

Eligible patients include women who decline or have persistent symptoms following a trial of conservative management. Women who have mixed urinary incontinence may be able to control their symptoms of urge incontinence and provide enough satisfaction that management of SUI is no longer necessary.

CONTRAINDICATIONS

- Patients with type III SUI (a fixed, nonfunctioning proximal urethra) are not candidates for a Burch procedure, as no hypermobility exists to correct
- Patients having cystocele, rectocele, or introital deficiency
- Patients not completed childbearing

LAPAROSCOPIC ANATOMY

The space of Retzius lies between the vesicoumbilical fascia posteriorly and the posterior rectus sheath and pubic bone anteriorly. This is the space first entered in Burch suspension.

Preoperative Evaluation

Postmenopausal women should receive at least 3 months of estrogen replacement therapy. Preoperative evaluation includes history, physical, gynecologic, and neurologic examinations. The routine tests include stress test, Q-tip test, urinalysis, urine culture, and sensitivity. All women should undergo an urodynamic evaluation, with emphasis on voiding time, voiding volume, and postvoid residual urine volume. Stress incontinence is diagnosed by a positive stress test in the absence of simultaneous detrusor contractions or pressure equalization on the stress urethral closure pressure profile.

Operative Technique

Following the induction of general endotracheal anesthesia, a Foley catheter should be applied in the bladder. A 10-mm operative video laparoscope is inserted infraumbilical and two 5 mm accessory trocars are inserted according to baseball diamond concept **(Fig. 3)**.

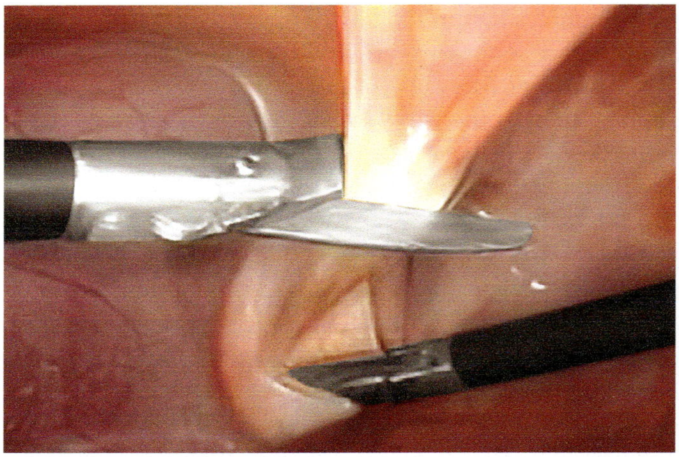

Fig. 4: Peritoneal incision in midline.

300 cc of methylene blue solution is filled into the bladder to keep the bladder weighted down and to allow the clear delineation of the dome of the bladder. Three-port techniques are used one in umbilicus and two 5 mm port 7.5 cm lateral and slightly below the umbilicus **(Fig. 3)**.

The anterior abdominal wall peritoneum 2 cm above the delineated dome of distended bladder is cut and pulled down. To enter the space of Retzius intra-abdominally, the umbilical ligaments are identified laterally **(Fig. 4)**.

The space of Retzius is developed using blunt and CO_2 dissection of fibrofatty tissue. Care is taken to avoid obturator nerve and aberrant obturator vessel injury. The midline trocar entry and anatomic landmarks, including the round ligament from the internal ring, are used to avoid bladder injury. Blunt dissection is used to expose the retropubic space. Surgeon should stay close to the back of the pubic bone, dropping the anterior bladder wall, vaginal wall, and urethra downward. Dissection is limited over the urethra in the midline, to approximately 2 cm lateral to the

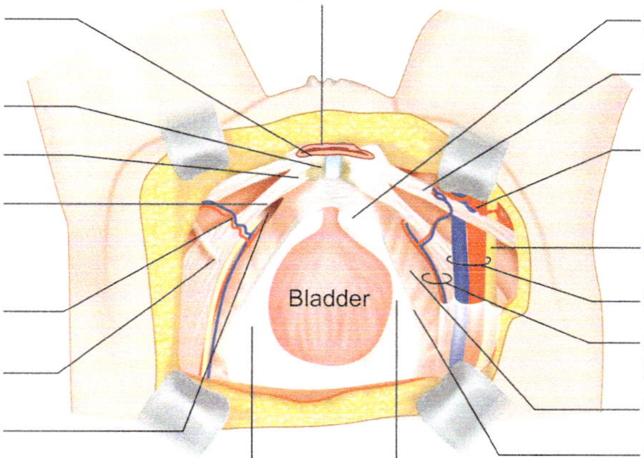

Fig. 5: Retropubic dissection to detect Cooper's ligament and tendinous arc of levator ani muscle.

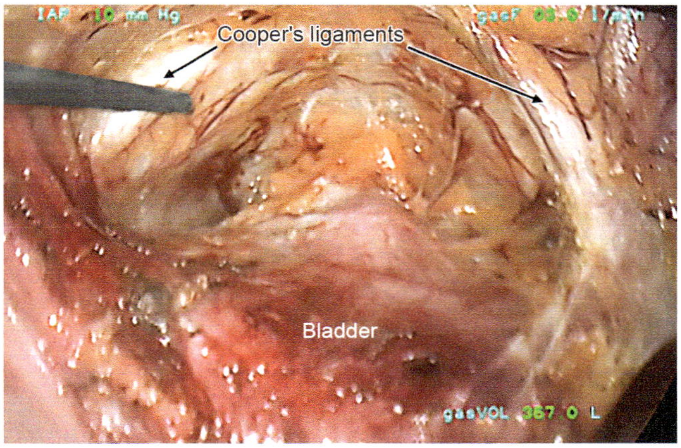

Fig. 6: Retropubic dissection to detect Cooper's ligament (arrows).

urethra, to protect its delicate musculature. An assistant should introduce one finger on each side of the catheterized urethra, elevating the lateral vaginal fornix. The overlying fibrofatty tissue is cleared laparoscopically from the anterior vaginal wall. The bladder is dissected medially from the paravaginal fascia from lateral to medial. Blunt dissection with atraumatic grasper is continued until the urethrovesical junction becomes apparent and the white glistening tissue of the paravaginal fascia appears.

Bladder muscle fibers of the urethrovesical junction should not be damaged at the time of dissection. Bleeding, if happens in this area, is controlled only with bipolar electrocoagulation because monopolar current can cause perforation of bladder or stricture of ureter. Retropubic dissection is continued until Cooper's ligament is clearly exposed **(Figs. 5 and 6)**.

Dissection in the space of Retzius is difficult in patients who have undergone previous laparotomy. Pneumoperitoneum pressure helps provide exposure of the space and its contents out to the obturator nerve.

The space of Retzius also can be entered with a preperitoneal approach just like total extraperitoneal hernia surgery. The balloon dissector consists of a cannula and balloon system. The dissector is inserted through a 10-mm infraumbilical incision. It is advanced between the rectus muscle and the anterior surface of the posterior rectus sheath toward the symphysis pubis **(Figs. 7A and B)**. The dissector's external sheath is removed and the balloon is inflated with approximately 500 mL of saline solution. During inflation, the balloon unrolls sideways and exerts a perpendicular force that separates tissue layers. A blunt dissection of the connective tissues is propagated as the balloon expands. Full dissection takes about 1 minute but surgeon should keep the balloon inflated for 5 minutes to achieve proper hemostasis. Lateral pressure of balloon will stop capillary bleeding, if kept for 5 minutes. When maximal volume is reached, the balloon is deflated and removed through the incision **(Figs. 8A and B)**.

The dissected space is insufflated with CO_2 at a pressure of 8–10 mm Hg. The predefined shape of the balloon, its nonelastomeric material, and the incompressible character of the saline assure a large, relatively bloodless working space of predictable size and shape. The space is adequate for identification of pertinent landmarks and unencumbered manipulation of endoscopic surgical instruments.

After complete dissection, the paravaginal fascia is identified as glistening fascia over the finger of assistant. Using a needle holder, a suture is placed over the paravaginal fascia at the level of the urethrovesical junction, approximately 1–1.5 cm from the urethra. The urethrovesical junction can be identified easily because of the Foley bulb with the catheter under gentle traction. This suture is placed perpendicular to the vaginal axis to include approximately 0.5–1 cm of tissue.

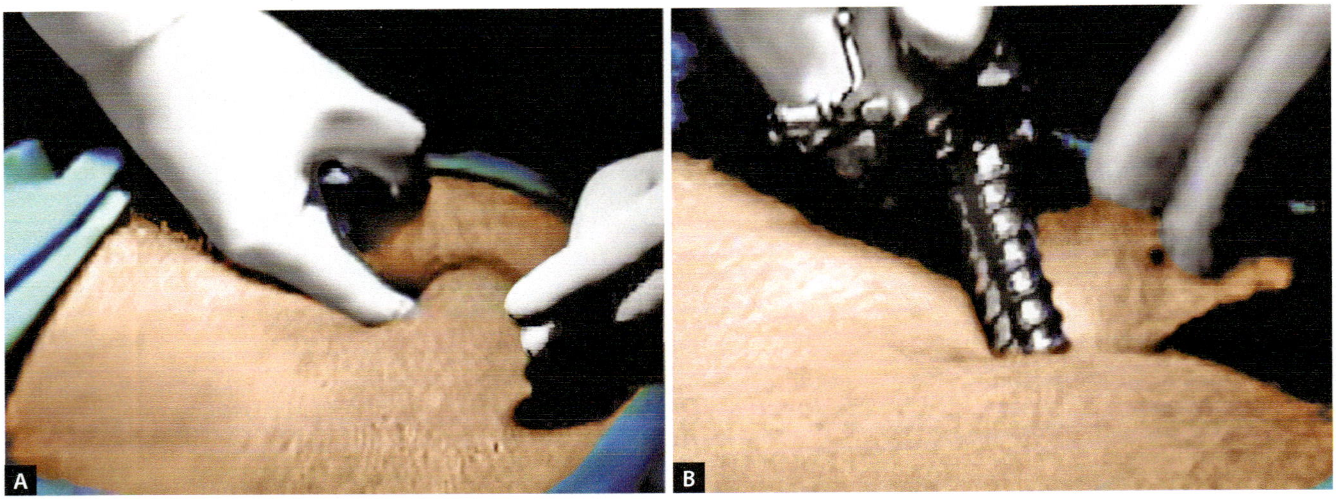

Figs. 7A and B: Extraperitoneal approach.

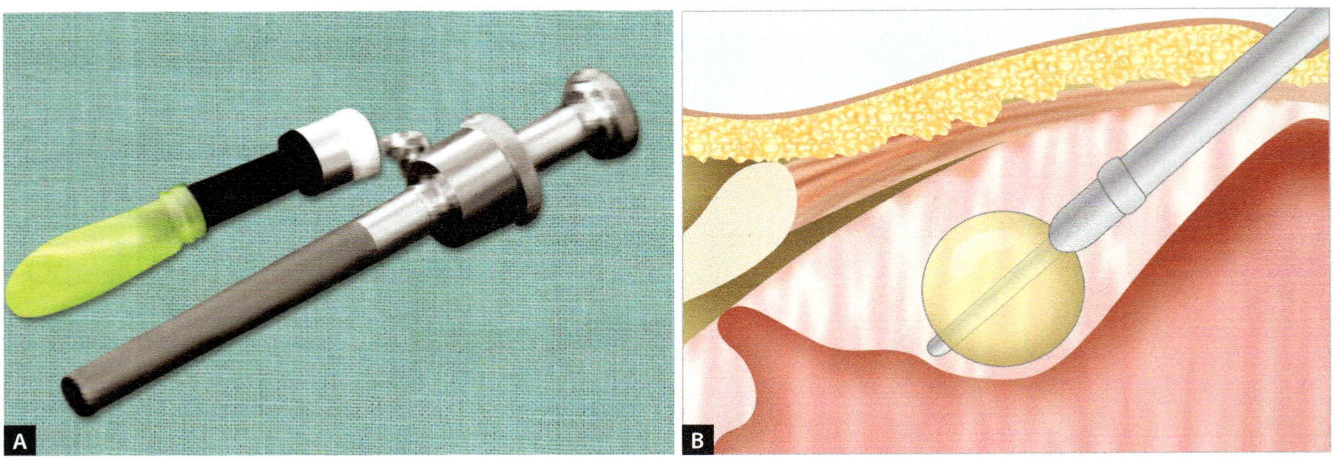

Figs. 8A and B: Balloon dilatation.

The complete vaginal fascia should be taken, so that it will not cut through. Precaution should be taken that suture does not penetrate the vaginal mucosa. Once the suture is placed over the paravaginal fascia, the suture is fixed to Cooper's ligament or the midline of the symphysis pubis.

The suture is tied either intracorporeally or extracorporeally with the help from an assistant who lifts the vagina upward and forward **(Fig. 9)**. The urethra is observed carefully to prevent it from being compressed against the pubic bone **(Fig. 10)**. This same suturing technique is repeated on the opposite side and the aim is to create a platform on which the bladder neck can rest **(Fig. 11)**. If the suspension is not enough with one suture, a second and rarely, a third set of sutures can be placed along the base of the bladder proximally.

After taking suture on both sides, cystoscopy should be performed to ensure that there is no suture pierced in the bladder. Cystoscopy also helps to assess the urethrovesical junction angle and to check uretheral patency.

Once the procedure is finished, the pneumoperitoneum pressure is decreased and the retropubic space is evaluated. If there is any bleeding, it is controlled with bipolar electrocoagulation. The peritoneal defect may be left open to heal spontaneously, or, if it is large, it should be closed laparoscopically with three to four interrupted or purse string sutures. The laparoscope is withdrawn from the abdomen and the procedure is concluded. The Foley catheter should be left in place for 2–3 days. If there is any fear of detrusor instability or bladder injury, the Foley catheter should be kept in place for 1 week or more.

Intercourse should be avoided for 6–8 weeks postoperatively and the patients are advised to avoid heavy lifting or strenuous exercise for at least 2 months.

POSTOPERATIVE COMPLICATIONS

- Anesthetic risks
- Wound complications including infection and hernia
- Bleeding/hematoma formation

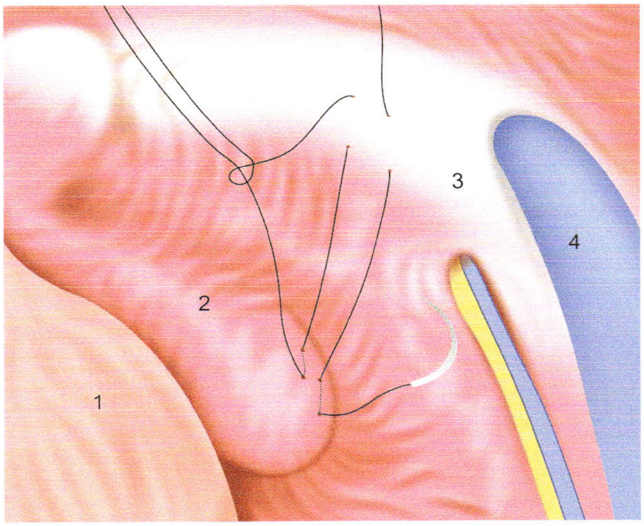

Fig. 9: Suturing of paravaginal fascia with Cooper's ligament with the help of assistant finger.

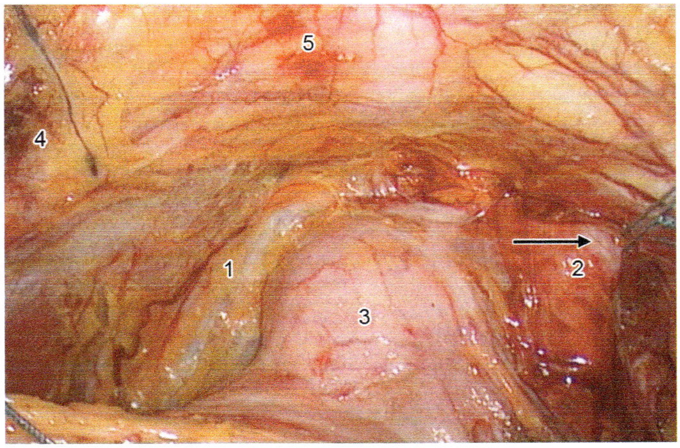

Fig. 10: Suturing of paravaginal fascia with Cooper's ligament (arrow). (1) Paravaginal fascia without suture applied; (2) Paravaginal fascia with suture applied; (3) Bladder; (4) Cooper's ligament of left side; (5) Pubic symphysis.

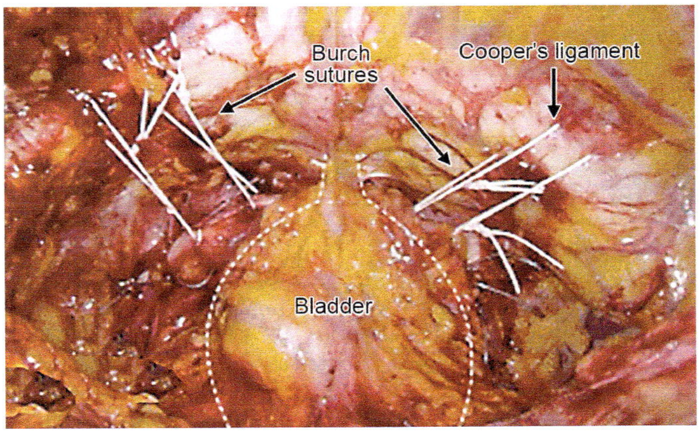

Fig. 11: Final view of suture placement in Burch suspension.

- Deep venous thrombosis
- Voiding difficulty
- Urinary retention, which may require catheter drainage or clean intermittent catheterization
- Development of urgency urinary incontinence
- Development of vaginal wall prolapse

Some of the less common problems are:

- New onset of intrinsic sphincteric deficiency
- Voiding pain
- Ureteral obstruction requiring reoperation
- Vesicovaginal fistula
- Vesicocutaneous fistula
- Foreign body erosion, if tacks were used for laparoscopic repair

CONCLUSION

Burch colposuspension has been shown to be a highly effective surgical treatment for SUI with low recurrence rates, although there is some loss of efficacy with time similar to other procedures. Concerning the laparoscopic approach, the conclusion from the Cochrane review was that the available evidence suggests that it may be as effective as open colposuspension 2 years postoperatively. The National Institute for Health and Care Excellence (NICE) guidelines include among their recommendations that laparoscopic Burch colposuspension is not recommended as a routine procedure for the treatment of SUI in women. In current recommendations, Burch colposuspension remains an option for secondary treatment. Because midurethral slings have recently become under scrutiny, it may return as a first-line treatment procedure. Laparoscopic Burch colposuspension should, therefore, nowadays be provided in fellowship programs worldwide.

BIBLIOGRAPHY

1. Alcalay M, Monga A, Stanton SL. Burch colposuspension: a 10–20 year follow up. Br J Obst Gynaecol. 1995;102:740-5.
2. Ankardal M, Ekerydh A, Crafoord K, Milsom I, Stjerndahl JH, Engh ME. A randomised trial comparing open Burch colposuspension using sutures with laparoscopic colposuspension using mesh and staples in women with stress urinary incontinence. BJOG. 2004;111:974-81.
3. Bo K, Talseth T, Holme I. Single blind, randomised, controlled trial of pelvic floor exercises, electrical stimulation, vaginal cones and no treatment in management of genuine stress incontinence in women. BMJ. 1999;318:487-93.
4. Boyles SH, Webber AM, Meyn L. Procedures for urinary incontinence in the United States 1979–1997. Am J Obstet Gynecol. 2003;189:70-5.

5. Burch JC. Urethro-vaginal fixation to Cooper's ligament for correction of stress incontinence, cystocoele and prolapse. Am J Obstet Gynecol. 1961;81:281-90.
6. Burton G. A five year prospective randomised urodynamic study comparing open and laparoscopic colposuspension. Neurourol Urodyn. 1999;18:295-6.
7. Cardozo L, Drutz HP, Baygani SK, Bump RC. Pharmacological treatment of women awaiting surgery for stress urinary incontinence. Obstet Gynecol. 2004;104:511-9.
8. Cardozo LD, Cutner AA. Surgical management of stress incontinence. Contemp Rev Obstet Gynaecol. 1992;4:36-41.
9. Chaliha C, Stanton SL. Complications of surgery for genuine stress incontinence. Br J Obst Gynaecol. 1999;106:1238-45.
10. Christofi N, Hextall A. Which procedure for incontinence? J Br Menopause Soc. 2005;11:23-7.
11. Delorme E. Transobturator urethral suspension: a mini-invasive procedure on the treatment of stress urinary incontinence in women. Prog Urol. 2001;11:1306-13.
12. Duckett JRA. The use of periurethral injectables in the treatment of genuine stress incontinence. Br J Obst Gynaecol. 1998;105:390-6.
13. Eckford SD, Abrams P. Para-urethral collagen implantation for female stress incontinence. Br J Urol. 1991;68:586-9.
14. Foldspang A, Mommsen S. Overweight and urinary incontinence in women. Ugeskr Laeger. 1995;157:5848-51.
15. Gorton E, Stanton S, Monga A, Wiskind AK, Lentz GM, Bland DR. Periurethral collagen injection: a long-term follow-up study. BJU Int. 1999;84:966-71.
16. Groutz A, Gordon D, Woman I, Jaffa AJ, David MP, Lessing JB. Tension-free vaginal tape for stress urinary incontinence: is there a learning curve? Neurourol Urodyn. 2002;21:470-2.
17. Henalla SM, Hall V, Duckett JR, Link C, Usman F, Tromans PM, et al. A multicentre evaluation of a new surgical technique for urethral bulking in the treatment of genuine stress incontinence. BJOG. 2000;107:1035-9.
18. Hilton P, Mayne C. The Stamey endoscopic bladder neck suspension: a clinical and urodynamic investigation including actuarial follow-up over four years. Br J Obstet Gynaecol. 1999;98:1141-9.
19. Huang KH, Kung FT, Liang HM, Huang LY, Chang SY. Concomitant surgery with tension-free vaginal tape. Acta Obstet Gynecol Scand. 2003;82:948-53.
20. Iosif CF, Bekassy Z, Ryhdestrom H. Prevalence of urinary incontinence in middle age women. Int J Gynecol Obstet. 1980;26:255-9.
21. Iosif CF, Bekassy Z. Prevalence of genitourinary symptoms in the menopause. Acta Obstet Gynecol Scand. 1984;63:257-60.
22. Jarvis GJ, Hall S, Stamp S, Millar DR, Johnson A. An assessment of urodynamic examination in incontinent women. Br J Obst Gynaecol. 1980;87:893-6.
23. Jarvis GJ. Surgery for genuine stress incontinence. Br J Obst Gynaecol. 1994;101:371-4.
24. Jolleys JV. Reported prevalence of urinary incontinence in a general practice. BMJ. 1988;296:1300-2.
25. Khullar V, Cardozo LD, Abbott D, Anders K. GAX collagen in the treatment of urinary incontinence in elderly women: a two year follow-up. Br J Obstet Gynaecol. 1997;104:96-9.
26. Kligman AM, Armstrong RC. Histologic response to intradermal Zyderm and Zyplast (glutaraldehyde cross-linked) collagen in humans. J Dermatol Surg Oncol. 1986;12:351-7.
27. Kondo A, Saito M, Yamada Y, Kato T, Hasegawa S, Kato K. Prevalence of hand-washing incontinence in females in comparison with stress and urge incontinence. Neurourol Urodyn. 1990;19:330-1.
28. Mommsen S, Foldspang A. Body mass index and adult urinary incontinence. World J Urol. 1994;12:319-22.
29. Monga AK, Robinson D, Stanton SL. Peri-urethral collagen injections for genuine stress incontinence: a two year follow-up. Br J Urol. 1995;76:156-60.
30. Mukherjee K, Constantine G. Urinary stress incontinence in obese women: tension-free vaginal tape is the answer. BJU Int. 2001;88:881-3.
31. National Institute for Clinical Excellence (NICE). Guidance on the Use of TVT for Stress Incontinence. Technology Appraisal Guidance No. 56. London: NICE; 2003.
32. National Institute for Clinical Excellence (NICE). Interventional Procedures Review of Transobturator Tape Insertion for Stress Urinary Incontinence. London: NICE; 2004.
33. Pickard R, Reaper J, Wyness L, Cody DJ, McClinton S, N'Dow J. Periurethral injection therapy for urinary incontinence in women. Cochrane Database Syst Rev. 2003;2:CD003881.
34. Rekers H, Drogendijk AC, Valkenburg H, Riphagen F. Urinary incontinence in women from 35 to 79 years of age: prevalence and consequences. Eur J Obstet Gynecol Reprod Biol. 1992;43:229-34.
35. Schultheiss D, Höfner K, Oelke M, Grünewald V, Jonas U. Percutaneous bladder neck suspension with bone anchors: an improvement in the therapy of female stress urinary incontinence. Neurourol Urodyn. 1998;17:457-8.
36. Ulmsten U, Petros P. Intravaginal salingoplasty: an ambulatory surgical procedure for the treatment of female urinary incontinence. Scand J Urol Nephrol. 1995;29:75-82.
37. Ulmsten U, Henriksson L, Johnson P, Varhos G. An ambulatory surgical procedure under local anaesthesia for treatment for female urinary incontinence. Int Urogynecol J. 1996;7:81-6.
38. Van Kerrebroeck P, Abrams P, Lange R. Duloxetine urinary incontinence study group. Br J Obst Gynaecol. 2004;111:249-57.
39. Vancaillie TG, Schuessler W. Laparoscopic bladderneck suspension. J Laparoendosc Surg. 1991;1:169-73.
40. Vetter NJ, Jones DA, Victor CR. Urinary incontinence in the elderly at home. Lancet. 1981;2:1275-7.
41. Ward K, Hilton P. Prospective multicentre randomised trial of tension-free vaginal tape and colposuspension for primary urodynamic stress incontinence: two year follow-up. Am J Obstet Gynecol. 2004;190:324-31.
42. Ward K, Hilton P. Prospective multicentre randomised trial of tension-free vaginal tape and colposuspension as primary treatment for stress incontinence. BMJ. 2002;325:67-70.

CHAPTER 37

Minimally Invasive Sling Operation for Stress Incontinence

INTRODUCTION

Female stress urinary incontinence (SUI) may be broadly subcategorized into types I, II, and III as follows:

- Type I SUI is defined as urine loss occurring in the absence of urethral hypermobility. This is the mildest form of SUI
- Type II SUI is defined as urine loss occurring due to urethral hypermobility. This is also known as genuine stress urinary incontinence (GSUI)
- Type III SUI is defined as urine leakage occurring from an intrinsic sphincter deficiency (ISD). ISD is a more complex form of female SUI

The subcategories of female SUI can be ascertained by direct physical examination and by measuring an abdominal leak point pressure (ALPP). ALPP, also known as the Valsalva or stress leak point pressure, is defined as the lowest abdominal pressure necessary to cause urine leakage.

An ALPP < 60 cm water is considered diagnostic of type III SUI, whereas an ALPP of 90–120 cm water is consistent with type II SUI. Values of 60–90 cm water reflect the presence of both type II and type III in combination. An ALPP > 120 cm water is considered diagnostic of type I SUI. Recent experience suggests that leak point pressures need not be stratified as they were in the past, as new slings manage all types of SUI.

Von Giordano is usually credited with performing the first pubovaginal sling operation in 1907, using a gracilis muscle graft around the urethra. In 1914, Frangenheim used rectus abdominis muscle and fascia for pubovaginal slings. In 1942, Aldridge, Millin, and Read corrected urinary incontinence using fascial slings. In 1965, Zoedler and Boeminghous first introduced synthetic slings.

Several different sling procedures are currently used to treat incontinence. Whatever sling surgery is performed, one should use the technique that produces the best outcomes in the hands of that particular surgeon.

Mesh sling procedures are currently the most common types of surgery performed to correct SUI. Based on industry estimates, there were approximately 250,000 of these procedures performed every year.

TENSION-FREE VAGINAL TAPE

Stress urinary incontinence or genuine stress incontinence is a problem of the urinary bladder where the urethral sphincter weakens and as a result cannot prevent the flow of urine through it when the intra-abdominal pressure rises such as in coughing, sneezing, lifting something heavy, or even standing or walking.

There are several causes of urethral sphincter weakness, most common being:

- Unattended pregnancy and childbirth
- Frequent heavy lifting
- Estrogen deficiency or menopause
- Obesity

Urinary incontinence is reported by 14% of women and urodynamic stress incontinence, the involuntary leakage of urine during increased abdominal pressure in the absence of a detrusor contraction, is diagnosed in over half of the women out of those presenting to hospital with urinary incontinence. Systematic reviews have shown that colposuspension has the best surgical results when compared with other treatments for urodynamic stress incontinence, with cure rates of up to 90% in women who have had no previous surgery for incontinence, although there are only limited data from randomized trials on which to base clinical practice. Although colposuspension remains the most popular choice for the treatment of stress incontinence, some authors have reported less than half of patients remaining dry and free of complications long term. Complications include hemorrhage, hematoma, bladder injury, and urinary tract infection. Up to 20% of women may develop *de novo* detrusor overactivity; voiding dysfunction has been reported in 3–32% of women and surgery for vaginal prolapse may be required in 2.5–26.7% after the procedure.

Minimally invasive suburethral sling procedures have nowadays become the most popular surgical treatment of SUI in women. Transvaginal tape is a minimally invasive procedure for women who suffer from SUI. In transvaginal tape, the urinary bladder and urethra are repaired, strengthened, and returned to its original position in the pelvis. Tension-free vaginal tape (also known as TVT) was first introduced in Sweden in the mid-1990s by Ulf Ulmsten and Papa Petros. The American Urological Association (AUA) had established a task force to determine the most effective operations for the treatment of SUI. They concluded with the most curative operations as published in the worldwide medically indexed literature as these: Burch urethral suspension procedure and the suburethral sling operation. Cure rates for both procedures were found to fall routinely between 80 and 90%. The TVT operation is a "sling" operation and its cure rate falls within the international standards of cure for other types of sling procedures. The TVT procedure is a relatively recent treatment for stress incontinence.

A polypropylene tape is inserted suburethrally under local anesthesia with sedation. The procedure is thought to work by providing a pubourethral "neoligament". Increased intraabdominal pressure results in a kink at the point of fixation, which prevents urine flow **(Fig. 1)**.

Surgical Technique

The patient should be placed in the lithotomy position taking care to avoid hip flexion >60°. The procedure can be carried out even under local anesthesia, but it may also be performed using regional or general anesthesia. The extent of dissection is minimal, i.e., a vaginal midline entry with a small paraurethral dissection to initially position the needle and two suprapubic skin incisions.

Using forceps, grasp the vaginal wall at each side of the urethra. Using a small scalpel, make a sagittal incision about 1.5 cm long starting approximately 1.0 cm from the outer urethral meatus. This incision will cover the midurethral zone and will allow for subsequent passage of the sling (tape).

With a small pair of blunt scissors, two small paraurethral dissections (approximately 0.5 cm) are made so that the tip of the needle can then be introduced into or passed through the paraurethral dissection **(Fig. 2)**.

Then, two abdominal skin incisions of 0.5–1 cm are made one on each side of the midline just above the symphysis not >4–5 cm apart. Incision placement and needle passage near the midline and close to the back of the pubic bone are important to avoid anatomic structures in the inguinal area and lateral pelvic sidewall.

The TVT rigid catheter guide is inserted into the channel of the Foley catheter (18 French). The handle of the guide is fixed around the catheter, proximal to its widening. The purpose of the guide is to move the bladder neck and urethra away from where the tip of the needle will pass into the retropubic space **(Figs. 3A and B)**.

Via use of the Foley catheter and the rigid catheter guide, the urethra and bladder are moved contralaterally to the side of the needle passage. During this maneuver, the bladder should be empty. Using the introducer, the needle is passed paraurethrally penetrating the urogenital diaphragm. Insertion and passage are controlled by using the long or index finger in the vagina under the vaginal wall on the ipsilateral side and fingertip control on the pelvic rim. The curved part of the needle should rest in the palm of the "vaginal" hand.

If you are right handed, this means that the left hand generally is the one to be used for needle guidance **(Figs. 4A to C)**. With the other hand, grip the handle of the introducer gently. Now introduce the needle tip into the retropubic space. Once again, observe that this should be done by the palm of the vaginal hand and with the needle tip horizontally, i.e., in the frontal plane. After passage of the urogenital diaphragm, you will feel that the resistance is significantly reduced. Immediately aim the tip of the needle

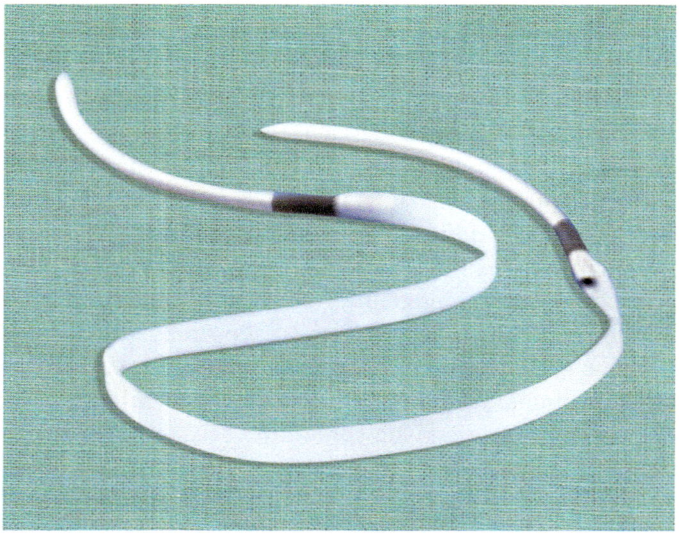

Fig. 1: Tension-free vaginal tape.

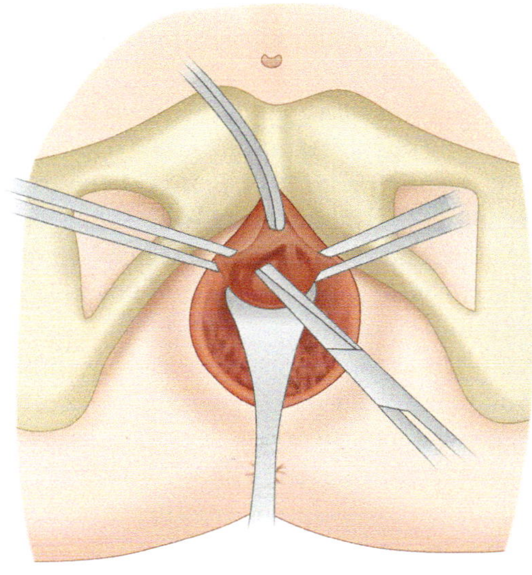

Fig. 2: Abdominal and vaginal incision for tension-free vaginal type (TVT).

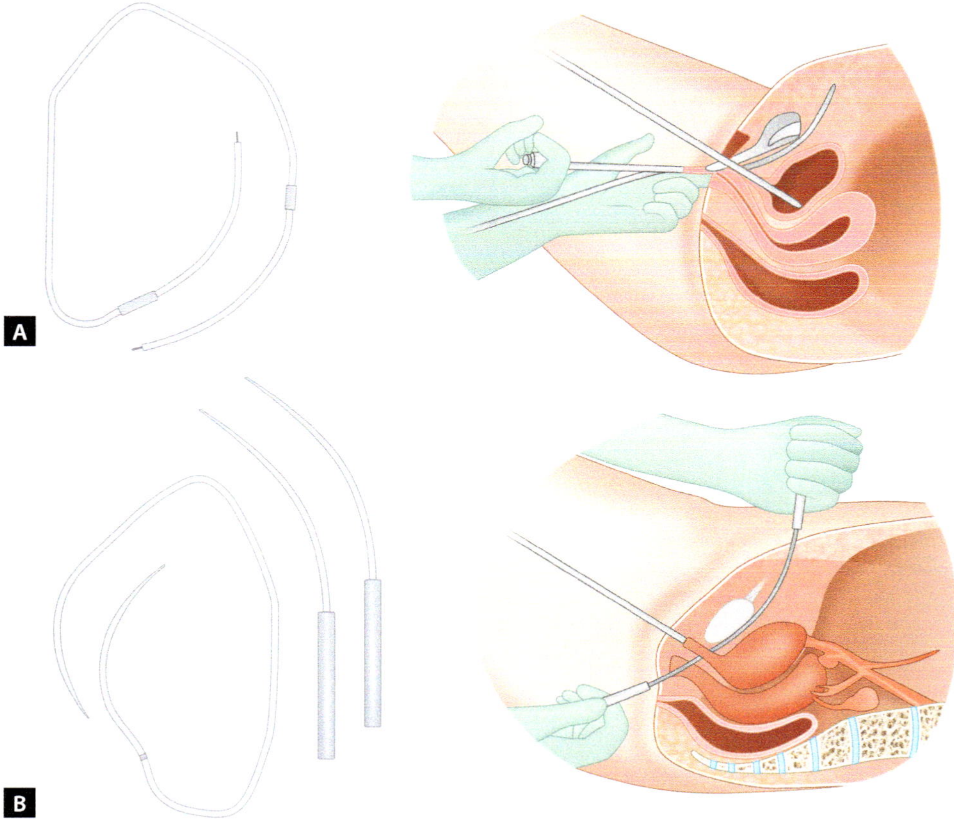

Figs. 3A and B: Passage of needle through retropubic space.

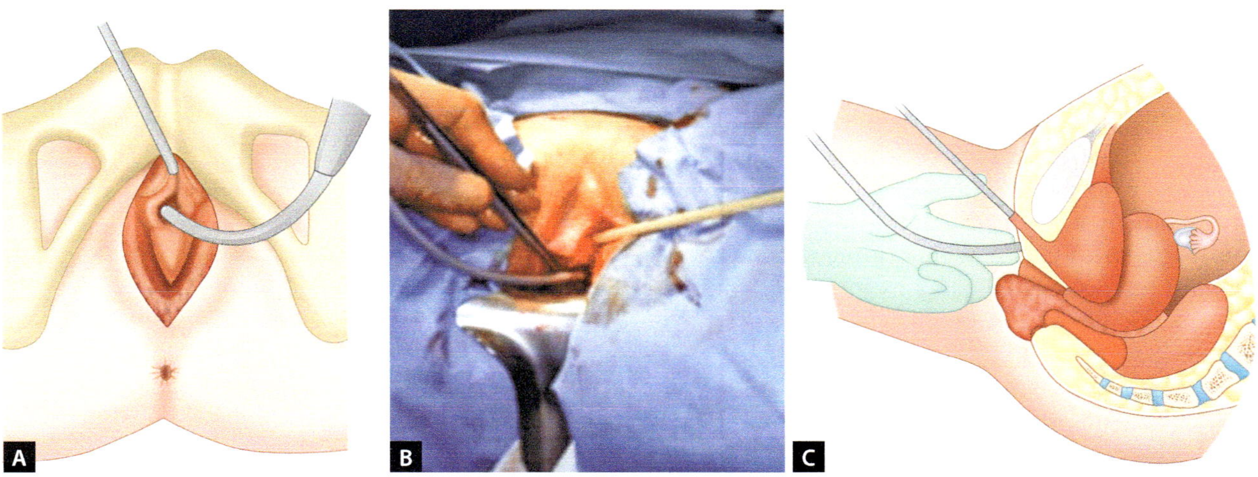

Figs. 4A to C: Safe entry of needle with use of urethral catheter guide.

toward the abdominal midline and lower the handle of the introducer thereby, pressing the tip of the needle against the back of the pubic bone. Now, move the needle tip upward to the abdominal skin incision, keeping in close contact with the pubic bone all the way. When the needle tip has reached the abdominal incision, cystoscopy is performed to confirm bladder integrity. The bladder must be emptied after the first cystoscopy. Disarticulate the reusable introducer and pull the remaining portion of the TVT needle through the abdominal incision. The procedure is then repeated on the other side.

The needles are then pulled upward to bring the tape (sling) loosely, i.e., without tension under the midurethra. Cut the tape close to the needles. Now, adjust the tape so that leakage is reduced allowing a few drops of urinary leakage to occur under stress. For this, use patient feedback, i.e.,

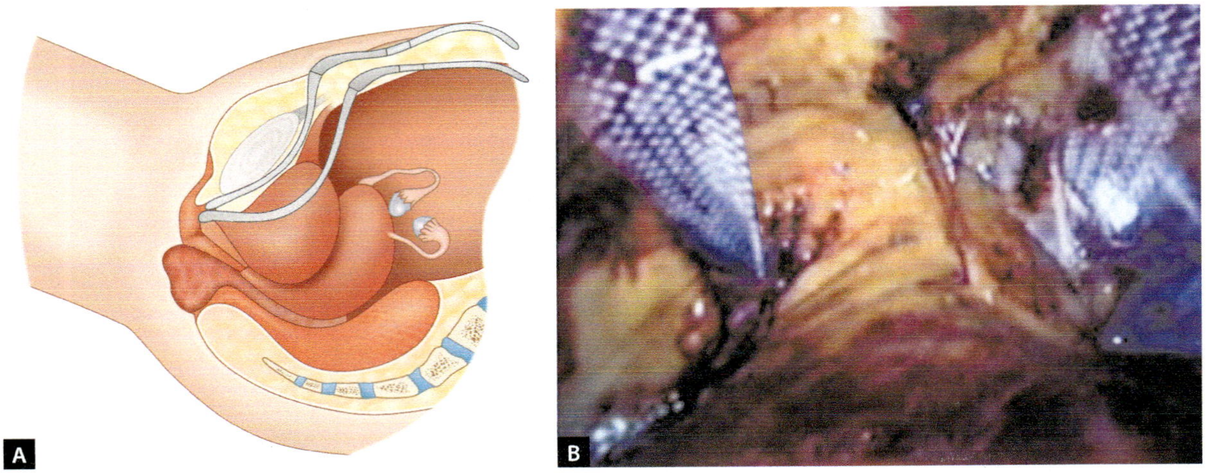

Figs. 5A and B: Completed application of tape with laparoscopic view.

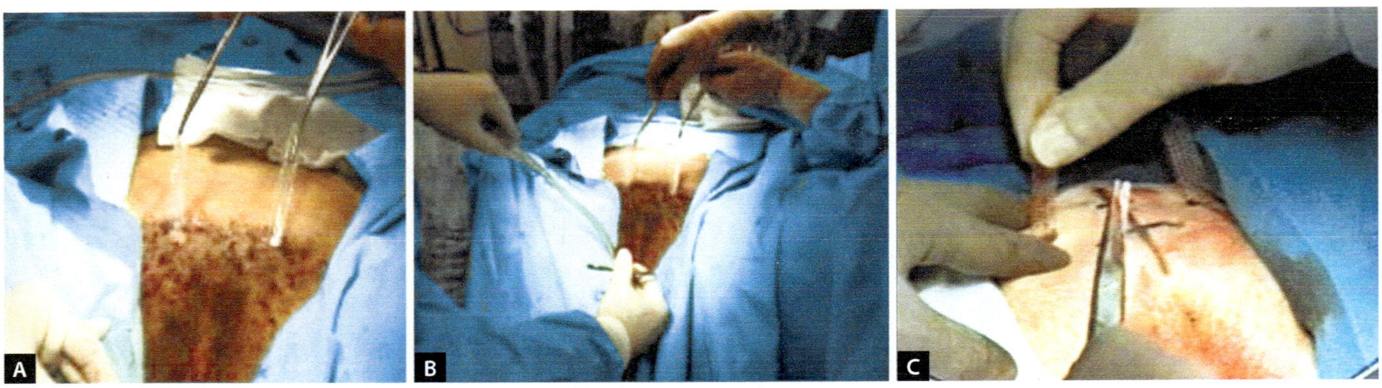

Figs. 6A to C: Removal of plastic tape with cutting the excessive mesh.

coughing with a full bladder (approximately 300 mL) and keep the vaginal incision temporarily closed by a gentle grip with small forceps **(Figs. 5A and B)**.

The plastic sheaths that surround the tape are then removed **(Figs. 6A to C)**. To avoid putting tension on the tape, a blunt instrument (scissors or forceps) should be placed between the urethra and the tape during removal of the plastic sheaths **(Fig. 7)**.

Premature removal of the sheath may make subsequent adjustments difficult. After proper adjustment of the tape, close the vaginal incision. The abdominal ends of the tape are then cut and left in subcutis. Do not suture them. Suture the skin incisions. Empty the bladder. Following this procedure, postoperative catheterization is not typically required. The patient should be encouraged to try to empty the bladder 2–3 hours after the operation.

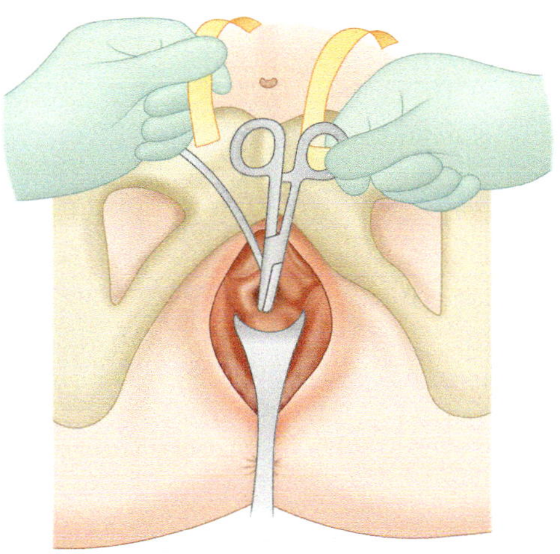

Fig. 7: Scissors or forceps should be placed between the urethra and the tape.

TRANSOBTURATOR TAPE

When TVT was first introduced into clinical practice in the mid- to late 1990s, the gold standard surgical procedure in the treatment of SUI was the Burch colposuspension. Several randomized controlled trials have compared the efficacy and safety of these two procedures and shown that TVT has a lower morbidity rate and equal or superior efficacy at mid-term follow-up. TVT has gradually replaced the colposuspension as the first choice of procedure, especially now that the long-term results (5–7 years outcome) are known (81.3% and 82% cure rate).

There are, however, concerns over the safety of TVT. A Finnish series of 1,455 women treated for SUI demonstrated several vascular injuries (venous lacerations were the most frequent injury reported), while Zilbert et al. reported a case of right external iliac artery injury. In addition, two deaths due to serious vascular injuries have been reported to the manufacturers as have bowel perforations. Most of these complications are related to the penetration of the retropubic space. In order to avoid these complications, but keep the principle of a minimally invasive procedure to reinforce the structures supporting the urethra, Delorme described the transobturator tape (TOT). In this technique a 2-cm incision is made through the vagina over the urethra and a tunnel created out to the obturator foramen on either side. A trocar is then passed from the thigh fold through the obturator foramen from the outside to the inside and brought round through the vaginal incision. A multifilament microporous tape is then fed through the trocar and brought through the obturator foramen. The procedure is repeated on both sides and the tape is left under no tension under the midurethra. De Leval et al. described a further modification to this surgical technique, which allows the passage of a trocar and tape through the obturator foramen from inside to out. The authors felt that this further reduced any risk of damage to the urethra and bladder; however, the long-term safety of this type of procedure is not known.

The TVT has revolutionized the surgical treatment of SUI, but remains an abdominal procedure with all of the potential complications therein. The TOT procedure described here produces the same end result, i.e., a tension-free tape left under the midurethra, but without the risks of a blind abdominal procedure.

Bladder perforation is the most common complication occurring during the TVT procedure with the incidence reported as between 0.8 and 21%. However, with the TOT procedure, the risk of bladder perforation is significantly reduced **(Fig. 8)**.

Functional Theories and Comparison with Tension-free Vaginal Tape

DeLancey's theories on pelvic support for the bladder and urethra help to explain the mechanism of action of the TOT in the treatment of SUI in that the position of the tape is similar to that of the natural hammock supporting the urethra. The TOT procedure using polypropylene tape satisfies most of the requirements for effective surgery.

In the medium term, the results are satisfactory and, unlike the retropubic tape (TVT), the purely perineal location of the TOT minimizes the risk of trauma to the bladder, intestine, major vessels, and nerves **(Figs. 9A and B)**.

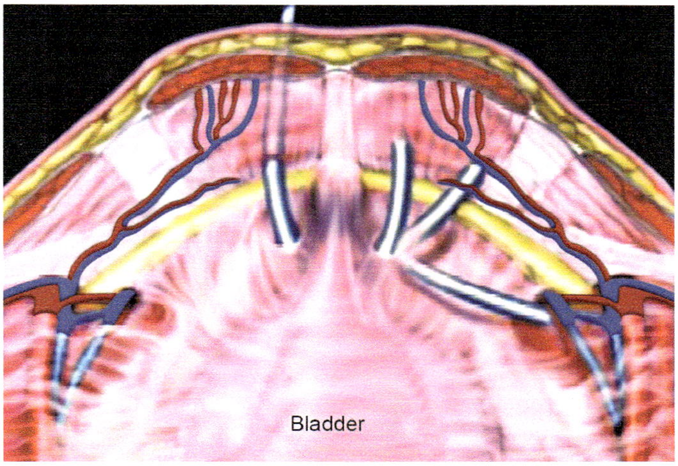

Fig. 8: Injuries in tension-free vaginal tape (TVT) procedure.

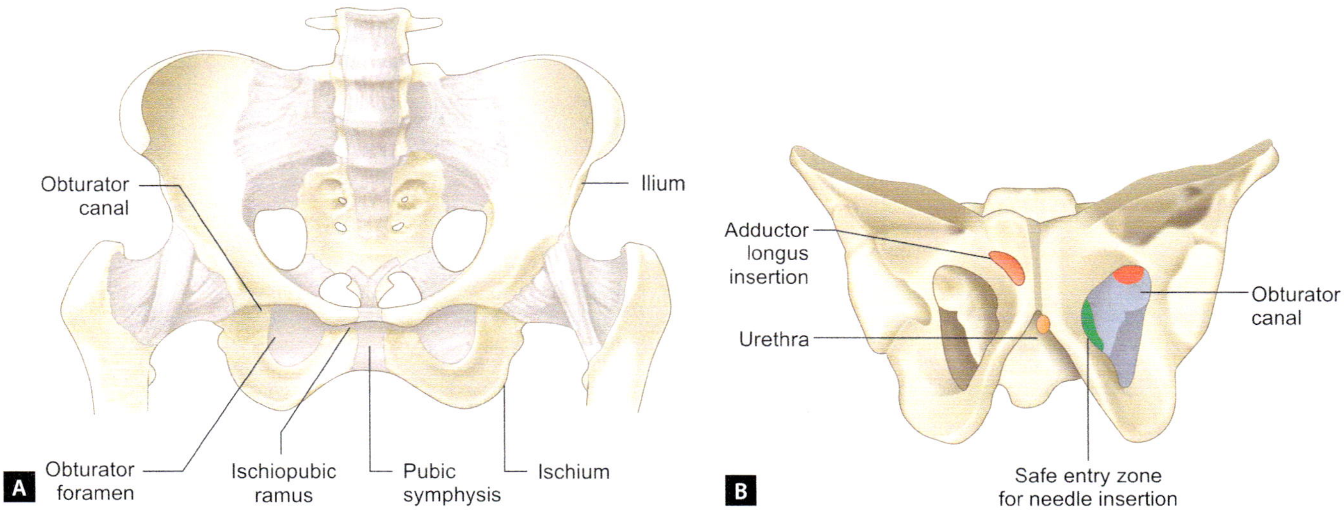

Figs. 9A and B: Pelvic anatomy demonstrating obturator foramen.

Operative Technique of Tension-free Vaginal Tape Obturator

Patient should be positioned in dorsal lithotomy with hips hyperflexed with buttock flush to the edge of the table. Make the exit points by tracing a horizontal line at the level of the urethral meatus and a second line parallel and 2 cm above the first line. Locate the exit points on the second line 2 cm lateral of the folds of the thigh. Using Allis clamps for traction, make a 1-cm midline vaginal incision starting 1 cm proximal to the urethral meatus **(Figs. 10A and B)**.

After initiating sharp dissection, continue by using a "push-spread" technique preferably using pointed curved scissor **(Figs. 11A and B)**. The path of the lateral dissection should be oriented at a 45° angle from the midline with the scissors oriented on the horizontal plane. Continue dissection toward the "junction" between the body of the pubic bone and the inferior pubic ramus and perforate the obturator membrane.

Winged guide should be inserted into the dissected trace and through the obturator membrane. Insert the TOT device tip with the helical pressure into the dissected tract following the channel of the winged guide. Push the direction of TOT device inward traversing and perforating the obturator membrane. Once in the TOT needle is in position, winged guide should be withdrawn **(Figs. 12A and B)**.

Once the winged guide has been removed, move the handle of TOT needle toward the midline to a near-vertical position. Then, rotate the handle of the helical passer counterclockwise for patient's right side and clockwise for patient's left side **(Figs. 13A and B)**.

The point of the helical passer should exit near the previously determined exit points. Slight skin manipulation may be required particularly in obese patients **(Figs. 14A and B)**.

When the tip of the plastic tube appears and passes at the skin opening, grasp the extreme point of the tip with a clamp and, while stabilizing the tube near the urethra, remove the helical passer by a reverse rotation of the handle **(Figs. 15A and B)**.

After removing the helical passer, the plastic tube should be pulled completely through the skin until the tape appears **(Figs. 16A and B)**.

Same procedure of TOT mesh insertion should be repeated for other side keeping in mind that there should not be twisting of mesh in the midline **(Figs. 17A and B)**.

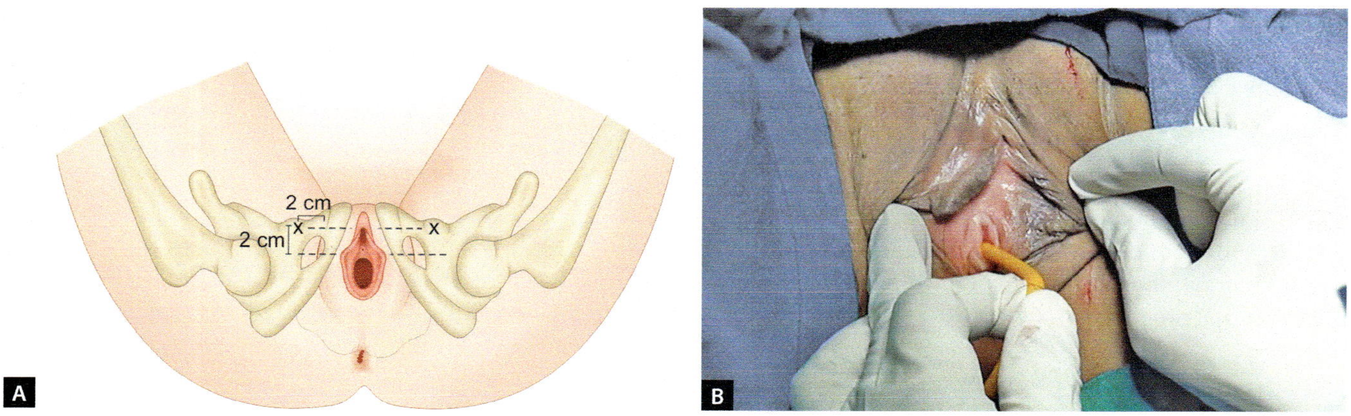

Figs. 10A and B: Position the patient, mark thigh exit point, and make vaginal midline incision.

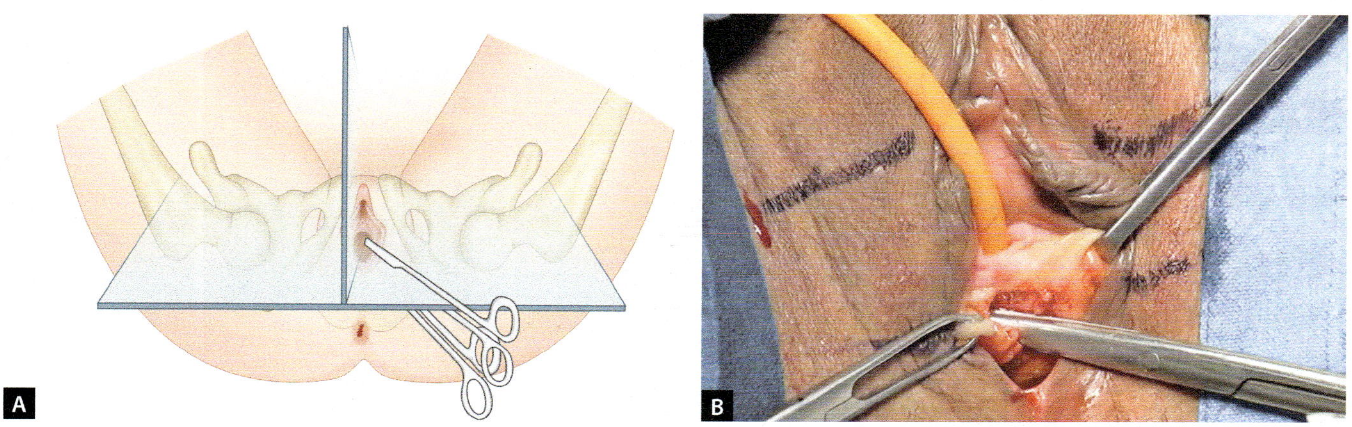

Figs. 11A and B: Dissect to the obturator membrane and perforate obturator membrane.

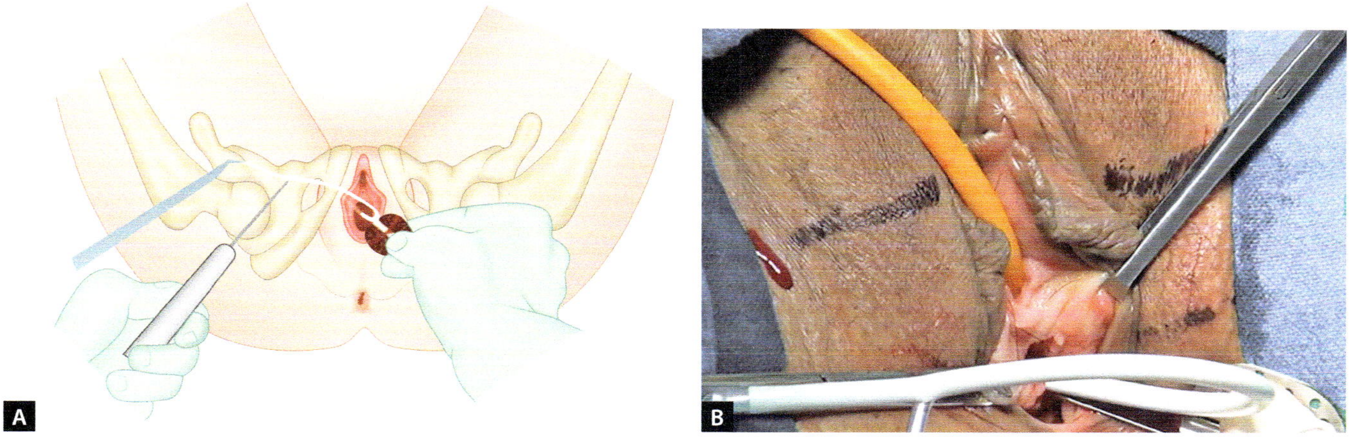

Figs. 12A and B: Insert winged guide and helical passer and then remove winged guide.

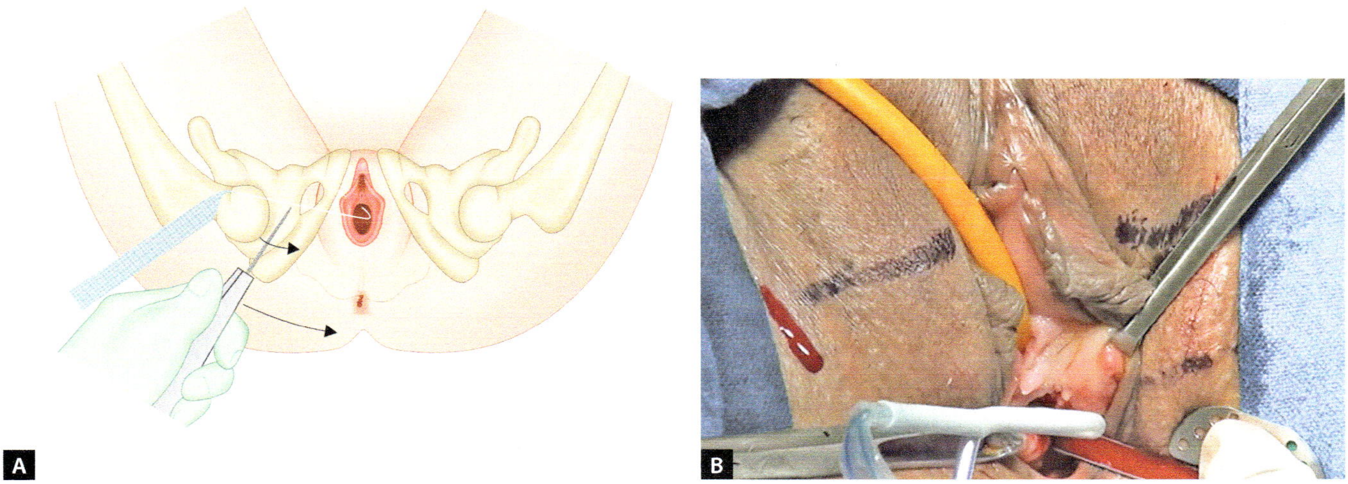

Figs. 13A and B: Rotate helical passer while moving the handle into midline.

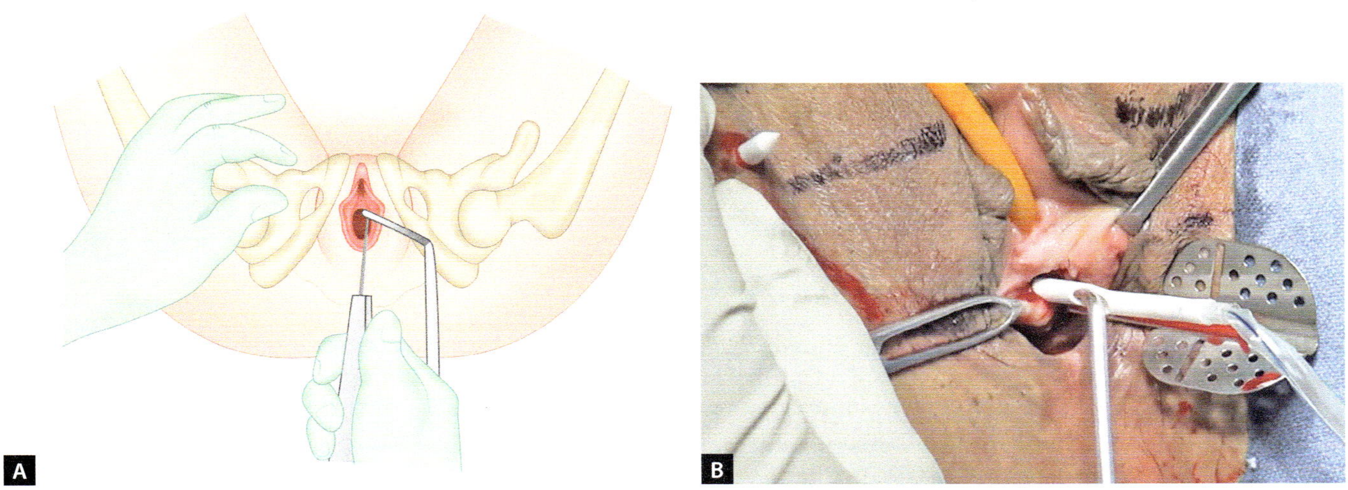

Figs. 14A and B: Facilitate passage of transobturator tape (TOT) through skin incision.

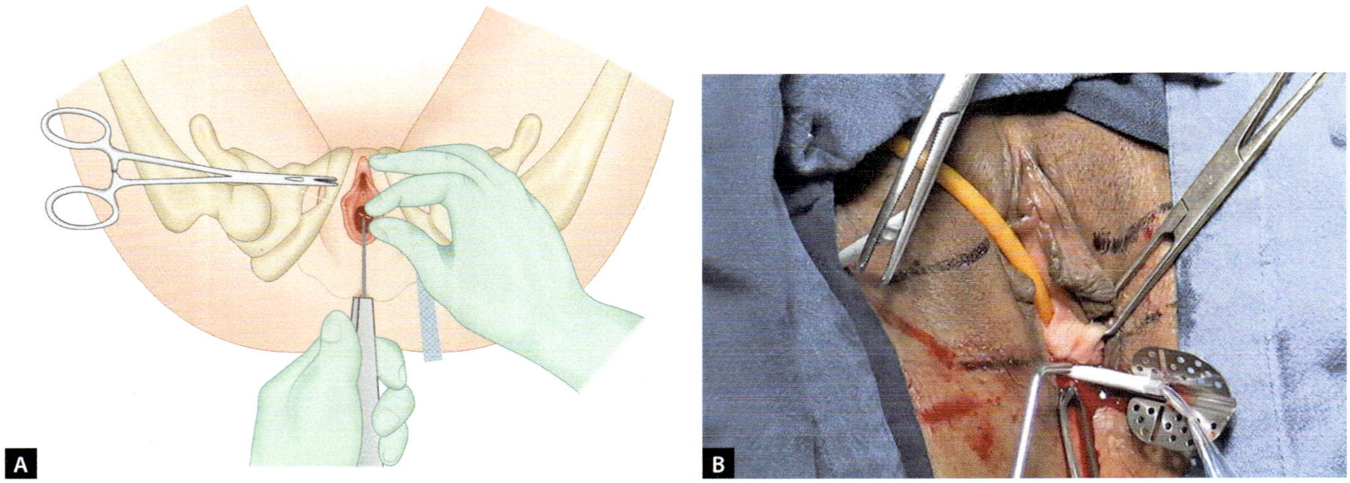

Figs. 15A and B: Grasp tip of plastic tube and then retract helical passer by reverse rotation.

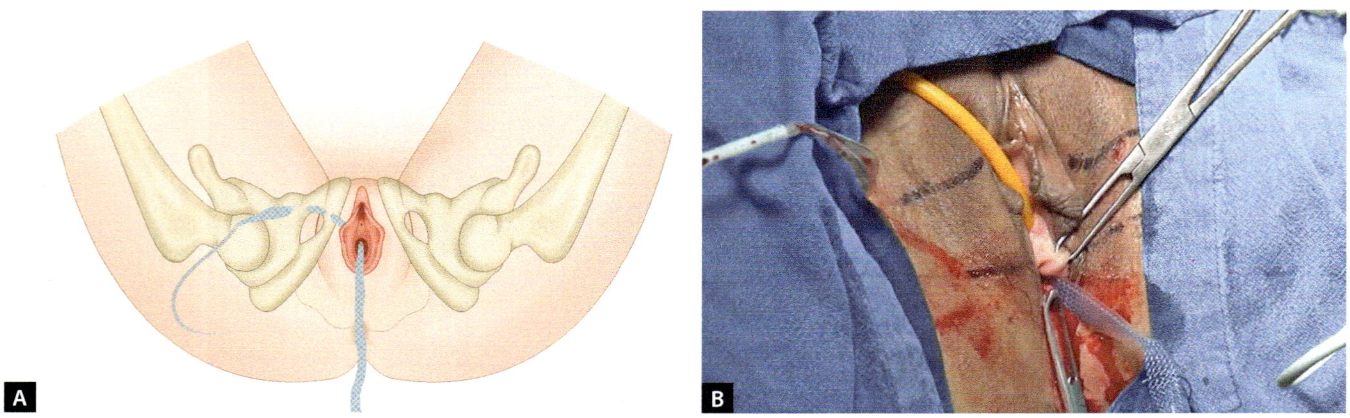

Figs. 16A and B: Pull plastic tube and tape completely through the skin.

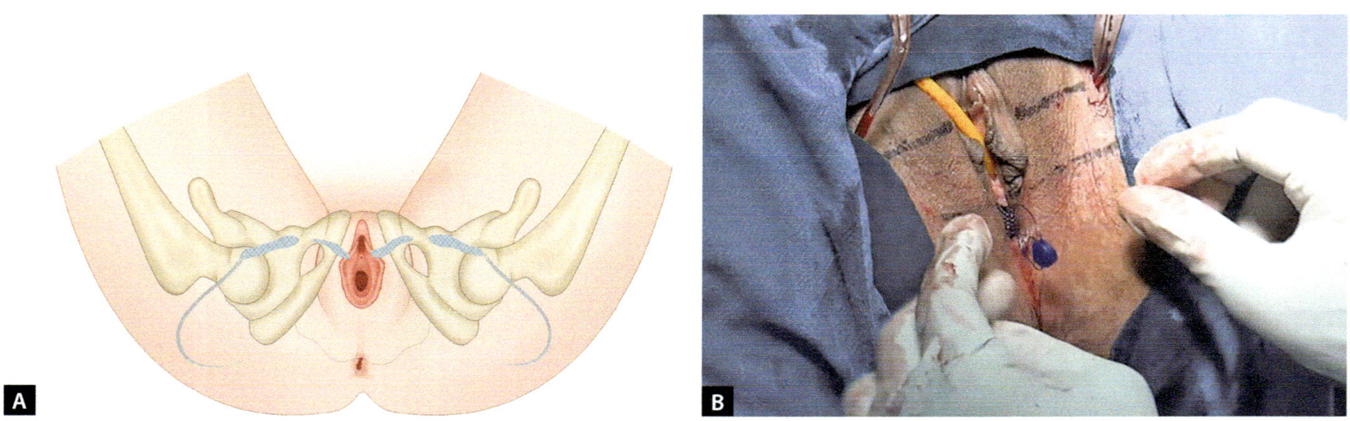

Figs. 17A and B: Steps of introduction of mesh should be repeated on patient's other side.

When the tape is in position, the plastic sheath that covers the tape should be removed **(Figs. 18A and B)**. One blunt instrument (e.g., scissors or forceps) should be placed between the urethra and the tape during removal of a plastic sheath, or use other suitable means during sheath removal, to avoid positioning the tape with tension. Following tape adjustment, close the vaginal incisions. Cut the tape ends at the exit points just below the skin on the inner thigh. Close the skin incisions with suture or surgical skin adhesive **(Figs. 18A and B)**. Surgeon should remember that "looser is better than tighter".

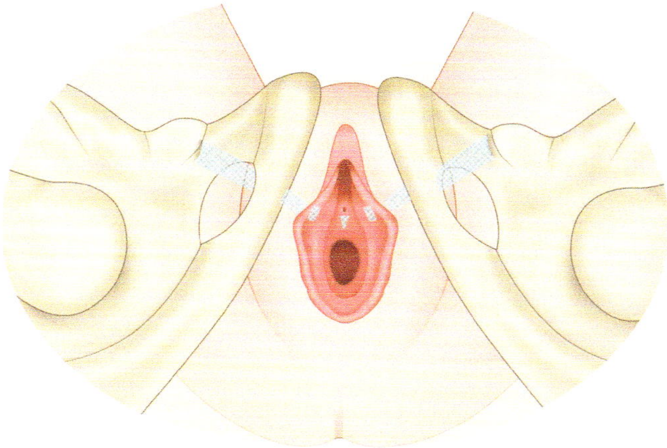

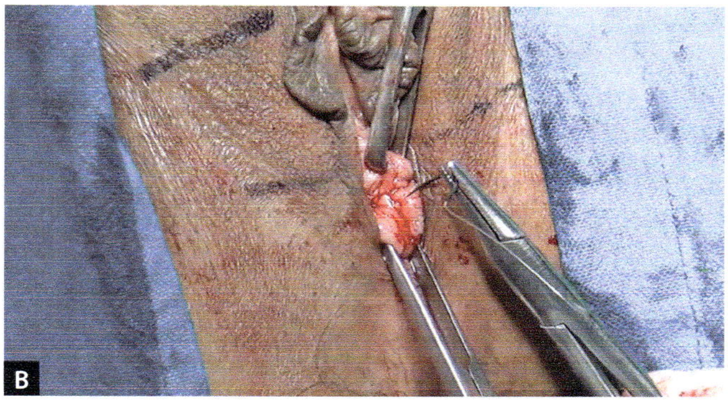

Figs. 18A and B: Adjust the tape, remove plastic sheath, and close vaginal incision.

CONTRAINDICATIONS OF TENSION-FREE VAGINAL TAPE AND TRANSOBTURATOR TAPE

As with any suspension surgery, these sling procedure should not be performed in pregnant patients. Additionally, because the prolene polypropylene mesh will not stretch significantly, it should not be performed in patients with future growth potential including women with plans for future pregnancy.

WARNINGS AND PRECAUTIONS

- Do not use TVT or TOT procedure for patients who are on anticoagulation therapy
- Do not use TVT or TOT procedure for patients who have a urinary tract infection
- Users should be familiar with surgical technique for bladder neck suspensions and should be adequately trained in the TVT or TOT implantation procedure before employing these devices. It is important to recognize that TVT or TOT is different from a traditional sling procedure in that the tape should be located without tension under midurethra
- Acceptable surgical practice should be followed for the TVT or TOT procedure as well as for the management of contaminated or infected wounds
- The TVT or TOT procedure should be performed with care to avoid large vessels, nerves, bladder, and bowel. Attention to local anatomy and proper passage of needles will minimize risks, especially in TVT
- Retropubic bleeding may occur postoperatively. Observe for any symptoms or signs before releasing the patient from hospital
- Cystoscopy should be performed to confirm bladder integrity or recognize a bladder perforation
- Do not remove the plastic sheath until the tape has been properly positioned
- Ensure that the tape is placed with minimal tension under midurethra
- Prolene mesh in contaminated areas should be used with the understanding that subsequent infection may require removal of the material
- The patient should be counseled that future pregnancies may negate the effects of the surgical procedure and the patient may again become incontinent
- Since no clinical experience is available with vaginal delivery following the TVT or TOT procedure, in case of pregnancy delivery via cesarean section is recommended
- Postoperatively, the patient is recommended to refrain from heavy lifting and/or exercise (i.e., cycling, jogging) for at least 3–4 weeks and intercourse for 1 month. The patient can return to other normal activity after 1 or 2 weeks
- Should dysuria, bleeding, or other problems occur, the patient is instructed to contact the surgeon immediately
- All surgical instruments are subject to wear and damage under normal use. Before use, the instrument should be visually inspected. Defective instruments or instruments that appear to be corroded should not be used and should be discarded
- As with other incontinence procedures, de novo detrusor instability may occur following the TVT procedure. To minimize this risk, make sure to place the tape tension-free in the midurethral position
- Punctures or lacerations of vessels, nerves, bladder, or bowel may occur during needle passage and may require surgical repair
- Transitory local irritation at the wound site and a transitory foreign body response may occur. This response could result in extrusion, erosion, fistula formation, and inflammation
- As with all foreign bodies, prolene mesh may potentiate an existing infection. The plastic sheath initially covering

the prolene mesh is designed to minimize the risk of contamination

- Overcorrection, i.e., too much tension applied to the tape, may cause temporary or permanent lower urinary tract obstruction

CONCLUSION

Mesh sling surgeries for SUI have been reported to be successful in approximately 70–80% of women at 1 year based on women's reports and physical examinations. Similar effectiveness outcomes are reported following nonmesh SUI surgeries such as Burch colposuspension. The use of mesh slings in transvaginal SUI repair introduces a risk that does not present in traditional nonmesh surgery for SUI repair, which is mesh erosion, also known as extrusion. Erosion of mesh slings through the vagina is the most commonly reported mesh-specific complication from SUI surgeries with mesh. The average reported rate of mesh erosion at 1 year following SUI surgery with mesh is approximately 2%. Mesh erosion is sometimes treated successfully with vaginal cream or an office procedure where the exposed piece of mesh is cut. In some cases of mesh erosion, it may be necessary to return to the operating room to remove part or all of the mesh.

BIBLIOGRAPHY

1. Andersson G, Johansson JE, Garpenholt O, Nilsson K. Urinary incontinence prevalence, impact on daily living and desire for treatment: a population-based study. Scand J Urol Nephrol. 2004;38:125-30.
2. Andonian S, Chen T, St-Denis B, Corcos J. Randomized clinical trial comparing suprapubic arch sling (SPARC) and tension-free vaginal tape (TVT): one-year results. Eur Urol. 2005;47:537-41.
3. Brophy MM, Klutke JJ, Klutke CG. A review of the tension-free vaginal tape procedure: outcomes, complications, and theories. Curr Urol Rep. 2001;2:364-9.
4. Brown JS, Vittinghoff E, Wyman JF, Stone KL, Nevitt MC, Ensrud KE, et al. Urinary incontinence: does it increase risk for falls and fractures? Study of Osteoporotic Fractures Research Group. J Am Geriatr Soc. 2000;48:721-5.
5. Burgio KL, Ives DG, Locher JL, Arena VC, Kuller LH. Treatment seeking for urinary incontinence in older adults. J Am Geriatr Soc. 1994;42:208-12.
6. Chaliha C, Stanton SL. The ethnic cultural and social aspects of incontinence: a pilot study. Int Urogynecol J Pelvic Floor Dysfunct. 1999;10:166-70.
7. Cindolo L, Salzano L, Rota G, Bellini S, D'Afiero A. Tension-free transobturator approach for female stress urinary incontinence. Minerva Urol Nefrol. 2004;56:89-98.
8. Costa P, Grise P, Droupy S, Monneins F, Assenmacher C, Ballanger P, et al. Surgical treatment of female stress urinary incontinence with a trans-obturator-tape (TOT) Uratape: short term results of a prospective multicentric study. Eur Urol. 2004;46:102-6.
9. Dargent D, Bretones S, George P, Mellier G. Insertion of a sub-urethral sling through the obturating membrane for treatment of female urinary incontinence. Gynecol Obstet Fertil. 2002; 30:576-82.
10. DeLeval, J. Novel surgical technique for the treatment of female stress urinary incontinence: transobturator vaginal tape inside-out. Eur Urol. 2003;44:724-30.
11. DeLancey JO. Structural support of the urethra as it relates to stress urinary incontinence: the hammock hypothesis. Am J Obstet Gynecol. 1994;170:1713-20.
12. Delorme E, Droupy S, de Tayrac R, Delmas V. Transobturator tape (Uratape): a new minimally invasive procedure to treat female urinary incontinence. Eur Urol. 2004;45:203-7.
13. Delorme E. Transobturator urethral suspension: mini-invasive procedure in the treatment of stress urinary incontinence in women. Prog Urol. 2001;11:1306-13.
14. Diokno AC, Burgio K, Fultz NH, Kinchen KS, Obenchain R, Bump RC. Medical and self-care practices reported by women with urinary incontinence. Am J Manag Care. 2004;10:69-78.
15. Dugan E, Roberts CP, Cohen SJ, Preisser JS, Davis CC, Bland DR, et al. Why older community-dwelling adults do not discuss urinary incontinence with their primary care physicians. J Am Geriatr Soc. 2001;49:462-5.
16. Fultz NH, Fisher GG, Jenkins KR. Does urinary incontinence affect middle-aged and older women's time, use and activity patterns? Obstet Gynecol. 2004;104:1327-34.
17. Goldberg RP, Kwon C, Gandhi S, Atkuru LV, Sand PK. Urinary incontinence after multiple gestation and delivery: impact on quality of life. Int Urogynecol J Pelvic Floor Dysfunct. 2005;16:334-6.
18. Grodstein F, Fretts R, Lifford K, Resnick N, Curhan G. Association of age, race, and obstetric history with urinary symptoms among women in the Nurses' Health Study. Am J Obstet Gynecol. 2003;189:428-34.
19. Hagen S, Hanley J, Capewell A. Test-retest reliability, validity, and sensitivity to change of the urogenital distress inventory and the incontinence impact questionnaire. Neurourol Urodyn. 2002;21:534-9.
20. Harvey MA, Kristjansson B, Griffith D, Versi E. The incontinence impact questionnaire and the urogenital distress inventory: a revisit of their validity in women without a urodynamic diagnosis. Am J Obstet Gynecol. 2001;185:25-31.
21. Heit M, Blackwell L, Thomas S, Ouseph R. Prevalence and severity of urinary incontinence in kidney transplant recipients. Obstet Gynecol. 2004;103:352-8.
22. Hermieu JF, Messas A, Delmas V, Ravery V, Dumonceau O, Boccon-Gibod L. Bladder injury after TVT transobturator. Prog Urol. 2003;13:115-7.
23. Holroyd-Leduc JM, Straus SE. Management of urinary incontinence in women: clinical applications. JAMA. 2004; 291:996-9.
24. Kinchen KS, Burgio K, Diokno AC, Fultz NH, Bump R, Obenchain R. Factors associated with women's decisions to seek treatment for urinary incontinence. J Women's Health (Larchmt). 2003;12:687-98.
25. Kuuva N, Nilsson CG. A nationwide analysis of complications associated with the tension-free vaginal tape (TVT) procedure. Acta Obstet Gynecol Scand. 2002;81:72-7.
26. Lagace EA, Hansen W, Hickner JM. Prevalence and severity of urinary incontinence in ambulatory adults: an UPRNet study. J Fam Pract. 1993;36:610-4.
27. Lukban JC. Suburethral sling using the transobturator approach: a quality-of-life analysis. Am J Obstet Gynecol. 2005;193:2138-43.
28. Melville JL, Delaney K, Newton K, Katon W. Incontinence severity and major depression in incontinent women. Obstet Gynecol. 2005;106:585-92.
29. Melville JL, Katon W, Delaney K, Newton K. Urinary incontinence in US women: a population-based study. Arch Intern Med. 2005;165:537-42.

30. Muir TW, Tulikangas PK, Paraiso FM, Walters MD. The relationship of tension-free vaginal tape insertion and the vascular anatomy. Obstet Gynecol. 2003;101:933-6.
31. Nilsson CG, Falconer C, Rezapour M. Seven-year follow-up of tension-free vaginal tape procedure for treatment of urinary incontinence. Obstet Gynecol. 2004;104:1259-62.
32. Novielli KD, Simpson Z, Hua G, Diamond JJ, Sultana C, Paynter N. Urinary incontinence in primary care: a comparison of older African-American and Caucasian women. Int Urol Nephrol. 2003;35:423-8.
33. Nygaard I, Turvey C, Burns TL, Crischilles E, Wallace R. Urinary incontinence and depression in middle-aged United States women. Obstet Gynecol. 2003;101:149-56.
34. Paraiso MF, Walters MD, Karram MM, Barber MD. Laparoscopic Burch colposuspension versus tension-free vaginal tape: a randomized trial. Obstet Gynecol. 2004;104:1249-58.
35. Peyrat L, Boutin JM, Bruyere F, Haillot O, Farfak H, Lanson Y. Intestinal perforation as a complication of tension-free vaginal tape procedure for urinary incontinence. Eur Urol. 2001;39:603-5.
36. Reymert J, Hunskaar S. Why do only a minority of perimenopausal women with urinary incontinence consult a doctor? Scand J Prim Health Care. 1994;12:180-3.
37. Sampselle CM, Harlow SD, Skurnick J, Brubaker L, Bondarenko I. Urinary incontinence predictors and life impact in ethnically diverse perimenopausal women. Obstet Gynecol. 2002; 100:1230-8.
38. Sandvik H, Seim A, Vanvik A, Hunskaar S. A severity index for epidemiological surveys of female urinary incontinence: comparison with 48-hour pad-weighing tests. Neurourol Urodyn. 2000;19:137-45.
39. Shaw C, Tansey R, Jackson C, Hyde C, Allan R. Barriers to help seeking in people with urinary symptoms. Fam Pract. 2001;18:48-52.
40. Shumaker SA, Wyman JF, Uebersax JS, McClish D, Fantl JA. Health-related quality of life measures for women with urinary incontinence: the Incontinence Impact Questionnaire and the Urogenital Distress Inventory: Continence Program in Women (CPW) Research Group. Qual Life Res. 1994;3:291-306.
41. Thom D. Variation in estimates of urinary incontinence prevalence in the community: effects of differences in definition, population characteristics, and study type. J Am Geriatr Soc. 1998;46:473-80.
42. Thom DH, Haan MN, Van Den Eeden SK. Medically recognized urinary incontinence and risks of hospitalization, nursing home admission and mortality. Age Ageing. 1997;26:367-74.
43. Thom DH, van den Eeden SK, Ragins AI, Wassel-Fyr C, Vittinghof E, Subak LL, et al. Differences in prevalence of urinary incontinence by race/ethnicity. J Urol. 2006;175:259-64.
44. Ulmsten U, Henriksson L, Johnson P, Varhos G. An ambulatory surgical procedure under local anesthesia for treatment of female urinary incontinence. Int Urogynecol J Pelvic Floor Dysfunct. 1996;7:81-5.
45. van Brummen HJ, Bruinse HW, van de Pol G, Heintz APM, van der Vaart CH. The effect of vaginal and cesarean delivery on lower urinary tract symptoms: what makes the difference? Int Urogynecol J Pelvic Floor Dysfunct. 2007;18:133-9.
46. Ward KL, Hilton P, UK and Ireland TVT Trial Group. A prospective multicenter randomized trial of tension-free vaginal tape and colposuspension for primary urodynamic stress incontinence: two-year follow-up. Am J Obstet Gynecol. 2004;190:324-31.
47. Zilbert AW, Farrell SA. External iliac artery laceration during tension-free vaginal tape procedure. Int Urogynecol J Pelvic Floor Dysfunct. 2001;12:141-3.

CHAPTER 38

Laparoscopic Repair of Pelvic Organ Prolapse

INTRODUCTION

Pelvic organ prolapse (POP) happens when the muscles and tissues supporting the pelvic organs (the uterus, bladder, or rectum) become weak or loose. This allows one or more of the pelvic organs to drop or press into or out of the vagina.

The different types of POP depend on the pelvic organ affected. The most common types include:

- *Cystocele*: This is the most common type of POP. This happens when the bladder drops into or out of the vagina
- *Rectocele*: This happens when the rectum bulges into or out of the vagina
- *Hysterocele*: This happens when the uterus bulges into or out of the vagina. Uterine prolapse is sometimes associated with small bowel prolapse (called enterocele), where part of the small intestine, or small bowel, bulges into the vagina

Apical prolapse is the descent of uterus, cervix, or vaginal vault. POP affects millions of women worldwide. It is estimated that approximately 200,000 inpatient surgical procedures for prolapse are performed annually. About 11–19% of women will undergo surgery for POP or incontinence by age 80–85 years and 30% of these women will require an additional POP or incontinence surgery. Anterior vaginal wall prolapses without concomitant apical prolapse are uncommon and apical prolapse repair should be included in the majority of pelvic reconstructive surgery procedures.

Vaginal vault prolapse occurs when the apex of the vagina descends below the introitus. It is sequelae of incorrectly performed hysterectomy and occurs due to disruption of the ligaments that maintain vaginal support. Numerous surgical techniques have been proposed to prevent and correct this condition, including abdominal sacral colpopexy with interposition of a mesh between the prolapsed vaginal vault and anterior surface of the sacrum. Traditionally, open surgical procedure usually requires a midline abdominal incision and extensive bowel manipulation.

INDICATIONS OF SURGERY

Symptomatic Prolapse

- Feeling of pelvic heaviness or full and low back pain
- Perception of lump at the opening of the vulva
- Mucosal erosion
- Bleeding
- Infection
- Splinting or digitation (the need to manually assist in reducing prolapse, often to void or defecate)

Concomitant symptoms may include the following:

- Urinary incontinence symptoms such as stress, urgency, or postural incontinence
- Bladder storage symptoms such as frequency, urgency, or overactive bladder syndrome
- Voiding symptoms such as hesitancy, slow stream, straining, incomplete emptying, or position-dependent voiding
- Sexual dysfunction symptoms such as dyspareunia or obstructed intercourse
- Anorectal dysfunction such as fecal incontinence, flatal incontinence, fecal urgency, straining to defecate, constipation, and incomplete evacuation

CONTRAINDICATIONS

Many of the general contraindications to laparoscopic sacral colpopexy are the same for any laparoscopic surgical procedure. These may include the following:

- Anemia
- Bleeding diathesis or the need for anticoagulation
- Significant cardiac or pulmonary comorbidities
- Active infection such as cystitis, bacterial or fungal vaginal infection, pelvic inflammatory disease, or active sexually transmitted disease
- Active venous thromboembolism
- Uncontrolled hyperglycemia.

Other contraindications specific to laparoscopic sacral colpopexy include the following:

- Vaginal cancer, cervical cancer, or uterine cancer that is untreated or cannot be adequately treated due to advanced stage
- Fistulas such as vesicovaginal, rectovaginal, vesicouterine, or urethral fistulas
- Previous pelvic prolapse repairs with infected or exposed foreign material and erosions.

Relative contraindications include the following:

- Pelvic irradiation
- Previous pelvic surgery or prolapse repair, depending on the nature of the operation and the subsequent pathology, side effects, or complications (the existence of such may warrant additional diagnostic evaluation and may require additional surgical intervention or change of approach to prolapse repair)
- Concomitant cystocele, rectocele, or urinary incontinence (the existence of such pathology may require additional surgery, a vaginal approach, or a combined approach).

The advantages of a laparoscopic sacral colpopexy include a better view of the pelvis, precise hemostasis, smaller incision, and less manipulation of the viscera. Sacral colpopexy involves placing a Hammock of polypropylene mesh between the prolapsed vaginal vault and the anterior surface of the sacrum. Multiple permanent sutures attach one end of the mesh to the apex of the vaginal vault and the opposite end to either the hollow of the sacrum or to the sacral promontory.

LAPAROSCOPIC SLING SURGERY FOR CYSTOCELE REPAIR

Factors that are linked to cystocele development include age, repeated childbirth, hormone deficiency, menopause, constipation, ongoing physical activity, heavy lifting, and prior hysterectomy **(Fig. 1)**. Symptoms of bladder prolapse include stress incontinence (inadvertent leakage of urine with physical activity), urinary frequency, difficult urination, a vaginal bulge, vaginal pressure or pain, painful sexual intercourse, and lower back pain. Urinary incontinence is the most common symptom of a cystocele.

Surgery is generally not performed unless the symptoms of the prolapse have begun to interfere with daily life. A staging system is used to grade the severity of a cystocele. A stage I, II, or III prolapse descends to progressively lower areas of the vagina. A stage IV prolapse descends to or protrudes through the vaginal opening. Surgery is generally reserved for stage III and IV cystoceles.

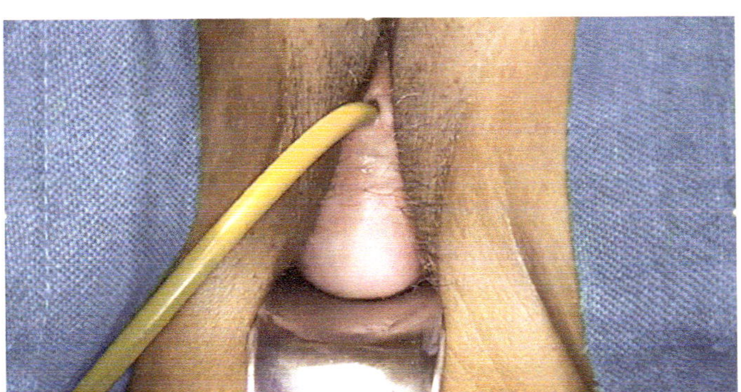

Fig. 1: Cystocele.

All surgical procedures were performed under general anesthesia. Every patient received a single dose of intravenous prophylactic antibiotics. The patients were placed in a lithotomy position. Laparoscopy was setup with the endoscope located at the 10-mm umbilical wound, two 5-mm trocar ports in the bilateral lower quadrant of the abdomen approximately 2 cm medial to the anterior superior iliac spine, and one 5-mm trocar port 7.5 cm left and lateral to the umbilicus. The peritoneum of anterior leaf of broad ligament should be opened on either side. In the midline, peritoneum should be opened at the uterovesical fold and bladder should be bluntly dissected to expose the anterior colpocervical junction **(Figs. 2A to D)**. Long mesh, a synthetic T-shaped prolene mesh, should be delivered into the pelvic cavity **(Fig. 3)**. The centerpiece of mesh should be fixed to the anterior vaginal fascia and cervix with 8–10 surgeons knot using polyester or silk suture **(Figs. 4A to D)**. An extraperitoneal tunnel was created along the left round ligament until it reached a location 2 cm medial to anterior superior iliac spine **(Figs. 5A to D)**. One arm of the long mesh was pulled out along the tunnel underneath the round ligament and fixed with the fascia of the abdominal oblique muscle. The same procedure was repeated on the contralateral side. The bilateral round ligaments and the mesh arms were sutured continuously with 2-0 Vicryl **(Figs. 6A to C)**. After fixing the mesh, peritoneum should be closed with continuous suture to hide the mesh completely. The tension of the mesh should be adjusted until the apical compartment is reduced to an appropriate position per the vaginal examination **(Fig. 7)**.

OPERATIVE PROCEDURE OF SACROCOLPOPEXY FOR VAULT PROLAPSE

Mechanical and antibiotic bowel preparation is given prior to the night of surgery. The vagina is thoroughly cleansed with an antiseptic before the procedure. The laparoscope is placed through the umbilicus and other instruments through three suprapubic 5 mm accessory trocars. The patient is placed in a steep Trendelenburg position and tilted to the left to move the bowel away from the operating field.

Before starting procedure, diagnostic laparoscopy is performed. The vagina is pushed up by a sponge on a ring forceps in the vaginal vault and adhesiolysis is performed as necessary. Peritoneum and connective tissue are removed from the vaginal apex until the vaginal fascia and scar are identified. While holding the vaginal apex with grasping forceps, the vesical peritoneum over the vaginal apex is incised using blunt dissection, hydrodissection, or scissors **(Figs. 8A to C)**. The bladder is dissected from the anterior vaginal wall and the rectum from the posterior vaginal wall to expose approximately 4 cm of the vaginal vault **(Figs. 9A to C)**. If a buttonhole gets made by mistake in the vagina, an inflated surgical glove is placed in the vagina to help maintain pneumoperitoneum.

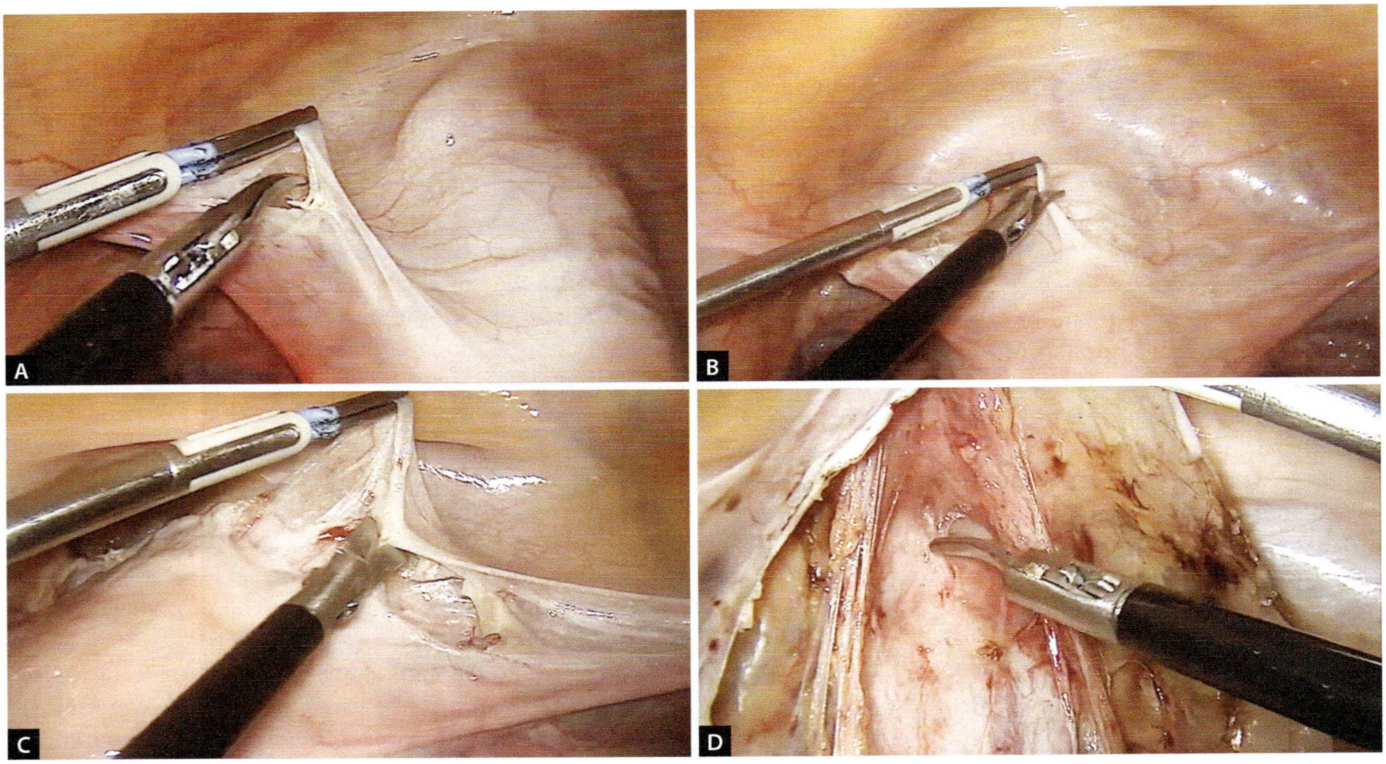

Figs. 2A to D: Anterior leaf of broad ligament should be opened on either side. In the midline, peritoneum should be opened at the UV fold and bladder is bluntly dissected to expose the anterior colpocervical junction.

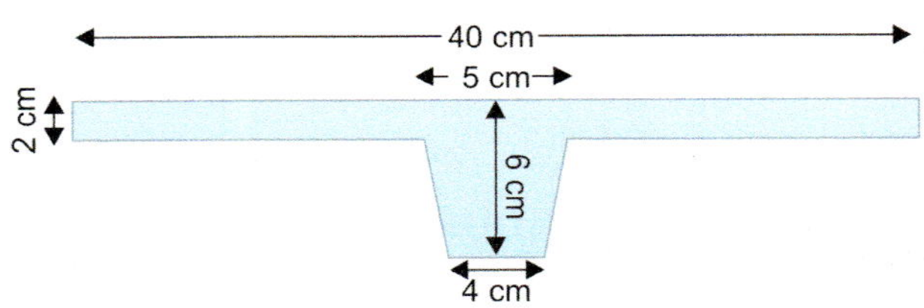

Fig. 3: Size of prolene mesh used to correct cystocele.

The posterior parietal peritoneum is lifted with grasping forceps and the anterior sacral fascia exposed **(Figs. 10A and B)**. Care is taken to avoid injuring the presacral vessels. Bleeding is controlled with bipolar electrodesiccation suture or clips. The peritoneal incision is extended downward to the vagina through the presacral space. The presacral space is entered through a vertical peritoneal incision at the right pararectal area using hydrodissection combined with the bipolar; this can be replaced by any cutting modality that the surgeon chooses. The peritoneal incision at the promontory is then extended along the rectosigmoid to continue over the deepest part of the cul-de-sac opening the recto- and vesicovaginal space. Some prefers to create a tunnel under the peritoneum avoiding later suturing. The lateral incision as well as the dissection downward toward the perineal body can be extended as far as required. This is the case when there is a large rectocele or when a concomitant rectopexy is required for rectal prolapse.

The following anatomic landmarks are identified to avoid bowel, ureter, and vessel injury is the right ureter, internal iliac artery and vein, descending colon, and presacral vessels. The sigmoid colon is reflected laterally to avoid injury to vessels in the sigmoid mesentery. The central 5 mm trocar above the symphysis pubis is replaced with a 10-mm trocar. The polypropylene mesh is rolled and introduced into the abdomen through the 10 mm suprapubic port. Three to five 1-0 nonabsorbable polybutilate coated polyester sutures are placed in a single row in the vaginal wall apex from one lateral fornix to the other. Each suture is placed through one end of the polypropylene mesh and tied loosely using extracorporeal or intracorporeal knot **(Figs. 11A to C)**.

Two permanent sutures or staples are placed in the periosteum of the sacrum over anterior longitudinal ligament apart in the midline over S3 and S4 **(Fig. 12)**. Care is taken to avoid vascular injury to paravertebral and perforating blood vessels in this area. Hemostasis is difficult even by laparotomy because of retraction of the severed vessels. The mesh is adjusted to hold the vaginal apex in the correct anatomic position without being tight. The excess mesh is trimmed from the strap **(Fig. 13)**. The peritoneum is closed over the strap using continuous suturing **(Fig. 14)**. Postoperatively, patients remain in bed for 24 hours. They are advised to avoid intercourse for 2 months. Their diet is advanced as tolerated and a mild laxative is prescribed to prevent constipation.

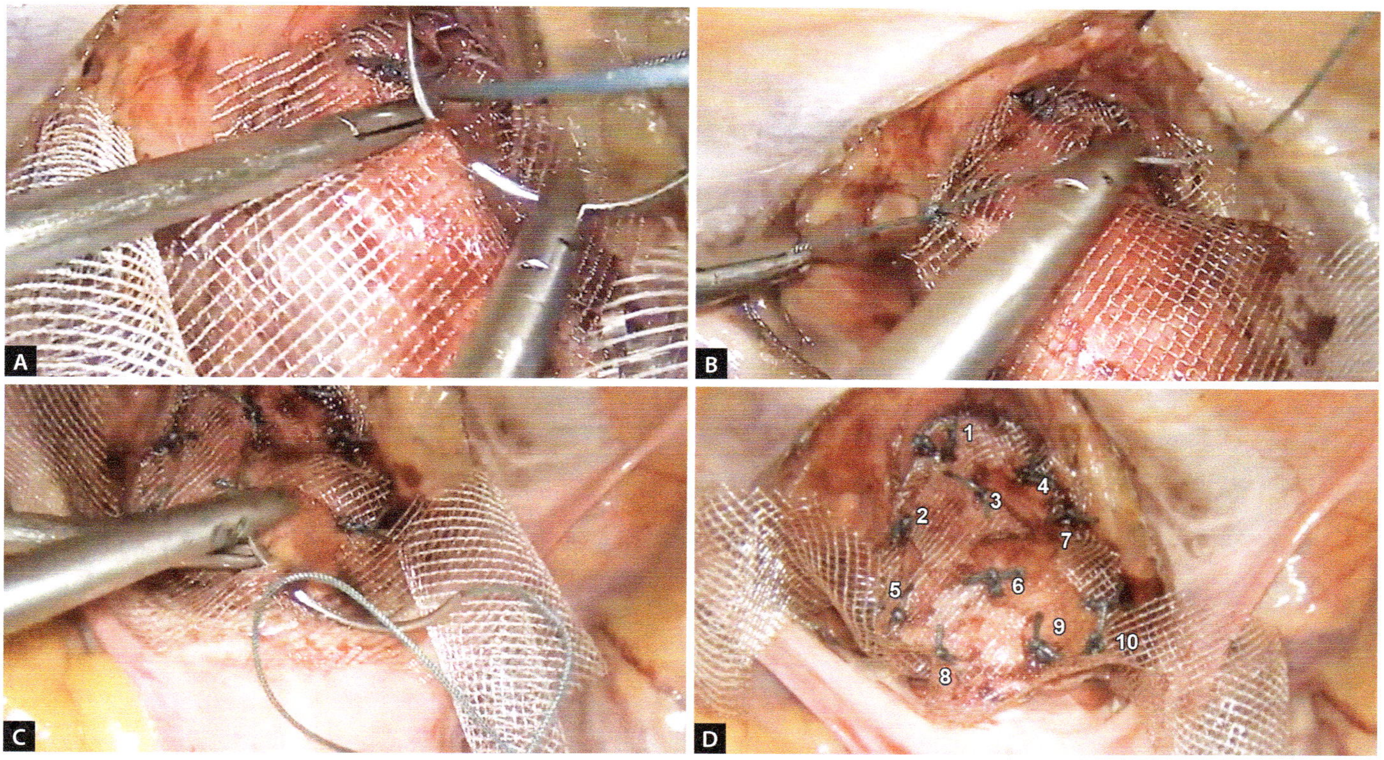

Figs. 4A to D: The centerpiece of mesh is fixed to the anterior vaginal fascia and cervix with 8–10 surgeons knot.

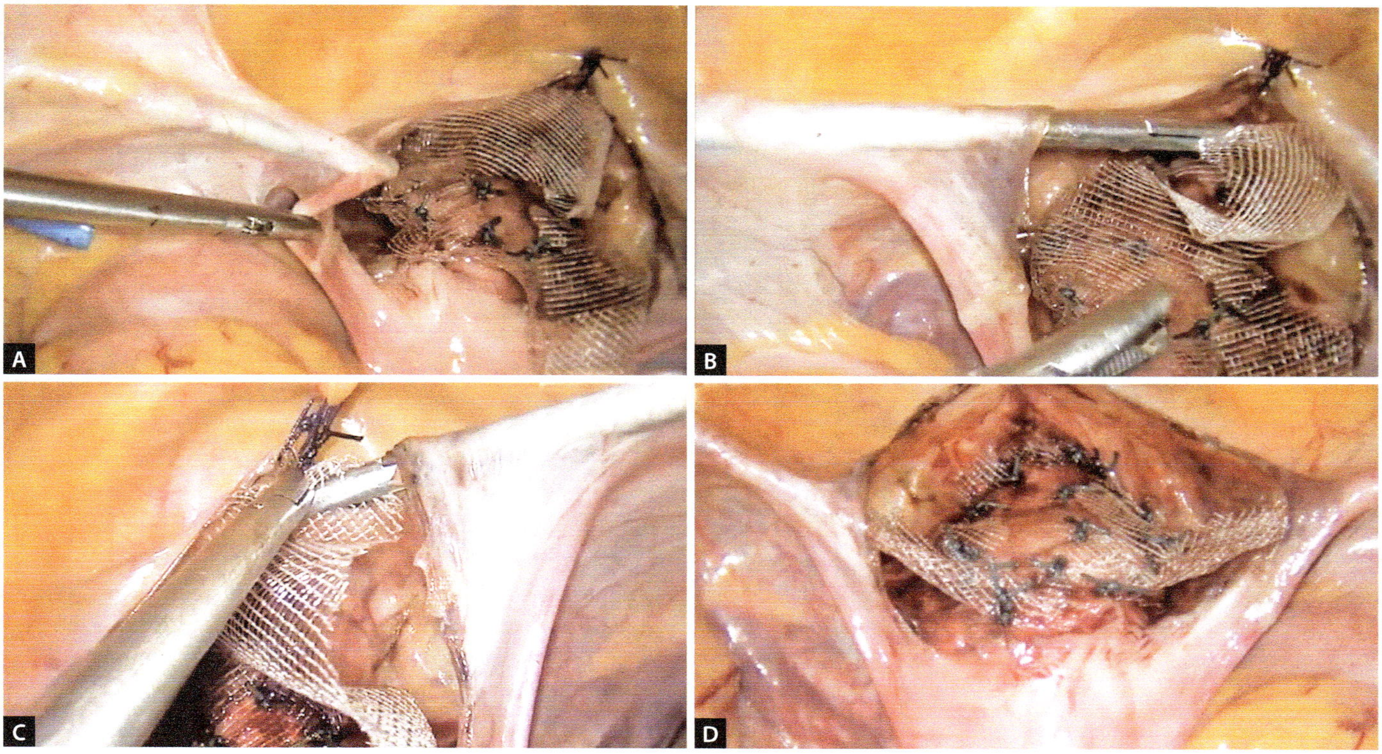

Figs. 5A to D: Pulling out along the tunnel underneath the round ligament.

Vaginal vault prolapse results from poor support of ligaments that normally maintain vaginal position. Several operative techniques are available to correct this problem. Abdominal colpopexy by suspending a mesh Hammock between the prolapsed vault and sacrum has been reported with good results. The laparoscopic modification of this operation combines the advantages of several procedures. Proper anatomic relationships are restored by correcting

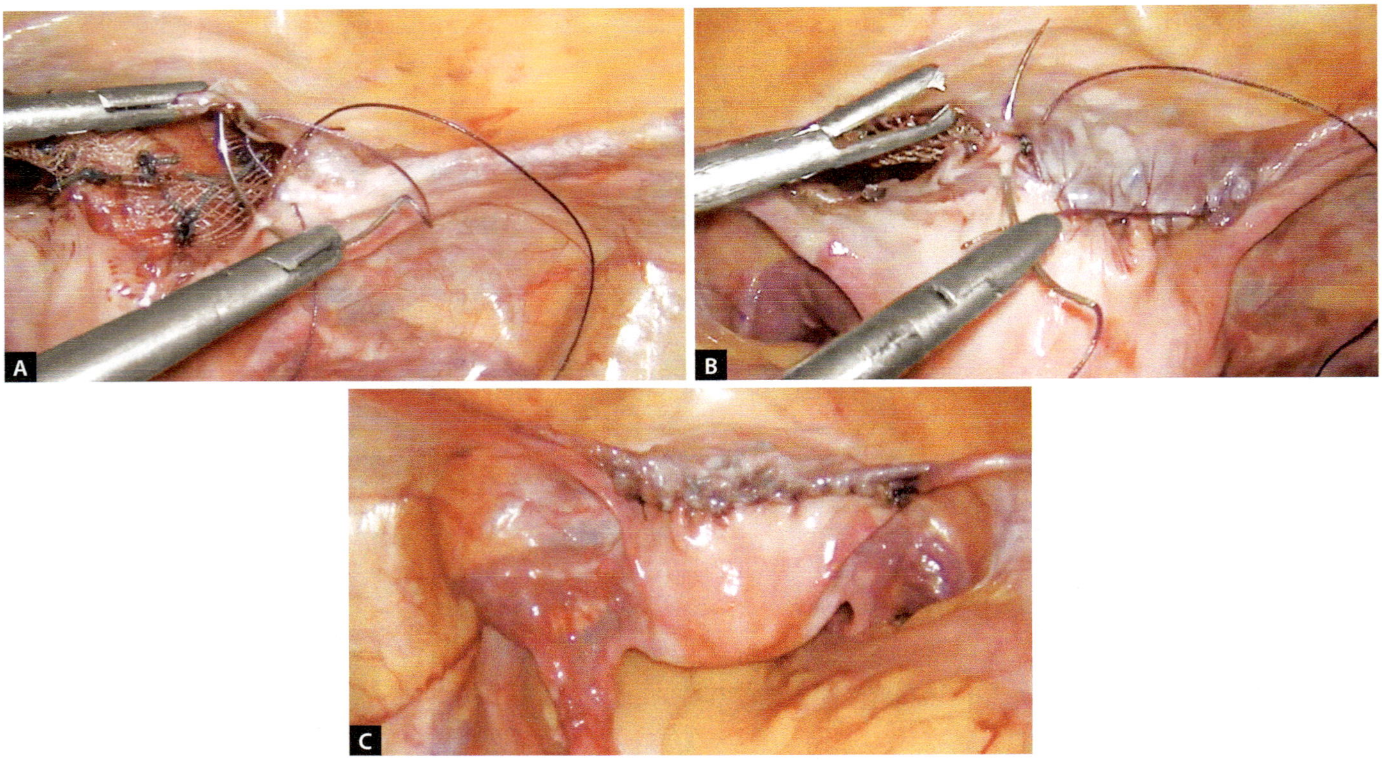

Figs. 6A to C: Closing of peritoneum to hide the mesh.

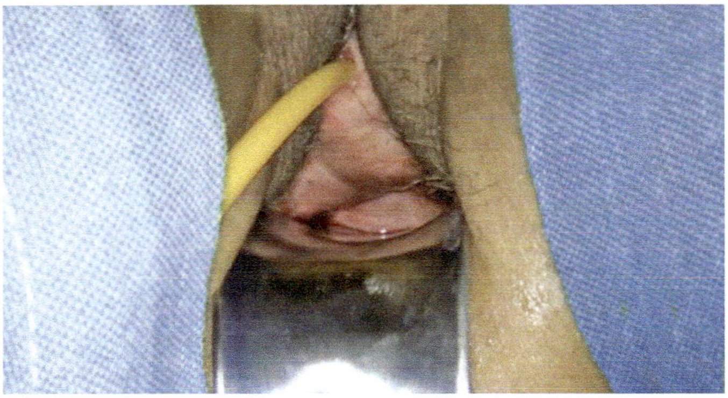

Fig. 7: Final look after repair of cystocele.

enterocele, reconstructing paracolpium fibers, and directing the vaginal axis toward S3 or S4 by evenly distributing tension over vaginal vault and the posterior cul-de-sac is obliterated using a Moschcowitz technique.

A laparoscopic approach has achieved favorable results with minimal blood loss, reduced hospitalization, and rapid recovery. An overall decrease in complications such as wound infection and dehiscence, deep vein thrombophlebitis, and small bowel ileus were noted when compared to laparotomy. Important patient selection factors include an ability to tolerate prolonged general anesthesia and pneumoperitoneum.

LAPAROSCOPIC PECTOPEXY

Although laparoscopic sacrocolpopexy has shown excellent anatomical and functional long-term results, laparoscopic pectopexy offers a feasible, safe, and comfortable alternative for apical prolapse surgery. Pectopexy may increase a surgeon's technical perspective for apical prolapse surgery. The pectopexy is performed under general anesthesia with endotracheal intubation and standard intramuscular cephalosporin antibiotics were used for prophylaxis. The patients were then placed in a modified lithotomy position with the hips at an approximate 180° extension, the knees flexed at almost 90°, and with the table tilted in a nearly 45° Trendelenburg position. Both arms were tucked along the patient's side. A 10-mm trocar was inserted directly from the umbilicus and pneumoperitoneum was generated until an intra-abdominal pressure of 14 mm Hg was achieved. Three additional 5 mm ports were inserted under direct visualization of the lower intra-abdominal area: median, left, and right from 2 cm medial and superior to the anterior superior iliac crests **(Figs. 15A and B)**. Following sterilization of the skin and covering of the patient, a RUMI uterine manipulator with a Koh Cup colpotomizer is transvaginally introduced at the beginning of the procedure. The surgeon stood on the patient's left and the first assistant handled the scope on the patient's right. The second assistant was positioned between the legs of the patient.

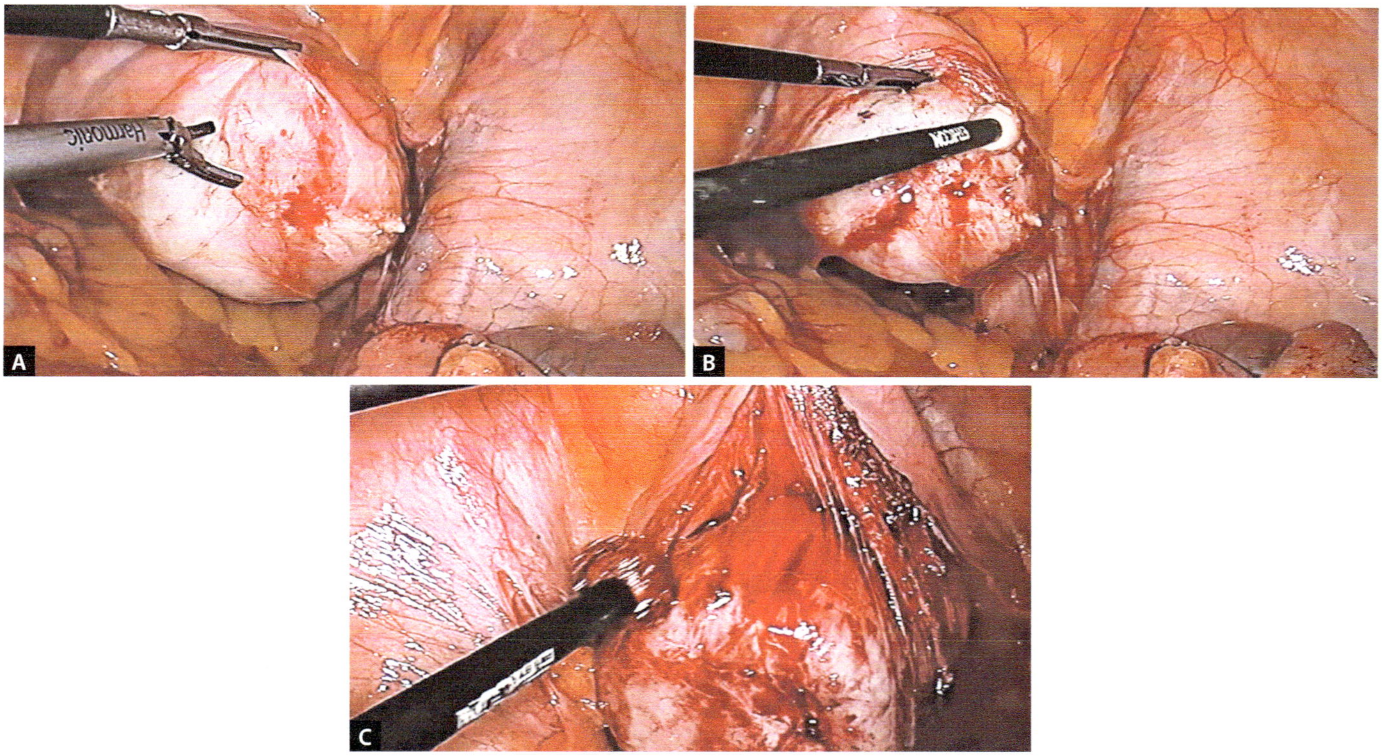

Figs. 8A to C: Dissection of bladder.

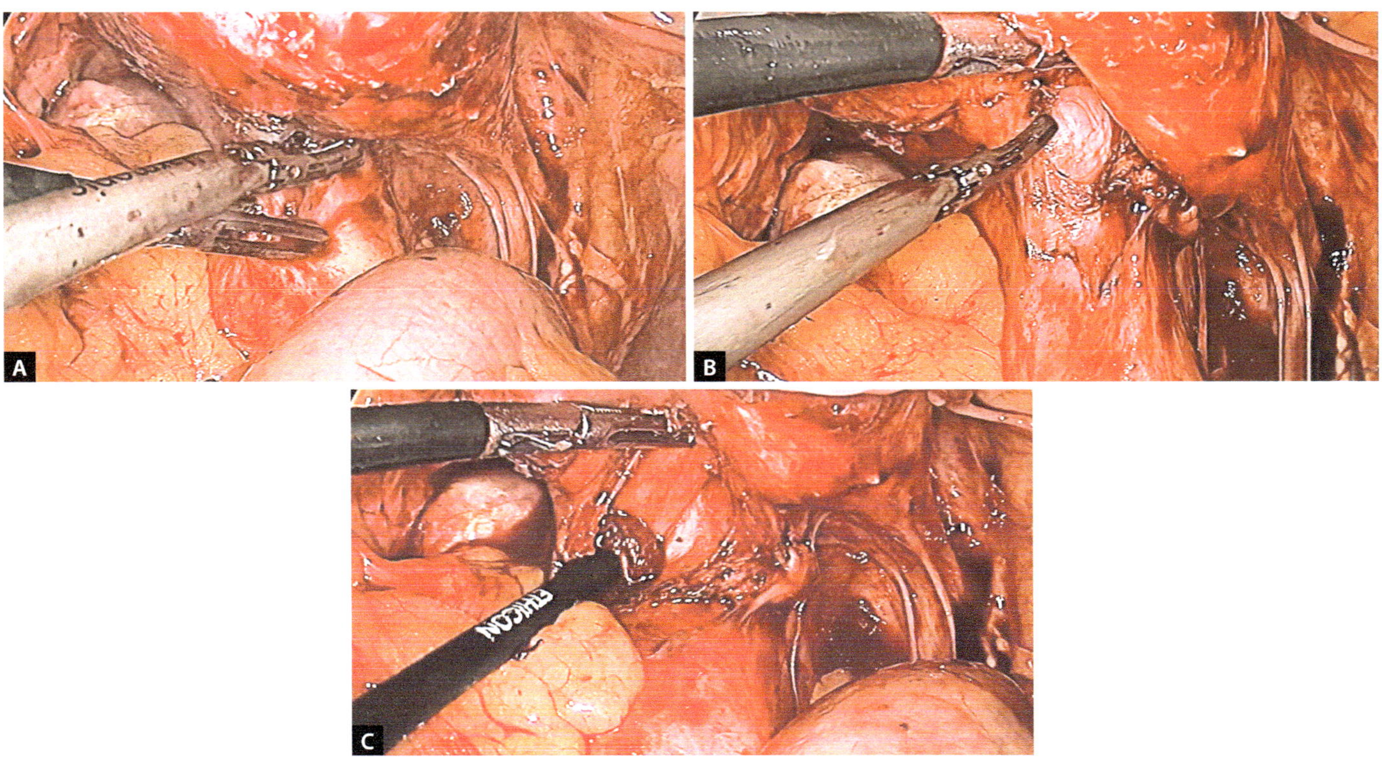

Figs. 9A to C: Dissection in between rectum and vagina.

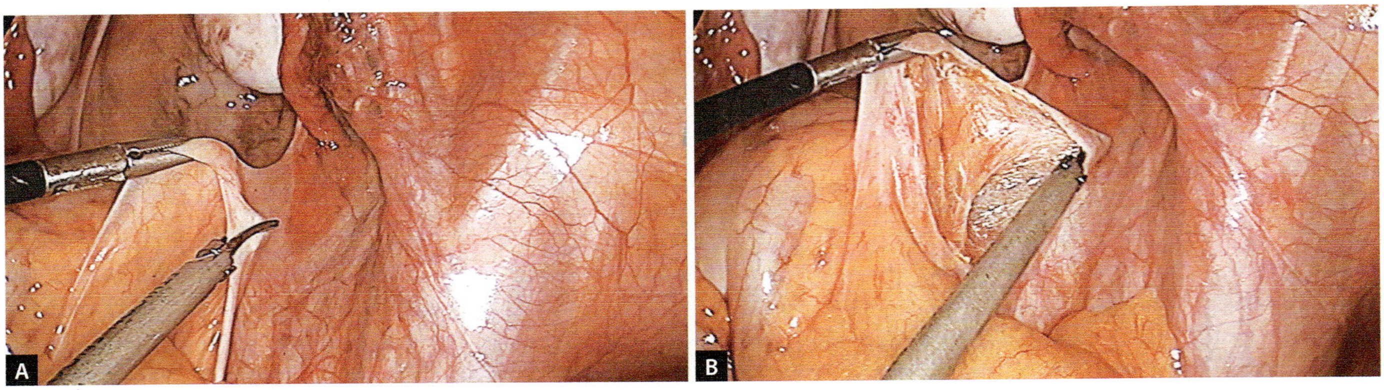

Figs. 10A and B: Opening of peritoneum over sacral promontory.

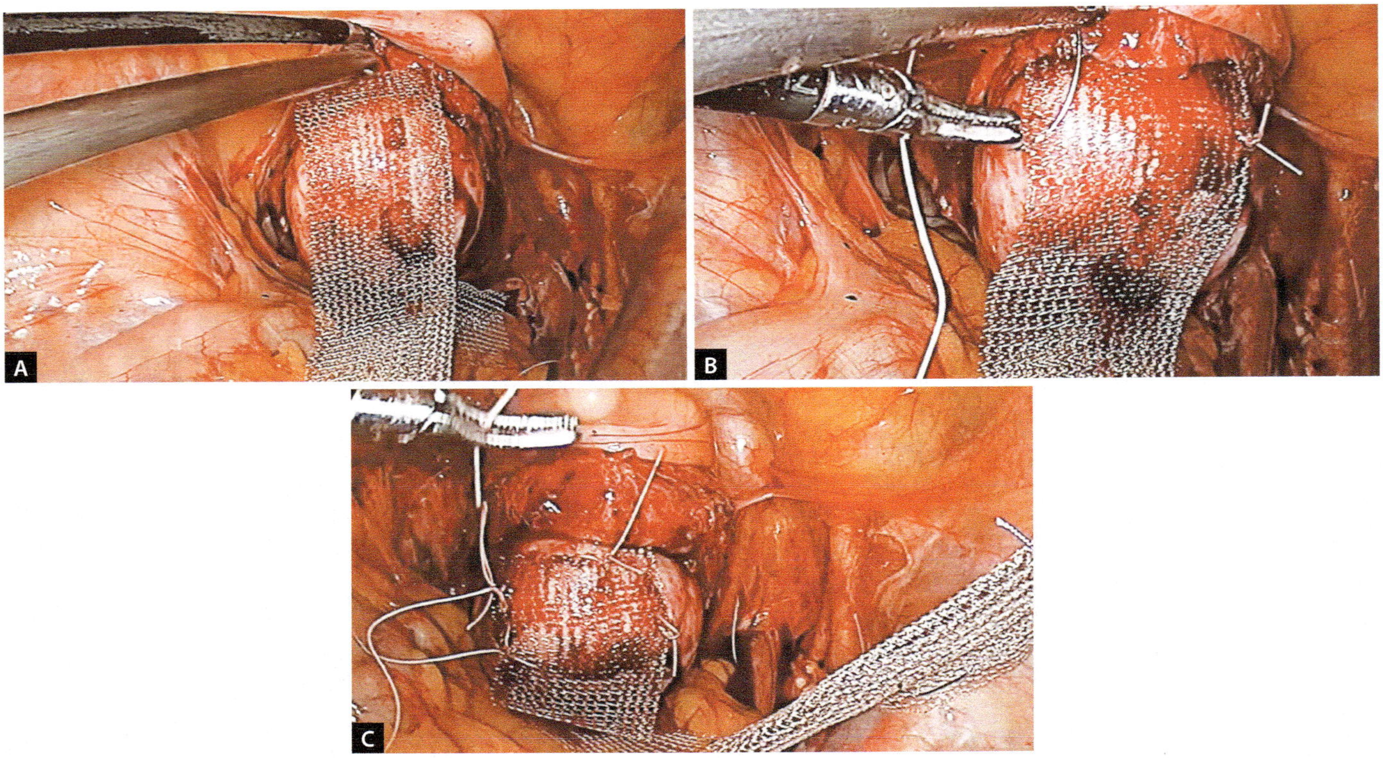

Figs. 11A to C: Fixation of mesh over vaginal cuff.

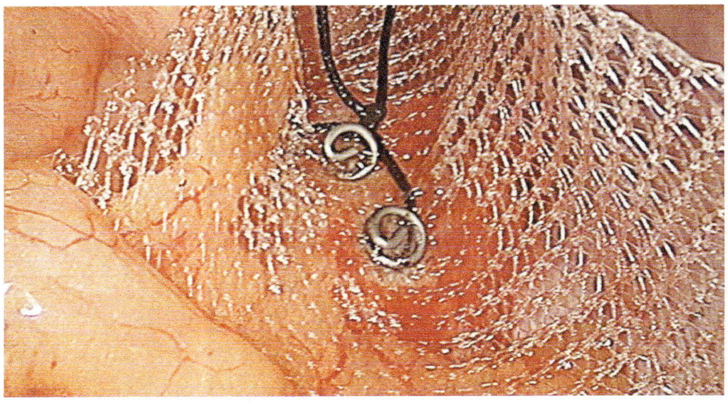

Fig. 12: Fixation of mesh to anterior longitudinal ligament.

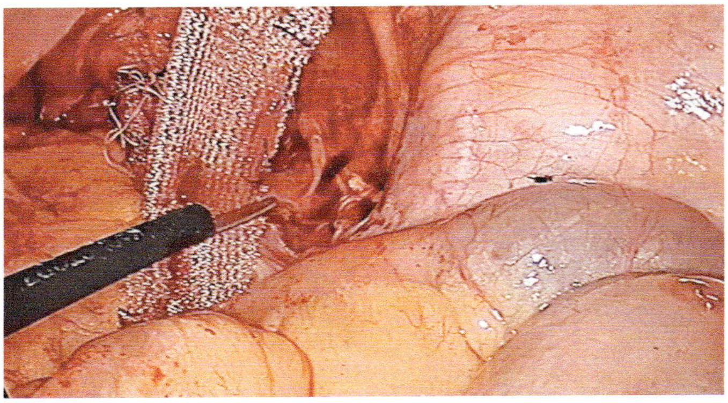

Fig. 13: Excess of the mesh is trimmed.

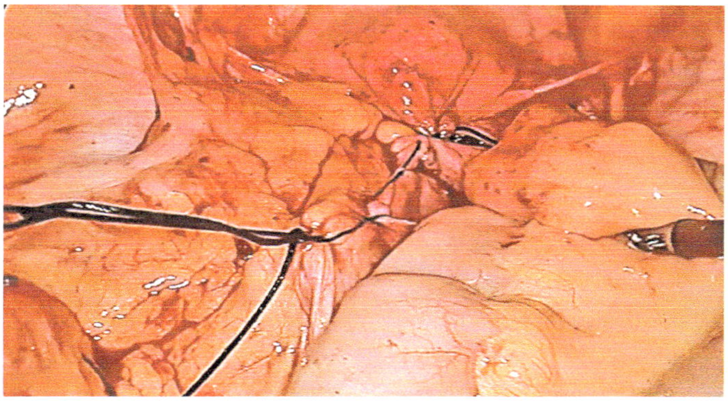

Fig. 14: Peritonization of mesh.

Pectopexy Technique

The peritoneum layer from midline is opened along the right round ligament toward the pelvic side wall and then same on left pelvic side wall. An incision in the medial and caudal direction was made with a harmonic scalpel **(Figs. 16A to D)**. Soft tissue in this area was dissected with blunt dissection, so an approximately 4–5 cm segment of the right iliopectineal ligament (Cooper's ligament) adjacent to the insertion of the iliopsoas muscle could be identified **(Figs. 17A and B)**. The same procedure was then repeated on the left side of the patient. The peritoneal layers on both sides were opened toward the vaginal apex and the anterior and posterior areas

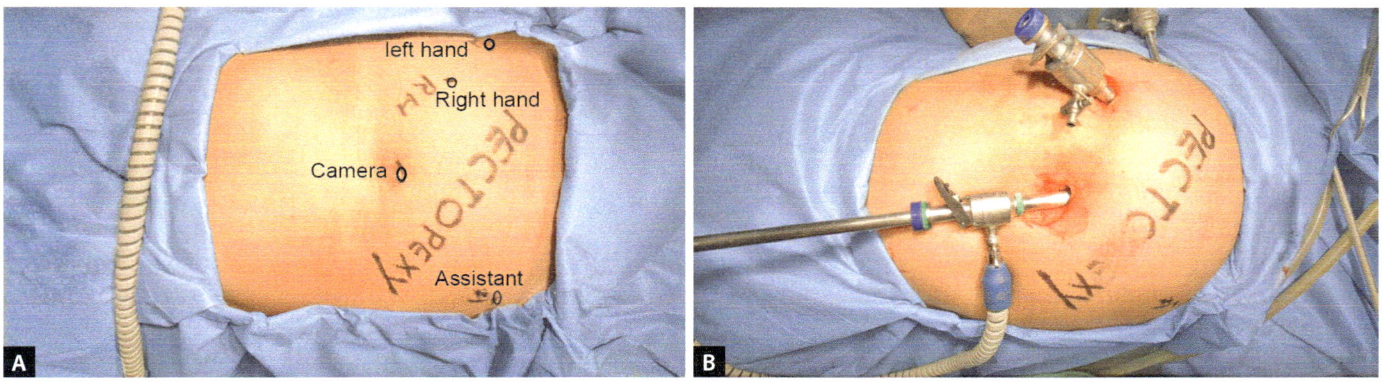

Figs. 15A and B: Port position in pectopexy.

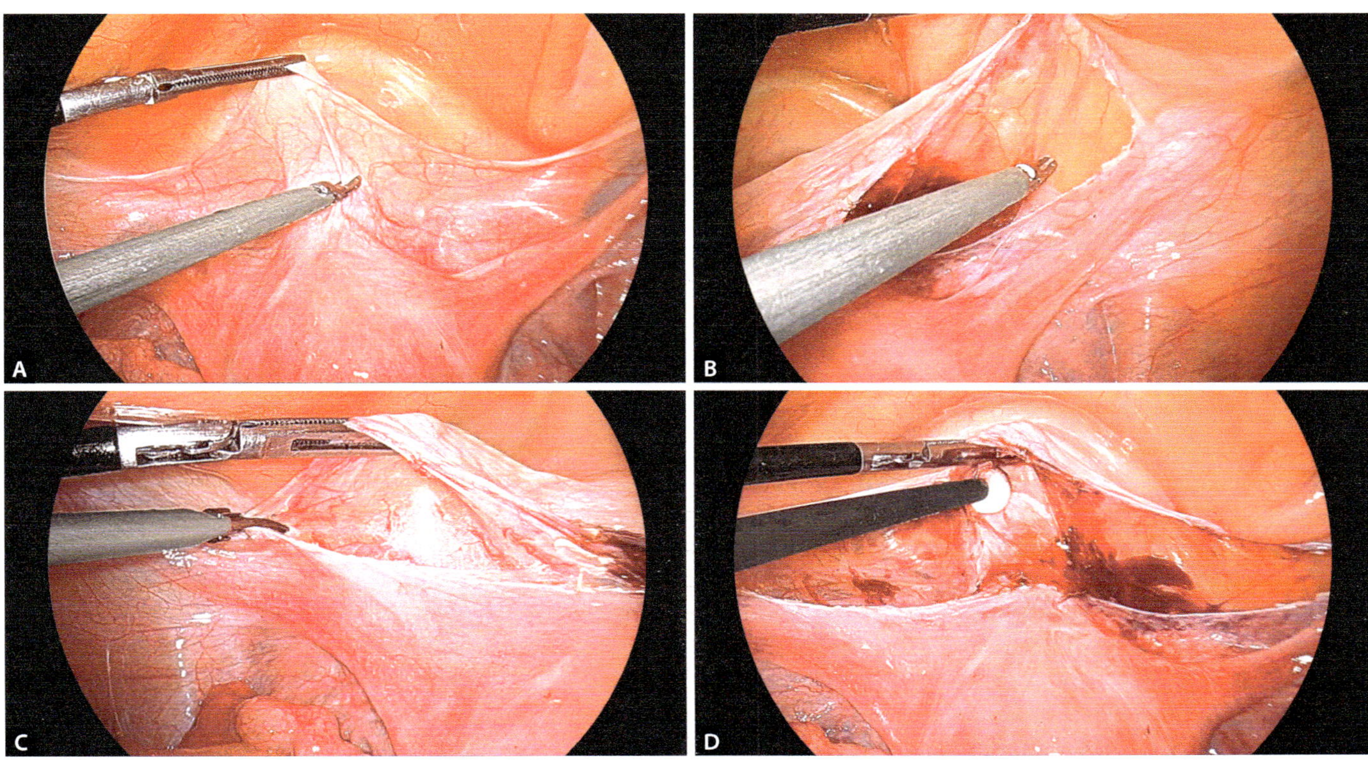

Figs. 16A to D: Opening of peritoneum on either side and separating bladder.

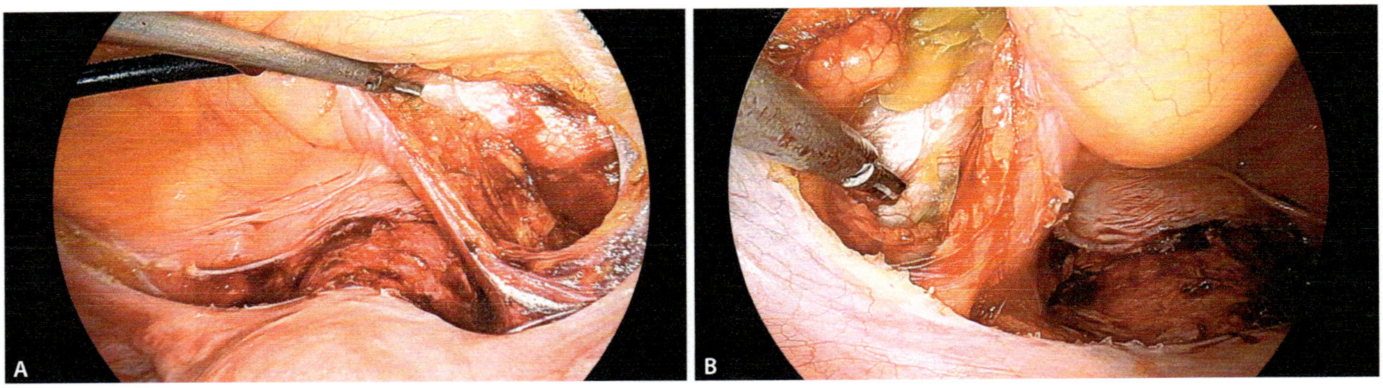

Figs. 17A and B: Exposing pectineal ligament of either side.

of the vaginal apex were prepared for the mesh fixation. In patients with a preserved uterus, the anterior peritoneum of the uterus was dissected and the lower anterior segment of the uterus was prepared for the mesh fixation. After completion of dissections, a polyvinylidene fluoride monofilament mesh is inserted into the abdominal cavity. The center of T-shaped mesh is fixed to the cervix and anterior vaginal fascia **(Fig. 18)**. The ends of the mesh were sutured to both iliopectineal ligaments via the intracorporeal suture technique using nonabsorbable suture or fixed with titanium tacker **(Figs. 19A and B)**. The mesh in the tension-free position was fixed to the vaginal apex or uterus with polydioxanone sutures and the vaginal apex or uterus was provided with a hammock-like fixation. Finally, the peritoneum above the mesh was sutured with an absorbable suture **(Figs. 20A to D)**.

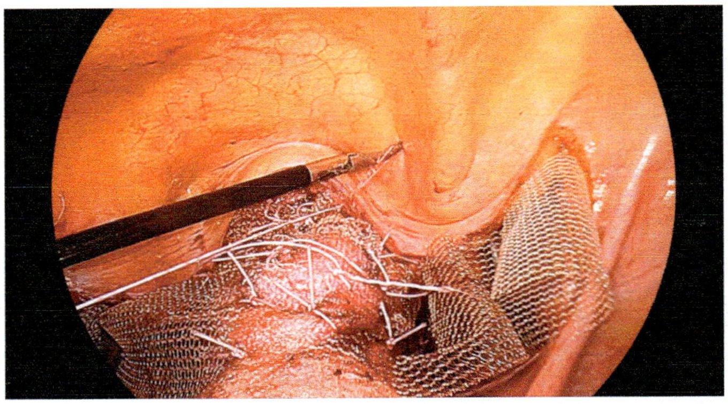

Fig. 18: Suturing middle of T-shaped mesh with cervix and vaginal fascia.

Laparoscopic pectopexy is an effective and alternative procedure for women with POP and a good option for preserving fertility. We found that pregnancy did not adversely affect the short-term success of laparoscopic pectopexy and vice versa.

POTENTIAL RISKS AND COMPLICATIONS

Although laparoscopic colposuspension has proven to be very safe, as in any surgical procedure, there are risks and potential complications. Potential risks include:

- *Bleeding*: Although blood loss during this procedure is relatively low compared to open surgery, a transfusion may still be required if deemed necessary either during the operation or afterward during the postoperative period.
- *Infection and erosion of bladder*: All patients are treated with intravenous antibiotics prior to the start of surgery to decrease the chance of infection from occurring within the urinary tract or at the incision sites. Women having vaginal erosion should be prescribed a vaginal estrogen cream two to three times daily for few weeks.
- *Adjacent organ injury*: Although uncommon, possible injury to surrounding tissue and organs including bowel, vascular structures, pelvic musculature, and nerves could require further procedures. Transient injury to nerves or muscles can also occur related to patient positioning during the operation.
- *Hernia*: Hernias at the incision sites rarely occur since all port entry incisions are closed under direct laparoscopic view.
- *Conversion to open surgery*: The surgical procedure may require conversion to the standard open operation, if extreme difficulty is encountered during the laparoscopic procedure (e.g., excess scarring or bleeding). This could result in a standard open incision and possibly a longer recuperation period.
- *Urinary incontinence*: Preexisting urinary incontinence will typically be addressed at the time of surgery with a bladder sling suspension; however, minor incontinence may still exist, which typically resolves with time. On occasion, medication may be required.
- *Urinary retention*: As with urinary incontinence, postoperative urinary retention is uncommon and usually is present in patients who undergo concurrent bladder sling suspension. Temporary intermittent self-catheterization may be required postoperatively.
- *Vesicovaginal fistula*: A fistula between the bladder and vagina is a rare complication of any pelvic surgery

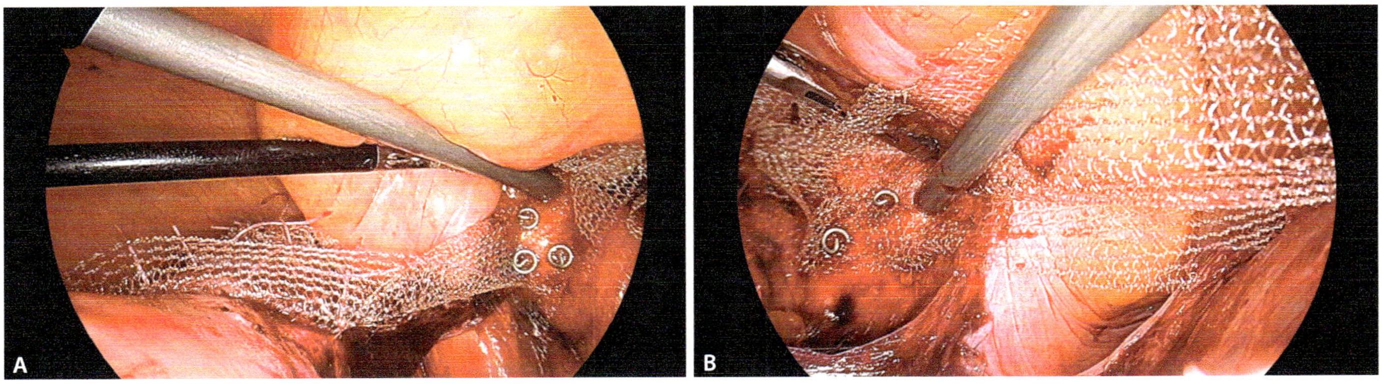

Figs. 19A and B: Mesh is fixed on either side of pectineal ligament.

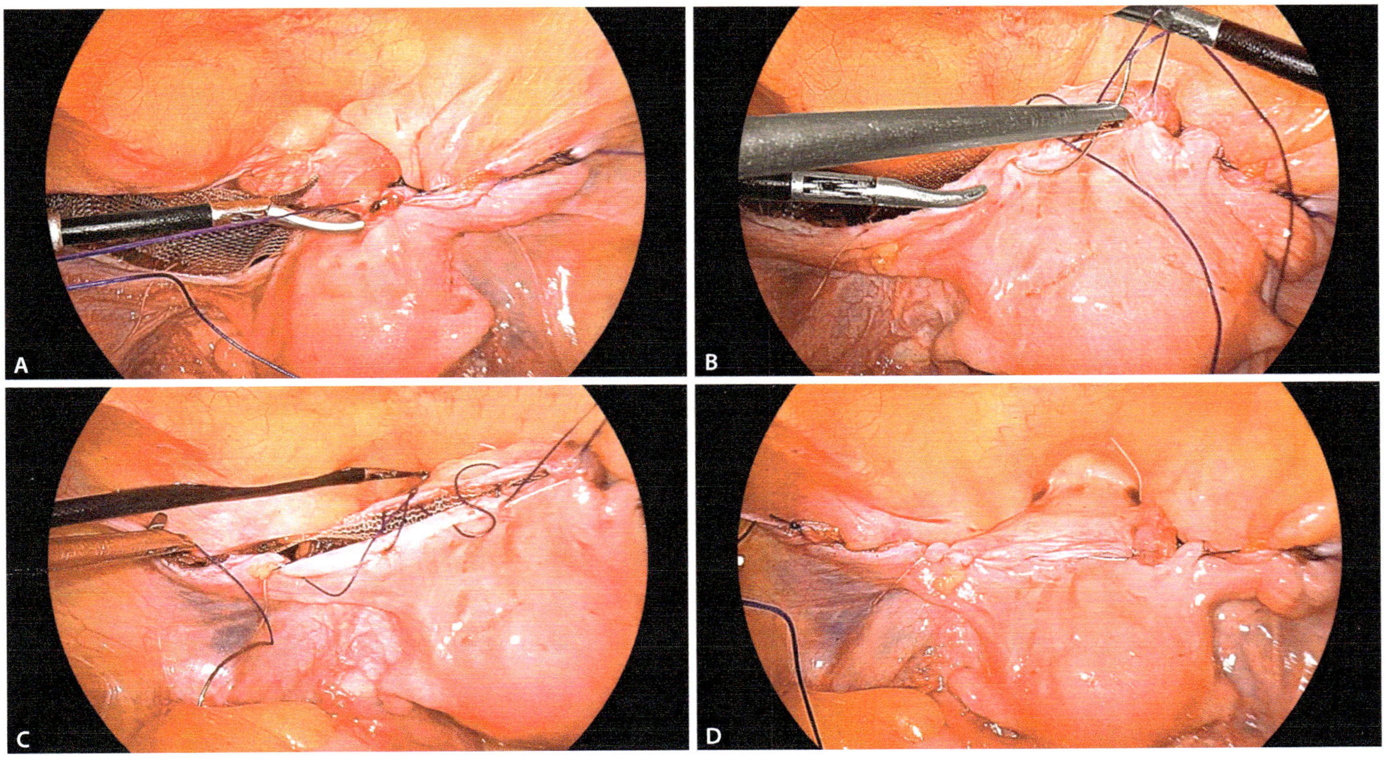

Figs. 20A to D: Peritonization of mesh.

involving the vagina, uterus, and bladder. A vesicovaginal fistula typically manifests with symptoms of continuous urinary leakage from the vagina. Although rare, these fistulas can be managed conservatively or by surgical repair through a vaginal incision.

Abdominal sacrocolpopexy, laparoscopic sacrocolpopexy, and laparoscopic pectopexy have comparable perioperative complications and short-term anatomical and subjective outcomes. Although the complication rates were not significantly different between the groups, the laparoscopic sacrocolpopexy and pectopexy groups had less morbidity. Moreover, laparoscopic pectopexy is a novel promising method for POP correction that offers some practical advantages such as shorter operating times when compared with laparoscopic sacrocolpopexy, so that it can be added to a surgeon's methods to more adequately react in complex presacral area dissections.

BIBLIOGRAPHY

1. Akladios CY, Dautun D, Saussine C, Baldauf JJ, Mathelin C, Wattiez A. Laparoscopic sacrocolpopexy for female genital organ prolapse: establishment of a learning curve. Eur J Obstet Gynecol Reprod Biol. 2010;149:218-21.
2. Alkatout I, Mettler L, Peters G, Noé G, Holthaus B, Jonat W, et al. Laparoscopic hysterectomy and prolapse: a multiprocedural concept. JSLS. 2014;18:89-101.
3. Baessler K, Schuessler B. Abdominal sacrocolpopexy and anatomy and function of the posterior compartment. Obstet Gynecol. 2001;97:678-84.

4. Banerjee C, Noé KG. Laparoscopic pectopexy: a new technique of prolapse surgery for obese patients. Arch Gynecol Obstet. 2011;284:631-5.
5. Beer M, Kuhn A. Surgical techniques for vault prolapse: a review of the literature. Eur J Obstet Gynecol Reprod Biol. 2005;119: 144-55.
6. Bundesministerium des Innern. Demography Report: Report of the German Federal Government on the Demographic Situation and Future Development of the Country. Berlin: German Federal Ministry of the Interior; 2011.
7. Cosson M, Boukerrou M, Lacaze S, Lambaudie E, Fasel J, Mesdagh H, et al. A study of pelvic ligament strength. Eur J Obstet Gynecol Reprod Biol. 2003;109:80-7.
8. El-Hamamsy D, Fayyad AM. New onset stress urinary incontinence following laparoscopic sacrocolpopexy and its relation to anatomical outcomes. Int Urogynecol J. 2015;26:1041-5.
9. Faure JP, Hauet T, Scepi M, Chansigaud JP, Kamina P, Richer JP. The pectineal ligament: anatomical study and surgical applications. Surg Radiol Anat. 2001;23:237-42.
10. Irvine L, Shaw R. The effects of patient obesity in gynaecological practice. Curr Opin Obstet Gynecol. 2003;13:179-84.
11. Kumar S, Malhotra N, Chumber S, Gupta P, Aruna J, Roy KK, et al. Control of presacral venous bleeding, using thumbtacks. Arch Gynecol Obstet. 2007;276:385-6.
12. LeClaire EL, Mukati MS, Juarez D, White D, Quiroz LH. Is de novo stress incontinence after sacrocolpopexy related to anatomical changes and surgical approach? Int Urogynecol J. 2014;25: 1201-6.
13. Lee RK, Mottrie A, Payne CK, Waltregny D. A review of the current status of laparoscopic and robot-assisted sacrocolpopexy for pelvic organ prolapse. Eur Urol. 2014;65:1128-37.
14. Maher C, Feiner B, Baessler K, Adams EJ, Hagen S, Glazener CM. Surgical management of pelvic organ prolapse in women. Cochrane Database Syst Rev. 2010;4:CD004014.
15. Noé KG, Schiermeier S, Alkatout I, Anapolski M. Laparoscopic pectopexy: a prospective, randomized, comparative clinical trial of standard laparoscopic sacral colpocervicopexy with the new laparoscopic pectopexy-postoperative results and intermediate-term follow-up in a pilot study. J Endourol. 2015;29:210-5.
16. Noé KG, Spüntrup C, Anapolski M. Laparoscopic pectopexy: a randomised comparative clinical trial of standard laparoscopic sacral colpo-cervicopexy to the new laparoscopic pectopexy: short-term postoperative results. Arch Gynecol Obstet. 2013;287:275-80.
17. North CE, Ali-Ross NS, Smith AR, Reid FM. A prospective study of laparoscopic sacrocolpopexy for the management of pelvic organ prolapse. BJOG. 2009;116:1251-7.
18. Nygaard IE, McCreery R, Brubaker L, Connolly A, Cundiff G, Weber AM, et al. Pelvic Floor Disorders Network Abdominal sacrocolpopexy: a comprehensive review. Obstet Gynecol. 2004;104:805-23.
19. Sarlos D, Brandner S, Kots L, Gygax N, Schaer G. Laparoscopic sacrocolpopexy for uterine and post-hysterectomy prolapse: anatomical results, quality of life and perioperative outcome—a prospective study with 101 cases. Int Urogynecol J Pelvic Floor Dysfunct. 2008;19:1415-22.
20. Sarlos D, Kots L, Ryu G, Schaer G. Long-term follow-up of laparoscopic sacrocolpopexy. Int Urogynecol J. 2014;25:1207-12.
21. Snyder TE, Krantz KE. Abdominal-retroperitoneal sacral colpopexy for the correction of vaginal prolapse. Obstet Gynecol. 1991;77:944-9.
22. Subak LL, Waetjen LE, van den Eeden S, Thom DH, Vittinghoff E, Brown JS. Cost of pelvic organ prolapse surgery in the United States. Obstet Gynecol. 2001;98:646-51.
23. Whitehead WE, Bradley CS, Brown MB, Brubaker L, Gutman RE, Varner RE, et al. Gastrointestinal complications following abdominal sacrocolpopexy for advanced pelvic organ prolapse. Am J Obstet Gynecol. 2007;197:78.e1-7.

CHAPTER 39

Essentials of Hysteroscopy

DEFINITION

Hysteroscopy is a procedure used to view the inside of the uterus through a telescope-like device called a hysteroscope. Hysteroscopy offers a valuable extension to the gynecologist's armamentarium. It can improve the diagnostic accuracy and can permit better treatment of uterine diseases. The hysteroscope is placed in the vagina and introduced into the uterus **(Figs. 1A and B)**. A hysteroscope is introduced in a sheath that provides an inflow and outflow channel for insufflation of the uterine cavity. In addition, an operative channel may be present to introduce scissors, graspers, or biopsy instruments. A hysteroscopic resectoscope is similar to a transurethral resectoscope and allows entry of an electric loop to shave off tissue, for instance, to eliminate a fibroid. A contact hysteroscope is a hysteroscope that does not use distension media.

INDICATIONS

- *Diagnostic hysteroscopy*: Hysteroscopy allows access to the uterotubal junction for entry into the fallopian tube; this is useful for tubal occlusion procedures for sterilization and for falloposcopy
- *Asherman's syndrome (i.e., intrauterine adhesions)*: Hysteroscopic adhesiolysis is the technique of lysing adhesions in the uterus using either microscissors (recommended) or thermal energy modalities. Hysteroscopy can be used in conjunction with laparoscopy or other methods to reduce the risk of perforation during the procedure
- *Endometrial polyp*: Polypectomy
- *Abnormal uterine bleeding*: In patients with abnormal uterine bleeding, hysteroscopy provides more accurate diagnosis than dilatation and curettage
- Adenomyosis
- Endometrial ablation (some newer systems specifically developed for endometrial ablation such as the NovaSure does not require hysteroscopy)
- Myomectomy for uterine fibroids
- Congenital uterine malformations (also known as Müllerian malformations)
- Evacuation of retained products of conception in selected cases
- Removal of embedded intrauterine devices (IUDs).

CONTRAINDICATIONS

- Pregnancy
- Heavy uterine bleeding
- Pelvic inflammatory disease
- Cervical malignancy
- Recent uterine perforation.

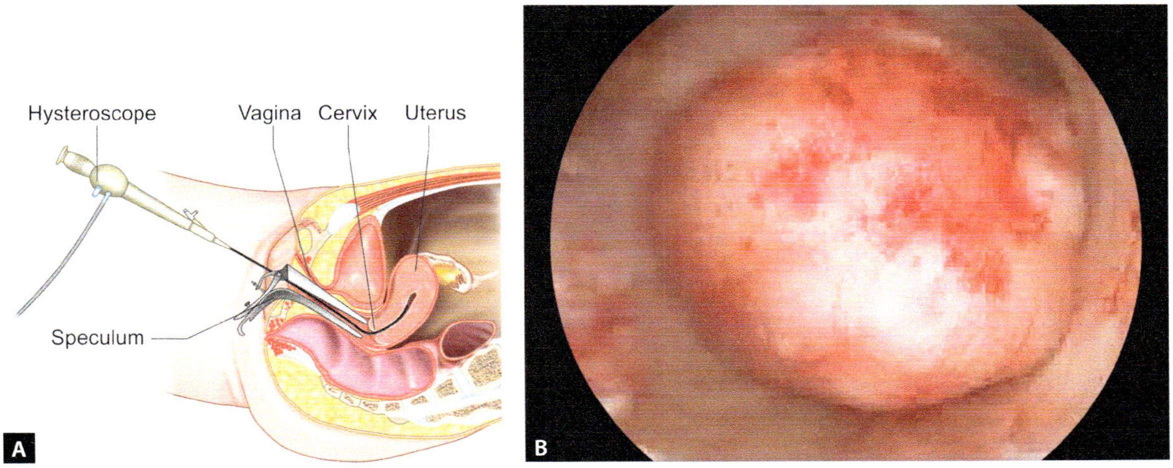

Figs. 1A and B: (A) Hysteroscopy; (B) Hysteroscopic visualization of submucous myoma.

HISTORY (FIGS. 2A AND B)

- First hysteroscope with cystoscope of Desormeaux by Pantaleoni in 1869
- First hysteroscope with built-in lens to magnify the image.

DELIVERY DEVICES

- Maximum recommended intrauterine operating pressure is 150 mm Hg
- Intrauterine pressure is a function of inflow pressure and outflow pressure
- Inflow pressure may be produced by gravity, pressured cuffs with (pressure) gauges, or approved pumps.

DISTENDING MEDIA

- *Group A*: Isotonic ionic solutions (normal saline and Ringer's lactate)
- *Group B*: 5% dextrose in water
- *Group C*: 1.5% glycine, sorbitol, and cytal
- *Group D*: Hyskon (32% dextran 70).

FLUID MONITORING

It is the role of the circulating nurse to maintain a flow sheet record of inflow and outflow of hysteroscopic media during the case.

For groups A, B, and C, the inflow and outflow must be estimated for every 500 cc of fluid used and measured at the conclusion of each bag of distending media.

For group D, the inflow and outflow must be measured for every 100 cc of fluid used.

The operating surgeon should be simultaneously informed of fluid balance status as it is recorded on the flow sheet. Spillage should be avoided.

Use of a table drape to collect excess fluid for accurate recording of fluid output is required.

EXCESSIVE FLUID ABSORPTION

The recommended volume of input to output discrepancy at which point the surgeon must assess serum electrolytes (especially sodium concentration) is:

- *Group A*: 1 L
- *Group B*: 1 L
- *Group C*: 1 L
- *Group D*: 250 mL

Once these volumes of discrepancy have been reached, serum electrolytes must be obtained and the operating surgeon has the option of:

Terminating the case: Awaiting the results of the electrolyte levels and proceeding accordingly.

Administering Lasix intravenous (IV) and judiciously proceeding with the case until the results are available.

RESECTOSCOPE

- The *resectoscope* has been used for male prostate surgery for over 50 years
- The resectoscope with in-built wire loop or other shape device uses high-frequency electrical current to cut or coagulate tissue **(Figs. 3A and B)**.

Procedure

Patient position is shown in **Figure 4**. Inside of the uterus is a potential cavity such as a collapsed air-dome and it is necessary to fill (distend) it with either a liquid or a gas (carbon dioxide) in order to see.

Diagnostic hysteroscopy and simple operative hysteroscopy can usually be done in an office setting. More complex operative hysteroscopy procedures are done in operating room setting **(Figs. 5A and B)**.

The volumes that are recommended in this section are not based on established "standards of care", since such

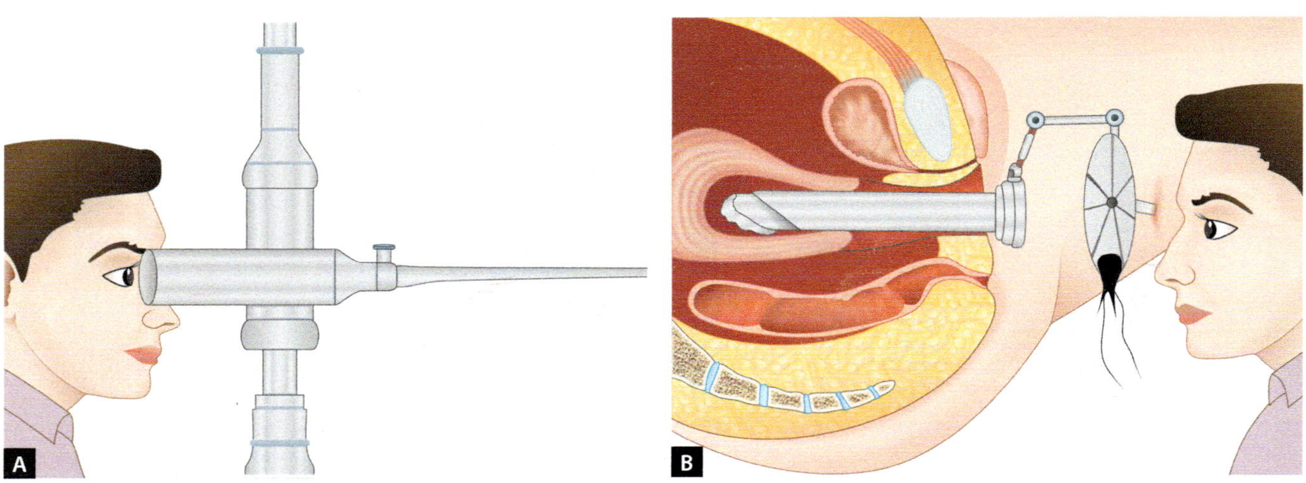

Figs. 2A and B: History of hysteroscopy. (A) First hysteroscope with cystoscope of Desormeaux by Pantaleoni; (B) First hysteroscope with built-in lens to magnify the image.

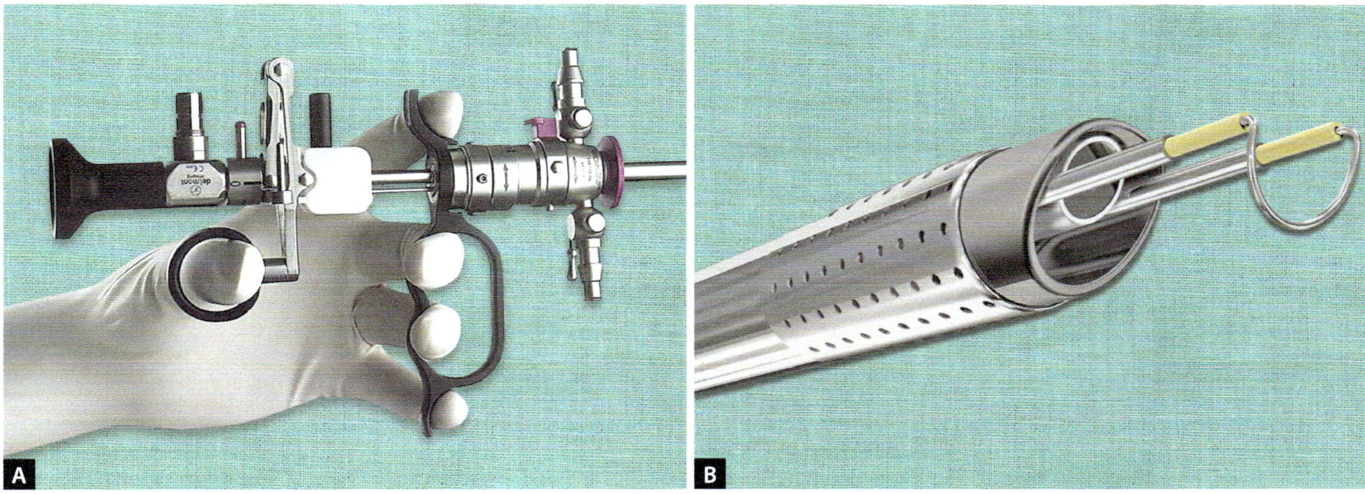

Figs. 3A and B: Resectoscope.

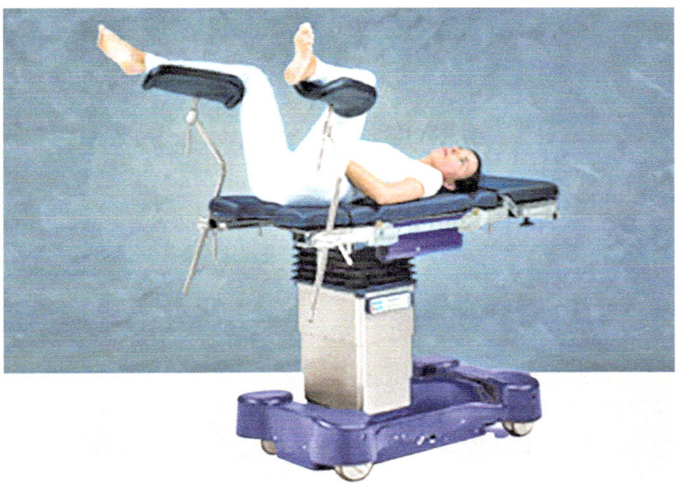

Fig. 4: Patient position in hysteroscopy.

standards have not yet been clearly formalized. For example, many surgeons use 1 L as a cutoff for 5% dextrose in water (D5W), while few others use 3 L. There is no established limit for the volume of D5W that can safely be given as an IV solution being directly infused into the circulation of a healthy person. No reports of major morbidity associated with the use of D5W have been reported in the literature.

Additional patient assessment following a large volume discrepancy between input and output may immediately involve determination of serum electrolytes. If a significant time has passed since the (presumed) absorption of fluid, other clinical parameters (if available) may become more informative (evidence of tissue edema, an increase in cardiac output associated with volume overload, change in pulse oximetry or ventilation parameters, and change in patient temperature, if room temperature fluid is used).

A resectoscope is used with continuous flow and a loop electrode to perform most of the hysteroscopic surgery. Any of the irrigation system for distending media available today is not sufficiently accurate. They are not rapid in response (so as to maintain a constant pressure), affordable, and easy to use. At present, many gynecologists use a simple system of placing a blood pressure cuff around each 1 L bag of normal saline solution to be used and apply 150 mm Hg pressure as measured on a gauge attached to the pressure cuff. This is connected to the inflow port on the resectoscope and flow is then adjusted using a stopcock on this port. Outflow from the resectoscope is via tubing that connects directly to a suction canister under full wall suction. The outflow port also has a stopcock that can be used to adjust the outflow.

The circulating nurse's primary responsibility during the operative hysteroscopy is to maintain pressure on the pressure cuff and watch the inflow and outflow balance. The nurse might appropriately report this balance to the surgeon and anesthesiologist every 15 minutes or whenever there is a significant volume of use (500 cc).

The resectoscope's monopolar electrocautery loop is attached to an electrical generator with variable power (wattage) settings. For any given power setting selected, there are also various blends of cutting or coagulation that can be chosen. It is advisable to use blend 1 which applies 80% current of the time and gives just a little coagulation as compared to pure cutting. For most cases, resectoscope is used at 50–80 W on blend 1 and to coagulate bleeders (if not initially controlled with the blend 1 settings), using 50 W at pure coagulation is recommended.

Once the hysteroscopic portion of the case is completed, a final tabulation of inflow and outflow volumes for the distending media is done. Direct your attention to the laparoscopy once the hysteroscopy is complete. A uterine manipulator is placed through the cervix.

Laparoscope should be inserted after that. For this, Veress needle is introduced. Insufflation of the abdomen with CO_2 gas so as to create a pneumoperitoneum is accomplished after "confirming the proper placement" of the Veress needle.

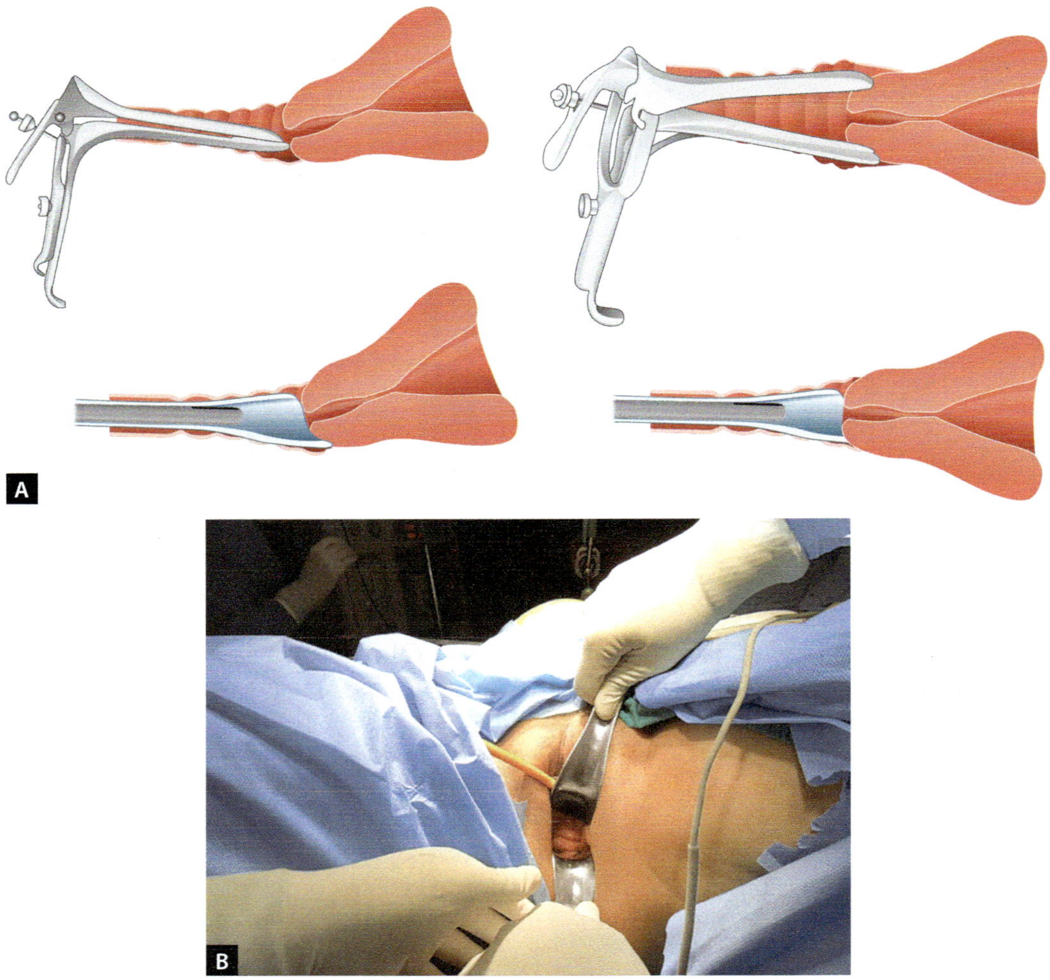

Figs. 5A and B: Vaginal speculum examination before hysteroscopy.

Once the pneumoperitoneum is created, the Veress needle is replaced by a trocar and sleeve. The diameter of the umbilical (main) trocar is 10–12 mm, so this instrument can cause considerable injury if not placed properly and atraumatically into the abdominal cavity. The presence of adhesions (scar) that adhere the bowel to the anterior abdominal wall is a consistent source of concern for laparoscopic surgeons.

If abundant adhesions are anticipated such that the surgeon believes that the complication rate with the blind Veress needle and trocar insertion is unacceptably high, then "open method" may be chosen. Hasson introduced this technique in which the direct insertion of the trocar without the creation of a prior pneumoperitoneum is accomplished by performing a cut down under direct observation of the layers of the abdominal wall. Suture holds the layers of the inner abdominal wall (fascia and peritoneum) to the trocar sleeve to prevent the release of gas through the incision site during the case. Extreme care must be exercised in making the peritoneal incision since bowel injury to adherent bowel may occur under direct observation as well.

Accessory trocar sites are usually required during the laparoscopic case. Typically, use two additional sites for placement of 5 mm (or uncommonly 10 mm) trocars in the suprapubic midline and left lower quadrant. All accessory trocars have the advantage of being able to be inserted under direct observation, so injury is less common. One injury associated with placement of the accessory trocars is laceration of the deep inferior epigastric vessels (which may be difficult to see either directly or via transillumination). Injury to the inferior epigastric vessels can be consistently avoided by placement of the additional trocars either lateral to the internal inguinal ring or medial to the umbilical ligaments (two structures that are usually easy to identify under direct laparoscopic observation).

Tools that are selected for the performance of the laparoscopic surgery should allow the surgeon to minimize postoperative adhesion formation. The surgical principles as discussed above are very important in terms of achieving the desired outcome. Gentle tissue handling during laparoscopy takes a great deal of time to develop. Avoidance of bleeding with gentle tissue handling is important and so is careful hemostasis using (selective) bipolar cautery. Continuous irrigation and aspiration of the tissues to remove char and minimize drying should be second nature to the laparoscopic infertility surgeon. Use of cutting instruments that minimize lateral tissue damage is also a primary importance.

Once the case has been completed, the instruments are removed from the abdomen allowing for the efflux of CO_2 gas. Usually, it takes additional 5 minutes to move the abdominal wall and contents about with only one remaining trocar sleeve is in place to try to allow any trapped gas to escape. Incisions are closed with subcuticular stitches, so as to avoid cosmetically unpleasant "railroad" type skin scars. The fascia is closed where incision in the fascia is >5 mm. In the immediate postoperative recovery time period, common problems include nausea and vomiting, most likely related to the CO_2 gas or the narcotic pain medications used perioperatively. Zofran is often the most effective antiemetic agent for postlaparoscopic vomiting. The nausea and vomiting do not typically persist for >12 hours postoperatively.

Shoulder pain due to retained CO_2 gas, which if trapped under the diaphragm (at base of the lungs), causes irritation of the phrenic nerve to cause the sensation of shoulder pain. Lying on one's abdomen with a pillow under the hips and lower abdomen (or the knee chest position) may allow the CO_2 gas to recollect in the pelvis rather than under the lungs and reduce this discomfort.

Subcutaneous crepitance (crackling) under the skin over the abdomen and extending superiorly to the chest and neck or inferiorly to the buttocks and thighs is typically a minor complication due to escape of the gas into the abdominal wall. A rare patient develops a very low blood pressure (not related to blood loss) and usually responds immediately to a bolus of IV fluid solution.

Incisional pain is usually mild but the internal (visceral) pain after surgery can be intense and may require narcotics or anti-inflammatory agents. Reportedly, a heating pad applied to the abdomen may also be helpful.

If a large volume of fluid is left in the abdomen at the conclusion of the case, then leakage through the incision sites is common for up to 2 days.

The surgeon should be called if there is a fever (>100°C) or chills, heavy or prolonged vaginal bleeding, heat or swelling of the incision sites, frequency or burning on urination, severe pelvic pain, persistent nausea or vomiting, faintness or dizziness, and inability to spontaneously urinate.

Postoperative urinary retention occurs more often in cases that last longer than 2 hours. If the patient is not able to void within 4–5 hours of postoperative period (and after removal of the Foley catheter), then patient should be straight catheterized again for the residual volume of urine and should try to void spontaneously once again. Do not allow patients to go home until either they can void spontaneously or they have an indwelling Foley catheter placed (for about 1 day).

COMPLICATIONS OF OPERATIVE HYSTEROSCOPY

- *Trauma*:
  - Cervical laceration
  - Uterine perforation
  - Injury to intra-abdominal viscera—rectum, bladder, and intestine
- *Intravasation*: Predisposing factors for venous intravasation of distending media:
  - Uterine tuberculosis
  - Submucous tumor
  - Hypoplastic uterus
  - Recently traumatized uterine cavity
  - Proximal tubal obstruction
  - Excessive pressure of instillation
  - Infection
- Exacerbate latent salpingitis
- Pelvic inflammatory disease (PID)
- Febrile reaction
- Bleeding
- Peritonitis.

A possible problem is uterine perforation when either the hysteroscope itself or one of its operative instruments breach the wall of the uterus. This can lead to bleeding and damage to other organs. If other organs such as bowel are injured during a perforation, the resulting peritonitis can be fatal. Furthermore, cervical laceration, intrauterine infection in prolonged procedures, electrical injuries, and complications caused by the distension media can be encountered.

The use of distending media can lead to serious and even fatal complications due to embolism or fluid overload with electrolyte imbalances. Particularly, the electrolyte-free insufflation media increase the risk of fluid overload with electrolyte imbalances, particularly hyponatremia, heart failure as well as pulmonary and cerebral edema.

The main factors contributing to fluid overload in hysteroscopy are:

- Hydrostatic pressure of the insufflation media
- Amount of exposed blood vessels such as being increased in endometrial ablation and submucous myomectomy
- Duration of the hysteroscopy procedure
- Women in fertile age are at increased risk of resultant hyponatremic encephalopathy, likely because of increased level of estrogens.

The overall complication rate for diagnostic and operative hysteroscopy was 2% with serious complications occurring in <1% of cases using older methods.

SAFETY MEASURES

Dilatation of the Cervix

The cervix must be dilated in order to enter into the uterine cavity with a hysteroscope. Most resectoscopes have an outer sheath diameter of about 9 mm, so that cervical dilation using mechanical dilators must be at least this amount. It is optimal to avoid overdilation of the cervix since leakage of the distending media through the cervix and around the hysteroscope (especially under pressures of about 150 mm Hg) then becomes possible.

Some cervical canals are difficult to negotiate with dilators. Different dilators have a variable amount of curvature to choose from. It is possible to perforate the lower uterine segments during dilation. Clinical situations in which perforation is more common include dilation of the pregnant uterus, fibroid uterus, uterus of a women exposed to diethylstilbestrol (DES) in utero, uterus after exposure to prostaglandins for cervical ripening, and infected uterus. Many cases of perforation occur at the onset of dilation and the subsequent dilators then continue to open the perforation site.

Occasionally, a rent in the lower uterine segment occurs during dilation. It is thought that rapid dilation or a difficult dilation involving a stenotic inflexible cervix may enhance the frequency of these tears. It is possible for a tremendous amount of distending media to become intravasated through these rents and into the large vessels of the lower uterine region if they are transected.

Cervical incompetence following hysteroscopic surgery is rarely reported but theoretically possible. The cervix is composed of a tough fibroconnective tissue and smooth muscle. Automatic closure of the internal os of the cervix is the general rule even following manual dilatation of up to 15 mm.

Bleeding

The pressure maintained in the uterine cavity may (but generally should not) exceed both the venous and the arterial pressures, so that active blood flow from transected vessels may not become apparent until the uterus is deflated. At lesser pressures, bleeding can be identified and usually controlled. If there is excessive bleeding following destructive procedures such as endometrial ablation, it can be frequently controlled by tamponade using an inflated Foley catheter balloon (10–30 mL for up to 16 hours) in the uterus. Sometimes, the excessive flow can be controlled with estrogen hormonal therapy (if due to denuding the lining).

Excessive Intravasation of Distending Media or Carbon Dioxide Gas

Whenever vessels get transected during hysteroscopic surgery and either fluid or gas gets entered into the uterine cavity under pressure, there is a possibility of intravasation (entry of these substances into the circulation).

Five percent dextrose in water is a good distending media for diagnostic hysteroscopy. Major complications with this solution are very rare. In fact, there are no reports in any of the world literature where major morbidity or mortality with the use of D5W at hysteroscopy is reported. Possible complications include water intoxication (a reduction in serum osmolality) with a dilutional reduction in sodium concentration, volume overload (when the circulating volume in the vascular system exceeds the ability of the heart to adequately pump this volume and the excess fluid typically begins to collect in the tissues of the lungs), hypothermia (significant reduction in body temperature) if room temperature solutions are used without warming, the patient with devices such as a "Bair Hugger", and hyperglycemia (significant excess in circulating glucose concentration that may not be rapidly metabolized, if the patient has insulin resistance or diabetes mellitus).

The major complication, that most hysteroscopic surgeon's focus on avoiding, is water intoxication. The risk of water intoxication from D5W in a healthy woman with normal renal function is very low, since the kidneys can typically produce in excess of 1,000 cc of dilute urine in response to a decrease in serum osmolarity.

Adhesions

Following hysteroscopic surgery, there is a chance of adhesion (scar) formation if significant electrocoagulation is used within the uterine cavity in the infertility patient.

Intraoperative estrogen IV (25 or 50 mg of Premarin) is given and at least a 30-day course of higher dose Premarin postoperatively (1.25 mg or preferably 2.5 mg, if tolerated) should be used.

Burn Injury to the Bowel

When resectoscopic electrosurgery is performed in the area of the uterine ostia (near the entry site of the fallopian tubes), there is a chance of thermal injury to adjacent tissue outside the uterine cavity. This is because the uterine wall in these regions is very thin and heat from the cautery can travel through the uterine wall and burn adjacent bowel.

Infection

Endometritis is uncommon after operative hysteroscopy and antibiotics are usually not "routinely" given. The potential benefits of antibiotics outweigh their risks when exposure to infection occurs.

HYSTEROSCOPY IN ABNORMAL UTERINE BLEEDING (FIG. 6)

Hysteroscopy in Cases of Infertility

Diagnostic laparoscopy in hysteroscopy is shown in **Figures 7 to 12**.

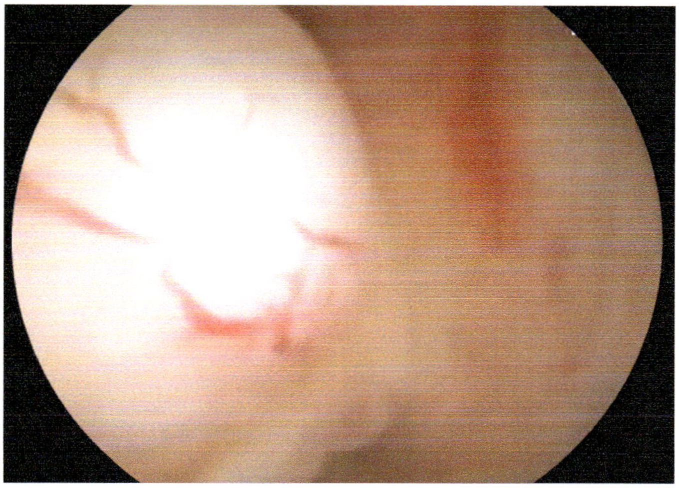

Fig. 6: Submucous myoma.

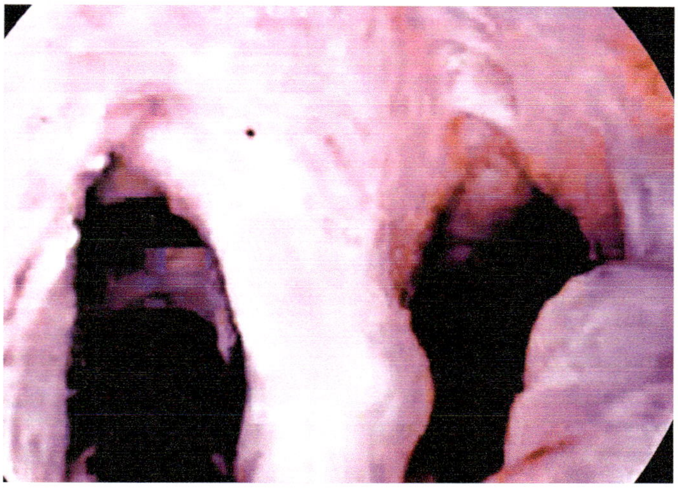

Fig. 7: Septate uterus.

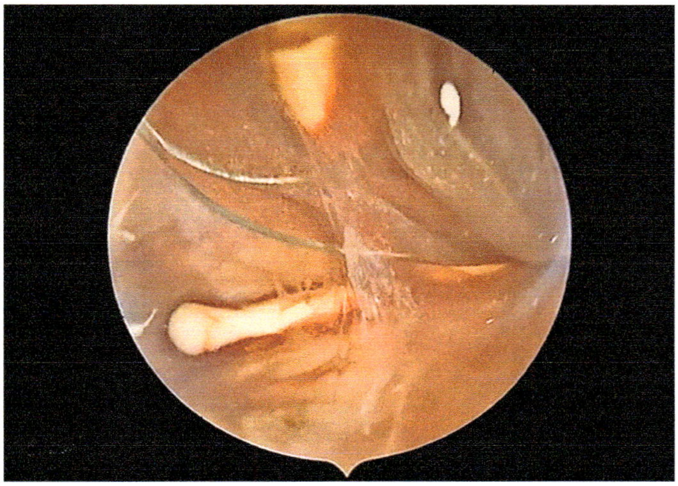

Fig. 8: Forgotten intrauterine device (IUD).

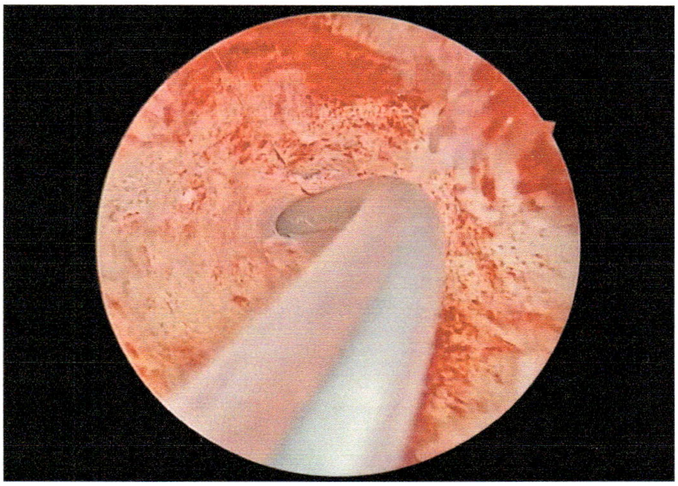

Fig. 9: Salpingo-catheterization.

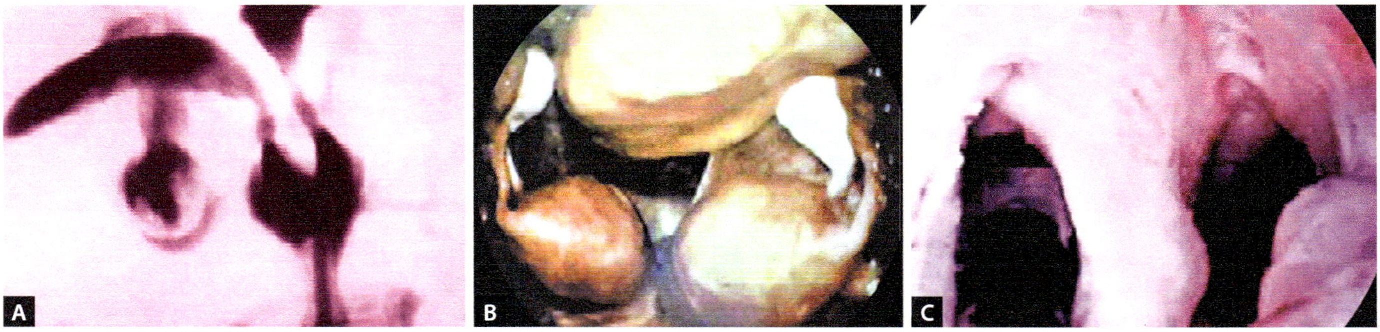

Figs. 10A to C: Bicornuate uterus.

CONCLUSION

Hysteroscopy is a valuable, simple, and low-risk technique, which allows an adequate exploration of the uterine cavity under visual control. It ensures speed and safety with the diagnosis and treatment. Hysteroscopic-guided biopsy and histopathology are considered as the "new gold standard" in evaluating a case of abnormal uterine bleeding. Hysteroscopy provides the possibility of immediate diagnosis and prompt and effective treatment. It allows finding out the source of bleeding and perform a directed biopsy of the suspected area.

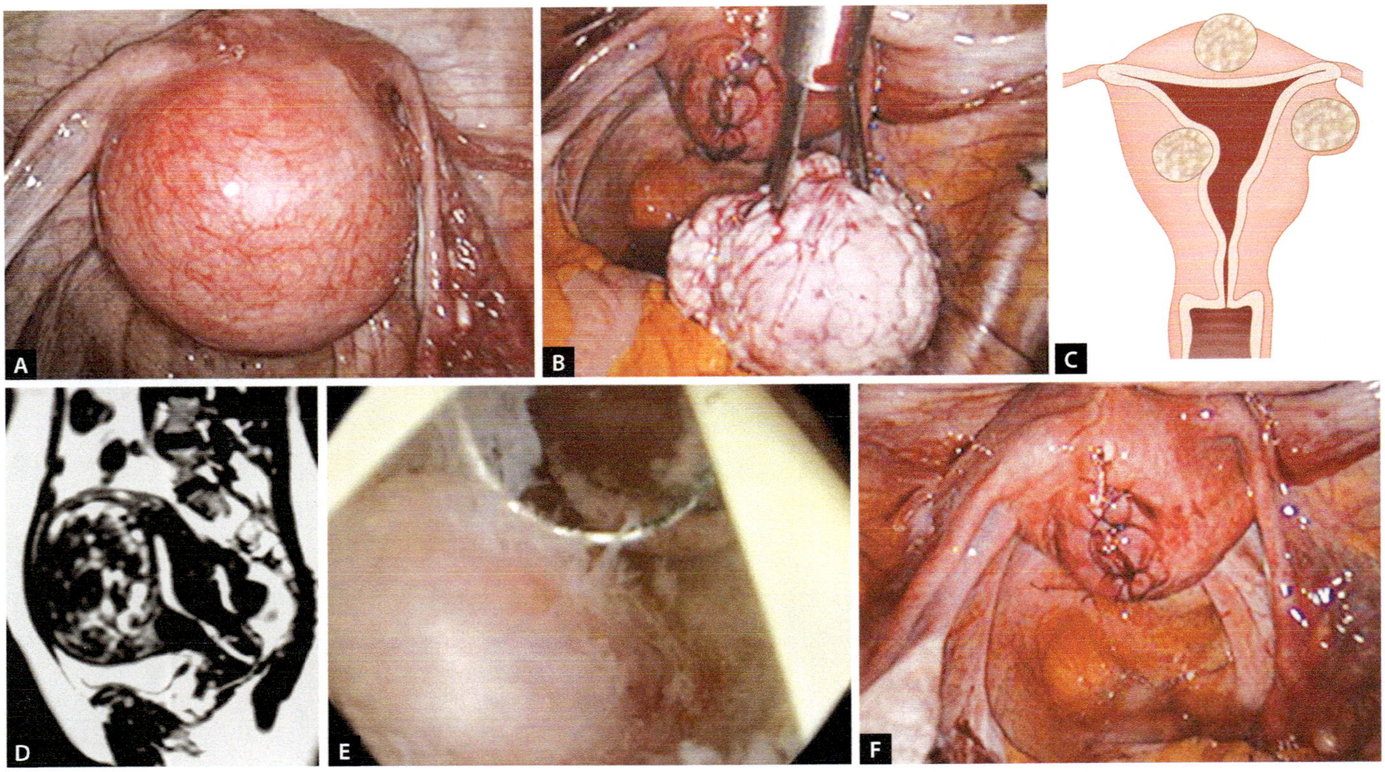

Figs. 11A to F: Intramural myoma.

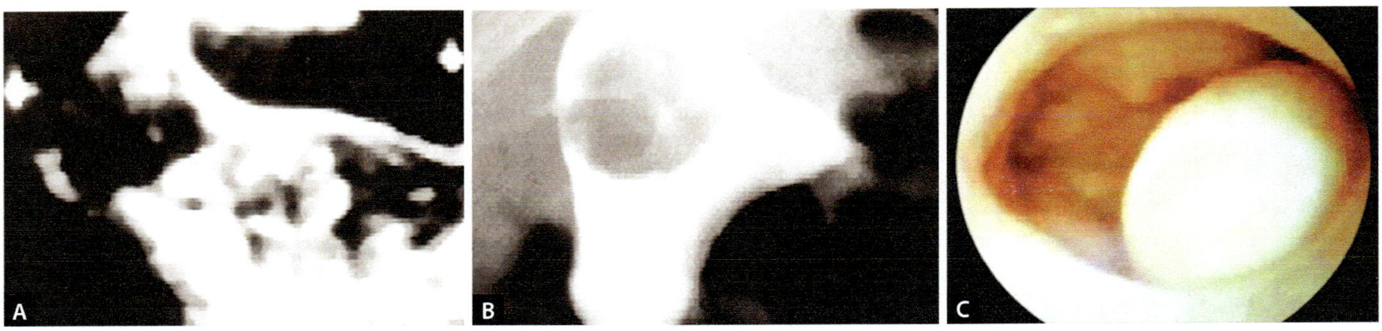

Figs. 12A to C: Submucous myoma.

It affords a more accurate diagnosis than dilatation and curettage for intrauterine pedunculated pathologies. But for hyperplasia and endometrium carcinoma, histopathology is 100% diagnostic. Endometrial polyps and pedunculated fibromyomas can be removed under direct vision with the hysteroscope. Endometrial atrophy diagnosis is best made by hysteroscopy. It is a very helpful technique in patients with intrauterine synechia. Since it can detect their presence, extension, and nature, these can also be removed. It can be concluded that hysteroscopy offers an invaluable advantage of direct visualization of any abnormality within the uterine cavity. It does not substitute other diagnostic procedures; rather, it complements them. Hysteroscopy is a safe, simple, quick, and economic technique, well-accepted by the patient, with great potential in gynecology.

BIBLIOGRAPHY

1. Acunzo G, Guida M, Pellicano M, Tommaselli GA, Di Spiezio Sardo A, Bifulco G, et al. Effectiveness of auto-cross-linked hyaluronic acid gel in the prevention of intrauterine adhesions after hysteroscopic adhesiolysis: a prospective, randomized, controlled study. Hum Reprod. 2003;18:1918-21.
2. Agostini A, Cravello L, Bretelle F, Shojai R, Roger V, Blanc B. Risk of uterine perforation during hysteroscopic surgery. J Am Assoc Gynecol Laparosc. 2002;9:264-7.
3. Alborzi S, Parsanezhad ME, Mahmoodian N, Alborzi S, Alborzi M. Sonohysterography versus transvaginal sonography for screening of patients with abnormal uterine bleeding. Int J Gynecol Obstet. 2007;96:20-3.
4. Aydeniz B, Gruber IV, Schauf B, Kurek R, Meyer A, Wallwiener D. A multicenter survey of complications associated with 21,676 operative hysteroscopies. Eur J Obstet Gynecol Reprod Biol. 2002;104:160-4.

5. Baumann R, Magos AL, Kay JD, Turnbull AC. Absorption of glycine irrigating solution during transcervical resection of endometrium. BMJ. 1990;300:304-5.
6. Benecke C, Kruger TF, Siebert TI, van der Merwe JP, Steyn DW. Effect of fibroids on fertility in patients undergoing assisted reproduction: a structured literature review. Gynecol Obstet Invest. 2005;59:225-30.
7. Berkeley AS, DeCherney AH, Polan ML. Abdominal myomectomy and subsequent fertility. Surg Gynecol Obstet. 1983;156:319-22.
8. Bernard G, Darai E, Poncelet C, Benifla JL, Madelenat P. Fertility after hysteroscopic myomectomy: effect of intramural fibroids associated. Eur J Obstet Gynecol Reprod Biol. 2000;88:85-90.
9. Bettocchi S, Ceci O, Di Venere R, Pansini MV, Pellegrino A, Marello F, et al. Advanced operative office hysteroscopy without anesthesia: analysis of 501 cases treated with a 5 Fr. bipolar electrode. Hum Reprod. 2002;17:2435-8.
10. Bettocchi S, Ceci O, Nappi L, Di Venere R, Masciopinto V, Pansini V, et al. Operative office hysteroscopy without anesthesia: analysis of 4863 cases performed with mechanical instruments. J Am Assoc Gynecol Laparosc. 2004;11:59-61.
11. Bettocchi S, Nappi L, Ceci O, Selvaggi L. What does 'diagnostic hysteroscopy' mean today? The role of the new techniques. Curr Opin Obstet Gynecol. 2003;15:303-8.
12. Bonnamy L, Marret H, Perrotin F, Body G, Berger C, Lansac J. Sonohysterography: a prospective survey of results and complications in 81 patients. Eur J Obstet Gynecol Reprod Biol. 2002;102:42-7.
13. Botsis D, Papagianni V, Makrakis E, Aravantinos L, Creatsas G. Sonohysterography is superior to transvaginal sonography for the diagnostic approach of irregular uterine bleeding in women of reproductive age. J Clin Ultrasound. 2006;34:434-9.
14. Bradley LD. Abnormal uterine bleeding. Nurse Pract. 2005;30:38-42.
15. Bradley LD. Complications in hysteroscopy: prevention, treatment and legal risk. Curr Opin Obstet Gynecol. 2002;14:409-15.
16. Bronz L, Suter T, Rusca T. The value of transvaginal sonography with and without saline instillation in the diagnosis of uterine pathology in pre- and postmenopausal women with abnormal bleeding or suspect sonographic findings. Ultrasound Obstet Gynecol. 1997;9:53-8.
17. Brooks PG, Loffer FD, Serden SP. Resectoscopic removal of symptomatic intrauterine lesions. J Reprod Med. 1989;34:435-7.
18. Brooks PG. Resectoscopic fibroid vaporizer. J Reprod Med. 1995;40:791-5.
19. Buttram VC, Reiter RC. Uterine leiomyomata: etiology, symptomatology, and management. Fertil Steril. 1981;36:433-45.
20. Campo S, Campo V, Gambadauro P. Short-term and long-term results of resectoscopic myomectomy with and without pretreatment with GnRH analogs in premenopausal women. Acta Obstet Gynecol Scand. 2005;84:756-60.
21. Cheng YM, Lin BL. Modified sonohysterography immediately after hysteroscopy in the diagnosis of submucous fibroid. J Am Assoc Gynecol Laparosc. 2002;9:24-8.
22. Cheong Y, Ledger WL. Hysteroscopy and hysteroscopic surgery. Obstet Gynecol Reprod Med. 2007;17:99-104.
23. Cicinelli E, Romano F, Anastasio PS, Blasi N, Parisi C, Galantino P. Transabdominal sonohysterography, transvaginal sonography, and hysteroscopy in the evaluation of submucous fibroids. Obstet Gynecol. 1995;85:42-7.
24. Clark TJ, Mahajan D, Sunder P, Gupta JK. Hysteroscopic treatment of symptomatic submucous fibroids using a bipolar intrauterine system: a feasibility study. Eur J Obstet Gynecol Reprod Biol. 2002;100:237-42.
25. Corson SL, Brooks PG, Serden SP, Batzer FR, Gocial B. Effects of vasopressin administration during hysteroscopic surgery. J Reprod Med. 1994;39:419-23.
26. Corson SL, Brooks PG. Resectoscopic myomectomy. Fertil Steril. 1991;55:1041-4.
27. Corson SL. Hysteroscopic diagnosis and operative therapy of submucous fibroid. Obstet Gynecol Clin North Am. 1995;22:739-55.
28. Cravello L, Agostini A, Beerli M, Roger V, Bretelle F, Blanc B. Results of hysteroscopic myomectomy. Gynecol Obstet Fertil. 2004;32:825-8.
29. Darwish A. Modified hysteroscopic myomectomy of large submucous fibroids. Gynecol Obstet Invest. 2003;56:192-6.
30. Derman SG, Rehnstrom J, Neuwirth RS. The long-term effectiveness of hysteroscopic treatment of menorrhagia and leiomyomas. Obstet Gynecol. 1991;77:591-4.
31. Dodson MG. Use of transvaginal ultrasound in diagnosing the etiology of menometrorrhagia. J Reprod Med. 1994;39:362-72.
32. Donnez J, Gillerot S, Bourgonjon D, Clerckx F, Nisolle M. Neodymium: YAG laser hysteroscopy in large submucous fibroids. Fertil Steril. 1990;54:999-1003.
33. Donnez J, Jadoul P. What are the implications of fibroids on fertility? A need for a debate? Hum Reprod. 2002;17:1424-30.
34. Donnez J, Nisolle M, Clerckx F, Gillerot S, Saussoy P. Hysteroscopic myomectomy. In: Donnez J, Nisolle M (Eds). An Atlas of Laser Operative Laparoscopy and Hysteroscopy. London: Parthenon Publishing; 1994. pp. 323-35.
35. Donnez J, Nisolle M, Grandjean P, Gillerot S, Clerckx F. The place of GnRH agonists in the treatment of endometriosis and fibroids by advanced endoscopic techniques. Br J Obstet Gynaecol. 1992;99:31-3.
36. Donnez J, Nisolle M, Grandjean P, Gillerot S, Clerckx F. The role of GnRH agonists in the endoscopic treatment of endometriosis and fibrofibroids. Contracept Fertil Sex. 1993;21:59-62.
37. Donnez J, Polet R, Smets M, Bassil S, Nisolle M. Hysteroscopic myomectomy. Curr Opin Obstet Gynecol. 1995;7:311-6.
38. Donnez J, Schrurs B, Gillerot S, Sandow J, Clerckx F. Treatment of uterine fibroids with implants of gonadotropin-releasing hormone agonist: assessment by hysterography. Fertil Steril. 1989;51:947-50.
39. Emanuel MH, Hart A, Wamsteker K, Lammes F. An analysis of fluid loss during transcervical resection of submucous fibroids. Fertil Steril. 1997;68:881-6.
40. Emanuel MH, Wamsteker K, Hart AA, Metz G, Lammes FB. Long-term results of hysteroscopic myomectomy for abnormal uterine bleeding. Obstet Gynecol. 1999;93:743-8.
41. Emanuel MH, Wamsteker K. The Intrauterine Morcellator: a new hysteroscopic operating technique to remove intrauterine polyps and fibroids. J Minim Invasive Gynecol. 2005;12:62-6.
42. Emanuel MH, Wamsteker K. Uterine leiomyomas. In: Brosens I, Wamsteker K (Eds). Diagnostic Imaging and Endoscopy in Gynecology. London: WB Saunders; 1997. pp. 185-98.
43. Farquhar C, Ekeroma A, Furness S, Arroll B. A systematic review of transvaginal ultrasonography, sonohysterography and hysteroscopy for the investigation of abnormal uterine bleeding in premenopausal women. Acta Obstet Gynecol Scand. 2003;82:493-504.
44. Farrugia M, McGurgan P, McMillan DL, O'Donovan PJ. Recent advances in electrosurgery. In: O'Donovan PJ, Downes EGR, McGurgan P (Eds). Advances in Gynaecological Surgery, 1st edition. London: Greenwich Medical Media; 2002.
45. Farrugia M, McMillan L. Versapoint^{TM} in the treatment of the focal intrauterine pathology in an outpatient clinic setting. Ref Gynecol Obstet. 2000;7:169-73.
46. Fedele L, Bianchi S, Dorta M, Brioschi D, Zanotti F, Vercellini P. Transvaginal ultrasonography versus hysteroscopy in the diagnosis of uterine submucous fibroids. Obstet Gynecol. 1991;77:745-8.

47. Fedele L, Vercellini P, Bianchi S, Brioschi D, Dorta M. Treatment with GnRH agonists before myomectomy and the risk of short-term fibroid recurrence. Br J Obstet Gynaecol. 1990;97:393-6.
48. Fernandez H, Sefrioui O, Virelizier C, Gervaise A, Gomel V, Frydman R. Hysteroscopic resection of submucosal fibroids in patients with infertility. Hum Reprod. 2001;16:1489-92.
49. Fried FA, Hulka JF. Transuterine resection of fibroids: a new approach to the management of submucous fibroids in selected patients. J Urol. 1987;138:1256-7.
50. Fukuda M, Shimizu T, Fukuda K, Yomura W, Shimizu S. Transvaginal hysterosonography for differential diagnosis between submucous and intramural fibroid. Gynecol Obstet Invest. 1993;35:236-9.
51. Gallinat A. Hysteroscopic treatment of submucous fibroids using the Nd:YAG laser and modern electrical equipment. In: Leuken RP, Gallinat A (Eds). Endoscopic Surgery in Gynecology. Berlin: Demeter Verlag; 1994. pp. 72-88.
52. Gallinat A. The master resectoscope. J Minim Invasive Gynecol. 2005;12:S31-2.
53. Garcia CR, Tureck RW. Submucosal leiofibroids and infertility. Fertil Steril. 1984;42:16-9.
54. Gianaroli L, Gordts S, D'Angelo A, Magli MC, Brosens I, Cetera C, et al. Effect of inner myometrium fibroid on reproductive outcome after IVF. Reprod Biomed Online. 2005;10:473-7.
55. Giatras K, Berkeley AS, Noyes N, Licciardi F, Lolis D, Grifo JA. Fertility after hysteroscopic resection of submucous fibroids. J Am Assoc Gynecol Laparosc. 1999;6:155-8.
56. Glasser MH, Zimmerman JD. The HydroThermAblator system for management of menorrhagia in women with submucous fibroids: 12- to 20-month follow-up. J Am Assoc Gynecol Laparosc. 2003;10:521-7.
57. Glasser MH. Endometrial ablation and hysteroscopic myomectomy by electrosurgical vaporization. J Am Assoc Gynecol Laparosc. 1997;4:369-74.
58. Goldenberg M, Sivan E, Sharabi Z, Bider D, Rabinovici J, Seidman DS. Outcome of hysteroscopic resection of submucous fibroids for infertility. Fertil Steril. 1995;64:714-6.
59. Goldrath MH, Fuller TA, Segal S. Laser photovaporization of endometrium for the treatment of menorrhagia. Am J Obstet Gynecol. 1981;140:14-9.
60. Guida M, Acunzo G, Di Spiezio Sardo A, Bifulco G, Piccoli R, Pellicano M, et al. Effectiveness of auto-crosslinked hyaluronic acid gel in the prevention of intrauterine adhesions after hysteroscopic surgery: a prospective, randomized, controlled study. Hum Reprod. 2004;19:1461-4.
61. Gutmann JN, Corson SL. GnRH agonist therapy before myomectomy or hysterectomy. J Minim Invasive Gynecol. 2005;12:529-37.
62. Hallez JP. Myomectomies by endouterine resection. Curr Opin Obstet Gynecol. 1996;8:250-6.
63. Hallez JP. Single-stage total hysteroscopic myomectomies: indications, techniques, and results. Fertil Steril. 1995;63:703-8.
64. Hamou J. Electroresection of fibroids. In: Sutton C, Diamond MP (Eds). Endoscopic Surgery for Gynecologists. London: WB Saunders; 1993. pp. 327-30.
65. Haney AF. Clinical decision-making regarding leiomyomata: what we need in the next millennium. Environ Health Perspect. 2000;108:835-9.
66. Hart R, Molnar BG, Magos A. Long-term follow-up of hysteroscopic myomectomy assessed by survival analysis. Br J Obstet Gynaecol. 1999;106:700-5.
67. Hickey M, Farquhar CM. Update on treatment of menstrual disorders. Med J Aust. 2003;178:625-9.
68. Hricak H. MRI of the female pelvis: a review. AJR Am J Roentgenol. 1986;146:1115-22.
69. Hunt JE, Wallach EE. Uterine factors in infertility—an overview. Clin Obstet Gynecol. 1974;17:44-64.
70. Indman PD. Hysteroscopic treatment of menorrhagia associated with uterine leiofibroids. Obstet Gynecol. 1993;81:716-20.
71. Indman PD. Hysteroscopic treatment of submucous fibroids. Clin Obstet Gynecol. 2006;49:811-20.
72. Indman PD. Use of carboprost to facilitate hysteroscopic resection of submucous fibroids. J Am Assoc Gynecol Laparosc. 2004;11:68-72.
73. Isaacson K. Hysteroscopic myomectomy: fertility-preserving yet underutilized. OBG Manag. 2003;15:69-83.
74. Istre O, Bjoennes J, Naess R, Hornbaek K, Forman A. Postoperative cerebral oedema after transcervical endometrial resection and uterine irrigation with 1.5% glycine. Lancet. 1994;344:1187-9.
75. Jansen FW, Vredevoogd CB, van Ulzen K, Hermans J, Trimbos JB, Trimbos-Kemper TC. Complications of hysteroscopy: a prospective, multicenter study. Obstet Gynecol. 2000;96:266-70.
76. Kanaoka Y, Hirai K, Ishiko O. Microwave endometrial ablation for an enlarged uterus. Arch Gynecol Obstet. 2003;269:30-32.
77. Kanaoka Y, Hirai K, Ishiko O. Microwave endometrial ablation for menorrhagia caused by large submucous fibroids. J Obstet Gynaecol Res. 2005;31:565-70.
78. Keltz M, Varasteh N, Levin B, Neuwirth R. Pregnancy rates following hysteroscopic polypectomy, myomectomy, and a normal cavity in infertile patients. Prim Care Update Ob Gyns. 1998;5:168.
79. Kolankaya A, Arici A. Fibroids and assisted reproductive technologies: when and how to act? Obstet Gynecol Clin North Am. 2006;33:145-52.
80. Laifer-Narin SL, Ragavendra N, Lu DS, Sayre J, Perrella RR, Grant EG. Transvaginal saline hysterosonography: characteristics distinguishing malignant and various benign conditions. AJR Am J Roentgenol. 1999;172:1513-20.
81. Lasmar RB, Barrozo PR, Dias R, Oliveira MA. Submucous fibroids: a new presurgical classification to evaluate the viability of hysteroscopic surgical treatment–preliminary report. J Minim Invasive Gynecol. 2005;12:308-11.
82. Lasmar RB, Barrozo PR. Histeroscopia: Uma Abordagem Pràtica. Brazil: Medsi, Rio de Janeiro; 2002. pp. 121-42.
83. Leone FP, Bignardi T, Marciante C, Ferrazzi E. Sonohysterography in the preoperative grading of submucous fibroids: considerations on three-dimensional methodology. Ultrasound Obstet Gynecol. 2007;29:717-8.
84. Leone FP, Lanzani C, Ferrazzi E. Use of strict sonohysterographic methods for preoperative assessment of submucous fibroids. Fertil Steril. 2003;79:998-1002.
85. Lethaby A, Vollenhoven B, Sowter M. Efficacy of preoperative gonadotropin hormone releasing analogues for women with uterine fibroids undergoing hysterectomy or myomectomy: a systematic review. BJOG. 2002;109:1097-108.
86. Lethaby A, Vollenhoven B, Sowter M. Preoperative GnRH analogue therapy before hysterectomy or myomectomy for uterine fibroids. Cochrane Database Syst Rev. 2001;2:CD000547.
87. Lin B, Akiba Y, Iwata Y. One-step hysteroscopic removal of sinking submucous fibroid in two infertile patients. Fertil Steril. 2000;74:1035-8.
88. Litta P, Vasile C, Merlin F, Pozzan C, Sacco G, Gravila P, et al. A new technique of hysteroscopic myomectomy with enucleation *in toto*. J Am Assoc Gynecol Laparosc. 2003;10:263-70.
89. Loffer FD. Endometrial ablation in patients with fibroids. Curr Opin Obstet Gynecol. 2006;18:391-3.
90. Loffer FD. Hysteroscopic endometrial ablation with the Nd:Yag laser using a nontouch technique. Obstet Gynecol. 1987;69:679-82.

91. Loffer FD. Improving results of hysteroscopic submucosal myomectomy for menorrhagia by concomitant endometrial ablation. J Minim Invasive Gynecol. 2005;12:254-60.
92. Loffer FD. Preliminary experience with the VersaPoint bipolar resectoscope using a vaporizing electrode in a saline distending medium. J Am Assoc Gynecol Laparosc. 2000;7:498-502.
93. Loffer FD. Removal of large symptomatic intrauterine growths by the hysteroscopic resectoscope. Obstet Gynecol. 1990;76:836-40.
94. Maher PJ, Hill DJ. Transcervical endometrial resection for abnormal uterine bleeding—report of 100 cases and review of the literature. Aust N Z J Obstet Gynaecol. 1990;30:357-60.
95. Maher PJ. Endoscopic management of fibro fibroidta. Rev Gynecol Pract. 2003;3:41-5.
96. Marziani R, Mossa B, Ebano V, Perniola G, Melluso J, Napolitano C. Transcervical hysteroscopic myomectomy: long-term effects on abnormal uterine bleeding. Clin Exp Obstet Gynecol. 2005;32:23-6.
97. Mazzon I, Sbiroli C. Miomectomia. In: Mazzon I, Sbiroli C (Eds). Manuale di Chirurgia Resettoscopica in Ginecologia. Torino, Italy: UTET; 1997. pp. 191-217.
98. Mazzon I. Nuova tecnica per la miometomia isteroscopica: enucleazione con ansa fredda. In: Cittadini E, Perino A, Angiolillio M, Minelli L (Eds). Testo-Atlante di Chirurgia Endoscopica Ginecologica. Palermo, Italy: COFESE Ed; 1995. p. 117.
99. Mencaglia L, Tantini C. GnRH agonist analogs and hysteroscopic resection of fibroids. Int J Gynaecol Obstet. 1993;43:285-8.
100. Munoz JL, Jimenez JS, Hernandez C, Vaquero G, Perez Sagaseta C, Noguero R, et al. Hysteroscopic myomectomy: our experience and review. JSLS. 2003;7:39-48.
101. Murakami T, Shimizu T, Katahira A, Terada Y, Yokomizo R, Sawada R. Intraoperative injection of prostaglandin F2 alpha in a patient undergoing hysteroscopic myomectomy. Fertil Steril. 2003;79:1439-41.
102. Murakami T, Tachibana M, Hoshiai T, Ozawa Y, Terada Y, Okamura K. Successful strategy for the hysteroscopic myomectomy of a submucous fibroid arising from the uterine fundus. Fertil Steril. 2006;86:1513.e19-22.
103. Murakami T, Tamura M, Ozawa Y, Suzuki H, Terada Y, Okamura K. Safe techniques in surgery for hysteroscopic myomectomy. J Obstet Gynaecol Res. 2005;31:216-23.
104. Nappi C, Di Spiezio Sardo A, Greco E, Guida M, Bettocchi S, Bifulco G. Prevention of adhesions in gynaecological endoscopy. Hum Reprod Update. 2007;13:379-94.
105. Narayan R, Rajat Goswamy K. Treatment of submucous fibroids and outcome of assisted conception. J Am Assoc Gynecol Laparosc. 1994;1:307-11.
106. Neuwirth RS, Amin HK. Excision of submucus fibroids with hysteroscopic control. Am J Obstet Gynecol. 1976;126:95-9.
107. Neuwirth RS. A new technique for and additional experience with hysteroscopic resection of submucous fibroids. Am J Obstet Gynecol. 1978;131:91-4.
108. Neuwirth RS. Hysteroscopic management of symptomatic submucous fibroids. Obstet Gynecol. 1983;62:509-11.
109. Neuwirth RS. Hysteroscopic submucous myomectomy. Obstet Gynecol Clin North Am. 1995;22:541-58.
110. Ng EH, Ho PC. Doppler ultrasound examination of uterine arteries on the day of oocyte retrieval in patients with uterine fibroids undergoing IVF. Hum Reprod. 2002;17:765-70.
111. Oliveira FG, Abdelmassih VG, Diamond MP, Dozortsev D, Melo NR, Abdelmassih R. Impact of subserosal and intramural uterine fibroids that do not distort the endometrial cavity on the outcome of *in vitro* fertilization-intracytoplasmic sperm injection. Fertil Steril. 2004;81:582-7.
112. Pace S. Transcervical resection of benign endocavitary lesions. Gynecol Endosc. 1993;2:165-9.
113. Parazzini F, Vercellini P, De Giorgi O, Pesole A, Ricci E, Crosignani PG. Efficacy of preoperative medical treatment in facilitating hysteroscopic endometrial resection, myomectomy and metroplasty: literature review. Hum Reprod. 1998;13:2592-7.
114. Parent B, Barbot J, Guedj H, Nordarian P. Hysteroscopic resection of uterine fibroids (in French). In: Parent B, Barbot J, Guedj H, Nordarian P (Eds). Hysteroscopie Chirurgicale. Laser et Techniques Classiques. Paris, France: Masson; 1994.
115. Perez-Medina T, Bajo JM, Martinez-Cortes L, Castellanos P, Perez de Avila I. Six thousand office diagnostic-operative hysteroscopies. Int J Gynaecol Obstet. 2000;71:33-8.
116. Perino A, Chianchiano N, Petronio M, Cittadini E. Role of leuprolide acetate depot in hysteroscopic surgery: a controlled study. Fertil Steril. 1993;59:507-10.
117. Phillips DR, Nathanson HG, Meltzer SM, Milim SJ, Haselkorn JS, Johnson P. Transcervical electrosurgical resection of submucous leiomyomas for chronic menorrhagia. J Am Assoc Gynecol Laparosc. 1995;2:147-53.
118. Polena V, Mergui JL, Perrot N, Poncelet C, Barranger E, Uzan S. Long-term results of hysteroscopic myomectomy in 235 patients. Eur J Obstet Gynecol Reprod Biol. 2007;130:232-7.
119. Preutthipan S, Theppisai U. Hysteroscopic resection of submucous fibroid: a result of 50 procedures at Ramathibodi Hospital. J Med Assoc Thai. 1998;81:190-4.
120. Pritts EA. Fibroids and infertility: a systematic review of the evidence. Obstet Gynecol Surv. 2001;56:483-91.
121. Propst AM, Liberman RF, Harlow BL, Ginsburg ES. Complications of hysteroscopic surgery: predicting patients at risk. Obstet Gynecol. 2000;96:517-20.
122. Richards PA, Richards PD, Tiltman AJ. The ultrastructure of fibromyomatous myometrium and its relationship to infertility. Hum Reprod Update. 1998;4:520-5.
123. Romer T, Schmidt T, Foth D. Pre- and postoperative hormonal treatment in patients with hysteroscopic surgery. Contrib Gynecol Obstet. 2000;20:1-12.
124. Romer T. Benefit of GnRH analogue pretreatment for hysteroscopic surgery in patients with bleeding disorders. Gynecol Obstet Invest. 1998;45:12-20.
125. Saidi MH, Sadler RK, Theis VD, Akright BD, Farhart SA, Villanueva GR. Comparison of sonography, sonohysterography, and hysteroscopy for evaluation of abnormal uterine bleeding. J Ultrasound Med. 1997;16:587-91.
126. Salim R, Lee C, Davies A, Jolaoso B, Ofuasia E, Jurkovic D. A comparative study of three-dimensional saline infusion sonohysterography and diagnostic hysteroscopy for the classification of submucous fibroids. Hum Reprod. 2005;20:253-7.
127. Seoud MA, Patterson R, Muasher SJ, Coddington CC. Effects of fibroids or prior myomectomy on *in vitro* fertilization (IVF) performance. J Assist Reprod Genet. 1992;9:217-21.
128. Serden SP, Brooks PG. Treatment of abnormal uterine bleeding with the gynecologic resectoscope. J Reprod Med. 1991;36:697-9.
129. Shokeir TA. Hysteroscopic management in submucous fibroids to improve fertility. Arch Gynecol Obstet. 2005;273:50-4.
130. Smets M, Nisolle M, Bassil S, Donnez J. Expansive benign lesions: treatment by laser. Eur J Obstet Gynecol Reprod Biol. 1996;65:101-5.
131. Smith DC, Uhlir JK. Myomectomy as a reproductive procedure. Am J Obstet Gynecol. 1990;162:1476-9.
132. Somigliana E, Vercellini P, Daguati R, Pasin R, De Giorgi O, Crosignani PG. Fibroids and female reproduction: a critical analysis of the evidence. Hum Reprod Update. 2007;13:465-76.
133. Stamatellos I, Apostolides A, Tantis A, Stamatopoulos P, Bontis J. Fertility rates after hysteroscopic treatment of submucous fibroids depending on their type. Gynecol Surg. 2006;3:206-10.
134. Stamatellos I, Bontis J. Hysteroscopic myomectomy. Eur Clin Obstet Gynecol. 2007;3:17-23.

135. Starks GC. CO_2 laser myomectomy in an infertile population. J Reprod Med. 1988;33:184-6.
136. Sudik R, Husch K, Steller J, Daume E. Fertility and pregnancy outcome after myomectomy in sterility patients. Eur J Obstet Gynecol Reprod Biol. 1996;65:209-14.
137. Surrey ES, Minjarez DA, Stevens JM, Schoolcraft WB. Effect of myomectomy on the outcome of assisted reproductive technologies. Fertil Steril. 2005;83:1473-9.
138. Sutton C. Hysteroscopic surgery. Best Pract Res Clin Obstet Gynaecol. 2006;20:105-37.
139. Takeda A, Manabe S, Hosono S, Nakamura H. Preoperative evaluation of submucosal fibroid by virtual hysteroscopy. J Am Assoc Gynecol Laparosc. 2004;11:404-9.
140. Taskin O, Sadik S, Onoglu A, Gokdeniz R, Erturan E, Burak F, et al. Role of endometrial suppression on the frequency of intrauterine adhesions after resectoscopic surgery. J Am Assoc Gynecol Laparosc. 2000;7:351-4.
141. Trew GH. Hysteroscopy and hysteroscopic surgery. Curr Obstet Gynaecol. 2004;14:183-90.
142. Tulandi T, Al-Took S. Endoscopic myomectomy: laparoscopy and hysteroscopy. Obstet Gynecol Clin North Am. 1999;26:135-48.
143. Tulandi T. Modern surgical approaches to female reproductive tract. Hum Reprod Update. 1996;2:419-27.
144. Turner RT, Berman AM, Topel HC. Improved demonstration of endometrial polyps and submucous fibroids using saline-enhanced vaginal sonohysterography. J Am Assoc Gynecol Laparosc. 1995;2:421-5.
145. Ubaldi F, Tournaye H, Camus M, van der Pas H, Gepts E, Devroey P. Fertility after hysteroscopic myomectomy. Hum Reprod Update. 1995;1:81-90.
146. Valle RF, Baggish MS. Hysteroscopic myomectomy. In: Baggish MS, Valle RF, Guedj H (Eds). Hysteroscopy: Visual Perspectives of Uterine Anatomy, Physiology and Pathology, 3rd edition. Philadelphia: Lippincott Williams and Wilkins; 2007. pp. 385-404.
147. Valle RF. Hysteroscopic removal of submucous leiomyomas. J Gynecol Surg. 1990;6:89-96.
148. Van Dongen H, Emanuel MH, Smeets MJ, Trimbos B, Jansen FW. Follow-up after incomplete hysteroscopic removal of uterine fibroids. Acta Obstet Gynecol Scand. 2006;85:1463-7.
149. Varasteh NN, Neuwirth RS, Levin B, Keltz MD. Pregnancy rates after hysteroscopic polypectomy and myomectomy in infertile women. Obstet Gynecol. 1999;94:168-71.
150. Vercellini P, Zaina B, Yaylayan L, Pisacreta A, De Giorgi O, Crosignani PG. Hysteroscopic myomectomy: long-term effects on menstrual pattern and fertility. Obstet Gynecol. 1999;94:341-7.
151. Verkauf BS. Myomectomy for fertility enhancement and preservation. Fertil Steril. 1992;58:1-15.
152. Vidal JJ. Patologl'a tumoral del cuerpo uterino. In: Usandizga JA, De la Fuente PY (Eds). Tratado de Ostetricia y Ginecologl'a Tomo II. Interamericana; 1998. p. 373.
153. Vilos GA, Abu-Rafea B. New developments in ambulatory hysteroscopic surgery. Best Pract Res Clin Obstet Gynaecol. 2005;19:727-42.
154. Walker CL, Stewart EA. Uterine fibroids: the elephant in the room. Science. 2005;308:1589-92.
155. Wamsteker K, Emanuel MH, de Kruif JH. Transcervical hysteroscopic resection of submucous fibroids for abnormal uterine bleeding: results regarding the degree of intramural extension. Obstet Gynecol. 1993;82:736-40.
156. West JH, Robinson DA. Endometrial resection and fluid absorption. Lancet. 1989;15:1387-8.
157. Wheeler JM, Taskin O. Second-look office hysteroscopy following resectoscopy: the frequency and management of intrauterine adhesions. Fertil Steril. 1993;60:150-6.
158. Wieser F, Tempfer C, Kurz C, Nagele F. Hysteroscopy in 2001: a comprehensive review. Acta Obstet Gynecol Scand. 2001;80:773-83.
159. Williams CD, Marshburn PB. A prospective study of transvaginal hydrosonography in the evaluation of abnormal uterine bleeding. Am J Obstet Gynecol. 1998;179:292-8.
160. Wortman M, Dagget A. Hysteroscopy myomectomy. J Am Assoc Gynecol Laparosc. 1995;3:39-46.
161. Yang JH, Lin BL. Changes in myometrial thickness during hysteroscopic resection of deeply invasive submucous fibroids. J Am Assoc Gynecol Laparosc. 2001;8:501-5.
162. Yaron Y, Shenhav M, Jaffa AJ, Lessing JB, Peyser MR. Uterine rupture at 33 weeks' gestation subsequent to hysteroscopic uterine perforation. Am J Obstet Gynecol. 1994;170:786-7.

SECTION

4 Laparoscopic Urology

CHAPTER 40

Ureteral Injury and Laparoscopy

URETERAL INJURIES

Ureteral injury is one of the most serious complications of gynecologic surgery. Ureteral injury during laparoscopic surgery has become more common as a result of the increased number of laparoscopic hysterectomies and retroperitoneal procedures that are being performed. Consequently, prevention of ureteral injuries should be a priority during laparoscopic gynecologic surgery. When a ureteral injury does occur, quick recognition of the problem and a working knowledge of its location and treatment are essential in providing patients with optimal medical care. Detailed anatomic knowledge of the retroperitoneum is necessary to prevent ureteral injuries.

The ureters are retroperitoneal tubular structures that extend from the renal pelvis, coursing medially and inferiorly to the bladder **(Fig. 1)**. Each ureter travels inferiorly along the psoas muscle and crosses the iliac vessels at approximately the level of the bifurcation of the common iliac arteries. In females, the ureter is crossed anteriorly by the ovarian vessels as they enter the pelvis. Inferiorly, they are crossed anteriorly by the uterine artery. At this point, they enter the cardinal ligament, approximately 1.5–2 cm lateral to the cervix before their insertion into the trigone of the bladder **(Fig. 1)**.

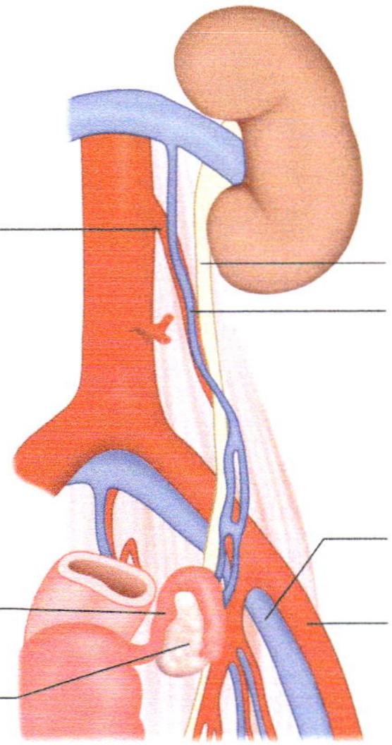

Fig. 1: Anatomy of ureter.

The ureters derive their blood supply from the renal artery, aorta, gonadal artery, and common iliac artery while they traverse intra-abdominally. These vessels approach the ureter from its medial side and course longitudinally within the periureteral adventitia. In the pelvis, the ureter derives its blood supply from the internal iliac artery or its branches. These vessels approach the ureter from its lateral side and also course longitudinally within the periureteral adventitia.

A significant ureteral injury is defined as any recognized or unrecognized iatrogenic trauma to the ureter that prevents it from functioning properly or effectively. The injury may lead to acute ureteral obstruction (e.g., a ureter that is inadvertently ligated) or discontinuity (i.e., inadvertent ureteral resection). If an injury to the ureter has occurred and is unrecognized, it may lead to chronic ureteral obstruction (i.e., crush injury, ischemia) or the formation of fistulas.

FREQUENCY OF URETERAL INJURY

The frequency of ureteral injury following gynecologic surgery is approximately 1% with a higher percentage of injuries occurring during abdominal hysterectomies and partial vaginectomies. Patients who have received pelvic radiation or who have advanced pelvic cancers requiring extensive surgical procedures are more likely to experience a ureteral injury **(Figs. 2A and B)**.

The rate of ureteral injuries in laparoscopic procedures varies. While some physicians report that laparoscopic procedures have an equivalent rate of ureteral stricture formation secondary to ureteral injury, other authors argue that the rate of ureteral strictures is significantly higher. More research is necessary before a definitive statement can be made regarding the rates of ureteral injury during laparoscopy.

ETIOLOGY

The seven most common mechanisms of operative ureteral injury are as follows:

1. Crushing from misapplication of a clamp
2. Ligation with a suture
3. Transection (partial or complete)
4. Angulation of the ureter with secondary obstruction

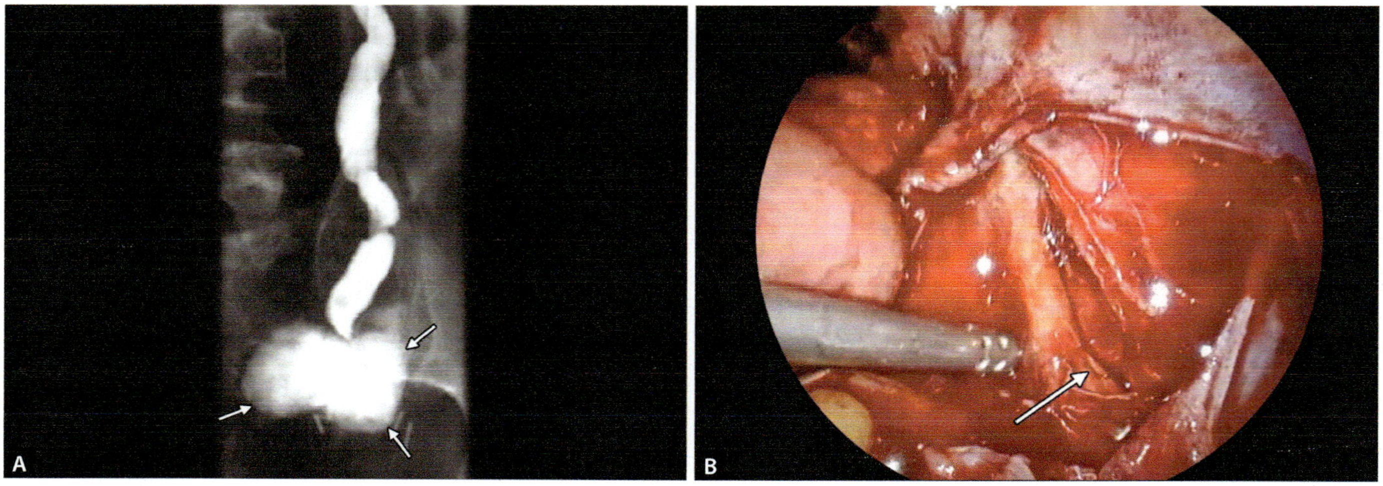

Figs. 2A and B: Ureteric injury during laparoscopic hysterectomy (arrows).

5. Ischemia from ureteral stripping or electrocoagulation
6. Resection of a segment of ureter
7. Excessive use of monopolar, which creates remote injury of ureter

Any combinations of these injuries may occur.

Several predisposing factors have been identified in iatrogenic urologic injury. These factors include uterus size larger than 12 weeks of gestation, ovarian cysts 4 cm or larger, endometriosis, pelvic inflammatory disease, prior intra-abdominal operation, radiation therapy, advanced state of malignancy, and anatomical anomalies of the urinary tract. Ureteral injuries can be either expected or unexpected and they may be the result of carelessness or due to a technically challenging procedure.

LEVEL OF URETERAL INJURIES

Intraoperative ureteral injury may result from transection, ligation, angulation, crush, ischemia, or resection **(Fig. 1)**.

There are three specific anatomic locations for potential ureteral injury during gynecologic laparoscopy:

1. At the infundibulopelvic ligament
2. At the ovarian fossa
3. In the ureteral canal

Among all the ureteral injuries, 14.3% occurred at or above the level of the pelvic brim, 11.4% occurred at or above the uterine artery, and 8.6% occurred at the level of the bladder **(Fig. 3)**. The initial procedure in 20% of these cases was laparoscopic-assisted vaginal hysterectomy. Alterations to normal anatomy may also hinder identification of the ureters as in severe endometriosis, which may involve the ureter and also cause intraperitoneal adhesions.

PREVENTION OF URETERAL INJURY

Injury to the ureters can be prevented by meticulous surgical technique and adequate visualization.

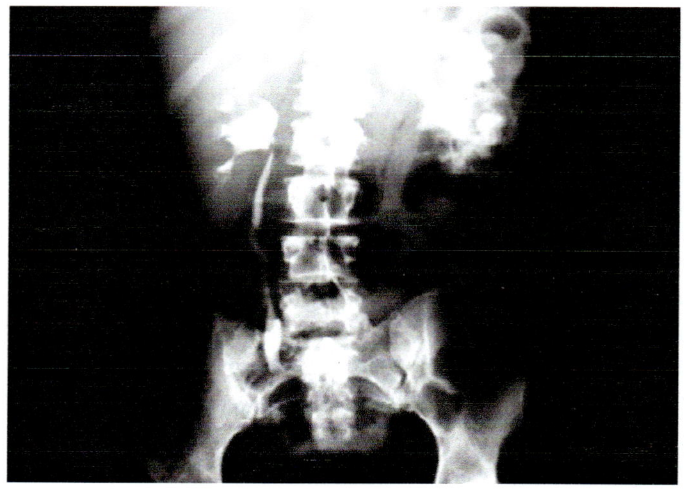

Fig. 3: Intravenous pyelogram (IVP) showing ureteric injury.

Techniques to enhance visualization include:

- *Ureteral catheterization with lighted stent*: Ureteral catheterization with lighted stents has been used to assist in identifying the location of the ureters during laparoscopic surgery to help prevent iatrogenic injury. If the lighted stents are not visible during laparoscopic surgery, four options are available as follows:
  1. Change the intensity of the laparoscopic lighting. By dimming the lights, the light from the stent may become visible
  2. Change the camera to a different port
  3. Identify the ureter where it is visible and follow it down to the surgical field
  4. Convert to an open procedure, so that the ureter can be palpated and identified

  Although ureteral catheterization helps to identify the ureters; however, in a large review of major gynecologic surgeries, Kuno et al. found that ureteral catheterization did not substantially reduce the risk of ureteral injury. The surgeon must practice meticulous surgical technique and have intimate knowledge of the ureter's course to prevent ureteral injury.

- *Hydrodissection*: By making a small opening in the peritoneum and injecting 50–100 mL of lactated Ringer's or normal saline solution along the course of the ureter, one can displace the ureter laterally and create a safe plane within which to operate.
- *Preoperative intravenous pyelogram (IVP)*: IVP has been used to locate the ureters in high-risk patients with potentially distorted anatomy; however, this did not decrease the risk of ureteral injury.

USE OF INFRARED URETERIC CATHETER

Several studies have been done to examine the advantages of the use of infrared or lighted ureteral stents in various procedures, including laparoscopic procedures. For instance, a study was conducted on the implications of the use of lighted ureteral stents on laparoscopic colectomy. The study was conducted between April 1996 and January 2000, where a total of 66 patients had infrared ureteral stents placed before laparoscopic colectomy was done. Among the total 66 patients, 32 of them were males and 34 of them were females. They had an average age of about 62.27 years.

A lot was discovered after the surgery and was reported. The researchers also identified the complications that were related to the use of the lighted ureteral stents. In the results, it was established that in spite of the use of the lighted ureteral stents, one man still suffered from an incomplete left ureteral injury during a sigmoid colectomy. However, the injury was managed by use of the conservative approach where the left ureteral stent was reinserted.

The value of the use of the infrared or lighted ureteral stents in laparoscopic colectomy was studied and several things were discovered. In some instances, there were ureteral injuries during the laparoscopic colectomy that were reported. Also, the injuries were reported in the laparoscopic hysterectomy.

Infrared Ureteral Stent

There are four types of ureteral injuries, including laceration, ligation, crush, and devascularization. All these types of injuries can be detected either intraoperatively or postoperatively. When the infrared ureteral stents are placed before laparoscopic surgery, they can help in detecting and identification of the ureteral injuries intraoperatively. This, therefore, helped the surgeon to take adequate and immediate action before the problem would become fatal.

In the same study, it was discovered that there was one patient who suffered from an incomplete ureteral injury during a sigmoid colectomy. For this to be detected, the diagnosis was done with retrograde cystourethrogram.

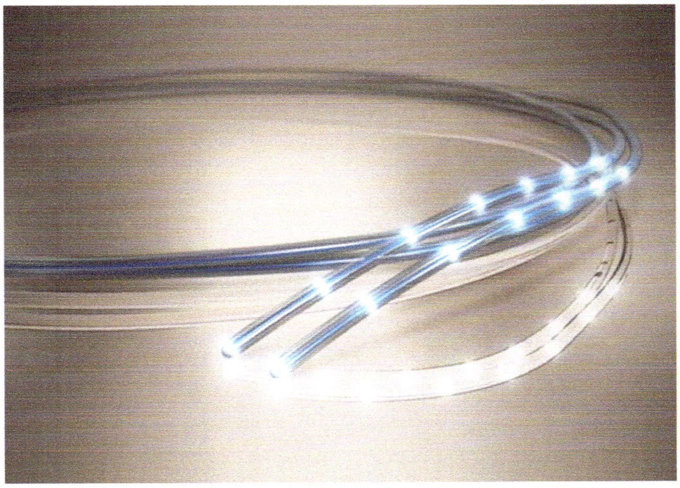

Fig. 4: Infrared ureteric catheter to prevent ureteric injury.

In fact, the injury was detected on postoperative 2 days after the procedure. The injury had some urinary ascites. The ureteral injury together with urinary ascites was managed by the reinsertion of the left ureteral stent temporarily. The temporary lighted ureteral stents were removed on the 11th day after the operation and the patient discharged. It is evident that use of the lighted ureteral stents in the laparoscopic colectomy led to a decrease in the number of patients with ureteral damage. The significant decrease in the number of patients who suffered from ureteral damage shows that the placement of infrared ureteral stents before laparoscopic surgery is done to reduce the risk of having the ureter damaged **(Fig. 4)**. In fact, in this study, out of the 66 patients, only one patient suffered from ureter damage. In addition, the placement of the lighted ureteral stent helped in the detection of the ureteral damage, which aided in the taking of immediate action to correct the problem. Actually, the problem could be solved postoperatively and even the patient got discharged after postoperative day 11. Therefore, the placement of the lighted ureteral stent during total laparoscopic hysterectomy does not only helps in the detection of damage to the ureter but also it helps in the taking of immediate action to correct the injury **(Figs. 5A to D)**.

The use of the ureteral stents is associated with an adverse effect, which is that it leads to postoperative gross hematuria in almost every patient that was in the study. Hematuria is normally known to last for an average of 3 days after the surgery; however, the placement of the bilateral ureteral stents led to a significant increase in the duration of the hematuria. Fortunately, hematuria is not associated with any clinical significance because it does not require a blood transfusion. In order to reduce the hematuria, there is one major thing that the surgeon would adopt and that is the use of unilateral stents rather than the bilateral stents. The unilateral stents can help to reduce the operative time as well as reduce the postoperative hematuria.

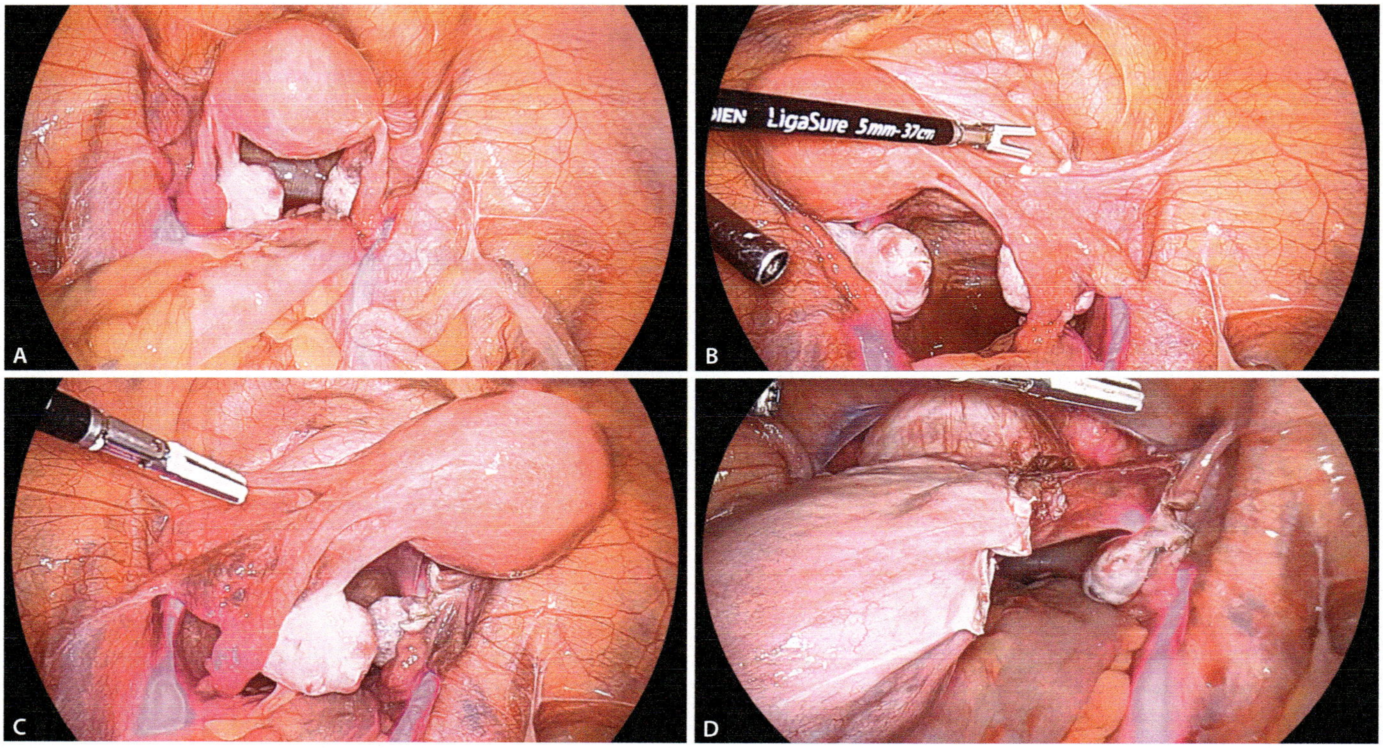

Figs. 5A to D: Use of infrared ureteric catheter during total laparoscopic hysterectomy.

Another adverse effect that was discovered in the study is that the use of lighted ureteral stent led to reflux anuria, which can be serious and even lead to an acute renal failure. Anuria is mostly linked to the result of neurogenic factors that are brought about by the manipulation of the ureter and mediated through the autonomic nervous system.

According to various studies, it was established that anuria that resulted after the placement of the ureteral stents was due to edema that is known to cause mechanical obstruction at the ureterovesical junction. The detection of this symptom is very important in order to take action immediately. Detection or recognition of such symptom would require repeated ureteral stents.

The role of infrared or lighted ureteral stent in laparoscopic colectomy can easily be seen. As it tries to improve vision for the identification of the ureter and, thus, reducing and preventing ureteral damage, the technique aims to make laparoscopic colectomy safe. Without the placement of the lighted ureteral stents, the risk of ureteral injury was high. Ureteral damage can lead to many problems to a patient that can also be very expensive to deal with, especially if it is not detected and recognized at an early stage. The best thing about the placement of the ureteral stents is that the surgeon can easily identify whether or not there is any ureteral damage. This allows the doctor to detect the injury early enough before it becomes fatal or difficult to deal with. When an injury is detected, immediate action is taken to correct the problem either intraoperatively or postoperatively.

The placement of the lighted ureteral stent requires special skills, which can actually be acquired through practice, in order to ensure that the stents are well placed so that it can effectively aid the surgeon during laparoscopic surgery. The use of infrared ureteral stents is a safe and cost-effective procedure that can aid in laparoscopic surgery, especially laparoscopic colectomy. The placement of the ureteral stents helps improve the vision, which, thus, helps avoid intraoperative ureteral injury. The ability to detect any ureteral injury using the procedure facilitates immediate action to be taken. Unilateral stent placement should always be the procedure to use rather than the bilateral procedure. Unilateral stent placement is associated with lower postoperative hematuria and can reduce operative time.

RECOGNITION OF URETERAL INJURY

Once a ureteral injury is suspected, the ureter must be identified to assess the severity of the injury. Ureteral injury should be suspected with the presence of hematuria or urinary extravasation. Intravenous indigo carmine may be given to aid in the diagnosis and localization of the site of injury. Unfortunately, the majority of ureteral injuries are diagnosed in the postoperative period. Patients who present with postoperative fever, flank pain, and leukocytosis should undergo evaluation for ureteral injury.

PATHOPHYSIOLOGY

The pathophysiology of ureteral injury depends on many factors, including the type of injury and the time when the injury is identified. Numerous consequences may occur after ureteral injury, including spontaneous resolution and healing of the injured ureter, hydronephrosis, ureteral necrosis with urinary extravasation, ureteral stricture formation, and uremia.

Spontaneous Resolution and Healing

If the injury to the ureter is minor, easily reversible, and noticed immediately, the ureter may heal completely and without consequence. Inadvertent ligation of the ureter is an example of such an injury. If this injury is noticed in a timely fashion, the suture can be cutoff the ureter without significant damage.

Hydronephrosis

If complete ligation of the ureter occurs, the urine from the ipsilateral kidney is prevented from draining into the bladder, leading to hydronephrosis and progressive deterioration of ipsilateral renal function. These events may occur with or without symptoms. If the urine in this obstructed system becomes infected, the patient will almost certainly become septic with pyonephrosis.

Ureteral Necrosis with Urinary Extravasation

In complete unrecognized ligation of the ureter, a section of the ureteral wall necrosis occurs because of pressure-induced ischemia. The ischemic segment of the ureter eventually weakens, leading to urinary extravasation into the periureteral tissues. If the urinary extravasation drains into the adjacent peritoneum, urinary ascites may develop. If the urinary ascites gets infected, peritonitis may ensue. If the peritoneum has remained intact, a urinoma may form in the retroperitoneum.

Ureteral Stricture

Ureteral stricture may occur when the adventitial layer of the ureter is stripped or electrocoagulated. When the adventitia, the outer layer of the ureter that contains the ureteral blood supply, is disturbed by either stripping or electrocoagulation, ischemia to a particular segment of ureter may result. Ischemic strictures of the ureter may then develop, leading to obstruction and hydronephrosis of the ipsilateral kidney.

Uremia

Uremia results when ureteral injury causes total urinary obstruction. This may result from a bilateral ureteral injury or from a unilateral ureteral injury occurring in a solitarily functioning kidney. Anuria is the only immediate sign of imminent uremia. These cases require immediate intervention to preserve renal function.

MANAGEMENT

Depending on the type, duration, and location of the ureteral injury, surgical treatment may range from simple removal of a ligature to ureteroneocystostomy **(Flowchart 1)**. The most common surgical treatments for ureteral injury are simple removal of a ligature, ureteral stenting, ureteral resection and ureteroureterostomy, transureteroureterostomy (TUU), and ureteroneocystostomy.

Observation

If a clamp or ligature constricting the ureter is discovered, the clamp or ligature should be removed immediately and the ureter should be examined. If ureteral peristalsis is preserved and it is believed that minimal damage has occurred, the ureter injury may be managed with observation.

Ureteral Stenting with or without Ureterotomy

If tissue ischemia or a partial transection of the ureteral wall is suspected, a ureteral stent should be placed. The purpose of the stent, which is typically placed cystoscopically, is to act as a structural backbone onto which the healing ureter may mold. It also guarantees drainage of urine from the renal pelvis directly to the urinary bladder. It also can work

Flowchart 1: Treatment logarithm of ureteric injuries.

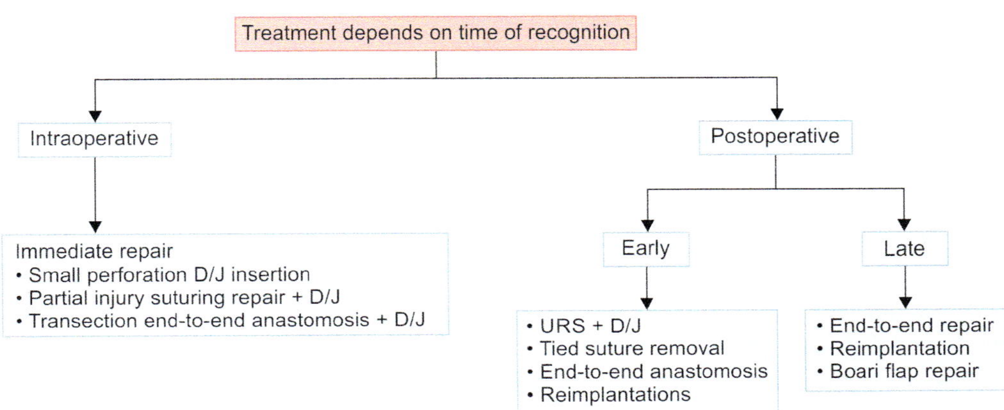

as a gentle dilator since it moves slightly in an up-and-down motion, associated with breathing, as the kidney unit moves. The use of the stent is thought to minimize the rate of obstruction of a ureteral stricture in the injured area.

Alternatively, a ureterotomy may be made along the length of the injured or strictured section of ureter before placement of a stent. Davis described this technique in 1943 (the Davis intubated ureterotomy) in which an ureterotomy is made and left open over the stent. The ureter eventually heals to form a watertight closure over the stent. The stent is withdrawn 6 weeks after it is placed, as it is estimated that all ureteral healing has occurred by that time.

The principles of the Davis intubated ureterotomy have been extended to endoscopic treatments of ureteral strictures. Ureteroscopic endoureterotomy and Acucise endoureterotomy are two modalities that are used to attempt to treat the segment of strictured ureter endoscopically by a longitudinal full-thickness ureteral incision, followed by a stent placement. The success of these procedures closely resembles the success of the open Davis intubated ureterotomy, which approaches 80% patency at 3 years.

Ureteral Resection and Ureteroureterostomy

The establishment of an anastomosis between two different ureters or between two segments of the same ureter may be required. This end-to-end anastomosis between two portions of a transected ureter can be done by open as well as laparoscopic surgery. If extensive ischemia or necrosis is the result of an injury, the ureter injury is best treated by excising the injured segment of the ureter and re-establishing continuity with the urinary system. If the ureteral injury occurred above the pelvic brim, the simplest reconstruction is a ureteroureterostomy, a procedure that is indicated for injuries to short segments of the ureter (i.e.,<2 cm), in which an anastomosis is performed between the two cut edges of the ureter.

Transureteroureterostomy

Transureteroureterostomy is a urinary reconstruction technique that is used to join one ureter to the other across the midline. It offers patients with distal ureteral obstruction, an option to live without external urostomy appliances or internal urinary stents. TUU is also used in undiversion procedures when the surgeon wants to avoid the pelvis because of previous trauma, surgery, or radiation therapy.

If ureteroureterostomy cannot be performed technically and the defect is too proximal in the ureter for ureteroneocystostomy, TUU may be performed. Absolute contraindications to TUU include urothelial cancer, contralateral reflux, pelvic irradiation, retroperitoneal fibrosis, or chronic pyelonephritis. Stone disease, which was once considered an absolute contraindication, is now considered a relative contraindication by some urologists, based on the current ability to prevent stone formation in over 90% of patients with medical therapy.

Ureteroneocystostomy

Ureteroneocystostomy is the operation to implant the upper end of a transected ureter into the bladder. If the ureteral injury occurred below the pelvic brim, where visualization of the ureter is difficult and where the vesical pedicles overlie the ureter, ureteroureterostomy is often too difficult to perform. In these cases, two types of ureteroneocystostomy procedures are indicated, either a psoas hitch or a Boari flap, in which the bladder is mobilized to reach the easily identifiable ureter proximal to the injury. Boari flaps are contraindicated in patients with prior pelvic radiation, a history of bladder cancer, or any condition with a thick, hypertrophied bladder wall.

Preoperative Details

If consultation with an urologist is indicated intraoperatively, the urologist dictates no specific preoperative preparation. If a ureteral injury is identified after the patient is stabilized following the initial gynecologic operation, a discussion is conducted regarding the possible treatment options. Preoperative antibiotics that target urinary organisms should be administered. If patients are persistently febrile secondary to a potentially infected and obstructed renal unit, percutaneous nephrostomy on the affected side may be indicated. Pertinent radiographic studies [e.g., intravenous urogram (IVU), CT scan] may be used to help define the location of ureteral injury preoperatively.

Intraoperative Details

Ureteral Stent Placement with or without Ureterotomy

The perineum of patient should be prepared and draped in the standard sterile manner and while the patient sedated adequately or anesthetized, a cystoscope should be inserted into the bladder.

After the bladder is examined and the ureteral orifices are identified, the ureteral orifice on the side of the injury should be cannulated with a ureteral catheter. A dilute cystografin-gentamicin mixture should be injected slowly through the ureteral catheter under fluoroscopy. Fluoroscopy should reveal the course of the ureter and identifying potential sites of injury.

A Teflon-coated guidewire should be placed under fluoroscopic guidance through the ureteral catheter and up the ureter into the renal pelvis. A double-J stent should be placed over the wire and pushed, so that its proximal J-hook is placed within the renal pelvis and its distal J-hook is within the bladder. Then, the wire is pulled and the stent position is reaffirmed fluoroscopically. Proper length of the stent can be estimated from the measured length of the ureter on retrograde pyelography from the ureteral orifice to the ureteropelvic junction. Allowing for roughly 10% magnification from the radiograph, subtract 2–3 cm and select that length of the ureteral stent. If, after placement, the stent is not well positioned because of inadequate or surplus length, it is best to replace it with a stent of proper dimensions **(Fig. 6)**.

If an endoscopic ureterotomy is to be made, prior to placing the stent, retrograde pyelography should be performed to delineate the ureteral anatomy and a Teflon-coated guidewire, acting as a safety wire, is positioned into the renal pelvis and out through the urethra.

With ureteroscopic endoureterotomy, a rigid ureteroscope should be placed through the ureteral orifice and into the ureter lumen until the ureteral lesion can be visualized. The ureteral stricture is then cut with a probe from a number of cutting modalities, including holmium laser or electrocautery. A full-thickness incision through the ureteral wall should be made until periureteral fat is visualized. Retrograde pyelography should be performed; extravasation of contrast outside the ureter should be seen. A wide-caliber ureteral stent should be then placed (usually 8F) in the fashion described above.

If Acucise endoureterotomy is performed, the Acucise device should be placed over the safety wire. Once position is confirmed via fluoroscopic guidance and the orientation of the cut is set, the Acucise balloon is inflated and electrocautery is instituted. The Acucise device should be withdrawn, retrograde pyelography should be performed to confirm extravasation, and a wide-caliber ureteral stent should be placed in the fashion described above.

The formal Davis intubated ureterotomy is typically performed intraoperatively only when consultation with an urologist is called for while the patient is open. In this case, the injured ureter is cut sharply in a longitudinal fashion.

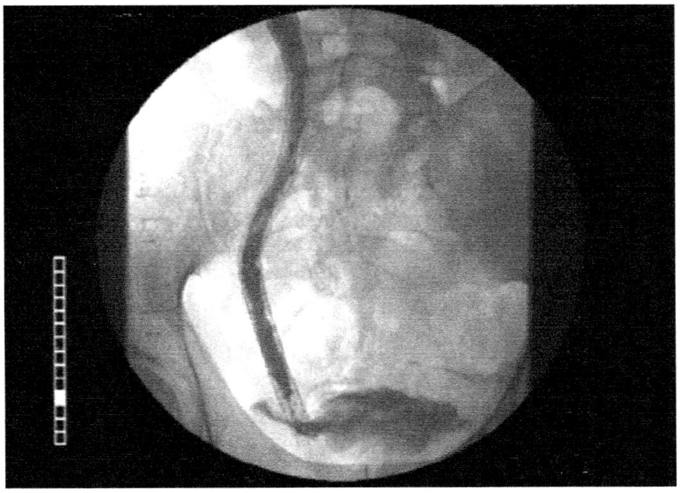

Fig. 6: Stent in the ureter.

A stent then can be placed to the kidney and bladder through the ureteral incision.

Ureteroureterostomy

It is end-to-end anastomosis of the two portions of a transected ureter. If the urologist is asked to evaluate the ureteral lesion intraoperatively, further dissection of the existing exposure is often necessary because the lack of exposure is the most likely contributor to the injury. Additional blunt and sharp dissection is often necessary to adequately identify the ureter and its course.

If the ureteral injury is discovered after the initial gynecologic procedure, the urologist must decide whether to enter through the original incision and approach the ureter transperitoneally or to make a new incision and approach the ureter using a retroperitoneal approach. Either approach is acceptable and each has distinct advantages and disadvantages.

If one decides to enter through a previous midline incision, intraperitoneal adhesions may complicate the dissection; however, this approach spares the patient an additional incision.

In contrast, if a modified Gibson incision is made to approach the ureter retroperitoneally, the dissection may be less challenging technically because it avoids the adhesions of the peritoneal cavity, but the patient is left with an additional incision.

Regardless of the approach, a Foley catheter is placed and the patient is prepared and draped in a sterile manner.

In the transperitoneal approach, an incision is made though the scar of the old incision. The dissection is extended down to the peritoneal cavity and once the small bowel and colon are identified, a vertical incision is made along the left side of the small bowel mesentery. Blunt dissection is performed in the retroperitoneum until the desired ureter is identified. If the inferior mesenteric artery (IMA) limits the exposure, it can be divided without consequence. If the left lower ureter is the area of the injury, the sigmoid can be mobilized medially to gain adequate exposure.

In the retroperitoneal approach, after the incision is made, the external oblique, internal oblique, and transversus abdominus muscles are dissected in a muscle-splitting manner. Once the transversalis fascia is incised, take care not to enter the peritoneal cavity. The peritoneum and its contents are retracted medially and the ureter is located in its extraperitoneal position.

The ureter is most consistently found at the bifurcation of the common iliac artery, but it is often difficult to identify, especially when dilated. Steps that can differentiate the ureter from a blood vessel with a similar appearance include pinching the structure with forceps and watching for peristalsis. If peristalsis occurs, the ureter has been identified. Additionally, a fine needle can be placed into the lumen of the questionable structure. If urine is retrieved through aspiration, the ureter has been identified; if blood is aspirated, then the structure is a blood vessel.

Once the ureter is identified and dissected from its surrounding tissues, the diseased segment is excised. Take particular care not to disrupt the adventitia of the ureter because its blood supply is contained within this layer. If difficulty is encountered in identifying the diseased segment, retrograde ureteropyelography can be performed to aid in localizing the lesion. Another option is to place a ureteral catheter cystoscopically up to the lesion; the ureteral catheter can then be palpated during the ureteral dissection.

Stay sutures are placed in each end of the ureter and the ureter is mobilized enough, so that tension-free anastomosis can be performed. Simple ureteroureterostomy is typically performed for ureteral lesions shorter than 2 cm. If the lesion is longer than 2 cm or if it appears that the ureteral ends will not come together without tension, seek an alternative surgical approach. Options include further mobilization of the ureter, mobilization of the ipsilateral kidney, TUU, ureteroneocystostomy, ileal ureter interposition, or a combination of the above.

Once the ureter appears to have enough length to be anastomosed without tension, both ureteral ends are spatulated. Two 5-0 absorbable sutures are placed in through the apex of the spatulated side of one ureter and out through the nonspatulated side of the opposite ureter. Each suture is tied and a running stitch is performed on one-half of the ureter. The same steps are performed to complete the anastomosis on the opposite half of the anastomosis.

Before completion of the second half, a double-J ureteral stent is placed by first placing a 0.038 cm Teflon-coated guidewire caudally and passing a standard 7F double-J stent over the wire. The wire is pulled after the position of the distal portion of the stent is confirmed within the bladder. Next, a small hole is made within the stent such that the wire can be passed cephalad, placed into the proximal tip of the stent, and comes out of the created hole in the side of the stent. Once the position of the cephalad tip in the renal pelvis is confirmed, the wire is pulled, leaving a well-positioned stent.

After the anastomosis is completed, a Penrose drain or a Jackson–Pratt (JP) drain is placed in the retroperitoneum and is brought out through the skin. Omentum may be retrieved from a small incision in the posterior peritoneum and can be used to wrap the repair. Adjacent retroperitoneal fat may be used. The anterior abdominal fascia and skin are closed.

Transureteroureterostomy

Transureteroureterostomy is a urinary reconstruction technique that is used to join one ureter to the other across the midline. It offers patients with distal ureteral obstruction, an option to live without external urostomy appliances or internal urinary stents. TUU is also used in undiversion procedures when the surgeon wants to avoid the pelvis because of previous trauma, surgery, or radiation therapy. A TUU is approached best via a midline incision and can be performed using both intraperitoneal and extraperitoneal approaches. A left-to-right intraperitoneal TUU is described.

After a Foley catheter is placed and the patient is prepared and draped in a sterile manner, a midline incision is made and the peritoneal cavity is opened. The small bowel is packed medially and the posterior peritoneum lateral to the sigmoid and descending colon is incised to expose the ureter. The ureter is dissected, preserving its adventitia. The diseased portion of the ureter is identified and a clamp is placed on the ureter proximal to the diseased portion. The diseased portion of ureter is excised, a stay stitch is placed on the proximal segment of the ureter, and the distal stump is ligated. The proximal ureter is dissected for a length of approximately 9–12 cm, while the adventitial vessels are preserved.

Attention is then turned to exposing the right ureter. The ascending colon is retracted medially, while an incision is made through the posterior peritoneum lateral to the colon. Blunt dissection aids in the identification of the ureter. Approximately 4–6 cm above the level of transection of the left ureter, the right ureter is exposed to make room for an anastomosis.

A retroperitoneal tunnel is created via blunt dissection and the left ureter is pulled through the tunnel by the stay suture. When the left ureter is pulled through, taking care not to wedge the ureter between the IMA and the aorta is important because obstruction may result. Instead, the ureter should be passed either over or under the IMA and should not be angulated or be under any tension. If the ureter is too short and a tension-free anastomosis can only be performed with the ureter firmly wedged between the IMA and the aorta, it is appropriate to consider ligation of the IMA. If this maneuver is not performed and the ureter is left firmly between the IMA and the aorta, a fibrous reaction of the ureter typically occurs, which causes an obstruction that must be treated later again with a surgical procedure.

The tip of the left ureter is spatulated and the medial wall of the right ureter is incised using a hook blade for a distance just longer than the diameter of the lumen of the left ureter. Using 4-0 or 5-0 absorbable suture material, a suture is placed at each end of the ureteral incision from the outside in. Each stitch is run over the course of one-half of the anastomosis. Before finishing the second side of the anastomosis, a stent is placed along the entire right ureter using the technique described in ureteral stent placement. The two stitches are tied to each other.

After the anastomosis is completed, a Penrose drain or a JP drain is placed in the retroperitoneum and is brought out through the skin. Omentum or any adjacent retroperitoneal fat may be used to wrap the repair. The anterior abdominal fascia and skin are closed.

Psoas Hitch

The psoas hitch ureteral reimplantation technique has been used with great success to bridge defects in ureteral length due to injury or planned resection. Several surgical principles have been historically stressed when performing this procedure, including adequate mobilization of the bladder, fixation of the bladder to the psoas tendon before reimplantation, the use of a submucosal nonrefluxing-type ureteral anastomosis, and a 6-week delay before attempting repair after a surgical injury.

After a Foley catheter is placed and the patient is prepared and draped in a sterile manner, various incisions are acceptable, including a midline, a Pfannenstiel, or a suprapubic V-shaped incision. A midline incision is preferred if the patient has a preexisting midline scar from a previous gynecologic operation. If entering the peritoneal cavity can be avoided, this incision is preferred.

The peritoneal reflection is dissected off the bladder. Some advocates saline installation in the subperitoneal connective tissue as a way of facilitating this portion of the dissection. If a peritoneal defect is encountered, it can be closed with a running chromic suture. Once the peritoneum is dissected off the bladder, the peritoneum can be reflected medially.

Attention is then turned to dissection and excision of the diseased ureteral segment. The diseased portion of the ureter is identified and a clamp is placed on the ureter proximal to it. The diseased portion of ureter is excised, a stay stitch is placed on the proximal segment of the ureter, and the distal stump is ligated.

The superior pedicle of the bladder is ligated on the ipsilateral side and the bladder wall is incised transversely, a little more than halfway around the bladder, in an oblique manner across the middle of its anterior wall at the level of its maximum diameter. When this horizontal incision is closed vertically, the effect of the incision is the elongation of the anterior wall of the bladder so that the apex of the bladder can be positioned and fixed above the iliac vessels.

After the bladder incision is made, two fingers are placed into the bladder to elevate it to the level of the proximal end of the ureter. If the bladder does not reach the proximal ureter, several steps can be performed for additional length. These steps include extending the bladder wall incision laterally to obtain further length or the peritoneum and connective tissue from the pelvic and lateral walls may be dissected from the contralateral side of the bladder. This dissection may require ligation and division of the superior vesical pedicle on the contralateral side too.

Once adequate mobilization of the bladder has occurred, the bladder is held against the tendinous portion of the psoas minor muscle without tension. Prolene sutures (2-0) are sutured into the bladder wall and to the tendon to fix the bladder in place.

With the bladder open, attention is turned to the ureteral reimplant. An incision is made in the bladder mucosa at the proposed site of the new ureteral orifice. A submucosal dissection occurs approximately 3 cm from the incision site, so that a tunnel is created. Lahey scissors may be used to facilitate this dissection. After achieving a 3-cm tunnel length, the scissors are inverted and the tips are pushed through the bladder wall. An 8F feeding tube is passed over the scissor blades and the stay suture on the proximal tip of the ureter is tied to the other end of the catheter, so that traction on the catheter draws the ureter into the bladder. The ureteral tip is trimmed obliquely and 4-6 absorbable sutures (4-0) are used to fix the ureter to the bladder mucosa. The ureteral adventitia is tacked to the extravesical bladder wall with several 4-0 absorbable sutures. A double-J ureteral stent may be placed at this time.

A nontunneled reimplant is also an acceptable choice in most adults, if ureteral length is insufficient. The end of the ureter can be reflected back after making a small longitudinal incision from the tip proximally about 1.5 cm. This will make the end of the ureter into a nonrefluxing nipple, which is useful when there is inadequate length for an antirefluxing submucosal tunnel.

After completing the reimplant, two fingers are placed within the bladder while five or six absorbable sutures (2-0) are placed within the bladder muscle, the psoas muscle, and the psoas minor tendon, paying specific attention not to suture the genitofemoral nerve. Alternatively, sutures may also take deep bites in the muscle itself. The bladder is closed with a 3-0 running absorbable suture on the mucosa and a running 2-0 suture incorporating the bladder muscle and adventitial layers. A Penrose drain or a JP drain is placed in the retroperitoneum next to the bladder closure. The anterior abdominal fascia and the skin then are closed.

Boari Flap

A Boari flap may be required to bridge long defects of the middle and lower ureter to the bladder. Laparoscopic construction of a Boari flap was performed in a patient with a ureteral stricture secondary to iatrogenic injury. The salient steps performed were spatulation of the transected ureteral end, fashioning of a Boari flap from the bladder, end-to-side anastomosis of the ureter to the flap, placement of a stent with the aid of a suction cannula, and closure of the flap over the stent. A Boari flap can be accomplished even laparoscopically with minimal morbidity.

After preparing and draping the patient, in open method, a midline or Pfannenstiel incision is made. Once the transversalis fascia is incised, the ureter may be approached either transperitoneally or retroperitoneally. In the transperitoneal approach, the peritoneal cavity is entered, the sigmoid or cecum is reflected medially, the posterior peritoneum is incised, and the ureter is identified.

In the retroperitoneal approach, care is taken not to enter the peritoneal cavity, the peritoneum is mobilized medially, and the ureter is identified and exposed. A stay stitch is placed in healthy ureter tissue just proximal to the injury. The remaining end of the ureter is tied off.

The peritoneum is then dissected from the wall of the bladder. This dissection may be facilitated with hydrodissection, in which saline is injected subperitoneally, separating the peritoneal layer from the muscle layers of the bladder.

The necessary length of the bladder flap (i.e., the distance between the posterior wall of the bladder and the end of the healthy proximal ureter) is measured with umbilical tape, the bladder is one-half full of saline, and the length and shape of the bladder flap are planned. To measure accurately on the dome of the bladder, several stay stitches are placed at the base of the proposed bladder flap and at the apex. The bladder flap should be planned with a large base because the base contains all the blood supply necessary for the flap. The length of the bladder flap (i.e., the distance between the base and apex) should equal the distance between the posterior wall of the bladder and the end of the healthy proximal ureter. The width of the apex should be at least three times the diameter of the ureter to prevent constriction after the flap is tubularized. Avoid scarred areas of the bladder.

After proper planning, an outline of the flap is made in the bladder wall with coagulating current and the bladder flap is remeasured. If the measurements are satisfactory, the bladder flap is cut via cutting current and the concomitant bleeding vessels are coagulated.

After the bladder flap is turned superiorly, Lahey scissors are used to prepare a ureteral tunnel. The tunnel should be at least 3 cm long and is created by placing the Lahey scissors submucosally at the apex of the flap, tunneling the appropriate distance and coming out through the mucosa. Submucosal injection of saline may aid in this dissection. An 8F feeding tube is pulled through the tunnel by the scissors and the stay suture on the proximal ureter is tied to the feeding tube after the ureteral end is spatulated. The feeding tube is pulled toward the bladder, followed by the ureter. The stay suture is cut after the ureter has traveled completely through the tunnel.

The bladder flap is sutured to the psoas tendon of the psoas minor with a few 2-0 absorbable sutures. These sutures fix the flap in place to prevent tension on the ureteral anastomosis.

The ureter is anastomosed to the bladder mucosa with several 4-0 absorbable sutures. A few of the sutures should include the muscle layer of the bladder to fix the ureter into place. An 8F feeding tube is passed up the ureter into the renal pelvis and out through the bladder and body wall.

Before closing the bladder, a large suprapubic tube is placed, i.e., either a 22-24F Malecot or Foley. Then, the bladder is closed by approximating the bladder mucosa with a 3-0 absorbable running suture followed by a second row of running sutures, which approximate the muscularis and adventitial layers. A few absorbable sutures (5-0) can be placed to approximate the distal end of the flap to the adventitia of the ureter. If a transperitoneal approach is used, close the peritoneum and then place a Penrose or a JP drain retroperitoneally adjacent to the bladder closure. The anterior abdominal fascia and skin are closed.

Postoperative Details

Ureteral Stent

After the patient has recovered from anesthesia and is in suitable condition, the patient may be discharged with instructions to return to the clinic in 14–21 days, when the stent will be removed. The patient is discharged with 3 days of antibiotics and oral analgesics for potential bouts of discomfort from the stent.

Ureteroureterostomy, Transureteroureterostomy, Psoas Hitch, and Boari Flap

Patients who undergo a transperitoneal approach are kept on a regimen of nothing by mouth (NPO) for the first day after surgery. Subsequently, signs of bowel function are monitored routinely. Once bowel sounds are present, the diet is advanced to clear liquids and when the patient passes flatus, a regular diet is instituted.

Patients who undergo a retroperitoneal approach are started on clear liquids on the first day after surgery unless they are nauseous. Their diets are also advanced when they have passed flatus.

All patients receive a patient-controlled analgesia (PCA) pump postoperatively, unless they had an epidural catheter placed intraoperatively. The latter are then given an epidural pump. Oral analgesics are administered after patients tolerate a regular diet.

All patients receive a 24-hour course of intravenous antibiotics to prevent wound infections.

Patients are encouraged to ambulate on the first day after surgery. Once the pain is controlled with oral analgesics and patients are tolerating a regular diet, they are eligible for discharge, with or without their drains. If drains are not removed while in the hospital, appointments are set to assess patients and their drains in the clinic.

Follow-up

In patients who do not require a cystotomy, the Foley catheter or suprapubic tube is left to drain the bladder until the drain output from the Penrose or JP drain is <30 mL/day. If this is achieved, the Foley catheter can be removed or the suprapubic tube can be clamped and the output from the Penrose or JP drain is monitored. If no drainage occurs, the drain can be removed. If drainage increases from the previous level, the Foley catheter is replaced or the suprapubic tube is unclamped. After several days, the same sequence of events occurs to determine whether the ureter has healed completely. If a stent or feeding tube is used, it can be removed 7–10 days after surgery.

In patients who require cystotomy, the Foley catheter or suprapubic tube is left in place for 7–10 days after surgery, at which time cystography is usually performed. If no extravasation is observed during the cystogram, the Foley catheter or suprapubic tube can be removed. At the same time, the outputs from the Penrose or JP drain are monitored. If no drainage occurs, the drain can be removed. If drain output increases from the previous level, the Foley catheter is replaced. After several days, the same sequence of events occurs to determine whether the ureter has healed completely. If a stent is used, the stent is removed 10–14 days after surgery.

Laparoscopic surgery has become a surgical discipline in its own right. Like any other surgical technique, it does involve a risk of complications. This risk of ureteral injury is related to the complexity of the laparoscopic procedure. The setup phase for laparoscopy must never be considered banal. The methods of postoperative monitoring must be adapted to take into account the shorter hospital stay and the fact that a considerable number of ureteral injuries go unnoticed intraoperatively.

CONCLUSION

- Awareness of risk factors and good experience in laparoscopy are the main factors in preventing and reducing the ureteric injuries
- Immediate and early diagnosis of ureteral injuries gives excellent outcome and minimal morbidity, while delayed diagnosis had prolong morbidity
- For any suspicious of ureteric injury, investigations should be done to rule out the injury
- Placement of stent is helpful especially in difficult cases and reduces rate of ureteric injury
- Intraoperative cystoscopy during laparoscopy leads to immediate diagnosis of ureteric injuries
- Excessive use of diathermy near the ureter may follow thermal injury to it

BIBLIOGRAPHY

1. Alleyassin A, Khademi A, Aghahosseini M, Safdarian L, Badenoosh B, Akbari HE. Comparison of success rates in the medical management of ectopic pregnancy with single-dose and multiple-dose administration of methotrexate: a prospective, randomized clinical trial. Fertil Steril. 2006;85:1661-6.
2. Ankum WM, Vander Veen F, Hamerlynck HV, Lammes FB. Suspected ectopic pregnancy. What to do when human chorionic gonadotropin levels are below the discriminatory zone. Suspected ectopic pregnancy. J Reprod Med. 1995;40:525-8.
3. Bender S. Fertility after tubal pregnancy. J Obstet Gynaecol Br Emp. 1956;63:400-3.
4. Boury-Heyler C, Madelenat P. Surgical treatment of 150 cases of extrauterine pregnancy. Chirurgie. 1983;109:395-8.
5. Bouyer J, Job-Spira N, Pouly J, Coste J, Germain E, Fernandez H. Fertility following radical, conservative-surgical or medical treatment for tubal pregnancy: a population-based study. BJOG. 2000;107:714-21.
6. Bruhat MA, Manhes H, Mage G, Pouly JL. Treatment of ectopic pregnancy by means of laparoscopy. Fertil Steril. 1980;33:411-4.
7. Carp MJ, Oelsner G, Serr DM, Mashiach S. Fertility after nonsurgical treatment of ectopic pregnancy. J Reprod Med. 1986;31:119-22.
8. Cartwright PS. Peritoneal trophoblastic implants after surgical management of pregnancy. J Reprod Med. 1991;36:523-4.
9. Chapron C, Querleu D, Crepin G. Laparoscopic treatment of ectopic pregnancy: a one hundred cases study. Eur J Obstet Gynecol Reprod Biol. 1991;41:187-90.
10. Clausen I. Conservative versus radical surgery for tubal pregnancy. Acta Obstet Gynecol Scand. 1996;75:8-12.
11. Colacurci N, De FP, Zarcone R, Fortunato N, Passaro M, Mollo A, et al. Time length of negativization of hCG serum values after either surgical or medical treatment of ectopic pregnancy. Panminerva Med. 1998;40:223-5.
12. Condous G, Okaro E, Khalid A, Timmerman DL, Zhou Y, van HS, et al. The use of a new logistic regression model for predicting the outcome of pregnancies of unknown location. Hum Reprod. 2004;19:1900-10.
13. Cutler SJ, Ederer F. Maximum utilization of life table methods in analyzing survival. J Chronic Dis. 1958;8:699-707.
14. DeChemey AH, Boyer SP. Laparoscopic salpingostomy for ectopic pregnancy. Obstet Gynecol. 1987;70:948-50.
15. Donnez J, Nisolle M. Laparoscopic treatment of ampullary tubal pregnancy. J Gynecol Surg. 1989;5:157-62.
16. Douglas J, Shingleton HM. Surgical management of tubal pregnancy: effect on subsequent fertility. South Med J. 1969; 62:954-5.
17. Dubuisson JB, Aubriot FX, Cardone V. Laparoscopic salpingectomy for tubal pregnancy. Fertil Steril. 1987;47:225-8.
18. Dubuisson JB, Aubriot FX, Foulot H, Bruel D, de Jolinière JB, Mandelbrot L. Reproductive outcome after laparoscopic salpingectomy for tubal pregnancy. Fertil Steril. 1990;53:1004-7.
19. Egarter C, Kiss H, Husslein P. Prostaglandin versus expectant management in early tubal pregnancy. Prostaglandins Leukot Essent Fatty Acids. 1991;42:177-9.
20. Elmoghazy DAM, Nour-El-Dine NM. Prevention of persistent ectopic pregnancy with single dose methotrexate after surgical conservation of the tube. Int J Gynecol Obstet. 2000;70:B57.
21. El-Sherbiny MT, El-Gharieb IH, Mera IM. Methotrexate versus laparoscopic surgery for the management of unruptured tubal pregnancy. Middle East Fertil Soc J. 2003;8:256-62.
22. Fedele L, Bianchi S, Tozzi L, Zanconato G, Silvestre V. Intramesosalpingeal injection of oxytocin in conservative laparoscopic treatment for tubal pregnancy: preliminary results. Hum Reprod. 1998;13:3042-4.
23. Fernandez H, Baton C, Lelaidier C, Frydman R. Conservative management of ectopic pregnancy: prospective randomized clinical trial of methotrexate versus prostaglandin sulprostone by combined transvaginal and systemic administration. Fertil Steril. 1991;55:746-50.
24. Fernandez H, Baton C. Treatment of ectopic pregnancy by transvaginal aspiration: prospective randomized clinical trial of Methotrexate versus Sulprostone by sonographic injection followed by systemic injection. Contracept Fertil Sex. 1990;18:261-5.

25. Fernandez H, Bourget P, Ville Y, Lelaidier C, Frydman R. Treatment of unruptured tubal pregnancy with methotrexate: pharmacokinetic analysis of local versus intramuscular administration. Fertil Steril. 1994;62:943-7.
26. Fernandez H, Pauthier S, Doumerc S, Lelaidier C, Olivennes F, Ville YY. Ultrasound-guided injection of methotrexate versus laparoscopic salpingotomy in ectopic pregnancy. Fertil Steril. 1995;63:25-9.
27. Fernandez H, Pauthier S, Sitbon D, Vincent Y, Doumerc S. Role of conservative therapy and medical treatment in ectopic pregnancy: literature review and clinical trial comparing medical treatment and conservative laparoscopic treatment. Contracept Fertil Sex. 1996;24:297-302.
28. Fernandez H, Yves VS, Pauthier S, Audibert F, Frydman R. Randomized trial of conservative laparoscopic treatment and methotrexate administration in ectopic pregnancy and subsequent fertility. Hum Reprod. 1998;13:3239-43.
29. Flamant DR, Lellouch J. Clinical Trials. London: Academic Press; 1980. pp. 214-23.
30. Foulot H, Chapron C, Morice P, Mouly M, Aubriot FX, Dubuisson JB. Failure of laparoscopic treatment for peritoneal trophoblastic implants. Hum Reprod. 1994;9:92-3.
31. Franklin EW, Zeiderman AM. Tubal ectopic pregnancy: etiology and obstetric and gynecologic sequelae. Am J Obstet Gynecol. 1973;117:220-5.
32. Fujishita A, Ishimaru T, Masuzaki H, Samejima T, Matsuwaki T, Chavez RO, et al. Local injection of methotrexate dissolved in saline versus methotrexate suspensions for the conservative treatment of ectopic pregnancy. Hum Reprod. 1995;10:3280-3.
33. Fujishita A, Masuzaki H, Newaz KK, Kitajima M, Hiraki K, Ishimaru T. Laparoscopic salpingotomy for tubal pregnancy: comparison of linear salpingotomy with and without suturing. Hum Reprod. 2004;19:1195-200.
34. Garbin O, de TR, de PL, Coiffic J, Lucot JP, Le-Goueff FF. Medical treatment of ectopic pregnancy; a randomized clinical trial comparing methotrexate mifepristone and methotrexate-placebo. J Gynecol Obstet Biol Reprod. 2004;33:391-400.
35. Gazvani MR, Baruah DN, Alfirevic Z, Emery SJ. Mifepristone in combination with methotrexate for the medical management of tubal pregnancy: a randomized controlled trial. Hum Reprod. 1998;13:1987-90.
36. Giana M. Trataments chirurgico conservative in caza digraviden zatubarica. Minerva Gynecol. 1979;30:51-99.
37. Gjelland K, Hordnes K, Tjugum J, Augensen K, Bergsjø P. Treatment of ectopic pregnancy by local injection of hypertonic glucose: a randomized trial comparing administration guided by transvaginal ultrasound or laparoscopy. Acta Obstet Gynecol Scand. 1995;74:629-34.
38. Gracia CR, Brown HA, Barnhart KT. Prophylactic methotrexate after linear salpingostomy: a decision analysis. Fertil Steril. 2001;76:1191-5.
39. Graczykowski JW, Mishell DR. Methotrexate prophylaxis for persistent ectopic pregnancy after conservative treatment by salpingostomy. Obstet Gynecol. 1997;89:118-22.
40. Gray DT, Thorburn J, Lundorff P, Strandell A, Lindblom B. A cost-effectiveness study of a randomized trial of laparoscopy versus laparotomy for ectopic pregnancy. Lancet. 1995;345:1139-43.
41. Hajenius P, Mol F, Mol B, Bossuyt P, Ankum W, van der Veen F. Interventions for tubal ectopic pregnancy. Cochrane Database Syst Rev. 2007;1:CD000324.
42. Hajenius PJ, Engelsbel S, Mol BWJ, van der Veen F, Ankum WM, Bossuyt PMM. Randomized trial of systemic methotrexate versus laparoscopic salpingostomy in tubal pregnancy. Lancet. 1997;350:774-9.
43. Hallatt JG. Tubal conservation in ectopic pregnancy: a study of 200 cases. Am J Obstet Gynecol. 1986;154:1216-21.
44. Hordnes K. Reproductive outcome after treatment of ectopic pregnancy with local injection of hypertonic glucose. Acta Obstet Gynecol Scand. 1997;76:703-5.
45. Hu CX, Han LX. Mifepristone in combination with methotrexate for the medical treatment of unruptured ectopic pregnancy. Acta Acad Med. 2003;12:171-2.
46. Hugues GJ. Fertility and ectopic pregnancy. Eur J Obstet Gynecol Reprod Biol. 1980;10:361-5.
47. Intramuscular. Fertil Steril. 1996;65:206-7.
48. Judlin P, Leguin T, Zaccabri A, Landes P. Avenir genital des patientes apres GEU: a proposd'une sine continue de 330 cas. J Gynecol Obstet Biol Reprod. 1988;17:58-9.
49. Kaya H, Babar Y, Ozmen S, Ozkaya O, Karci M, Aydin AR. Intratubal methotrexate for prevention of persistent ectopic pregnancy after salpingostomy. J Am Assoc Gynecol Laparosc. 2002;9:464-7.
50. Klauser CK, May WL, Johnson VK, Cowan BD, Hines RS. Methotrexate for ectopic pregnancy: a randomized single dose compared with multiple doses. Obstet Gynaecol. 2005;105:64S.
51. Koninckx PR, Witters K, Brosens J, Stemers N, Oosterlynck D, Meuleman C. Conservative laparoscopic treatment of ectopic pregnancies using the CO_2 laser. Br J Obstet Gynaecol. 1991;98:1254-9.
52. Korhonen J, Stenman U, Ylostalo P. Low-dose oral methotrexate with expectant management of ectopic pregnancy. Obstet Gynecol. 1996;88:775-8.
53. Laatikainen T, Tuomivaara L, Kaar K. Comparison of a local injection of hyperosmolar glucose solution with salpingostomy for the conservative treatment of tubal pregnancy. Fertil Steril. 1993;60:80-4.
54. Landstrom G, Bryman I, Ekstrom P, Engman M, Gunnarsson J, Hjersing MM. Ectopic pregnancy: local medical treatment versus oral methotrexate therapy—a multicentre pilot study. Hum Reprod. 1998;13:38.
55. Lang PF, Weiss PA, Mayer HO, Haas JG, Honigl W. Conservative treatment of ectopic pregnancy with local injection of hyperosmolar glucose solution or prostaglandin F2a: a prospective randomised study. Lancet. 1990;336:78-81.
56. Langebrekke A, Somes T, Umes A. Fertility after treatment of tubal pregnancy by laparoscopic laser surgery. Acta Obstet Gynecol Scand. 1993;72:547-9.
57. Langer R, Raziel A, Ron-El R, Golan A, Bukovsky I, Caspi E. Reproductive outcome after conservative surgery for unruptured tubal pregnancy—a 15-year experience. Fertil Steril. 1990;53:227-31.
58. Lund J. Early ectopic pregnancy; comments on conservative treatment. J Obstet Gynecol Br Emp. 1955;62:70-6.
59. Lundorff P, Hahlin M, Sjöblom P, Lindblom B. Persistent trophoblast after conservative treatment of tubal pregnancy: prediction and detection. Obstet Gynecol. 1991;77:129-33.
60. Lundorff P, Thorburn J, Hahlin M, Kallfelt B, Lindblom B. Laparoscopic surgery in ectopic pregnancy: a randomized trial versus laparotomy. Acta Obstet Gynecol Scand. 1991;70:343-8.
61. Lundorff P, Thorburn J, Lindblom B. Fertility after conservative surgical treatment of ectopic pregnancy evaluated in a randomized trial. Ugeskr Laeger. 1993;155:3282-6.
62. Lundorff P, Thorburn J, Lindblom B. Fertility outcome after conservative surgical treatment of ectopic pregnancy evaluated in a randomized trial. Fertil Steril. 1992;57:998-1002.
63. Lundorff P, Thorburn J, Lindbloom B. Second-look laparoscopy after ectopic pregnancy. Fertil Steril. 1990;53:604-9.
64. Lundorff P. Laparoscopic surgery in ectopic pregnancy. Acta Obstet Gynecol Scand. 1997;164:81-4.
65. Lundorff P. Treatment of ectopics and subsequent adhesion formation. Prog Clin Biol Res. 1993;381:139-47.
66. Makinen JI, Salmi TU, Nikkanen VPJ, Koskinen EYJ. Encouraging rates of fertility after ectopic pregnancy. Int J Fertil. 1989;34:46-51.

67. Manhes H, Mage G, Pouly JL. Treatment, coelioscopique de la grossesse tubaire: ameliorations techniques. Presse Med. 1983;12:1431.
68. Mathieu J, Soulerin A. Le pronostic obstetrical après grossesse extra uterine. Rev Fr Gynecol Obstet. 1957;52:167-76.
69. Mol BW, Hajenius PJ, Ankum WM, van der Veen F, Bossuyt PM. Conservative versus radical surgery for tubal pregnancy. Acta Obstet Gynecol Scand. 1996;75:866-7.
70. Mol BW, Hajenius PJ, Engelsbel S, Ankum WM, Hemrika DJ, van der Veen F. The treatment of tubal pregnancy in the Netherlands: an economic evaluation of systemic methotrexate and laparoscopic salpingostomy. Am J Obstet Gynecol. 1999;181:945-51.
71. Mol BW, Hajenius PJ, Engelsbel S, Ankum WM, van der Veen F, Hemrika DJ, et al. Serum human chorionic gonadotropin measurement in the diagnosis of ectopic pregnancy when transvaginal sonography is inconclusive. Fertil Steril. 1998; 70:972-81.
72. Mol BW, Matthijsse HM, Tinga DJ, Huynh VT, Hajenius PJ, Ankum WM, et al. Fertility after conservative and radical surgery for tubal pregnancy. Hum Reprod. 1998;13:1804-9.
73. Mol BW, van der Veen F, Bossuyt PM. Implementation of probabilistic decision rules improves the predictive values of algorithms in the diagnostic management of ectopic pregnancy. Hum Reprod. 1999;14:2855-62.
74. Mottla GL, Rulin MC, Guzick DS. Lack of resolution of ectopic pregnancy by intratubal injection of methotrexate. Fertil Steril. 1992;57:685-7.
75. Murphy AA, Nager CW, Wujek JJ, Kettel LM, Torp VA, Chin HG. Operative laparoscopy versus laparotomy for the management of ectopic pregnancy: a prospective trial. Fertil Steril. 1992;57:1180-5.
76. Murphy AA. Operative laparoscopy. Fertil Steril. 1987;47:1-18.
77. Nagamani M, London S, St Amand P. Factors influencing fertility after ectopic pregnancy. Am J Obstet Gynecol. 1984;149:533-5.
78. Nieuwkerk PT, Hajenius PJ, Ankum WM, van der Veen F, Wijker W, Bossuyt PM. Systemic methotrexate therapy versus laparoscopic salpingostomy in patients with tubal pregnancy. Part I. Impact on patients' health-related quality of life. Fertil Steril. 1998;70:511-7.
79. Nieuwkerk PT, Hajenius PJ, van der Veen F, Ankum WM, Wijker W, Bossuyt PM. Systemic methotrexate therapy versus laparoscopic salpingostomy in tubal pregnancy. Part II. Patient preferences for systemic methotrexate. Fertil Steril. 1998;7:518-22.
80. Oelsner G, Goldenberg M, Admon D, Pansky M, Tur-Kaspa I, Rabinovitch O, et al. Salpingectomy by operative laparoscopy and subsequent reproductive performance. Hum Reprod. 1994;9:83-6.
81. Paavonen J, Varjonen-Toivonen M, Komulainen M, Heinonen PK. Diagnosis and management of tubal pregnancy: effect on fertility outcome Int J Gynecol Obstet. 1985;23:123-33.
82. Palmer R. Resultats et indications de la chirurgie conservatrice au cours de la grossesse extra utirine. CR Soc Fr Gynecol. 1972;42:317-20.
83. Peng LX. The comparison of three conservative treatments for ectopic pregnancy; analysis of 97 cases. Guangxi Med J. 1997;19:752-4.
84. Pereira GD, Hajenius PJ, Mol BW, Ankum WM, Hemrika DJ, Bossuyt PM, et al. Fertility outcome after systemic methotrexate and laparoscopic salpingostomy for tubal pregnancy. Lancet. 1999;353:724-5.
85. Ploman L, Wicksell F. Fertility after conservative surgery in tubal pregnancy. Acta Obstet Gynecol Scand. 1960;39:143-52.
86. Porpora MG, Oliva MM, De CA, Montanino G, Cosmi EV. Comparison of local methotrexate and linear salpingostomy in the conservative laparoscopic treatment of ectopic pregnancy. J Am Assoc Gynecol Laparosc. 1996;3:271-6.
87. Pouly JL, Chapron C, Manhes H, Canis M, Wattiez A, Bruhat MA. Multifactorial analysis of fertility after conservative laparoscopic treatment of ectopic pregnancy in a series of 223 patients. Fertil Steril. 1991;56:453-60.
88. Pusey J, Taylor PJ, Leader A, Pattinson HA. Outcome and effect on medical intervention in women experiencing infertility following removal of an ectopic pregnancy. Am J Obstet Gynecol. 1984;148:524-7.
89. Querleu D, Lenain F, Hennion A. Feconditi apres grossesse extrauterine. Contracept Fertil Sex. 1988;16:131-5.
90. Reich H, Jones DA, De Caprio J. Laparoscopic treatment of 109 consecutive ectopic pregnancies. J Reprod Med. 1988;33:885-90.
91. Rozenberg P, Chevret S, Camus E, de TR, Garbin O, Poncheville LL. Medical treatment of ectopic pregnancies: a randomized clinical trial comparing methotrexate-mifepristone and methotrexate-placebo. Hum Reprod. 2003;18:1802-8.
92. Sadan O, Ginath S, Debby A, Rotmensch S, Golan A, Zakut HH. Methotrexate versus hyperosmolar glucose in the treatment of extrauterine pregnancy. Arch Gynecol Obstet. 2001;265:82-4.
93. Saraj AJ, Wilcox JG, Najmabadi S, Stein SM, Johnson MB, Paulson RJ. Resolution of hormonal markers of ectopic gestation: a randomized trial comparing single-dose intramuscular methotrexate with salpingostomy. Obstet Gynecol. 1998;92:989-94.
94. Seifer DB, Gutmann JN, Grant WD, Kamps CA, DeCherney AH. Comparison of persistent ectopic pregnancy after laparoscopic salpingostomy versus salpingostomy at laparotomy for ectopic pregnancy. Obstet Gynecol. 1993;81:378-82.
95. Sharma JB, Gupta S, Malhotra M, Arora R. A randomized controlled comparison of minilaparotomy and laparotomy in ectopic pregnancy cases. Indian J Med Sci. 2003;57:493-500.
96. Shea RT, Thompson GR, Harding A. Intra-amniotic methotrexate versus CO_2 laser laparoscopic salpingotomy in the management of tubal ectopic pregnancy: a prospective randomized trial. Fertil Steril. 1994;62:876-8.
97. Sherman A, Langer R, Sadovsky G, Bukovsky I, Caspi E. Improved fertility following ectopic pregnancy. Fertil Steril. 1982;37:497-502.
98. Shulman A, Maymon R, Zmira N, Lotan M, Holtzinger M, Bahary C. Conservative treatment of ectopic pregnancy and its effect on corpus luteum activity. Gynecol Obstet Invest. 1992;33:161-4.
99. Silva PD, Schaper AM, Rooney B. Reproductive outcome after 143 laparoscopic procedures for ectopic pregnancy. Obstet Gynecol. 1993;81:710-15.
100. Skulj V, Pavlic Z, Stoilkovic C, Bacic G, Drazancic A. Conservative operative treatment of tubal pregnancy. Fertil Steril. 1964;15:634-9.
101. Sowter MC, Farquhar CM, Gudex G. An economic evaluation of single-dose systemic methotrexate and laparoscopic surgery for the treatment of unruptured ectopic pregnancy. Br J Obstet Gynaecol. 2001;108:204-12.
102. Sowter MC, Farquhar CM, Petrie KJ, Gudex G. A randomized trial comparing single-dose systemic methotrexate and laparoscopic surgery for the treatment of unruptured ectopic pregnancy. Br J Obstet Gynaecol. 2001;108:192-203.
103. Stovall TG, Ling FW, Gray LA, Carson SA, Buster JE. Methotrexate treatment of unruptured ectopic pregnancy: a report of 100 cases. Obstet Gynecol. 1991;77:749-53.
104. Su Y, Sun Y, Ma L. Observation on treatment of ecotopic pregnancy by combination therapy of Chinese herbal medicine with mifepristone or methotrexate. Zhongguo Zhong Xi Yi Jie He Za Zhi. 2002;22:417-9.
105. Sultana CJ, Easley K, Collins RL. Outcome of laparoscopic versus traditional surgery for ectopic pregnancies. Fertil Steril. 1992;57:285-9.
106. Thorburn J, Philipson M, Lindblom B. Fertility after ectopic pregnancy in relation to background factors and surgical treatment. Fertil Steril. 1988;49:595-601.
107. Timonen S, Nieminen U. Tubal pregnancy: choice of operative method of treatment. Acta Obstet Gynecol Scand. 1967;46:327-39.

108. Tulandi T, Guralnick M. Treatment of tubal ectopic pregnancy by salpingotomy with or without tubal suturing and salpingectomy. Fertil Steril. 1991;55:53-5.
109. Tuomivaara L, Kaupilla A. Radical or conservative surgery for ectopic pregnancy? A follow-up study of fertility of 323 patients. Fertil Steril. 1988;50:580-3.
110. Tzafettas J, Anapliotis S, Zournatzi V, Boucklis A, Oxouzoglou N, Bondis J. Transvaginal intra-amniotic injection of methotrexate in early ectopic pregnancy: advantages over the laparoscopic approach. Early Hum Dev. 1994;39:101-7.
111. Ugur M, Yesilyurt H, Soysal S, Gokmen O. Prophylactic vasopressin during laparoscopic salpingotomy for ectopic pregnancy. J Am Assoc Gynecol Laparosc. 1996;3:365-8.
112. Vehaskari A. The operation of choice for ectopic pregnancy to subsequent fertility. Acta Obstet Gynecol Scand. 1960; 39:1-7.
113. Vermesh M, Presser SC. Reproductive outcome after linear salpingostomy for ectopic gestation: a prospective 3-year follow-up. Fertil Steril. 1992;57:682-4.
114. Vermesh M, Silva PD, Rosen GF, Stein AL, Fossum GT, Sauer MV. Management of unruptured ectopic gestation by linear salpingostomy: a prospective, randomized clinical trial of laparoscopy versus laparotomy. Obstet Gynecol. 1989;73:400-4.
115. Wang J, Yang Q, Yu Z. Clinical study of tubal pregnancy treated with integrated traditional Chinese and Western medicine. Zhongguo Zhong Xi Yi Jie He Za Zhi. 1998;18:531-3.
116. Wei FY, Chen HF. Clinical analysis of 82 cases of ectopic pregnancy treated by methotrexate combined with traditional Chinese recipe. Zhong Xi Yi Jie He Xue Bao. 2003;1:267-92.
117. Weinstein M, Morris MB, Dutters D. Ectopic pregnancy: a new surgical epidemic. Obstet Gynecol. 1983;61:698-701.
118. Yalcinkaya TM, Brown SE, Mertz HL, Thomas DW. A comparison of 25 mg/m^2 vs. 50 mg/m^2 dose of methotrexate (MTX) for the treatment of ectopic pregnancy (EP). J Soc Gynecol Invest. 2000;7:179A.
119. Zilber U, Pansky M, Bukovsky I, Golan A. Laparoscopic salpingostomy versus laparoscopic local methotrexate injection in the management of unruptured ectopic gestation. Am J Obstet Gynecol. 1996;175:600-2.

CHAPTER 41

Laparoscopic Urological Procedures

INTRODUCTION

Laparoscopic urological surgery can be divided into three areas:

1. Diagnostic
2. Extirpative
3. Reconstructive

Because much of urologic surgery is reconstructive and radiologic imaging techniques continue to refine the accuracy of urologic diagnoses, the role of laparoscopy in urologic practice has decreased in the past few years. However, there are specific areas of urologic surgery in which laparoscopic applications have expanded. Laparoscopy is used extensively in pediatric urology for the diagnosis and operative correction of undescended testicles as well as the laparoscopic removal of obstructed or poorly functioning kidneys. Another major surgery is laparoscopic adrenalectomy for both benign and malignant conditions of the adrenal gland.

LAPAROSCOPIC VARICOCELECTOMY

Laparoscopic varicocele ligation has been performed by many urologists and reports from several medical centers have been published. The data suggest that laparoscopic varicocele ligation is therapeutically superior to open surgical and radiographic (embolization) techniques. Laparoscopic varicocelectomy appears to reduce postoperative morbidity. Whether it is necessary to identify and preserve the testicular artery during laparoscopic varicocelectomy, it remains controversial. Loughlin and Brooks reported on the use of a laparoscopic Doppler probe that they believe facilitates the identification and preservation of the testicular artery. Matsuda et al. claim that the testicular artery does not have to be preserved; they clip the testicular artery and veins en bloc. Further, multicenter experience is needed to resolve whether the testicular artery should be preserved during laparoscopic varicocele ligation. Because the testicular artery is preserved during open surgical repair or radiographic embolization procedures, we generally preserve the testicular artery during varicocelectomy.

Operative Technique

The technique of laparoscopic varicocele ligation is straightforward. The procedure is usually performed using general anesthesia. A urethral catheter is placed to empty the bladder and a Veress needle is placed at the umbilicus to inflate the peritoneal cavity with carbon dioxide. Alternatively, Hasson technique can be performed at the inferior margin of the umbilicus and the trocar can be placed into the peritoneum under direct vision. Three laparoscopic ports are placed for varicocelectomy according to baseball diamond concept.

The intra-abdominal vas deferens can be identified as structure joining the spermatic cord above the internal inguinal ring **(Fig. 1)**. The gonadal vessels are visualized easily in the retroperitoneum. The posterior peritoneum is excised with cautery, laser, or endoscopic scissors. The gonadal vessels are then mobilized; however, reliably identifying the spermatic artery and its branches is sometimes difficult through the laparoscope **(Figs. 2A and B)**. Therefore, many surgeons prefer to use the laparoscopic Doppler probe to facilitate identification of the spermatic artery during laparoscopic varicocele ligation.

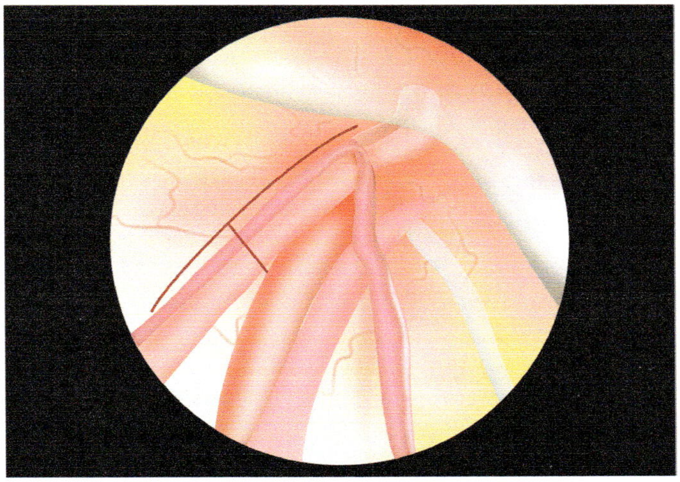

Fig. 1: Laparoscopic varicocelectomy.

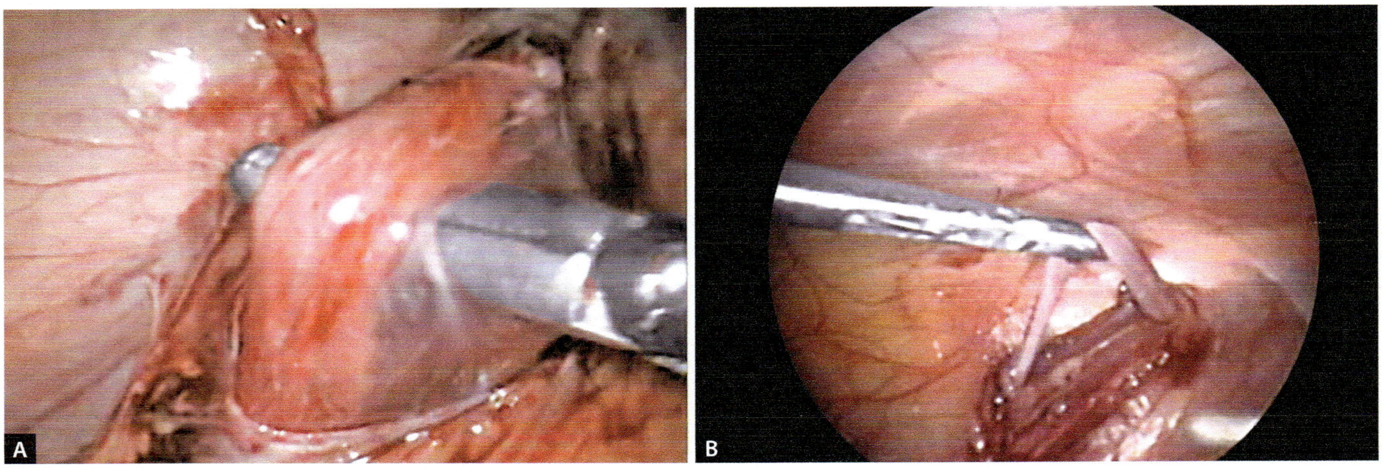

Figs. 2A and B: The spermatic vein is identified.

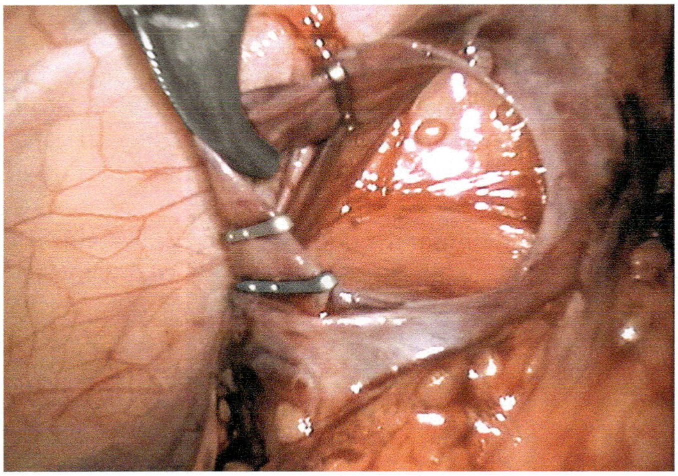

Fig. 3: Clips applied around spermatic vein.

The Doppler probe is 28.58 cm long and fits through a 5-mm laparoscopic port. After identifying the gonadal artery, the surgeon isolates the gonadal vein or veins using blunt dissection with atraumatic graspers.

Endoscopic clip applier is used to secure it or intracorporeal suturing is used to ligate the gonadal vein or veins while sparing the artery **(Fig. 3)**.

LAPAROSCOPIC RETROPERITONEAL NODE DISSECTION

The laparoscopic retroperitoneal node dissection in the management of testicular cancer is still not very frequently performed. Increased operating time is a consideration in applying laparoscopic techniques to a procedure. As with pelvic node dissection, the question has also been raised as to the completeness of the laparoscopic retroperitoneal node dissection. Laparoscopic dissection of the nodal tissue behind the aorta and vena cava is difficult laparoscopically.

Laparoscopic retroperitoneal node dissection appears, at least for now, best applied to patients without evidence of bulky disease in the retroperitoneum, who would otherwise be candidates for observation rather than surgical exploration. Although the laparoscopic procedure does not currently appear to be as through a dissection as the open node dissection, it offers the opportunity to have some pathologic documentation of nodal status in patients considered for observation. The technique for laparoscopic retroperitoneal node dissection has not been standardized and is still evolving; therefore, the reader is referred to the case reports for the author's individual techniques.

LAPAROSCOPIC MANAGEMENT OF LYMPHOCELES

Lymphoceles are not uncommon after renal transplantation; an incidence of 0.6–18% has been reported. It can also occur after pelvic lymphadenectomy and an incidence of 5.6% has been reported in these circumstances. Most of these patients are asymptomatic and do not require much aggressive treatment. When the lymphocele becomes symptomatic or is associated with fever and potential infection, however, drainage of the lymphocele is indicated. Several investigators have reported successful laparoscopic drainage of lymphoceles.

Operative Technique

The technique of lymphocele drainage is described as follows: After the induction of general endotracheal anesthesia, the surgeon places a urethral catheter to drain the bladder and a nasogastric tube is then inserted. A Veress needle is inserted into the peritoneal cavity in the left upper quadrant to avoid the transplant allograft. A pneumoperitoneum is achieved in the usual manner and 10 mm trocar sheath is inserted through the same site into the peritoneal cavity. The video endoscope is placed through this port and two additional 5 mm ports are inserted under direct vision in the periumbilical area in the right upper quadrant at the level of the midclavicular line.

The abdomen is carefully inspected and the renal transplant and associated lymphocele are visualized. They appear as two extrinsic bulges in the retroperitoneum. The lymphocele is distinguishable by its superolateral location to the graft and the soft consistency on probing. The lymphocele also transmits light readily when the light source is placed at its wall. The patient is placed in Trendelenburg position to allow the small bowel to fall cephalad and to facilitate the visibility of the lymphocele. The lymphocele is then entered using electrocautery. The peritoneum and its attached lymphocele wall are grasped and the incision is extended circumferentially using laparoscopic scissors. An ellipse of lymphocele wall is removed, thereby creating a window. After careful marsupialization of the edges of the window, the lymphocele is inspected and all internal loculations are lysed and excised to create a single cavity. At the end of surgery, the cavity is irrigated and inspected for adequate hemostasis prior to the usual completion of the laparoscopic procedure.

LAPAROSCOPIC URETEROLYSIS

Usually, the patient undergoes laparoscopic ureterolysis via a transperitoneal approach. An external ureteral stent should be placed to help identify the ureter as it is done with laparoscopic nephrectomy. The ureter is identified by a close-up vision of telescope and then successfully mobilized laparoscopically. Laparoscopic biopsy forceps should be used to obtain multiple biopsy specimens of the periureteral tissue. Laparoscopic ureterolysis is not a very frequently performed procedure. Additional experience will help determine how applicable laparoscopic ureterolysis will become in the future.

LAPAROSCOPIC ILEAL CONDUIT

In many centers, laparoscopic surgeons are performing laparoscopic ileal loop conduit. This procedure is commonly performed for palliation of obstruction in old man with fibrosarcoma of the prostate. The ileal loop itself is fashioned laparoscopically using endoscopic stapling devices. To perform the ureteral anastomosis, however, the distal ureters and a portion of the conduit have to be brought in through a trocar site and an extracorporeal and handsewn ureteroileal anastomosis is performed on each side.

The report emphasizes the limitations of laparoscopic instrumentation at this time. Laparoscopic suturing is cumbersome and the ureteroileal anastomosis could not have been completed easily laparoscopically. Until either tissue welding techniques or better suturing techniques are available, only limited applications are available for laparoscopic reconstructive surgery such as that outlined in this case report.

LAPAROSCOPIC PELVIC LYMPHADENECTOMY

Laparoscopic pelvic lymphadenectomy has the potential to aid in the staging of prostate cancer. Most urologists embrace the philosophy that if the pelvic lymph nodes are involved in prostate cancer, cure cannot be achieved with radical prostatectomy or radiation therapy and hormonal therapy is indicated in these patients for palliation.

Vascular injuries are most common complication during dissection. Adherence to good laparoscopic technique and familiarity with the anatomy are the most reliable ways to avoid complications.

Operative Technique

The pneumoperitoneum is established in the standard manner. Trocar placement is then performed. The size and location of trocar sites for the procedure vary with the surgeon's preference. Most use the diamond configuration. An alternative used by some surgeons is the so-called fan configuration for trocar placement. This configuration allows the surgeon and the surgical assistant to manipulate instruments with both hands during the dissection. It is also helpful in obese patients or in those with a prominent urachus. The size of the trocars used at each site may vary. A 10-mm port is usually placed in the umbilicus for the laparoscope. An additional 10 mm port is placed in at least one other site for tissue removal. Another 10 mm port is used for the endoscopic clip applier. Usually, 5 mm ports are used for the remaining trocar sites. After completion of trocar placement, the laparoscopic landmarks for pelvic node dissection are identified. These landmarks include the medial umbilical ligament (remnant of the obliterated umbilical artery), urachus, bladder, vas deferens, iliac vessels, spermatic vessels, and internal ring. The next maneuver is to incise the posterior peritoneum parallel and lateral to the medial umbilical ligament. Early identification of the ureter is important to avoid ureteral injury. The vas deferens is then divided to facilitate operative access to the obturator space. Using primarily blunt dissection, the iliac vein and artery are identified. The nodal tissue overlying the external iliac vein is then teased medially to expose the internal obturator muscle. A laparoscopic vein retractor can be used to retract the external iliac vein laterally and permit easier, more complete dissection of the nodal tissue beneath the vein. The dissection proceeds with removing tissue off the vein distally until Cooper's ligament and the pubic bone are identified.

Electrosurgery is used to fulgurate small vessels and lymphatics and the distal extent of the packet is freed from the pubic bone. The packet is pulled proximally and freed from the underside of the pubic bone. At this point, the obturator nerve is identified. Because nodal tissue can be quite bulky and difficult to grasp, adequate forceps can ensure a more reliable grasp of the specimen. With blunt dissection, the obturator nerve is cleaned off proximally and endoscopic clips are used to divide the distal portion of the dissection. At the completion of the laparoscopic pelvic lymphadenectomy, the iliac artery, vein, pubic bone, and obturator nerve can be seen clearly. The field is checked for hemostasis and the dissection is performed in an identical manner on the opposite side. The trocars are removed and the puncture sites are closed in the usual manner.

LAPAROSCOPIC NEPHRECTOMY

Anterior Relation of Kidney (Fig. 4)

Right Kidney

- Inferior surface of liver (1)
- Second part of duodenum (2)
- Hepatic flexor of colon (3)

Left Kidney

- Inferior surface of spleen (5)
- Tail of pancreas (4)
- Splenic flexor of colon (6)

Posterior Relation of Kidney (Fig. 5)

- Psoas muscle (1)
- Quadratus lumborum muscle (2)

Several obstacles are preventing laparoscopic nephrectomy technique from being more widely embraced. The first is the time factor which is considerably longer than for an open nephrectomy. The second is the handling of the renal pedicle. Clayman et al. have used titanium clips to secure the renal artery and vein. Ehrlich et al. used an endoscopic linear stapler to secure the pedicle. Despite the fact that Clayman et al. group did not report any significant intraoperative or postoperative bleeding because of inadequate pedicle control, many urologists are uneasy with this aspect of the operation. The third and perhaps most serious concern is the applicability of this technique to cases of renal malignancy. Currently, the adrenal gland is not included in the laparoscopic radical nephrectomy; although this exclusion is probably more a theoretical concern in lower pole and midpole tumors, it would be a limiting factor in upper pole tumors.

Tumor spillage during any laparoscopic procedure is an obvious practical concern. Several reports documented tumor implantation during laparoscopy. Clayman et al. tried to solve this problem by developing an entrapment system for the kidney and the lymph nodes. These systems consist of impermeable bags inserted through the laparoscopic trocar. The surgical specimen is placed within the bag or pouch and a drawstring around the opening of the bag allows for closure and acts as a handle to remove the pouch from the abdominal cavity through the laparoscopic trocar. In nephrectomy, the renal specimen is fragmented and aspirated using an especially designed electrical tissue morcellator placed through the neck of the kidney sac. The development of this type of technology decreases, but does not eliminate the potential for tumor spillage. Undoubtedly, more work is needed to address the concern of tumor implantation, if this technique is to be applied to malignant renal tumors.

Operative Technique

The patient is kept nil by mouth for 8 hours. Initially, positioned the patient in supine for the anesthesia and placement of orogastric tube and 18 Fr Foley catheter. After this, patient is positioned in a modified lateral decubitus position with the umbilicus placed over the break in the operating table. Flexed the table as needed or put a balloon under the patient at the level of the umbilicus. Support the buttocks and the dorsum with padding and all the potential pressure points. The surgeon is positioned in the abdominal

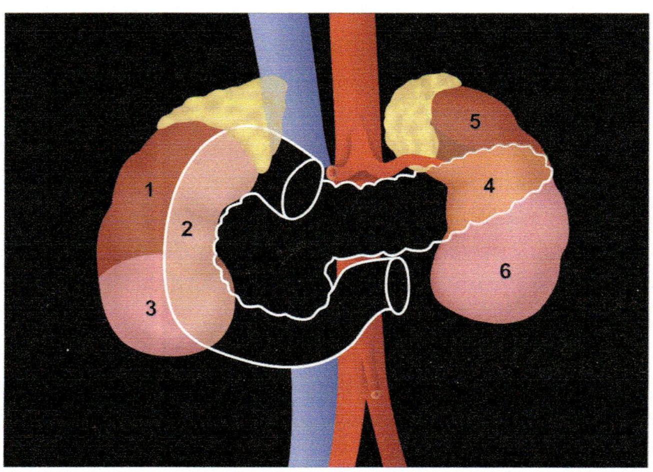

Fig. 4: Anterior relation of kidney.

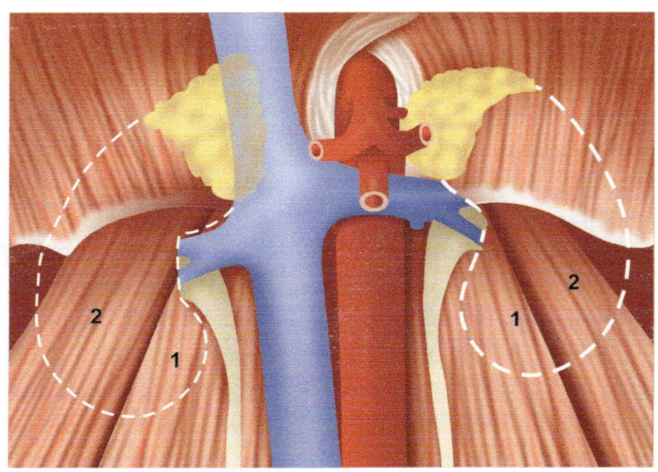

Fig. 5: Posterior relation of kidney.

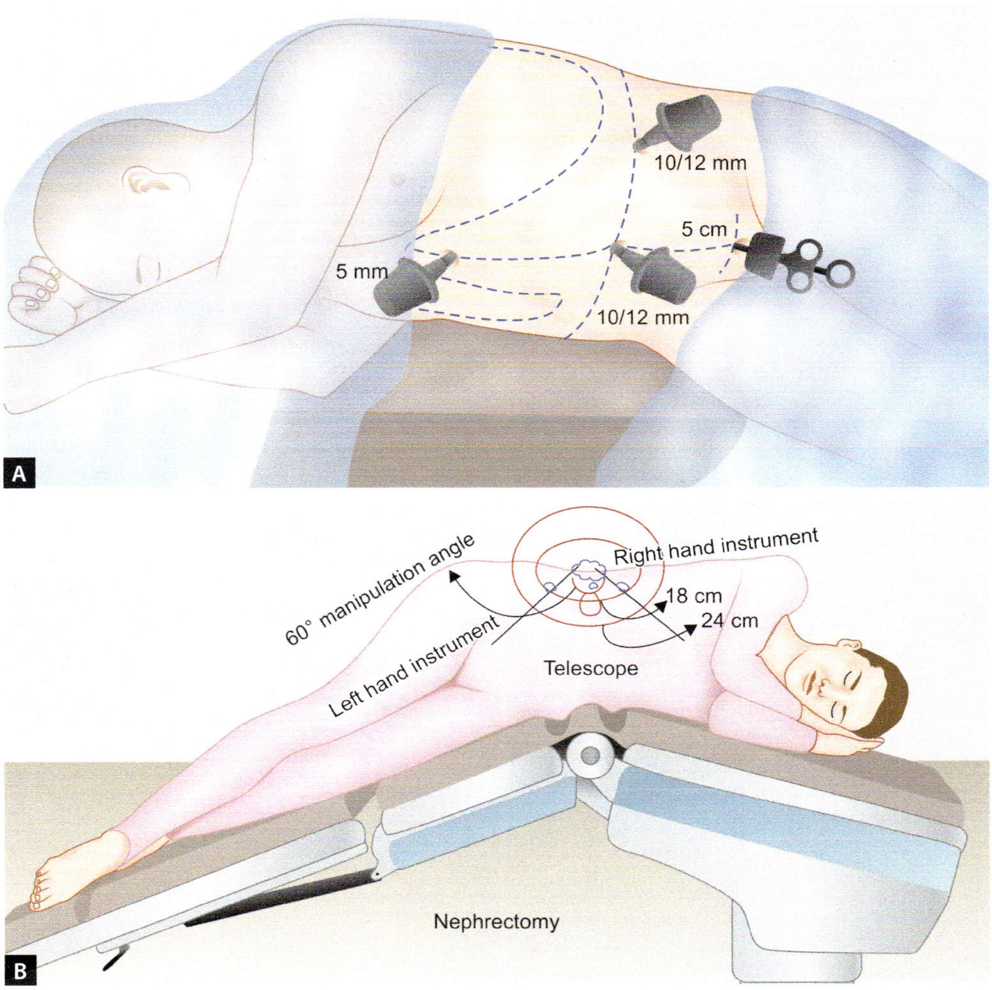

Figs. 6A and B: Port position in laparoscopic nephrectomy.

side of the patient and the first assistant is placed caudally to the surgeon. The laparoscopic cart is positioned at the back of the patient's chest with the operative team facing the video monitor. The instrument table is positioned behind the operative team. A cutaneous incision is made two fingerbreadths below the costal margin arch at the level of the lateral border of the rectus muscle. The Veress needle is introduced through the incision and after that surgeon should establish the pneumoperitoneum. After 10-mm paraumbilical port, camera port for the 30° telescope and another 10-mm right hand working port are introduced in the epigastrium pararectally **(Figs. 6A and B)**. A 5-mm left hand working port is introduced in the hypogastric region pararectally. One or two 5-mm ports are placed as per requirement for bowel and liver retraction.

Laparoscopic radical nephrectomy is done medial to lateral through a transperitoneal approach. The retraction of the liver is required to improve the visualization of the renal hilum and this is done by atraumatic grasper placed through an extra 5-mm trocar below the ribs in the anterior axillary line. The dissection of peritoneum over the right renal vein (RRV) in relation to inferior vena cava (IVC) is done by using the Harmonic Ace or any similar energy source such as thunderbeat in transperitoneal approach **(Fig. 7)**.

Kocherization is done anterior and leftward mobilization of the second part (C loop) of the duodenum after incision of the parietal peritoneum on its right aspect; the IVC and left renal vein (LRV) are encountered posteriorly **(Fig. 8)**.

The RRV is dissected circumferentially with the blunt dissection. The right renal artery which lies inferior and posterior to the RRV is dissected and stapled **(Figs. 9A and B)**.

The tributaries of the renal vein are clipped with titanium clips doubly and divided. The renal artery is divided first with Harmonic Ace and all fibrofatty tissues with lymph nodes around the renal hilum are dissected upward toward the specimen. The kidney is mobilized with Gerota's fascia from surrounding structures. The separation of the kidney from the lateral abdominal wall is done at last, so that the specimen does not fall on the operative field.

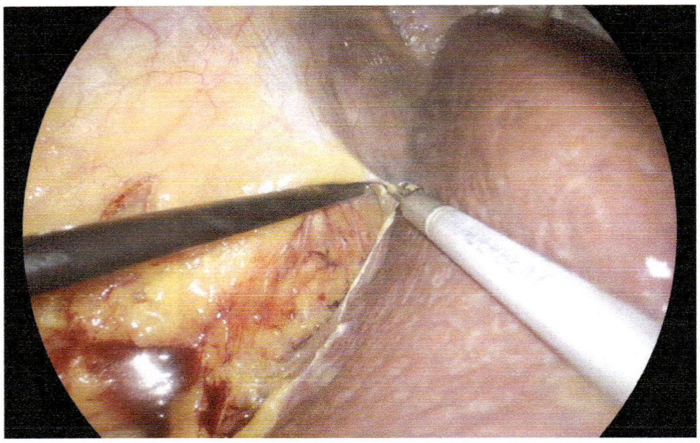

Fig. 7: Start of dissection in nephrectomy.

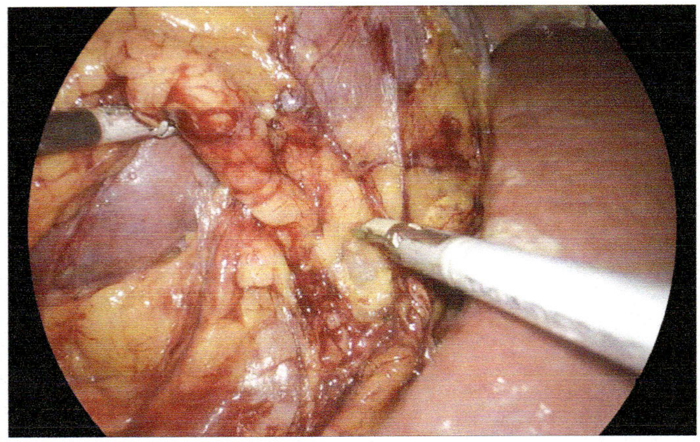

Fig. 8: Kocherization of duodenum and colon.

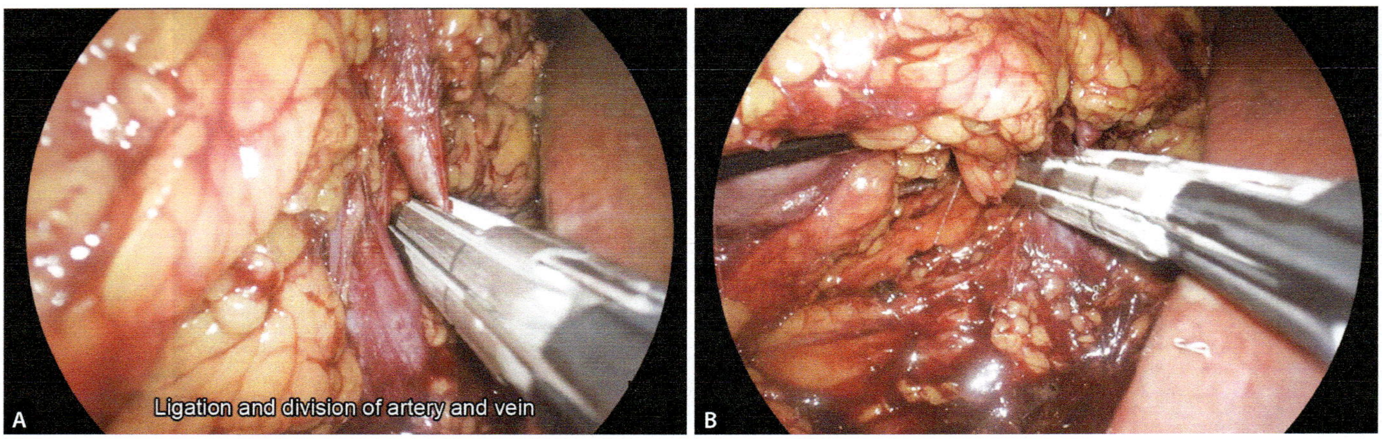

Figs. 9A and B: Stapling of renal artery and vein.

Dissection of the Ureter

The psoas tendon is a reliable landmark when searching for the gonadal vein and ureter. Once located, the ureter is elevated from the psoas muscle, clipped, and cut **(Figs. 10A to D)**. The gonadal vein may be visualized at an early stage during the dissection of Gerota's fascia, if the bowel is properly retracted medially. The hemostasis is checked with the irrigation of a normal saline solution and also by reducing CO_2 pressure to reduce the tamponade effect on bleeding veins. Number 32 French drain is kept at the renal hilum.

The specimen is kept in a large size Endobag to prevent port site metastasis and delivered through a small muscle-splitting incision in the right iliac fossa or through an incision between two trocars **(Fig. 11)**. All port sites are irrigated with betadine and closed with Vicryl.

Complications of Laparoscopic Nephrectomy

The complication rate of laparoscopic transperitoneal nephrectomy is 5.64%.

The most frequent complications are:
- Bleeding (2.5%)
- Retroperitoneal hematoma (1.2%)
- Bowel injury (1%)

There were no statistically significant differences in complications rate by age, sex, or surgical access: transperitoneal versus retroperitoneal. The complications rate was similar for both the laparoscopic and hand-assisted technique. Laparoscopic nephrectomy has established its role as a standard of care for the management in a patient who required nephrectomy. Long-term follow-up has demonstrated that laparoscopic nephrectomy has shorter patient hospitalization time and effective outcome.

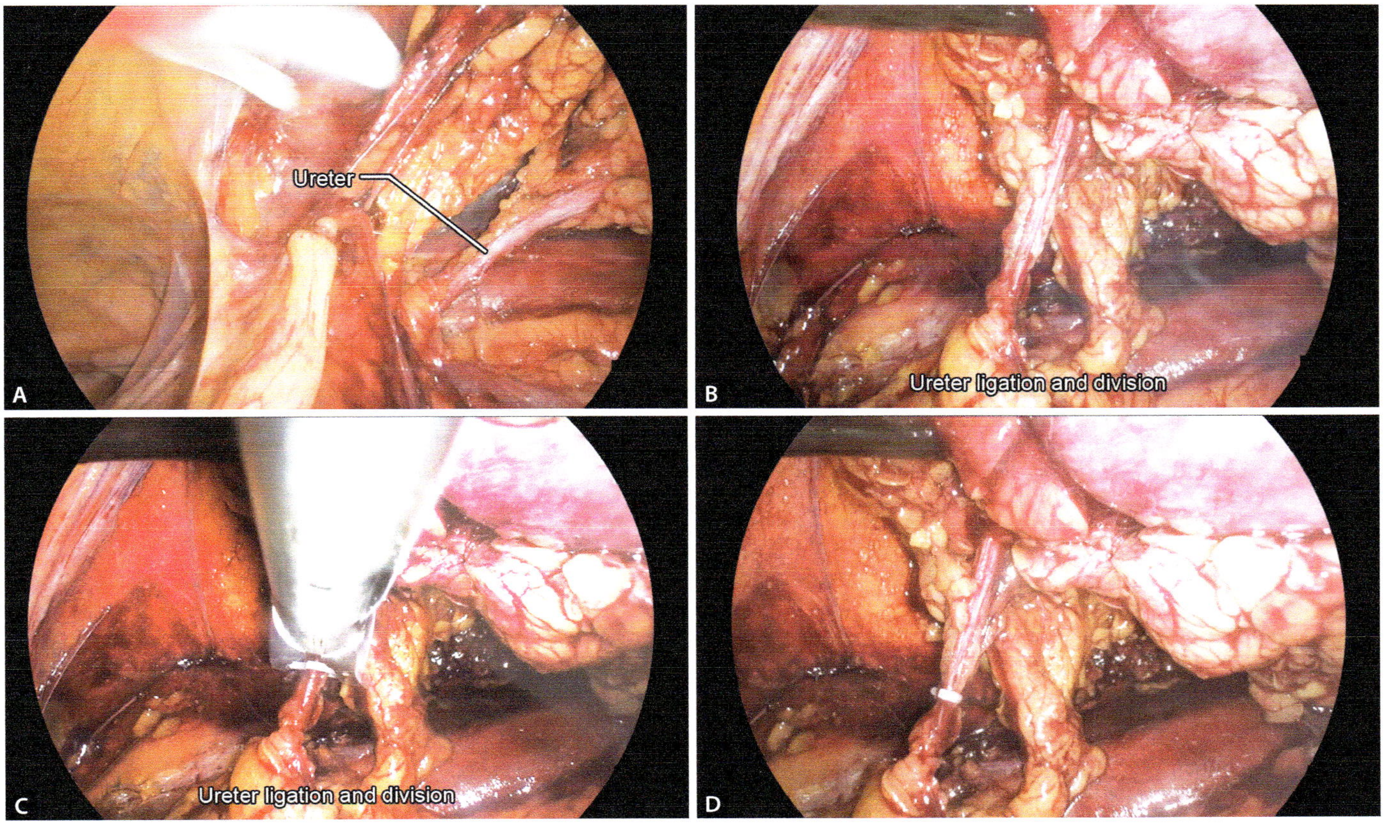

Figs. 10A to D: Clipping of ureter during nephrectomy.

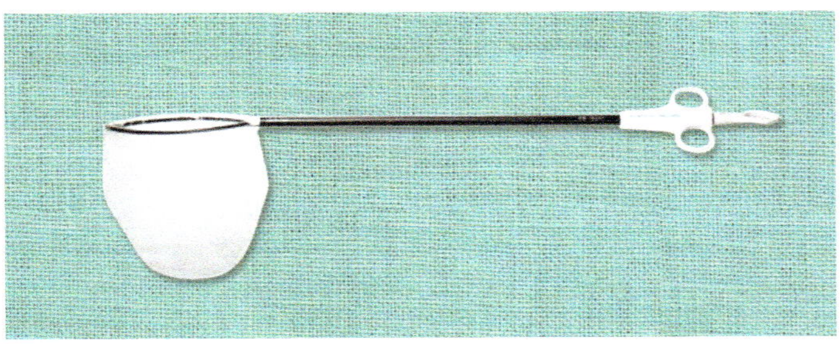

Fig. 11: Large size Endobag for kidney removal.

BIBLIOGRAPHY

1. Berends FJ, den Hoed PT, Bonjer HJ, Kazemier G, van Riemsdijk I, Weimar W, et al. Technical considerations and pitfalls in laparoscopic live donornephrectomy. Surg Endosc. 2002;16:893-8.
2. Buell JF, Lee L, Martin JE, Dake NA, Cavanaugh TM, Hanaway MJ, et al. Laparoscopic donor nephrectomy vs open live donor nephrectomy: a quality of life and functional study. Clin Transplant. 2005;19:102-9.
3. De Klerk M, Keizer KM, Claas FH, Witvliet M, Haase-Kromwijk BJ, Weimar W. The Dutch national living donor kidney exchange program. Am J Transplant. 2005;5:2302-5.
4. Dunker MS, Bemelman WA, Slors JF, van Duijvendijk P, Gouma DJ. Functional outcome, quality of life, body image, and cosmesis in patients after laparoscopic-assisted and conventional restorative proctocolectomy: a comparative study. Dis Colon Rectum. 2001;44:1800-7.
5. Govani MV, Kwon O, Batiuk TD, Milgrom ML, Filo RS. Creatinine reduction ratio and 24-hour creatinine excretion on posttransplant day two: simple and objective tools to define graft function. J Am Soc Nephrol. 2002;13:1645-9.
6. Guillonneau B, Jayet C, Tewari A, Vallancien G. Robot-assisted laparoscopic nephrectomy. J Urol. 2001;166:200-1.
7. Horgan S, Vanuno D, Sileri P, Cicalese L, Benedetti E. Robotic-assisted laparoscopic donor nephrectomy for kidney transplantation. Transplantation. 2002;73:1474-9.
8. Hoznek A, Hubert J, Antiphon P, Gettman M, Hemal AK, Abbou CC. Robotic renal surgery. Urol Clin North Am. 2004;31:731-6.
9. Hsu THS, Su L, Ratner LE, Kavoussi LE. Renovascular complications of laparoscopic donor nephrectomy. Urology. 2002;60:811-5.
10. Ingelfinger JR. Risks and benefits to the living donor. N Engl J Med. 2005;353:447-9.
11. Johansson M, Thune A, Nelvin L, Stiernstam M, Westman B, Lundell L. Randomized clinical trial of open versus laparoscopic cholecystectomy in the treatment of acute cholecystitis. Br J Surg. 2005;92:44-9.
12. Joshi GP. Anesthesia for minimally invasive surgery: laparoscopy, thoracoscopy, hysteroscopy. Anesthesiol Clin North Am. 2001; 19:89-105.
13. Kok NF, Alwayn IP, Lind MY, Tran KT, Weimar W, Ijzermans JN. Donor nephrectomy: mini-incision muscle-splitting open approach versus laparoscopy. Transplantation. 2006;81:881-7.

14. Kuang W, Ng CS, Matin S, Kaouk JH, El-Jack M, Gill I. Rhabdomyolysis after laparoscopic donor nephrectomy. Urology 2002;60:911.
15. Leventhal JR, Deeik RK, Joehl RJ, Rege RV, Herman CH, Fryer JP, et al. Laparoscopic live donor nephrectomy—is it safe? Transplantation. 2000;70:602-6.
16. Lewis GR, Brook NR, Waller JR, Bains JC, Veitch PS, Nicholson ML. A comparison of traditional open, minimal-incision donor nephrectomy and laparoscopic donor nephrectomy. Transpl Int. 2004;17:589-95.
17. Lind MY, Hazebroek EJ, Hop WC, Weimar W, Bonjer HJ, IJzermans JN. Right-sided laparoscopic live-donor nephrectomy: is reluctance still justified? Transplantation. 2002;74:1045-8.
18. Lind MY, Liem YS, Bemelman WA, Dooper PM, Hop WC, Weimar W, et al. Live donor nephrectomy and return to work: does the operative technique matter? Surg Endosc. 2003;17:591-5.
19. London E, Rudich S, McVicar J, Wolfe B, Perez R. Equivalent renal allograft function with laparoscopic versus open live donor nephrectomies. Transplant Proc. 1999;31:258-60.
20. Majeed AW, Troy G, Nicholl JP, Smythe A, Reed MW, Stoddard CJ, et al. Randomised, prospective, single-blind comparison of laparoscopic versus small-incision cholecystectomy. Lancet. 1996;347:989-94.
21. Najarian JS, Chavers BM, McHugh LE, Matas AJ. 20 years or more of follow-up of living kidney donors. Lancet. 1992;340:807-10.
22. Nogueira JM, Cangro CB, Fink JC, Schweitzer E, Wiland A, Klassen DK, et al. A comparison of recipient renal outcomes with laparoscopic versus open live donor nephrectomy. Transplantation. 1999;67:722-8.
23. Novotny MJ. Advanced urologic laparoscopy. Laparoscopic live donor nephrectomy. Urol Clin North Am. 2001;28:127-35.
24. Oyen O, Andersen M, Mathisen L, Kvarstein G, Edwin B, Line PD, et al. Laparoscopic versus open living-donor nephrectomy: experiences from a prospective, randomized, single-center study focusing on donor safety. Transplantation. 2005;79:1236-40.
25. Perry KT, Freedland SJ, Hu JC, Phelan MW, Kristo B, Gritsch AH, et al. Quality of life, pain and return to normal activities following laparoscopic donor nephrectomy versus open mini-incision donor nephrectomy. J Urol. 2003;169:2018-21.
26. Philosophe B, Kuo PC, Schweitzer EJ, Farney AC, Lim JW, Johnson LB, et al. Laparoscopic versus open donor nephrectomy: comparing ureteral complications in the recipients and improving the laparoscopic technique. Transplantation. 1999;68:497-502.
27. Ratner LE, Ciseck LJ, Moore RG, Cigarroa FG, Kaufman HS, Kavoussi LR. Laparoscopic live donor nephrectomy. Transplantation. 1995;60:1047-9.
28. Ratner LE, Montgomery RA, Maley WR, Cohen C, Burdick J, Chavin KD, et al. Laparoscopic live donor nephrectomy: the recipient. Transplantation. 2000;69:2319-23.
29. Rodrigo E, Ruiz JC, Piñera C, Fernández-Fresnedo G, Escallada R, Palomar R, et al. Creatinine reduction ratio on post-transplant day two as criterion in defining delayed graft function. Am J Transplant. 2004;4:1163-9.
30. Simforoosh N, Basiri A, Tabibi A, Shakhssalim N, Moghaddam SMH. Comparison of laparoscopic and open donor nephrectomy: a randomized controlled trial. Br J Urolog Int. 2005;95:851-5.
31. Smets EM, Garssen B, Cull A, de Haes JC. Application of the multidimensional fatigue inventory (MFI-20) in cancer patients receiving radiotherapy. Br J Cancer. 1996;73:241-5.
32. Srivastava A, Tripathi DM, Zaman W, Kumar A. Subcostal versus transcostal mini donor nephrectomy: is rib resection responsible for pain related donor morbidity. J Urol. 2003;170:738-40.
33. Subramonian K, DeSylva S, Bishai P, Thompson P, Muir G. Acquiring surgical skills: a comparative study of open versus laparoscopic surgery. Eur Urol. 2004;45:346-51.
34. Sundqvist P, Feuk U, Häggman M, Persson AEG, Stridsberg M, Wadstro MJ. Hand-assisted retroperitoneoscopic live donor nephrectomy in comparison to open and laparoscopic procedures: a prospective study on donor morbidity and kidney function. Transplantation. 2004;78:147-53.
35. Sung GT, Gill IS. Robotic renal and adrenal surgery. Surg Clin North Am. 2003;83:1469-82.
36. Troppmann C, Ormond DB, Perez RV. Laparoscopic (vs open) live donor nephrectomy: a UNOS database analysis of early graft function and survival. Am J Transplant. 2003;3:1295-301.
37. Wadstrom J. Hand-assisted retroperitoneoscopic live donor nephrectomy: experience from the first 75 consecutive cases. Transplantation. 2005;80:1060-6.
38. Ware JE, Snow KK, Kosinski M, Gandek B. SF-36 Health Survey: Manual and Interpretation Guide. Boston: Health Institute, New England Medical Center; 1993.
39. Wolf JS, Merion RM, Leichtman AB, Campbell DA, Magee JC, Punch JD, et al. Randomized controlled trial of hand-assisted laparoscopic versus open surgical live donor nephrectomy. Transplantation. 2001;72:284-90.
40. Yang SL, Harkaway R, Badosa F, Ginsberg P, Greenstein MA. Minimal incision living donor nephrectomy: improvement in patient outcome. Urology. 2002;59:673-7.
41. Yilmaz S, Paavonen T, Havry P. Chronic rejection of rat allografts. II. The impact of prolonged ischaemia time on transplant histology. Transplantation. 1992;53:823-7.

SECTION

5 Pediatric Laparoscopy

CHAPTER 42

Laparoscopic Pediatric Surgery

"There are no great discoveries or advances as long as there are unhappy children in the world".

—Albert Einstein

LAPAROSCOPY IN INFANTS AND CHILDREN

When widespread use of laparoscopy and thoracoscopy in adult patients occurred in the first part of the 1990s, it did not transfer into widespread application in the pediatric population for a number of reasons. One of the strong reasons was the fact that pediatric surgeons did not have a commonly performed procedure, such as cholecystectomy, in which to refine their endoscopic skills. The most common intra-abdominal procedure performed in infants and children is appendectomy and fundoplication and it is difficult initially to learn these skills. In addition, the small intra-abdominal working space in infants and young children makes the operations more difficult and time-consuming. Children seem to recover more rapidly than adults because of the fact that there is no underlying heart or lung disease **(Fig. 1)**. In the early 1990s, it was unclear whether there would be further benefits to an already faster healing process and recovery time. The main advantage of laparoscopy is the fact that it enables a magnified view of the abdominal cavity and the treatment of more than one pathology, even if located in different parts of the abdominal cavity, without enlarging the abdominal incision as in case of open surgery and during the same anesthesia. Moreover, the laparoscopy permits identification and treatment of clinically silent pathologies or discovery of a rare associated pathology while performing surgery for a different indication.

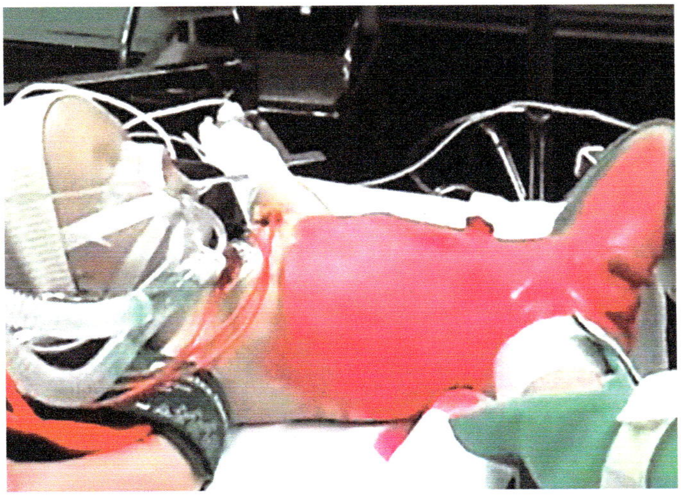

Fig. 1: All the vital parameter should be strictly monitored in pediatric age group.

Many of the leaders in pediatric surgery were not skilled in this new technology and, therefore, pediatric surgeons finishing their training program were not being trained in this laparoscopic approach. When information and documentation of the benefits of minimal access surgery have been published, this technology is used more today as compared to the mid-1990s. Intra-abdominal procedures such as fundoplication, splenectomy, appendectomy, and cholecystectomy are being commonly performed by pediatric surgeons. In addition, many pediatric surgeons use diagnostic laparoscopy through a known unilateral inguinal hernia sac to determine whether there is a contralateral patent processus vaginalis, which might indicate the need for contralateral repair under the same anesthesia. Laparoscopic primary pull-through procedures in the neonatal period for correction of Hirschsprung's disease are popular among many pediatric surgeons. The cutting edge of laparoscopy in pediatric surgery is procedures such as intestinal resection for Crohn's disease and colectomy with J-pouch reconstruction for ulcerative colitis. In the chest, many operations in children are applicable for the thoracoscopic route as thoracoscopic repair of esophageal atresia with tracheoesophageal fistula, but the thoracoscopic approach remains in its infancy with this congenital anomaly at this time.

A number of pediatric surgeons utilizes laparoscopic fundoplication following open gastrostomy in children. Regarding recurrence of gastroesophageal reflux following partial anterior fundoplication, many of these recurrences can simply be converted to a Nissen fundoplication with good results. Usually, there is much less inflammation and adhesion formation following the initial laparoscopic procedure than occurs following an open operation.

Laparoscopic Appendectomy in Children

Below the age of 1 year, the port for the telescope is inserted through the abdominal wall 1 cm to the left of the umbilicus. In small children, the umbilical ring is too loose to keep the trocar airtight. In older children, the umbilicus is chosen for the telescopic port. Before advancing the trocar, a skin incision is made slightly smaller than the trocar in order to secure gastight skin closure around the trocar shaft. Too small incision is risky because it results in too forceful trocar insertion. A Veress needle is inserted and carbon dioxide (CO_2) is insufflated up to an intra-abdominal pressure of 12 mm Hg. The smaller the child, the slow the insufflation flow rate should be. With practice, the pressure can be estimated by palpating the abdomen. Insufflation and pressure control are executed through valves at the trocars. A second and third trocar is inserted in the right lower hypochondria and left iliac fossa according to baseball diamond concept. Its site is chosen by pressing the abdominal wall from outside. In pediatric age, the surgeon should try to stay lateral to the umbilical ligaments. Trocars may get caught in a ligament and may, therefore, be difficult to advance. The right trocar is used for the grasper forceps and also to take in the appendix for later removal. In children up to 8–10 years, the appendix will usually fit a 7.5-mm trocar. If the child is over 10 years, a 10-mm port suffices. A 5-mm trocar in the left lower abdomen will provide access for the cautery, scissors, and a second forceps. Expiratory capnography is mandatory for the anesthesiologist in all children. They are prepared to ventilate with decreased residual functional capacities, decreased tidal volumes, and increased frequencies during laparoscopy.

Urinary catheters and nasogastric tubes or drainages were never used. The fascia was approximated with a single absorbable suture. The appendix stump was simply ligated with a Roeder's or Meltzer's knot just like adult patient. No purse string or Z suture is required. In the beginning, laparoscopy took considerably longer than an open approach (up to 90 minutes vs. 25 minutes). Practice decreased the time consumed, which is now nearly identical to that required for open procedures (25 minutes).

Other Causes of Pain in Abdomen in Pediatric Age Group

Hydatids can easily be exposed and removed laparoscopically. We have seen a few cases in pediatric group that mimicked acute appendicitis. The ovaries can be trapped within dense adhesions; sometimes, other additional signs of previous inflammatory processes are demonstrated as well. Such adhesions can be transected laparoscopically, although we are not sure it is worth the trouble. A Meckel's diverticulum can be identified and removed by laparoscopy. Congenital and acquired adhesions and ligaments are also found frequently in children. New aspects may be added to clinical symptoms. Laparoscopy can be used in children with incidentally discovered inguinal hernia.

Laparoscopic Cholecystectomy in Children

Laparoscopic cholecystectomy is the procedure of choice for the treatment of adults with gallbladder stone disease. However, cholelithiasis is rare in children; for this reason, it is difficult to evaluate the validity of this procedure in a large case series of pediatric patients. The presence of gallbladder stones is generally idiopathic in children and their discovery is sometimes incidental during a sonographic examination performed to search for other abdominal pathologies. However, there are well-known predisposing factors to the developing gallbladder stones in children. Among infants affected by hemolytic disease such as hemolytic anemia, for instance, the incidence of gallbladder stones is much higher than the normal population. Its reported incidence ranges from 10 to 40% in various series. The management of children with cholelithiasis requires great caution; an accurate hematological study is always necessary to detect a possible underlying hematological disease. In cases of gallstones discovered incidentally, an accurate follow-up is suggested, since a spontaneous resolution of the pathology is possible. Generally, noncalcified gallbladder stones in children disappear within 3–6 months. By contrast, surgery is needed for calcified stones in both nonsymptomatic and symptomatic children. Laparoscopic cholecystectomy rather than open cholecystectomy is the procedure of choice in symptomatic infants. Laparoscopy in infants should be performed using very small instruments (3 or 5 mm in diameter). Technically, this approach is similar to the one employed for adults, although careful consideration of a child's anatomical difference is essential to avoid complications. It is important to keep in mind that in pediatric patients, there may be biliary tree anomalies such as gallbladder duplication, ductal abnormalities, accessory bile duct, or accessory cystic artery. These findings do not represent a contraindication to the laparoscopic procedure, if the surgeon is able to perform a delicate and accurate dissection of the elements at the level of Calot's triangle. Bile duct injuries, which are often reported in adults, are very rare in children and may be due to more clear anatomy and less fat. The junction between the cystic duct and the common bile duct is much more visible in children due to the scarcity of fatty tissue and adhesions at the level of Calot's triangle at this age. This improved visualization makes the dissection of the cystic duct easier and less dangerous than in adult patients. The presence of common bile duct stones in children is an extremely rare event in the pediatric population. At any rate, the presence of jaundice, dilatation of the biliary tree at ultrasonography, alkaline phosphatase and total bilirubin above the normal range by >5 mg/dL, and/or a history of pancreatitis are indications for a cholangiography or an endoscopic retrograde cholangiopancreatography (ERCP). In addition, we believe that intraoperative cholangiograms can also be performed in infants.

With respect to the ERCP, the sequential approach of endoscopic sphincterotomy and stone extraction followed by laparoscopic cholecystectomy is a safe and effective method in children as well as in adults. One important advantage is that laparoscopic cholecystectomy in children can be associated, if necessary, with other technical procedures such as the closure of a peritoneal vaginal duct in cases of inguinal hernia; thus, a second operation or another incision can be avoided. However, if another procedure is required, laparoscopic expertise on the part of the surgeon is fundamental to avoid additional morbidity. We performed a concomitant splenectomy in infants affected by spherocytosis and one with thalassemia. Based on our experience, laparoscopic cholecystectomy is as valid and effective procedure in pediatric patients as it is in adults. In children, it is important to perform a complete preoperative evaluation to search for the possible coexistence of hematological disease.

Laparoscopic Splenectomy in Children

The preliminary results and the retrospective comparison help to establish the safety and efficacy of laparoscopic splenectomy in children. Although the peritoneal cavities of the children are limited, there are no special risks in the pediatric patients. As many splenectomies are now being performed for cytopenic/anemic disease in children, pediatric patients requiring splenectomy may benefit from this minimally access approach. Decreased postoperative pain and recovery time are anticipated in these patients, just as for thousands of patients undergoing laparoscopic splenectomy.

Absolute contraindications to laparoscopic splenectomy include contraindications to general anesthesia. Extensive inflammation and adhesions in the left upper quadrant may be a relative contraindication because of the increased possibility of hemorrhage. Significant splenomegaly may also be a relative contraindication caused by increased difficulty of dissection and the need for more complex extraction procedures. A large spleen compared to small abdomen is a problem in pediatric laparoscopic splenectomy. Especially in patients with HS, the spleen size is usually large.

Bleeding tendency is a contraindication to laparoscopic procedures. Many patients requiring splenectomy are coagulopathic from thrombocytopenia or qualitative platelet dysfunction. Preoperative use of intravenous immunoglobulin G (IgG) should be considered for the patients with idiopathic thrombocytopenic purpura (ITP). The response to IgG is generally as efficacious as the response to steroids with the added advantage of fewer associated side effects.

The surge on performing splenectomy must be cognizant of this fact and have a low threshold for conversion to an open procedure in the event of a hemorrhage that is not easily visualized or controlled through the operating ports. As laparoscopic splenectomy is an advanced technique, we recommend that anyone attempting the procedure be fully experienced in laparoscopic surgical techniques and instrumentation. Understanding the limitations of minimal access surgery, in addition to possessing the ability to convert to the open procedure to assure safe splenectomy and patient safety, is also important. Laparoscopic splenectomy may prove at least as safe as the open approach, if performed by experienced surgeons.

The disadvantage is increased operative time. However, this may diminish with experience and introduction of the Endo Catch II. With more experience and advances in technology, laparoscopic splenectomy may become easier and surgeon may be able to reduce their operative time and anesthetic risks. Several other aspects of the operative technique developed in pediatric patients deserve emphasis. Early mobilization of the spleen significantly increases the difficulty of exposing the hilum. The splenic artery and vein are individually clipped and divided and a linear stapler is not necessary in pediatric patients. As superior branches of the short gastric vessels are difficult to clip at the early phase of procedure, those branches should be left and divided at the end. Accessory spleen should be searched in patients with hematologic disease requiring splenectomy for hypersplenism. Although these may occur within the attaching ligaments of the spleen and in the mesentery and omentum, they most frequently occur in the hilum along the splenic vessels. Four accessory spleens were found in our series and they were successfully removed under laparoscopic guidance. The magnified view afforded during laparoscopy can allow for easier identification of accessory spleens, especially in the hilar region. The inability to identify accessory spleens by palpation is one limitation of laparoscopic surgery.

Thorough evaluation for accessory splenic tissue is essential intraoperatively. Traditional splenectomy, performed through a midline or subcostal incision, is associated with a number of complications, including hemorrhage, atelectasis, pneumonia, ileus, subdiaphragmatic abscess, and incisional hernias. These may prolong the hospital stay and convalescence.

Because the small incisions of laparoscopic surgery are less painful than upper abdominal incisions, patients use fewer narcotics, have fewer respiratory complications, and have improved return of pulmonary function. Patients treated laparoscopic splenectomy ambulated the same day and a decrease in postoperative hospital stay was seen compared to those who underwent open surgery. Most of the patients returned to unrestricted activities within 1 week after being discharged.

LAPAROSCOPIC REPAIR OF PEDIATRIC HERNIA

The first use of laparoscopy in cases of inguinal hernia in children was for diagnosis. Laparoscopic or transinguinal laparoscopic evaluation for a contralateral patent vaginalis process has been previously reported as a means of avoiding metachronous hernias. In these cases, the internal examination has been performed by laparoscopic technique, placing the optical trocar through the umbilicus. The main problem is to decide whether or not to treat the contralateral hernia sac immediately. Is the contralateral vaginalis process wide and deep enough to be responsible in the short term for a metachronous contralateral hernia?

During laparoscopy for inguinal hernia repair, surgeon often encounters an unexpected bilateral hernia. This situation underscores the importance of laparoscopy as a means of improving the diagnosis of bilateral hernias. Femoral hernias are often misdiagnosed and treated as inguinal hernias. Thus, laparoscopic groin exploration is valuable means of evaluating children with presumed recurrent inguinal hernias. Less than 1% of all groin masses seen in children are due to femoral hernias. Because these hernias are so uncommon, they are often overlooked, misdiagnosed, or even treated as inguinal hernias. In fact, the correct diagnosis of femoral hernia is often made at the time of groin re-exploration for a presumed recurrent inguinal hernia. The laparoscopic approach may offer better diagnostic ability than conventional open exploration because all potential hernial defects in both groins can be examined under direct laparoscopic vision. Furthermore, unilateral or simultaneous bilateral tension-free repair can be done using the laparoscopic technique. Laparoscopy is helpful to diagnose a femoral hernia. It enables an accurate identification of the nature of the groin defect. However, the technical details of laparoscopic femoral hernia repair are still under discussion, even in adult series. The role of laparoscopy in the management of suspected recurrent pediatric hernias has been described. For patients with a patent processus vaginalis, laparoscopy is efficient for diagnosis and treatment.

Which laparoscopic procedure is most efficient in pediatric surgery cases?

- Ligature alone of the hernia sac without dividing the peritoneum. It has a high recurrence rate; this may due to the use of absorbable sutures or to the continuity of the peritoneum, which is left intact. Furthermore, the risk of injury to the vas deferens or the vessels from the needle running under the peritoneum without previous dissection seems to be high.
- Performing the procedure without ligature of the hernia sac, while only dividing the peritoneum on the site of the inner inguinal ring, seems to be enough to avoid early complications and to achieve a low recurrence rate. But, it may lead to intraperitoneal adhesions.
- To avoid such adhesions, many surgeons operate the patent processus vaginalis just like open surgery. The vaginalis process is divided by separating the sac, which remains in the scrotal pouch or in the labia majora and the peritoneum at the internal inguinal ring. This procedure does not require opening of the inguinal canal. Dissection of the vas deferens and spermatic vessels is done at the level of the internal inguinal ring, where these elements are more easy to spare from the peritoneum, whereas more adhesions may be encountered in the inguinal canal. The peritoneum is ligated. At the end of the procedure, one should pay close attention to the testis position, so as to avoid a secondary occurrence at an ectopic site. Pain and discomfort resolve very quickly.

Laparoscopic herniorrhaphy in children is gaining increasing acceptance in pediatric surgery. The essential step in the conventional method for inguinal hernia repair in children is the simple ligation of the hernial sac without narrowing the open ring **(Figs. 2A to C)**. The internal inguinal ring is reached by opening the inguinal canal and dissecting

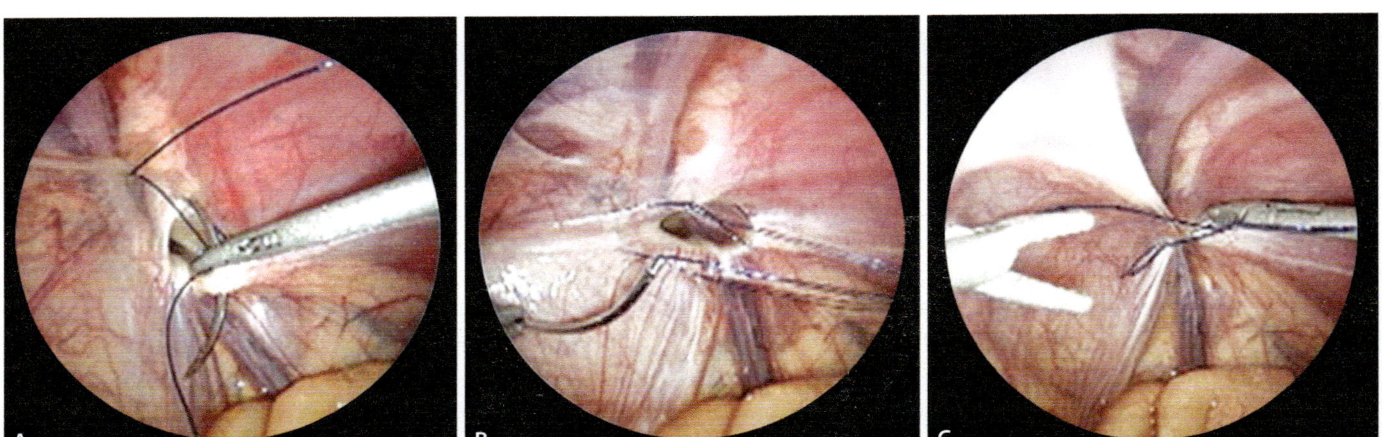

Figs. 2A to C: Purse-string suture for pediatric inguinal hernia repair.

the hernial sac from the cord structures. Postoperatively, the major damage from which the patient has to recover is not the ligature of the hernial sac, but the trauma of access itself. Therefore, the clinical goal is to leave the abdominal wall as intact as possible. Laparoscopy is most appropriate for this purpose to gain access to the abdominal cavity in order to close the inner inguinal ring from within.

The laparoscopic repair of pediatric hernia requires 2 mm instruments; the use of larger instruments would lead to an increase in the size of the incision that would make it equivalent to a conventional groin incision **(Fig. 3)**. Bilateral inguinal hernias, as well as indirect and direct hernias, are of no concern in laparoscopic herniorrhaphy. There is no difference between the access and treatment for unilateral and bilateral laparoscopic hernia repair and the laparoscopic repair of a direct hernia. Needle for intracorporeal suturing is introduced through abdominal wall in case of pediatric patient **(Figs. 4A and B)**.

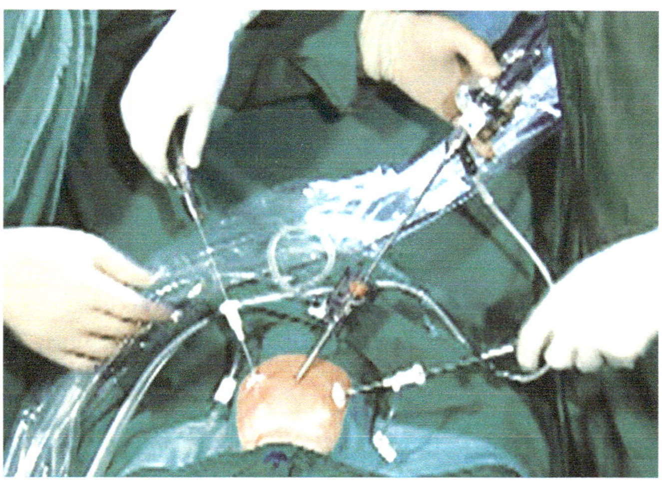

Fig. 3: Port position for pediatric appendicectomy.

Because it remains unclear whether a small open processus vaginalis develops subsequently into a hernia, we choose to close open inner inguinal rings down to a 2-mm width whether they are unilateral or bilateral. In many of patients, the contralateral side was found to be open as well; by closing these openings, it is assumed to exclude the possibility that hernias would occur.

The recurrence rate of inguinal hernias in children is slightly higher with laparoscopic herniorrhaphy than with the conventional technique. In patients with recurrences after laparoscopic herniorrhaphy, the surgeon has an undisturbed anatomy for groin incision; the risk of an injury to the vas deferens, subsequent testicular atrophy, and the risk of superior displacement of the testicle seem less likely. In cases of hernia recurrence after conventional hernia repair, laparoscopy allows us to clearly differentiate an indirect hernia from a direct one. Direct inguinal hernias in children are not that rare. The cosmetic results are excellent. Once the technique of intracorporeal suturing in a limited space is mastered, laparoscopic herniorrhaphy is safe, reproducible, and technically easy for experienced laparoscopists. If there is any uncertainty about the contralateral side, whether it is a direct or an indirect hernia, and in cases of inguinal hernia recurrence, the laparoscopic procedure is highly preferable as a primary technique that combines diagnosis and the potential for immediate treatment.

Laparoscopic Pediatric Fundoplication

Gastroesophageal fundoplication currently is one of the three most common major operations performed on infants and children by pediatric surgeons. With the advent of laparoscopic surgery, the number of gastroesophageal fundoplications has virtually exploded. Morbidity always was substantial with this operation and laparoscopy has not changed this.

In recent years, laparoscopic Nissen fundoplication has been performed with increasing frequency in pediatric

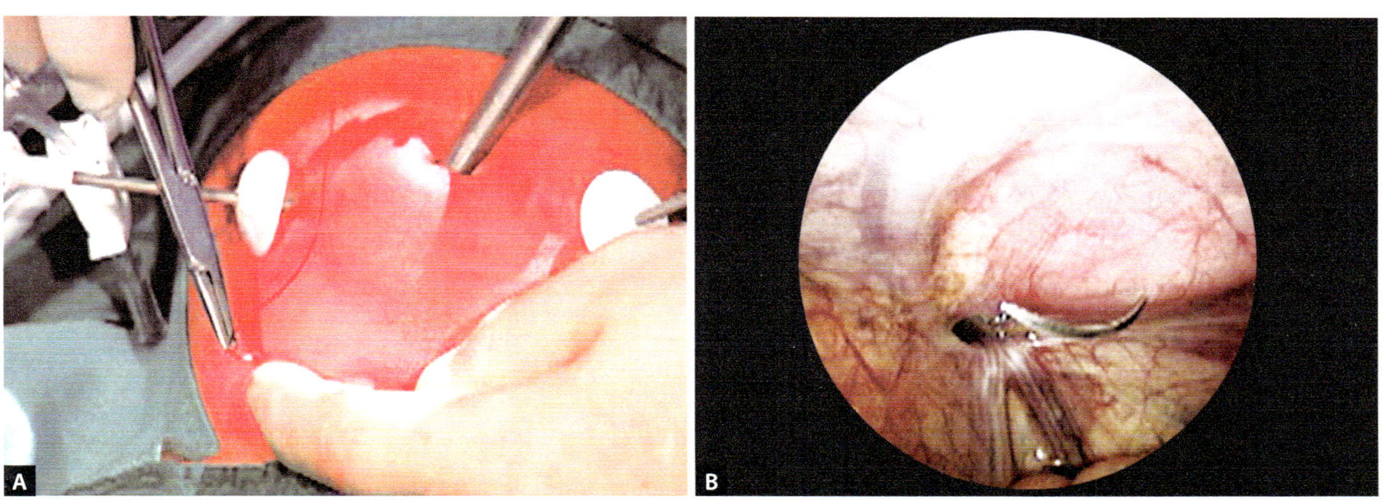

Figs. 4A and B: Needle should be introduced percutaneous in pediatric age group.

patients with symptomatic gastroesophageal reflux disease (GER) because it causes minimal trauma to the abdominal wall and supposedly eases patient recovery. Initial experience demonstrates that Nissen fundoplication can be accomplished successfully and safely using the laparoscopic approach in very small babies suffering from severe GER. Infants and children who are candidates for antireflux procedure differ in many aspects from the adult population. In adults, GER is typically associated with hiatal hernia and is usually unrelated to any other abnormality. In children, on the other hand, there is usually no hiatal hernia, but clinically significant GER is often associated with neurological impairment, metabolic abnormality, or some other severe underlying disease. Therefore, even after successful surgical resolution of GER, these babies often remain very sick due to their primary disease.

Many children undergoing antireflux operation are at increased risk because of chronic parenchymal lung damage due to recurrent episodes of pneumonia and because they are often severely malnourished. Operative risk is especially high in children with familial dysautonomia. Concomitant impairment of gastrointestinal motility is also unique to the pediatric population. In particular, impairment of the swallowing mechanism and delayed gastric emptying should be taken into account by the surgeon. Hence, when the swallowing mechanism is impaired, gastrostomy should be constructed for postoperative feeding or fluid administration to prevent persistent aspirations. Likewise, the surgeon should consider pyloroplasty when there is preoperative evidence of delayed gastric emptying. In this case, it is usually preferable to do an open procedure, although a pyloroplasty can be accomplished through a small laparotomy incision at the end of the laparoscopic procedure. There are several technical concerns in laparoscopic Nissen fundoplication that are unique to infants and small children. Because the operating space is very small, it is necessary to use especially designed short instruments and to handle them with great care. To prevent dislocation, the trocars need to be secured to the skin by stitches.

The pneumoperitoneum should be maintained at pressure as low as 10 mm Hg. Elevation of pressure may cause difficulty in ventilation, with resultant hypercarbia. It is sometimes necessary even in pediatric age group to increase the pneumoperitoneum pressure temporarily, for example, during suturing, and to immediately deflate the abdomen, if expiratory CO_2 increases or any difficulty in ventilation is encountered. At the same time, the minimal fat around the esophagus in these small babies and the absence of hiatus hernia make the definition of the dissection planes clearer. Thus, the dissection itself, including mobilization of the esophagus, identification of the vagus nerves, and construction of the fundic wrap, are easier in small children than in adults. Furthermore, it is usually unnecessary to divide the short gastric vessels to achieve a tension-free wrap. Small children who need an antireflux operation often suffer from chronic lung disease, which makes them especially susceptible to postoperative lung complications. The laparoscopic approach seems to minimize these complications. The minimal trauma to the upper abdominal wall in this approach results in less impairment of respiration and, thus, minimizes the need for narcotics and sedatives postoperatively in pediatric patients. Recent reports suggested that recovery was smoother following laparoscopic antireflux operations than after open procedures, with comparable short-term results. Laparoscopic Nissen fundoplication is feasible and safe in very small children and infants and that it appears to offer some advantages over the standard open technique.

LAPAROSCOPIC PEDIATRIC UROLOGY

The major advances in laparoscopic urologic surgery began with pediatric applications. Laparoscopy has raised great interest in the past few years in the field of pediatric urology. It has evolved from a simple diagnostic maneuver to complex operative procedures. With respect to current indication for laparoscopy in pediatric urology, several well-established clinical procedures such as treatment of varicocele and nonpalpable testis, the current data suggest that laparoscopic surgery is a safe and feasible technique in pediatric urology, if performed by expert surgeons, and that it certainly will develop further in the next few years.

The first laparoscopic urologic applications were in the localization of an impalpable undescended testicle. This technique became the definitive diagnostic and first operative step in management of this condition. Laparoscopy offered a 97% chance of finding a testicle or proving its absence. Recent advances in endoscopic and accessory instrumentation have allowed the urologist to expand the role of laparoscopy in the pediatric population. In some respects, children may be better suited for laparoscopic procedures than adults because of their decreased intra-abdominal and retroperitoneal fat.

The main problem in pediatric laparoscopic urology is the choice of the most suitable way to reach the urinary tract. Until a few years ago, the transperitoneal route was the only route to the kidney and the urinary tract. In general, surgeons prefer the transperitoneal approach at the beginning of their experience in pediatric laparoscopic urology because of the well-known and wide peritoneal chamber. Usually, four to five ports are necessary and, after the colic angle is detached and Toldt's fascia is opened, the kidney and upper urinary tract are easily identifiable. The lower urinary tract, the testis, and the spermatic vessels also can be treated using this approach. Retroperitoneoscopy, also called lumboscopy, follows all the criteria of open renal surgery, respecting the integrity of the peritoneal cavity.

Currently, laparoscopy has been used in pediatric urology for:

- Localization and evaluation of impalpable undescended testicles
- Gonadal examination and biopsy in patients with intersex disorders
- Orchiectomy for undescended testicles
- Diagnosis and treatment of pediatric inguinal hernias
- Staged orchiopexy
- Spermatic vein ligation in patients with a varicocele
- Retarded testicular growth
- Nephrectomy
- Nephroureterectomy
- Pyeloplasty.

There are several important factors to consider when operating in the pediatric patient. First, there is a relatively short distance between the anterior abdominal wall and the great vessels. Thus, the margin for error in pediatric laparoscopy is inversely proportional to the age and size of the patient. Trocars and needles must not be passed too deeply to avoid vascular injury. Also, the child has a thinner abdominal fascia requiring less pressure to introduce the Veress needle and trocars into the abdomen. In addition to this, the pelvic anatomy differs in infants and young children. A large portion of the bladder is located outside the bony pelvis. Prompt decompression of the bladder with a catheter before a Veress needle is essential to avoid a bladder perforation. Also, much less CO_2 gas is required in the child, as the peritoneal cavity is small compared to that of an adult.

Children's dimensions are well suited to laparoscopy. Landmarks are readily identifiable and palpable. For example, the bifurcation of the great vessel as well as the sacral promontory is usually easily felt. In addition, abdominal or pelvic masses are easily detected in most children.

LAPAROSCOPY FOR THE IMPALPABLE UNDESCENDED TESTICLE OR INTERSEX EVALUATION

Cryptorchidism is the most common disorder of male sexual differentiation, affecting 0.8% of infants at 1 year of age, 3% of full-term newborns, and 21% of premature babies. Approximately, 20% of undescended testicles are nonpalpable, either in the scrotum or in the inguinal area, and in 20–50% of children with nonpalpable testis, the testis is absent. Early investigation and treatment of nonpalpable testis are essential to decrease the incidence of infertility and to allow adequate follow-up for possible testicular malignancies.

Diagnostic laparoscopy is indicated for patients with nonpalpable testis or an intersex problem. After a thorough physical examination has been accomplished, laparoscopy may be used and has a direct impact on any subsequent surgical procedure. For example, if the testis is absent and blind-ending vessels are seen, an open exploration can be avoided. If, however, a testicle is present, the precise location with laparoscopy determines the optimal incision for any open procedure. If an orchiopexy is considered, the first part of a Fowler–Stephens procedure may be performed laparoscopically. This results in minimal manipulation of the testicle. Furthermore, if the testicle is dysplastic, it may be removed laparoscopically.

A testicle that cannot be located and palpated on careful physical examination of the inguinal or scrotal areas is defined as *nonpalpable*. In such a case, intra-abdominal location, true agenesis, the "vanishing testis", hypoplasia, and ascent of a canalicular testicle on examination are all possibilities that have to be investigated.

Abdominal inspection starts with assessment of the insertion site to evaluate the safety of using a 5-mm port and continues with evaluation of the spermatic vessels and vas deferens on the normal side. Only the affected side is assessed and the spermatic vessels and vas deferens are followed to the internal inguinal ring. When both the spermatic vessels and the vas deferens meet and enter the internal inguinal ring, the intervention is concluded. If a small intra-abdominal testis is observed, two additional trocars are inserted in the two sides of the lower abdomen and laparoscopic orchiectomy is performed after clipping of the spermatic vessels and the vas deferens. When an apparently normal testis is observed inside the abdomen, the spermatic vessels are clipped as high as possible from the testicle, in order to avoid inadvertent production of ischemia. In this way, the first stage of the Fowler–Stephens procedure is accomplished. In the second stage, performed 6 months later, the laparoscope is inserted as in the first stage. When an atrophic testis is found, laparoscopic orchiectomy is performed, as described before. When a normal-sized intra-abdominal testicle is observed, laparoscopic-guided orchiopexy follows, without difficulty. In this way, fruitless inguinal explorations are avoided.

Laparoscopy has gradually become the gold standard for the diagnosis and proper treatment of the nonpalpable testis in children. At diagnosis, laparoscopy allows precise location of an undescended testicle and is the only diagnostic modality capable of establishing the definitive diagnosis of testicular absence. Laparoscopy precisely defines the intra-abdominal anatomy with an accuracy rate of 99%.

Complications following laparoscopy for diagnosis and treatment of intra-abdominal testicles are infrequent. Preperitoneal insufflation is undoubtedly the most common and may be as high as 5%. More serious complications, including intestinal or vascular injuries as well as injuries to the urinary bladder and ureter, have been reported but are rare. They may be reduced or avoided by the "open" introduction of a Hasson blunt trocar, thus avoiding blind puncture with a Veress needle.

Operative Technique

After placement of the Veress needle into the abdominal cavity, insufflation is begun. During insufflation, the intra-abdominal pressure should rise slowly at a rate of 0.5 L/min in pediatric patient and the abdomen of the child should become diffusely tympanic. Most children require CO_2 volumes between 0.5 and 2.0 L. Following proper insufflation, the Veress needle is removed and trocars are placed. When placing trocars, it is important not to advance these too deeply in the abdomen in order to avoid injury to the underlying bowel and vascular structures. After placement of the umbilical 10 mm trocar, the laparoscope is introduced into the abdominal cavity. Actual pressure of 10 mm Hg suffices for diagnostic procedures. For more complex procedures, pressure of 12–15 mm Hg is desirable and allows for better maintenance of an adequate pneumoperitoneum.

The abdomen is inspected in the midline between the obliterated umbilical arteries in the urachus. On the pelvic sidewall, the spermatic vessels may be seen coursing toward the internal inguinal ring. If a testicle is palpable in the scrotum, the vas deferens on that side is usually quite obvious as it travels through the inguinal ring to the retrovesical recess. In most children, the external iliac vessels are easily seen as there is minimal extraperitoneal pelvic fat. The cord structures may be further identified by placing slight traction on the spermatic cord and pulling down on the descended testicle. This will cause a dimpling of the peritoneum and the spermatic vessels are easily seen near the internal ring. In direct hernias and patent processus vaginalis, it may also be noted.

After inspecting the side of the normal testicle, attention is focused on the side with the undescended, impalpable gonad. If a patent processus vaginalis is noted, gonads or remnants may be present distally. However, absence of a patent processus vaginalis does not eliminate the possibility of a gonadal remnant in the inguinal area. If the cord structures are seen extending through the inguinal ring with a patent processus vaginalis, the testicle may not be visible initially. Gentle pressure on the external canal will push a canalicular testicle back through the internal ring. Although canalicular testes may be managed with a standard, open inguinal orchidopexy, the benefit of laparoscopy in these cases is to assess cord length and testicular mobility. This will have a direct impact on the planned surgical approach.

During diagnostic laparoscopy, an atraumatic grasper may be placed under direct vision to allow manipulation of bowel loops. In most cases, only two ports are needed. If the testicular absence is suspected, the inspection is accomplished by direct observation of blind-ending spermatic vessels. Often, the vas deferens may end blindly at the same site or nearby, but it is the determination of the spermatic vessels that is pathognomonic for a nonexistent gonad. In those patients with a blind-ending vas deferens, it is important that inspection can be carried as high up along the sidewall toward the lower pole of the kidney as possible. If blind-ending vessels are not seen, close observation of this area is necessary. Laparoscopic inspection of the lower pole of the kidney suffices to rule out rare, high-placed gonads. Inspection of the abdominal cavity is not necessary in these patients whose spermatic vessels are blind ending, in order to declare testicular absence.

In patients with an intersex condition, biopsy should be taken from dysplastic gonad or it may be removed. A biopsy may be accomplished with a biopsy needle passed directly into the abdomen under laparoscopic control. If an orchiectomy is to be performed, the dysplastic gonad is isolated. The spermatic vessels are identified and clipped. The vessels are then cut and the stump inspected to insure adequate hemostasis. If a testicle is seen, it may be brought down into the scrotum with a Fowler–Stephens procedure. When performing a Fowler–Stephens procedure, the technique is similar to removing a testicle. Once the testicle is clearly identified, the dissection is limited to the cephalad surface of the testicle to identify the spermatic artery.

This dissection will not disturb the vessels of the vas deferens, which will form the major blood supply of the testicle. Initially, the spermatic artery is identified and a window is created around the vessel. A clip applier is placed through a 10-mm trocar site that has access to the spermatic artery. Two clips are placed proximal and two clips are placed distally on the artery. The artery is then cut with scissors. In some circumstances, electrocautery may be used to coagulate the spermatic artery before the vessel is cut. This maneuver is the first step of a Fowler–Stephens procedure and can be accomplished with minimal amount of interabdominal dissection. During next stage of surgery, the testicle is brought down into the scrotum on its enhanced blood supply. This two-stage procedure has been successful not only in patients with long vasal loops but also in patients with high abdominal testis and short vas deferens.

In some patients, an impalpable testicle may be proximal to the internal ring in such a way that its vessels allow adequate mobilization. In these instances, a single-stage orchidopexy may be performed. This is done laparoscopically using three ports. Two 5 mm ports are placed in a lateral position and one 10 mm trocar is placed in the midline. A peritoneal incision lateral to the spermatic cord is made. The spermatic cord is rolled medially and elevated from the retroperitoneal tissues. The gubernaculum is opened adjacent to the patent processus vaginalis. The anterior peritoneum of the gubernaculum is then opened laterally. If a loop of the vas deferens is identified, it is reflected in the cephalad direction. The testicle is grasped and the gubernacular attachments are cauterized and divided. The vas deferens is then mobilized by opening the peritoneum medially. With adequate dissection, the testicle will be able to be moved around the pelvis.

A small transverse skin incision is created at the base of the hemiscrotum and carried down through dartos fascia. A subcutaneous pouch is created and the testicle is pulled down into the pouch. A small clamp is passed through the canal that has been developed into the peritoneal cavity. The gubernacular reflections of the lower pole of the testis can then be grasped and the testicle brought down the hemiscrotum without tension. The testicle is secured in the dartos pouch and the skin incision is closed. The Foley catheter and nasogastric tube may be removed in the operating room. Patients are usually given oral antibiotics for 24 hours and discharged from the hospital on the same day. Diets are advanced as tolerated.

Laparoscopy now constitutes the reference technique for the diagnosis and treatment of the nonpalpable testis. It is a simple procedure, allowing a definitive diagnosis and two-stage relocation without increasing the risk of testicular atrophy. Diagnostic laparoscopy also identifies the specific location of the intra-abdominal testicle, facilitating the development of an optimal surgical strategy. The good results reported in most series have established the laparoscopic management of the nonpalpable testis as "state-of-the-art," with results superior to those achieved with open surgical techniques regarding morbidity, complication rate, and length of hospital stay.

OTHER LAPAROSCOPIC PEDIATRIC UROLOGICAL PROCEDURES

Many other pediatric conditions may be treated using the laparoscopy. If nephrectomy in the pediatric patient is planned, a retroperitoneal approach may have a distinct advantage in certain older children. Laparoscopic pyeloplasty for ureteropelvic junction obstruction has also been performed with very encouraging result. Bladder autoaugmentation, another innovative procedure, is performed by incising the detrusor muscle to increase the capacity of the bladder. Other laparoscopic pediatric procedures such as hernia repairs and partial nephrectomy also have been performed. In pediatric laparoscopy, the greatest risk of complications occurs at the time of access. Some surgeons have eliminated this risk by using the Hasson trocar technique rather than the Veress needle technique. In children, the peritoneal space is small and the surgeon should be familiar with working in a smaller environment. The safety of pediatric laparoscopy is well established and more and more pediatric surgeons are nowadays switching over to laparoscopy.

Laparoscopic Pediatric Nephrectomy

It is, perhaps, the most popular urologic indication for the laparoscopic procedure. The first cases reported in the international literature were managed using the transperitoneal approach, but the subsequent reports of nephrectomy in children were based on retroperitoneoscopy. In children, the indications denote exclusively benign diseases such as multicystic or dysplastic kidneys causing renal hypertension, nonfunctioning kidneys associated with reflux nephropathy or obstructive uropathy, xanthogranulomatous pyelonephritis, protein-losing nephropathy, and occasionally, nephrolithiasis or nephropathy causing uncontrollable hypertension. The relative contraindications are malignant renal tumors, previous intra-abdominal or retroperitoneal surgery, renal trauma attributable to poor endoscopic vision into the perinephric hematoma, severe cardiopulmonary disease or severe coagulopathy, and morbid obesity with a high- positioned kidney attributable to difficult renal access retroperitoneally.

In cases of vesicoureteral reflux associated with a grossly refluxing megaureter, the ureter must be sectioned near the ureterovesical junction at the level of the bladder whereas in the absence of a grossly refluxing megaureter, the ureter can be divided either by electrocautery or between ligatures or clips at a convenient distance from the renal tissue. The extraction of the kidney can be achieved by using Endobag.

Stone Removal

Retroperitoneoscopic stone removal is another procedure that presents several advantages for children. The indications are large stones entrapped at the level of the pelvis unresponsive to medical treatment. Three ports are generally necessary, one for the telescope, two for the working instruments, and sometimes a fourth trocar for a retractor to lift the renal parenchyma. The first step of the operation is to place an uretheral probe first via cystoscopy and then lumboscopy. The pelvis then is opened with scissors, after which the stone extracted and removed with an Endobag.

Renal Biopsy

Renal biopsy can be performed with only one trocar, using a 10-mm operative telescope with an operative channel to introduce the biopsy instrument; if necessary, another 5 mm port can be introduced.

Adrenalectomy

Resection of the adrenal glands can be performed laparoscopically or via retroperitoneoscopy. It has various advantages over conventional open surgery. With regard to tumor size, in cases of adrenal masses <5–6 cm, laparoscopy or lumboscopy provides an excellent access route. If the mass is >6 cm, the open approach is preferable. Although the specific indications will continue to be defined, they generally include adrenal benign cysts, pheochromocytoma, adenoma, and aldosteronoma. In the case of neuroblastoma or other malignant tumors affecting children, it is preferable to adopt an open approach. A good knowledge of the adrenal pathophysiology and surgical anatomy is fundamental to the success of this procedure. Moreover, it is important to keep in mind the potential bleeding risk during dissection, especially on the right side, where the dissection may be more difficult because of the short adrenal vein and proximity of the vena cava.

Dismembered Pyeloplasty

Open pyeloplasty has been widely accepted as the surgical treatment of choice for pyeloureteral junction obstruction in children. The success rate for this procedure exceeds 90%. With the rapid advent of minimally access surgical techniques, laparoscopic dismembered pyeloplasty through a transperitoneal route has been described for both adults and children. Although the procedure is technically demanding and requires advanced laparoscopic surgical suturing techniques for meticulous pelviureteric anastomosis, encouraging results projecting success rates comparable with those achieved through an open approach have been reported. The first laparoscopic dismembered pyeloplasty used to treat ureteropelvic junction obstruction was described in 1992. Since then, other reports have been published describing the use of either laparoscopy or lumboscopy.

The first step of the procedure is to identify the pyeloureteral junction and the planned line of pelvic reduction. A 4/0 polydioxanone suture over a straight needle then is passed percutaneously through the abdominal wall to the upper pole of the renal pelvis and then passed back through the abdominal wall again at the same point. This serves as a "hitch stitch" to stabilize and present in the pelvis. The pyeloureteral junction is dismembered, the pelvis is trimmed, and the upper ureter is spatulated. Pelviureteric anastomosis then is performed using continuous 6/0 polydioxanone sutures for infants and younger children and 5/0 polydioxanone sutures for older patients. A double pigtail transanastomotic ureteric stent usually is left in situ for a few weeks postoperatively. Certainly, well-performed laparoscopy and intracorporeal suturing and knotting are necessary in the performance of this procedure. Currently, videosurgical pyeloplasty is performed only in few centers with extensive experience in pediatric laparoscopic urology.

Bladder Autoaugmentation

Bladder autoaugmentation by seromyotomy via laparoscopic technique has been used in selected cases to treat poor bladder capacity. This technique is easy to perform using laparoscopy, but in pediatric urology, an enterocystoplasty or a gastrocystoplasty generally is preferred for the treatment of patients with decreased bladder capacity.

Ureteral Reimplantation

The bladder is first drained and then insufflated with CO_2 to 10–12 mm Hg pressure. The bladder is anchored to the anterior abdominal wall with one or two separated stitches inserted percutaneously under cystoscopic guidance. Under cystoscopic vision, a camera port is first inserted over the dome of the bladder. Two other working ports with an umbrella mechanism then are inserted on either side of the bladder's lateral wall over the suprapubic skin crease. The refluxing ureter is isolated and dissected free as with the Cohen procedure. The ureteric hiatus is repaired with interrupted 5/0 polydioxanone sutures. After the creation of a submucosal channel, an ureteroneocystostomy is performed according to the Cohen procedure using separated 6/0 stitches. A urethral catheter is left *in situ* only for 24 hours postoperatively.

Excision of Prostatic Utricles

The prostatic utricles, an enlarged diverticulum in the posterior urethra of males, were first described by Englisch in 1874.

Although most prostatic utricles are asymptomatic and do not need any surgical intervention. Some patient manifest symptoms as a result of infection or enlarged utricles and have been associated with recurrent urinary tract infections, stone formation, disturbed urination, recurrent epididymitis, infertility, and neoplastic degeneration. Surgical excision is the recognized treatment of choice. Surgical access to the prostatic utricle always has been a major hurdle because it lies deep within the pelvis. The first step in the operation consists of a cystourethroscopy for cannulation of the prostatic utricle. The cystoscope is left in situ inside the prostatic utricle to facilitate subsequent identification during laparoscopy.

The bladder dome is hitched upward to the anterior abdominal wall by a 4/0 polydioxanone suture inserted percutaneously under laparoscopic vision. The peritoneal reflection is incised using electrocautery, starting immediately behind the bladder. The prostatic utricle is easily identified with the guidance of illumination from the cystoscope. Using a 5-mm ultrasonic scalpel, the prostatic utricle is completely mobilized and divided at its confluence with the urethra. The urethral defect is either closed by intracorporeal suturing using fine vicryl or simply by coagulation. The excised prostatic utricle is removed through the supraumbilical camera port.

Complicated Urachal Disease

The urachus is an obliterated fibrous cord extending from the allantoic duct remnant at the umbilicus to the apex of the bladder. Traditional surgical management of benign urachal disease involves the radical excision of all anomalous tissue with a cuff of bladder tissue via the open approach. Some authors advocate the use of such aggressive surgery only for persistent and recurrent cases. However, there is the potential for malignant change and a high risk of recurrent symptoms in conservatively managed cases. The laparoscopic approach to the complete excision of urachal abnormalities is performed via a three-port approach. The cyst is identified and removed with a cuff of bladder dome. The bladder defect is closed in two layers and the indwelling urinary catheter is removed after 2 days.

Laparoscopic procedures have evolved greatly in pediatric urology during the past few years. With time and greater experience, surgeons began to prefer retroperitoneoscopy for cases of urologic pathology, despite the major difficulties associated with the smaller operating chamber. Moreover, lumboscopy meets all the criteria of open renal surgery, according to which all urologic interventions are performed via the retroperitoneal route without transgressing the abdominal cavity. One main problem with retroperitoneal approach is that access to the bladder base or the ureterovesical junction may be difficult in older children. In addition, the retroperitoneal approach does not allow a thorough search of the peritoneal cavity for a small dysplastic and ectopic kidney, nor does it accommodate a complex ureterocele excision or bladder base reconstruction. To overcome these problems, a selective approach to the diseased kidney and ureter depending on the involved pathology is necessary. The position of the diseased kidney, the presence or absence of a refluxing ureter, and the need for ureterocelectomy and bladder base reconstruction are the main determining factors. Nephrectomy for nonfunctioning reflux nephropathy kidneys or duplex moiety necessitating resection of a grossly dilated megaureter, especially in children older than 5 years preferably is undertaken via a lateral extraperitoneal approach. Finally, nephrectomy for small dysplastic kidneys associated with ureteric ectopia and urinary incontinence as well as complex duplex excision with extensive ureterocelectomy and lower urinary tract reconstruction should be performed via a transperitoneal laparoscopic approach. The possible urologic indications for laparoscopic surgery can be divided into diagnostic, ablative, and reconstructive procedures. For cases of nonpalpable testis, laparoscopy is considered a better diagnostic examination and operative procedure for an orchidopexy. With regard to operative laparoscopic urologic procedures, most well-established clinical indications concern ablative procedures. To date, laparoscopic nephrectomy seems to be the procedure most frequently applied in pediatric urology.

The rapid advent of robotic technology will greatly enhance the dexterity and precision control of surgical manipulation in a small confined space of pediatric patient. It may significantly shorten the learning curve for advanced laparoscopic procedures.

BIBLIOGRAPHY

1. A prospective analysis of 1518 laparoscopic cholecystectomies. The Southern Surgeons Club. N Engl J Med. 1991;324:1073-8.
2. Allen SR, Lawson L, Garcia V, Inge TH. Attitudes of bariatric surgeons concerning adolescent bariatric surgery (ABS). Obes Surg. 2005;15:1192-5.
3. Ancona E, Anselmino M, Zaninotto G, Costantini M, Rossi M, Bonavina L, et al. Esophageal achalasia: laparoscopic versus conventional open Heller-Dor operation. Am J Surg. 1995; 170:265-70.
4. Antonoff MB, Kreykes NS, Saltzman DA, Acton RD. American Academy of Pediatrics Section on Surgery hernia survey revisited. J Pediatr Surg. 2005;40:1009-14.
5. Apelgren KN, Molnar RG, Kisala JM. Laparoscopic is no better than open appendectomy. Am Surg.1995;61:240-3.
6. Baker LA, Docimo SG, Surer I, Peters C, Cisek L, Diamond A, et al. A multi-institutional analysis of laparoscopic orchidopexy. BJU Int. 2001;87:484-9.
7. Barkun JS, Wexler MJ, Hinchey EJ, Thibeault D, Meakins JL. Laparoscopic versus open inguinal herniorrhaphy: preliminary results of a randomized controlled trial. Surgery. 1995;118:703-10.
8. Cass DL. Ovarian torsion. Semin Pediatr Surg. 2005;14:86-92.
9. Chan KL, Hui WC, Tak PK. Prospective randomized single-center, single-blind comparison of laparoscopic vs open repair of pediatric inguinal hernia. Surg Endosc. 2005;19:927-32.
10. Chen LE, Langer JC, Dillon PA, Foglia RP, Huddleston CB. Management of late-stage parapneumonic empyema. J Pediatr Surg. 2002;37:371-4.
11. Coran AG, Teitlebaum DH. Recent advances in the management of Hirschsprung's disease. Am J Surg. 2000;180:382-7.
12. Diamond IR, Langer JC. Laparoscopic-assisted versus open ileocolic resection for adolescent Crohn disease. J Pediatr Gastroenterol Nutr. 2001;33:543-7.
13. Diaz DM, Gibbons TE, Heiss K, Wulkan ML, Ricketts RR, Gold BD. Antireflux surgery outcomes in pediatric gastroesophageal reflux disease. Am J Gastroenterol. 2005;100:1844-52.
14. Dubois F, Icard P, Berthelot G, Levard H. Coelioscopic cholecystectomy—preliminary report of 36 cases. Ann Surg. 1990;211:60-2.
15. Eshraghi N, Farahmand M, Soot SJ, Rand-Luby L, Deveny CW, Sheppard BC. Comparison of outcomes of open versus laparoscopic Nissen fundoplication performed in a single practice. Am J Surg.1998;175:371-4.
16. Esposito C, Corcione F, Garipoli V, Ascione G. Pediatric laparoscopic splenectomy: are there real advantages in comparison with the traditional open approach? Pediatr Surg Int. 1997;12:509-10.
17. Gans SL, Berci G. Advances in endoscopy of infants and children. J Pediatr Surg. 1971;6:199-233.
18. Gans SL, Berci G. Peritoneoscopy in infants and children. J Pediatr Surg. 1973;8:399-405.
19. Georgeson KE, Inge TH, Albanese CT. Laparoscopically-assisted anorectal pull-through for high imperforate anus: a new technique. J Pediatr Surg. 2000;35:927-30.
20. Georgeson KE. Laparoscopic-assisted total colectomy with pouch reconstruction. Semin Pediatr Surg. 2002;11:233-6.
21. Gibeily GJ, Ross MN, Manning DB, Wherry DC, Kao TC. Late-presenting appendicitis. Surg Endosc. 2003;17:725-9.
22. Gilchrist BF, Lobe TE, Schropp KP, Kay GA, Hixson SD, Wrenn EL, et al. Is there a role for laparoscopic appendectomy in pediatric surgery? J Pediatr Surg. 1992;27:209-12.
23. Goldstein AM, Cho NL, Mazziotti MV, Zitsman JL. Pneumatically-assisted laparoscopic reduction of intussusception. Pediatr Endosurg Innov Tech. 2003;7:33-7.

24. Golub R, Siddiqui F, Pohl D. Laparoscopic versus open appendectomy: a meta-analysis. J Am Coll Surg. 1998;186:545-53.
25. Gorsler CM, Schier F. Laparoscopic herniorrhaphy in children. Surg Endosc. 2003;17:571-3.
26. Grewal H, Sweat J, Vazquez WD. Laparoscopic appendectomy in children can be done as a fast-track or same-day surgery. JSLS. 2004;8:151-4.
27. Hall NJ, Van Der Zee J, Tan HL, Pierro A. Meta-analysis of laparoscopic versus open pyloromyotomy. Ann Surg. 2004;240:774-8.
28. Horgan S, Holterman MJ, Jacobsen GR, Browne AF, Berger RA, Moser F, et al. Laparoscopic adjustable gastric banding for the treatment of adolescent morbid obesity in the United States: a safe alternative to gastric bypass. J Pediatr Surg. 2005;40:86-90.
29. Ikeda H, Ishimaru Y, Takayasu H, Okamura K, Kisaki Y, Fujino J. Laparoscopic versus open appendectomy in children with uncomplicated and complicated appendicitis. J Pediatr Surg. 2004;39:1680-5.
30. Inge TH, Krebs NF, Garcia VF, Skelton JA, Guice KS, Strauss RS, et al. Bariatric surgery for severely overweight adolescents: concerns and recommendations. Pediatrics. 2004;114:217-23.
31. Iwanaka T, Arai M, Yamamoto H, Fukuzawa M, Kubota A, Kouchi K, et al. No incidence of port-site recurrence after endosurgical procedure for pediatric malignancies. Pediatr Surg Int. 2003;19:200-3.
32. Johnson AB, Peetz ME. Laparoscopic appendectomy is an acceptable alternative for the treatment of perforated appendicitis. Surg Endosc. 1998;12:940-3.
33. Kadamba P, Habib Z, Rossi L. Experience with laparoscopic adrenalectomy in children. J Pediatr Surg. 2004;39:764-7.
34. Kato Y, Yamataka A, Miyano G, Tei E, Koga H, Lane GJ, et al. Tissue adhesives for repairing inguinal hernia: a preliminary study. J Laparoendosc Adv Surg Tech A. 2005;15:424-8.
35. Kenyon TA, Lenker MP, Bax TW, Swanstrom LL. Cost and benefit of the trained laparoscopic team: a comparative study of a designated nursing team vs a nontrained team. Surg Endosc. 1997;11:812-4.
36. Kia KF, Mony VK, Drongowski RA, Golladay ES, Geiger JD, Hirschl RB, et al. Laparoscopic vs open surgical approach for intussusception requiring operative intervention. J Pediatr Surg. 2005;40:281-4.
37. Kim SS, Lau ST, Lee SL, Waldhausen JH. The learning curve associated with laparoscopic pyloromyotomy. J Laparoendosc Adv Surg Tech A. 2005;15:474-7.
38. Koyle MA, Oottamasathien S, Barqawi A, Rajimwale A, Furness PD. Laparoscopic palomovaricocele ligation in children and adolescents: results of 103 cases. J Urol. 2004;172:1749-52.
39. Laerman LA, Grimes DA. Rapid hospital discharge following laparoscopy for ectopic pregnancy: a promise unfulfilled? West J Med. 1997;167:145-8.
40. Lawrence K, McWhinnie D, Goodwin A, Doll H, Gordon A, Gray A, et al. Randomised controlled trial of laparoscopic versus open repair of inguinal hernia: early results. BMJ. 1995;311:981-5.
41. Lejus C, Delile L, Plattner V, Baron M, Guillou S, Héloury Y, et al. Randomized, single-blinded trial of laparoscopic versus open appendectomy in children: effects on postoperative analgesia. Anesthesiology. 1996;84:801-6.
42. Martin LC, Puente I, Sosa JL, Bassin A, Breslaw R, McKenney MG, et al. Open versus laparoscopic appendectomy. A prospective randomized comparison. Ann Surg. 1995;222:256-62.
43. Meehan JJ, Georgeson KE. The learning curve associated with laparoscopic antireflux surgery in infants and children. J Pediatr Surg. 1997;32:426-9.
44. Memon MA, Fitzgibbons RJ. Assessing risks, costs and benefits of laparoscopic hernia repair. Ann Rev Med. 1998;49:95-109.
45. Muehlstedt SG, Pham TQ, Schmeling DJ. The management of pediatric appendicitis: a survey of North American pediatric surgeons. J Pediatr Surg. 2004;39:875-9.
46. Ortega AE, Hunter JG, Peters JH, Swanstrom LL, Schirmer B. A prospective, randomized comparison of laparoscopic appendectomy with open appendectomy. Am J Surg. 1995;169:208-13.
47. Parikh MS, Shen R, Weiner M, Siegel N, Ren CJ. Laparoscopic bariatric surgery in super-obese patients (BMI_50) is safe and effective: a review of 332 patients. Obes Surg. 2005;15:858-63.
48. Ransom SB, McNeely SG, White C, Diamond MP. A cost-effectiveness evaluation of laparoscopic disposable versus nondisposable infraumbilical cannulas. J Am Assoc Gynecol Laparosc. 1996;4:25-8.
49. Reddy VS, PhanHH, O'Neill JA, Neblett WW, Pietsch JB, Morgan WM, et al. Laparoscopic versus open splenectomy in the pediatric population: a contemporary single-center experience. Am Surg. 2001;67:859-63.
50. Richards KF, Fisher KS, Flores JH, Christensen BJ. Laparoscopic Nissen fundoplication: cost, morbidity and outcome compared with open surgery. Surg Laparosc Endosc. 1996;6:140-3.
51. Rothenberg SS. Laparoscopic intestinal resection. Semin Pediatr Surg. 2002;11:211-6.
52. Rothenberg SS. The first decade's experience with laparoscopic Nissen fundoplication in infants and children. J Pediatr Surg. 2005;40:142-6.
53. Sandoval C, Strom K, Stringel G. Laparoscopy in the management of pediatric intra-abdominal tumors. JSLS. 2004;8:115-8.
54. Somme S, Rodriguez JA, Kirsch DG, Liu DC. Laparoscopic versus open fundoplication in infants. Surg Endosc. 2002;16:54-6.
55. Spurbeck WW, Davidoff AM, Lobe TE, Rao BN, Schropp KP, Shochat SJ. Minimally invasive surgery in pediatric cancer patients. Ann Surg Oncol. 2004;11:340-3.
56. Spurbeck WW, Prasad R, Lobe TE. Two-year experience with minimally invasive herniorrhaphy in children. Surg Endosc. 2005;19:551-3.
57. Templeman C, Fallat ME, Blinchevsky A, Hertweck SP. Noninflammatory ovarian masses in girls and young women. Obstet Gynecol. 2000;96:229-33.
58. Watson DI, Coventry BJ, Chin T, Fill PG, Malycha P. Laparoscopic versus open splenectomy for immune thrombocytopenic purpura. Surgery. 1997;121:18-22.
59. Wenner J, Graffner H, Lindell G. A financial analysis of laparoscopic and open cholecystectomy. Surg Endosc. 1995;9:702-5.

SECTION

6 Miscellaneous

- Other Minimal Access Surgical Procedures
- Minimal Access Bariatric Surgery
- Complications of Minimal Access Surgery
- Role of Training in Minimal Access Surgery
- Minimal Access Robotic Surgery
- Transanal Endoscopic Microsurgery
- Future of Minimal Access Surgery
- Troubleshooting and Checklist

CHAPTER 43

Other Minimal Access Surgical Procedures

TWO-PORT CHOLECYSTECTOMY

Laparoscopic cholecystectomy is the gold standard for the treatment of gallstone disease. The operation is routinely performed using four or three ports of entry into the abdomen. At laparoscopy hospital, we frequently perform cholecystectomy by two-port method using modified extracorporeal knot **(Fig. 1)**.

With this technique, we can give traction over the gallbladder in any direction for proper exposure. This new innovative two-port method of gallbladder removal can be used only for simple uncomplicated cholelithiasis cases by experienced surgeon, but it has definite advantage over conventional three- or four-port cholecystectomy. In two-port cholecystectomy, fundus is retracted by help of strategically passed suture **(Figs. 2 and 3)**.

Once the proper exposure of cystic pedicle is achieved, Maryland is used for dissection **(Figs. 4A to D)**.

Extracorporeal knot can be applied for cystic duct without any problem after nice dissection of cystic pedicle **(Figs. 5A to D)**.

The knot, which is tied over the cystic pedicle, is used to pull the neck of the gallbladder up and with the help of hook, gallbladder is separated from the liver **(Figs. 6 and 7)**.

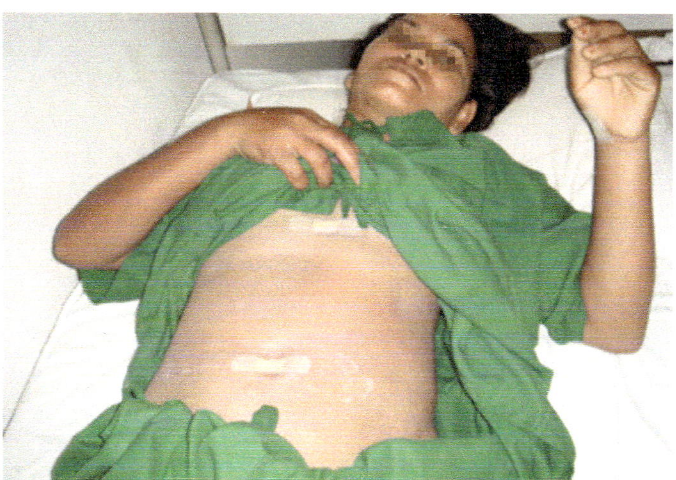

Fig. 1: Port position for two-port cholecystectomy.

Patients undergoing cholecystectomy by two-port method had a better resumption of diet and less postoperative pain. Two-port cholecystectomy is technically feasible and may further improve the surgical outcomes in terms of postoperative pain and better cosmetic value. The two-port cholecystectomy should be performed by experienced laparoscopic surgeon because skilled choreographic hand movement is very important in this surgery. Bimanual skill and correct interpretation of anatomy are must before proceeding for this technique. We do not recommend two-port cholecystectomy as a routine procedure.

Ending of the Operation

The instruments and ports are removed. Telescope should be removed leaving gas valve of umbilical port open to let out all the gas. At the time of removing umbilical port, telescope should be again inserted and umbilical port should be removed over the telescope to prevent any entrapment of omentum. The wound is then closed with suture. Vicryl should be used for rectus and unabsorbable intradermal or stapler for skin. A single suture is used to close the umbilicus and upper midline fascial opening. Many laparoscopic surgeons routinely leave this fascial defect without ill effect. Some surgeon likes to inject local anesthetic agent over port site to avoid postoperative pain. Sterile dressing over the wound should be applied.

TWO-PORT REPAIR OF VENTRAL HERNIA

Two-port ventral hernia is one of the options in case of small uncomplicated ventral hernia surgery. Patient should be under general anesthesia, nasogastric tube is introduced, and there should not be any organomegaly, if surgeon is planning two-port laparoscopic repair of ventral hernia. Access is performed through Palmer's point. Veress needle or open technique both can be used for access from the Palmer's point. All the safety indicators should be used and checked at the time of access. A 10-mm port should be introduced carefully through Palmer's point. It should be introduced perpendicular not oblique toward anus to avoid injury of splenic flexor of colon. Telescope should be introduced and the size, extent, and content of hernia are assessed.

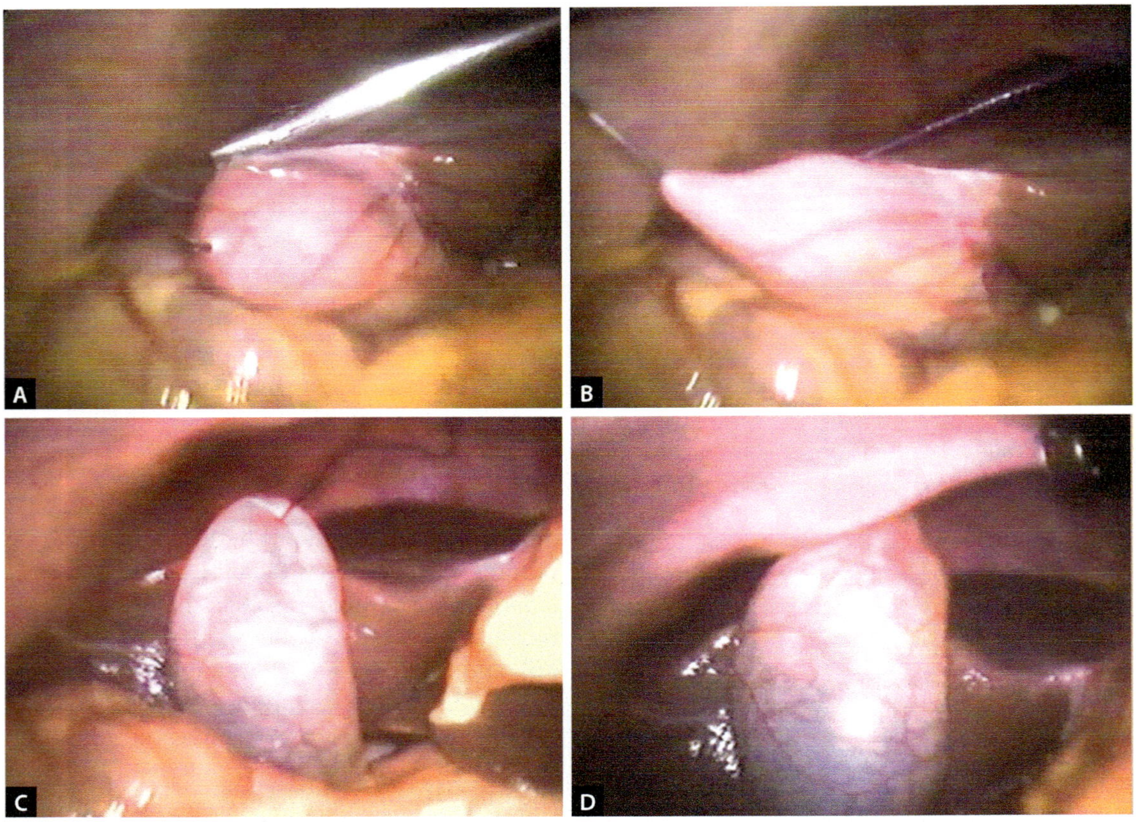

Figs. 2A to D: Fundus is retracted up with the help of needle and thread is passed through intercostals space under vision.

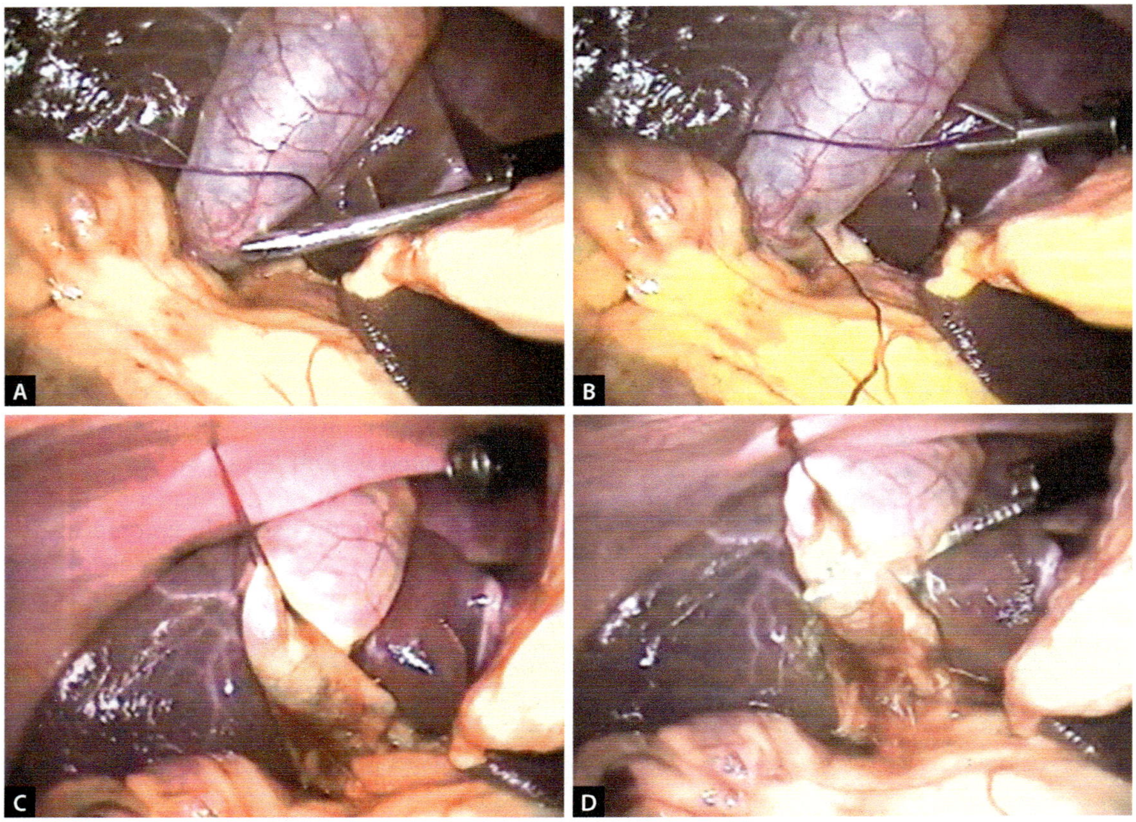

Figs. 3A to D: Another Vicryl is applied over Hartmann's pouch to provide anterolateral traction. Any leak from the gallbladder is irrigated and sucked nicely with the help of suction irrigation instrument.

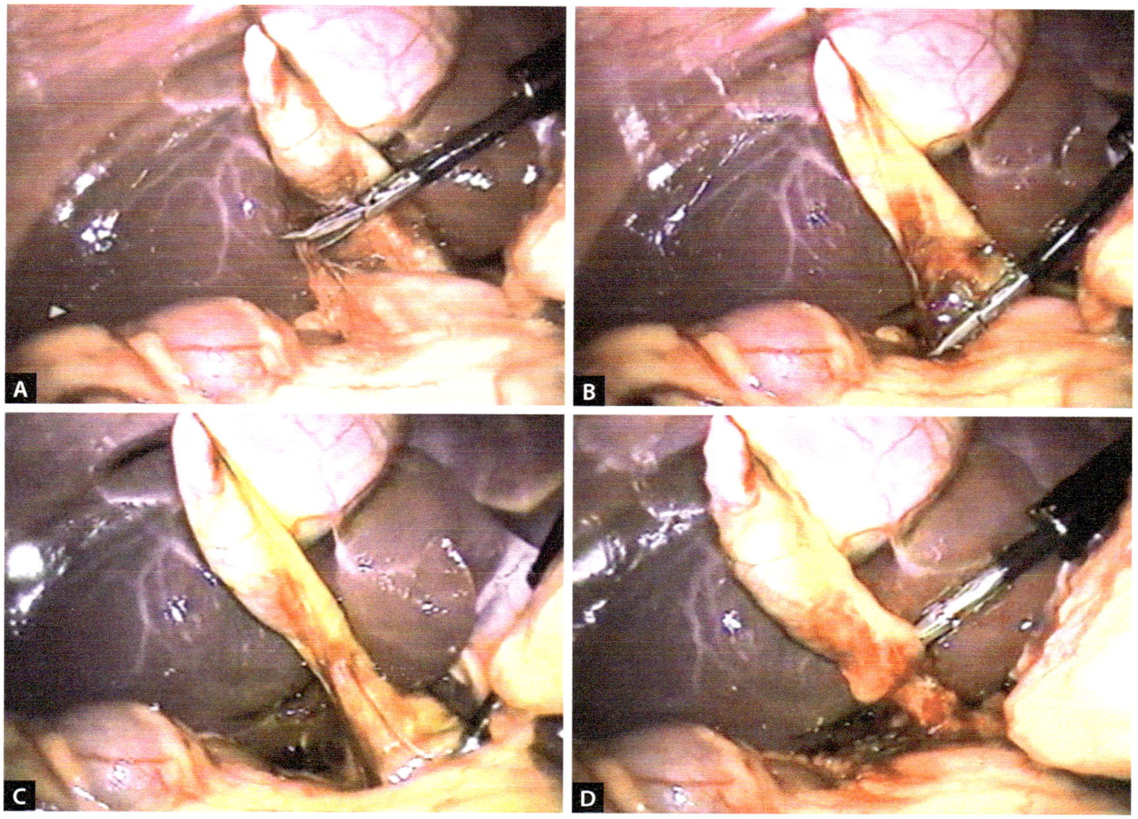

Figs. 4A to D: Dissection of cystic pedicle is performed by Maryland.

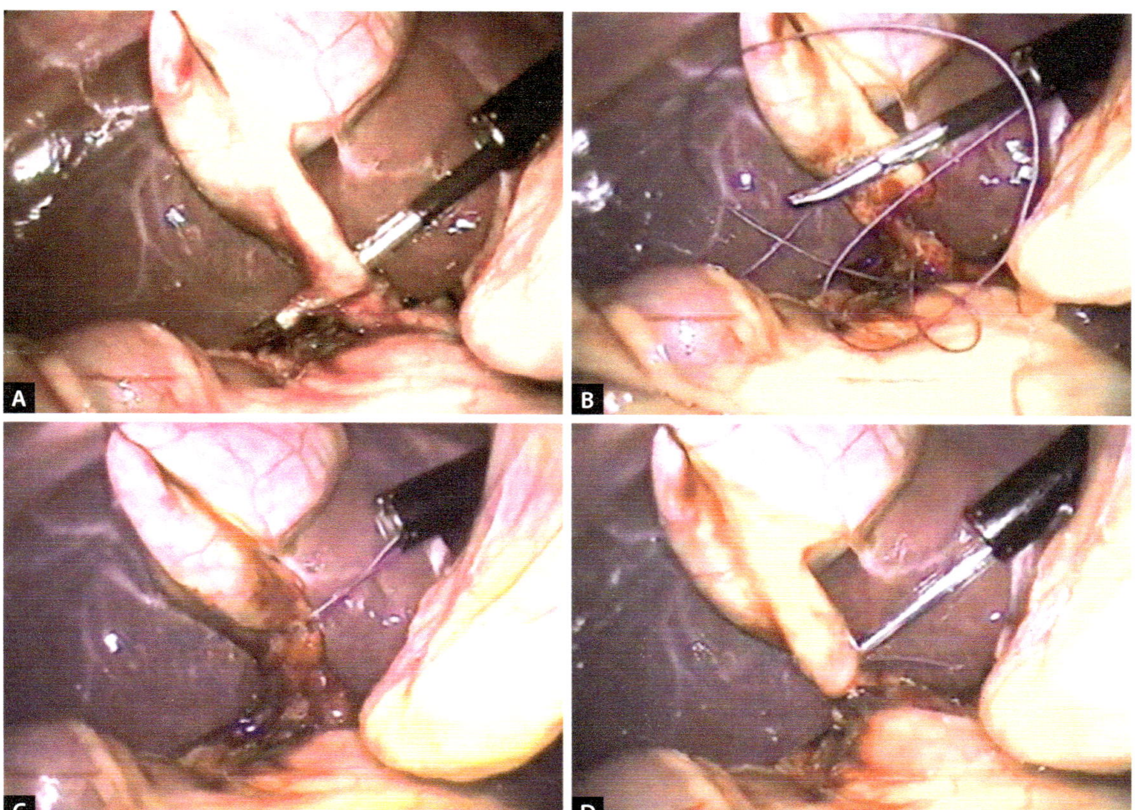

Figs. 5A to D: Clip or extracorporeal Meltzer's knot is applied over cystic artery and duct.

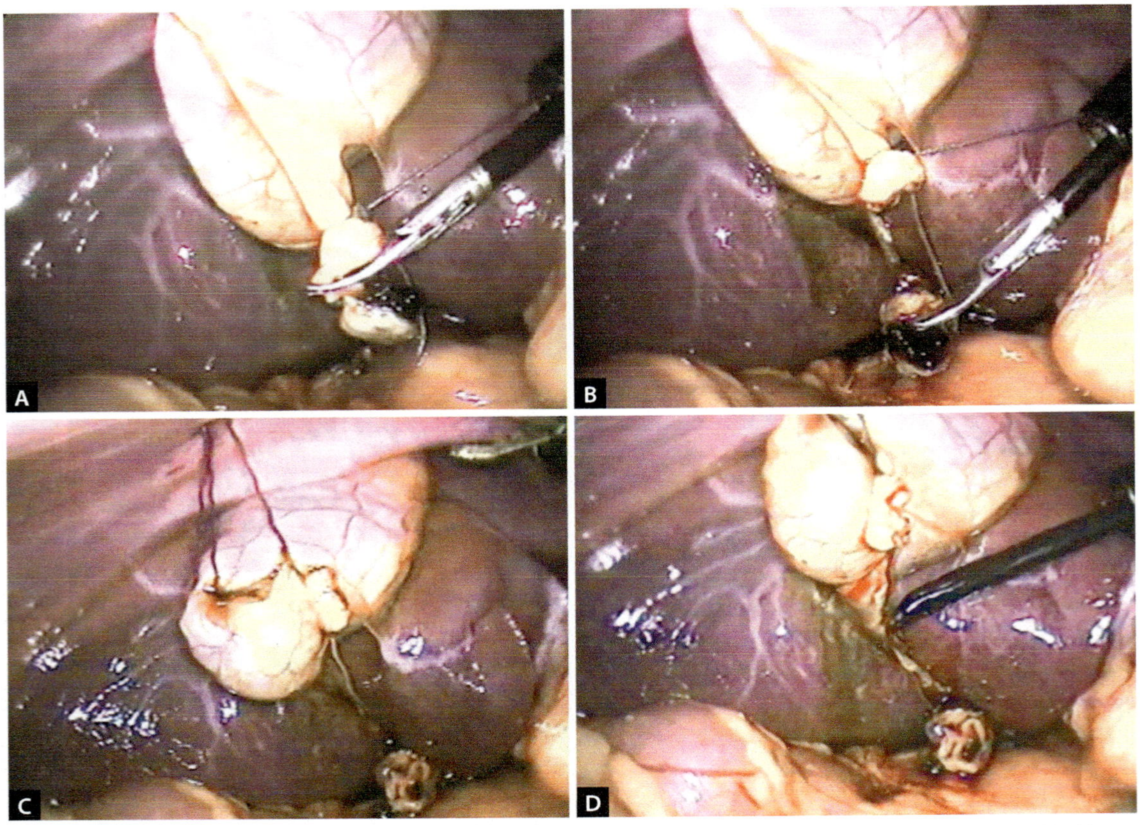

Figs. 6A to D: The extracorporeal knot of cystic duct is used to pull the neck up and to expose bed of the gallbladder.

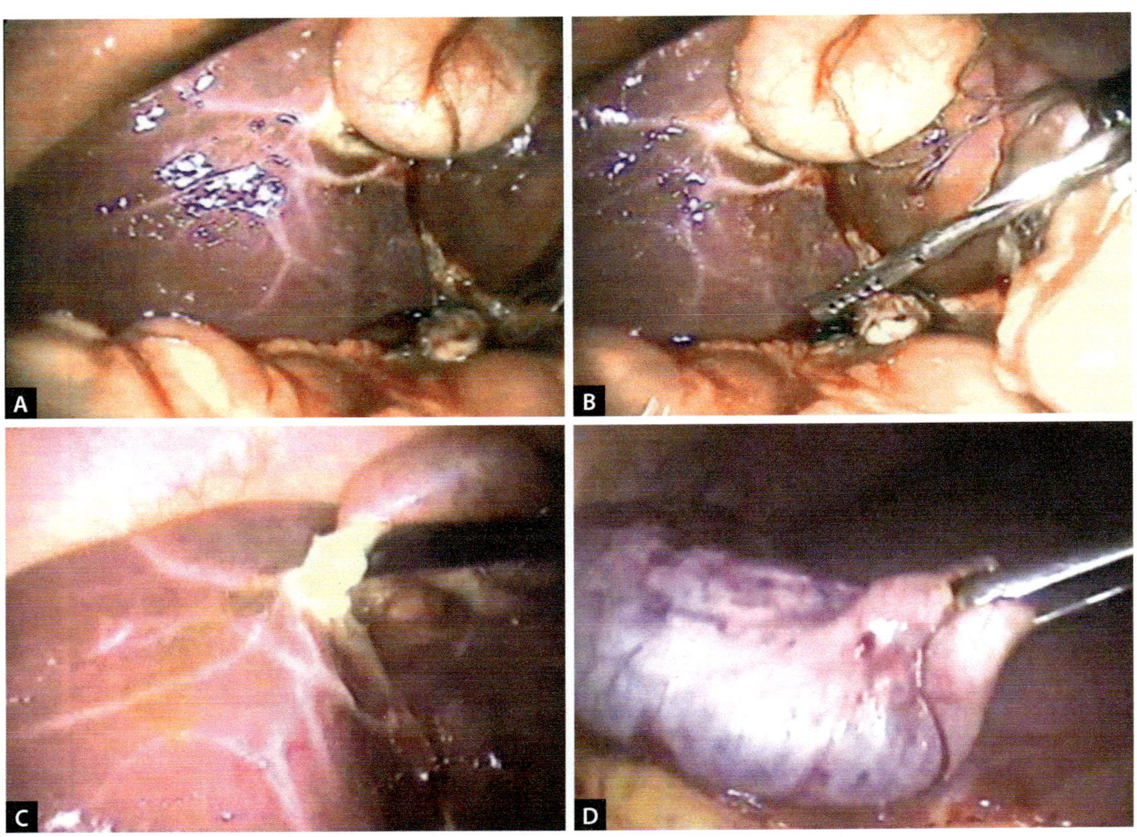

Figs. 7A to D: Any leak should be sucked and gallbladder is separated with the help of hook.

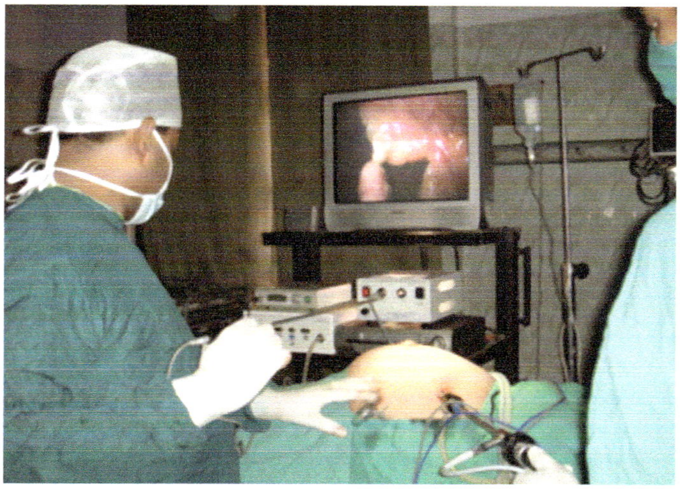

Fig. 8: Access is done through the Palmer's point.

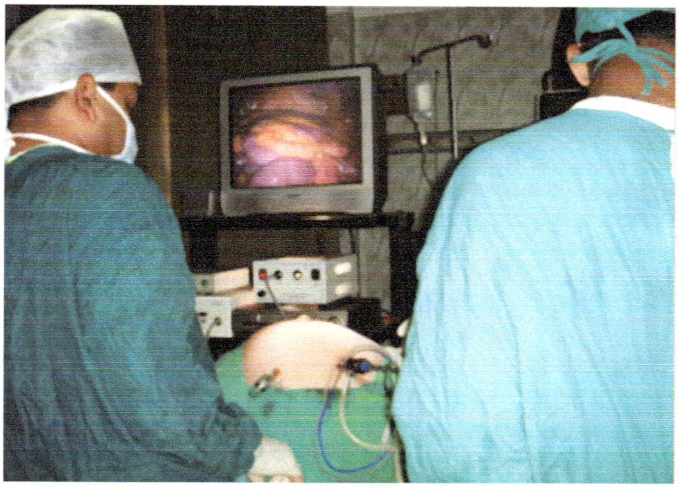

Fig. 9: 45° azimuth angle is kept for second port.

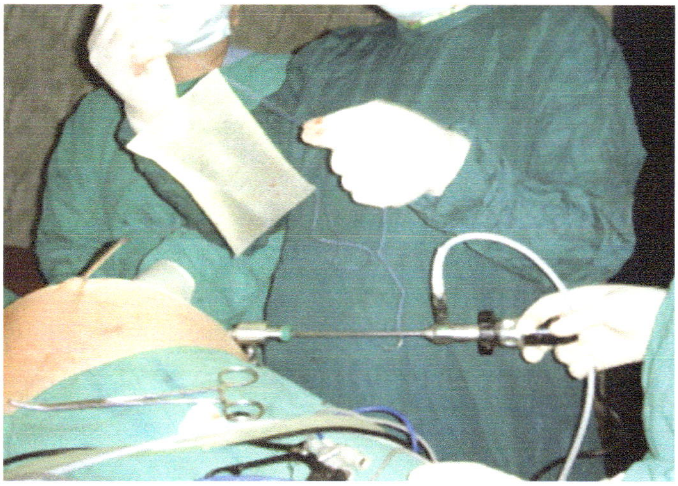

Fig. 10: 12 cm long Prolene is tied at three corner of the mesh keeping 6 cm long pair of free suture at each end.

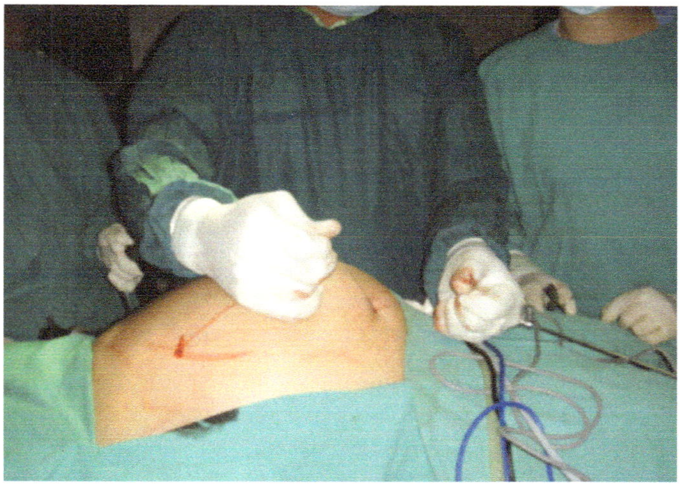

Fig. 11: Each pair of suture is pulled out through the same skin incision but different rectus and muscle layer.

After initial assessment of ventral hernia, one more port is introduced according to baseball diamond concept but keeping the azimuth angle (angle between telescope and instrument) 45° **(Figs. 8 and 9)**.

Content of hernia is reduced and adhesiolysis should be performed for any possible omental or bowel adhesion. Size of the mesh is selected in such a way that at least it should cover 4 cm all around beyond the healthy margin of defect. A 1-mm wide, just skin, deep stab incision should be given at all the four corner of mesh.

A 12-cm long Prolene is tied around three corner of the mesh and one of the remaining corners should be tied through the needle and thread introduced through one of the stab wound of skin **(Fig. 10)**. The thread which was introduced percutaneously will help to stabilize the mesh and it will act as the third port **(Fig. 11)**.

Both the end of Prolene is pulled out through the same skin puncture side but keeping rectus and peritoneum in between **(Fig. 12)**.

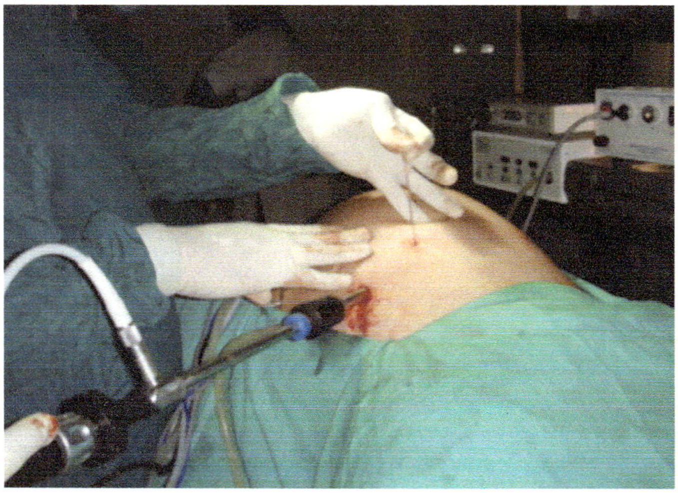

Fig. 12: Both end of suture is tied outside the skin. Skin is lifted to slip the knot subcutaneously.

The end of both the thread should be ligated using Tumble Square knot and it should be slipped inside skin

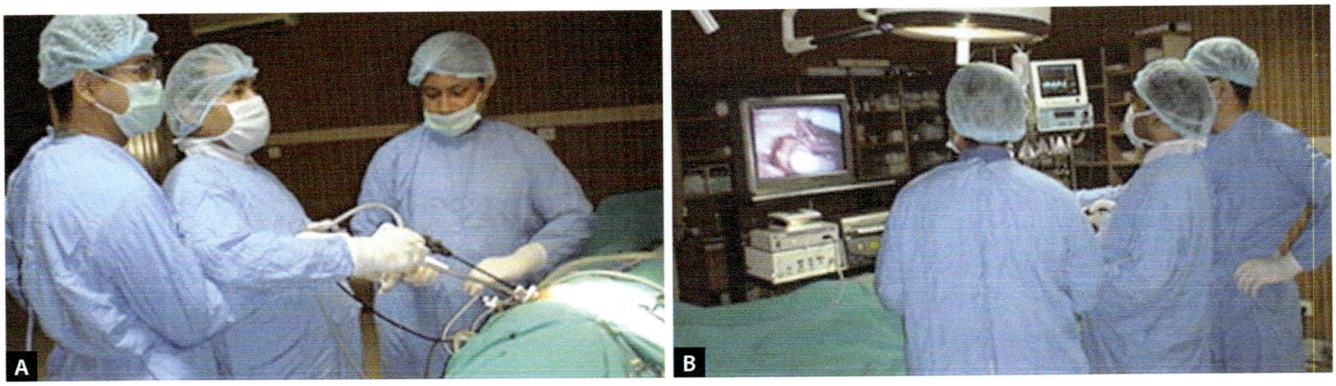

Figs. 13A and B: Single-incision laparoscopic surgery.

depth before locking to avoid loosening. This two-port technique can be accomplished with the help of Anchor or ProTack or Tacker, if patient can afford. Two-port technique using Prolene is safe and economical method of performing laparoscopic repair of ventral hernia. Although using strategically placed knot, we have performed one-port repair of ventral hernia also with the help of suture passer but if adhesions are present, one-port technique is not possible. Two-port techniques should be included in the practice of repair of ventral hernia surgery laparoscopically because in case of any difficulty, the third port can be introduced any time without any difficulty.

SINGLE-INCISION LAPAROSCOPIC SURGERY

Usually, when a new surgical technique is introduced, the focus will be on the feasibility, safety, and clinical advantage of the method. On the other hand, safety is highly dependent on how easily the new technique can be learned by average surgeons. It is a well-known fact that the implementation phase of new techniques is associated with an increased risk of complications emphasizing the importance of thorough training and education for the operating surgeon. The first report of single-incision laparoscopic surgery (SILS) was by Navarra et al. who performed an SILS cholecystectomy in 1997. Since then, there have been many reports regarding the use of SILS for appendectomy, splenectomy, nephrectomy, prostatectomy, colectomy, sleeve gastrectomy, adrenalectomy, and adjustable gastric band. However, there have been no reported randomized clinical trials with direct comparison between SILS to conventional laparoscopic surgery.

Despite the lack of evidence demonstrating any superiority of SILS, it is being increasingly performed unfortunately in a largely unregulated fashion without formal training. Concern has been raised that this new procedure is more technically challenging and is likely associated with a significant learning curve and also its own disadvantage and complication.

Single-incision laparoscopic surgery is a new technique that has now been utilized in many centers for minimal access surgery (MAS) **(Figs. 13A and B)**. The major difficulty with this new technique is the sacrifice that has to be made in terms of comfort and ergonomics. One of the great advantage of SILS is patients are very satisfied with their single scar and particularly enthusiastic in regard to the cosmetic outcome of single incision approach.

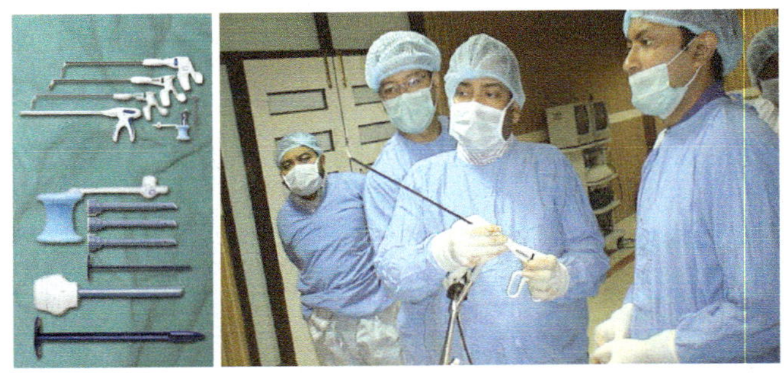

Fig. 14: Articulating instruments used in single-incision laparoscopic surgery.

Single-incision laparoscopic surgery was first performed for the treatment of appendicitis at Department of Pediatric Surgery, Dokuz Eylül Medical School University, Izmir, Turkey and first presented at—The Annual Congress of Turkish Association of Pediatric Surgeons, October 2005.

Synonym

All over the world, SILS is called by following names:
- *SPL*: Single Port Laparoscopy
- *SPA*: Single Port Access Surgery
- *SILS*: Single-incision Laparoscopic Surgery
- *LESS*: Laparoendoscopic Single-site Surgery
- *OPUS*: One-port Umbilical Surgery
- *NOTUS*: Natural Orifice Transumbilical Surgery.

Equipment

Many companies are making SILS equipment **(Figs. 14 and 15)**. Few of the famous brands are:
- *SILS device from*: Covidien
- *GelPOINT system from*: Applied Medical
- *R-Port and TriPort from*: Advanced Surgical Concepts
- *Uni-X from*: Pnavel.

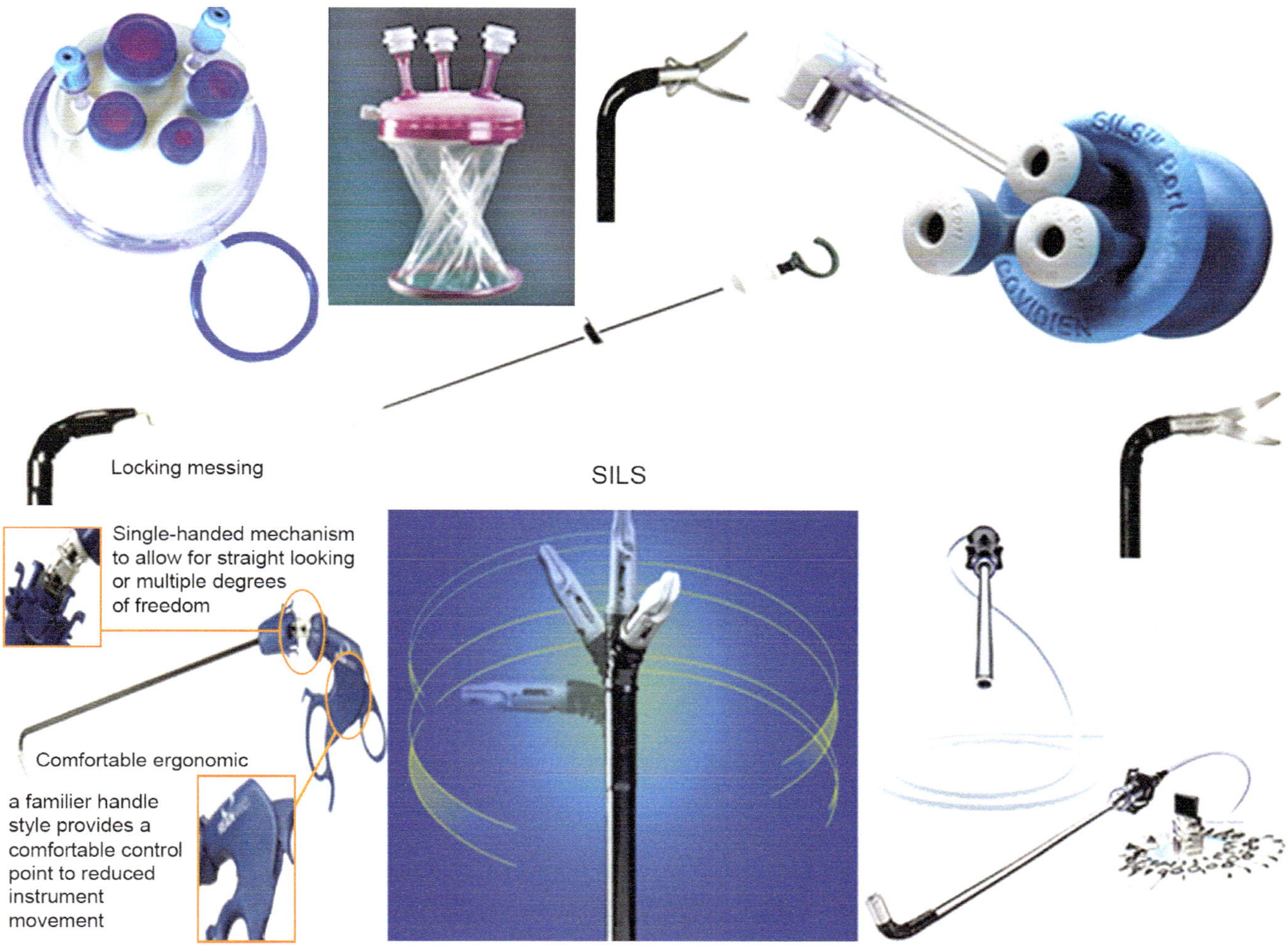

Fig. 15: Some of the popular single-incision laparoscopic surgery (SILS) equipment.

Case selection is paramount for the success of SILS and at world laparoscopy hospital, we performed SILS for the cases, which is not complicated and has minimum risk. Good ergonomics in SILS need articulating instrument and high end energy sources such as tissue response generator (LigaSure) and ultrasonic dissector (Harmonic).

Advantages of Single-incision Laparoscopic Surgery

- Cosmesis +++ **(Figs. 16 and 17)**
- Ease of tissue retrieval ++++
- Combination procedure +++
- Patient acceptance ++++
- Quality of life analysis ++
- Standard equipment ++
- Do not violate natural orifices ++++
- Surgeon's domain +++.

Disadvantages of Single-incision Laparoscopic Surgery

- More pain compared to laparoscopic surgery
- Violating principles of ergonomics

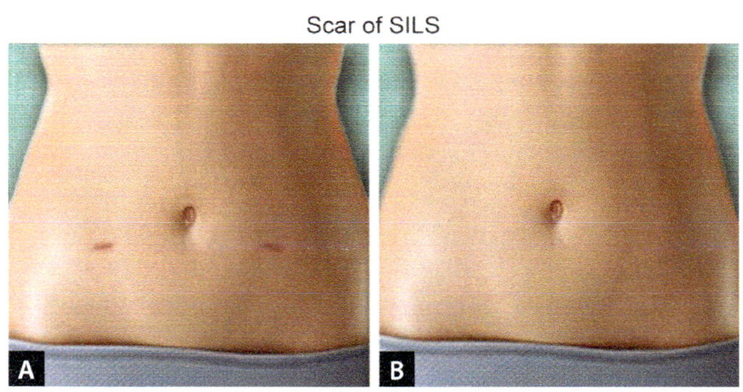

Figs. 16A and B: Comparison of scar of single-incision laparoscopic surgery (SILS) and conventional laparoscopic surgery.

- Incisional hernia chances are more compared to laparoscopic surgery
- More wound infection compared to laparoscopic surgery
- Bigger learning curve compared to laparoscopic surgery
- Not cost-effective compared to laparoscopic surgery.

The evolution of surgery toward less invasive approaches has act as stimulant effect toward the development of new less invasive techniques in entering the abdominal cavity. An example of such technique is the use of a single skin incision through which multiple instruments can be

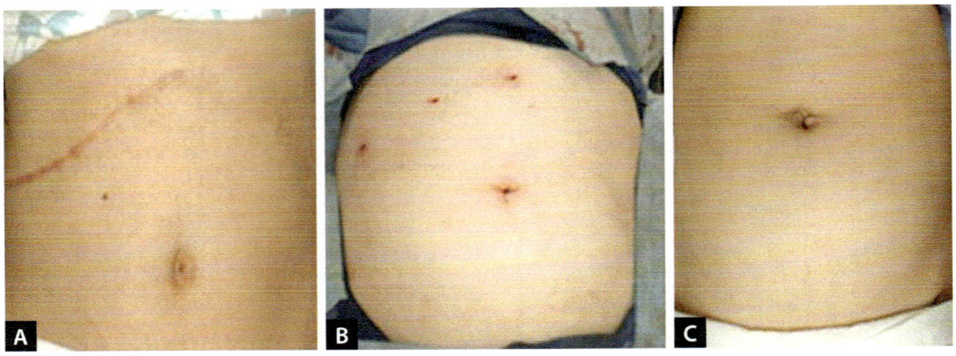

Figs. 17A to C: Comparison of scar of single-incision laparoscopic surgery (SILS), laparoscopic surgery, and open surgery.

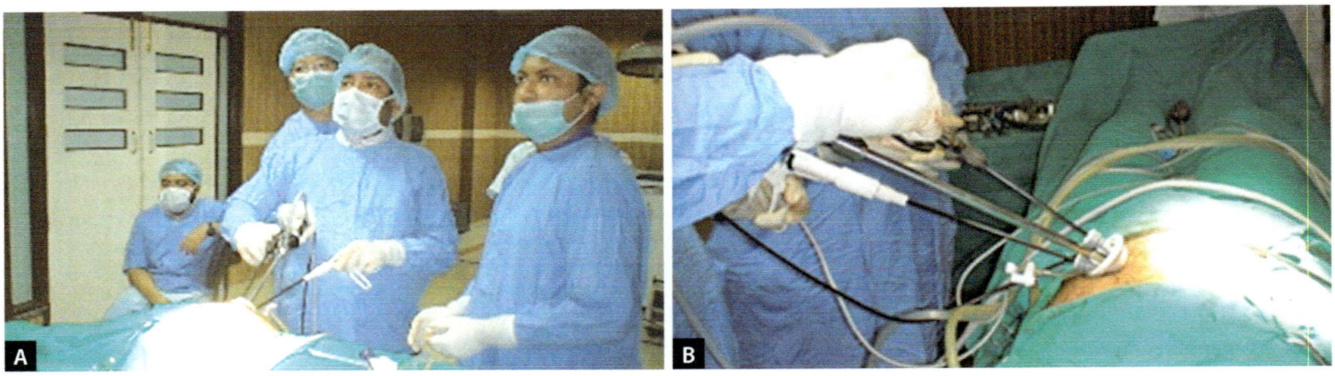

Figs. 18A and B: Position of surgical team in single-incision laparoscopic surgery (SILS).

inserted into the abdomen. This single-incision laparoscopic technique has been described by a variety of names as we have discussed earlier. With this single incision of entry, SILS is theoretically less invasive approach compared to the standard multiport laparoscopic surgery. However, SILS may not allow the same level of manual dexterity and technical performance compared to conventional laparoscopic surgery that in certain aspect, it even violates the principle of laparoscopic surgery **(Figs. 18A and B)**.

Laparoscopic cholecystectomy (LC) has become the standard procedure for treating gallstones, cholecystitis, or gallbladder polyps. Traditionally, LC has involved four ports. Many laparoscopic techniques happen to be developed using this four-port LC and it has become possible to do these techniques safely. Now, having established the security of LC, our interest centered on lowering the invasiveness and scarring brought on by the procedure. Cuesta et al. reported single-incision laparoscopic cholecystectomy (SILC), in which two 5 mm ports were introduced through the umbilicus, along with a Kirschner wire hook was introduced with the right subcostal area to pull in an upright direction in order to visualize Calot's triangle.

Several surgeons have described performing SILC using three 5 mm ports in the umbilicus. Meanwhile, Merchant et al. also performed SILS by inserting a GelPort (Applied Medical, Rancho Santa Margarita, CA, USA) to stretch the umbilical fascia incision for simple access with instruments into the abdominal cavity. Furthermore, a method involving several transumbilical-placed ports for SILS was newly developed and SILS by way of the ASC TriPort (Advanced Surgical Concepts, Wicklow, Ireland) continues to be described successively. On the other hand, a fascinating new instrument named SPIDER (TransEnterix, Inc., Research Triangle Park, NC) to be used in single-incision surgery was created and its use in SILS in an animal experiment has been reported. As a result of these clinical studies, using SILC has spread rapidly. Various ports and instruments are available and various surgical methods utilized in performing SILS can be found in many institutions; however, it is necessary to develop a great method that can be performed safely such as the conventional four-port LC and it is also essential to balance safety, operability, and economy in this new technique.

Under general anesthesia, an approximately 25 mm vertical skin incision is made through the center of the umbilicus, the peritoneal cavity should be entered with the open method, and then the SILS port inserted **(Figs. 19A to E)**. Three exclusive 5 mm ports were inserted through the SILS port and one 5 mm port changeable for an exclusive 12 mm port. The pneumoperitoneum should set at 12–15 mm and flexible scope (Olympus, Tokyo, Japan) should be used, if possible for that intra-abdominal visualization. A couple of loop-type retractor (Mini-loop retractor II; Covidien) should inserted directly within the right subcostal area.

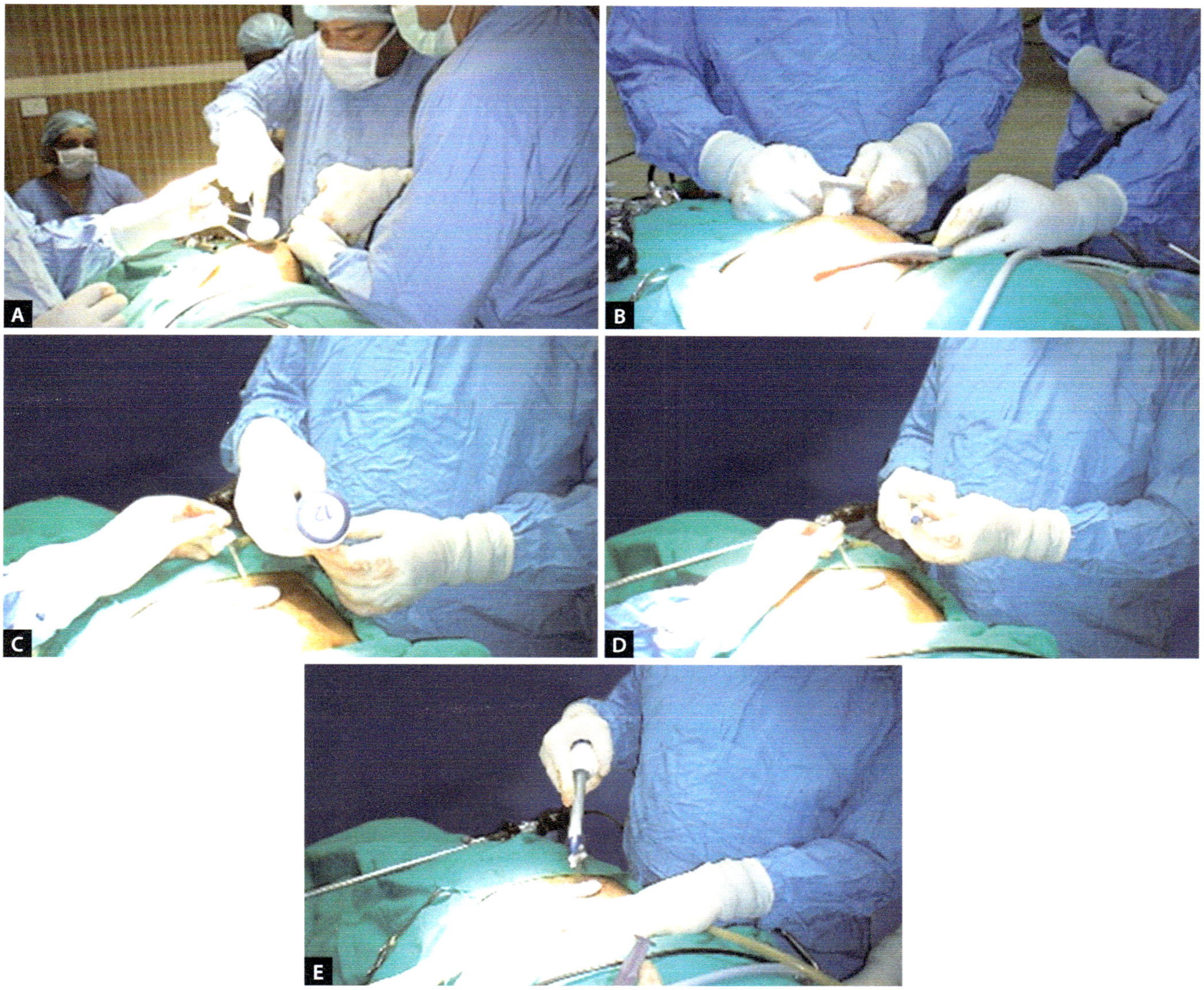

Figs. 19A to E: Single-incision laparoscopic surgery (SILS) port and its access.

Following the patient should be put into the reverse Trendelenburg position and slightly rotated to the left, the fundus of the gallbladder should tightened by way of this loop-type retractor and also the gallbladder thereafter suspended. In dissecting the gallbladder, a curved grasper, bipolar forceps, or monopolar hooks should be utilized in the two remaining apertures. The cystic duct and artery should be exposed and clipped having a 5-mm clip applier (Endo Clip; Covidien) after which divided with laparoscopic scissors. The gallbladder should be extracted by having an endoscopic retrieval bag (Endo Catch Gold; Covidien).

Easy replacing a 5-mm port having a 12-mm port is one of the advantages of this port. Actually, SILS, while using SILS port, was proven as safe as conventional four-port LC and complications, for example, bile duct injury or uncontrolled bleeding did not occur. However, the issue areas where improvements are needed would be that the umbilical scar through the SILS port is larger than that of conventional four-port LC. Concretely, the umbilical scar length when it comes to conventional four-port LC involved 15 mm; however, while using SILS port, it was approximately 25 mm and furthermore in instances where the umbilicus bottom was shallow, the scar may be unexpectedly large. Conflict between your operative instruments and also the scope is inevitable and also the procedure seemed to be inconvenient to do since the surgeon and also the assistant needed to stand in the same side from the patient.

The fundus from the gallbladder may be tightened with the Roeder's or Meltzer's knot and so the straight needle was inserted from the abdominal cavity right subcostal abdominal wall. The gallbladder should be elevated by raising this nylon suture and a good surgical field obtained. The surgeon operated both one instrument and also the 5 mm flexible scope by hand and the assistant designed a good surgical field such as Calot's triangle through the traction of the gallbladder utilizing a fine loop retractor and nylon suture. This technique relieved the interference between your surgeon and also the assistant and between your forceps themselves. To extract the exfoliated gallbladder, one 5 mm port should be removed and an endoscopic retrieval bag should be inserted directly with an original hole and the gallbladder ended up being extracted.

The fascial defect of the umbilicus incision should be repaired with approximately two stitches and an intradermal suture should be performed on the skin **(Figs. 20A and B)**. It should be noted that during MAS, generally, we do not shave the hair of skin around the port site. If it is required, just trimming of hair should be done on the operation table itself. Shaving of hair many hours before the surgery is liable to bring the bacteria on the surface and may increase the chances of skin infection. This method represents noninvasive surgery that mixes low invasiveness with a scarless outcome. The surgeon operates one instrument along with a 5-mm flexible scope and the assistant pulls or pushes the fine loop retractor and the nylon suture. This straightforward transition is also an advantage of our two-port technique, since it can be created in any case of cholecystitis or intraperitoneal adhesion.

With the global growth of using SILS, large series of cases happen to be reported in many institutes. Curcillo et al. reported that within their multi-institutional 297 case series, the utilization of one more port away from umbilicus occurred in only 34 cases plus they concluded that SILS was safe and can serve as an alternative choice to multiport therapy with fewer scars and cosmesis. Erbella and Bunch surprisingly reported that their mean operative time was 30 minutes (from 22 to 75 minutes) in 100 consecutive SILS cases. Rivas et al. reported that they observed surgeons in training and located that experienced laparoscopic surgeons may not have to undergo a steep learning curve plus they concluded that SILS was becoming the conventional process of most elective patients with gallbladder disease. Other reports also concluded that SILS was safe; however, Hernandez et al. reported that biliary complication (cystic duct stump leak) took place among 100 SILS cases and Edwards et al. described that biliary complications occurred in 3.7% of the SILS patients (cystic duct stump leak; 1 and accessory duct leak; 2). Moreover, iatrogenic combined bile duct and right hepatic artery injury during SILS has already been reported and the authors recommended that surgeons should have a low threshold to add additional ports at the appropriate interval to make sure that procedures were completed safely, especially in their early stages.

As described, SILS is really a useful technique; however, it is important to make sure that the procedure is as safe as conventional four-port LC. In our department, to secure the safety, acute cholecystitis is excluded in the indication for SILS for that present. Comparative studies between SILS and conventional four-port LC regarding operating time, operative cost, complications, postoperative pain, cosmetic result, and time for you to go back to normal activity have been performed gradually with time. Fronza et al. reported that the operating time was significantly longer in SILS and 12% of SILS patients were readmitted within 24 hours after the operation, although these readmissions were due to complications similar to those present in four-port LC. Similarly, Chang et al. figured that there is a substantial difference in operative time (SILS was approximately 1.6 times longer) as well as in operative cost (SILS was 1.29 times more expensive), but no difference in postoperative discomfort was observed. However, they result that patients who underwent SILS returned to normal activity 1.8 days earlier than four-port LC patients seem to demonstrate the usefulness of SILS. Furthermore, two randomized controlled trials (RCTs) that compared SILS with conventional four-port LC have already been published. One of these trials included 70 patients and the other included 40 patients. Inside a result present with both trials, the operating amount of time in SILS was more than that in four-port LC, although it was discovered that the two methods differed with regard to the patients' postoperative pain. According to the conventional reports, the benefit of SILS has not yet become clear; therefore, well-designed RCTs are essential to judge the corrective operative outcomes and also the necessity of SILS.

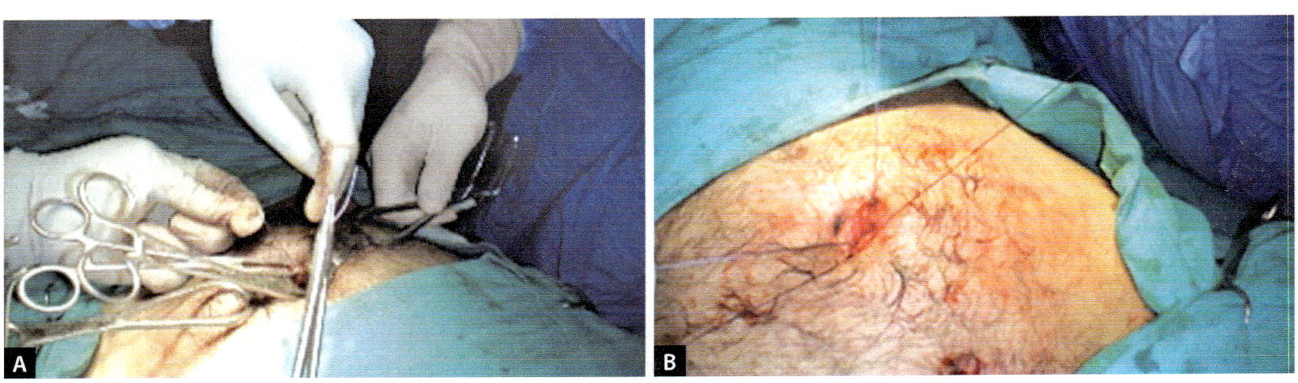

Figs. 20A and B: Port closure technique in single-incision laparoscopic surgery (SILS).

RETROPERITONEOSCOPY

Traditionally, laparoscopic surgeries are performed by transperitoneal approach following establishment of pneumoperitoneum by closed technique using the Veress needle or by the open mini-laparotomy. The parietal peritoneum is then secondarily incised and dissected to obtain access to the retroperitoneal target organs such as kidneys, ureters, adrenals, and lymph nodes. Transperitoneal laparoscopy, although seemingly expeditious, invites the potential calamities of possible vascular and bowel injuries. On the other hand, retroperitoneal laparoscopy has its own difficulty due to working in a contained limited space. However, with technical refinements, several recent reports of successful retroperitoneoscopic surgeries have proved the feasibility and distinct advantages of this approach.

Historical Perspective

Retroperitoneoscopy has experienced a delayed development and acceptance compared with peritoneoscopy. Difficulties in providing adequate visualization and room for surgical maneuvering as well as concerns about deleterious effects of insufflating the retroperitoneal space account for this retarded progression. Although pneumoretroperitoneum has been used safely for >50 years to aid in radiographic visualization of the kidneys and adrenals, the conjunctive use of endoscopes has only recently been attempted.

Retroperitoneoscopy through the flank in a human was pioneered by Wickham, who performed an extraperitoneal laparoscopic ureterolithotomy in 1978.

Earliest techniques, termed pelviscopy, utilized a telescope to bluntly dissect within the pelvic retroperitoneum to sample pelvic lymph nodes. The obvious disadvantage of such technique has been the difficulty in exposing the obturator nodes, precluding the performance of an adequate staging lymphadenectomy. In the initial series reported by Hald and Rasmussen, many of the patients had no lymph nodes found in their surgical specimen. With refinements of surgical techniques, subsequently more complete pelviscopic node dissections have been reported.

Surgical Technique

Probably, the most important initial step in retroperitoneoscopy is the expansion and distention of the retroperitoneal space by an expanding balloon device. A balloon device modified fingers of a latex rubber glove is tied off and the glove is secured over the distal end of the sheath of cannula **(Fig. 21)**.

The device is placed in the retroperitoneum and expanded by injecting saline. Special trocars are available with transparent balloons at their inner end that can be inflated with air or fluid to allow laparoscopic visibility of retroperitoneum through the clear distended balloon.

Retroperitoneoscopy through the Flank

This approach is applicable to surgery on adrenals, kidneys, and upper ureters. The patient is placed in a lateral decubitus position with slight forward tilt. A small incision is made about 2 cm below the 12th rib, just lateral to the sacrospinalis. The incision is deepened through the fused lamellae of lumbar fascia to enter the perinephric space **(Fig. 22)**.

The space is further dissected by blunt digital exploration. The expanding device is introduced into the retroperitoneal space and about 800–1,000 mL saline are injected to inflate the balloon. The balloon is then deflated and removed **(Figs. 23A and B)**.

Laparoscope in 11 mm trocar is introduced into the retroperitoneal space and carbon dioxide (CO_2) insufflation is continued to maintain a pressure of about 14 mm Hg. With the posterior parietal peritoneum pushed away by the expanding device, the retroperitoneal space is widely opened

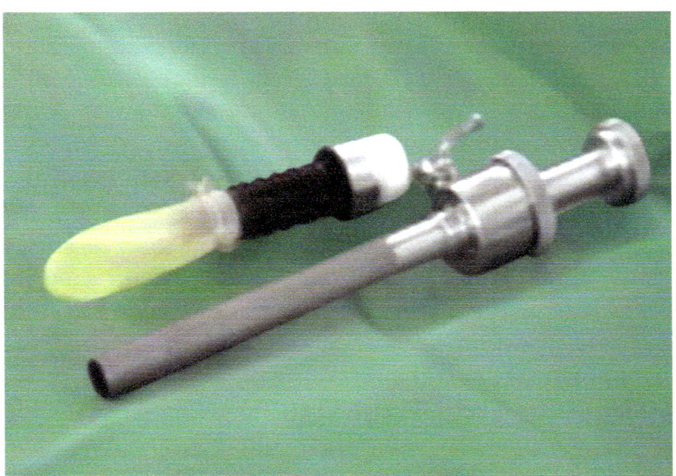

Fig. 21: Finger of glove over sheath of cannula.

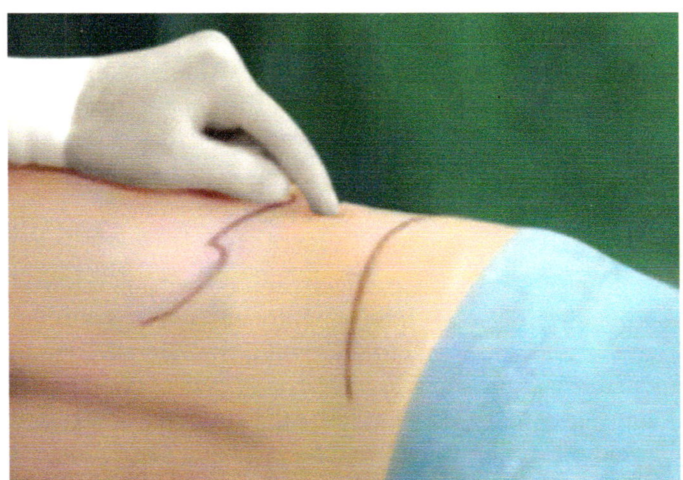

Fig. 22: Place for primary trocar insertion in retroperitoneoscopy.

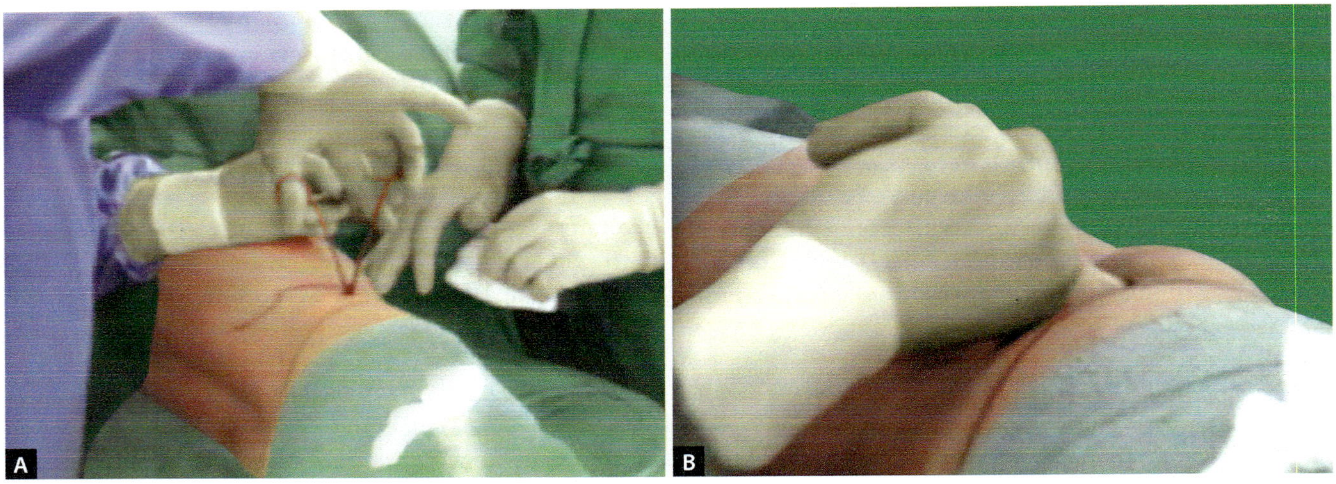

Figs. 23A and B: Finger dissection of retroperitoneal space.

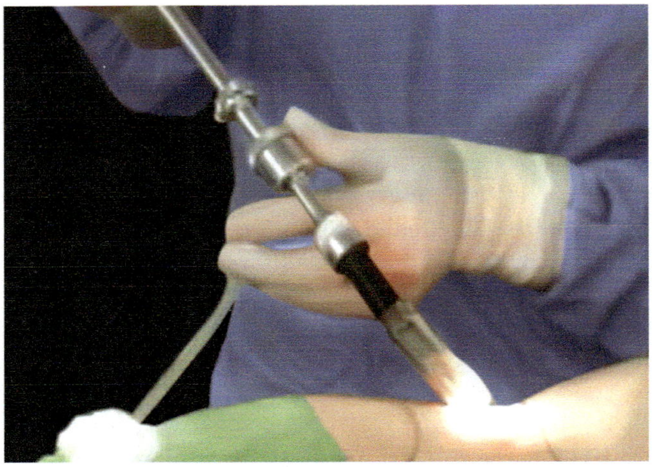

Fig. 24: Laparoscope with balloon cannula system.

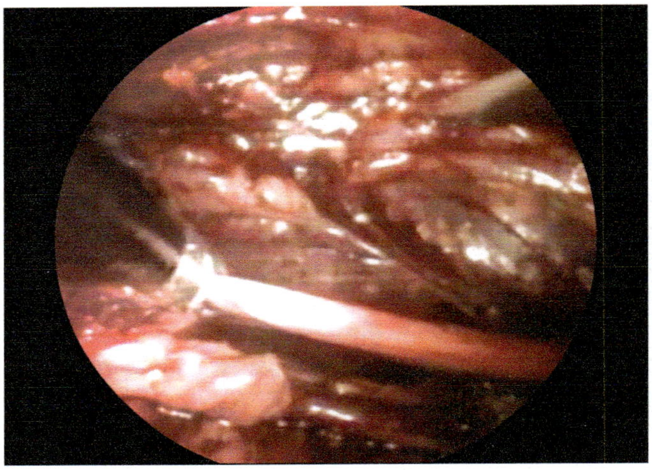

Fig. 25: Ureter as seen during retroperitoneoscopy.

by continued insufflation and subsequent working ports are established under camera vision. The number and location of accessory ports are determined by the surgical procedure to be undertaken. However, it is usually advisable to keep the ports posterior to the anterior axillary line to avoid puncture of the lateral peritoneal reflection. During laparoscopic dissection, it is often helpful to move the laparoscope to the anterior ports for better visibility as the situation may dictate **(Fig. 24)**.

Retroperitoneoscopy: Anterolateral

For surgery on mid and lower ureters and for internal spermatic vein ligation, the retroperitoneoscopy is performed by a small incision at McBurney's point. The external oblique aponeurosis is incised and underlying fibers of the internal oblique and transverse muscles of the abdomen are split to reach the extraperitoneal space. Following careful digital dissection, the expanding device is introduced and inflated in the retroperitoneum **(Figs. 25 and 26)**.

Retroperitoneoscopy for Pelvic Lymph Node

Pelvic retroperitoneoscopy is ideal for bilateral staging pelvic lymph node dissection and bladder neck suspension procedures. A small midline incision is made about 2 cm below the umbilicus. The linea alba is opened and underlying extraperitoneal space is developed by digital dissection behind the rectus muscle of the abdomen. The expanding device is introduced and expanded by injecting about 1,200 mL saline solution. The balloon is decompressed and removed. The laparoscope is introduced with high-flow CO_2 insufflation. Anatomic landmarks of the symphysis pubis, superior pubic rami, bladder neck, and external iliac vein pulsations in the pelvis are easily identified. Complete bilateral staging lymphadenectomy is accomplished by en bloc dissection of the fibrofatty lymphatic tissue from the triangular area bounded laterally by the external iliac vein, proximally by the hypogastric artery, and inferiorly by the endopelvic fascia **(Figs. 27 and 28)**.

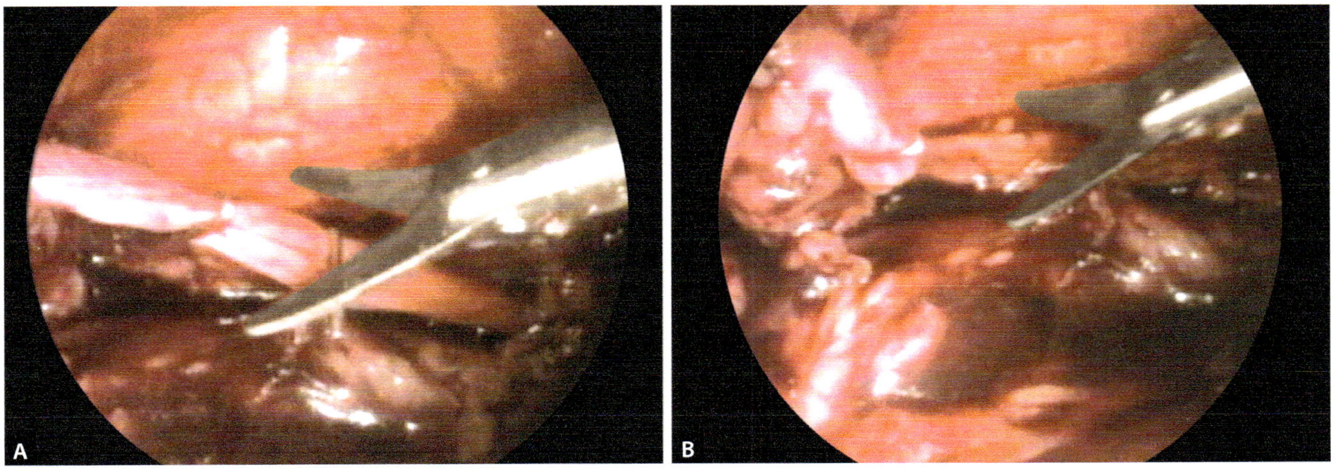

Figs. 26A and B: Two clips are applied over ureter and cut in between.

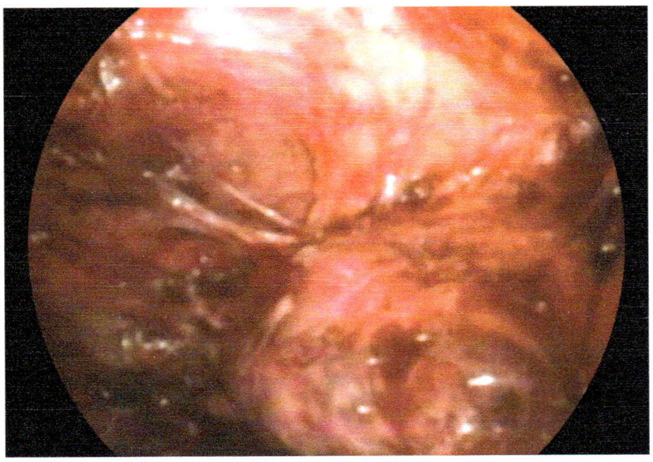

Fig. 27: Posterior dissection of left kidney.

Conclusion

The pioneering concept of retroperitoneal expansion by Gaur and coworkers has led to the resurgence of retroperitoneoscopy. Artificial balloon expansion creates the necessary space and retraction of neighboring viscera, so that subsequent insufflation can maintain the open space for surgical maneuvering. In a way, this technique simulates the steps of dissection and retraction traditionally used during open surgery.

Aside from preventing the potential hazards of transperitoneal access and intraperitoneal dissection, there are certain distinct advantages of retroperitoneoscopy in patient positioning, intestinal retraction, anatomic approach to the renal hilum, and postoperative wound drainage. For retroperitoneal approaches to the adrenals, kidneys, and ureters, the patient is placed in the lateral decubitus position, as opposed to the supine position for laparoscopy. The intestines contained within the intact peritoneal envelope remain displaced during retroperitoneal dissection, thereby avoiding extensive colonic mobilization and constant retraction of bowel. During nephrectomy, the renal hilum is approached from the posterior aspect, allowing easier initial control of the renal arteries. Similarly, exposure of other retroperitoneal structures such as the adrenal gland in the right side is relatively easier than with the anterior approach.

The closed extraperitoneal space allows more effective postoperative drainage, especially following reconstructive and reparative surgery such as pyeloplasty, partial nephrectomy, pyelolithotomy, and ureterolithotomy. The perceived difficulties of surgical dissection of kidneys and adrenal glands in a restricted environment during retroperitoneoscopy have not proved true with the present technique or initial balloon expansion. However, organ entrapment, especially of large specimens, in the limited space is difficult.

The anterolateral extraperitoneal approach allows access for ureterolithotomy on the lower ureter at and above the pelvic inlet. Internal spermatic vein ligation extraperitoneally is done for treatment of varicocele. The extraperitoneal dissection appears, however, to be more extensive and such an approach will not be suitable for bilateral variocele surgery. In the pelvis, the excellent anatomic appearance of the bladder, bladder neck, and symphysial structures makes the extraperitoneal approach ideally suited for procedures such as laparoscopic bladder-neck suspension and surgery for urachal pathologies. The majority of bladder diverticula are located posterolaterally and are, therefore, not often amenable to extraperitoneal excision.

For the bilateral staging of pelvic lymphadenectomy, the extraperitoneal approach has proved its safety and feasibility. The lymph node dissection is anatomically precise, simulating the standards of open pelvic lymphadenectomy.

The advantage of retroperitoneal CO_2 insufflation is that by avoiding CO_2 contact with the peritoneal membrane, there is less hypothermia and reduced postoperative pain from diaphragmatic irritation. In conclusion, retroperitoneoscopy offers another viable option in the

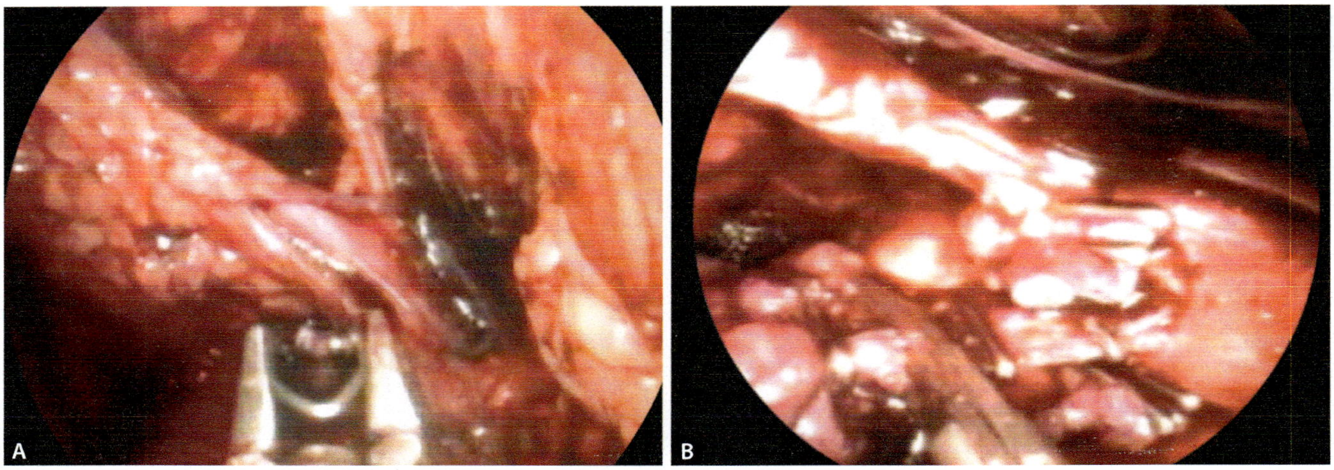

Figs. 28A and B: Dissection of hilum of kidney and application of clips before cutting.

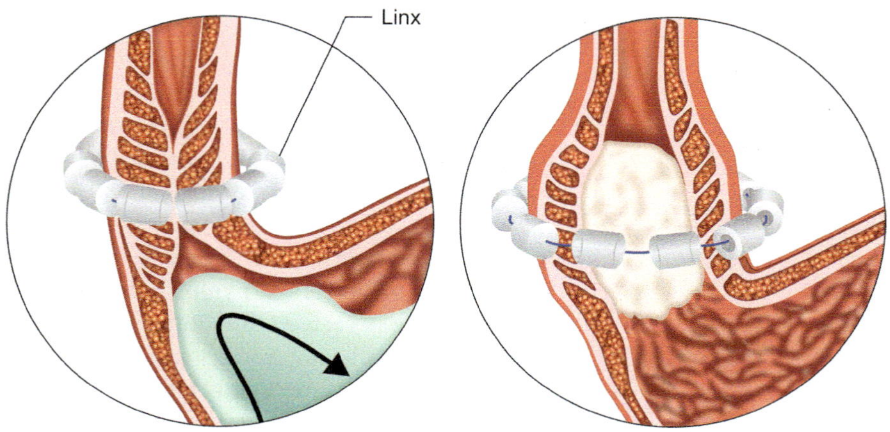

Fig. 29: LINX® procedure for gastroesophageal reflux disease (GERD).

developing field of laparoscopy. The surgical indications that warrant an extraperitoneal approach in open surgery hold true for retroperitoneoscopy as well. As a minimally invasive technique, retroperitoneoscopy emulates the established standards and principles of open urologic procedures without compromising surgical efficiency and patient safety.

MINIMAL ACCESS LINX PROCEDURE

Northwestern Medicine has launched LINX®, a new laparoscopic procedure to treat gastroesophageal reflux disease (GERD). This procedure involves a string of metal beads that are drawn together by a magnet. When this string is placed around the lower esophagus, the magnet pulls the beads together and closes off the esophagus from the stomach. When the patient swallows, the beads separate to allow food to pass into the stomach. The magnet then draws the beads back together to keep acid from going up into the esophagus **(Fig. 29)**.

The success rate for LINX® is very high. Of the patients who undergo this procedure, 90–95% are able to stop taking medication completely and the remaining 5–10% rarely take medication. There are also several advantages to this procedure over the previous approaches used to treat GERD. Recovery time is typically quick, with patients commonly going home the same day. Patients are also encouraged to eat right away after the LINX® procedure, whereas previous surgical approaches have required patients to follow a liquid diet for up to 2 weeks.

MINIMAL ACCESS TRANSORAL INCISIONLESS FUNDOPLICATION PROCEDURE

The transoral incisionless fundoplication (TIF) is a minimally invasive treatment for GERD. The TIF procedure is performed from inside the patient's stomach without incisions. This procedure delivers patient outcomes similar to those provided by conventional antireflux surgical procedures, but is less invasive, has fewer adverse effects, and does not limit future treatment options. Following the principles of antireflux surgery for GERD, the TIF procedure repairs the antireflux barrier by reducing a hiatal hernia (≤2 cm) and creating a valve 2–4 cm in length and >270° circumferential wrap, thus restoring the dynamics of the angle of His **(Fig. 30)**.

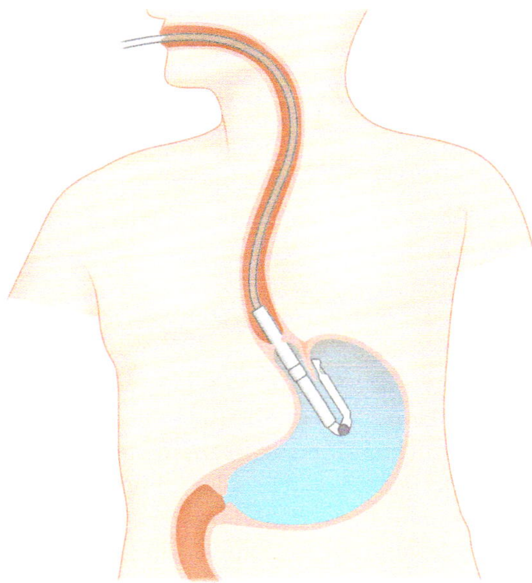

Fig. 30: Transoral incisionless fundoplication.

MINIMAL ACCESS NECK SURGERY

One of the newest frontiers is in minimally invasive soft-tissue surgery performed outside an established body cavity. The neck has been one of the soft tissue spaces of considerable interest and endoscopic or endoscopic-assisted techniques have recently been used to perform both thyroidectomy and parathyroidectomy. Several technical advances have facilitated the development of these new procedures, including the availability of balloon dilator for making artificial space, external lifts, ultrasonic coagulators, and smaller 2–3 mm diameter endoscopic instrumentation.

Background

In whole world, thyroidectomy and parathyroidectomy are the two most commonly performed endocrine surgical procedures. The most common indication for thyroidectomy is a solitary nodule that is not clearly benign on fine-needle biopsy. Parathyroidectomy is most commonly performed for primary hyperparathyroidism, in which a single enlarged gland or adenoma accounts for maximum number of cases. The principles of neck exploration for these two disorders are well established and the morbidity of operation is low when carried out by an experienced minimal access surgeon. Unlike many open abdominal operations, recovery is also rapid and most patients are discharged from the hospital the day after surgery and return to unlimited physical activity within fortnight.

Already many surgeons are attempting to perform thyroidectomy and parathyroidectomy through smaller and smaller open incisions to achieve better cosmetic results. However, as open incisions become smaller, surgical exposure, access, ease of dissection, and even safety may be compromised. Further evidence is that parathyroidectomy, for example, is viewed as an invasive procedure by patients and by referring endocrinologists is the reluctance of many individuals with asymptomatic or minimally symptomatic disease to undergo a definitive and curative operation, despite the cumulative risks of hyperparathyroidism over time, including osteoporosis and other metabolic sequelae.

In parathyroid surgery, there has also been interest in a focused, unilateral exploration of the neck rather than the accepted gold standard of bilateral neck exploration with identification and biopsy of all four parathyroids. Exploration of both sides of the neck avoids the problem of missed multiple adenomas or asymmetric hyperplasia, which can occur in up to 5–15% of cases and eliminates the need for preoperative localization studies. However, the advantages of unilateral neck exploration are that it results in less dissection and operative times are shorter. There may also be fewer injuries to the recurrent laryngeal nerve and the other parathyroid glands from leaving the contralateral neck undisturbed. Improvements in the accuracy of parathyroid imaging, such as ^{99m}Tc sestamibi scanning and intraoperative assessment of curative resection with the quick parathyroid hormone assay, have led to better outcomes from and wider application of the unilateral approach. These considerations become increasingly important in the current economic environment in health care.

Under these circumstances, minimal access approach to neck exploration may offer certain possible benefits, including improved visualization due to magnification, better cosmesis, less trauma to the neck musculature, less pain, and a more rapid recovery. Disadvantages of this approach might include longer operative times, increased hospital costs, possible risk of injury to the recurrent laryngeal nerve, potential tumor spillage, inability to localize the parathyroids, and adverse effects of neck insufflation. Consideration of an endoscopic approach to neck exploration, at the least, presents several challenges from an anatomic standpoint. Unlike the abdominal cavity, in which there is an easily distensible space for laparoscopy, the area that must be expanded and maintained to allow endoscopic access in the neck is composed of only potential spaces between soft tissue and muscle planes and the trachea. The thyroid and parathyroid glands are situated within the pretracheal space and are covered by the strap muscles anteriorly and laterally, which also limits exposure and access.

The absence of a discrete anatomic compartmental boundary in the neck adds further problems, if insufflation is used because of the potential for gaseous diffusion subcutaneously and into the mediastinum. The thyroid and parathyroids are also highly vascular structures and are intimately related to the recurrent laryngeal nerve and inferior thyroid artery. Further, the location of the parathyroids, especially the inferior glands, is often variable.

Several technologic advances have been necessary to facilitate the development of endoscopic neck exploration. Miniature 2–3 mm endoscopic instruments have been constructed suitable for smaller working space and the more delicate structures in the neck. Many balloon space maker devices have been invented, just like used in laparoscopic hernia repair, could be adapted to create a working space. Gasless laparoscopy has been used with mechanical lifts and retractors to maintain the working space and, thus, eliminate the need for insufflation of the neck. Ultrasonic coagulators and small clip appliers may be more appropriate for obtaining hemostasis in the neck rather than monopolar cautery. Endoscopic ultrasound also aids in intraoperative localization of the parathyroid adenoma, which is localized preoperatively by sestamibi scanning. These considerations led our group to first explore the possibility of an endoscopic approach to neck exploration in an experimental animal model.

Endoscopic Parathyroidectomy

Endoscopic parathyroidectomy in humans was first performed successfully by Gagner in 1995. The patient had familial hyperparathyroidism and initially presented with acute pancreatitis for which he required laparoscopic pancreaticojejunostomy with stone extraction as well as LC. A preoperative sestamibi scan showed four-gland uptake consistent with generalized parathyroid hyperplasia and a subtotal parathyroidectomy was performed endoscopically. Access to the neck was obtained with four 5 mm ports placed 1 cm above the clavicle and sternal notch. Exposure was achieved by insufflation of the subplatysmal space with 15 mm Hg^{2+} pressure, which was maintained throughout the operation. Operative time was 5 hours and intraoperatively, the patient experienced tachycardia and hypercarbia. Postoperatively, he had subcutaneous emphysema from the eyelids to the scrotum. He recovered uneventfully, however, and was discharged on the fourth postoperative day with a normal serum calcium level.

Since this initial report, endoscopic parathyroidectomy has been carried out by a small number of surgeons using either low-level gas insufflation of the neck or external retractors without CO_2 gas. Gagner has excised parathyroid adenomas in several cases, but uses a lower CO_2 insufflation pressure (7–10 mm Hg^{2+}) to reduce the adverse effects of this technique. Duluq has also successfully performed endoscopic parathyroidectomy in several patients with low-level (7 mm Hg^{2+}) CO_2 insulation for exposure. Norman and Albrink attempted parathyroidectomy in four patients after preoperative localization with sestamibi imaging. Initial access to the pretracheal space was achieved via a 1.5-cm incision, but CO_2 at a low insulation pressure (8 mm Hg^{2+}) was used to maintain a working space. Although the parathyroid adenoma was visualized in three of the four cases, endoscopic excision was successful in only two patients and only one normal parathyroid was identified out of these four explorations. At the conclusion of the endoscopic procedure, all patients were converted to open exploration via a 3.5-cm incision, through which the ipsilateral remaining parathyroids, both normal and adenomatous, were identified and either biopsied or removed. Postoperatively, there was subcutaneous air in the anterior neck, but no other sequela of CO_2 insulation was noted.

We recently performed endoscopic parathyroidectomy in two patients with primary hyperparathyroidism using a gasless technique. Preoperative localization of the parathyroid adenoma was carried out with ^{99m}Tc sestamibi scanning, which identified abnormal uptake in the left neck of both patients. Following the induction of general anesthesia, the parathyroid adenoma was more precisely localized with transcutaneous ultrasound and in each case was posterior to the thyroid lobe. A 1.5-cm incision was then made at the sternal notch and the strap muscles were divided in the midline to enter the pretracheal space under direct vision. In the first patient, a modified space maker balloon was inserted into this space and inflated to 60 mL volume. After removal of the balloon, a working space was maintained with a handheld S-shaped retractor. The strap muscles were further separated from the left lobe of the thyroid and the thyroid was retracted medially with a Babcock clamp placed through the open insertion site. Endoscopic visualization was achieved with a 3-mm 30° arthroscope. Two 4-mm ports were placed in the neck anterior to the sternocleidomastoid muscle.

A normal inferior parathyroid was identified and biopsied and the adenoma was localized to the superior position with the aid of laparoscopic ultrasound. The enlarged gland was posterior to the thyroid lobe and wedged between two branches of the inferior thyroid artery and the recurrent laryngeal nerve, which led to a lengthy and tedious dissection. Excision was accomplished by blunt dissection with 3 mm endoscopic instruments and the ultrasonic scalpel. Small Ligaclips placed through the open insertion site were used to ligate the vascular pedicle. The second patient was approached in a similar fashion, but a small lift ring attached to a mechanical retractor was used to maintain exposure. A left superior adenoma was removed that weighed 1.7 g. The recurrent laryngeal nerve and inferior thyroid artery were identified during the dissection, but it is difficult to locate the inferior parathyroid despite careful examination of the region of the thyrothymic ligament. Total operative time in our two patients has averaged approximately 4 hours. Exposure was suboptimal at times due to the small space and there was difficulty in retracting the strap muscles laterally and the thyroid gland medially. Very small amounts of bleeding or fluid accumulation obscured the operative field and required frequent sponging through the open insertion site. Manipulation and retraction of the parathyroid with the small instruments was sometimes difficult as well. Parathyroid tissue was confirmed in all specimens and serum calcium levels have been normal postoperatively.

Miccoli used an endoscopic-assisted approach in approximately 20 patients. Handheld retractors are used to maintain exposure and the dissection has been carried out with one or two lateral ports. A brief period of insufflation is used initially to aid in expanding the pretracheal space, but the remainder of the operation is carried out, with gasless retraction. Preliminary results have been favorable, but not all patients have had a normal ipsilateral parathyroid identified. Confirmation of successful excision of the parathyroid adenoma was made intraoperatively with use of the quick parathyroid hormone assay.

Alternatives to Endoscopic Parathyroidectomy

Minimally invasive or less invasive approaches to parathyroidectomy have been described recently that do not require endoscopic techniques or instrumentation. Norman and Chheda performed parathyroidectomy through a minimal 2–3 cm open incision after precise preoperative localization of the adenoma with sestamibi imaging. The technique used for parathyroid localization is analogous to that used for sentinel node mapping with radiolymphoscintigraphy. The ^{99m}Tc sestamibi scanning is carried out 3 hours prior to surgical exploration. The operation is then directed with an 11-mm Neoprobe, which is used to scan and quantitate radioactivity in all four quadrants of the neck. A 2–3 cm incision is made over the site of maximal gamma activity and the adenoma is excised through this minimal incision. The authors have used this technique in 14 patients, 13 of whom had adenomas and one who was correctly predicted to have parathyroid hyperplasia. The adenomas were located operatively on average in just 19 minutes. Nine cases were carried out under local anesthesia and 11 (79%) patients were discharged the same day as surgery. Serum calcium levels were normal postoperatively and there were no operative complications. This approach is potentially very attractive because it requires minimal dissection and can be carried out under local anesthesia as strictly as outpatient procedure. Both operative and recovery times should be short, which may result in lower hospital costs, despite the use of preoperative scintigraphic localization. Frozen section examination by pathology may also become unnecessary if, after excision, all radioactivity is confined to the resected specimen. The limitations of this approach currently are that neither the ipsilateral parathyroid nor the recurrent laryngeal nerves have been routinely identified in these dissections. Further, the accuracy of "sentinel" mapping of the parathyroid adenoma must be confirmed by other investigators.

Thoracoscopic Parathyroidectomy

Video-assisted thoracoscopy should be considered as an alternative to median sternotomy in patients with ectopic mediastinal parathyroid adenomas. Prim and coworkers reported the use of thoracoscopic techniques to successfully excise mediastinal parathyroids in four patients with persistent hyperparathyroidism after failed cervical exploration. All glands were localized preoperatively by a combination of radionuclide scintigraphy and CT scan. The location of the abnormal glands in these four cases included the aortopulmonary window, near the ascending aorta, the aortic arch, and the region of the main pulmonary artery. Three thoracoscopic ports were used, including a 10-mm initial access port placed in the midaxillary line at the 6th intercostal space. Operative times averaged 3.25 hours and all patients became normocalcemic postoperatively, although one patient with secondary hyperparathyroidism developed recurrent hypercalcemia 9 months after surgery. A subxiphoid laparoscopic approach has also been used to excise a mediastinal parathyroid adenoma, but this technique would appear to provide access to glands in the anterior mediastinum only.

Endoscopic Thyroidectomy

Endoscopic excision of the thyroid is more technically demanding because of the more complex blood supply and the intimate relationship of the thyroid gland to the recurrent laryngeal nerve. A lateral approach is used in which three laparoscopic trocars are placed in the subplatysmal space along the anterior border of the sternocleidomastoid muscle from the jugular notch to the angle of the mandible. Both low pressure CO_2 and a wall lifter inserted at the jugular trocar site are used to maintain a working space. Division of the strap muscles is necessary to access the thyroid. The thyroid vessels are divided with clips and an ultrasonic dissector is used to dissect the thyroid from the recurrent laryngeal nerve. In addition, both parathyroids are identified and preserved as is the external branch of the superior laryngeal nerve.

Conclusion

Early experience with endoscopic neck exploration prevents any definitive conclusions about its role in the management of patients with either hyperparathyroidism or thyroid disorders. Published experiences have to date been limited to small case reports and results and outcomes have not been reported in detail. The minimally invasive open approach of "sentinel" parathyroidectomy reported by Norman and Chheda has much to commend it, including accurate localization, rapid operative times, and improved cosmesis, and it is an outpatient operation that can be performed under local anesthesia.

Although the laparoscope provides optical magnification of important neurovascular structures, including the recurrent laryngeal nerve, better methods for exposure, and retraction of the strap muscles and thyroid, it would greatly facilitate visualization and dissection. Improved instruments are needed that allow safe manipulation of the parathyroid to lower the risk of parathyroid rupture as well as to speed the operative dissection. Suction and irrigation devices designed specifically for small spaces such as the neck would help maintain a dry operative field. Surgeons will also need flexibility in the exposure and operative approach to deal successfully with variations in parathyroid anatomy.

Patient selection should be careful for endoscopic approach until there is further experience and improved operative technique. Individuals, who are obese, have a nodular goiter, have had previous neck surgery, or who are likely to have generalized parathyroid hyperplasia, should not be considered as a good candidate for an endoscopic exploration. Despite these limitations and challenges, the search for less invasive means for performing neck exploration will undoubtedly continue and has already led to renewed interest in a unilateral operative approach in patients with primary hyperparathyroidism.

MINIMAL ACCESS SURGERY IN ORTHOPEDIC SURGERY

Introduction

Conventional (open) methods result in high amount of morbidity. To reduce the morbidity during the secondary injury, i.e., the surgical procedures while opening to reach the site of pathology, encourage the clinician to use the MAS or endoscopic techniques in orthopedic surgery. MAS with endoscope in orthopedic practice is useful in the following fields:

- Arthroscopic surgery in sports-related injuries and other pathologies in shoulder, elbow, wrist, hip, knee, foot, and ankle
- Arthroscopic-assisted surgery in orthopedic trauma
- Spine surgery
- Benign bone tumors.

Arthroscopy is a minimally invasive surgical procedure in which a physical examination of the interior of a joint is performed using an arthroscope, a type of endoscope that is inserted into the joint through a small incision. The advantage of arthroscopy over traditional open procedures is that the joint does not have to be opened up fully and surgery is performed with two small incisions—one for the arthroscope and other for the surgical instruments. This reduces the recovery time for the patient and may increase the rate of surgical success due to lesser trauma to the connective tissue. It is especially useful for professional athletes, who frequently injure joints and require faster healing. There is also less scarring because of the smaller incisions. In procedures where endoscope or arthroscope is used, the advantage increases manifold by providing magnified view. The advantages of magnification and minimal scarring are extended also to the management of fracture fixation, carpal tunnel release at wrist joint, and spinal surgeries. As technology becomes more and more advanced, a greater number of minimally invasive surgical interventions have evolved. With the increase in proficiency of arthroscopic or endoscopic surgery, surgeons are now using the same technique for intramedullary lesion and tumor surgery also.

BOX 1: The benefits of minimal access surgery (MAS) in orthopedics.

- Less painful
- Faster rehabilitation
- Better visualization of the pathology
- Shorter hospital stay
- Cheaper (long term)
- Esthetic
- More precise

Clinical effectiveness of MAS procedures over open procedures was proven beyond doubt. Hundreds of controlled randomized trials of procedures using the MAS techniques were published in the 1970s and 1980s. The advantages of MAS over conventional open surgery are listed in **Box 1**.

In an era of rising healthcare costs, MAS offers a significant economic advantage over conventional open surgery. Decreased hospital time, decreased rehabilitation time, and a rapid return to normal activities all add up to a significant "savings" in economic and social costs. Many surgical procedures require a combination of both minimal invasive and open techniques. Therefore, the use of MAS must be tempered with knowledge of its limitations.

History

Medical endoscopy for internal organs has begun in the early 1800s by Bozzini. In 1918, Prof Kenji Takagi reported the arthroscopic examination in cadaveric knee at Tokyo University with the cystoscope. Dr Eugen Bircher was the first to perform and publish the first arthroscopy on live patients to diagnose tuberculosis. Initially, internal examination was done by direct visualization through the eyepiece till the advent of fiberoptic light source and camera. On the other hand, the surgical skills in arthroscopy surgery have improved with fine instrumentation. Since, then the developments in arthroscopy have become manifold.

As with any other surgical technique, arthroscopic surgery continues to evolve, improvements in fiberoptics, video reproduction, and miniaturization, it will enhance and widen its application. During the past two decades, arthroscopic procedures have been replacing traditional, more invasive orthopedic surgical procedures. Today arthroscopy is being done in almost all joints. High performance athletes need a minimal surgical exposure for a faster recovery and quick return to the field with very minimal morbidity. Recently, training simulators (virtual reality) have come into vogue to teach the skills necessary for arthroscopy, especially the knee.

ARTHROSCOPIC SURGERY IN SPORTS-RELATED INJURIES AND OTHER PATHOLOGY

Knee Joint

Diagnosis

Knee arthroscopy, with the advantage of direct and magnified view inside joint, makes it an excellent diagnostic tool. Its diagnostic accuracy rate of 95% has considerable advantages as compared with the 75% accuracy rate of clinical evaluation alone. The high sensitivity of MRI for arthroscopically remediable lesions in cases of internal derangement of the knee indicates that it could be used as a screening test before arthroscopy. Comparison of magnetic resonance imaging and arthroscopy confirmed the higher accuracy of magnetic resonance imaging in the diagnosis of internal derangement, but the results for articular cartilage lesions were much less good. Intra-articular fracture, chondral injury, and meniscal and ligamentous injuries (partial or complete) can be diagnosed and treated simultaneously.

Trauma

Anatomic reduction, typically obtained by direct visualization through an arthrotomy and internal fixation (open reduction and internal fixation), is the traditional treatment method for displaced intra-articular condylar fractures of the distal femur and proximal tibia. Arthroscopic-assisted reduction and internal fixation, of a displaced, malrotated intra-articular fracture fragment involving the tibia or femur, have benefits of decreased blood loss, shortened operative time, excellent intra-articular visualization, decreased soft-tissue dissection, and shortened postoperative recovery.

Ligamentous Injury

In acute ligamentous injuries, arthroscopy has limited or no role for repair of these ligamentous structures. Once the acute stage subsides, the ligamentous structures can be reinforced or reconstructed. Arthroscopic-assisted ligamentous reconstruction is the gold standard treatment for ruptured ligament.

Meniscal Injury

Meniscal injury is caused due to meniscal tear.

Chondral Injury

According to recent research, up to 10–12% of individuals present with chondral injuries. When symptomatic, chondral lesions manifest as swelling and knee pain. The loss of cartilage may be partial or complete and it may affect one or multiple locations. Nonsurgical treatment modalities include analgesics, knee brace, and physiotherapy. Surgical treatment varies from arthroscopic debridement to implantation of autologous chondrocytes beneath a periosteal patch covering the lesion. Autologous chondrocyte transplantation has a durable outcome for as long as 11 years.

Osteoarthritis

Arthroscopic debridement in early osteoarthritic patients may provide early symptomatic relief to pain. The long-term results are comparable with conservative management.

Hip Joint

Hip arthroscopy is technically demanding, with a steep learning curve, and requires special distraction tools and operating equipment. Access to the hip joint is difficult because of the resistance to distraction resulting from the large muscular envelope, the strength of the iliofemoral ligament, and the negative intra-articular pressure. This operation should not be done without specific education in its methods. Hip arthroscopy allows thorough visualization of the acetabular labrum, femoral head, and acetabular chondral surfaces as well as of the fovea, ligamentum teres, and adjacent synovium. Microsurgical tools developed specifically for arthroscopic hip surgery can be used to provide the least intrusive means of diagnosis and treatment of conditions involving the above mentioned structures (**Box 2**).

No radiographic study, including high-contrast gadolinium-enhanced arthrography and magnetic resonance imaging, is entirely sensitive or specific for the diagnosis of labral tears or chondral lesions. Thus, a high level of clinical suspicion based on the patient's symptoms and positive physical findings is paramount for the clinician to recognize subtle abnormalities in the hip joint.

BOX 2: Indications for hip arthroscopy.

- Labral tears
- Loose bodies
- Acetabular and femoral head chondral flap lesions
- Foreign body removal
- Synovial chondromatosis
- Collagen diseases with impinging synovitis
- Crystalline hip arthropathies
- Ruptured or impinging ligamentum teres
- Capsular shrinkage (Ehlers–Danlos syndrome)
- Posttraumatic conditions (e.g., Pipkin fracture)
- After total hip arthroplasty
- Osteonecrosis (early stages prior to collapse)
- Extra-articular conditions

Ankle Joint

The advantages and experiences of arthroscopy in large joints were extended to the small joints such as ankle and wrist. Arthroscopy of the ankle is a relatively new discipline but has in recent years been increasingly applied to the diagnostic and therapeutic treatment of ankle disorders. Indications for arthroscopy in ankle joint are given in **Box 3**.

About 30° wide angles, 2.7 mm arthroscope with a 3.5-mm shaver is used for ankle joint. Ankle joint is also distended, maximum up to 50 mm Hg pressure with the help of pump. To distract the ankle joint, ankle strap can also be used for manual traction. Standard portals are anteromedial, medial to the tibialis and anterior tendon, and located about 5 mm proximal to the medial malleolus and anterolateral, just lateral to the peroneus tertius tendon. Initial arthroscopy is performed with the scope in the anteromedial portal, but for the majority of the case, this portal will be used for instrumentation. Possible complications with anterior approach are injury to greater saphenous nerve and vein and injury to the dorsal lateral branch of the peroneal nerve.

Recent studies suggest that, with the patient in the prone position, arthroscopic equipment may be introduced into the posterior aspect of the ankle without gross injury to the posterior neurovascular structures.

Shoulder Joint

The shoulder joint is well encapsulated with muscular covering throughout its circumference. Open surgical procedures lead to bleeding and high morbidity; hence, minimal access procedures are preferred with the use of arthroscope. Indications for shoulder arthroscopy are enumerated in **Box 4**.

Beach chair position is comfortable for both the patient and the surgeon as it allows free access to shoulder joint and the option of converting to an open procedure. Standard portals for shoulder joint are posterior, anterior, and lateral.

BOX 3: Indications for ankle arthroscopy.

- *Soft tissue*:
  - Soft-tissue impingement
  - Synovitis (diagnosis and biopsy)
  - Arthrofibrosis
- Osteochondral defect of the talus
- Intra-articular fracture and occult intra-articular injury
- Arthrodesis of ankle joint

BOX 4: Indications for shoulder arthroscopy.

- *Soft tissue*:
  - Soft-tissue impingement
  - Synovitis (diagnosis and biopsy)
  - Arthroscopic-assisted lysis of adhesion
- Arthroscopic subacromial decompression (ASAD) and acromioplasty
- Arthroscopic reconstruction (Bankart lesion repair and slap lesions)

Complication for shoulder arthroscopy and its position are brachial plexus strain and hypoglossal nerve injury.

Elbow Joint

Arthroscopic surgery for elbow joint is still in primitive stage and limited to arthroscopic synovectomy. Arthroscopic synovectomy is a reliable procedure to alleviate pain in early grades of rheumatoid arthritis. The fundamental of arthroscopy is visualization and access. Visualization and access to the ulnohumeral and radiocapitellar articulation are rather difficult. Recent study has come out with a joint jack to widen the ulnohumeral joint space to work better posteriorly.

Wrist Joint

Wrist arthroscopy is the third most common joint after knee and shoulder joint to be examined by arthroscope.

MINIMAL ACCESS SURGERY IN ORTHOPEDIC TRAUMA

Opening of the fracture site during exposure further jeopardize the vascularity at the fracture site, which adversely effects the healing at the fracture site. The involvement of intra-articular fracture needs minimal tissue stripping to further jeopardize the vascularity. This principle leads to the foundation of the minimal access surgical principle in orthopedic trauma surgery. This principle helps to maintain the biology around the fracture site, so this fixation is also known as biological fixation. Biological fixation or MAS is extremely useful at the site of fractures with comminution or areas with doubtful vascularity.

SPINE SURGERY AND ARTHROSCOPY

Spinal surgeries are thought to be risky due to the vicinity of the important structures and high vascularity (venous plexus) around the spine. The conventional (open) exposure to reach the site of pathology needs wide exposure, which, in turn, leads to large amount of morbidity and prolongs the period of recovery, especially in the thoracic spine surgeries. The advantage of endoscopy such as precision, magnification, and small incision for exposure has lead to the endoscopic spinal surgery to the great advantage than conventional open procedure.

The endoscope allows the surgeon to use a "keyhole" incision to access the herniated disk. Muscle and tissue are dilated rather than being cut when accessing the disk. This leads to less tissue destruction, less postoperative pain, quicker recovery times, earlier rehabilitation, and avoidance of general anesthesia. Thermal annuloplasty is an adjunctive procedure that uses bipolar electrothermal energy (radiofrequency and/or laser) to ablate or depopulate the sensitized pain nociceptors in the annulus, ablate any inflammatory/granulation tissue that has grown into the annulus, and to shrink and tighten the stretched or torn collagen fibers of the annulus.

Scoliosis is a three-dimensional problem. The aim of surgery is to try to restore the normal contour of the back from both the front view and the side view. A technique to assist in getting a maximum of correction with a minimum of scar and morbidity by releasing the contacted anterior tissue with the use of the endoscope to go into the chest (similar to the way surgeon stakes out gallbladders now) in front where the actual vertebra is and take out the disks in front, thus relaxing up the spine so we can get better correction and the fusion in back. This method goes in through the chest using three or four small incisions to reach the front of the spine. Once inside the chest, the spine is clearly visible and "soft" tissues can be cleaned off exposing the spine. The disks are easily seen and can be removed.

BONE ENDOSCOPY AND TUMORS

With the increasing experience of seeing inside the soft cavities such as joint, the same arthroscope is now used to see inside the bony cavities. The initial results are equal than the open surgical procedure with added advantages of minimal invasive, no immobilization, quick hospital discharge, minimal chances of pathological fracture, and very small surgical scar. This is especially useful for benign cystic lesion of bone such as giant cell tumor, simple bone cyst, or enchondroma. With the endoscopic technique, curettage of the cystic lesion and filling of the cavity by morselized autologous bone or bone cement can be done effectively. This minimal invasive technique allows the lesion to heal at much faster rate and with minimal scaring. This technique is being in practice for the management of these cystic lesions in soft bones or in cancellous bones.

BIBLIOGRAPHY

1. Abbou CC, Cicco A, Gasman D, Hoznek A, Antiphon P, Chopin DK, et al. Retroperitoneal laparoscopic versus open radical nephrectomy. J Urol. 1999;161(6):1776-80.
2. Abolyosr A. Laparoscopic versus open orchidopexy in the management of abdominal testis: a descriptive study. Int J Urol. 2006;13(11):1421-4.
3. American Society of Anesthesiologists. New classification of physical status. Anesthesiology. 1963;24(1):111.
4. Ashton RC, McGinnis KM, Connery CP, Swistel DG, Ewing DR, DeRose JJ. Totally endoscopic robotic thymectomy for myasthenia gravis. Ann Thorac Surg. 2003;75(2):569-71.
5. Azagra JS, Goergen M, Gilbart E, Jacobs D. Laparoscopic anatomical (hepatic) left lateral segmentectomy—technical aspects. Surg Endosc. 1996;10(7):758-61.
6. Baba S, Ito K, Yanaihara H, Nagata H, Murai M, Iwamura M. Retroperitoneoscopic adrenalectomy by a lumbodorsal approach: clinical experience with solo surgery. Word J Urol. 1999;17(4):54-8.
7. Berkmen F, Alagol H. Germinal cell tumors of the testis in cryptorchids. J Exp Clin Cancer Res. 1998;17(4):409-12.
8. Bisgaard T, Klarskov B, Trap R, Kehlet H, Rosenberg J. Pain after microlaparoscopic cholecystectomy. A randomized double-blind controlled study. Surg Endosc. 2000;14(6):340-4.
9. Bode CO, Nwawolo CC, Giwa-Osagie OF. Surgical education at the West African College of Surgeons. World J Surg. 2008;32(6):2162-6.
10. Carmignani L, Morabito A, Gadda F, Bozzini G, Rocco F, Colpi GM. Prognostic parameters in adult impalpable ultrasonographic lesions of the testicle. J Urol. 2005;174(30):1035-8.
11. Chandrasekharam VVSS. Laparoscopy vs inguinal exploration for the nonpalpable undescended testis. Indian J Pediatr. 2005;72(12):1021-3.
12. Charny CK, Jarnagin WR, Schwartz LH, Frommeyer HS, DeMatteo RP, Fong Y, et al. Management of 155 patients with benign liver tumors. Br J Surg. 2001;88(6):808-13.
13. Cheah WK, Lenzi JE, So JB, Kum CK, Goh PM. Randomized trial of needlescopic versus laparoscopic cholecystectomy. Br J Surg. 2001;88(5):45-7.
14. Cherqui D, Husson E, Hammoud R, Malassagne B, Stéphan D, Bensaid S, et al. Laparoscopic liver resections: a feasibility study in 30 patients. Ann Surg. 2000;232(6):753-62.
15. Cherqui D, Rahmouni A, Charlotte F, Boulahdour H, Métreau JM, Meignan M, et al. Management of focal nodular hyperplasia and hepatocellular adenoma in young women: a series of 41 patients with clinical, radiological, and pathological correlations. Hepatology. 1995;22(6):1674-81.
16. Cherqui D. Laparoscopic liver resection. Br J Surg. 2003;90(6): 644-6.
17. Cleary K, Nguyen C. State of the art in surgical robotics: clinical applications and technology challenges. Comput Aided Surg. 2001;6(6):312-28.
18. Cortes D, Thorup J, Visfeldt J. Multinucleated spermatogonia in cryptorchid boys: a possible association with an increased risk of testicular malignancy later in life? APMIS. 2003;111(1):25-30.
19. Cortez D, Thorup J, Peterson BL. Testicular neoplasia in undescended testes of cryptorchid boys—does surgical strategy have an impact on the risk of invasive testicular neoplasia? Turk J Pediatr. 2004;46 Suppl:35-42.
20. Corvin S, Sturm W, Anastasiadis A, Kuczyk M, Stenzl A. Laparoscopic management of adult nonpalpable testicle. Urol Int. 2005;75(4):337-9.
21. Cuschieri A, Shimi S, Banting S, Nathanson LK, Pietrabissa A. Intraoperative cholangiography during laparoscopic cholecystectomy. Routine vs selective policy. Surg Endosc. 1994; 8(4):302-5.
22. Delaunay L, Bonnet F, Cherqui D, Rimaniol JM, Dahan E, Atlan G. Laparoscopic cholecystectomy minimally impairs postoperative cardiorespiratory and muscle performance. Br J Surg. 1995;82(3):373-6.
23. DeRose JJ, Swistel DG, Safavi A, Connery CP, Ashton RC. Mediastinal mass evaluation using advanced robotic techniques. Ann Thorac Surg. 2003;75(6):571-3.
24. Desai CS, Prabhu RY, Supe AN. Laparoscopic orchidectomy for undescended testis in adults. J Postgrad Med. 2002;48(5):25-6.
25. Descottes B, Glineur D, Lachachi F, Valleix D, Paineau J, Hamy A, et al. Laparoscopic liver resection of benign liver tumors. Surg Endosc. 2003;17(1):23-30.
26. Descottes B, Lachachi F, Sodji M, Valleix D, Durand-Fontanier S, de Laclause BP, et al. Early experience with laparoscopic approach for solid liver tumors: initial 16 cases. Ann Surg. 2000;232(5):641-5.
27. Dunlap KD, Wanzer L. Is the robotic arm a cost-effective surgical tool? Assoc Oper Room Nurs J. 1998;68(4):265-72.
28. El-Anany F, Gad El-Moula M, Abdel Moneim A, AbdallahA, Takahashi M, Kanayama H, et al. Laparoscopy for impalpable testis: classification-based management. Surg Endosc. 2007; 21(3):449-545.
29. Elder JS. Ultrasonography is unnecessary in evaluating boys with a nonpalpable testis. Pediatrics. 2002;110(4):748-51.

30. Farges O, Jagot P, Kirstetter P, Marty J, Belghiti J. Prospective assessment of the safety and benefit of laparoscopic liver resections. J Hepatobiliary Pancreat Surg. 2002;9(2):242-8.
31. Farrer JH, Walker AH, Rajfer J. Management of the postpubertal cryptorchid testis: a statistical review. J Urol. 1985;134(4):1071-6.
32. Fong Y, Jarnagin W, Conlon KC, Dematteo R, Dougherty E, Blumgart LH. Hand-assisted laparoscopic liver resection. Arch Surg. 2000;135(7):854-9.
33. Ford TF, Parkinson MC, Pryor JP. The undescended testis in adult life. Br J Urol. 1985;57(2):181-4.
34. Gagner M, Rheault M, Dubuc J. Laparoscopic partial hepatectomy for liver tumor [abstract]. Surg Endosc. 1992;6(2):99.
35. Hamdorf JM, Hall JC. Acquiring surgical skills. Br J Surg. 2000;87(5):28-37.
36. Hrebinko RL, Bellinger MF. The limited role of imaging techniques in managing children with undescended testes. J Urol. 1993; 150(2 Pt 1):458-60.
37. Hüscher CG, Lirici MM, Chiodini S. Laparoscopic liver resections. Semin Laparosc Surg. 1998;5(3):204-10.
38. IHPBA Brisbane 2000 terminology of liver anatomy and resections. HPB Surg. 2000;2(3):333-9.
39. Ivanov A, Dewey C, Fahlenkamp D, Luning M. MRT in nonpalpable testes. Rofo. 1994;160(3):249-53.
40. Jarnagin WR, Gonen M, Fong Y, DeMatteo RP, Ben-Porat L, Little S, et al. Improvement in perioperative outcome after hepatic resection: analysis of 1,803 consecutive cases over the past decade. Ann Surg. 2002;236(4):397-406.
41. Kammula US, Buell JF, Labow DM, Rosen S, Millis JM, Posner MC. Surgical management of benign tumors of the liver. Int J Gastrointest Cancer. 2001;30(3):141-6.
42. Kaneko H, Takagi S, Shiba T. Laparoscopic partial hepatectomy and left lateral segmentectomy: technique and results of a clinical series. Surgery. 1996;120(3):468-75.
43. Katkhouda N, Hurwitz M, Gugenheim J, Mavor E, Mason RJ, Waldrep DJ, et al. Laparoscopic management of benign solid and cystic lesions of the liver. Ann Surg. 1999;229(4):460-6.
44. Kavoussi LR, Moore RG, Adams JB, Partin AW. Comparison of robotic versus human laparoscopic camera control. J Urol. 1995;154(6):2134-6.
45. Kneebone R, ApSimon D. Surgical skills training: simulation and multimedia combined. Med Educ. 2001;35(9):909-15.
46. Kondraske GV, Hamilton EC, Scott DJ, Fischer CA, Tesfay ST, Taneja R, et al. Surgeon workload and motion efficiency with robot and human laparoscopic camera control. Surg Endosc. 2002;16(6):1523-7.
47. Kucheria R, Sahai A, Sami TA, Challacombe B, Godbole H, Khan MS, et al. Laparoscopic management of cryptorchidism in adults. Eur Urol. 2005;48(3):453-7.
48. Laurent A, Cherqui D, Lesurtel M, Brunetti F, Tayar C, Fagniez PL. Laparoscopic liver resection for subcapsular hepatocellular carcinoma complicating chronic liver disease. Arch Surg. 2003;138(7):763-9.
49. Le Bartz G, Petit T, Ravasse P. Is there any interest to perform ultrasonography in boys with undescended testis? Arch Pediatr. 2006;13(5):426-8.
50. Leggett PL, Churchman-Winn R, Miller R. Minimizing ports to improve laparoscopic cholecystectomy. Surg Endosc. 2000;14(7):32-6.
51. Lesurtel M, Cherqui D, Laurent A, Tayar C, Fagniez PL. Laparoscopic versus open left lateral hepatic lobectomy: a case-control study. J Am Coll Surg. 2003;196(2):236-42.
52. Leung KF, Lee KW, Cheung TY, Leung LC, Lau KW. Laparoscopic cholecystectomy: two-port technique. Endoscopy. 1996;6(4):505-7.
53. Lomanto D, De Angelis L, Ceci V, Dalsasso G, So J, Frattaroli FM, et al. Two-trocar laparoscopic cholecystectomy: a reproducible technique. Surg Laparosc Endosc Percutan Tech. 2001;11(4):248-51.
54. Mcheik JN, Levard G. Laparoscopic treatment of the nonpalpable testis. Results. Prog Urol. 2002;12(2):294-7.
55. Menconi GF, Melfi FAM, Givigliano F, Angeletti CA. Robotic pulmonary lobectomy: early operative experience and preliminary clinical results. Eur Surg. 2002;34(5):173-6.
56. Merola S, Weber P, Wasielewski A, Ballantyne GH. Comparison of laparoscopic colectomy with and without the aid of a robotic camera holder. Surg Laparosc Endosc Percutan Tech. 2002;12(6):46-51.
57. Moher D, Schulz KF, Altman DG. The CONSORT statement: revised recommendations for improving the quality of reports of parallel-group randomised trials. Lancet. 2001;357(6):1191-4.
58. Morgan JA, Thornton BA, Peacock JC, Hollingsworth KW, Smith CR, Oz MC, et al. Does robotic technology make minimally invasive cardiac surgery too expensive? A hospital cost analysis of robotic and conventional techniques. J Card Surg. 2005;20(4):246-51.
59. Morino M, Morra I, Rosso E, Miglietta C, Garrone C. Laparoscopic vs open hepatic resection: a comparative study. Surg Endosc. 2003;17(12):1914-8.
60. Nijs SM, Eijsbouts SW, Madern GC, Leyman PM, Lequin MH, Hazebroek FW. Nonpalpable testes: is there a relationship between ultrasonographic and operative findings? Pediatr Radiol. 2007;37(4):374-9.
61. Panait L, Doarn CR, Merrell RC. Applications of robotics in surgery. Chirurgia (Bucur). 2002;97(5):549-55.
63. Perniceni T, Slim K. What are the validated indications for laparoscopy in digestive surgery? Gastroenterol Clin Biol. 2001;25(4 Suppl):B57-70.
63. Poon CM, Chan KW, Ko CW, Chan KC, Lee DW, Cheung HY, et al. Two-port laparoscopic cholecystectomy: initial results of a modified technique. J Laparoendosc Adv Surg Tech A. 2002;12(5):259-62.
64. Poon RT, Fan ST, Lo CM, Liu CL, Lam CM, Yuen WK, et al. Improving perioperative outcome expands the role of hepatectomy in management of benign and malignant hepatobiliary diseases: analysis of 1222 consecutive patients from a prospective database. Ann Surg. 2004;240(4):698-710.
65. Raina V, Shukla NK, Gupta NP, Deo S, Rath GK. Germ cell tumours in uncorrected cryptorchid testis at Institute Rotary Cancer Hospital, New Delhi. Br J Cancer. 1995;71(2):380-2.
66. Ramachandran CS, Arora V. Two-port laparoscopic cholecystectomy: an innovative new method for gallbladder removal. J Laparoendosc Adv Surg Tech A. 1998;8(3):303-8.
67. Rangarajan M, Jayakar SM. Laparoscopic orchidectomy for the adult impalpable testis—experiences in a rural teaching hospital. Surg Endosc. 2007;21(1):66-9.
68. Rodriguez MDA, Freire AU, Orpez AR, Lorenzo CG. Diagnostic and therapeutic laparoscopy for nonpalpable testis. Surg Endosc. 2003;17(11):1756-8.
69. Rau HG, Buttler E, Meyer G, Schardey HM, Schildberg FW. Laparoscopic liver resection compared with conventional partial hepatectomy—a prospective analysis. Hepatogastroenterology. 1998;45(24):2333-8.
70. Ruurda JP, Hanlo PW, Hennipman A, Broeders IA. Robot-assisted thoracoscopic resection of a benign mediastinal neurogenic tumor: technical note. Neurosurgery. 2003;52(4):462-4.
71. Satar N, Bayazit Y, Doran S. Laparoscopy in the management of impalpable testicle. Acta Chir Belg. 2005;105(6):662-6.
72. Shin D, Lemack GE, Goldstein M. Induction of spermatogenesis and pregnancy after adult orchiopexy. J Urol. 1997;158(6):2242.
73. Siemer S, Humke U, Hildebrandt U, Karadiakos N, Ziegler M. Diagnosis of nonpalpable testes in childhood: comparison of magnetic resonance imaging and laparoscopy in a prospective study. Eur J Pediatr Surg. 2000;10(2):114-8.

74. Soper NJ, Brunt LM, Kerbl K. Laparoscopic general surgery. N Engl J Med. 1994;330(6):409-19.
75. Soper NJ, Dunnegan DL. Routine versus selective intra-operative cholangiography during laparoscopic cholecystectomy. World J Surg. 1992;16(6):1133-40.
76. Terkivatan T, de Wilt JH, de Man RA, van Rijn RR, Zondervan PE, Tilanus HW, et al. Indications and long-term outcome of treatment for benign hepatic tumors: a critical appraisal. Arch Surg. 2001;136(9):1033-8.
77. Vibert E, Perniceni T, Levard H, Denet C, Shahri NK, Gayet B. Laparoscopic liver resection. Br J Surg. 2006;93(1):67-72.
78. Waseem T. Technologic advances in robotic surgery. J Coll Physicians Surg Pak. 2005;15(9):559-61.
79. Weimann A, Ringe B, Klempnauer J, Lamesch P, Gratz KF, Prokop M, et al. Benign liver tumors: differential diagnosis and indications for surgery. World J Surg. 1997;21(9):983-90.
80. Welvaart K, Tijssen JGP. Management of the undescended testis in relation to the development of cancer. J Surg Oncol. 2006;173(4):219-23.
81. Wolverson MK, Houttuin E, Heiberg E, Sundaram M, Shields JB. Comparison of computed tomography with high-resolution real-time ultrasound in the localization of the impalpable undescended testis. Radiology. 1983;146(1):133-6.
82. Yoshino I, Hashizume M, Shimada M, Tomikawa M, Tomiyasu M, Suemitsu R, et al. Thoracoscopic thymomectomy with the da Vinci computer-enhanced surgical system. J Thorac Cardiovasc Surg. 2001;122(5):783-5.

CHAPTER 44 Minimal Access Bariatric Surgery

INTRODUCTION

Obesity has become an epidemic. Over 36% of the population of the USA is morbidly obese. Since 1980, the incidence of morbid obesity has quadrupled. Obesity is now the second leading cause of preventable death. Morbid obesity is responsible for approximately >500,000 deaths per year. 14% of all cancer deaths in men and 20% of all cancer deaths in women are due to morbid obesity. Current definition of obesity is body mass index (BMI): Weight (kg)/Height (m^2).

- Normal weight—BMI ≥ 18.5–24.9 kg/m^2
- Overweight—BMI ≥ 25–29.9 kg/m^2
- Obesity—BMI ≥ 30 kg/m^2
- Morbid obesity—BMI ≥ 40 kg/m^2 (or ≥35 kg/m^2 in the presence of comorbidities)
- Supermorbid obesity—BMI ≥ 50 kg/m^2

Obesity results into many comorbidities, which ultimately leads to early death. Most of the comorbidities are shown in **Figure 1**.

LAPAROSCOPIC TREATMENT FOR MORBID OBESITY

Indications of surgical treatment of obesity are:

- Body mass index of 35 kg/m^2 or over with any comorbidity
- Body mass index of 40 kg/m^2 or greater without comorbidity

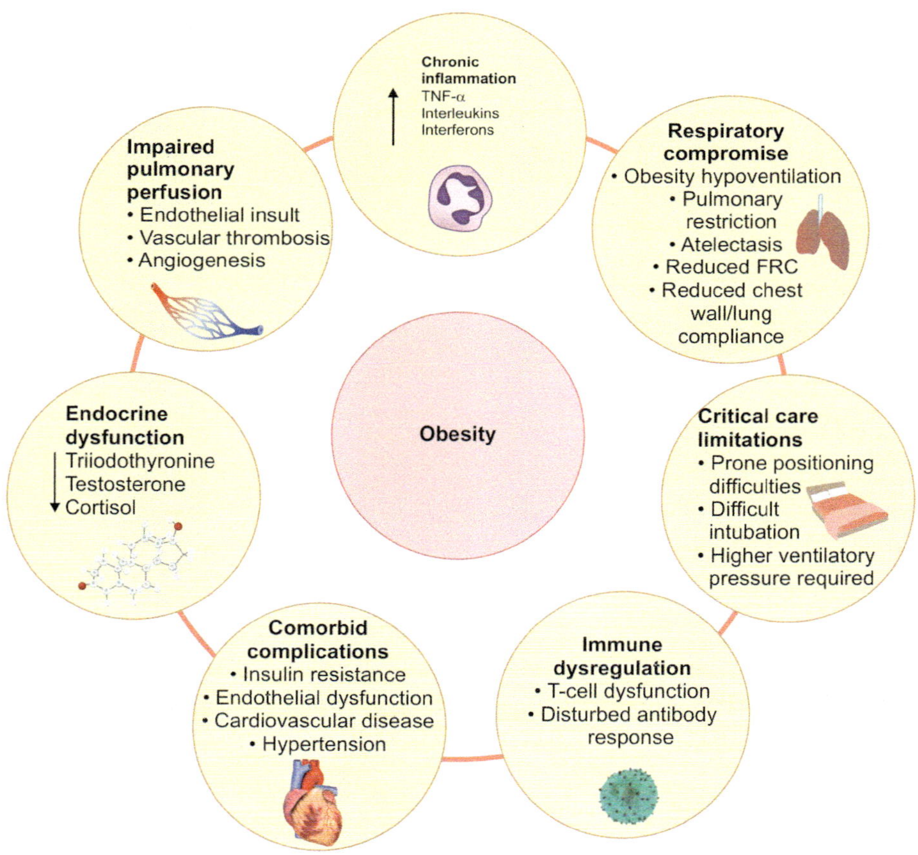

Fig. 1: Obesity-related diseases.
(FRC: functional residual capacity; TNF-α: tumor necrosis factor-α)

- Traditionally, age should be 18–60-year-old
- Nonendocrine-related cause of obesity
- Patients dedicated to permanent lifestyle changes and long-term follow-up

There are many types of surgical option available to treat morbid obesity, most common are:

- *Restrictive procedures*:
  - Lap-Band
  - Vertical-banded gastroplasty (VBG)
  - Sleeve gastrectomy/Gastric plication
- *Malabsorptive procedure*:
  - Jejunoileal (JI) bypass
- *Combination procedures*:
  - Roux-en-Y gastric bypass (RYGB)/Mini gastric bypass (MGB)
  - Biliary pancreatic diversion/duodenal switch

The most frequently performed gastric procedures for morbid obesity today include the sleeve gastrectomy and MGB. However, four basic approaches have been traditionally used for the treatment of obesity. The first operation done for obesity was the JI bypass. This operation was aimed to bypass 90% of the jejunum and ileum to induce malabsorption. This operation was abandoned due to a high incidence of severe complications such as hepatic failure, cirrhosis, nephropathy, and numerous other metabolic complications. The gastroplasty was developed to limit the amount of oral intake per meal. This operation involves partitioning the stomach into a small upper pouch that empties through a restricted stoma. The VBG was popular version of the gastroplasty but now abandoned. The third approach to obesity was RYGB. This operation also involves formation of a small upper gastric pouch that is anastomosed to a Roux-en-Y jejunal limb. The operation both limits oral intake per meal as well as induces dumping syndrome. Lastly, the partial biliopancreatic bypass induces a selective maldigestion and malabsorption. This operation involves a partial gastrectomy and diversion of the biliary and pancreatic secretions to the distal 50 cm of ileum; it is primarily performed in the "super" obese population (BMI > 60 kg/m^2). There was a time of modification of the adjustable silicone gastric band developed by Kuzmak. This gastric banding device has been modified for laparoscopic placement and is a form of gastric restriction or gastroplasty, but this procedure has also lost its popularity.

RESULTS OF DIFFERENT BARIATRIC SURGERY

The goals of surgery are to induce and maintain weight loss. Outcome from surgery is usually expressed as the amount or percent of excess weight loss. Several trials have compared the effect of gastric restriction versus gastric bypass. Subsequently, these trials have confirmed that RYGB and MGB result in more weight loss compared with gastric banding. The early complications following RYGB operation for obesity include subphrenic abscess or leak from an anastomosis or staple line. This complication is usually amenable to percutaneous aspiration and drainage; however, a small number of patients may require reoperation. The majority of early postoperative complications are minor wound infections and seromas. Late complications of the RYGB include vitamin B_{12} and iron deficiency. On the other hand, vitamin B_{12} and iron deficiency anemia are uncommon after VBG. Incisional hernia is another complication of morbidly obese patients undergoing laparotomy. Other late complications include failure to lose weight, late weight regain, and outlet stenosis. Staple line disruption has been a common problem and has prompted the use of four rows of staples instead of two. Another approach has been to divide the stomach to produce an isolated gastric pouch.

LAPAROSCOPIC VERTICAL-BANDED GASTROPLASTY

To perform laparoscopic VBG, the patient is placed in reverse Trendelenburg position with the legs separated in low stirrups. The surgeon stands between the patient's legs. An alternative approach is to place the patient supine with a footrest in the reverse Trendelenburg position. The surgeon stands on the patient's right side with an assistant on the left side. Five trocars are placed in the standard manner for gastric surgery. The telescope is placed through the 10 mm midepigastric port and the liver retractor is placed through a right subcostal port **(Figs. 2A and B)**.

There are two operating ports, one in each paramedian position (right, 10–33 mm; left, 15 mm). A window is created at the lesser curve of the stomach in an avascular plane using harmonic shears. The posterior stomach wall is freed of any adhesions. An alternative approach to the lesser sac is made by dividing the gastroepiploic vessels along the greater curvature. A 32-F dilator is placed via the mouth into the stomach. A site on the anterior stomach 4–5 cm from the gastroesophageal junction and 3 cm from the lesser curve is marked with the electrocautery. This site will be the center of the circular stapler. The right paramedian port is upsized to a 33-mm port to allow introduction of the circular stapling device. The anvil of the circular stapler is then placed posterior to the stomach. The pointed trocar is inserted through the stomach at the site previously marked with the cautery. The stapler is then connected and fired **(Fig. 2C)**.

The attachments from the diaphragm to the fundus of the stomach are divided and the fundus is dissected inferiorly using blunt technique. A linear 60 mm, four-row, noncutting stapler is introduced through the left paramedian port. The stapler is inserted through the circular window along the dilator and fired. A linear cutter is applied lateral to the previously placed rows of staples. At the circular window, a strip of polypropylene or polytetrafluoroethylene (1.5 × 5 cm) is brought around the stoma. The band is sutured into place

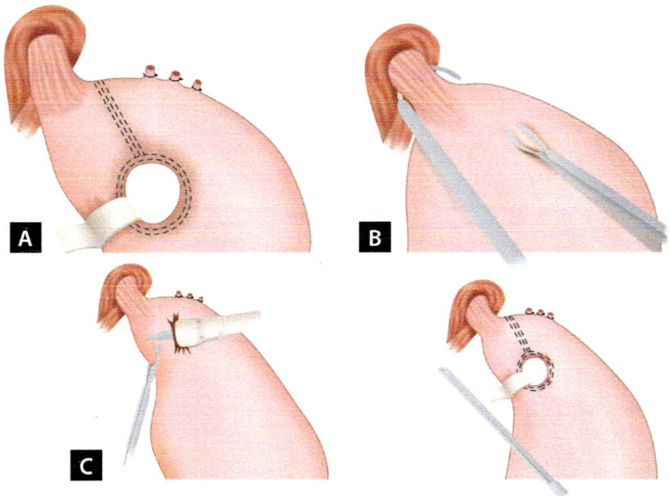

Figs. 2A to C: Laparoscopic vertical-banded gastroplasty.

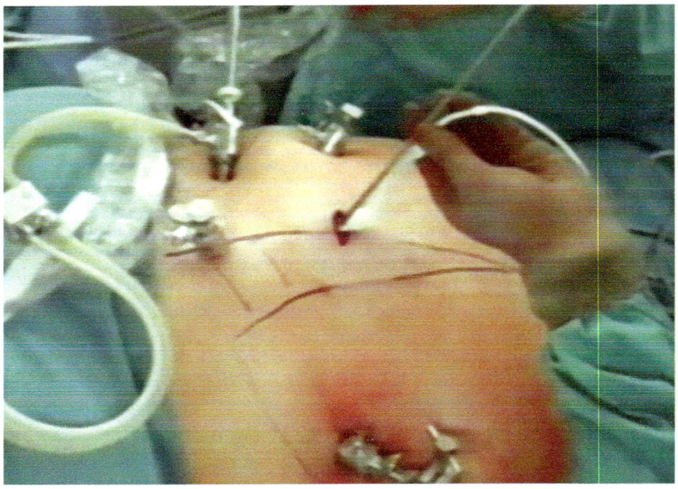

Fig. 3: Port position of laparoscopic gastric banding.

around the dilator. A nasogastric tube is not mandatory with this procedure.

LAPAROSCOPIC ROUX-EN-Y GASTRIC BYPASS

Patient positioning and port placement are as for other gastric procedures. The dissection starts at the fundus of the stomach with division of the phrenicogastric ligament. The fundus is mobilized in an inferior direction by blunt dissection. On the anterior wall of the stomach, an electrocautery mark is made 4–5 cm distal to the angle of His to serve as a landmark for the size of the gastric pouch. The lesser omentum is then opened adjacent to the mark at 4–5 cm inside the nerve of Latarjet. Dissection is carried through the lesser sac to an opening near the angle of His. The medial subcostal port is changed to an 18-mm port and a straight, four-row, cutting 60 mm stapler is used to divide the stomach. A standard 60 mm Roux limb is fashioned by dividing the proximal jejunum with a 60-mm linear stapler. The limb is brought up in a retrocolic, retrogastric path to the small (15 mL) proximal gastric pouch. A circular stapler is used for the gastrojejunostomy. The anvil is inserted via the oral cavity by endoscopic approach and using a percutaneous pull wire technique. An anastomosis is fashioned by connecting the anvil to the stapler introduced through the 18 mm port. A stapled side-to-side enteroenterostomy is then done to restore gastrointestinal continuity.

LAPAROSCOPIC ADJUSTABLE GASTRIC BANDING

An alternative gastric restrictive operation is the adjustable silicone gastric banding (ASGB) procedure. It was first introduced for placement through laparotomy by Kuzmak in 1986. This operation has the advantage of being the least invasive operation as it is completely reversible and allows for adjustment of the gastric pouch outlet.

The main steps of laparoscopic ASGB are given in **Figure 3**.

The patient is placed in a lithotomy position and in reverse Trendelenburg position as for the most gastric operations. A total of six ports are placed. The liver retractor is placed through a right subcostal one; the telescope is inserted through a subxiphoid positioned port. The main operating ports are in the right and left paramedian positions. The assistant uses a left subcostal and an epigastric port. The left paramedian port is 15 mm for introduction of the band device. All of the other ports are 10 mm.

A gastric calibration tube is placed via the mouth into the stomach. The balloon is inflated to 15 cc and pulled up through the gastroesophageal junction.

A site on the lesser curve is chosen to begin dissection that corresponds to the widest circumference of the balloon inside stomach. The balloon is deflated and the tube is withdrawn back into the esophagus **(Figs. 4A and B)**.

A retrogastric tunnel is then created using blunt dissection, staying close to the gastric wall. The posterior gastric wall should be easily recognized to prevent injury. A small opening in the phrenicogastric ligament is made with electrocautery **(Figs. 5A and B)**.

A grasping instrument is then placed through the retrogastric tunnel. The band is then introduced into the abdomen and grasped with the instrument. The band is pulled into position around the stomach **(Figs. 6A and B)**.

The calibration tube is then reinserted into the proper position and the band closed around the tube. The calibration tube allows for proper stoma calibration **(Figs. 7A to D)**.

At least four sutures are then placed in the seromuscular layer of the stomach just proximal and distal to the band to keep it in the proper position, otherwise the chances of displacements are there. The injection port is then connected to the band tubing and implanted into the left rectus sheath at the paramedian port site **(Figs. 8A to D)**.

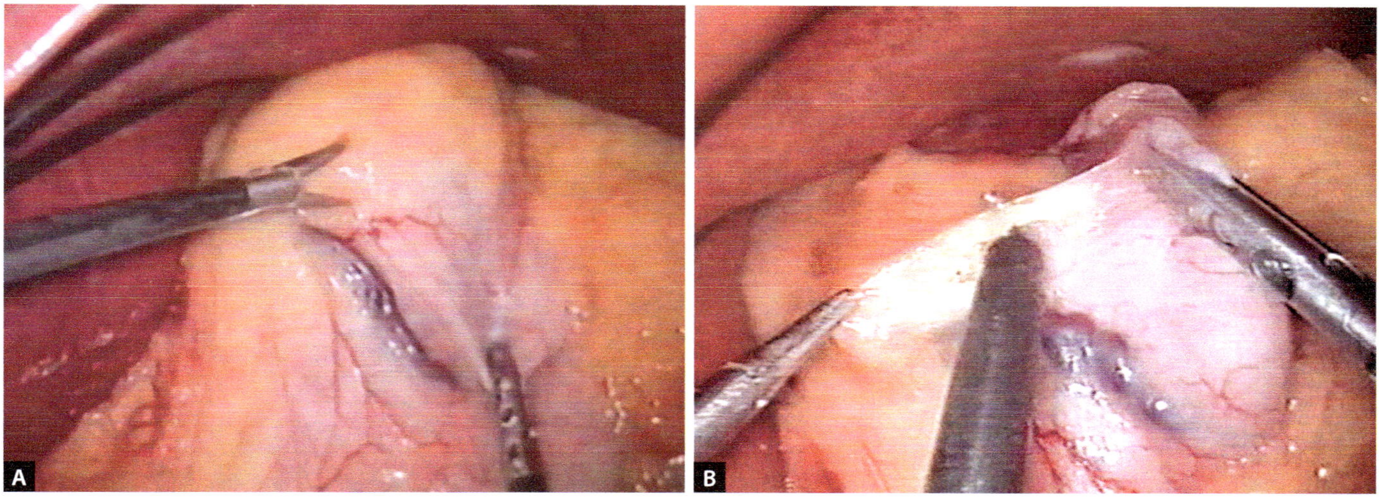

Figs. 4A and B: Lesser curvature, a site chosen to start dissection.

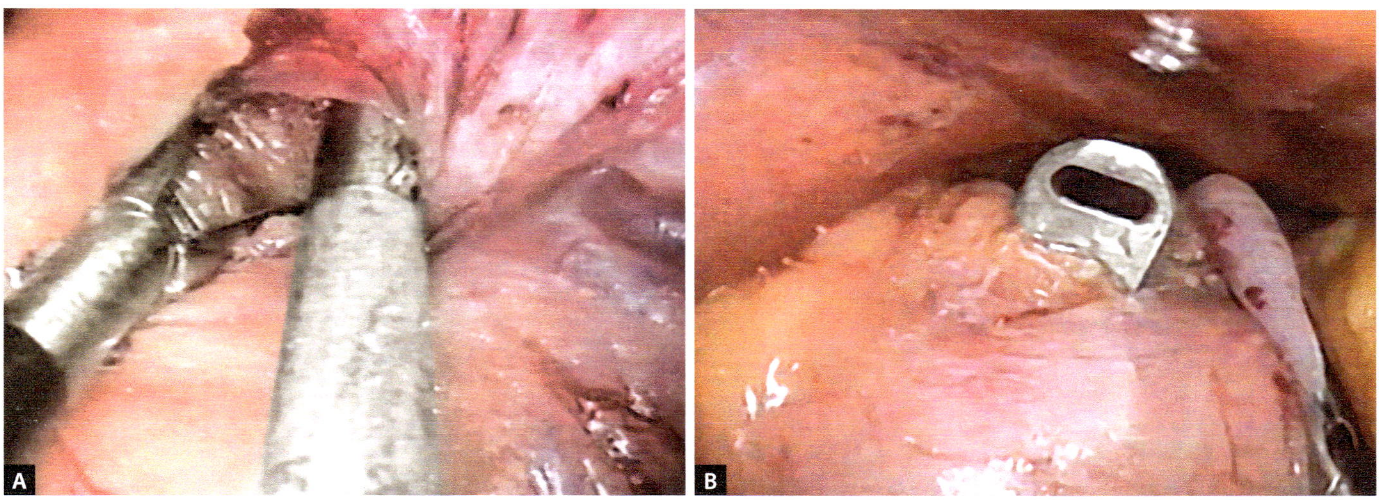

Figs. 5A and B: Grasping instrument coming from behind through retrogastric tunnel.

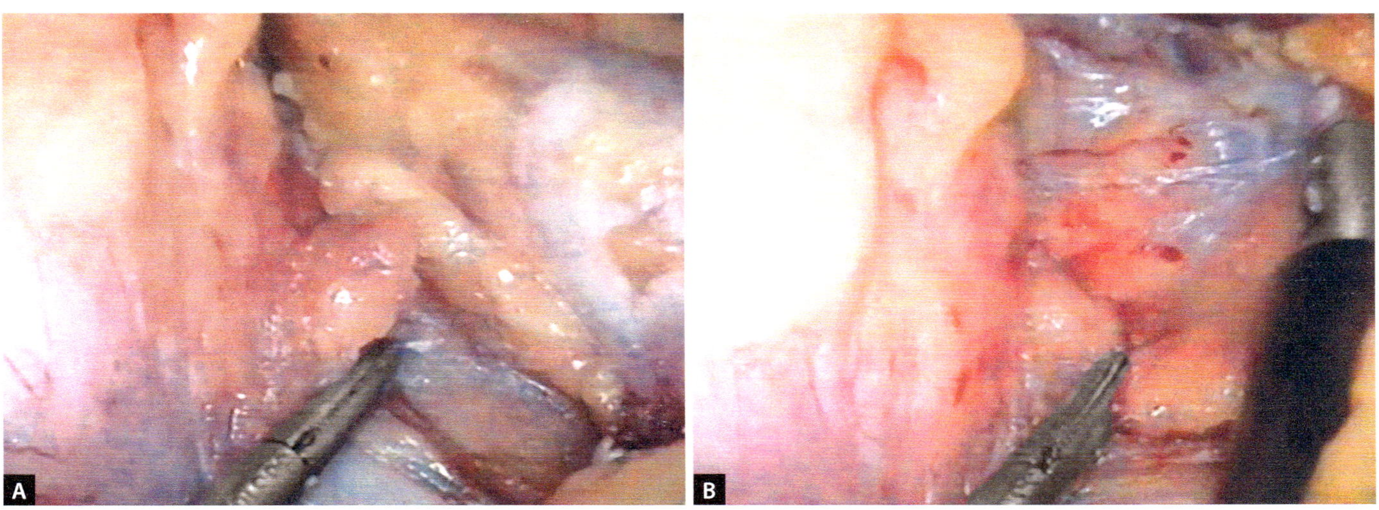

Figs. 6A and B: Creation of a retrogastric tunnel.

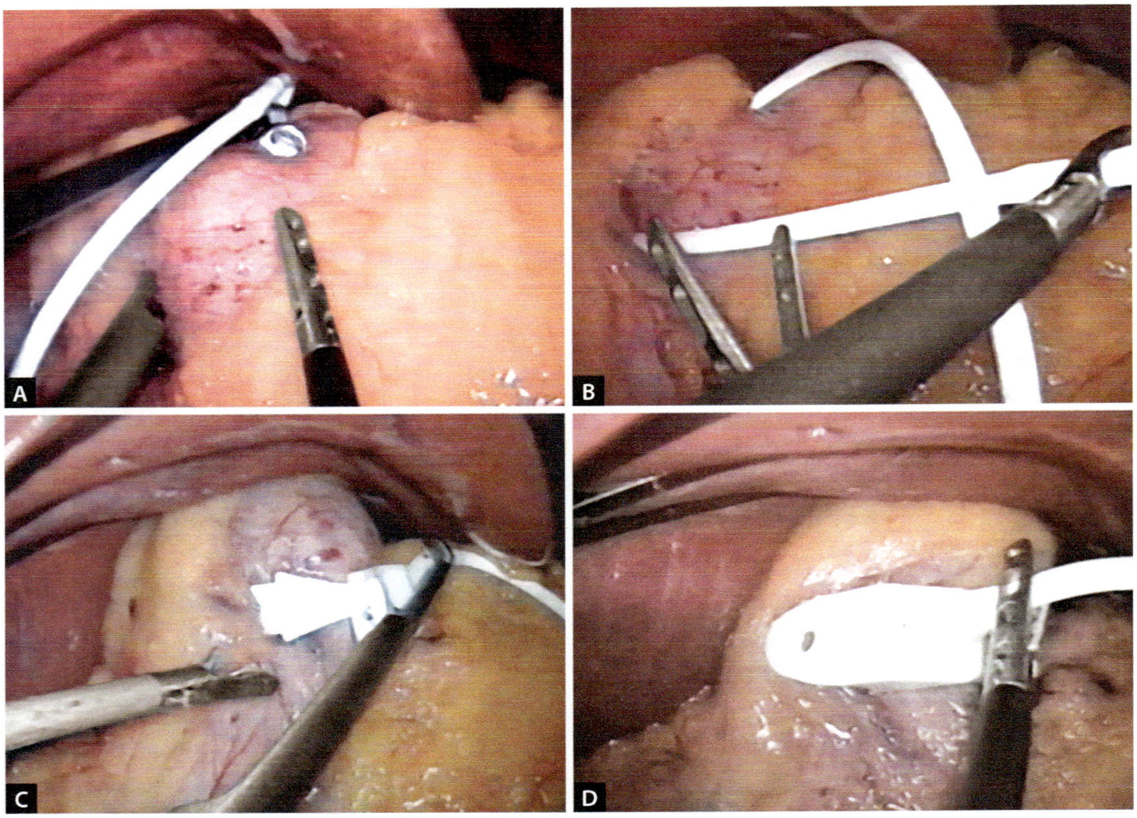

Figs. 7A to D: Band is pulled from below the stomach through retrogastric tunnel and is tightened leaving 15 mL volume of stomach above.

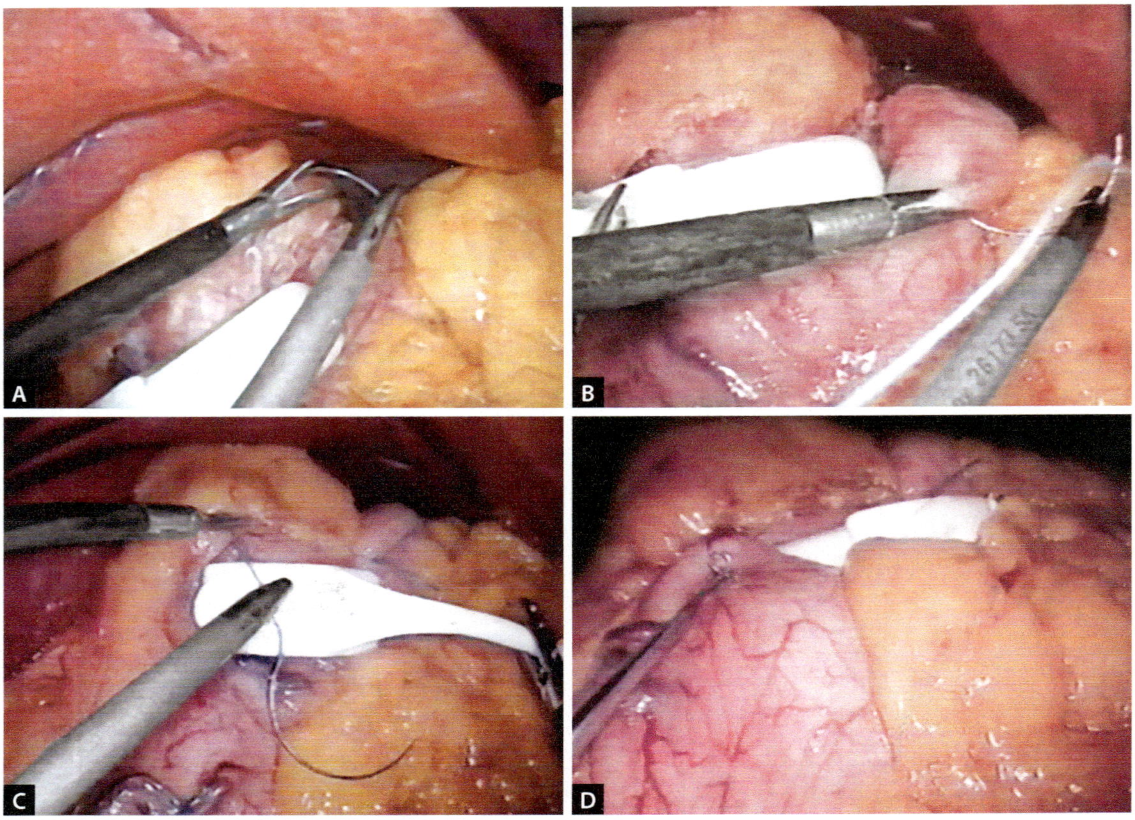

Figs. 8A to D: Suture is placed to fix the band in position.

SLEEVE GASTRECTOMY, MINI GASTRIC BYPASS, AND ROUX-EN-Y GASTRIC BYPASS

Refer Chapter 21: Laparoscopic Bariatric Surgery.

COMPLICATIONS

Adjustable Gastric Banding

Early complications of the adjustable gastric band procedure are as follows:

- Injury of the stomach or esophagus
- Bleeding
- Food intolerance (most common immediate post-operative complication)
- Wound infection
- Pneumonia

Late complications are as follows:

- Food intolerance or noncompliance to band
- Band slippage (stomach prolapse)
- Pouch dilatation
- Band erosion into the stomach
- Port complications
- Reoperation rate
- Esophageal dilatation
- Failure to lose weight
- Port infection and band infection
- Leakage of the balloon or tubing
- Mortality

Gastric Bypass

Early complications of RYGB are as follows:

- Anastomotic leak
- Pulmonary embolism and deep vein thrombosis (DVT)
- Wound infection (more common with open approach)
- Gastrointestinal hemorrhage and bleeding
- Respiratory insufficiency and pneumonia
- Acute distention of the distal stomach

Late complications (less frequent and less dramatic than with gastric banding) of the RYGB procedure are as follows:

- Stomal stenosis, most common
- Bowel obstruction, small bowel obstruction
- Internal hernia
- Cholelithiasis
- Micronutrient deficiencies
- Marginal ulcer
- Staple line disruption
- Ventral hernia formation (more prevalent after open approach)

Biliopancreatic Diversion with Duodenal Switch

This procedure is less well known, so the complications are potentially more problematic if the surgeon is unfamiliar with the procedure.

Fat malabsorption results in diarrhea and foul-smelling gas in approximately 30% of patients.

The potential nutritional deficiencies mandate frequent follow-up visits with close monitoring and supplementation of multivitamins and minerals.

- Malabsorption of fat-soluble vitamins (vitamins A, D, E, and K)
- Vitamin A deficiency, which causes night blindness
- Vitamin D deficiency, which causes osteoporosis
- Iron deficiency (similar incidence to RYGB procedure)
- Protein-energy malnutrition (may require a second operation to lengthen the common channel)

CONCLUSION

In developed world, obesity is a major national health problem. It is clear that morbidly obese patients suffer from significant comorbidity and die at younger age than healthy weight individuals. Weight loss and maintenance of normal weight correct the majority of weight-related morbidity and return life expectancy to that of the general population. All the laparoscopic surgeons should remember that morbidly obese patients are at an increased risk of significant morbidity and mortality with laparoscopic surgery. However, strict attention to detail allows for proper selection of patients for surgery with reduction in the perioperative risk.

BIBLIOGRAPHY

1. Adams TD, Gress RE, Smith SC, Halverson RC, Simper SC, Rosamond WD, et al. Long-term mortality after gastric bypass surgery. N Engl J Med. 2007;357:753-61.
2. Alexander CI, Liston WA. Operating on the obese woman—a review. BJOG. 2006;113:1167-72.
3. Amorim AR, Rössner S, Neovius M, Lourenco PM, Linné Y. Does excess pregnancy weight gain constitute a major risk for increasing long-term BMI? Obesity. 2007;15:1278-86.
4. Angrisani L, Favretti F, Furbetta F, Iuppa A, Doldi SB, Paganelli M, et al. Italian Group for Lap-Band System: results of multicenter study on patients with BMI < or =35 kg/m^2. Obes Surg. 2004;14:415-8.
5. Angrisani L, Lorenzo M, Borrelli V. Laparoscopic adjustable gastric banding versus Roux-en-Y gastric bypass: 5-year results of a prospective randomized trial. Surg Obes Relat Dis. 2007;3:127-32.
6. Baughcum AE, Burklow KA, Deeks CM, Powers SW, Whitaker RC. Maternal feeding practices and childhood obesity: a focus group study of low-income mothers. Arch Pediatr Adolesc Med. 1998;152:1010-4.
7. Baughcum AE, Powers SW, Johnson SB, Chamberlin LA, Deeks CM, Jain A, et al. Maternal feeding practices and beliefs and their relationships to overweight in early childhood. J Dev Behav Pediatr. 2001;22:391-408.
8. Baxter J. Obesity surgery. Lancet. 2008;371:557.
9. Baxter J. Obesity surgery—another unmet need. BMJ. 2000;321:523-4.
10. Bessesen DH. Update on obesity. J Clin Endocrinol Metab. 2008;93:2027-34.
11. Buchwald H, Avidor Y, Braunwald E, Jensen MD, Pories W, Fahrbach K, et al. Bariatric surgery: a systematic review and meta-analysis. JAMA. 2004;292:1724-37.

12. Buchwald H, Varco RL, Matts JP, Long JM, Fitch LL, Campbell GS, et al. Effect of partial ileal bypass surgery on mortality and morbidity from coronary heart disease in patients with hypercholesterolemia. Report of the Program on the Surgical Control of the Hyperlipidemias (POSCH). N Engl J Med. 1990;323:946-55.
13. Busetto L, Angrisani L, Basso N, Favretti F, Furbetta F, Lorenzo M, et al. Safety and efficacy of laparoscopic adjustable gastric banding in the elderly. Obesity (Silver Spring). 2008;16:334-8.
14. Cannizzo F, Kral JG. Obesity surgery: a model of programmed undernutrition. Curr Opin Clin Nutr Metab Care. 1998;1:363-8.
15. Centre for Public Health Excellence at NICE (UK), National Collaborating Centre for Primary Care (UK). Obesity: The Prevention, Identification, Assessment and Management of Overweight and Obesity in Adults and Children. London: National Institute for Health and Clinical Excellence (NICE); 2006.
16. Chapman IM. Obesity in old age. Front Horm Res. 2008;36:97-106.
17. Cho GJ, Lee JH, Park HT, Shin JH, Hong SC, Kim T, et al. Postmenopausal status according to years since menopause as an independent risk factor for the metabolic syndrome. Menopause. 2008;15:524-9.
18. Christou NV, Sampalis JS, Liberman M, Look D, Auger S, McLean APH, et al. Surgery decreases long-term mortality, morbidity, and health care use in morbidly obese patients. Ann Surg. 2004;240:416-23.
19. Cohen RV, Schiavon CA, Pinheiro JS, Correa JL, Rubino F. Duodenal-jejunal bypass for the treatment of type 2 diabetes in patients with body mass index of 22–34 kg/m^2: a report of 2 cases. Surg Obes Relat Dis. 2007;3:195-7.
20. DeMaria EJ. Bariatric surgery for morbid obesity. N Engl J Med. 2007;356:2176-83.
21. Dennis KE. Postmenopausal women and the health consequences of obesity. J Obstet Gynecol Neonatal Nurs. 2007;36:511-9.
22. Dixon JB, O'Brien PE, Playfair J, Chapman L, Schachter LM, Skinner S, et al. Adjustable gastric banding and conventional therapy for type 2 diabetes: a randomized controlled trial. JAMA. 2008;299:316-23.
23. Eckel RH. Clinical practice: nonsurgical management of obesity in adults. N Engl J Med. 2008;358:1941-50.
24. Fatima J, Houghton SG, Iqbal CW, Thompson GB, Que FL, Kendrick ML, et al. Bariatric surgery at the extremes of age. J Gastrointest Surg. 2006;10:1392-6.
25. Favretti F, Sagato G, Ashton D, Busetto L, De Luca M, Mazza M, et al. Laparoscopic adjustable gastric banding in 1,791 consecutive obese patients: 12-year results. Obes Surg. 2007;17:168-75.
26. Fernandez AZ, Demaria EJ, Tichansky DS, Kellum JM, Wolfe LG, Meador J, et al. Multivariate analysis of risk factors for death following gastric bypass for treatment of morbid obesity. Ann Surg. 2004;239:698-702.
27. Ferro-Luzzi A, Toth MJ, Elia M, Schurch B. Report of the ODECG Working Group on body weight and body composition of the elderly. Eur J Clin Nutr. 2000;54:S160-1.
28. Finkelstein EA, Fiebelkorn IC, Wang G. State-level estimates of annual medical expenditures attributable to obesity. Obes Res. 2004;12:18-24.
29. Flum DR, Salem L, Elrod JAB, Dellinger EP, Cheadle A, Chan L. Early mortality among Medicare beneficiaries undergoing bariatric surgical procedures. JAMA. 2005;294:1903-8.
30. Folsom AR, Kushi LH, Anderson KE, Mink PJ, Olson JE, Hong CP, et al. Associations of general and abdominal obesity with multiple health outcomes in older women: the Iowa Women's Health Study. Arch Intern Med. 2000;160:2117-28.
31. Fontaine KR, Barofsky I. Obesity and health-related quality of life. Obes Rev. 2001;2:173-82.
32. Fontaine KR, Redden DT, Wang C, Westfall AO, Allison DB. Years of life lost due to obesity. JAMA. 2003;289:187-93.
33. Fried M, Hainer V, Basdevant A, Buchwald H, Deitel M, Finer N, et al. Interdisciplinary European guidelines for surgery for severe (morbid) obesity. Obes Surg. 2007;17:260-70.
34. Gagner M, Milone L, Yung E, Broseus A, Gumbs AA. Causes of early mortality after laparoscopic adjustable gastric banding. J Am Coll Surg. 2008;206:664-9.
35. Gastrointestinal surgery for severe obesity: National Institutes of Health Consensus Development Conference Statement. Am J Clin Nutr. 1992;55:615S-9.
36. Greendale GA, Unger JB, Rowe JW, Seeman TE. The relation between cortisol excretion and fractures in healthy older people: results from the MacArthur studies—Mac. J Am Geriatr Soc. 1999;47:799-803.
37. Hallowell PT, Stellato TA, Schuster M, Graf K, Robinson A, Jasper JJ. Avoidance of complications in older patients and Medicare recipients undergoing gastric bypass. Arch Surg. 2007;142:506-10.
38. Harris TB, Launer LJ, Madans J, Feldman JJ. Cohort study of effect of being overweight and change in weight on risk of coronary heart disease in old age. Br Med J. 1997;314:1792-4.
39. Hawkes K. The grandmother effect. Nature. 2004;428:128-9.
40. Holmes E, Loo RL, Stamler J, Bictash M, Yap IKS, Chan Q, et al. Human metabolic phenotype diversity and its association with diet and blood pressure. Nature. 2008;453:396-400.
41. Kral JG, Biron S, Simard S, Hould FS, Lebel S, Marceau S, et al. Large maternal weight loss from obesity surgery prevents transmission of obesity to children who were followed for 2 to 18 years. Pediatrics. 2006;118:1644-9.
42. Kral JG, Sjöström L, Gustafson A. Effects of jejuno-ileal bypass on serum lipoproteins and glucose tolerance in severely obese patients. Eur J Clin Invest. 1980;10:363-7.
43. Kral JG. A stitch in time versus a life in misery. Surg Obes Relat Disord. 2007;3:2-5.
44. Kral JG. ABC of obesity. Management: Part III–surgery. Br Med J. 2006;333:900-3.
45. Kral JG. Effects of truncal vagotomy on body weight and hyperinsulinemia in morbid obesity. Am J Clin Nutr. 1980;33:416-9.
46. Kral JG. Morbid obesity and related health risks. Ann Int Med. 1985;103:1043-7.
47. Kral JG. Morbidity of severe obesity. Surg Clin North Am. 2001;81:1039-61.
48. Kral JG. Preventing and treating obesity in girls and young women to curb the epidemic. Obes Res. 2004;12:1539-46.
49. Lahdenperä M, Lummaa V, Helle S, Tremblay M, Russell AF. Fitness benefits of prolonged post-reproductive lifespan in women. Nature. 2004;428:178-81.
50. Linné Y, Dye L, Barkeling B, Rössner S. Long-term weight development in women: a 15-year follow-up of the effects of pregnancy. Obes Res. 2004;12:1166-78.
51. Livingston EH, Huerta S, Arthur D, Lee S, Shields SD, Heber D. Male gender is a predictor of morbidity and age a predictor of mortality for patients undergoing gastric bypass surgery. Ann Surg. 2002;236:576-82.
52. Loos RJF, Lindgren CM, Li S, Wheeler E, Zhao JH, Prokopenko I, et al. Common variants near MC4R are associated with fat mass, weight and risk of obesity. Nat Genet. 2008;40:768-75.
53. Marceau P, Hould FS, Simard S, Lebel S, Bourque RA, Potvin M, et al. Biliopancreatic diversion with duodenal switch. World J Surg. 1998;22:947-54.
54. Mark A. Dietary therapy for obesity: an emperor with no clothes. Hypertension. 2008;51:1426-34.
55. McLean JA, Barr SI, Prior JC. Cognitive dietary restraint is associated with higher urinary cortisol excretion in healthy premenopausal women. Am J Clin Nutr. 2001;73:7-12.

56. McMahon MM, Sarr MG, Clark MM, Gall MM, Knoetgen J, Service FJ, et al. Clinical management after bariatric surgery: value of a multidisciplinary approach. Mayo Clin Proc. 2006;81:S34-45.
57. McTigue K, Larson JC, Valoski A, Burke G, Kotchen J, Lewis CE, et al. Mortality and cardiac and vascular outcomes in extremely obese women. JAMA. 2006;296:79-86.
58. Miller ME, Kral JG. Surgery for obesity in older women. Menopause Int. 2008;14:155-62.
59. Moo TA, Rubino F. Gastrointestinal surgery as treatment for type 2 diabetes. Curr Opin Endocrinol Diabetes Obes. 2008;15: 153-8.
60. National Center for Health Statistics (US). Health, United States, 2004: With Chartbook on Trends in the Health of Americans. Hyattsville (MD): US Department of Health and Human Services, Centers for Disease Control and Prevention; 2004.
61. Nguyen NT, Paya M, Stevens CM, Mavandadi S, Zainabadi K, Wilson SE. The relationship between hospital volume and outcome in bariatric surgery at academic medical centers. Ann Surg. 2004;240:586-94.
62. NHS Digital. (2020). The NHS Information Centre. [online] Available from http://www.ic.nhs.uk/. [Last accessed May, 2021].
63. O'Brien PE, Dixon JB, Laurie C, Skinner S, Proietto J, McNeil J, et al. Treatment for mild to moderate obesity with laparoscopic adjustable banding or an intensive medical program: a randomized trial. Ann Intern Med. 2006;144:625-33.
64. O'Brien PE, Dixon JB. Laparoscopic adjustable gastric banding in the treatment of morbid obesity. Arch Surg. 2003;138:376-82.
65. OECD. (2005). OECD Factbook 2005: Economic, Environmental, and Social Statistics. [online] Available from https://www.oecd-ilibrary.org/docserver/factbook-2005-en.pdf?expires=162 0730800&id=id&accname=guest&checksu m=AAC30EA7644980 500 2FABBDA1A58853A. [Last accessed May, 2021].
66. Ogden CL, Carroll MD, Flegal KM. High body mass index for age among US children and adolescents, 2003-2006. JAMA. 2008;299:2401-5.
67. Oster G, Thompson D, Edelsberg J, Bird AP, Colditz GA. Lifetime health and economic benefits of weight loss among obese persons. Am J Public Health. 1999;89:1536-42.
68. Perry CD, Hutter MM, Smith DB, Newhouse JP, McNeil BJ. Survival and changes in comorbidities after bariatric surgery. Ann Surg. 2008;247:21-7.
69. Pories WJ, MacDonald KG, Morgan EJ, Sinha MK, Dohm GL, Swanson MS, et al. Surgical treatment and its effect on diabetes: 10-year follow-up. Am J Clin Nutr. 1992;55:582S-5.
70. Poulose BK, Griffin MR, Moore DE, Zhu Y, Smalley W, Richards WO, et al. Risk factors for postoperative mortality in bariatric surgery. J Surg Res. 2005;127:1-7.
71. Puhl R, Brownell KD. Bias, discrimination and obesity. Obes Res. 2001;9:788-805.
72. Raftopoulos Y, Gatti GG, Luketich JD, Courcoulas AP. Advanced age and sex as predictors of adverse outcomes following gastric bypass surgery. JSLS. 2005;9:272-6.
73. Rand CSW, Macgregor AMC. Successful weight loss following obesity surgery and the perceived liability of morbid obesity. Int J Obes. 1991;15:577-9.
74. Reeves GK, Pirie K, Beral V, Green J, Spencer E, Bull D, et al. Cancer incidence and mortality in relation to body mass index in the Million Women Study: cohort study. BMJ. 2007;335: 1134-45.
75. Rehfeld JF, Juhl E, Quaade F. Effect of jejunoileostomy on glucose and insulin metabolism in ten obese patients. Metabolism. 1970;19:529-38.
76. Reid IR. Glucocorticoid osteoporosis—mechanisms and management. Eur J Endocrinol. 1997;137:209-17.
77. Rideout CA. High cognitive dietary restraint is associated with increased cortisol excretion in postmenopausal women. J Gerontol A Biol Sci Med Sci. 2006;61:628-33.
78. Rooney BL, Schauberger CW. Excess pregnancy weight gain and long-term obesity: one decade later. Obstet Gynecol. 2002;100:245-52.
79. Rubino F, Forgione A, Cummings DE, Vix M, Gnuli D, Mingrone G, et al. The mechanism of diabetes control after gastrointestinal bypass surgery reveals a role of the proximal small intestine in the pathophysiology of type 2 diabetes. Ann Surg. 2006;244:741-9.
80. Sabeti PC, Varilly P, Fry B, Lohmueller J, Hostetter E, Cotsapas C, et al. Genome-wide detection and characterization of positive selection in human populations. Nature. 2007;449:913-8.
81. Schauer P, Chand B, Brethauer S. New applications for endoscopy: the emerging field of endoluminal and transgastric bariatric surgery. Surg Endosc. 2007;21:347-56.
82. Schilling PL, Davis MM, Albanese CT, Dutta S, Morton MD. National trends in adolescent bariatric surgical procedures and implications for surgical centers of excellence. J Am Coll Surg. 2008;206:1-12.
83. Scopinaro N, Gianetta E, Adami GF, Friedman D, Traverso E, Marinari GM, et al. Biliopancreatic diversion for obesity at eighteen years. Surgery. 1996;119:261-8.
84. Seehra H, MacDermott N, Lascellesb RG, Taylor TV. Lesson of the week: Wernicke's encephalopathy after vertical banded gastroplasty for morbid obesity. Br Med J. 1996;312:434.
85. Shanley DP, Sear R, Mace R, Kirkwood TBL. Testing evolutionary theories of menopause. Proc R Soc B. 2007;274:2943-9.
86. Sjöström L, Lindroos AK, Peltonen M, Torgerson J, Bouchard C, Carlsson B, et al. Lifestyle, diabetes, and cardiovascular risk factors 10 years after bariatric surgery. N Engl J Med. 2004;351:2683-93.
87. Sjöström L, Narbro K, Sjöström CD, Karason K, Larsson B, Wedel H, et al. Effects of bariatric surgery on mortality in Swedish obese subjects. N Engl J Med. 2007;357:741-52.
88. Srinivasan M, Patel MS. Metabolic programming in the immediate postnatal period. Trends Endocrinol Metab. 2007;19:146-52.
89. St Peter SD, Craft RO, Tiede JL, Swain JM. Impact of advanced age on weight loss and health benefits after laparoscopic gastric bypass. Arch Surg. 2005;140:165-8.
90. Stettler N, Zemel BS, Kumanyika S, Stallings VA. Infant weight gain and childhood overweight status in a multicenter, cohort study. Pediatrics. 2002;109:194-9.
91. Sugerman HJ, DeMaria EJ, Kellum JM, Sugerman EL, Meador JG, Wolfe LG. Effects of bariatric surgery in older patients. Ann Surg. 2004;240:243-7.
92. Taylor C, Layani L. Laparoscopic adjustable gastric banding in patients > or = 60 years old: is it worthwhile? Obes Surg. 2006;16:1579-83.
93. Tsai AG, Wadden TA. Systematic review: an evaluation of major commercial weight loss programs in the United States. Ann Intern Med. 2005;142:56-66.
94. van Baal PHM, Polder JJ, de Wit GA, Hoogenveen RT, Feenstra TL, Boshuizen HC, et al. Lifetime medical costs of obesity: prevention no cure for increasing health expenditure. PLoS Med. 2008;5:e29.
95. Vincent RP, Ashrafian H, le Roux CW. Mechanisms of disease: the role of gastrointestinal hormones in appetite and obesity. Nat Clin Pract Gastroenterol Hepatol. 2008;5:268-77.
96. Whitmer RA, Gustafson DR, Barrett-Connor E, Haan MN, Gunderson EP, Yaffe K. Central obesity and increased risk of dementia more than three decades later. Neurology. 2008;71:1057-64.
97. Zaninotto P, Wardle H, Stamatakis E, et al. Forecasting obesity to 2010. Department of Health, London, 2006. [online] Available from http://www.dh.gov.uk/en/Publicationsandstatistics/Publications/PublicationsStatistics/DH_4138630. [Last accessed May, 2021].

CHAPTER 45

Complications of Minimal Access Surgery

INTRODUCTION

Initial development of "minimal access surgery" began in the animal laboratory and was later studied in selected academic centers. It was imported to the community hospitals only when its benefits and safety were established. The development of laparoscopic cholecystectomy was not designed to enhance the safety of the procedure, but rather to reduce the discomfort associated with the surgical incision. The fierce economical competition in medicine fueled by the managed care movement led to the rapid adoption of laparoscopic surgery among surgeons and gynecologist in community hospitals who were not formally trained in this technique and acquired their knowledge by subscribing to short courses.

Low complication rates were reported by centers specializing in laparoscopic surgery, mostly in academic centers. These centers were able to reduce the complication rate to minimum by developing proficiency in this surgery. Regrettably, many inexperienced surgeons perform this technique within sufficient training and are responsible for the majority of complications seen during the performance of laparoscopic surgery.

Physicians who performed <100 such procedures reported 14.7 complications per 1,000 patients. In contrast, experienced surgeon reported a complication rate of only 3.8 complications per 1,000 procedures. The Southern Surgeons Club Survey reported that the incidence of bile duct injury was 2.2% when the surgeon had previously performed <13 procedures. As surgeons gained experience, the incidence of bile duct injury dropped to 0.1% afterward.

ANESTHETIC AND MEDICAL COMPLICATIONS IN LAPAROSCOPY

Although all types of anesthesia involve some risk, major side effects and complications from anesthesia in laparoscopy are uncommon. Anesthetic complications include those that are more common in association with laparoscopic surgery as well as those that can occur in any procedure requiring general anesthetics. One-third of the deaths associated with minor laparoscopic procedures such as sterilization or diagnostic laparoscopy are secondary to complication of anesthesia.

Among the potential complications of all general anesthetics are:

- Hypoventilation
- Esophageal intubation
- Gastroesophageal reflux
- Bronchospasm
- Hypotension
- Narcotic overdose
- Cardiac arrhythmias
- Cardiac arrest.

Laparoscopy results in multiple postoperative benefits including fewer traumas, less pain, less pulmonary dysfunction, quicker recovery, and shorter hospital stay. These advantages are regularly emphasized and explained. With increasing success of laparoscopy, it is now proposed for many surgical procedures. Intraoperative cardiorespiratory changes occur during pneumoperitoneum and partial pressure of arterial carbon dioxide ($PaCO_2$) increases due to carbon dioxide (CO_2) absorption from peritoneal cavity. Laparoscopy poses a number of inherent features that can enhance some of these risks. For example, the Trendelenburg position, in combination with the increased intraperitoneal pressure provided by pneumoperitoneum by CO_2, exerts greater pressure on the diaphragm, potentiating hypoventilation, resulting hypercarbia, and metabolic acidosis. This position, combined with anesthetic agents that act as muscle relaxant opens the esophageal sphincter, facilitates regurgitation of gastric content, which, in turn, often leads to aspiration and its attendant complications of bronchospasm, pneumonitis, and pneumonia. Intraoperative aspiration pneumonia is very common in laparoscopy, but postoperative pneumonia is common after open surgery.

Various parameters of cardiopulmonary function associated with CO_2 insufflation include reduced partial pressure of arterial oxygen (PaO_2), oxygen (O_2) saturation, tidal volume and minute ventilation as well as an increased respiratory rate. The use of intraperitoneal CO_2 as a distension medium is associated with an increase in $PaCO_2$

and a decrease in pH. Increased abdominal pressure and elevation of the diaphragm may be associated with basilar atelectasis, which can result into right-to-left shunt and a ventilation-perfusion mismatch.

Although during laparoscopy, the patient's anesthetic care is in the hands of the anesthesiologist, it is important for the laparoscopic surgeon to understand the prevention and management of anesthetic complications by proper knowledge of risk involved with pneumoperitoneum.

Carbon Dioxide Embolism

Several case reports and experimental data suggest that the first finding during a CO_2 embolism may be a rapid increase in end-tidal CO_2 ($EtCO_2$) tension as some of the CO_2 injected into the vascular system is excreted into the lungs. As more gas is injected, a vapor lock is formed in portions of the lungs. Areas of the lung are ventilated but not perfused (i.e., become dead space) and the end-tidal CO_2 rapidly falls. In contrast, during an air embolism, the end-tidal CO_2 tension falls immediately. Other findings of a massive CO_2 embolism include a harsh, mill-wheel murmur, a marked decrease in blood pressure, and a decrease in hemoglobin-O_2 saturation. In minimal access surgery, the use of CO_2 was started just to minimize the risk of CO_2 embolism. CO_2 is the most widely used peritoneal distension medium. Part of the reason for this selection is the ready absorption of CO_2 in blood. It is 20 times more absorbable than room air; consequently, the vast majority of frequent microemboli that do occur are absorbed, usually by the splanchnic vascular system quickly and without any incident. However, if large amounts of CO_2 gain access to the central venous circulation, if there is peripheral vasoconstriction, or if the splanchnic blood flow is decreased by excessively high intraperitoneal pressure, severe cardiorespiratory compromise may result. The reported incidence of death due to CO_2 embolism is not clearly and authentically mentioned in any of the published article but it is assumed to be 1:10,000.

Diagnosis of Carbon Dioxide Embolism

Carbon dioxide embolism is difficult to diagnose clinically. Among the presenting signs of CO_2 embolus are sudden, otherwise unexplained hypotension, cardiac arrhythmia, cyanosis, and the development of the classical "mill-wheel" or "water-wheel" heart murmur. The end-tidal CO_2 may increase and findings consistent with pulmonary edema may manifest. Accelerating pulmonary hypertension may also occur resulting in right-sided heart failure.

Prevention of Carbon Dioxide Embolism

Because gas embolism may occur as a result of direct intravascular injection via an insufflation needle, the surgeon should ensure that blood is not emanating from the needle prior to the initiation of insufflation. Gynecologic surgeons can uniformly reduce the risk of CO_2 embolus by operating in an environment where the intraperitoneal pressure is maintained at <20 mm Hg. In most instances, excepting the initial placement of trocar in an insufflated peritoneum, the surgeon should be able to function comfortably with the intraperitoneal pressure between 8 and 12 mm Hg, maximum 15 mm Hg. Such pressures may also provide protection from many of the other adverse cardiopulmonary events. The risk of CO_2 embolus is also reduced by the meticulous maintenance of hemostasis and avoiding open venous channels, which are the portal of entry for gas into the systemic circulation. Another option in high-risk patient is the use of "gasless" or "apneumic" laparoscopy, where extra- or intraperitoneal abdominal lifting mechanisms are used to create a working space for the laparoscopic surgeon. However, limitations of these devices have, to date, precluded their wide acceptance by most of the surgeons.

The anesthesiologist should continuously monitor the patient's skin colors, blood pressure, heart sounds, electrocardiogram, and end-tidal CO_2, so that the signs of CO_2 embolus are recognized early and can be managed.

Management of Carbon Dioxide Embolism

If a CO_2 embolism should occur:

- The patient should receive 100% O_2
- Insufflation should be stopped and the abdomen decompressed
- The patient should be placed with the right side elevated in the Trendelenburg position to avoid further entrapment of CO_2 in the pulmonary vasculature
- A central venous catheter, if placed rapidly, may allow aspiration of CO_2
- Full inotropic support should be instituted.

Cardiopulmonary bypass may be required to evacuate the gas lock and help remove the CO_2.

If CO_2 embolus is suspected or diagnosed, the operating room team must act quickly. The surgeon must evacuate CO_2 from the peritoneal cavity and should place the patient in the Durant or left lateral decubitus position, with the head below the level of the right atrium. A large bore central venous line should be immediately established to allow aspiration of gas from the heart. Because the findings are nonspecific, other causes of cardiovascular collapse should be considered.

Periodically, gases other than CO_2 are investigated for use for laparoscopy. Argon, air, helium, and nitrous oxide have all been used in an attempt to eliminate the problems associated with hypercarbia and peritoneal irritation seen with CO_2. The lack of solubility of air, helium, and argon effectively prevents hypercarbia that occurs with insufflation with CO_2, but increases the lethality many fold, if gas embolism occurs. Deaths from argon gas embolism, when the argon beam coagulator has been used during laparoscopy, suggest that this concern is real. Nitrous oxide has solubility similar to that of CO_2, but unfortunately it can support combustion. Explosions, when electrocautery was used following insufflation with nitrous oxide, have occurred. An intra-abdominal fire, when nitrous oxide was intended to be used for insufflation, has also been reported.

Cardiovascular Complications

Laparoscopic surgery requires the insufflation of CO_2 into the abdominal cavity. Complications associated with CO_2 insufflation include:

- Escape of CO_2 into the heart or pleural cavity
- Effects of the resultant increased intra-abdominal pressure on cardiac, renal, and liver physiology
- Effects of the absorbed CO_2 on cardiorespiratory function.

The fatal complication of CO_2 embolization to the heart and lung was discussed earlier. CO_2 is insufflated under 12–15 mm Hg pressure to elevate the abdominal wall and allow the camera the necessary distance to the organ operated on. Depending on the intra-abdominal pressure used and the position the patient is placed—head up or head down—several potential harmful physiologic derangements may occur.

Cardiac arrhythmias occur relatively frequently during the performance of laparoscopic surgery and are related to a number of factors, the most significant of which is hypercarbia and the resulting acidemia. Early reports of laparoscopy-associated arrhythmia were in association with spontaneous respiration. Consequently, most anesthesiologists have adopted the universal practice of mechanical ventilation during laparoscopic surgery. There are also a number of pharmacological considerations that lead the anesthesiologist to select agents that limit the risk of cardiac arrhythmia. The surgeon may aid in reducing the incidence of hypercarbia by operating with intraperitoneal pressures that are <15 mm Hg.

The use of an alternate intraperitoneal gas is another method by which the risk of cardiac arrhythmia may be reduced. However, while nitrous oxide is associated with a decreased incidence of arrhythmia, it increases the severity of shoulder tip pain, and, more importantly, is insoluble in blood. External lifting systems (apneumic laparoscopy) are another option that can provide protection against cardiac arrhythmia.

Hypotension can also occur secondary to excessively increased intraperitoneal pressure resulting in decreased venous return and resulting decreased cardiac output. This undesirable result may be potentiated, if the patient is volume depleted. Hypotension secondary to cardiac arrhythmias may also be a consequence of vagal discharge in response to increased intraperitoneal pressure. All of these side effects will be more dangerous for the patient with preexisting cardiovascular compromise.

Gastric Reflux during Laparoscopy

Patients undergoing laparoscopy are usually considered at high risk of acid aspiration syndrome due to gastric regurgitation, which might occur due to the rise in intragastric pressure consequent to the increased IAP. However, during pneumoperitoneum, the lower esophageal sphincter tone far exceeds the intragastric pressure and the raised barrier pressure limits the incidence of regurgitation.

Many study aimed to evaluate whether or not the use of intermittent positive pressure ventilation via the laryngeal mask airway that is associated with a higher risk of gastroesophageal reflux when compared with intermittent positive pressure ventilation via a tracheal tube in patients undergoing day-case gynecological laparoscopy in the head-down position.

Generally, gastric regurgitation and aspiration are complications potentiated by laparoscopic surgery. Some patients are at increased risk, including those with obesity, gastroparesis, hiatal hernia, or any type of gastric outlet obstruction. In such patients, it is important to quickly secure the airway with a cuffed endotracheal tube and to routinely decompress the stomach with a nasogastric or orogastric tube. The surgeon can contribute to aspiration prophylaxis by operating at the lowest necessary intraperitoneal pressure. Patients should be taken out of the Trendelenburg position prior to being extubated. The adverse effects of aspiration may be minimized with the routine preoperative administration of metoclopramide, H2 blockers, and nonparticulate antacids.

Extraperitoneal Gas

During laparoscopic surgery, a number of the complications associated with pneumoperitoneum or its achievement are described in the vascular, gastroenterologic, urologic, and anesthetic sections. However, the problem of extraperitoneal placement or extravasation of gas has not been considered. In some instances, this complication occurs as a result of deficient technique (incorrect placement of insufflation needles; excessive intraperitoneal pressure); while in others, the extravasation is related to gas tracking around the ports or along the dissection planes themselves.

Subcutaneous emphysema may occur if the tip of the Veress needle does not penetrate the peritoneal cavity prior to insufflation of gas. The gas may accumulate in the subcutaneous tissue or between the fascia and the peritoneum. Extraperitoneal insufflation, which is associated with higher levels of CO_2 absorption than intraperitoneal insufflation, is reflected by a sudden rise in the $EtCO_2$, excessive changes in airway pressure, and respiratory acidosis.

Subcutaneous emphysema most commonly results from preperitoneal placement of an insufflation needle or leakage of CO_2 around the cannula sites, the latter frequently because of excessive intraperitoneal pressure. The condition is usually mild and limited to the abdominal wall. However, subcutaneous emphysema can become extensive, involving the extremities, the neck, and the mediastinum. Another relatively common location for emphysema is the omentum or mesentery, a circumstance that the surgeon may mistake for preperitoneal insufflation.

Diagnosis

Usually, the diagnosis will not be a surprise for the surgeon that will have had difficulty in positioning the primary cannula within the peritoneal cavity. Subcutaneous emphysema may be readily identified by the palpation of crepitus, usually in the abdominal wall. In some instances, it can extend along contiguous fascial planes to the neck, where it can be visualized directly. Such a finding may reflect the development of mediastinal emphysema. If mediastinal emphysema is severe or if pneumothorax is developing, the anesthesiologist may report difficulty in maintaining a normal pCO_2, a feature that may indicate impending cardiovascular collapse.

Prevention

The risk of subcutaneous emphysema during laparoscopic surgery is reduced by proper positioning of an insufflation needle. Prior to insertion, it is important to check the insufflation needle for proper function and patency and to establish the baseline flow pressure by attaching it to the insufflation apparatus. The best position for insertion is at the base of the umbilicus, where the abdominal wall is the thinnest. The angle of insertion varies from 45° to near 90°, depending upon the patient's weight, the previous abdominal surgery, and type of anesthesia as described in the section on prevention of vascular injuries. The insertion action should be smooth and firm until the surgeon observing and listening to the device passing through the layers—two (fascia and peritoneum) in the umbilicus and three (two layers of fascia; one peritoneum) in the left upper quadrant feels that placement is intraperitoneal.

No one test is absolutely reliable at predicting intraperitoneal placement. Instead, a number of tests should be used. Of course, aspiration of the insufflation needle should precede all other evaluations. Two tests depend upon the preinflation intraperitoneal pressure. If a drop of water is placed on the open end of the insufflation needle, it should be drawn into the low-pressure intraperitoneal environment of the peritoneal cavity. Although some disagree, the elevation of the anterior abdominal wall is a reasonable way of creating a negative intraperitoneal pressure. Perhaps, a more quantitative way of demonstrating the same principle is to attach the tubing to the needle after insertion but prior to initiating the flow of gas. Elevation of the abdominal wall should result in creation of a low or negative intraperitoneal pressure (1–4 mm Hg). Insufflation should be initiated at a low flow rate of about 1 L/min until the surgeon has confidence that proper placement has been achieved. Loss of liver dullness should occur when about 500 mL of gas has entered the peritoneal cavity. The measured intraperitoneal pressure should be below 10 mm Hg but up to 14 mm Hg, if the patient is obese. Abdominal distension should be symmetrical. If, at any time, the surgeon feels that the needle is not located intraperitoneally, it should be withdrawn and reinserted. Once the peritoneal cavity has been insufflated with an adequate volume of gas, the primary trocar is introduced. The laparoscope is introduced, and, if the cannula is satisfactorily located, the tubing is attached to the appropriate port.

The risk of subcutaneous emphysema may be reduced by maintaining a low intraperitoneal pressure following the placement of the desired cannulas operate below 15 mm Hg and usually work at about 10 mm Hg. Although primary blind insertion of sharp trocar has been demonstrated to be as safe as secondary insertion following pneumoinsufflation, the relative incidence of subcutaneous emphysema is unknown.

Management

Subcutaneous emphysema often presents a management dilemma. Rarely, subcutaneous emphysema has pathophysiologic consequences. More often, it is extremely uncomfortable for the patient and is often disfiguring and alarming for patients and family. When subcutaneous emphysema is severe, physicians may feel compelled to treat it, but the currently described techniques are often invasive or ineffective.

If the surgeon finds that the insufflation has occurred extraperitoneally, there exists a number of management options. While removing the laparoscope and repeating the insufflation is possible, it may be made more difficult because of the new configuration of the anterior peritoneum. Open laparoscopy or the use of an alternate sites such as the left upper quadrant should be considered. One attractive approach is to leave the laparoscope in the expanded preperitoneal space while the insufflation needle is reinserted through the peritoneal membrane, caudal to the tip of the laparoscope under direct vision.

For mild cases of subcutaneous emphysema, no specific intra- or postoperative therapy is required, as the findings, in at least mild cases, quickly resolve following evacuation of the pneumoperitoneum. When the extravasation extends to involve the neck, it is usually preferable to terminate the procedure, as pneumomediastinum, pneumothorax, hypercarbia, and cardiovascular collapse may result. Following the end of the procedure, it is prudent to obtain a chest X-ray. The patient should be managed expectantly unless a tension pneumothorax results, when immediate evacuation must be performed, using a chest tube or a wide bore needle (14–16 gauge) inserted in the second intercostal space in midclavicular line.

ELECTROSURGICAL COMPLICATIONS

Unlike open surgery where hemostasis (control of bleeding) is accomplished by pressure and careful application of fine clamps and ligatures, laparoscopic surgery must rely on electrosurgery to achieve hemostasis. Excessive use of energy can burn a hole in the wall of the organ involved. Current can also cause injury to adjacent organs and even distant organs. Complications of electrosurgery occur secondary to thermal injury from one of three basic causes. The first is thermal trauma from unintended or inappropriate use of the active electrode(s). The second from current diverting to another, undesirable path, causing injury remote from the immediate operative field. Third is injury at the site of the "return" or dispersive electrode. Active electrode injury can occur with either unipolar or bipolar instruments, while trauma secondary to current diversion or dispersive electrode accidents only occur with the unipolar technique. Complications of electrosurgery are reduced with strict adherence to safety protocols coupled with a sound understanding of the circumstances that can lead to undesirable effects on tissue.

Active Electrode Trauma

Unintended activation in open space without touching the tissue is one of the more common mechanisms by which the active electrode causes complications. Such a complication frequently occurs when an electrode, left untended within the peritoneal cavity, is inadvertently activated by compression of the hand switch or depression of the foot pedal. Control of the electrosurgical unit (ESU) or generator by someone other than the operating surgeon is also a source of accidental activation of the electrode.

Direct extension is another mechanism by which the active electrode(s) cause complications. The zone of vaporization or coagulation may extend to involve large blood vessels or vital structures such as the bladder, ureter, or bowel. Bipolar current reduces, but does not eliminate, the risk of thermal injury to adjacent tissue. Consequently, care must be taken to isolate blood vessels prior to desiccation, especially when near vital structures and to apply appropriate amounts of energy in a fashion that allows an adequate margin of noninjured tissue.

Diagnosis

During minimal access surgery, the diagnosis of direct thermal visceral injury may be suspected or confirmed intraoperatively. Careful evaluation of nearby intraperitoneal structures should be made if unintended activation of the electrode occurs. The visual appearance will depend upon a number of factors including the type of the electrode, its proximity to tissue, the output of the generator, and the duration of its activation. High power density activations will often result in vaporization injury and will be more easily recognized than lower power density lesions that result in desiccation and coagulation.

The diagnosis of visceral thermal injury is often delayed until the signs and symptoms of fistula or peritonitis present. This will be particularly true with desiccation injury. Because these complications may not present until 2 to at least 10 days following surgery, long after discharge, both the patient and the physician must be made aware of the possible consequences. Consequently, patients should be advised to report any fever or increasing abdominal pain experienced postoperatively.

Prevention

Electrosurgical injuries are largely prevented if: (a) the surgeon is always in direct control of electrode activation and (b) all electrosurgical hand instruments are removed from the peritoneal cavity when not in use. When removed from the peritoneal cavity, the instruments should be detached from the electrosurgical generator or they should be stored in an insulated pouch near to the operative field. These measures prevent damage to the patient's skin, if the foot pedal is accidentally depressed.

Management

Once diagnosed, thermal injury to bowel, bladder, or ureter, recognized at the time of laparoscopy, should immediately be managed appropriately, considering the potential extent of the zone of coagulative necrosis. The extent of thermal trauma will depend upon the characteristics of the energy transferred to tissue. An electrosurgical incision made with the focused energy from a pointed electrode will be associated with a minimal amount of surrounding thermal injury and may be repaired in a fashion identical to one created mechanically. However, with desiccation injury created as a result of prolonged contact with a relatively large caliber electrode, the thermal necrosis may extend centimeters from the point of contact. In such instances, wide excision or resection will be necessary.

Remote Injury

Remote injury due to current diversion can occur when an electrical current finds a direct path out of the patient's body via grounded sites other than the dispersive electrode. Alternatively, the current can be diverted directly to other tissue before it reaches the tip of the active electrode. In either instance, if the power density becomes high enough, unintended and severe thermal injury can result.

These injuries can only occur with ground-referenced ESUs because they lack an isolated circuit. In such generators, when the dispersive electrode becomes detached, unplugged, or otherwise ineffective, the current will seek any grounded conductor. If the conductor has a small surface area, the current or power density may become high enough to cause thermal injury. Examples include electrocardiograph patch electrodes or the conductive metal components of the operating table.

Modem ESUs are designed and built with isolated circuits and impedance monitoring systems or active electrode monitoring system. Consequently, if any part of the circuit is broken, an alarm sounds, and/or the machine "shuts down", thereby preventing electrode activation. Since the widespread introduction of such generators, the incidence of burns to alternate sites has become largely confined to cases involving the few remaining ground-referenced machines.

Insulation Failure

Failure in the insulation coating the shaft of a laparoscopic electrosurgical electrode can allow current diversion to adjacent tissue. The high power density resulting from such small points of contact fosters the creation of a significant injury. During laparoscopic surgery, bowel is frequently the tissue near to, or in contact with, the shaft of the electrode, making it the organ most susceptible to this type of electrosurgical injury. The fact that the whole shaft of the electrode is frequently not encompassed by the surgeon's visual field at laparoscopy makes it possible that such an injury can occur unaware to the operator.

Prevention of complication of insulation failure starts with the selection and care of electrosurgical hand instruments. Loose instrument bins should be replaced with containers designed to keep the instruments from damaging each other. The instruments should be examined prior to each case, searching for worn or obviously defective insulation. When found, the damaged instrument should be removed and repaired or replaced. Despite all efforts, unobserved breaks in insulation may rarely occur. While the use of disposable instruments is often claimed as a way of reducing the incidence of insulation failure, there is no guarantee that this is the case, as invisible defects may occur in the manufacturing process. Furthermore, the insulation on disposable electrodes is thinner and more susceptible to trauma. Consequently, when applying unipolar electrical energy, the shaft of the instrument should be kept free of vital structures and, if possible, totally visible in the operative field.

Direct Coupling

During minimal access surgery, direct coupling occurs when an activated electrode touches and energizes another metal conductor such as a laparoscope, cannula, or other instrument. If the conductor is near to, or in contact with, other tissue, a thermal injury can result. Such accidents often happen following unintentional activation of an electrode. Prevention of direct coupling is facilitated by removal of the electrodes when not in use and visually confirming that the electrode is not in inappropriate contact with other conductive instruments prior to activation.

Capacitive Coupling

Many capacitive coupling of diathermy current have been reported as causes of occult injury during surgical laparoscopy. Capacitance reflects the ability of a conductor to establish an electrical current in an unconnected but nearby circuit. An electrical field is established around the shaft of any activated laparoscopic unipolar electrode, a circumstance that makes the electrode a capacitor. This field is harmless if the circuit is completed via a dispersive, low power density pathway. If capacitive coupling occurs between the laparoscopic electrode and a metal cannula positioned in the abdominal wall, the current without any complication returns to the abdominal wall where it traverses to the dispersive electrode. However, if the metal cannula is anchored to the skin by a nonconductive plastic retaining sleeve or anchor (a hybrid system), the current will not return to the abdominal wall because the sleeve acts as an insulator. Instead, the capacitor will have to search elsewhere to complete the circuit. Consequently, bowel or any other nearby conductor can become the target of a relatively high power density discharge. The risk is greater with high voltage currents such as the coagulation output on an electrosurgical generator. This mechanism is also more likely to occur when a unipolar electrode is inserted through an operating laparoscope that, in turn, is passed through a plastic laparoscopic port. In this configuration, the plastic port acts as the insulator. If the electrode capacitively couples with the metal laparoscope, nearby bowel will be at risk for significant thermal injury.

During minimal access surgery, prevention of capacitive coupling can largely be accomplished by avoiding the use of hybrid laparoscope cannula systems that contain a mixture of conductive and nonconductive elements. Instead, it is preferred that all plastic or all metal cannula systems be used. When and if operating laparoscopes are employed, all metal cannula systems should be the rule unless there is no intent to perform unipolar electrosurgical procedures through the operating channel.

Risk of this injury is very much minimized if low voltage radiofrequency current (cutting) is used and when the high voltage outputs are avoided.

Dispersive Electrode Burns

The use of isolated circuit generators with return electrode monitors has all but eliminated dispersive electrode-related thermal injury. Return electrode monitoring (REM) is actually accomplished by measuring the impedance (sometimes called resistance) in the dispersive electrode, which should always be low because of the large surface area. To accomplish this, most return electrode monitors, actually, are divided into two electrodes, allowing the generator to compare the impedance from the two sides of the pad. If the overall impedance is high or if there is a significant difference between the two sides, as is the case with partial detachment, the active electrode cannot be activated. Without such devices, partial detachment of the patient pad could result in a thermal injury because reducing the surface area of the electrode raises the current density. It is important for the surgeon to establish what type of ESU is being used in each case. Absence of an REM system is a reason for increased scrutiny of the positioning of the dispersive electrode, both before the surgery begins, and as the operation progresses.

Electrode Shields and Monitors

A United States-based company (Electroscope Inc.) markets a system that helps to reduce further the chance of director capacitive coupling. A reusable shield is passed over the shaft of the laparoscopic electrode prior to its insertion into the peritoneal cavity. This shield protects against insulation failure and detects the presence of significant capacitance. Should an insulation break occur or when capacitance becomes threatening, the integrated monitoring system automatically shuts down the generator. The shield enlarges the effective diameter of the electrode by about 2 mm, making it necessary to use larger caliber laparoscopic ports.

Despite perceptions to the contrary, electrosurgery has been rendered a safe modality for use in surgical procedures. However, safe and effective application of electrical energy requires an adequate understanding and implementation of basic principles as well as the availability of modern electrosurgical generators and appropriate education of medical and support staff. Care and prudence must be exercised when utilizing electricity within the peritoneal cavity. The zone of significant thermal injury usually extends beyond that of the visible injury, a feature that must be borne in mind when operating in close proximity to vital structures such as bowel bladder, ureter, and large and important blood vessels. It is equally important to impart the minimal amount of thermal injury (if any) necessary to accomplish the task at hand, even around nonvital structures, by using the ideal power output and the appropriate active electrodes.

HEMORRHAGIC COMPLICATIONS

Hemorrhagic complications may occur as a consequence of entry into the peritoneal cavity or as a result of trauma incurred to blood vessels encountered during the course of the procedure.

Hemorrhage Associated with Access Technique

Great Vessel Injury

During access, the most dangerous hemorrhagic complications of entry are to the great vessels, including the aorta and vena cava as well as the common iliac vessels and their branches, the internal and external iliac arteries and veins. The incidence of major vascular injury is probably underreported, but has been estimated to range widely from 0.93 to 9 per 10,000 cases. The trauma most often occurs secondary to insertion of an insufflation needle, but may be created by the tip of the trocar. However, not uncommonly, the injury is associated with the insertion of ancillary laparoscopic ports into the lower quadrants. The vessels most frequently damaged are the aorta and the right common iliac artery, which branches from the aorta in the midline. The anatomically more posterior location of the vena cava and the iliac veins provides relative protection, but not immunity, from injury. While most of these injuries are small amenable to repair with suture, some have been larger, requiring ligation with or without the insertion of a vascular graft. Not surprisingly, death has been reported in a number of instances.

Diagnosis: If great vessels are injured, most often the problem presents as profound hypotension with or without the appearance of a significant volume of blood within the peritoneal cavity. In some instances, the surgeon aspirates blood via the insufflation needle, prior to introduction of distension gas. Frequently, the bleeding may be contained in the retroperitoneal space, a feature that usually delays the diagnosis. Consequently, the development of hypovolemic shock in the recovery room may well be secondary to otherwise unrecognized laceration to a great vessel. To avoid the late recognition, it is important to evaluate the course of each great vessel prior to completing the procedure.

Prevention: There are a number of ways by which the incidence of large vessel trauma can be minimized. Certainly, it is essential that the positioning of ancillary or secondary trocar in the lower quadrants be performed under direct vision. This is more difficult for the primary cannula. It has been suggested that the use of "open laparoscopy" for the initial port entirely avoids the issue of great vessel injury secondary to insufflation needles and trocars. However, open laparoscopy has its own potential drawbacks such as increased operating time, the need for larger incisions, and a greater chance of wound infection, all without eliminating the incidence of bowel injury at entry.

The risk of large vessel injury should be reduced if careful attention is paid to access technique and equipment used. If used, both insufflation needles and the trocar should be kept sharp and surgeon should use same instrument each time. The safety sheath of the insufflation needle should be checked to ensure that both the spring and the sliding mechanism are functioning normally. Many disposable trocar-cannula systems are constructed with a safety mechanism that covers or retracts the trocar following passage through the fascia and peritoneum. However, there are currently no available data that demonstrate a reduction in the incidence of major vessel injury with the use of these devices.

The application of appropriate technique is based upon a sound understanding of the normal anatomic relationships between the commonly used entry points and the great vessels. A "safety zone" exists inferior to the sacral promontory in the area bounded superiorly by the bifurcation of the aorta, posteriorly by the sacral curve, and laterally by the iliac vessels. Safe insertion of the insufflation needle mandates that the instrument be maintained in a midline, sagittal plane while the operator directs the tip between the iliac vessels, anterior to the sacrum but inferior to the bifurcation of the aorta and the proximal aspect of the vena cava. Such positioning requires elevation of the abdominal wall while angling the insufflation needle about 45º to horizontal. The tactile and visual feedback created when the needle passes through the fascial and peritoneal layers of the abdominal wall, if recognized and heeded, may prevent overaggressive insertion attempts. Such proprioceptive feedback is diminished with disposable needles as compared to the classic Veress model. Instead, the surgeon must listen to the "clicks" as the needle obturator retracts when it passes through the rectus fascia and the peritoneum. The needle should never be forced.

It is critical to note that these anatomic relationships may vary with body type and with the orientation of the patient to the horizontal position. In women of normal weight and body habitus, in the horizontal recumbent position, the bifurcation of the aorta is located immediately beneath the umbilicus. However, in obese individuals, the umbilicus may be positioned up to 2 or more cm below bifurcation. Fortunately, this circumstance allows the insufflation needle to be directed in a more vertical position—those between 160 and 200 pounds between 45 and 90°, while those women over 200 pounds at nearly 90°. Women placed in a head-down position (Trendelenburg position) will shift their great vessel more superiorly and anteriorly in a fashion that may make them more vulnerable to an entry injury. Consequently, positioning of the insufflation needle, and at least the initial trocar and cannula, should be accomplished with the patient in a horizontal position. This approach additionally facilitates the evaluation of the upper abdomen, an exercise that is limited if the intraperitoneal content is shifted cephalad by the patient's head-down position.

The risk of great vessel injury is likely reduced by insufflating the peritoneal cavity to adequate pressure. An intraperitoneal pressure of 20 mm Hg, while not desirable for prolonged periods of time, can aid in separating the abdominal wall from the great vessels during the process of insertion of a sharp trocar.

Management: If blood is withdrawn from the insufflation needle, it should be left in place while immediate preparations are made to obtain blood products and perform laparotomy. If the diagnosis of hemoperitoneum is made upon initial visualization of the peritoneal cavity, a grasping instrument may be used, if possible, to temporarily occlude the vessel. While it is unlikely that significant injury can predictably be repaired by laparoscopically directed technique, if temporary hemostasis can be obtained, and the laceration visualized, selected, localized lesions can be repaired, with suture, under laparoscopic guidance. Such an attempt should not be made by any other than experienced and technically adept surgeons. Even if such an instance exists, fine judgment should be used so as not to delay the institution of lifesaving, open surgical repair.

Most surgeons should gain immediate entry into the peritoneal cavity and immediately compress the aorta and vena cava just below the level of the renal vessels, gaining at least temporary control of blood loss. At that juncture, the most appropriate course of action, including the need for vascular surgical consultation, will become more apparent.

Abdominal Wall Vessels

Most commonly injured abdominal wall vessels are the inferior epigastric and superior epigastric vessel. They are invariably damaged by the initial passage of an ancillary trocar or when a wider device is introduced later in the procedure. The problem may be recognized immediately by the observation of blood dripping along the cannula or out through the incision. However, it is not uncommon for the cannula itself to obstruct the bleeding until withdrawal at the end of the case.

More sinister are injuries to the deep inferior epigastric vessels, branches of the external iliac artery and vein that also course cephalad, but are deep to the rectus fascia and often deep to the muscles themselves. More laterally located are the deep circumflex iliac vessels that are uncommonly encountered in laparoscopic surgery. Laceration of these vessels may cause profound blood loss, particularly when the trauma is unrecognized and causes extraperitoneal bleeding.

Diagnosis: Diagnosis of abdominal wall vasculature injury is by visualization of the blood dripping down the cannula or by the postoperative appearance of shock, abdominal wall discoloration, and/or a hematoma located near to the incision. In some instances, the blood may track to a more distant site, presenting as a pararectal or vulvar mass. Delayed diagnosis may be prevented at the end of the procedure by laparoscopically evaluating each peritoneal incision following removal of the cannula.

Prevention: With the help of telescope, transillumination of the abdominal wall from within will, at least in most thin women, allow for identification of the superficial inferior epigastric vessels. However, the deep inferior epigastric vessels cannot be identified by this mechanism because of their location deep to the rectus sheath. Consequently, prevention of deep inferior epigastric vessel injury requires that the surgeon understand the anatomic course of these vessels.

The most consistent landmarks are the median umbilical ligaments (obliterated umbilical arteries) and the entry point of the round ligament into the inguinal canal. At the pubic crest, the deep inferior epigastric vessels begin their course cephalad between the medially located medial umbilical ligament and the laterally positioned exit point of the round ligament. The trocar should be inserted medial or lateral to the vessels, if they are visualized. If the vessels cannot be seen and it is necessary to position the trocar laterally, it should be positioned 3–4 cm lateral to the median umbilical ligament or lateral to the lateral margin of the rectus abdominis muscle. Too lateral an insertion will endanger the deep circumflex epigastric artery. The operator may further limit risk of injury by placing a No. 22 spinal needle through the skin at the desired location, directly observing the entry via the laparoscope. This not only provides more reassurance that a safe location has been identified, but the easily visualized peritoneal needle hole gives the surgeon a target for inserting the trocar with greater precision.

A common mistake is to fashion the incision appropriately, only to direct the trocar medially in its course through the abdominal wall, thereby injuring the vessels. Another factor that may contribute to the risk of injury is the use of large diameter trocar. Consequently, for this and other reasons, the surgeon should use the smallest trocar necessary for performance of the procedure.

Management: Superficial inferior epigastric artery lacerations usually respond to expectant management. Rotation of the cannula to a position where compression is possible is also helpful. Rarely is a suture necessary.

We have found that the use of a straight suture passer is most useful for the ligation of lacerated deep inferior epigastric vessels. A number of other devices and techniques have been introduced that facilitate the accomplishment of this task. To summarize, the trocar and cannula are removed. Then, under laparoscopic visualization and using a ligature carrier, a ligature is placed through the incision and directed laterally and inferiorly, where it is held by a grasping forceps. The ligature carrier is removed and subsequently passed through the incision again, without a suture, but this time medial and inferior to the lacerated vessels. The suture is threaded into the carrier from within the peritoneal cavity and is then externalized and tied. For small incisions, narrower than the diameter of the surgeon's finger, the knot may be tightened with a knot manipulator.

There are other less uniformly successful methods for attaining hemostasis from a lacerated deep inferior epigastric vessel. The most obvious is the placement of large, through-and-through mattress sutures. These are usually removed about 48 hours later. Electrodesiccation may be successful. Either a unipolar or bipolar grasping forceps is passed through another ancillary cannula taking care to identify, grasp, and adequately desiccate the vessel. Either continuous or "blended" current is used at appropriate power outputs for the machine and the electrode. Another method that has enjoyed some success is temporary compression with the balloon of a Foley catheter, passed through the incision into the peritoneal cavity, then secured and tightened externally with a clamp. While some suggest that the balloon should be left in place for 24 hours, the delicate channel may be damaged by the clamp, making it impossible to deflate the balloon. For this reason, we not recommend this option.

Intraperitoneal Vessel Injury

The bleeding may result from inadvertent entry into a vessel failure of a specific occlusive technique or human error in the application of the selected technique. Furthermore, in addition to the problem of delayed hemorrhage inherent in transection of arteries, there may be further delay in diagnosis at laparoscopy because of the restricted visual field and the temporary occlusive pressure exerted by the CO_2 within the peritoneal cavity.

Diagnosis: During laparoscopy, inadvertent division of an artery or vein will usually become immediately self-evident. However, in some instances, transected arteries will go into spasm only to begin bleeding minutes to hours later, an event that may temporarily go unnoticed due to the limited field of view presented by the laparoscope. Consequently, at the end of the procedure, all areas of dissection should be carefully examined. In addition, the CO_2 should be vented, decreasing the intraperitoneal pressure to about 5 mm Hg, allowing recognition of vessels occluded by the higher pressure.

Prevention: Attention to meticulous technique is at least as important in laparoscopically-directed surgery as it is for open or vaginal cases. During dissection, vessels should be identified and occluded prior to division, a task made simpler by the magnification afforded by the laparoscope. If suture is used to occlude a vessel, it must be, of the appropriate caliber, positioned with an adequate pedicle and tied snugly with a secure knot. Electrosurgery, if used, should be applied in the appropriate waveform and power density and for a time adequate to allow for sufficient tissue desiccation. Clips should be of a size appropriate for the vessel and they must be applied in a secure fashion, also with an adequate pedicle of tissue. Care should be exercised to avoid manipulation of pedicles secured with clips or suture, as such trauma could adversely affect the security of the closure. When linear stapling devices are employed, the appropriate staple size should be selected and the tissue encompassed in the staple line should be of uniform thickness. Failure to maintain relatively uniform tissue thickness may result in inadequate compression of blood vessels that course through the thinner areas of the pedicle.

Management: Transected vessels should be secured immediately. If electrosurgical desiccation is used to maintain or achieve hemostasis, the use of a serial ammeter is useful to demonstrate the endpoint of energy application. There is evidence that artery larger in diameter than 3 mm is less reliably occluded with desiccation than are those 3 mm or less. Care must be exerted to avoid blind clamping and electrosurgical desiccation, even with bipolar instruments, especially when <1 cm from ureter or bowel. When a vessel is in such a location, it is usually preferable to secure it with a clip.

Identification of small vessel bleeding and ooze is often facilitated by the use of copious irrigation and even underwater examination. Capillary ooze may be managed with higher voltage fulguration currents using electrodes with a bulbous tip. When using electrosurgery for this purpose, the use of electrolyte-containing solutions should be avoided, as they disperse current, rendering the technique ineffective. Instead, the low viscosity fluids such as glycine are recommended as, in addition to being nonconductive, they may facilitate localization of the vessels.

GASTROINTESTINAL COMPLICATIONS

Following laparoscopy, it is not uncommon for the patient to experience nausea. However, in some instances, the problem becomes severe. Gastrointestinal viscera potentially injured during the performance of gynecologic laparoscopy and include the stomach, the small bowel, and the colon.

Insufflation Needle Injuries

Needle entry into the stomach almost invariably happens in the presence of gastric distension. While this may occur secondary to aerophagia, the complication is frequently related to difficult or improper intubation or to the use of mask induction with an inhalation anesthetic. Mechanical entry into large or small bowel may occur in any instance, but is up to 10 times more common when laparoscopy is performed on patients with previous intraperitoneal inflammation or abdominal surgery. In such instances, loops of intestine can adhere to the abdominal wall under the insertion site. Perforation may also occur following an overly aggressive attempt to insert the insufflation needle.

Recognition

Recognition of gastric entry by the insufflation needle may follow identification of any or all of the signs of extraperitoneal entry, including increased filling pressure, asymmetric distension of the peritoneal cavity, or the aspiration of gastric particulate matter through the lumen of the needle. However, the hollow, capacious nature of the stomach may allow the initial insufflation pressure to remain normal. Unfortunately, in some instances, the problem is not identified until the trocar is inserted and the gastric mucosa identified by direct vision. Recognition of bowel entry usually follows observation of the signs described above for gastric injury, with the addition of feculent odor to the list of findings. Prevention of insufflation needle injury to the gastrointestinal tract is important because such measures largely eliminate the risk of more sinister trocar trauma. Gastric perforation can largely be eliminated with the selective use of preoperative oral or nasogastric suction. The surgeon should request that this can be performed if there has been difficulty with intubation or when the needle is intentionally inserted near to the stomach in the left upper quadrant.

Many have suggested that open laparoscopy is the most appropriate and effective way to reduce the incidence of intestinal injury in a patient at risk because of previous lower abdominal surgery. However, there are no studies that prove this to be the case. Indeed, there exists evidence that open laparoscopy is itself associated with intestinal injury. Consequently, many surgeons have suggested the use of left upper quadrant insertion with a properly decompressed stomach.

Although not strictly a prophylactic measure, the routine use of preoperative mechanical bowel preparation, at least in selected, high-risk cases, will diminish the need for laparotomy and/or colostomy, if large bowel entry occurs.

Management

The management of any trauma to the gastrointestinal tract depends in part upon the nature of the injury and in part upon the organ(s) involved. In general, insufflation needle punctures that have not resulted in a defect significantly larger than their diameter may be handled expectantly. Larger defects should be repaired or resected, by laparoscopic- or a laparotomy-based technique, depending upon extent of the lesion.

If, following insertion of an insufflation needle, particulate debris is identified, the needle should be left in place and an alternate insertion site identified such as the left upper quadrant. If the insufflation needle possesses a removable obturator, an arrow caliber optical fiber or laparoscope may be passed to evaluate the location of the tip and to aid in later identification of the puncture site. Immediately following successful entry into the peritoneal cavity, the site of injury is identified. Unless significant injury or bleeding is identified, the situation may be handled expectantly. If there is unexpected extension of the laceration, it should be managed similarly to a trocar injury.

Trocar Injuries

During access technique, damage caused by sharp trocar penetration is usually more serious than when needle injury occurs. Most often, the injury is created by the primary trocar because of its blind insertion. However, inadequate attention paid to the insertion of ancillary cannulas may also result in visceral injury.

Diagnosis

If a primary trocar penetrates bowel, the diagnosis is usually made when the surgeon visualizes the mucosal lining of the gastrointestinal structure following insertion of the laparoscope. If large bowel is entered, feculent odor may be noted. However, in some instances, the injury may not immediately be recognized as the cannula may not stay within or it may pass through the lumen and out the other side of the viscus. Such injuries usually occur when a single loop of bowel is adhered to the anterior abdominal wall near to the entry point. Consequently, it is important at the end of the procedure to directly view the removal of the primary cannula, either through the cannula itself or via an ancillary port. Routine direct visualization of primary port incisional closure will facilitate the accomplishment of this task. Unfortunately, the injury may go unrecognized until it presents postoperatively as peritonitis, abscess, enterocutaneous fistula, or death.

Prevention

The following measures were reported to reduce the incidence of trocar injuries:

- Disposable laparoscopes are usually sharper. They require less force to insert and, thus, there is less chance of compressing the trocar against the bowel or blood vessels
- Some manufacturers provide a plastic sheath, which springs and covers the sharp edge of the trocar after insertion. Safety shields will not prevent injury, however, in case of bowel adhesions
- The use of ultrasound to "map" the abdominal wall for safe entry area is recommended, especially when adhesions are present
- The smaller 5 mm cannula is safer as it requires less pressure to insert. Equipped with a camera, it allows safe placement of the larger cannula under vision
- Hasson described an open surgical approach to placement of the cannula, thus reducing the risk of perforation by the blind closed technique
- Before the conclusion of surgery, a thorough search for bowel injuries must be performed as delay in recognition of such injury can be catastrophic. Thus, review of the videotapes can ascertain if safety measures were taken during this critical part of the procedure.

Despite the widespread use of retractable trocars or safety sheaths, injury to bowel or other structures may occur. As stated above, many employ, routinely or selectively, the concept of "open" laparoscopy, where the peritoneal cavity is entered directly via an infra- or intraumbilical incision. Despite the apparent virtues of this approach, bowel entry may still occur. An alternative approach, especially when entering an abdomen with previous laparotomy scars, is the insertion of an arrow caliber cannula in the left upper quadrant following decompression of the stomach. It is unusual for a patient to have had previous surgery in this location. Following placement of the cannula, usually just below the costal margin in the midclavicular line, an arrow diameter laparoscope may be passed, allowing a direct view of the abdominal wall under the umbilicus or other planned site of insertion. If necessary, the small laparoscope may be used to direct the dissection of intestine from under the insertion site. This approach gains additional value with the introduction of a fiber laparoscope small enough to fit through the lumen of an insufflation needle.

Stomach injuries most frequently occur when there has been difficulty in intubation and may be more common following left upper quadrant insertion if the stomach has not previously been decompressed. Consequently, liberal use of oral or nasogastric decompression will likely reduce the incidence of trocar injury to the stomach.

Most common cause of bowel injuries usually is when the intestine is adherent to the abdominal wall under the site of trocar insertion. Adherence is usually secondary to previous surgery. Consequently, in such patients, open laparoscopy or left upper quadrant entry may be used. Preoperative mechanical bowel preparation should be employed in high-risk patients to facilitate repair of colonic defects without the need to perform a laparotomy.

Management

Trocar injuries to small bowel require repair. If it can be ascertained that the injury is isolated and if the operator is capable, the lesion may be sutured under laparoscopic guidance with a double layer of running 2-0 or 3-0 synthetic absorbable suture. Extensive lesions may require resection and reanastomosis. In well-trained and experienced hand, this may be performed under laparoscopic direction. However, in most instances, laparotomy will be required. Regardless of the method of repair, copious irrigation should be employed and the patient admitted for postoperative observation. The patient is kept without oral intake and nasogastric decompression should be liberally used at the discretion of the surgeon.

If the injury is to the sigmoid colon, primary repair may be attempted if the bowel has been mechanically prepared preoperatively. Otherwise, colostomy should be considered, with the possible exception of ascending colon lesions. If uncertainty exists regarding the extent of injury, laparotomy is always indicated.

INJURY TO BLADDER

Laparoscopy-associated damage to the bladder or ureter may occur secondary to mechanical or thermal trauma. Vesical injury is often secondary to a trocar entering the undrained bladder, but may also occur during dissection of the bladder, either from other adhered structures or from the anterior aspect of the uterus. The proliferation of laparoscopically-directed retropubic suspension for urinary incontinence will likely be associated with bladder injury. Ureteric injury is more commonly encountered secondary to thermal damage. However, more recently, there have been descriptions of ureteric trauma secondary to other causes such as mechanical dissection or the use of linear stapling devices.

Diagnosis

If urinary bladder is injured, intraoperative identification of the injury is the most important aspect of management. The surgeon may be cognizant of entering a hollow viscus or may note the presence of urine in the operative field. If an indwelling catheter is in place, hematuria or pneumaturia (CO_2 in the indwelling drainage system) may be noted. Existence of a bladder laceration may be confirmed with the injection of sterile milk or a dilute methylene blue solution via a catheter. Thermal injury to the bladder may not be initially apparent, presenting later in the patient's postoperative course.

Unfortunately, although intraoperative recognition of ureteric injury has been described, diagnosis is usually delayed until sometime following the procedure. Ureteric lacerations may be proven intraoperatively with the injection of indigo carmine. Thermal injury will present, 24 hours to 14 days, following surgery with one or a combination of fever, abdominal or flank pain, and the clinical findings of peritonitis. A leukocytosis may be present and an intravenous pyelogram (IVP) will demonstrate extravasation of urine or urinoma. Intraoperative recognition of mechanical obstruction, with staples or a suture, will be made only by direct visualization. Not surprisingly, cases of laparoscopy-associated ureteric obstruction seem to present at a time similar to those that follow laparotomy-based procedures a few days to a week following the operation. These patients present with flank pain and may have fever. The diagnosis may be suggested by abdominal ultrasound, but an IVP can be more precise at identifying the site and completeness of the obstruction.

Uretero- or vesicovaginal fistula will present in a delayed fashion with incontinence or discharge. Confirmation of bladder fistula will be by direct visualization and/or the leakage of instilled methylene blue onto a tampon. Ureterovaginal fistula will not pass the methylene blue from the bladder, but will be demonstrated with the intravenous injection of indigo carmine.

Prevention

Before start of surgery, patient should void urine. Trocar-related cystotomies are generally preventable with routine preoperative bladder drainage. Additional caution must be exercised in the patient previously exposed to abdominal or pelvic surgery, where there is a tendency for the bladder to be pulled above the level of the symphysis pubis. The urachus, although rarely present, should be avoided, if possible. It is likely that the placement of an indwelling catheter, at least for prolonged or difficult cases, will reduce the incidence of injury resulting from dissection. Surgical separation of the bladder from the uterus or other adherent structures requires good visualization, appropriate retraction, and excellent surgical technique. Sharp mechanical dissection is preferred, particularly when relatively dense adhesions are present.

If the surgeon cannot, with assurance, steer a wide path from its course, the ureter must be directly visualized. This is especially true when laser, electrosurgical, or stapling techniques are employed. Frequently, the ureter can be seen through the peritoneum of the pelvic sidewall between the pelvic brim and the attachment of the broad ligament. However, because of patient variation or the presence of pathology, the location of the ureter can become obscured. In such instances, the ureter can usually be visualized through the peritoneum at the pelvic brim, although the maneuver is slightly more difficult on the left because of the location of the sigmoid mesentery. If CO_2 laser energy is to be employed, fluid injected at an appropriate location between the peritoneal surface and the ureter can provide a degree of protection from thermal injury.

If entry into the retroperitoneal space is required for exposure, there should be no hesitation to undertake such dissection. The surface of the peritoneum should be breached with scissors at the closest level proximal, and anterior, to the most distal site of planned dissection where the location of the ureter is known or anticipated. If the ureter is seen through the peritoneum, it may be grasped with a Babcock forceps to minimize trauma while the peritoneum is incised. Careful sharp and blunt dissection then may be applied to provide adequate exposure in the operative field. If the ureter cannot be seen through the peritoneal surface, a fine, toothed forceps should be employed to grasp and elevate the peritoneum allowing careful entry into the retroperitoneal space.

The techniques used for retroperitoneal dissection are also important in reducing the risk of ureteric injury. Blunt dissection can be facilitated with the instillation of fluid into the retroperitoneal space under pressure. Others have advocated the selective preoperative placement of ureteric stents including those that are illuminated to provide additional safety. We prefer instead the use of mechanical (sharp or blunt) dissection with sharp-curved scissors and a narrow, pointed grasping forceps attached to an electrosurgical generator. The assistant is provided with a narrow, pointed, and toothed grasping forceps as well as a suction irrigation system to use, as requested, through an ancillary cannula. Dissection proceeds, respecting the blood supply of the ureter, by minimizing direct manipulation and by preserving the integrity of its sheath. If electrical energy is used, it must be applied judiciously at safe distances from the ureter and its blood supply. The narrow, pointed grasping forceps facilitate precise and safe desiccation of small caliber blood vessels.

Treatment

Most of the injury of the bladder can be managed conservatively. Small caliber injuries to the bladder (1–2 mm) may be treated expectantly, with prolonged catheterization for 7–14 days. However, in such cases, the duration of catheterization can be reduced or eliminated if repair is undertaken intraoperatively. When a more significant injury to the bladder is identified, it may often be repaired under laparoscopic direction, provided the presence of adequate surgical skill and a location that is amenable to laparoscopic technique. Further evaluation of the location and extent of the laceration may be provided by direct laparoscopic examination of the mucosal surface of the bladder. Should the laceration be near to or involve the trigone, open repair may be preferable. In making this evaluation, the mechanism of injury should be considered, as desiccation resulting from electrical energy may extend beyond the visible limits of the lesion.

A purse string closure may be fashioned using any of a number of synthetic absorbable sutures of 2-0 to 3-0 caliber, tying the knot either intra- or extracorporeally. For linear lacerations, the defect is preferably closed in two layers. If there is significant thermal injury, it may be valuable to excise the coagulated segment. Postoperative catheterization with either a large caliber urethral or suprapubic catheter should be maintained for 5–7 days for simple fundal lacerations and for 2 weeks for those closer to the trigone, the vaginal vault, or those that may be associated with significant thermal injury.

During minimal access surgery, intraoperative diagnosis of ureteric injury provides the opportunity for intraoperative management. If damage is less, it may respond adequately to the passage of a ureteric stent for about 10–20 days. However, in most instances, repair is indicated. The principles should follow those previously established for open cases. While laparoscopically-directed repair of ureteric lacerations and transections have been described, such maneuvers should be practiced only by those with exceptional surgical skill and experience. Even in these cases, it is advisable to consult intraoperatively with a specialist in urology.

When the diagnosis of ureteral injury is delayed until following surgery, the imperative is to establish drainage. Some obstructions or lacerations, if incomplete or small, may be successfully treated with either the retrograde or anterograde passage of a ureteral stent. Urinomas may be drained percutaneously. If a stent cannot be successfully manipulated across the lesion, a percutaneous nephrostomy should be created and plans should be made for operative repair.

NEUROLOGIC INJURY

The incidence of nerve injury associated with laparoscopy is more common in obese patient, but has been estimated at 0.5 per 1,000 cases. Peripheral neurologic injury is usually related either to inappropriate positioning of the patient or occurs secondary to pressure exerted by the surgeon or assistants. During laparoscopy, nerve injury may happen rarely as a result of the surgical dissection.

In the lower extremity, the trauma may be direct such as compression of the perineal nerve against stirrups. Alternatively, the femoral nerve or the sciatic nerve or its branches may be overstretched and damaged by inappropriate positioning of the hip or the knee joint.

Brachial plexus injuries may occur secondary to the surgeon or assistants leaning against the abducted arm during the procedure. Alternatively, if the patient is placed in steep Trendelenburg position, the brachial plexus may be damaged because of the pressure exerted on the shoulder joint.

Diagnosis

If nerve is damaged in most instances, the patient is found to have sensory and/or motor deficit as they emerge from the effects of the anesthesia. The diagnosis can usually be suspected by clinical examination. Injuries to the perineal nerve will be reflected by loss of sensation in the lateral aspect of the leg and foot together with a foot drop. Brachial plexus injuries may be variable, but usually involve damage to the C5-C6 roots manifesting in loss of flexion of the elbow and adduction of the shoulder. Electromyography can be used to further define the extent and location of the lesion by testing nerve conduction and recording the electrical potential for various muscles. This evaluation should be delayed for 3 weeks to allow for complete degeneration of injured nerves.

Prevention

During laparoscopic procedure, if nerve injury has to be prevented, then surgeon should must achieve a good ergonomics of patient. The incidence of brachial plexus injury can be reduced by placing the arms in an adducted position, which also facilitates the performance of pelvic surgery by allowing the surgeon to stand in a more comfortable position. Should it be necessary to leave the arm in an abducted position, adequate padding and support of the arms and shoulders are necessary and can be facilitated with the use of shoulder supports, preventing the slippage of the patient up the table when placed in Trendelenburg position. Furthermore, in such a position, the surgeon may not lean on the patient's arm.

Sciatic and perineal nerve injury is minimized with the use of appropriate stirrups and careful positioning protocols. Those stirrups that combine both knee and foot support are probably best. Additional measures include simultaneous raising and lowering of the legs, flexion of the knees before flexion of the hips, and limitation of external rotation of the hip. Assistants should be admonished to avoid placing undue pressure on the inner thighs.

Injury to the obturator and genitofemoral nerves is uncommon, but will likely increase as greater numbers of retroperitoneal dissections are performed. In such cases, it will be important to clearly understand the anatomy, maintain hemostasis, and to exert the utmost care in performing the dissections, carefully identifying the neural structures as they are encountered.

Management

Most injuries to peripheral nerves recover spontaneously. The time to recovery depends upon the site and severity of the lesion. For most peripheral injuries, full sensorineural recovery occurs in 3–6 months. Recovery may be facilitated with physical therapy, appropriate braces, and electrical stimulation of the affected muscles. Transection of major intrapelvic nerves will require open microsurgical repair.

DISSECTION AND THERMAL INJURY

Recognition

Diagnosis of injury to the bowel incurred during the course of dissection may be more straightforward. Any length of dissected bowel should be carefully examined prior to proceeding further with the procedure. This is, if anything, more important during laparoscopic operations in comparison to those performed via laparotomy, for comprehensive "running" of the bowel near the end of the case is far more difficult under endoscopic guidance.

There has been confusion in the past regarding the frequency of thermal injury to bowel following the use of electrical energy. Formerly, many injuries actually caused by mechanical trauma were erroneously attributed to electrosurgical accidents.

Thermal injury to bowel may be more difficult to diagnose intraoperatively, particularly if created with electrical or laser energy, a feature that makes careful adherence to safety protocols a surgeon's imperative. Even if thermal injury is recognized, it is difficult to estimate the extent of the damage by visual inspection, as the zone of desiccation may exceed the area of visual damage. An understanding of the differing impacts of the various types of electrical current is essential for estimation of the extent of injury. In some instances, diagnosis is delayed until the development of peritonitis and fever, usually a few days later, but occasionally not for several weeks.

Prevention

Total prevention of dissection or thermal injury is impossible, but the incidence of penetrating or energy-based enteric complications may be reduced with patience, prudence, and meticulous technique. A sound understanding of the principles of electrosurgery is critical to reducing the incidence of electrical trauma.

When dissecting, exposure of the operative field must be accomplished with a combination of good visualization and adequate traction and, if necessary, countertraction applied by forceps. In many instances, it will be necessary to enlist the aid of a competent assistant. Dissection close to bowel should be performed mechanically, using sharp scissors, not with electrical or laser energy sources. Occlusion of blood vessels near to bowel is preferably accomplished with clips, but may be performed with bipolar current provided that there is an adequate margin of tissue, a circumstance that usually requires skeletonization of the vessel.

There is no certainty about the proper distance to maintain between the electrode and the bowel serosa. Animal histological studies, using the rather large caliber Kleppinger forceps, have demonstrated that desiccation injury begins to affect bowel serosa and muscularis between 5 and 10 mm away. It is likely that the zone of safety is less for instruments that compress tissue well or that use electrodes with a smaller surface area. Regardless, if the difficulty of the dissection makes the surgeon uncomfortable, alternative methods for hemostasis should be used. If this is not feasible, the aid of more experienced colleagues should be sought the procedure abandoned or converted into an open case.

Management

The treatment of mechanical bowel trauma recognized during the dissection follows the principles described above for trocar injury. If the diagnosis is delayed until the postoperative recognition of peritonitis, surgical consultation should be obtained and laparotomy arranged.

Thermal injury may be handled expectantly, if the lesion is superficial and confined. It is possible to estimate the degree of tissue injury, if the nature of the current and other parameters is known, such as the wattage, current density, and duration of contact with tissue. For example, fulguration current, arcing to bowel, is unlikely to cause thermal injury >1 mm deep, even with rather prolonged exposure. On the other hand, the high power density provided by a sharp electrode will quickly cause penetrating injury of the bowel. Such lesions will have relatively little collateral thermal injury and may be repaired as if they were created by mechanical means. This is a circumstance vastly different from that occurring when there is direct and even relatively short, duration of contact (seconds) with a low power density electrode. The significant thermal injury that results will often mandate wide excision of the lesion or local resection of the injured segment of bowel.

INCISIONAL HERNIA

It is not that the incidence of laparoscopic incisional hernia is unknown, it is clear that the complication has been underreported. Recent reports of incisional hernia after laparoscopy have stressed the relationship of this complication with the use of ports 10 mm in diameter or larger. In our opinion, this can probably be attributed to increased operating times which result in excessive manipulation of the port site, thereby widening the fascial and peritoneal defects.

While no incision is immune to the risk of herniation, those defects that are 10 mm or more in diameter are particularly vulnerable. The increasing number and size of the incisions, ID combination with the surgeon's variable propensity to close them, will likely further contribute to the increasing incidence. Another important contributing factor may be the use of cannula anchoring devices that effectively increase the diameter of the incision by 2–3 mm.

Diagnosis

After laparoscopy, the most common hernia appears to occur in the immediate postoperative period where bowel or omentum passes through the unopposed or inadequately repaired defect. The patient may be symptomatic or can present with any or a combination of pain, fever, periumbilical mass, obvious evisceration, and the symptoms and signs of mechanical bowel obstruction, often within hours and usually within the first postoperative week. Consequently, the surgeon should take care not to casually disregard the patients who talk about symptoms consistent with herniation.

Because Richter's hernias contain only a portion of the circumference of the bowel wall in the defect, the diagnosis is often delayed. It is likely that such lesions most commonly occur in incisions that are made away from the midline. The initial presenting symptom is usually pain, since the incomplete obstruction and still allows the passage of intestinal content. Fever can present if incarceration occurs and peritonitis may result from the subsequent perforation. The diagnosis is difficult to make and requires a high index of suspicion. Ultrasound or CT scanning may be useful in confirming the diagnosis.

While many defects likely remain asymptomatic, late presentation may occur if bowel or omentum becomes trapped. The symptoms and findings are similar to that described for earlier presentations.

Prevention

The underlying fascia and peritoneum should be closed not only when using trocars of 10 mm and larger as previously suggested, but also when extensive manipulation is performed through a 5-mm trocar port, causing extension of the incision.

There are a number of unproven but seemingly logical preemptive strategies. First, it is desirable to use the smallest possible cannula whenever possible recognizing that hernia has even been reported in conjunction with the use of 5 mm trocars. Second, the "Z-track" insertion method, particularly applied, in the umbilicus, may be of value. This approach offsets the skin and fascial incisions by entering the subcutaneous tissue, then sliding the conically-tipped trocar along the fascia for a short distance prior to penetrating it. Such a track is purported to close like a curtain, reducing the incidence of hernia. Third, all ancillary cannula should be removed under direct vision to ensure that bowel is not drawn into the incision. Insertion of an obturator (or a laparoscope) into the cannula may further prevent suction from drawing bowel or omentum into the incision. Fourth, at least those incisions 10 mm or greater in diameter should undergo fascial closure under direct laparoscopic vision, thereby preventing incorporation of bowel. This may be accomplished by using a small caliber diameter laparoscope through one of the narrow cannula to direct incisional closure. A narrow diameter, three-quarter round, needle (Ethicon UR-6) facilitates such a closure, as does the use of one of the newer devices. Finally, the laparoscope cannula should be removed with the laparoscope in position, preventing accidental incorporation of bowel.

If the final incision is of sufficiently large diameter to require closure, blind insertion of needles may be avoided by prepositioning sutures. They are placed when the laparoscope is in another location and tied following removal of the final cannula. The sutures should be used to elevate the abdominal wall as the laparoscope and cannula are simultaneously removed, looking down the endoscope to ensure that bowel or omentum are not inadvertently drawn into the wound.

Management

Management of postoperative development of incisional hernia after laparoscopy is same as that of open surgery. Management of laparoscopic incisional defects depends upon the timing of the presentation and the presence or absence of entrapped bowel and its condition. Evisceration will always require surgical intervention. If the diagnosis is made in the recovery room, the patient may be returned to the operating room, the bowel or omentum replaced in the peritoneal cavity (provided there is no evidence of necrosis or suture incorporation), and the incision repaired, usually under laparoscopic guidance. However, if the diagnosis is delayed, it is likely that the bowel is incarcerated and at risk for perforation. In such circumstances, resection will likely be necessary, usually via laparotomy. Most gynecologic surgeons should request general surgical consultation.

INFECTION

Wound infection following laparoscopy is less but not rare. Even a case of postoperative wound infection due to *Mycobacterium chelonae* also has been reported. A 35-year-old woman presented with multiple erythematous nodules, plaques, and discharging sinuses over the abdomen, 45 days after she had undergone laparoscopic ovarian cystectomy. The seropurulent discharge from the wound showed acid-fast bacilli on Ziehl–Neelsen stain and culture yielded *Mycobacterium chelonae*. The patient responded to clarithromycin and doxycycline. The source of infection was probably contaminated water or disinfectant solution used for sterilization of laparoscopic instruments. In the urologic and general surgical wound infection, rates seem to range from 5 to 6 per 1,000 cases. While the vast majority of wound infections are handled successfully with expectant management, drainage, or antibiotics, severe necrotizing fasciitis has been reported.

Many other types of postlaparoscopy infection have been reported including bladder infection, pelvic cellulitis, and pelvic abscess. While bacteremia has been described, there have been no reports of disseminated infection following laparoscopic surgery.

This is true that the risk of infection associated with laparoscopy is low, much lower than that associated with open abdominal or vaginal surgery. Nevertheless, until clinical studies dictate otherwise, it is prudent to continue to practice strict sterile technique and to offer appropriate prophylactic antibiotics to selected patients. These could include those with enhanced risk for bacterial endocarditis as well as those who are to undergo procedures (e.g., laparoscopic hysterectomy), suspected of increasing the chance of wound, or vault infection. Patients should be instructed to routinely take their temperature following discharge and to immediately report fever of 38°C or more.

BIBLIOGRAPHY

1. Azagra JS, Goergen M, Gilbart E, Jacobs D. Laparoscopic anatomical (hepatic) left lateral segmentectomy—technical aspects. Surg Endosc. 1996;10:758-61.
2. Belli G, Fantini C, D'Agostino A, Belli A, Cioffi L, Russolillo N. Laparoscopic left lateral hepatic lobectomy: a safer and faster technique. J Hepatobiliary Pancreat Surg. 2006;13:149-54.
3. Berci G, Cuschieri A. Creation of pneumoperitoneum and trocar insertion. In: Berci G, Cuschieri A (Eds). Practical Laparoscopy. London: Baillière Tindall; 1986. pp. 44-64.
4. Berci G, Cuschieri A. Practical Laparoscopy. London: Baillière Tindall; 1986.
5. Berci G, Dunkelman D, Michel SL, Sanders G, Wahlstrom E, Morgenstern L. Emergency minilaparoscopy in abdominal trauma: an update. Am J Surg. 1983;146:261-5.
6. Berci G, Sackier J, Paz-Partlow M. Emergency laparoscopy. Am J Surg. 1991;161:332-5.
7. Berci G, Wahlstorm E. Emergency laparoscopy. In: Dent L (Eds). Surgical Endoscopy. Chicago: Chicago Year Book; 1985. pp. 478-83.
8. Berci G. Complications of laparoscopy. In: Berci G, Cuschieri A (Eds). Practical Laparoscopy. London: Baillière Tindall; 1986. pp. 165-77.
9. Berci G. Laparoscopy for oncology. In: Moosa AR, St Schimpff C, Robson MC (Eds). Textbook of Oncology. Baltimore: Williams & Wilkins; 1991. pp. 210-9.
10. Berci G. Laparoscopy in general surgery. In: Berci G (Ed). Endoscopy. Norwalk, CT: Appleton-Century-Crofts; 1976. pp. 382-400.
11. Boyce WN, Cammerer RC, Anderson DL. Laparoscopy and hepatology. In: Berci G, (Ed). Endoscopy. Norwalk, CT: Appleton-Century-Crofts; 1976. pp. 401-11.
12. Cadeddu JA, Wolfe JS, Nakada S, Chen R, Shalhav A, Bishoff JT. Complications of laparoscopic procedures after concentrated training in urological laparoscopy. J Urol. 2001;166:2109-11.
13. Cadiere GB, Torres R, Dapri G, Capelluto E, Himpens J. Multimedia article: laparoscopic left lateral hepatic lobectomy for metastatic colorectal tumor. Surg Endosc. 2005;19:152.
14. Caione P, Micali S, Rinaldi S, Capozza N, Lais A, Matarazzo E, et al. Retroperitoneal laparoscopy for renal biopsy in children. J Urol. 2000;164:1080-5.
15. Carnevale N, Baron N, Delaney HM. Peritoneoscopy as an aid in the diagnosis of abdominal trauma: a preliminary report. J Trauma. 1977;17:634-41.
16. Castilho LN, Castillo OA, Denes FT, Mitre AI, Arap S. Laparoscopic adrenal surgery in children. J Urol. 2002;168:221-4.
17. Chee-Awai RA, Chandhoke PS, Koyle MA. Laparoscopic nephrectomy in children. Semin Laparosc Surg. 1998;5:47-54.
18. Chen HW, Lin GJ, Lai CH, Chu SH, Chuang CK. Minimally invasive extravesical ureteral reimplantation for vesicoureteral reflux. J Urol. 2002;167:1821-3.
19. Cherqui D, Husson E, Hammoud R, Malassagne B, Stephan F, Bensaid S, et al. Laparoscopic liver resections: a feasibility study in 30 patients. Ann Surg. 2000;232:753-62.
20. Colodny AH. Laparoscopy in pediatric urology: too much of a good thing? Semin Pediatr Surg. 1996;5:23-9.
21. Critchley LA, Critchley JA, Gin T. Haemodynamic changes in patients undergoing laparoscopic cholecystectomy: measurement by transthoracic electrical bioimpedance. Br J Anaesth. 1993;70:681-3.
22. Cuschieri A, Berci G. Laparoscopic Biliary Surgery. London: Blackwell Publishing; 1990.
23. Cuschieri A. Value of laparoscopy in hepatobiliary disease. Ann R Coll Surg Engl. 1975;57:33-8.
24. Delarue A, Guys JM, Louis-Borrione C, Simeoni J, Esposito C. Pediatric endoscopic surgery: pride and prejudice. Eur J Pediatr Surg. 1994;4:323-6.
25. DeSouza G, Lewis MC, TerRiet MF. Severe bradycardia after remifentanil. Anesthesiology. 1997;87:1019-20.
26. Dexter SP, Vucevic M, Gibson J, McMahon MJ. Hemodynamic consequences of high- and low-pressure capnoperitoneum during laparoscopic cholecystectomy. Surg Endosc. 1999;13:376-81.
27. Docimo SG, Moore RG, Adams J, Kavoussi LR. Laparoscopic bladder augmentation using stomach. Urology. 1995;46:565-9.
28. Dorsay DA, Greene FL, Baysinger CL. Hemodynamic changes during laparoscopic cholecystectomy monitored with transesophageal echocardiography. Surg Endosc. 1995;9:128-33.
29. Duckett JW. Pediatric laparoscopy: prudence please. J Urol. 1994;151:742.
30. Eguchi D, Nishizaki T, Ohta M, Ishizaki Y, Hanaki N, Okita K, et al. Laparoscopy-assisted right hepatic lobectomy using a wall-lifting procedure. Surg Endosc. 200;20:1326-8.

31. El-Ghoneimi A, Valla JS, Steyaert H, Aigrain Y. Laparoscopic renal surgery via a retroperitoneal approach in children. J Urol. 1998;160:1138-41.
32. Esposito C, Ascione G, Garipoli V, DeBernardo G, Esposito G. Complications of pediatric laparoscopic surgery. Surg Endosc. 1997;11:665-7.
33. Esposito C, Damiano R, Gonzalez-Sabin MA, Savanelli A, Centone A, Settimi A, et al. Laparoscopy-assisted orchidopexy: an ideal treatment for children with intra-abdominal testes. J Endourol. 2002;16:659-62.
34. Esposito C, Garipoli V, Di Matteo G, De Pasquale M. Laparoscopic management of ovarian cysts in newborns. Surg Endosc. 1998;12:1152-4.
35. Esposito C, Monguzzi G, Gonzalez-Sabin MA, Rubino R, Mantinaro L, Papparella A, et al. Laparoscopic treatment of pediatric varicocele: a multicenter study of the Italian society of video surgery in infancy. J Urol. 2000;163:1944-6.
36. Esposito C, Monguzzi G, Gonzalez-Sabin MA, Rubino R, Montinaro L, Papparella A, et al. Results and complication of laparoscopic surgery for pediatric varicocele. J Pediatr Surg. 2001;36:767-9.
37. Gaisford W. Peritoneoscopy: a valuable technique for surgeons. Am J Surg. 1975;130:671-7.
38. Galizia G, Prizio G, Lieto E, Castellano P, Pelosio L, Imperatore V, et al. Hemodynamic and pulmonary changes during open, carbon dioxide pneumoperitoneum and abdominal wall-lifting cholecystectomy. A prospective, randomized study. Surg Endosc. 2001;15:477-83.
39. Gaur DD, Agarwal DK, Purohit KC. Retroperitoneal laparoscopic nephrectomy: initial case report. J Urol. 1993;149:103-5.
40. Gazzaniga AB, Slanton WW, Barlett RH. Laparoscopy in the diagnosis of blunt and penetrating injuries to the abdomen. Am J Surg. 1976;131:315-8.
41. Gettman MT, Peschel R, Neururer R, Bartsch G. A comparison of laparoscopic pyeloplasty performed with the daVinci robotic system versus standard laparoscopic techniques: initial clinical results. Eur Urol. 2002;42:453-7.
42. Gill SI, Kavoussi LR, Clayman RV, Ehrlich R, Evans R, Fuchs G, et al. Complications of laparoscopic nephrectomy in 185 patients: a multi-institutional review. J Urol. 1995;154:479-83.
43. Godje O, Friedl R, Hannekum A. Accuracy of beat-to-beat cardiac output monitoring by pulse contour analysis in hemodynamical unstable patients. Med Sci Monit. 2001;7:1344-50.
44. Grady RW, Mitchell ME, Carr MC. Laparoscopic and histologic condition of the inguinal vanishing testis. Urology. 1998;52:866-9.
45. Guilloneau B, Ballanger P, Lugagne PM, Valla JS, Vallancien G. Laparoscopic versus lumboscopic nephrectomy. Eur Urol. 1996;29:288-91.
46. Henning H, Look D. Complications. In: Henning H, Look D (Eds). Laparoscopy. Stuttgart: Thieme Medical Publishers; 1985.
47. Henning H, Look D. Laparoskopie. Stuttgart, Thieme Medical Publishers; 1985.
48. Hirvonen EA, Nuutinen LS, Kauko M. Hemodynamic changes due to Trendelenburg positioning and pneumoperitoneum during laparoscopic hysterectomy. Acta Anaesthesiol Scand. 1995;39:949-55.
49. Hofer CK, Zalunardo MP, Klaghofer R, Spahr T, Pasch T, Zollinger A. Changes in intrathoracic blood volume associated with pneumoperitoneum and positioning. Acta Anaesthesiol Scand. 2002;46:303-8.
50. Hopkins HH. Optical principles of the endoscopies. In: Berci G (Ed). Endoscopy. Norwalk, CT: Appleton-Century-Crofts; 1976. pp. 3-26.
51. Jacobeus HC. Kurze Obersich tubermeine Erfahrungen mit der Laparosckopie. Munch Med Wochenschr. 1911;58:2017.
52. Joris JL, Noirot DP, Legrand MJ, Jacquet NJ, Lamy ML. Hemodynamic changes during laparoscopic cholecystectomy. Anesth Analg. 1993;76:1067-71.
53. Kalk H, Bruhl W. Leitfadender Laparoskopie. Stuttgart: Theime Medical Publishers; 1951.
54. Kallipolitis GK, Milingos SD, Creatsas GK, Deligeoroglou EK, Michalas SP. Laparoscopic gonadectomy in a patient with testicular feminization syndrome. J Pediatr Adolesc Gynecol. 2000;13:23-6.
55. Kaneko H. Laparoscopic hepatectomy: indications and outcomes. J Hepatobiliary Pancreat Surg. 2005;12:438-43.
56. Kaneko H, Takagi S, Shiba T. Laparoscopic partial hepatectomy and left lateral segmentectomy: technique and results of a clinical series. Surgery. 1996;120:468-75.
57. Kelling G. Verhand lungdeutscher Natur forscherund Aerzte. Leipzig: Vogel; 1902.
58. Khurana S, Borzi PA. Laparoscopic management of complicated urachal disease in children. J Urol. 2002;168:1526-8.
59. Machado MA, Makdissi FF, Bacchella T, Machado MC. Hemihepatic ischemia for laparoscopic liver resection. Surg Laparosc Endosc Percutan Tech. 2005;15:180-3.
60. McCallum RW, Berci G. Laparoscopy in hepatic disease. Gastroint Endosc. 1976;23:20-4.
61. Meininger D, Byhahn C, Bueck M, Binder J, Kramer W, Kessler P, et al. Effects of prolonged pneumoperitoneumon hemodynamics and acid-base balance during totally endoscopic robot-assisted radical prostatectomies. World J Surg. 2002;26:1423-7.
62. Meininger D, Byhahn C, Mierdl S, Westphal K, Zwissler B. Positive end-expiratory pressure improves arterial oxygenation during prolonged pneumoperitoneum. Acta Anaesthesiol Scand. 2005;49:778-83.
63. Merrot T, Ordorica-Flores R, Steyeart H, Ginier C, Valla JS. Is diffuse xanthogranulomatous pyelonephritis a contraindication to retroperitoneoscopic nephroureterectomy? A case report. Surg Laparosc Endosc. 1998;8:366-9.
64. Meynol F, Steyaert H, Valla JS. Adnexa torsion in children: earlier diagnosis and treatment by laparoscopy. Arch Pediatr. 1997;4:416-9.
65. Miller OF, Bloom TL, Smith LJ, McAleer IM, Kaplan GW, KolonTF. Early hospital discharge for intravesical ureteroneocystostomy. J Urol. 2002;167:2556-9.
66. Millward-Sadler GH, Whorwell PJ. Liver biopsy. In: Wright R (Ed). Liver and Biliary Disease. London: Baillière Tindall; 1985. pp. 496-514.
67. Morgenstern L, Shapiro SJ. Techniques of splenic conservation. Arch Surg. 1979;14:449-54.
68. Nyirady P, Kiss A, Pirot L, Sarkozy S, Bognar Z, Csontai A, et al. Evaluation of 100 laparoscopic varicocele operations with preservation of testicular artery and ligation of collateral vein in children and adolescent. Eur Urol. 2002;42:594-7.
69. O'Rourke N, Fielding G. Laparoscopic right hepatectomy: surgical technique. J Gastrointest Surg. 2004;8:213-6.
70. Odeberg S, Ljungqvist O, Svenberg T, Gannedahl P, Bäckdahl M, von Rosen A, et al. Haemodynamic. effects of pneumoperitoneum and the influence of posture during anaesthesia for laparoscopic surgery. Acta Anaesthesiol Scand. 1994;38:276-83.
71. Pauli C, Fakler U, Genz T, Henning M, Lorenz HP, Hess J. Cardiac output determination in children: equivalence of the transpulmonary thermodilution method to the direct Fick principle. Intensive Care Med. 2002;28:947-52.
72. Paz-Partlow M. Documentation of laparoscopy. In: Berci G, Cuschieri A (Eds). Practical Laparoscopy. London: Baillière Tindall; 1986. pp. 1-32.
73. Peters CA. Complications in pediatric urological laparoscopy: results of a survey. J Urol. 1996;155:1070-3.

74. Peters CA. Laparoendoscopy renal surgery in children. J Endourol. 2000;14:841-7.
75. Reid JE, Mirakhur RK. Bradycardia after administration of remifentanil. Br J Anaesth. 2000;84:422-3.
76. Robinson BC, Snow BW, Cartwright PC, De vries CR, Hamilton BD, Anderson JB. Comparison of laparoscopic versus open partial nephrectomy in a pediatric series. J Urol. 2003;169: 638-40.
77. Root HO, Hauser CW, McKinley CR, La Fave JW, Mendiola RP. Diagnostic peritoneal lavage. Surgery. 1965;57:633-7.
78. Ruddock C. Peritoneoscopy. Surg Gynecol Obstet. 1937;65: 623-9.
79. Sakka SG, Reinhart K, Meier-Hellmann A. Comparison of pulmonary artery and arterial thermodilution cardiac output in critically ill patients. Intensive Care Med. 1999;25:843-6.
80. Sandham JD, Hull RD, Brant RF, Knox L, Pineo GF, Doig CJ, et al. A randomized, controlled trial of the use of pulmonary-artery catheters in high-risk surgical patients. N Engl J Med. 2003;348:5-14.
81. Sherwood R, Berci G, Austin E, Morgenstern L. Minilaparoscopy for blunt abdominal trauma. Arch Surg. 1980;115:672-3.
82. Stubbe H, Schmidt C, Hinder F. [Invasive cardiovascular monitoring—four methods compared]. Anaesthesiol Intensivmed Notfallmed Schmerzther. 2006;41:550-5.
83. Takasaki K. Glissonean pedicle transection method for hepatic resection: a new concept of liver segmentation. J Hepatobiliary Pancreat Surg. 1998;5:286-91.
84. Takasaki K, Kobayashi S, Tanaka S, Saito A, Yamamoto M, Hanyu F. Highly anatomically systematized hepatic resection with Glissonean sheath code transection at the hepatic hilus. Int Surg. 1990;75:73-7.
85. Veress J. Neues Instrument zurausfurung von brustoder Bauchpunktionen. Dtsch Med Wochenschr. 1938;41:1480-1.
86. Vibert E, Perniceni T, Levard H, Denet C, Shahri NK, Gayet B. Laparoscopic liver resection. Br J Surg. 2006;93:67-72.
87. von Spiegel T, Wietasch G, Bürsch J, Hoeft A. [Cardiac output determination with transpulmonary thermodilution. An alternative to pulmonary catheterization?]. Anaesthesist. 1996;45:1045-50.
88. Wittgen CM, Andrus CH, Fitzgerald SD, Buadendistel LJ, Dahms TE, Kaminski DL. Analysis of the hemodynamic and ventilatory effects of laparoscopic cholecystectomy. Arch Surg. 1991;126:997-1000.
89. Wood RAB, Cuschieri A. Laparoscopy for chronic abdominal pain. Br J Surg. 1979;60:900-2.
90. Yamanaka N, Tanaka T, Tanaka W, Yamanaka J, Yasui C, Ando T, et al. Laparoscopic partial hepatectomy. Hepatogastroenterology. 1998;45:29-33.
91. Zoeckler SJ. Peritoneoscopy: a reevaluation. Gastroenterology. 1958;34:969.
92. Zuckerman R, Gold M, Jenkins P, Rauscher LA, Jones M, Heneghan S. The effects of pneumoperitoneum and patient position on hemodynamics during laparoscopic cholecystectomy. Surg Endosc. 2001;15:562-5.

CHAPTER 46

Role of Training in Minimal Access Surgery

INTRODUCTION

The popularity of laparoscopic techniques has led to a new domain in surgical training, with a move away from the apprenticeship model, toward structured programs of teaching new skills outside the operating room. Hands-on courses enable young surgeons to practice techniques on synthetic, porcine, or more recently, virtual-reality (VR) models are now common place. The aim has been to ensure trainees are armed with basic laparoscopic skills such as hand-eye coordination and depth perception prior to entering the operating room **(Fig. 1)**. The success of these initial courses led to the development of similar courses for the advanced laparoscopic skills required for gastric and colonic surgery.

Compared to aviation, where VR training has been standardized and simulators have proven their definite benefit in increasing skill, the objectives, needs, and means of VR training in minimally invasive surgery (MIS) are established **(Fig. 2)**.

Rasmussen distinguishes three levels of human behavior:

1. Skill-based behavior
2. Rule-based behavior
3. Knowledge-based behavior

SKILL-BASED BEHAVIOR

This represents surgeon's behavior that takes place without conscious control. Task execution is highly automated at this level of behavior and is based on fast selection of motor programs, which control the appropriate muscles. The motor programs are based on an accurate internal representation of the task, the system dynamics, and the environment at hand (e.g., learned by training and experience). An example of an everyday skill is walking. Many tasks in surgery can be considered as a sequence of skilled acts. For example, an experienced surgeon performs a suture task smoothly, without conscious control over his or her movements.

In MIS, suturing canal so be considered as skill-based behavior. However, because of the indirect access to the tissue, it is a much more complicated skill because of reduced depth perception and difficult hand-eye coordination **(Fig. 3)**.

RULE-BASED BEHAVIOR

At the next level of human behavior, rule-based behavior is applied. During rule-based behavior, task execution is controlled by stored rules or procedures. These may have been derived empirically from previous occasions or

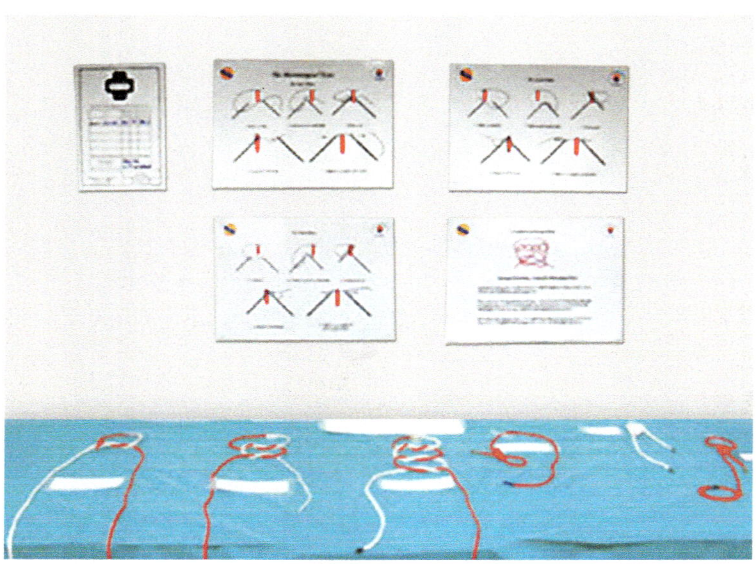

Fig. 1: Demonstration of different types of knot to keep them in memory.

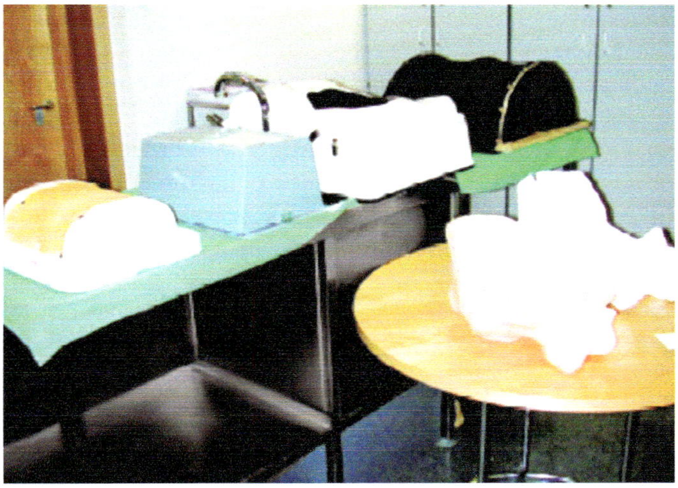

Fig. 2: Different types of simple pelvitrainers.

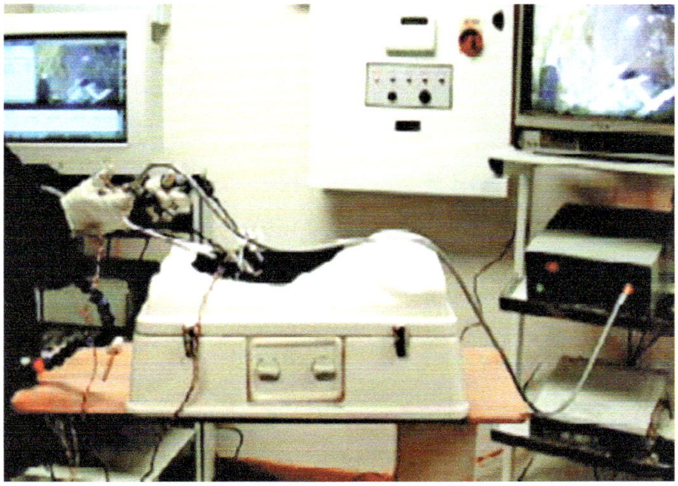

Fig. 3: Pelvitrainer exercises to improve skill.

communicated from other persons' expertise as instructions or as a cookbook recipe. Appropriate rules are selected according to their "success" in previous experiences. For example, procedural steps and the recognition of anatomy and pathology in MIS require rule-based behavior. At the rule-based level, the information is typically perceived as discrete signs. A sign serves to activate or to trigger a stored rule. Stopping your car in front of a red light is a good example of a sign (red light) that triggers a stored rule (stop car). In laparoscopic cholecystectomy, having fully established, the critical view of safety is the sign that triggers the rule that the appropriate structures may be clipped next.

KNOWLEDGE-BASED BEHAVIOR

In unfamiliar situations, faced with a task for which no rules are available from previous encounters, human behavior is knowledge based. During knowledge-based behavior, the goal is explicitly formulated, based on an analysis of the overall aim. Different plans are developed and their effects mentally tested against the goal. Finally, a plan is selected. Serious complications that occasionally occur during surgery demand a great deal of knowledge-based behavior from the surgeon. He or she has to analyze the complication and the aim of the surgical procedure in order to develop strategies to counter the complication. Then, he or she has to select the best strategy and consequently take the appropriate actions.

At the knowledge-based level, information is perceived as symbols. Symbols refer to chunks of conceptual information, which are the basis for reasoning and planning. Pathological symptoms are a good example of symbols in medical practice.

Training in laparoscopic surgery is beginning to evolve into a stepwise, curricular approach that is not organ or procedure specific. Instead, it is necessary to learn manipulative skills, which are then combined to achieve proficiency in tasks such as laparoscopic suturing or division of a vessel. The constituent parts can then be combined with anatomical knowledge to enable completion of a specific procedure. Basic psychomotor skills can be learnt with a simple, cheap version of a video-box trainer. Higher level skills such as dissection and use of high-energy instruments will necessitate the use of more realistic tissues, which can be achieved on porcine or human cadaveric models. Recent advances in VR simulation are also beginning to produce realistic simulations of complete procedures, for example, laparoscopic cholecystectomy.

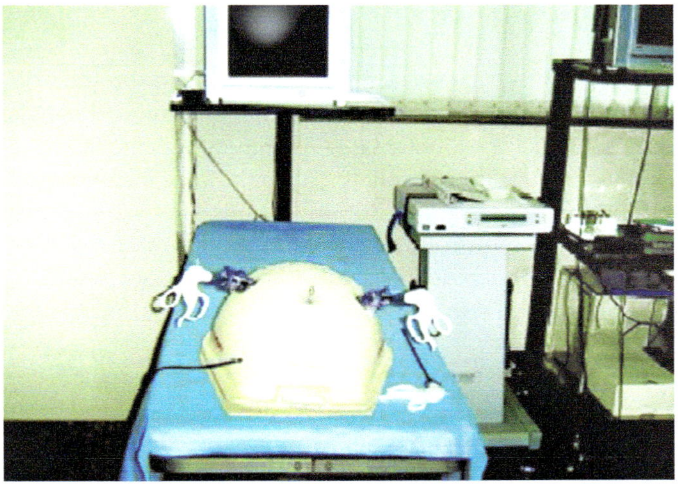

Fig. 4: The simple pelvitrainer can be used for improving suturing skill.

It would be rational to assume that a high-fidelity simulation model, such as anesthetized animal tissue, would be superior in terms of training outcome to a synthetic plastic model **(Fig. 4)**.

In fact, a study comparing two groups learning to perform microanastomotic repair of a transected spermatic cord on either the animal or synthetic model found no difference in eventual outcome of the two groups. The synthetic model is obviously cheaper and does not require specialized storage facilities. It can be assumed that as the subjects were using real sutures and instruments, the nature of the task was learnt regardless of the fidelity of the simulated tissue.

TRAINING: OBJECTIVES, NEEDS, AND MEANS

To enable the design and evaluation of an effective and efficient training method, it is of utmost importance to determine the training objectives, needs, and means, since they provide an answer to the questions:

1. What is the end goal of the training?
2. What should be trained?
3. How can we train it?

The objectives represent the level of competence that is expected of the trainee after he or she has completed the training. Training needs are the difference between the initial level of competence of the trainees and the required level of competence after successful completion of the training defined in the objectives. Ultimately, demands for effectivity and efficiency on the one hand, and the state-of-the-art in technology on the other hand, determine the tools and methods for training, i.e., the training means. Effective training ensures that all training objectives are met. Efficient training ensures that the training means are cost-effective and that the required training time is minimized. Since safety and patient outcome are the most important criteria in surgery, training effectivity should be of primary importance **(Fig. 5)**.

The complexity and the costs of the training means are largely determined by the training objectives that have been set. Fulfilling all training needs of laparoscopic residents with only one training method will require a highly complex and probably very expensive trainer in which all three levels of behavior can be trained. Such a trainer is not yet available. The complexity and the cost of a training means are relatively low if the training objectives comprise skill-based behavior only, since this can be trained with simple models such as pelvitrainers **(Fig. 6)**. Evidently, the cost and complexity of a training means increase when the training objectives advance from the training of skill-based behavior to the training of knowledge-based behavior. Fortunately, the overall effectivity of training increases as well when higher levels of behavior, such as knowledge-based behavior, are incorporated in the training objectives.

PRESENT TRAINING IN LAPAROSCOPY

A closer look at the training program of laparoscopic residents provides an indication of the training needs that are addressed and the training means that are available today. Much as in conventional surgery, the laparoscopic surgeon must effectively combine the three levels of behavior. Instrument handling and dissection techniques require skill-based behavior, whereas the recognition of surgical anatomy requires a great deal of rule-based behavior. Complications such as uncontrollable bleeding or unsuspected situations such as the encountering of aberrant anatomy require problem solving on a knowledge-based level.

Obviously, training of skill-based behavior in laparoscopic surgery is highly desired as laparoscopy combines unusual hand-eye coordination with the use of complex instruments. Surgical residents are usually trained in laparoscopic surgery during 2 days introduction course. Basic skill-based behaviors such as instrument tissue handling and minimally invasive suturing are trained. Additionally, rule-based behavior is trained through lectures, textbooks, and video instructions. After the resident has successfully completed this course, he or she will receive training in the operating room. It is only in operating room that most knowledge-based behavior necessary to deal with complications and emergencies is acquired. Currently, a living animal model provides the only

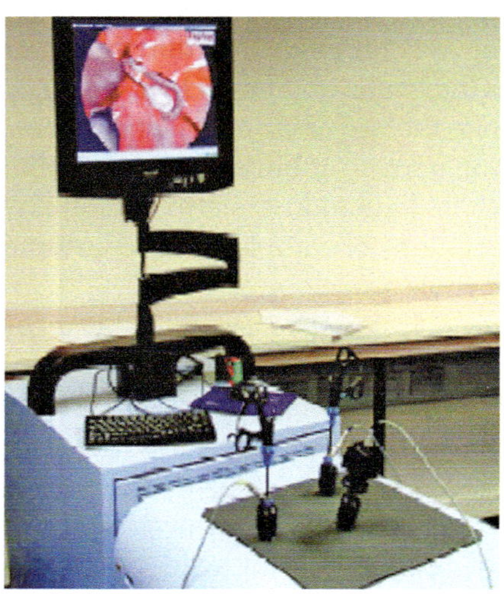

Fig. 5: The programming of virtual reality simulator will increase rule-based level.

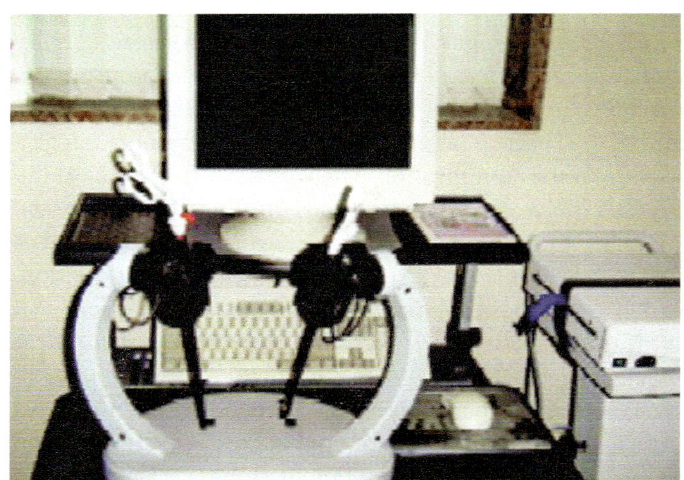

Fig. 6: Prototype virtual reality pelvitrainers.

way to effectively train rule- and knowledge-based behavior outside the operating room. Training on living animal models is very useful in the training curriculum of resident surgeons. However, at the same time, the use of laboratory animals for training is discouraged by many government policies. Technological innovations, such as VR simulation, will change the way laparoscopic surgery is trained. Current accomplishments in surgical simulation envision the dawning of the next-generation surgical education. In this respect, aviation industry provides excellent examples of the effectiveness and efficiency of VR simulators as a means of training.

Simulator training in aviation in contrast to surgery, the training needs in aviation, has explicitly been defined by regulatory authorities such as Federal Aviation Administration (FAA) and the training means are certified accordingly. The training objectives, needs, and means in pilot training have been investigated in depth and models of pilot behavior have been developed as a tool to design, to evaluate, and to optimize training methods. Half a century of extensive research has resulted in many training tools, from basic flight training devices to the high-tech full flight simulator (FFS) **(Figs. 7 and 8)**.

After the introduction of VR training methods in the 1990s, the training of surgeons has often been compared to the training of pilots. The training of laparoscopic residents can best be compared to type conversion training of pilots. During type conversion training, young pilots who have finished flight training at the academies and have recently joined an airline are trained to fly a particular type of aircraft. The general objective of type conversion training is to teach the trainee how to safely control, navigate, and manage a particular operational aircraft. Since the trainees have already acquired much of the skill-based behavior required to fly a multiengine aircraft, the training needs mainly consist of acquiring additional rule- and knowledge-based behavior. The trainees have to learn the new checklists and the specific procedures during takeoff and landing and they have to become familiar with all the aircraft systems such as electronics and hydraulics. Furthermore, they have to train all sorts of emergency scenarios that may occur during actual flight. Training of this knowledge-based behavior is very important since it significantly improves flight safety. This training provides an excellent training tool to accomplish all the specified training needs. The high level of realism during training of a pilot has even made zero flight time training possible, during which type conversion training takes place completely outside a real aircraft.

For the sake of proper training and for the safety of our patients, the objectives, needs, and means in laparoscopy training should be defined. Along this guideline, VR simulators should be developed. An explicit formulation of the training objectives facilitates the development and certification of a simulator since it determines what the simulator should be capable of. For example, pilots spend many hours in training on low-cost simulator **(Fig. 9)**.

The laparoscopy simulators that have been developed during the past decade can all be considered as laparoscopy training devices. Most of these simulators specifically aim at training skill-based behavior such as endoscopic manipulation and endoscopic camera navigation. However, performing safe laparoscopy also requires a professional level of rule- and knowledge-based behavior from the surgeon. Ideally, these should also be trained outside the operation theater. Currently, the training of rule- and knowledge-based behavior outside the operation theater is only possible on living animal models. However, technological innovations such as increasing computing power, detailed anatomical models, soft tissue modeling, and force feedback will enable the integration of all levels of behavior in a VR training simulator for laparoscopy. In the future, this might result in a full-scale laparoscopy simulator (FLS), comparable to the

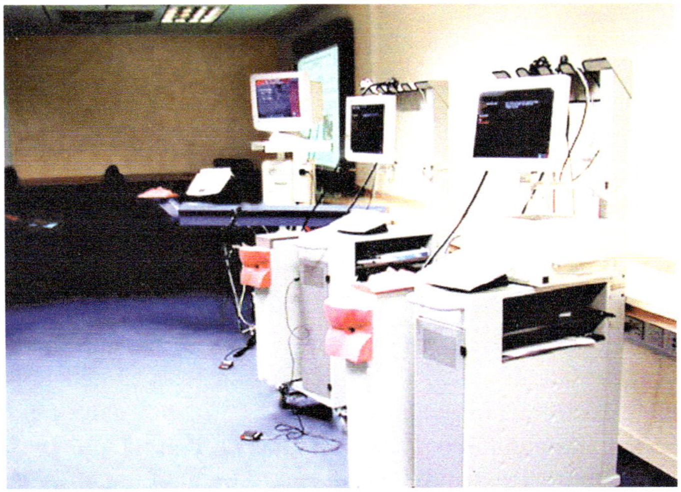

Fig. 7: Different types of virtual reality systems for endoscopy.

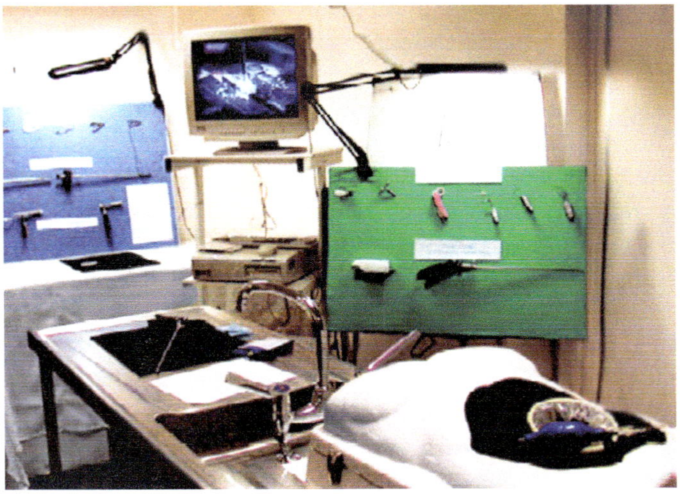

Fig. 8: Hand-assisted laparoscopic surgery (HALS) training box.

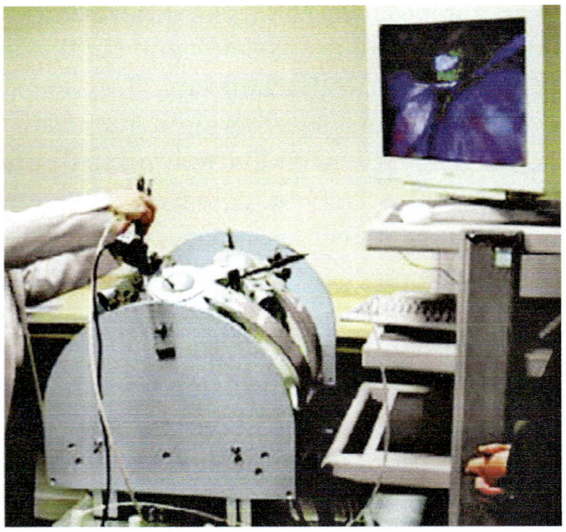

Fig. 9: Virtual reality trainer with programmable circuit.

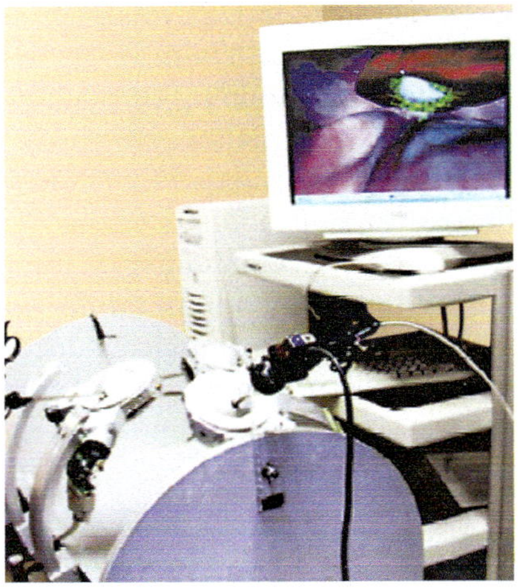

Fig. 10: Virtual reality trainer with software control.

FFS in pilot training. Perhaps, an FLS even introduces zero operating time training as the ultimate objective.

The medical society should establish detailed objectives of training. Recently, experts have begun to investigate what level of professional behavior is required to perform safe laparoscopy. In addition, they are establishing the training needs of laparoscopic residents by determining what should be trained to accomplish the training objective. The question of which aspects of skill-, rule-, and knowledge-based behavior should be trained is addressed. Currently, there is no such standard available. Once the training objectives have been standardized and the training needs at the different levels of behavior have been identified, the simulator society will have clear guidelines as to what their training devices should be capable of.

One of the most obvious training needs of laparoscopic residents is the training of manual skills. The manual skills required during laparoscopy are rather different from those in conventional surgery. Training of skill-based behavior is feasible with basic trainers such as a pelvitrainer. The VR basic skill trainers that are commercially available usually simulate a generic abdomen and endoscopic instruments on a computer monitor. Basic tasks, such as pick and place tasks, are implemented to train endoscopic manipulation. The training of skill-based behavior does not require a highly realistic anatomical environment, e.g., the organs do not necessarily have to be simulated realistically. For example, the VR trainer simulates basic manipulation tasks in a highly simplified environment similar to the pelvitrainer box. Several studies have reported that training on the VR facilitated the learning of skill-based behavior **(Fig. 10)**.

An advantage of VR simulators over simple pelvitrainers is the capability to easily extend the training to the rule-based level of behavior, since textbook theory, instructions, and training videos can easily be integrated in the simulator software. Much textbook material and many training videos

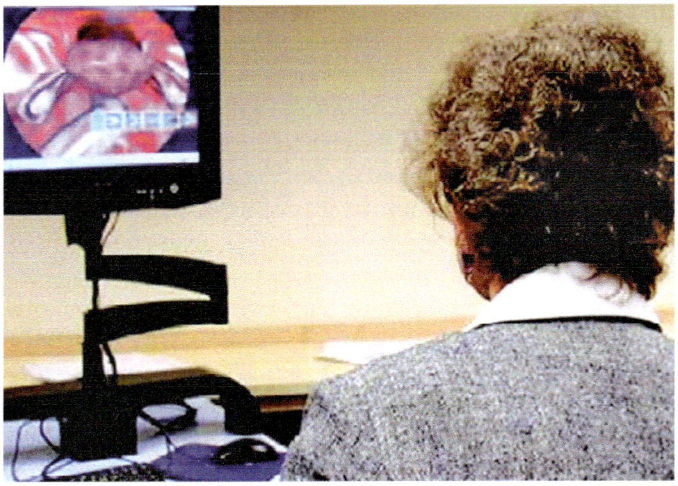

Fig. 11: Virtual reality trainer for laparoscopic-assisted vaginal hysterectomy (LAVH).

that provide rule-based behavior training have been made available on the internet. Laparoscopy simulators are capable of training skill- and rule-based behavior. To train knowledge-based behavior, a laparoscopy simulator should be capable of accurately imitating the surgical environment encountered during laparoscopic surgery **(Fig. 11)**.

The perceived information from the environment should be simulated accurately to ensure effective training. The training of knowledge-based behavior on a simulator still poses a huge challenge. Two fundamental problems occur. Whereas the physics that determines the behavior of an aircraft is fairly well known and described mathematically, the physics that describes the behavior of soft-tissue organs is highly complicated and many parameters are simply still missing. Additionally, each aircraft roughly has the same flight characteristics and cockpit layout, but each new patient has a different anatomical layout than the previous one. Laparoscopy simulators have to be able to generate "random" patients **(Fig. 12)**.

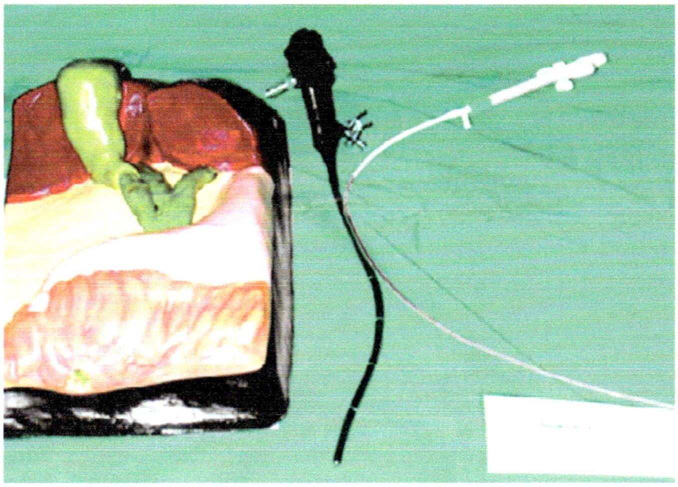

Fig. 12: Simulated models of GB and CBD to improve choledochoscopic skill. (CBD: common bile duct; GB: gallbladder)

The integration of knowledge-based behavior training in a future simulator would enhance safety levels in laparoscopy, since then every possible surgical complication could be trained beforehand. As in aviation, intensive training can reduce a situation that at first required improvising at a knowledge-based behavior level from the trainee to a situation that can be solved by applying trained rules.

LEARNING CURVE IN LAPAROSCOPY

TP Wright originally introduced the concept of a learning curve in aircraft manufacturing in 1936. He described a basic theory for costing the repetitive production of airplane assemblies. The term was introduced to medicine in the 1980s after the advent of minimal access surgery. It also caught the attention of the public and the legal profession when a surgeon told a public enquiry in Britain that a high death rate was inevitable while surgeons were on a learning curve. Recently, it has been labeled as a dangerous curve with a morbidity, mortality, and unproven outcomes. Yet there is no standardization of what the term means. In an endeavor to help laparoscopic surgeons toward evidence-based practices, this commentary will define and describe the learning curve, its drawing followed by a discussion of the factors affecting it, statistical evaluation, effect on randomized controlled trials (RCTs) and clinical implications for both practice and training, the limitations and pitfalls, ethical dilemmas, and some thoughts to pave the way ahead.

Definition and Description

For the Wright learning curve, the underlying hypothesis is that the direct man-hours necessary to complete a unit of production will decrease by a constant percentage each time the production quantity is doubled. In manufacturing, the learning curve applies to the time and cost of production. Can a surgeon's learning curve be described on similar lines? A simple definition would be: The time taken and/or the number of procedures an average surgeon needs to be able to perform a procedure independently with a reasonable outcome. But, then who is an average surgeon? Another definition may be that a learning curve is a graphic representation of the relationship between experience with a new procedure or technique and an outcome variable such as operation time, complication rate, hospital stay, or mortality. A learning curve may also be operationally defined as an improvement in performance over time. Although learning theorists often disagree about what learning is, they agree that whatever the process is, its affects are clearly cumulative and may, therefore, be plotted as a curve. By cumulative, it is meant that somehow the effects of experience carry over to aid later performance. This property is fundamental to the construction of learning curves. The improvement tends to be most rapid at first and then tails off. Hence, there are three main features of a learning curve. First, the initial or starting point defines where the performance of an individual surgeon begins. Secondly, the rate of learning measures how quickly the surgeon will reach a certain level of performance and thirdly, the asymptote or expert level measures where the surgeon's performance stabilizes. This has implications for the laparoscopic surgeon—it suggests that practice always help improve performance, but the most dramatic improvement happens first. Also, with sufficient practice, surgeons can achieve comparable levels of performance.

Drawing of Learning Curves

There is a variety of methods of constructing learning curves. They all assume that successive exposures in a learning series may be plotted on the X-axis, response characteristics on Y-axis, and the data points distributed in the XY plane may be legitimately connected by a curve. This is the Cartesian method. More recently, the cumulative sum method has been applied for the construction of these curves for basic skills in an esthetic procedures—the method consists of relatively simple calculations that can be easily performed on an electronic spreadsheet. Statistical inferences can be made from observed success and failure. The method also provides both numerical and graphical representation of the learning process.

The multimode learning curve is useful because several factors can be put into one graph. The earlier used method of the performance analysis with its on the spot appraisals at certain time intervals has been replaced by continuous assessment. For continuous data such as operation time, the moving average method is useful.

Factors Affecting Learning Curves

Complex hierarchies of factors are involved here **(Fig. 13)**. Factors such as guidelines, protocols, and standards for clinical governance agreed upon by the medical

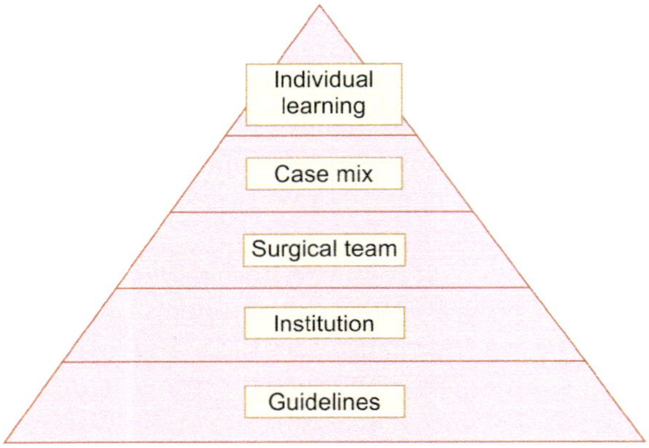

Fig. 13: Hierarchy of factors affecting learning curve.

fraternity are vital. Next, the institutional policies and cost-effectiveness are contributory. Needless to say, the surgical team, the case mix, and public awareness are relevant. The final level in the hierarchy that can influence individual learning is the characteristics of the surgeon such as attitude, capacity for acquiring new skills, and previous experience.

Among the latter, i.e., the characteristics of the surgeon, the learning curve may depend on the manual dexterity of the individual surgeon and the background knowledge of surgical anatomy. The type of training the surgeon has received is also important as training on inanimate trainers and animal tissue has been shown to facilitate the process of learning. The slope of the curve depends on the nature of the procedure and frequency of procedures performed in specific time period. Many studies suggest that complication rates are inversely proportional to the volume of the surgical workload. However, rapidity of learning is not significantly related to the surgeon's age, size of practice, or hospital setting. Another important factor that affects the learning curve is the supporting surgical team. A recent observational study to investigate the incidence of technical equipment problems during laparoscopic procedures reported that in 87% of procedures, one or more incidents with technical equipment or instruments occurred. Hence, improvement and standardization of equipment combined with incorporation of checklists to be used before surgery have been recommended.

Statistical Evaluation of Learning Curves

Various statistical methods have been reported in the assessment of the learning curve. Commonly, data are split into arbitrary groups and the means compared by chi-squared test or ANOVA. Some studies had data displayed graphically with no statistical analysis. Others used univariate analysis of experience versus outcome. Some studies used multivariate analysis techniques such as logistic regression and multiple regression to adjust for confounding factors. A systematic review concluded that the statistical methods used for assessing learning curves have been crude and the reporting of studies poor. Recognizing that better methods may be developed in other nonclinical fields where learning curves are present (psychology and manufacturing), a systematic search was made of then on clinical literature to identify novel statistical methods for modeling learning curves. A number of techniques were identified including generalized estimating equations and multilevel models. The main recommendation was that given the hierarchical nature of the learning curve data and the need to adjust for covariant, hierarchical statistical models should be used.

Effect of Learning Curve on Randomized Controlled Trials

The learning curve can cause difficulties in the interpretation of RCTs by distorting comparisons. The usual approaches to designing trials of new surgical techniques have been either to provide intensive training and supervision or require participating surgeons to perform a fixed number of procedures prior to participation in a trial. Surgeons have been reluctant to randomize until they are proficient in a technique but once convinced of its worth, argue that it is too late to randomize. However, the best way to address the problem is to have a statistical description of the learning curve effect within a trial and various methods can then be used, for example, Bayesian hierarchical model.

IMPLICATIONS FOR PRACTICE AND TRAINING

In the current era of evidence-based medicine, enthusiasm for laparoscopic surgery is rapidly gaining momentum. There is an immense amount of literature showing advantages of minimal access surgery and acceptance by the public. The learning curve from any procedures has been documented. As far as training is concerned, the introduction of laparoscopic techniques in surgery led to many unnecessary complications. This led to the development of skills laboratories involving use of box trainers with either innate or animal tissues, but lacks objective assessment of skill acquisition. VR simulators have the ability to teach psychomotor skills. However, it is a training tool and needs to be thoughtfully introduced into the surgical training curriculum. A recent prospective RCT showed that virtual simulator combined with inanimate box training leads to better laparoscopic skill acquisition. An interesting finding reported is that in skills training, every task should be repeated at least 30–35 times for maximum benefit. The distribution of training over several days has also been shown to be superior to training in 1 day. Other factors enhancing training are fellowship programmer or playing video games. One can also obtain feedback for improvement of training program. In one such study, the deficiency factors identified were lack of knowledge, lack of synchronized movement of the nondominant hand, and easy physical fatigue.

Incorporation of intensive, well-planned in vitro training into the curriculum was made and the programmed reassessed.

What are the limitations or pitfalls?

"Steep" learning curves are usually used to describe procedures that are difficult to learn. However, this is a misnomer as it implies that large gains in proficiency are achieved over a small number of cases. Instead, the curve for a procedure that requires a lot of cases to reach proficiency should be described as "flattened".

As long as no valid scoring system concerning the complexity of a surgical intervention exists, the learning curve cannot be used as benchmarks to compare different surgeons or clinics as legitimate instruments to rank surgeons or different hospitals. Limitations of long learning curves, facilities for training, mistakes of pioneers, and surgical techniques not being described in books are some of the limitations. There are other limitations due to the nature of laparoscopic surgery such as the lack of three-dimensional (3D) vision and of tactile sensations, difficult hand-eye coordination, and long instruments.

ETHICAL DILEMMAS

Many dilemmas exist and many questions will always be with us—who bears the burden of the learning curve? Are the patients aware of the risks? Many reports validate the impression that a patient operated upon during the learning curve takes greater risks and incurs more adverse circumstances than the patient operated upon later. The issue of how informed the informed consent should be needed to be addressed. Is the integrity and conscience of a surgeon measurable? Should the forces of marketing be curtailed or regulated?

THE WAY FORWARD

Laparoscopic surgery is here to stay and success in it is determined by how quickly and effectively we learn. However, certain measures may be taken to lessen some of the adverse effects of the learning curve and others to help laparoscopic surgeons ease into the specialist. Setting up of minimal standards and credentialing is a must. Current guidelines in many countries are vague and general. The evidence for training is well documented. The message for individual surgeons is to identify their deficiencies and chart a way forward for their personal graph of progress. Evaluation and monitoring in a systematic scientific manner will benefit the surgeon with a satisfactory learning curve that will ensure that patient welfare is not compromised.

CONCLUSION

In this chapter, it has been pointed out that it is important to establish the training objectives, needs, and means, since they provide an answer to the questions—What is the end goal of the training?, What should be trained?, and How can we train it? Rasmussen's model of human behavior provides a practical framework for the definition of the training objectives, needs, and means in MIS, and the evaluation thereof.

IMPORTANT RESOURCES

http://www.bjssoc.com
http://www.laparoscopyhospital.com
http://www.obgyn.net
http://www.laparoscopy.net
http://www.medscape.com
http://www.websurg.com
http://www.ivf.com/laprscpy.html
http://www.sages.org
http://www.edu.rcsed.ac.uk
http://www.webmd.com

BIBLIOGRAPHY

1. Aggarwal R, Grantcharov T, Moorthy K, Hance J, Darzi A. A competency-based virtual reality training curriculum for the acquisition of laparoscopic psychomotor skill. Am J Surg. 2006;191(1):128-33.
2. Aggarwal R, Grantcharov TP, Eriksen JR, Blirup D, Kristiansen VB, Funch-Jensen P, et al. An evidence-based virtual reality training program for novice laparoscopic surgeons. Ann Surg. 2006; 244(2):310-4.
3. Baldwin PJ, Paisley AM, Brown SP. Consultant surgeons' opinion of the skills required of basic surgical trainees. Br J Surg. 1999;86(8):1078-82.
4. Bridges M, Diamond DL. The financial impact of teaching surgical residents in the operating room. Am J Surg. 1999;177(1):28-32.
5. Broe D, Ridgway PF, Johnson S, Tierney S, Conlon KC. Construct validation of a novel hybrid surgical simulator. Surg Endosc. 2006;20(6):900-4.
6. Brunner WC, Korndorffer JR, Sierra R, Dunne JB, Yau CL, Corsetti RL, et al. Determining standards for laparoscopic proficiency using virtual reality. Am Surg. 2005;71(1):29-35.
7. Brunner WC, Korndorffer JR, Sierra R, Massarweh NN, Dunne JB, Yau CL, et al. Laparoscopic virtual reality training: are 30 repetitions enough? J Surg Res. 2004;122(2):150-6.
8. Carter FJ, Schijven MP, Aggarwal R, Grantcharov T, Francis NK, Hanna GB, et al. Consensus guidelines for validation of virtual reality surgical simulators. Surg Endosc. 2005;19(12):1523-32.
9. Champion HR, Gallagher AG. Surgical simulation—a 'good idea whose time has come'. Br J Surg. 2003;90(7):767-8.
10. Chang L, Petros J, Hess DT, Rotondi C, Babineau TJ. Integrating simulation into a surgical residency program: is voluntary participation effective? Surg Endosc. 2007;2(3):418-21.
11. Cuschieri A, Francis N, Crosby J, Hanna GB. What do master surgeons think of surgical competence and revalidation? Am J Surg. 2001;182(2):110-6.
12. Dent TL. Training, credentialling, and granting of clinical privileges for laparoscopic general surgery. Am J Surg. 1991; 161(3):399-403.
13. Deziel D, Millikan KW, Economou SG, Doolas A, Ko ST, Airan MC. Complications of laparoscopic cholecystectomy: a national survey of 4,292 hospitals and an analysis of 77,604 cases. Am J Surg. 1993;165(1):9-14.
14. Eriksen JR, Grantcharov T. Objective assessment of laparoscopic skills using a virtual reality stimulator. Surg Endosc. 2005; 19(9):1216-9.

15. European Community. Directive 2000/34/EC of the European Parliament and of the Council of 22 June 2000 amending Council Directive 93/104/EC concerning certain aspects of the organization of working time to cover sectors and activities excluded from that Directive. J Eur Commun. 2000;195(2):41-5.
16. Figert PL, Park AE, Witzke DB, Schwartz RW. Transfer of training in acquiring laparoscopic skills. J Am Coll Surg. 2001;193(5): 533-7.
17. Gallagher AG, McClure N, McGuigan J, Ritchie K, Sheehy NP. An ergonomic analysis of the fulcrum effect in the acquisition of endoscopic skills. Endoscopy. 1998;30(7):617-20.
18. Gallagher AG, Ritter EM, Satava RM. Fundamental principles of validation, and reliability: rigorous science for the assessment of surgical education and training. Surg Endosc. 2003;17(10): 1525-9.
19. Grantcharov TP, Kristiansen VB, Bendix J, Bardram L, Rosenberg J, Funch-Jensen P. Randomized clinical trial of virtual reality simulation for laparoscopic skills training. Br J Surg. 2004;91(2):146-50.
20. Grantcharov TP, Rosenberg J, Pahle E, Funch-Jensen P. Virtual reality computer simulation: an objective method for the evaluation of laparoscopic surgical skills. Surg Endosc. 2001;15(5):242-4.
21. Hackethal A, Immenroth M, Burger T. Evaluation of target scores and benchmarks for the traversal task scenario of the Minimally Invasive Surgical Trainer-Virtual Reality (MIST-VR) laparoscopy simulator. Surg Endosc. 2006;20(4):645-50.
22. Hanna GB, Cuschieri A. Influence of the optical axis-to-target view angle on endoscopic task performance. Surg Endosc. 1999;13(4):371-5.
23. Hanna GB, Shimi SM, Cuschieri A. Randomised study of influence of two-dimensional versus three-dimensional imaging on performance of laparoscopic cholecystectomy. Lancet. 1998;351(9098):248-51.
24. Hyltander A, Liljegren E, Rhodin PH, Lonroth H. The transfer of basic skills learned in a laparoscopic simulator to the operating room. Surg Endosc. 2002;16(9):1324-8.
25. Jakimowicz JJ, Cuschieri A. Time for evidence-based minimal access surgery training—simulate or sink. Surg Endosc. 2005;19(12):1521-2.
26. Kolkman W, Wolterbeek R, Jansen FW. Gynecological laparoscopy in residency training program: Dutch perspectives. Surg Endosc. 2005;19(6):1498-502.
27. Korndorffer JR, Dunne JB, Sierra R, Stefanidis D, Touchard CL, Scott DJ. Simulator training for laparoscopic suturing using performance goals translates to the operating room. J Am Coll Surg. 2005;201(1):23-9.
28. Korndorffer JR, Scott DJ, Sierra R, Brunner WC, Dunne JB, Slakey DP, et al. Developing and testing competency levels for laparoscopic skills training. Arch Surg. 2005;140(1):80-4.
29. Moore MJ, Bennett CL. The learning curve for laparoscopic cholecystectomy. The Southern Surgeons Club. Am J Surg. 1995;170(6):55-9.
30. Rosser JC, Rosser LE, Savalgi RS. Skill acquisition and assessment for laparoscopic surgery. Arch Surg. 1997;132(2):200-4.
31. Sakorafas GH, Tsiotos GG. New legislative regulations, problems, and future perspectives, with a particular emphasis on surgical education. J Postgrad Med. 2004;50(5):274-7.
32. Schijven M, Jakimowicz J. Face-, expert, and referent validity of the Xitact LS500 laparoscopy simulator. Surg Endosc. 2002;16(12):1764-70.
33. Schijven M, Jakimowicz J. Construct validity: experts and residents performing on the Xitact LS500 laparoscopy simulator. Surg Endosc. 2003;17(8):803-10.
34. Schijven M, Jakimowicz J. Virtual reality surgical laparoscopic simulators: how to choose. Surg Endosc. 2003;17(6):1943-50.
35. Schijven MP, Berlage JT, Jakimowicz JJ. Minimal-access surgery training in the Netherlands: a survey among residents-in-training for general surgery. Surg Endosc. 2004;18(12):1805-14.
36. Schijven MP, Jakimowicz J. The learning curve on the Xitact LS500 laparoscopy simulator: profiles of performance. Surg Endosc. 2004;18:121-7.
37. Schijven MP, Jakimowicz JJ. Introducing the Xitact LS500 laparoscopy simulator: toward a revolution in surgical education. Surg Technol Int. 2003;11:32-6.
38. Schijven MP, Jakimowicz JJ, Broeders IAMJ, Tseng LNL. The Eindhoven laparoscopic cholecystectomy training course—improving operating room performance using virtual reality training: results from the first E.A.E.S. accredited virtual reality trainings curriculum. Surg Endosc. 2005;19(9):1220-6.
39. Schijven MP, Jakimowicz JJ, Carter FJ. How to select aspirant laparoscopic surgical trainees: establishing concurrent validity comparing Xitact LS500 index performance scores with standardized psychomotor aptitude test battery scores. J Surg Res. 2004;121(1):112-9.
40. Scott DJ, Bergen PC, Rege RV, Laycock R, Tesfay ST, Valentine RJ, et al. Laparoscopic training on bench models: better and more cost-effective than operating room experience? J Am Coll Surg. 2000;191(3):272-83.
41. Seymour NE, Gallagher AG, Roman SA, O'Brien MK, Bansal VK, Andersen DK, et al. Virtual reality training improves operating room performance: results of a randomized, double- blinded study. Ann Surg. 2002;236(4):458-63.
42. Taffinder N, Sutton C, Fishwick RJ, McManus IC, Darzi A. Validation of virtual reality to teach and assess psychomotor skills in laparoscopic surgery: results from randomized controlled studies using the MIST VR laparoscopic simulator. Stud Health Technol Inform. 1998;50:124-30.
43. Torkington J, Smith SG, Rees B, Darzi A. The role of the basic surgical skills course in the acquisition and retention of laparoscopic skill. Surg Endosc. 2001;15(7):1071-5.
44. Van Sickle KR, McClusky DA, Gallagher AG, Smith CD. Construct validation of the ProMIS simulator using a novel laparoscopic suturing task. Surg Endosc. 2005;19(9):1227-31.
45. Verdaasdonk EG, Stassen LP, Monteny LJ, Dankelman J. Validation of a new basic virtual reality simulator for training of basic endoscopic skills: the SIMENDO. Surg Endosc. 2006;20(3):511-8.
46. Verdaasdonk EG, Stassen LP, Schijven MP, Dankelman J. Construct validity and assessment of the learning curve for the SIMENDO endoscopic simulator. Surg Endosc. 2007;21(8):1406-12.
47. Wilson MS, Middlebrook A, Sutton C, Stone R, McCloy RF. MIST VR: a virtual reality trainer for laparoscopic surgery assesses performance. Ann R Coll Surg Engl. 1997;79(6):403-4.
48. Woodrum DT, Andreatta PB, Yellamanchilli RK, Feryus L, Gauger PG, Minter RM. Construct validity of the LapSim laparoscopic surgical simulator. Am J Surg. 2006;191(1):28-32.

CHAPTER 47 Minimal Access Robotic Surgery

INTRODUCTION

On July 11, 2000, the Food and Drug Administration (FDA) approved the first completely robotic surgery device, the da Vinci surgical system from Intuitive Surgical (Mountain View, CA). The system enables surgeons to remove gallbladders and perform other general surgical procedures while seated at a computer console and three-dimensional (3D) video imaging system across the room from the patient. The surgeons operate controls with their hands and fingers to direct a robotically controlled laparoscope **(Fig. 1)**.

This system and other robotic devices developed or under development by companies such as Computer Motion (Santa Barbara, CA) and Integrated Surgical Systems (Davis, CA) have the potential to revolutionize surgery and the operating room. They provide surgeons with the precision and dexterity necessary to perform complex, minimally invasive surgery (MIS) procedures, such as beating-heart single- or double-vessel bypass and neurological, orthopedic, and plastic surgery, among many other future applications. Manufacturers believe that their products will broaden the scope and increase the effectiveness of MIS; improve patient outcomes; and create a safer, more efficient, and more cost-effective operating room. It is the vision of these companies that robotic systems will one day be applicable to all surgical specialties, although it is too early to tell the full extent to which they will be used.

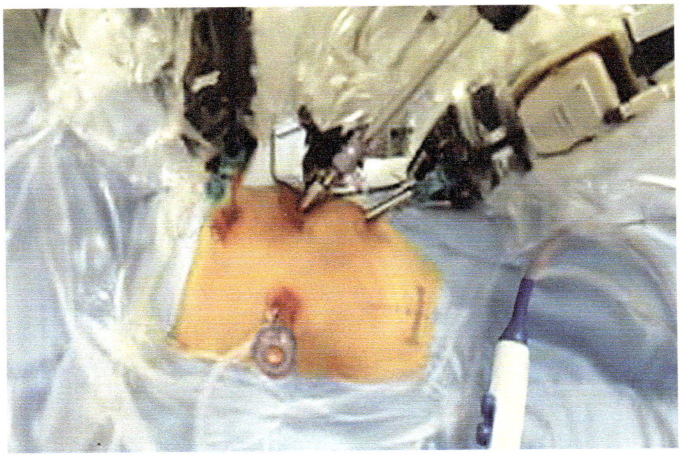

Fig. 1: Robotic surgery port placement for nephrectomy.

The first generation of surgical robots is already being installed in a number of operating rooms around the world. These are not true autonomous robots that can perform surgical tasks on their own, but they are lending a mechanical helping hand to surgeons. These machines still require a human surgeon to operate them and input instructions. Remote control and voice activation are the methods by which these surgical robots are controlled. Robotics are being introduced to minimal access surgery because they allow for unprecedented control and precision of surgical instruments. So far, these machines have been used to position an endoscope, perform gallbladder surgery, and correct gastroesophageal reflux and heartburn. The ultimate goal of the robotic surgery field is to design a robot that can be used to perform closed-chest, beating-heart surgery.

Recently, transatlantic surgery between USA and Strasbourg is a revolution in transatlantic minimal access surgery. In this surgery, there was slight delay (66 ms) in transfer of data but in future, this delay can easily minimized. In the future, remote handling technology will overcome the manipulative restriction in the current instruments. There is no doubt 10 years from now that some surgeons will be operating exclusively via a computer interface controlling a master-slave manipulation. *If computer-controlled machinery can mimic the awareness, adaptability, and knowledge of a human surgeon, such a takeover in the operating theater is actually realistic.*

In the operating room of the future, physicians will use tiny high-tech tools to travel inside the body with dexterity and precision beyond imaging. The future of any new technology depends upon the training.

Three surgical robots that have been recently developed are:

1. da Vinci surgical system
2. ZEUS robotic surgical system
3. Automated Endoscopic System for Optimal Positioning (AESOP) robotic system.

The "da Vinci" system has seven degree of freedom movement, so it can perform more complex task. The "da Vinci" system has been used to perform a number of general surgical procedures such as cholecystectomy and fundoplication. Robotic fundoplication allows easier passage around and behind the esophagus during its dissection and easier mobilization of the curvature of the stomach. Suturing the wrap and the crural approximation are also easier with the help of these robots.

The $1 million da Vinci system consists of two primary components:

1. A viewing and control console
2. A surgical arm unit **(Figs. 2A to C)**.

In using da Vinci for gallbladder surgery, three incisions, no larger than the diameter of a pencil, are made in the patient's abdomen, which allows for three stainless-steel rods to be inserted. The rods are held in place by three robotic arms. One of the rods is equipped with a camera, while the other two are fitted with surgical instruments that are able to dissect and suture the tissue of the gallbladder. Unlike in conventional surgery, these instruments are not directly touched by the doctor's hands.

Effect or tips of the da Vinci surgical system incorporate miniature wrists that allow them to mimic any movement made by the surgeon at the control console. Sitting at the control console, a few feet from the operating table, the surgeon looks into a viewfinder to examine the 3D images being sent by the camera inside the patient. The images show the surgical site and the two surgical instruments mounted on the tips of two of the rods. Joystick-like controls, located just underneath the screen, are used by the surgeon to manipulate the surgical instruments. Each time one of the joysticks is moved, a computer sends an electronic signal to one of the instruments, which moves in synchronization with the movements of the surgeon's hands.

Another robotic system is the ZEUS system, made by Computer Motion, which is already available in Europe. However, both the da Vinci and ZEUS systems must receive governmental approval for each procedure that a surgeon plans to use it for. The $750,000 ZEUS has a similar setup to that of the da Vinci. It has a computer workstation, a video display, and hand controls that are used to move the table-mounted surgical instruments. While the ZEUS system has not yet been cleared for American use beyond clinical trials, German doctors have already used the system to perform coronary bypass surgery.

The ZEUS system employs the assistance of the AESOP robotic system. Released by Computer Motion in 1994, AESOP was the first robot to be cleared by the FDA for assisting surgery in the operating room. AESOP is much simpler than the da Vinci and ZEUS systems. It is basically just one mechanical arm, used by the physician to position the laparoscope. Foot pedals or voice-activated software allows the surgeon to position the camera, leaving his or her hands free to continue operating on the patient **(Fig. 3)**. The use of a computer console to perform operations from a distance opens up the idea of telesurgery, which would involve a doctor performing delicate surgery thousands of

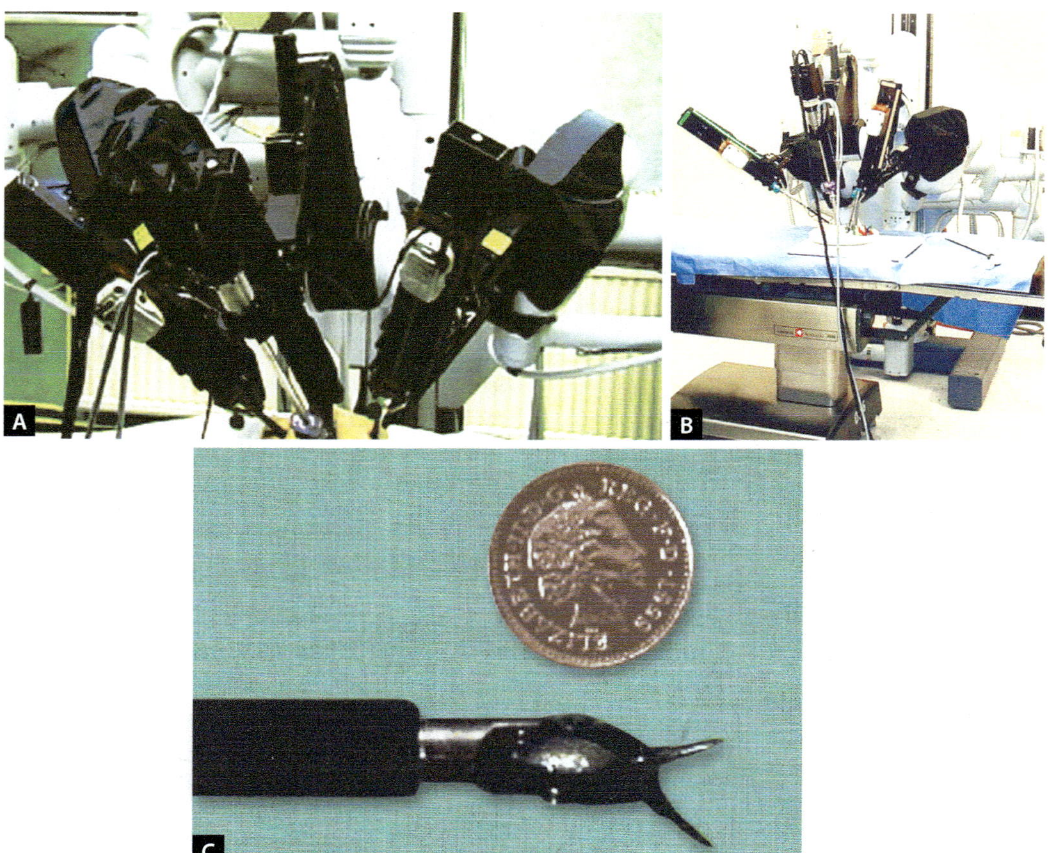

Figs. 2A to C: (A and B) Robotic arms of da Vinci surgical system; (C) Effector tips of the da Vinci surgical system.

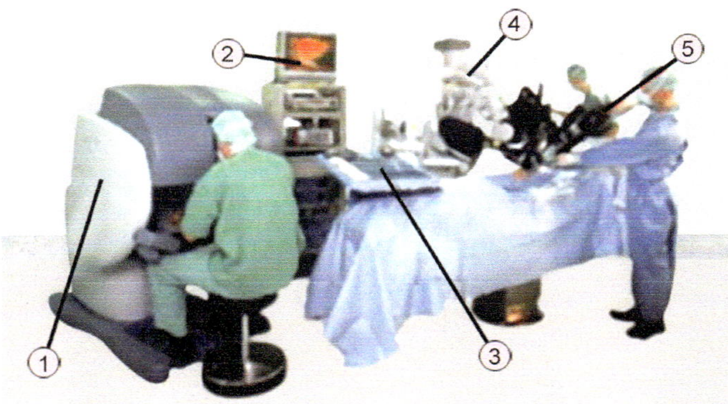

Fig. 3: Robotic surgery. (1) Surgeon console; (2) Image processing equipment; (3) EndoWrist instruments; (4) Surgical arm cart; and (5) High-resolution three-dimensional (3D) endoscope.

miles away from the patient. If it were possible to use the computer console to move the robotic arms in real time, then it would be possible for a doctor in New Delhi to operate on a patient in New York. A major obstacle in telesurgery has been the time delay between the doctor moving his or her hands to the robotic arms responding to those movements. Currently, the doctor must be in the room with the patient for robotic systems to react instantly to the doctor's hand movements.

Having fewer personnel in the operating room and allowing doctors the ability to operate on a patient, long distance could lower the cost of health care. In addition to cost-efficiency, robotic surgery has several other advantages over conventional surgery, including enhanced precision and reduced trauma to the patient. For instance, heart bypass surgery now requires that the patient's chest 30.48 cm long incision. However, with the da Vinci or ZEUS systems, it is possible to operate on the heart by making three small incisions in the chest, each only 10 mm in diameter. The patient would experience less pain and less bleeding, which means a faster recovery.

Robotics also decreases the fatigue that doctors experience during surgeries that can last several hours. Surgeons can become exhausted during those long surgeries and can experience hand tremors as a result. Even the steadiest of human hands cannot match those of a surgical robot. The da Vinci system has been programmed to compensate for tremors, so if the doctor's handshakes, the computer ignores it and keeps the mechanical arm steady. While surgical robots offer some advantages over the human hand, we are still a long way from the day when autonomous robots will operate on people without human interaction. But, with advances in computer power and artificial intelligence, it could be that in this century a robot will be designed that can locate abnormalities in the human body, analyze them, and operate to correct those abnormalities without any human guidance.

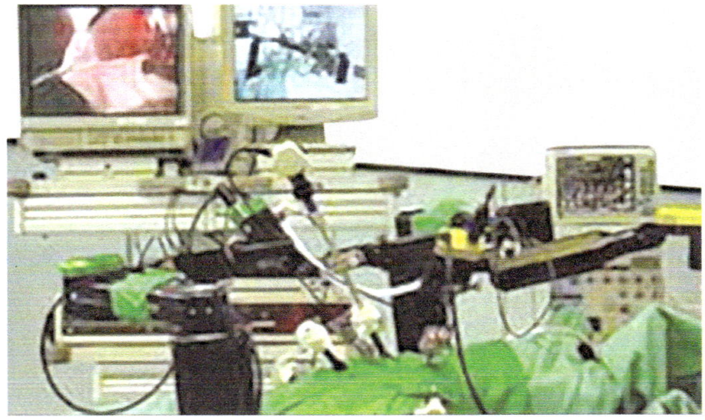

Fig. 4: Robotic surgery via master-slave manipulator.

The fallopian tube reconnection procedure, referred to as tubal reanastomosis, was performed by Dr Tommaso Falcone, who is Head of the Reproductive Endocrinology and Infertility Section at the Cleveland Clinic. Dr Falcone used Computer Motion's ZEUS robotic surgical system as part of a clinical trial, approved by the United States FDA.

The patient, a 38-year-old woman, and her healthy 10-day-old son are both in excellent condition and have returned to their Cleveland-area home. The mother had originally undergone a tubal ligation sterilization operation in her 20s. She and her partner later wished to have a child together and began preparing for a reversal operation. The patient saw an advertisement for the ZEUS study and consulted with trial leader Dr Falcone. The lady was informed in detail of the investigational protocol and agreed to have the robotically-assisted procedure.

In addition to the ZEUS System, Computer Motion markets the AESOP 3000, a voice-controlled endoscope positioning system, and the HERMES Control Center, a centralized system, which enables the surgeon to voice control a network of "smart" medical devices. Currently, the ZEUS system is under an FDA-approved investigational device exemption and is also CE marked for commercial sale in Europe.

Robotics is rapidly developing in surgery, although the word is slightly misused in this connection. None of the systems under development involves a machine acting autonomously. Instead, the machine acts as a remote extension of the surgeon. The correct term for such a system is a "master-slave manipulator," although it seems unlikely that this term will gain general currency.

Minimal invasive surgery is itself a form of telemanipulation because the surgeon is physically separated from the workspace. Telerobotics is an obvious tool to extend the surgeons capabilities. The goal is to restore the tactile cues and intuitive dexterity of the surgeon, which are diminished by MIS. A slave manipulator, controlled through a spatially consistent and intuitive master with a force feedback system, could replace the tactile sensibilities and restore dexterity **(Fig. 4)**.

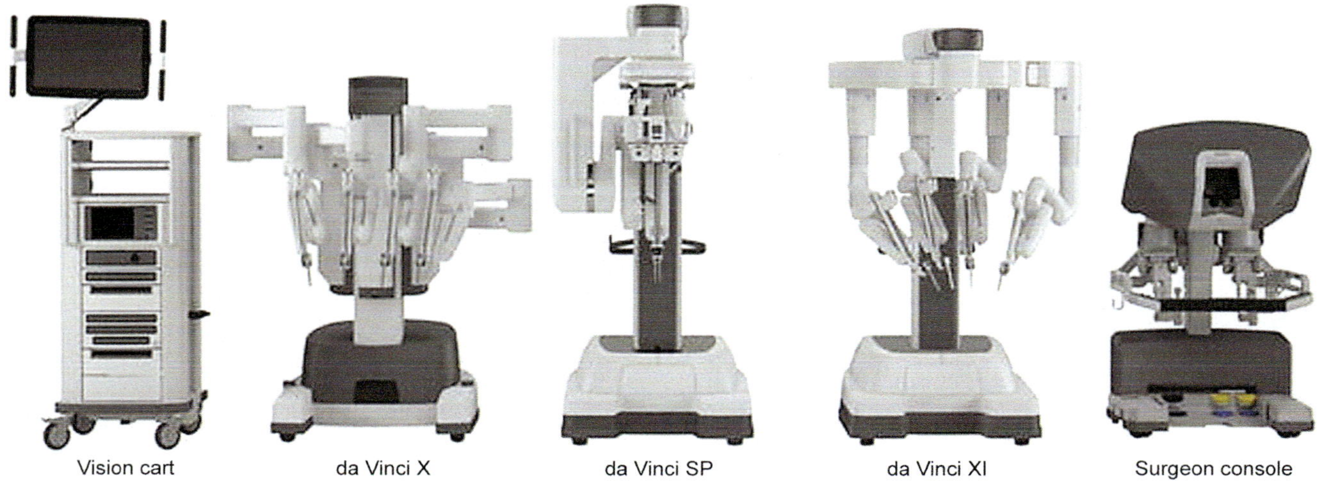

Fig. 5: Master-slave manipulator.

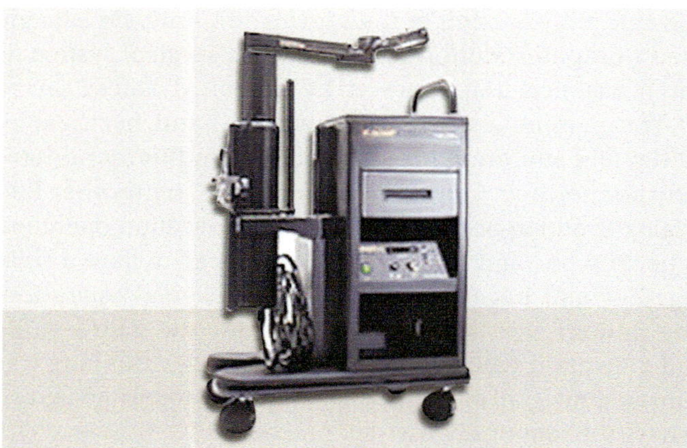

Fig. 6: Robotic console.

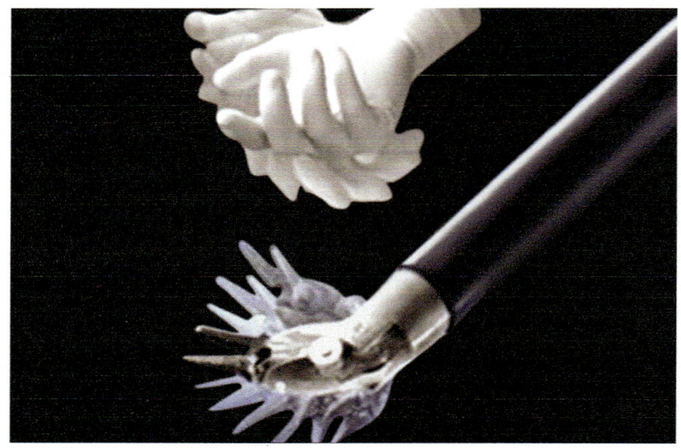

Fig. 7: Robotic arm.

Although the potential of robotic surgery is just beginning but progress may come quickly. Laparoscopic gallbladder surgery was first done in 1987, but it became standard within 5 years. Just think about a surgeon! He picks up this black box and waves it over your body and you are fixed. How is that going to happen? One day, a surgeon may use robotic devices to enter the body through its own orifices. They could carry medical instruments inside the body, where they would be manipulated by simple computer commands **(Figs. 5 to 7)**.

The robotic arm after addition of wrists permits the surgeon to mimic his own movements, rather than experience limitations of the rigid long cylindrical laparoscopic instrument and has obvious advantages in terms of dexterity and complexity of instrument **(Fig. 8)**.

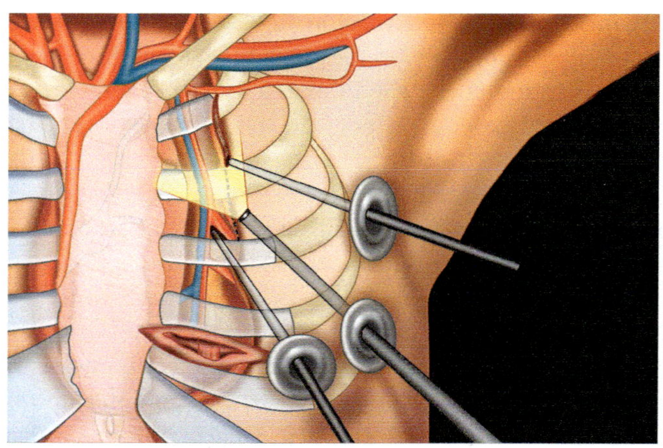

Fig. 8: Ports in cardiac minimal access surgery.

INSTRUMENTS OF ROBOTIC SURGERY

da Vinci Surgical System (Figs. 9 to 20)

Using the most advanced technology available today, the da Vinci surgical system enables surgeons to perform delicate and complex operations through a few tiny incisions with increased vision, precision, dexterity, and control. The da Vinci surgical system consists of several key components, including: an ergonomically designed console where the surgeon sits while operating, a patient-side cart where the patient lays during surgery, four interactive robotic arms, a high-definition 3D vision system, and proprietary EndoWrist instruments.

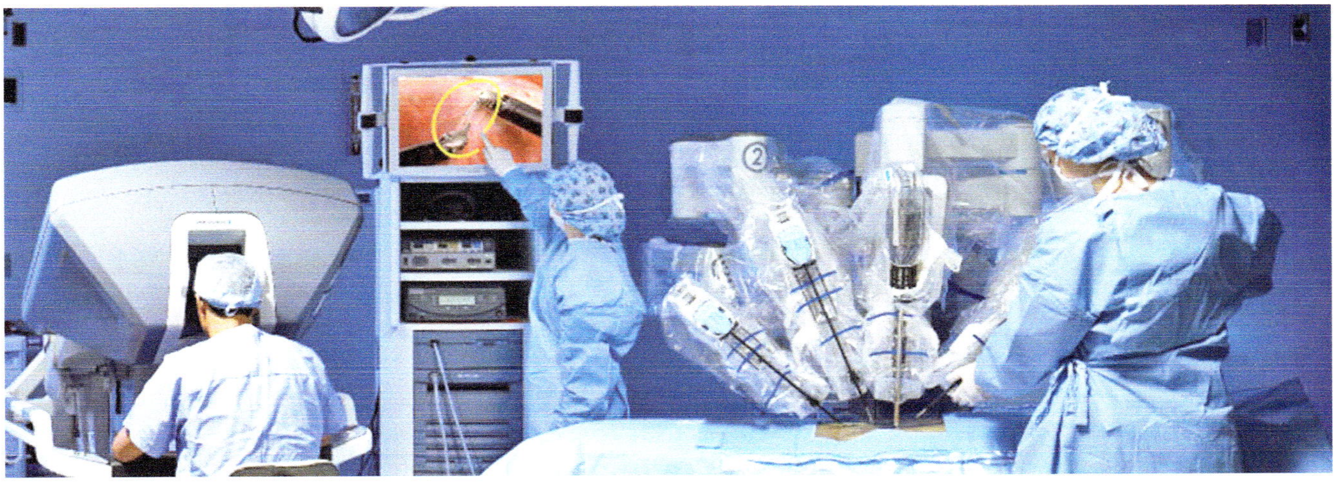

Fig. 9: da Vinci high-definition surgical robot.

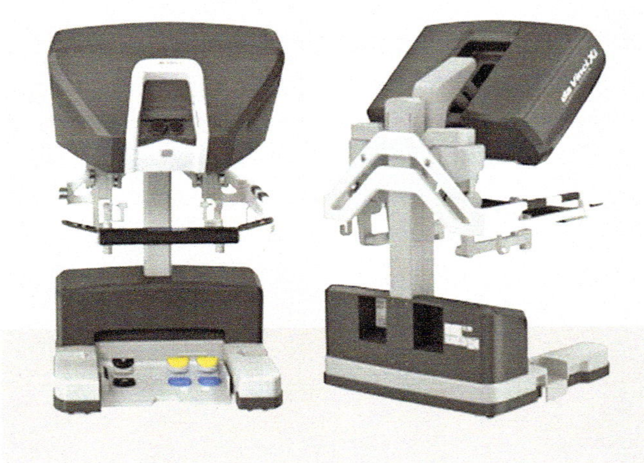

Fig. 10: da Vinci surgeon console.

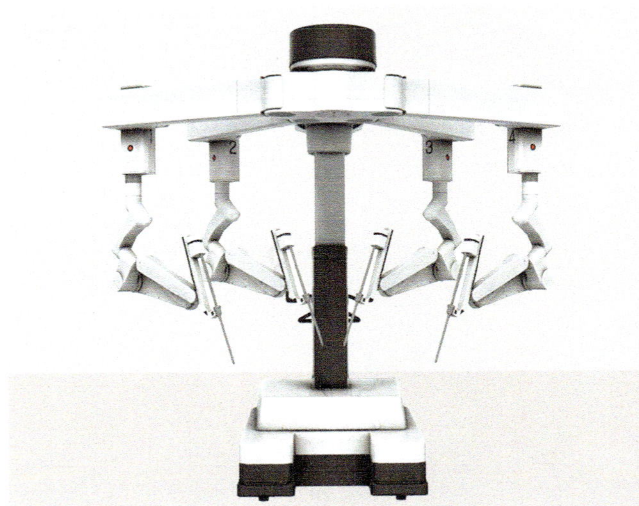

Fig. 11: Patient cart.

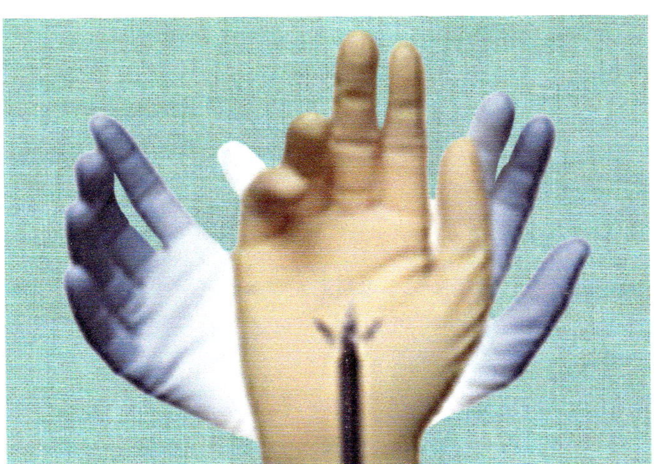

Fig. 12: Seven-degree movement is possible.

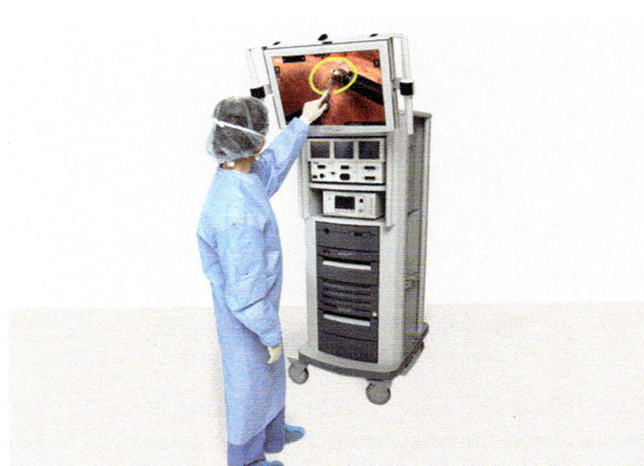

Fig. 13: da Vinci vision cart.

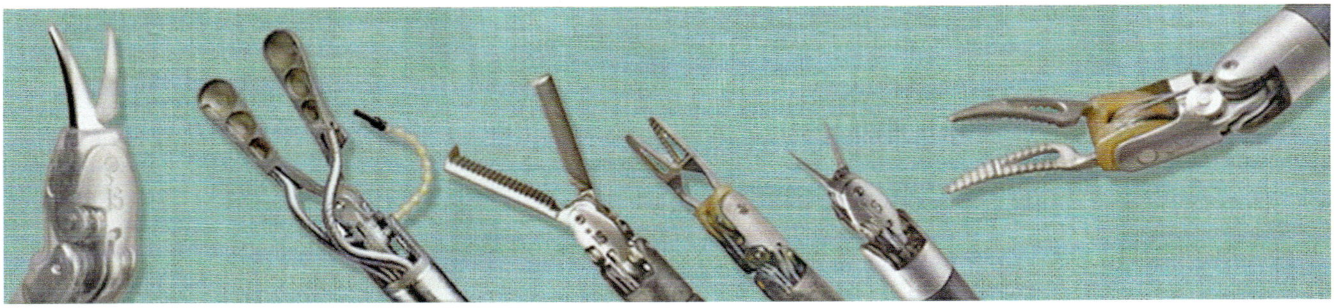

Fig. 14: Robotic EndoWrist instruments.

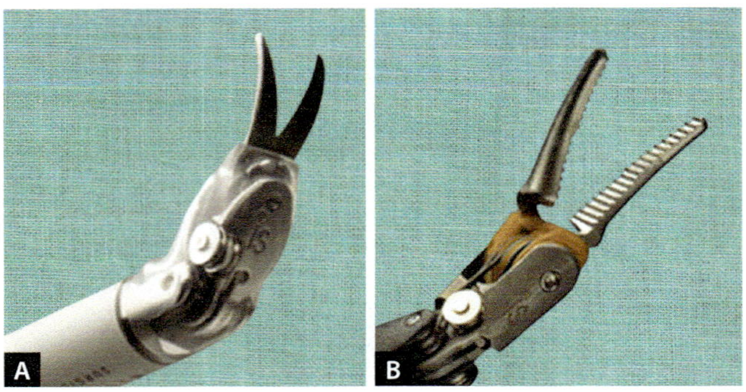

Figs. 15A and B: Robotic scissors and bipolar dissector.

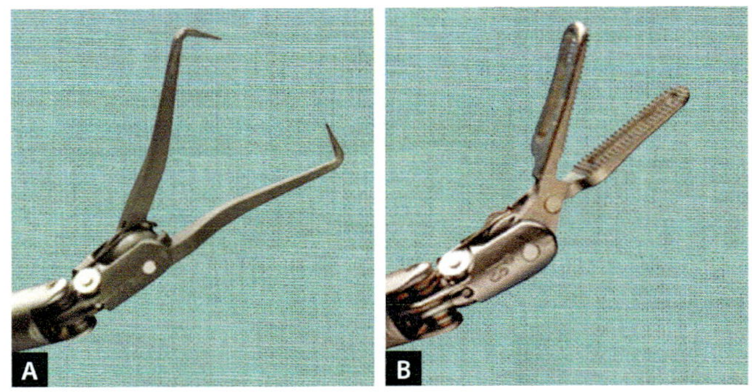

Figs. 16A and B: Robotic tenaculum and grasper.

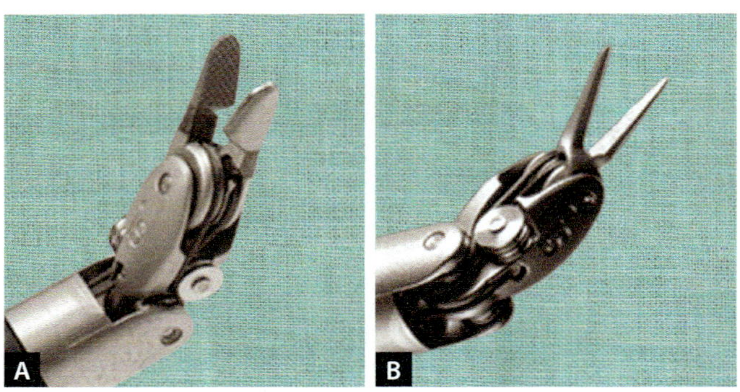

Figs. 17A and B: Robotic needle holder.

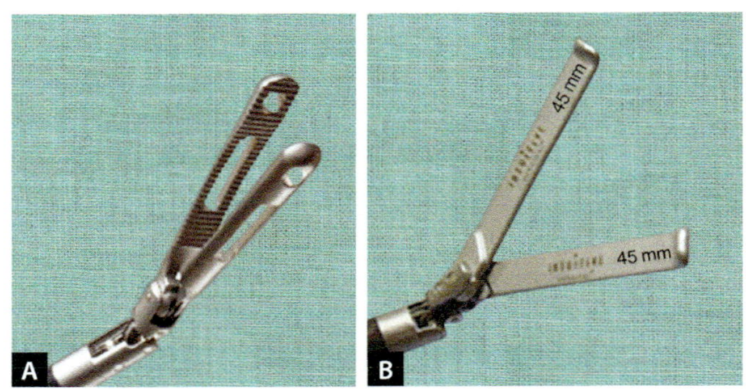

Figs. 18A and B: Robotic atraumatic grasper.

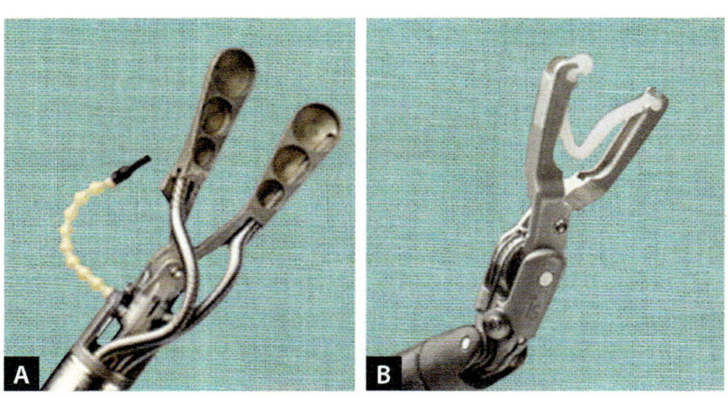

Figs. 19A and B: Robotic clip applicator.

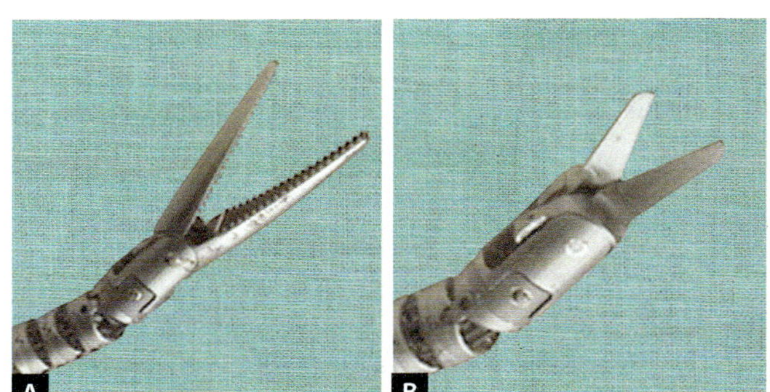

Figs. 20A and B: Robotic scissor and Maryland.

da Vinci is powered by state-of-the-art robotic technology that allows the surgeon's hand movements to be scaled, filtered, and translated into precise movements of the EndoWrist instruments working inside the patient's body.

Core Technology

- System components
- Three-dimensional high-definition (HD) vision.

Instrumentation

Using the da Vinci surgical system, the surgeon operates seated comfortably at a console while viewing an HD, 3D image inside the patient's body.

- The surgeon's fingers grasp the master controls below the display with hands and wrists naturally positioned relative to his or her eyes
- The system seamlessly translates the surgeon's hand, wrist, and finger movements into precise, real-time movements of surgical instruments
- The patient-side cart is where the patient is positioned during surgery. It includes either three or four robotic arms that carryout the surgeon's commands
- The robotic arms move around fixed pivot points, which reduce trauma to the patient, improve the cosmetic outcome, and increase overall precision
- The system requires that every surgical maneuver be under the direct control of the surgeon. Repeated safety checks prevent any independent movement of the instruments or robotic arms
- A full range of EndoWrist instruments is available to the surgeon while operating
- The instruments are designed with seven degrees of motion—a range of motion even greater than the human wrist
- Each instrument has a specific surgical mission such as clamping, suturing, and tissue manipulation
- Quick-release levers speed instrument changes during surgery
- The vision system is equipped with an HD, 3D endoscope (flexible tube with a camera and light at the tip) and image processing equipment that provides true-to-life images of the patient's anatomy
- A view of the operating field is available to the entire operative room (OR) team on a large viewing monitor (vision cart). This widescreen view provides the surgical assistant at the patient's side with a broader perspective and visualization of the procedure.

INSTRUMENTS AND ACCESSORIES

Intuitive surgical's exclusive EndoWrist instruments are designed to provide surgeons with natural dexterity and full range of motion for precise operation through tiny incisions. Modeled after the human wrist, EndoWrist instruments can offer an even greater range of motion than the human hand. They truly allow the da Vinci® system to take surgical precision and technique beyond the limits of the human hand. Similar to human tendons, an EndoWrist instrument's internal cables provide maximum responsiveness, allowing rapid and precise suturing, dissection, and tissue manipulation. EndoWrist instruments provide enhanced dexterity, precision, and control:

- 7° of freedom
- 90° of articulation
- Intuitive motion and finger-tip control
- Motion scaling and tremor reduction.

The wrist-like movement, responsiveness, and robotic control afforded by the da Vinci system and its exclusive EndoWrist instruments provide surgeons fluid ambidexterity and unparalleled precision. The EndoWrist instruments are available in a wide selection of specialized tip designs to enable a broad range of da Vinci procedures. As da Vinci surgery is adopted in new specialties, our engineers work side-by-side with surgeons to develop new EndoWrist instruments to address new clinical needs. The following is a list of instrument categories for which intuitive offers specialized tip designs.

Energy instruments are used by the da Vinci surgeon to provide coagulation, cutting, and dissection of tissues. These include monopolar and bipolar cautery instruments (electrical energy), the *Harmonic*™ ACE (mechanical energy), the *PK*™ dissecting forceps (advanced bipolar), and laser.

Grasping instruments allow for manipulation of a wide range of tissues, from fine, thin tissues such as peritoneum to dense, fibrous tissues such as uterus. Needle drivers provide the ability to suture with the finest of needles used in cardiovascular surgery as well as the thickest needles used in repair of uterine defects. *Suture Cut*™ needle drivers include an integral cutting blade for efficient cutting of suture after knot tying and increased surgeon autonomy and efficiency. Retracting instruments allow the surgeon to dynamically provide exposure of the surgical field. This minimizes dependency on the patient-side assistant, providing the da Vinci surgeon with full control of the operative field.

Clip appliers, probe graspers, and cardiac stabilizers are available to allow the da Vinci surgeon to perform specialized procedures such as vessel clipping, cryoablation, and beating-heart surgery.

A selection of 5 mm EndoWrist instruments provides the surgeon with the ability to use smaller access ports. Some surgeons prefer smaller access ports when performing pediatric, thoracic, bariatric, gynecologic, and general surgery.

OPERATING ROOM CONFIGURATION, PORT PLACEMENT, AND DOCKING

Before any procedure, the robot has to be prepared for surgery. It includes the connection of all necessary parts such as sterile drapes and connectors needed for surgery and the calibration process. These steps are conducted by a core team of scrub nurses specifically trained in handling the robot while the patient is in preparation for surgery. Currently, the only available system for laparoscopic surgery is the da Vinci surgical system, developed by Intuitive Surgical (Sunnyvale, CA, USA).

Any robotic procedure is performed by a team of surgeons and nurses. It includes the console surgeon, patient-side assistant surgeon, and the scrub nurse. Although console surgeon is the leader of the team, a trained assistant surgeon is of paramount importance as he/she is the person responsible for robot docking, instrument change, manipulation of laparoscopic instruments, application of hemostatic instruments/clips, lavage and aspiration, specimen extraction, drainage, and closure of abdominal wall. A trained scrub nurse is also important in draping the robotic arms, attaching the optics, instrument changes, and undocking of the robot.

Operating Room Configuration

This topic includes the optimum positioning of the following components in the operating room (OR) so as to allow for maximum functionality:
- Surgeon console positioning
- Patient cart positioning
- Vision cart positioning.

Surgeon Console Positioning

The surgeon console is placed outside of the sterile field. It should be oriented in such a position so that the surgeon has a clear view of the operative field, vision cart, and able to communicate directly with the assistant surgeon and the scrub nurse.

For moving or positioning the surgeon console, only the handle **(Fig. 21)** on the back of the console is used. It should never be pushed or pulled by the console body or armrest to maneuver the console into place. Wheel locks located on the rear wheels of the surgeon console should be locked after positioning of console for the surgery.

Patient Cart Positioning

The patient cart is placed in the sterile field. It should be draped in a separate area in the room prior to moving it into place for surgery. This should be an area of the room where it will not easily come into contact with nonsterile objects or impede traffic. Once the patient cart is draped and the patient is positioned, prepared, and draped, ports are placed. Then, use the patient cart motor drive to help move the cart into the sterile field.

The patient cart brakes are designed to automatically engage when the motor drive is not in use.

Motor drive operation: The motor drive interface consists of the following components **(Fig. 22)**:
- Throttle
- Throttle enable switch
- Shift switches.

To operate the motor drive:
- Ensure that the patient cart is powered on
- Ensure the shift switches are in the drive position **(Figs. 23A and B)**
- Throttle enable switch is to be held and throttle rotated away from the operator or toward him/her depending on the intended direction of movement
    - The cart power light-emitting diode (LED) will flash green whenever the throttle enable switch is activated
    - The drive speed of the cart can be controlled by rotating the throttle to different extent in each direction.

The motor drive will not engage whenever cannulas or instruments are installed on the system. A yellow LED on motor drive interface labeled "cannula installed: cart drive disabled" will indicate when cannulas or instruments are installed and motor drive is nonoperational. This has been done for safety purpose.

Shift switches: The patient cart can be moved without the use of the motor drive (for example, during a power loss) by rotating the shift switches **(Fig. 23B)** to the neutral (N) position. The cart can then be moved manually. When the cart has been moved, shift switches should be placed in the drive (D) position to set the patient cart brakes.

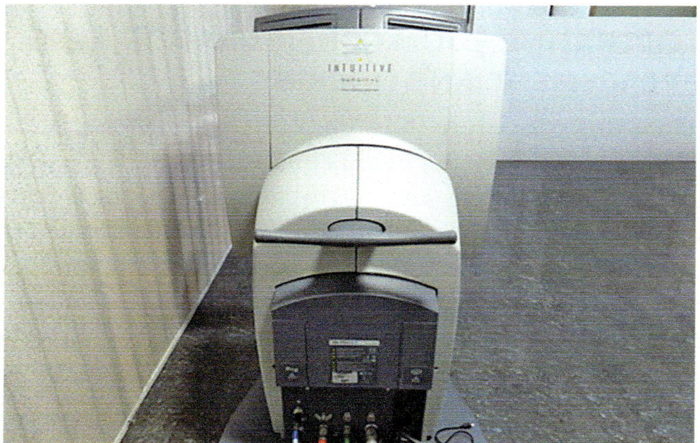

Fig. 21: Surgeon console handle.

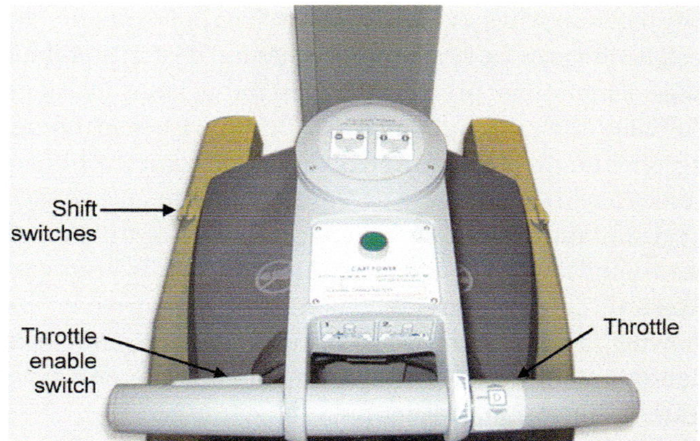

Fig. 22: Location of throttle, throttle enable switch, and shift switches.

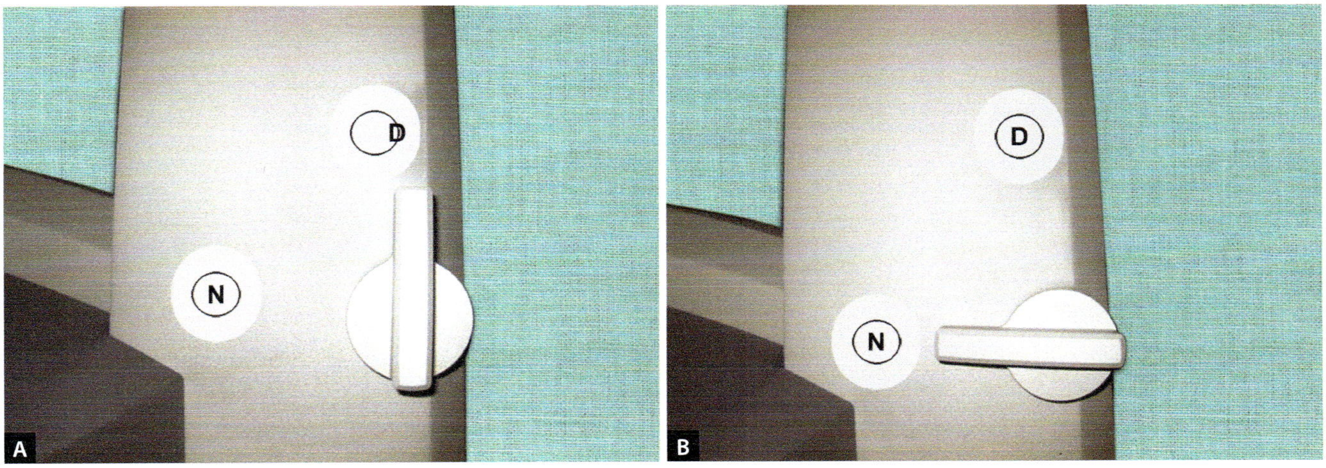

Figs. 23A and B: (A) Drive motor engaged; (B) Drive motor disengaged. (D: drive; N: neutral)

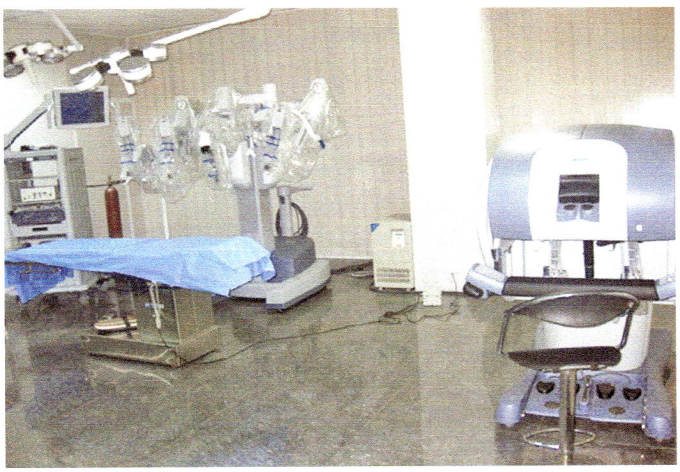

Fig. 24: Position of vision cart.

For patient safety, the shift switches must be kept in the drive (D) position so that the motor drive remains engaged during surgery **(Fig. 23A)**.

Vision Cart Positioning

The vision cart is placed adjacent to the patient cart, just outside of the sterile field, to allow the patient cart operator to see the component displays **(Fig. 24)**.

- The vision cart should be close enough to the patient cart to allow unrestricted camera cable movement during surgery
- Wheel locks are located on the rear wheels of the vision cart. These should be locked after the cart is positioned for surgery.

Steps of docking:

- Position patient and OR table, including table tilt
- Position patient cart over patient
- Set patient cart brakes
- Docking the camera arm
- Docking the instrument arms
- Check system setup.

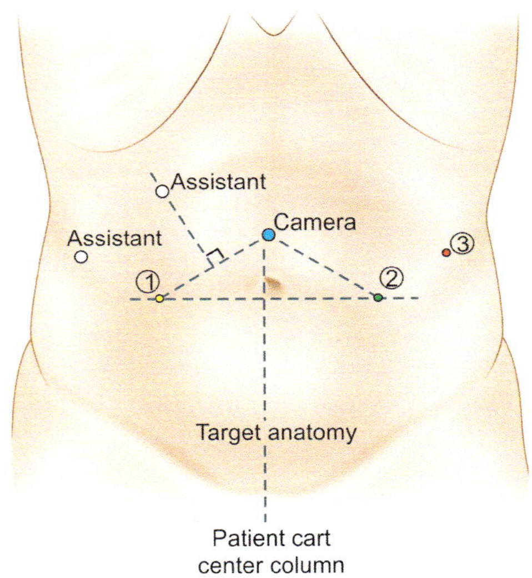

Fig. 25: Camera port positioning.

The patient table should be positioned according to surgeon preference (depending on the contemplated procedure) before docking the robotic arms. Once the arms are docked to the ports and instruments are placed, patient position should not be changed. The pneumoperitoneum is created and the ports are inserted by either the lead surgeon or the patient-side assistant surgeon.

Port Placement

The port positions vary from patient-to-patient, procedure-to-procedure, and surgeon-to-surgeon. It is very difficult to form guidelines-specific position of ports, but broad guidelines are framed to maximize endoscopic view, instrument reach, and to minimize external arm clashing.

Camera port is inserted keeping following principles in mind **(Fig. 25)**:

- Should be in line with the target anatomy (TA)
- Should beat 10–20 cm distance from the TA

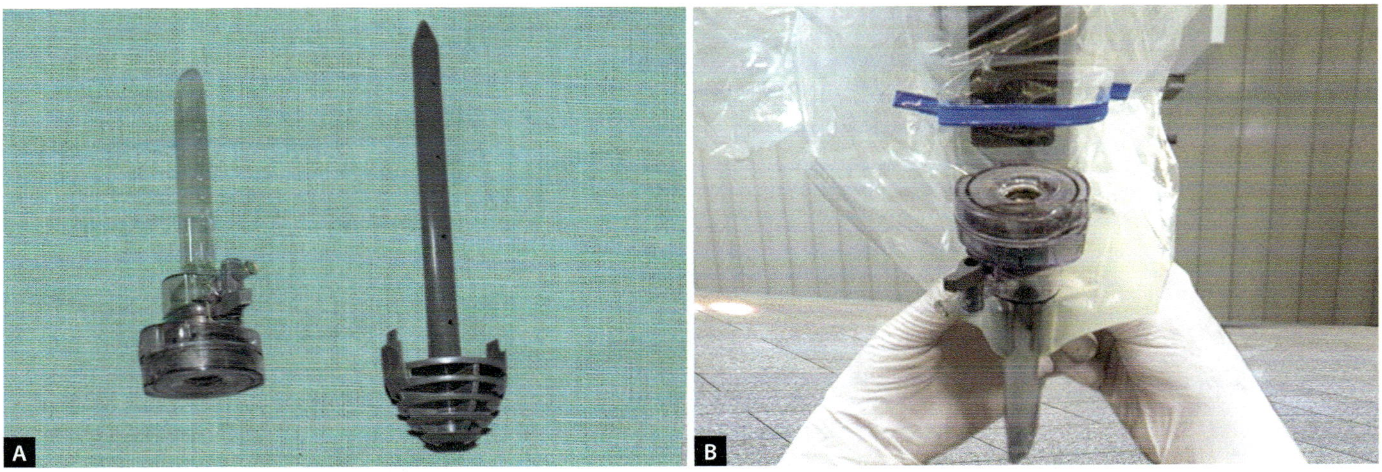

Figs. 26A and B: (A) Disposable 12 mm trocar cannula assembly for camera port; (B) Camera port being mounted on the camera arm.

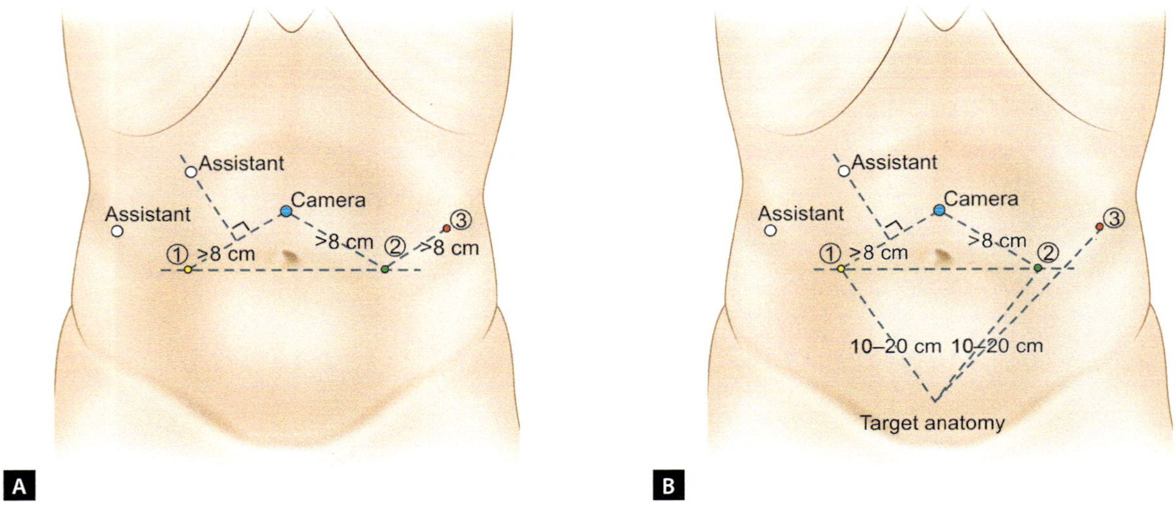

Figs. 27A and B: Port placement.

- Should be in line with the center column of the patient cart. A diagnostic laparoscopy is done after insertion of the camera port to look for safe entry, any adhesions, and surgical feasibility.

A disposable 12 mm trocar cannula assembly is used as the camera port **(Figs. 26A and B)**. There are specialized camera arm cannula mounts (on the patient cart camera arm) corresponding to each validated third-party cannula.

Working Ports

An 8 mm da Vinci ports are inserted for robotic arms that are inserted keeping in mind the following principles:

- >8 cm distance between the da Vinci ports **(Fig. 27A)**
- 10–20 cm distance should be maintained between the da Vinci ports and TA **(Fig. 27B)**.

A 10 cm distance from TA is good but 20 cm distance is better. Ports placed closed to the TA impede the view of the surgical site and make the operation technically challenging. Conversely, ports placed >20 cm from TA make it difficult to see or reach with robotic instruments.

Assistant port, if needed, is inserted 5–10 cm away from the da Vinci ports in the desirable position. 5 or 10 mm ports can be used according to the intended function of the port.

The da Vinci provides 8 mm reusable cannulas with disposable seals for the robotic arms. They come with bladeless obturator for insertion.

These come in two lengths **(Fig. 28)**:

1. Short (11 cm cannula)
2. Long (16 cm cannula) for high body mass index (BMI) patients.

Remote Center Technology

Remote center is the fixed point in the space around which surgical arm and cannula move. It helps in maneuvering instruments/endoscopes in surgical site while exerting minimal force on the abdominal or thoracic wall **(Figs. 29A and B)**.

It is marked on the da Vinci cannulas at a point to minimize stress to the patient. Remote center can be adjusted on patient side at the patient cart using the clutch button.

Positioning the Patient Cart

Once the patient is positioned and the ports are inserted, it is time to attach patient cart instrument arms to the patient in a process called docking. Before moving patient cart into position over the patient, it is important to align the OR table and the patient. Then, push the patient cart over the patient using the motor drive on the cart.

Motor drive can be used in integrated mode when patient cart is connected to the rest of the system or in standalone mode as well. The *shift switches* on the base of the patient cart need to be set in drive (D) position **(Fig. 30)**. Then, the cart can be moved by pressing the *throttle enable switch* and throttling either forward or backward **(Fig. 31)**. It can be moved manually if the shift switch is set in neutral (N) position.

Two people should be used to move the cart, one pushes or pulls the cart and the second person verbally directs regarding the direction of movement. When the cart is in position, shift switch should be set to drive position for locking the cart. Installing the camera or instrument arm locks the patient cart automatically for patient safety.

Care should be taken to align the camera port, TA, and the center column **(Fig. 32)**.

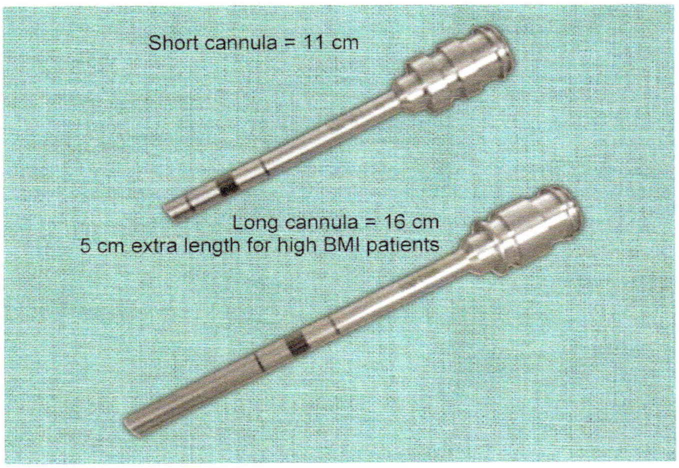

Fig. 28: The da Vinci cannula.
(BMI: body mass index)

Docking the Camera Arm

Camera arm should be docked first after positioning the patient cart. Align the camera port, TA, and the center column of the patient cart. Use clutch button to change the angle of camera arm to match the angle of cannula so that it points to TA **(Fig. 33)**.

Stabilize the cannula at the port site with one hand pointing it toward the TA. Bring cannula into the cannula mount on the camera arm and clip both wings shut to hold the cannula in place **(Fig. 34)**.

Camera arm setup joint #2 is placed opposite the instrument arm 3 **(Fig. 35)**. Setup joints are numbered starting from the joint closest to the center column. Setting the system in this position allows maximum range of motion for all instrument arms.

There is a thick blue line and a blue arrow on setup joint #2 on the camera arm indicating the *sweet spot* **(Fig. 36)**. Sweet spot should be aligned by lining up the blue arrow within the boundaries of blue line. Setting sweet spot gives patient cart arms maximum range of motion ensuring instrument and endoscope reach of all parts of TA.

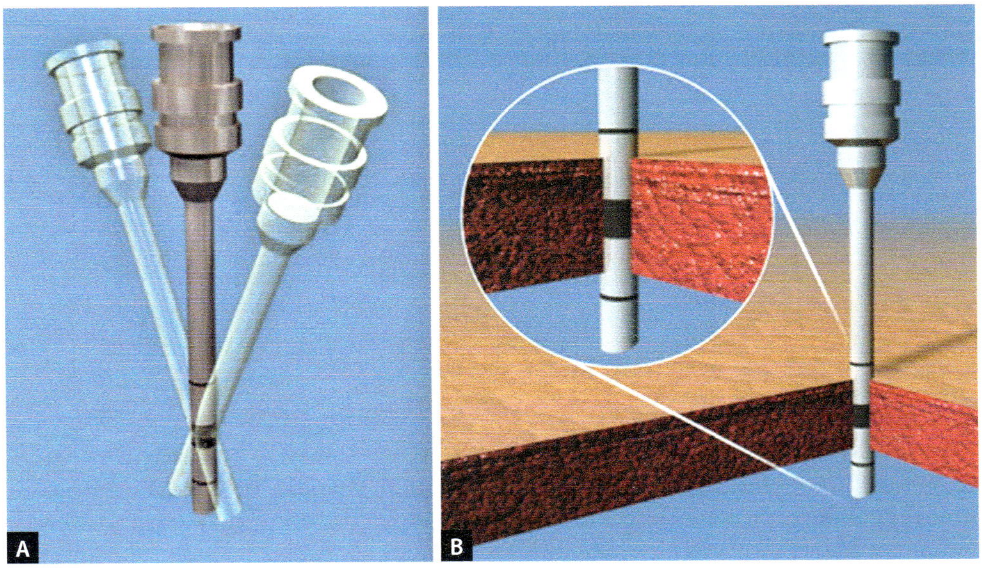

Figs. 29A and B: Remote center technology.

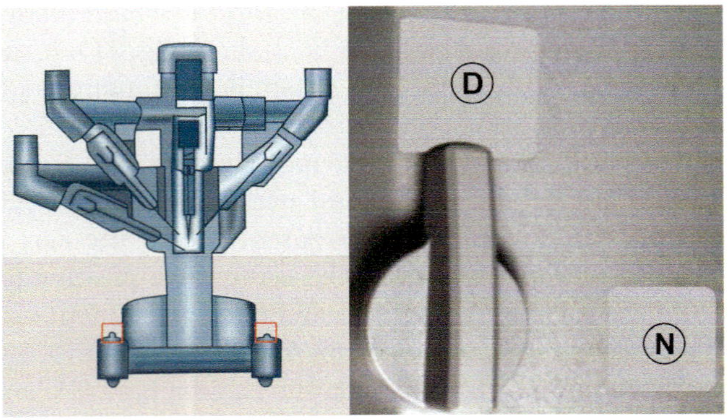

Fig. 30: Shift switch.

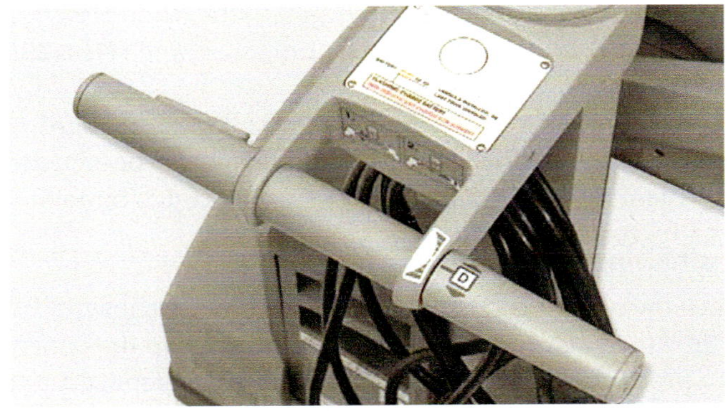

Fig. 31: Throttle with throttle enable switch.

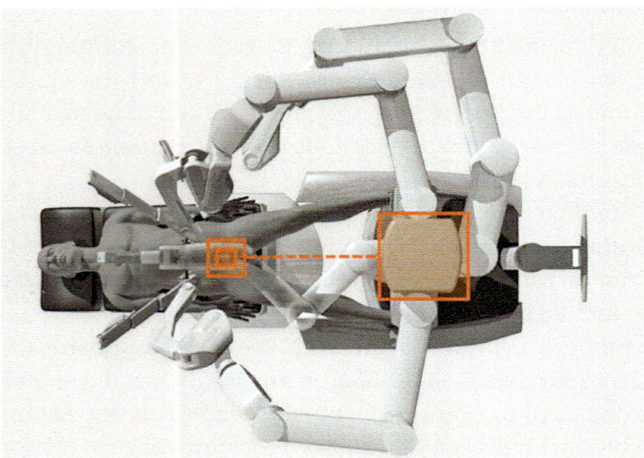

Fig. 32: Alignment of camera arm, target anatomy, and center column of patient cart.

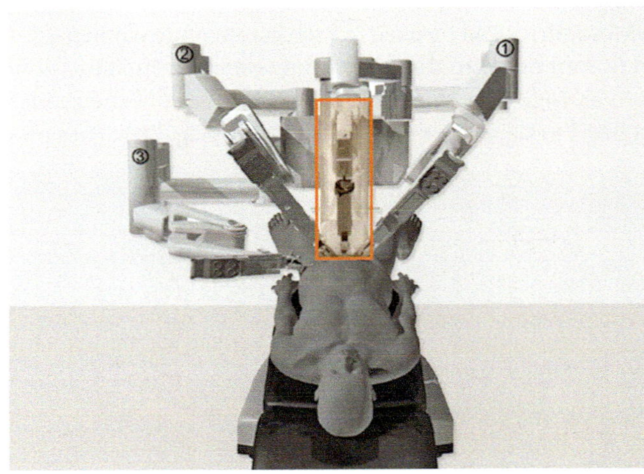

Fig. 33: Docking the camera arm.

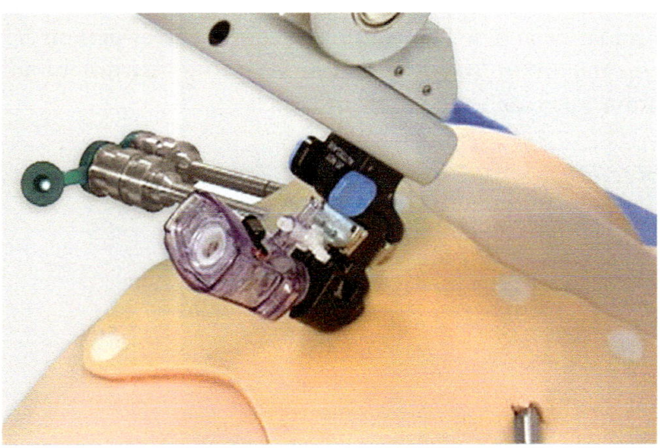

Fig. 34: Mounting cannula to camera arm.

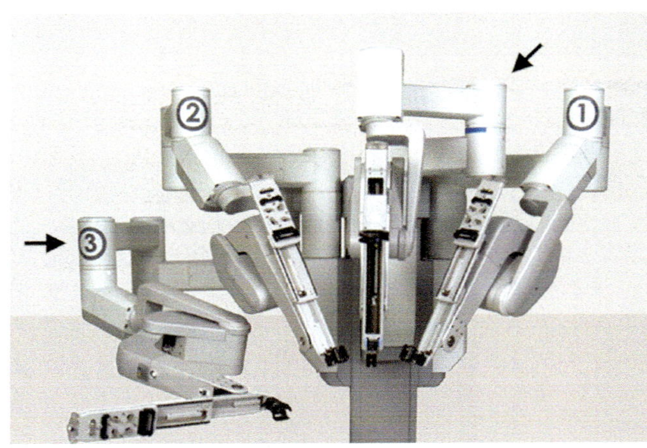

Fig. 35: Camera arm setup joint #2 facing opposite instrument arm 3 (arrow).

Remember that overextending or not extending the camera arm enough will limit the instrument range of motion.

Align the camera arm clutch button, third setup joint, and the center column **(Fig. 37)**. Strive to maintain the sweet spot and alignment of the camera arm throughout the docking process.

Docking of Instrument Arms

After docking the camera arm, instrument arms are positioned in place so as to allow maximum range of motion of the arms. It is done in following steps:

- Position the instrument arm with the arm number and sterile adaptor facing forward **(Fig. 38)**

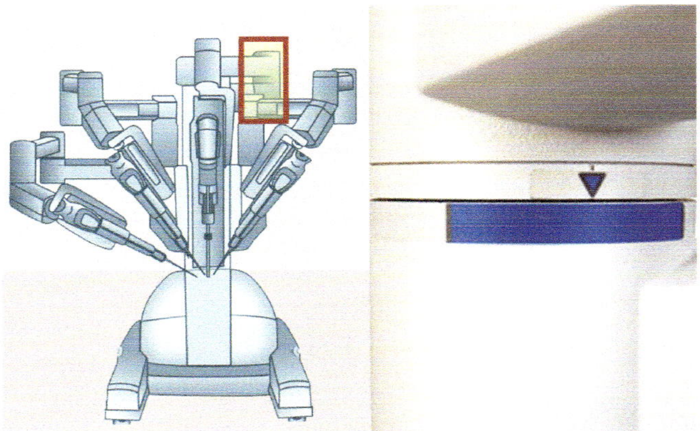

Fig. 36: Sweet spot and its alignment.

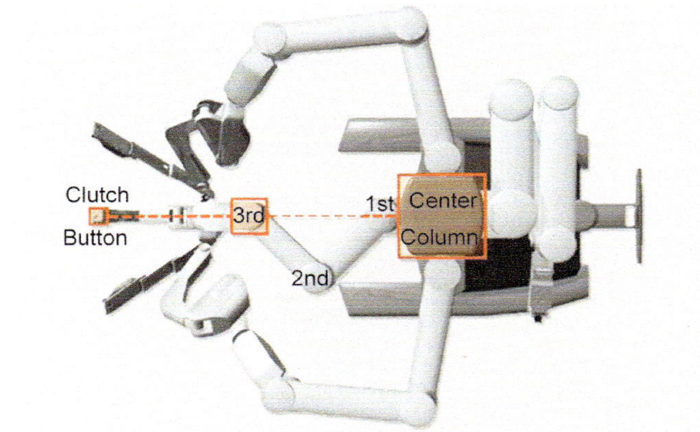

Fig. 37: Alignment of camera arm clutch button, third setup joint, and the center column.

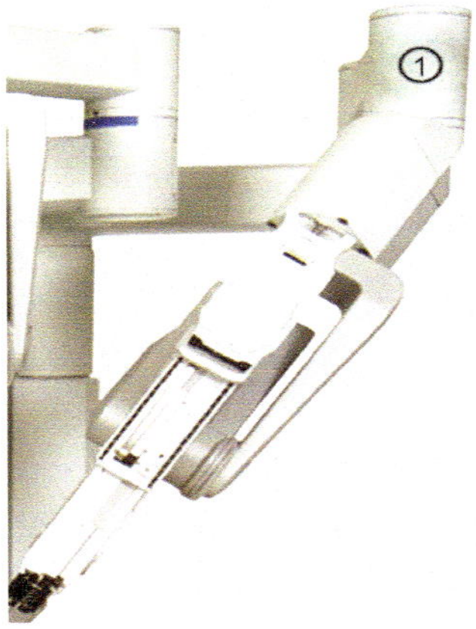

Fig. 38: Positioning of instrument arm.

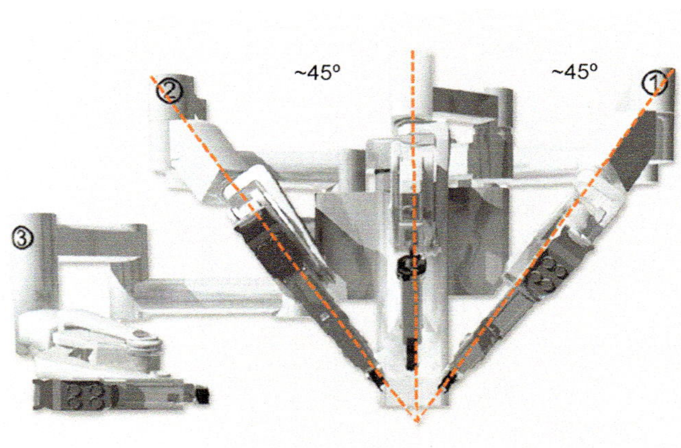

Fig. 39: Alignment of instrument arms with respect to camera arm and each other.

- Allow approximately 45° angle between each arm **(Fig. 39)**. Note that the position of instrument arm 3 can vary according to patient body habitus and the procedure. After positioning, ensure that the arms will not collide with the patient or interfere with each other
- Dock the instrument arms by bringing them to the cannula using the port clutch button. Bring the instrument arm to the cannula and lock the wings of the quick click cannula mount on the arm to clip the arm to the cannula **(Fig. 40)**.

Confirm that the remote center of the port is present at the desired place in the abdominal wall. Remember to stabilize the cannula with one hand at the port site while docking the instrument arm.

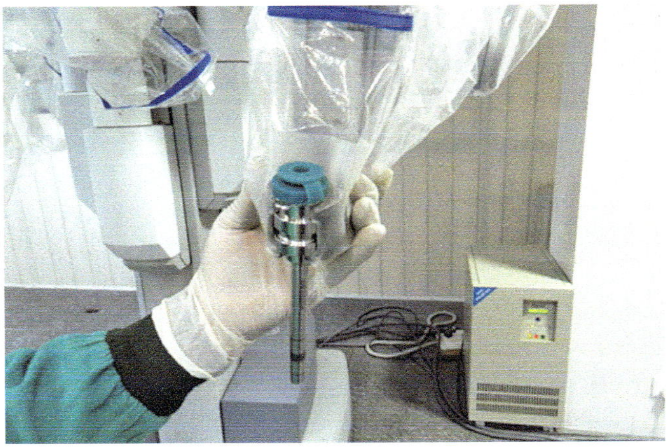

Fig. 40: Example of mounting instrument arm onto the cannula.

Check System Setup

After docking the instrument arms, check the arm setup. Start by confirming that the sweet spot of the camera arm is in right position (i.e., arrow is pointing toward the thick blue line). If needed, move the arm back into position taking care to stabilize the cannula at the port site.

Next, check the alignment of the camera port, TA, and the center column of the patient cart.

Now check the instrument arm setup. Separate the instrument arms to maximize the range of motion **(Fig. 41)**. Check the setup joint angles to minimize potential collisions.

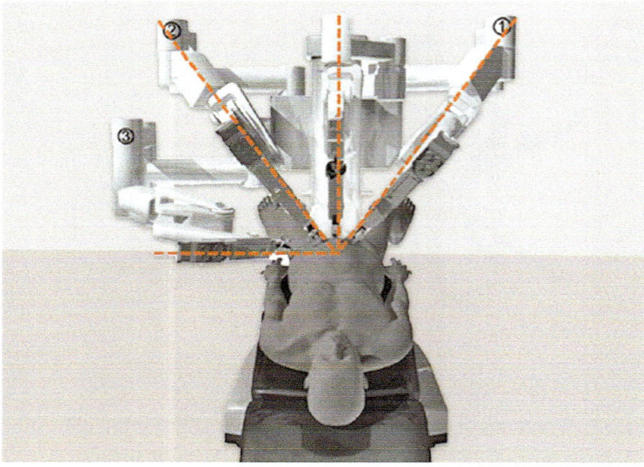

Fig. 41: Relative positions of the instrument arms.

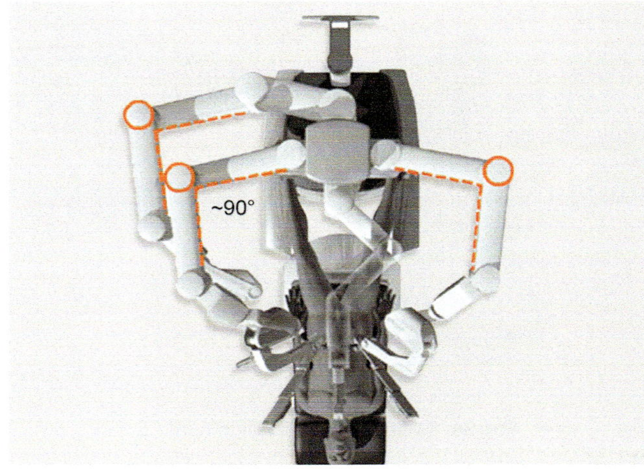

Fig. 42: Right angle at setup joint #2.

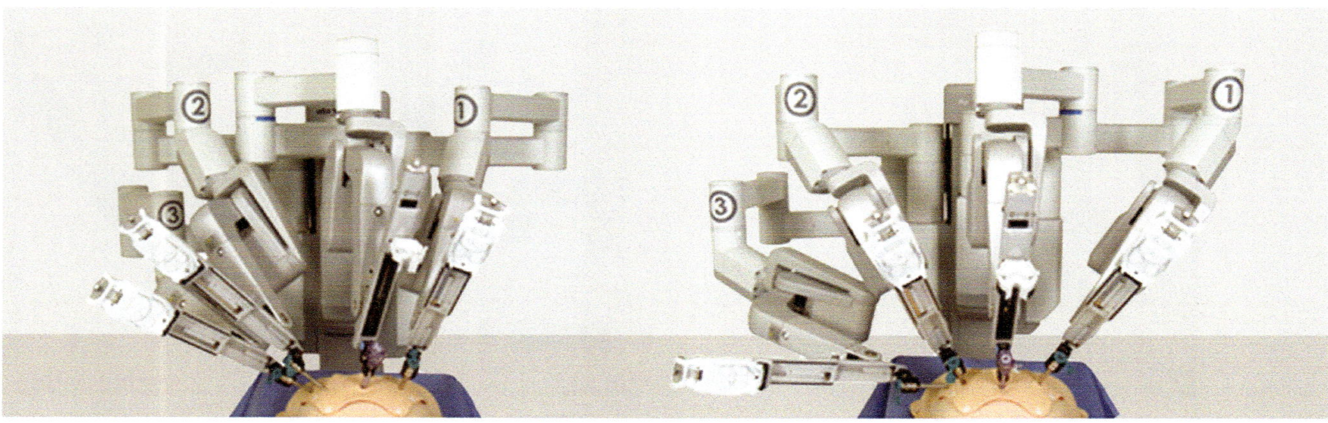

Incorrect Correct

Fig. 43: Depiction of the correct method of docking of patient cart.

The angle at the setup joint #2 should be approximately 90° **(Fig. 42)**. **Figure 43** depicts the correct method of docking the patient cart.

Endoscope Insertion and Removal

First, insert the endoscope into the cannula keeping the intuitive logo on the camera head facing the camera arm. Place the body of the endoscope into the camera arm sterile adaptor making sure that the body of endoscope is fully connected **(Fig. 44)**. Give it a gentle turn to ensure it is locked in place.

Next, secure the camera cable using the camera cable clip and drape the cable across the instrument arm **(Fig. 45)**.

Push the endoscope into the cannula by pressing the camera arm clutch button till it is past the cannula tip toward the TA. Press the clutch button again to lock the camera assembly into place.

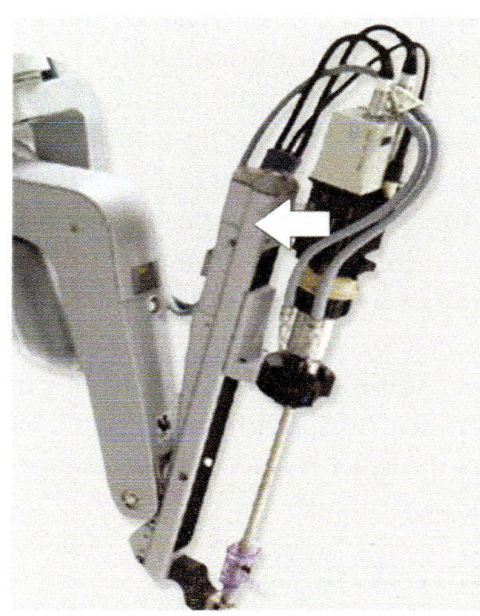

Fig. 44: Endoscope insertion into camera arm sterile adaptor of the camera arm.

To remove the endoscope, remove the camera cables from the clip on the camera arm. Then, unlock the endoscope by opening the two latches on the camera arm sterile adaptor. Then, remove the endoscope.

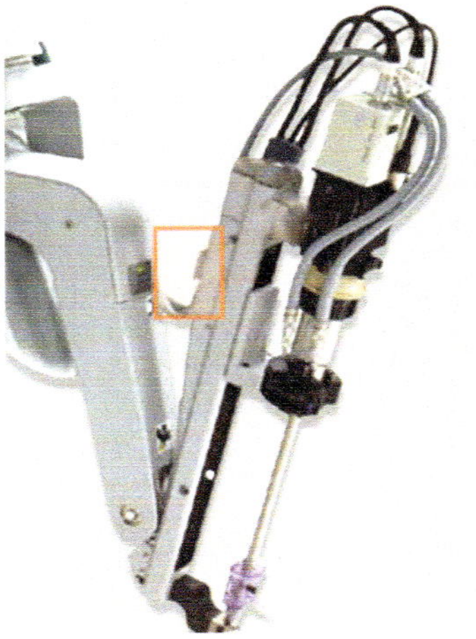

Fig. 45: Camera cable clip highlighted.

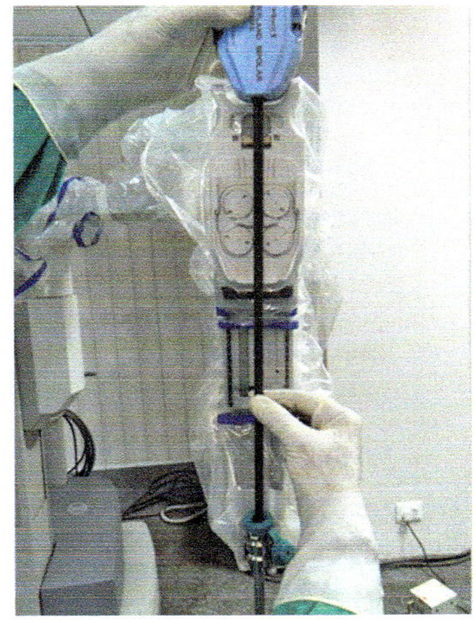

Fig. 46: Inserting the instrument into the cannula.

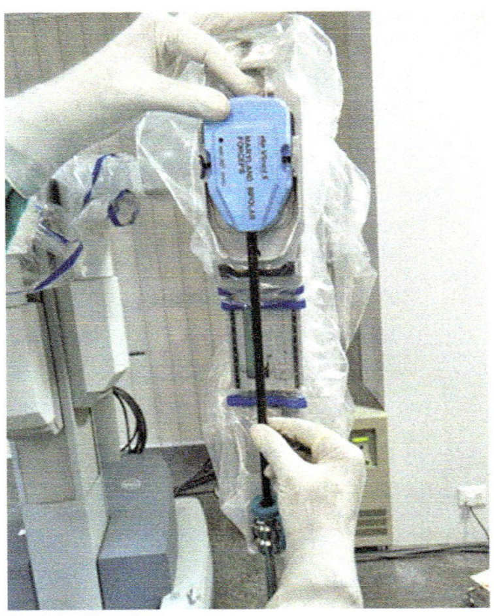

Fig. 47: Sliding the instrument into sterile adaptor on the instrument arm.

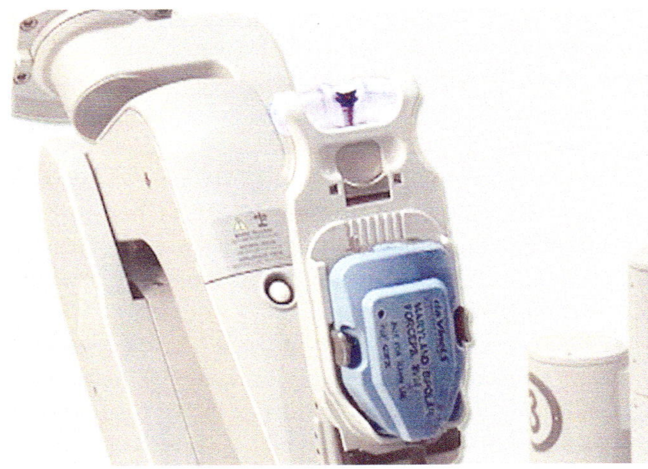

Fig. 48: Light-emitting diode (LED) turning blue indicating proper insertion.

Instrument Insertion

Begin by straightening the instrument tip. Insert the instrument into the cannula **(Fig. 46)**. Slide the instrument housing into the sterile adaptor **(Fig. 47)** sandwiching the instrument housing and the instrument arm between both hands. Press the arm clutch button and push the instrument into the surgical field, keeping the tip under endoscopic vision.

If there is any resistance while inserting the instrument, one should stop and check for the reason. When the LED lights turn blue **(Fig. 48)**, the surgeon can take control of the instrument and start operating.

Instrument Removal and Guided Tool Change

For removing the instruments, surgeon should straighten the instrument tip and open the jaws of the instrument to ensure that it does not hold any tissue **(Fig. 49)**. Then, press the release levers on the instrument housing and simply pull off the instrument **(Fig. 50)**.

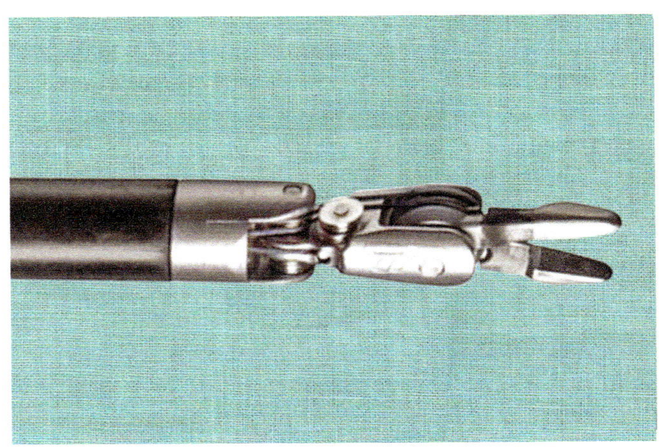

Fig. 49: Straightening the instrument tip and opening of jaws of the instrument before removal.

Removal of the instrument should be done with utmost care and with complete knowledge of the operating surgeon, so as to prevent any inadvertent injury to the tissues.

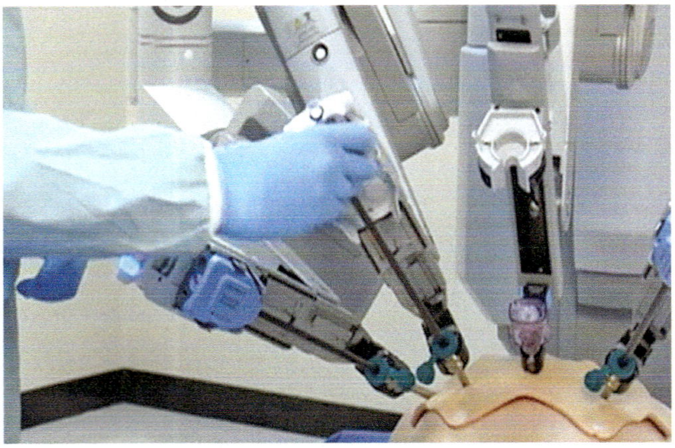

Fig. 50: Pressing the levers to remove the instrument.

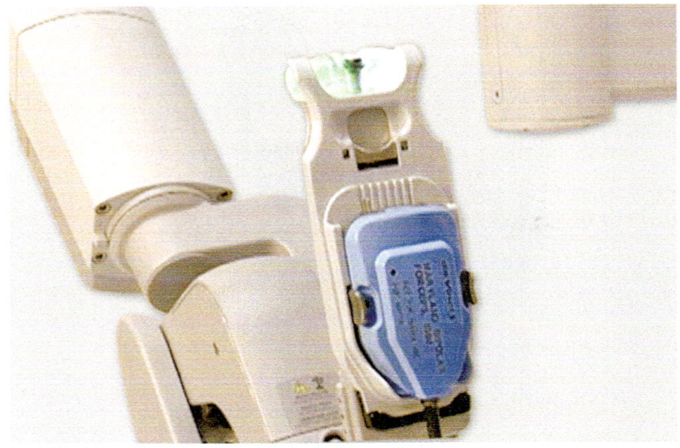

Fig. 51: Light-emitting diode (LED) blinking alternately white and green indicating activation of guided tool change.

Guided Tool Change

This feature helps in aligning a new instrument in the same position as the previous one removed. It adapts the replaced instrument tip just short of the position of previously placed instrument tip.

When this feature is activated, the LEDs on the instrument arm alternately blink white and green **(Fig. 51)**. Just push the instrument with one finger **(Fig. 52)** and guided tool change (GTC) will guide it into correct position. Stop as soon as you encounter any resistance.

This function is disabled when there is a change in the position of instrument arm during changing the instrument. This is because the position memory of the instrument arm is reset when the position is changed.

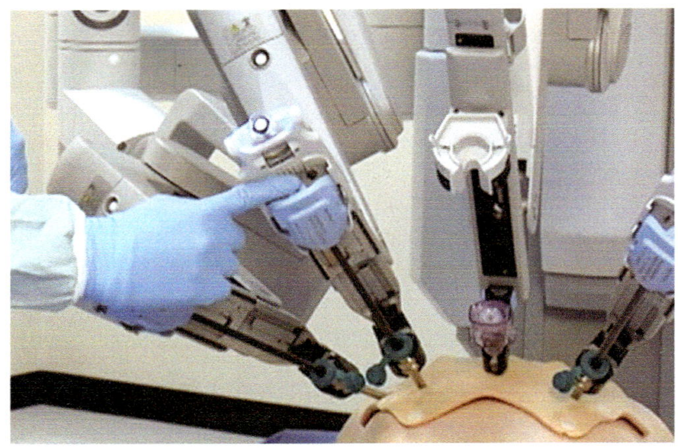

Fig. 52: Pushing the instrument with one finger.

ROBOTIC CHOLECYSTECTOMY

Introduction

In general surgery, advanced robotics will likely find its place in the most complex laparoscopic procedures where the enhanced dexterity and superior visualization will extend the feasibility of the minimally invasive approach, particularly in patients requiring advanced suturing and precise tissue dissection. Robot-assisted laparoscopic cholecystectomy is a safe and effective bridge to advanced robotics in general surgery.

Laparoscopic cholecystectomy is a prime operation with which to begin robot applications for several reasons. First, gallstone disease is the most common of all abdominal diseases for which patients undergo a laparoscopic procedure. Moreover, it is an operation with a very standardized approach to prevent complications. This standardized approach has an added advantage of having aspects that may be more broadly applied to other more complex minimally invasive operations. For example, the dissection of the Calot's triangle is analogous to dissection and isolation of vasculature, the cystic duct and artery can be tied instead of using clips, and removal of the gallbladder from the gallbladder fossa requires a vascular dissection and the appreciation of tissue planes. Therefore, robotic cholecystectomy may allow general surgeons to acquire clinical da Vinci experience in a familiar setting.

Segments of Robotic Cholecystectomy

Segment Operative Tasks

- Skin incision, port placement, exploration, adhesiolysis, patient positioning, and robotic arm draping
- Positioning of da Vinci, docking of robot arms, and camera
- Initial dissection of gallbladder until placement into endoscopic bag
- Gallbladder extraction, performance of additional procedures, and incision closure.

Preoperative Preparation

Indications and preoperative preparation are similar to conventional laparoscopic procedure. An informed consent is to be taken from the patient explaining the new technology and its possible complications. A prophylactic dose of intravenous antibiotic is given just prior to commencement of surgery.

An orogastric or nasogastric tube is placed prior to creation of pneumoperitoneum to decompress stomach. Sequential compression devices are placed on legs for deep vein thrombosis (DVT) prophylaxis. Footboard is placed to keep patient from sliding off table. A seat belt is tied at midthigh region.

Patient Position

Patient is placed in a supine position and right arm is tucked by the side of the patient. Standard surgical preparation is done from nipple line to thigh. A standard protection bar over the patient's head may easily block the robotic arms, giving protection to the head. Convex protection shields or bars that protect the patient's nose and the ventilation tube are good protection for robotic-assisted surgical interventions.

Pneumoperitoneum is created with closed (Veress needle) or open technique. A 12-mm camera port is inserted at the umbilicus, which should be around 20 cm away from the TA (cystic pedicle). A diagnostic laparoscopy is done. Then, a mild left tilt of the table is done with reverse Trendelenburg position.

Port Position (Fig. 53)

Three 8 mm da Vinci ports are inserted at least 10 cm apart for the robotic arm placement. The remote centers of the ports are placed at the level of abdominal wall.

- *Robotic arm 1*: Left midclavicular line, below the subcostal margin
- *Robotic arm 2*: Right midclavicular line, 5–10 cm below the subcostal margin
- *Robotic arm 3*: 10 cm below and lateral to robotic arm 2 (optional, some surgeons use a 5/12 mm assistant port rather than a robotic arm as the third port).

Docking and Operating Room Setup

The arms are draped with disposable sterile drapes. The patient cart is brought over the patient's right shoulder **(Fig. 54)**. This implies that the robot is located behind the operating field and that the robotic arms cross this area and seem to work in a backward direction. The center column of the robotic cart acts as the vertical central axis of the robot. This column should be positioned at the far end of an axis running from the umbilicus through the hilar region of the liver.

The patient table should be tilted according to the surgeon's choice before docking. Align the "sweet spot" for proper camera arm positioning. Align the clutch button, third setup joint, and the center column. Allow 45° angle between each arm. Dock the camera arm and other arms to the respective ports. Camera and the instruments are placed in the ports.

The operating room setup is shown in **Figure 55**.

Operative Technique

Step 1 (Diagnostic Laparoscopy and Port Position)

Patient is kept in supine position. Parts cleaned and draped from nipple line to midthigh. Pneumoperitoneum is created with Veress needle at umbilical position. A 12-mm camera port is inserted at the umbilicus using Optiview cannula **(Fig. 56)**.

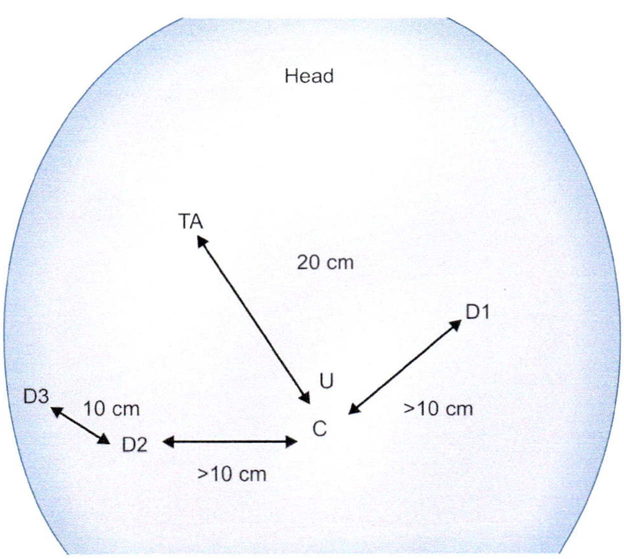

Fig. 53: Port positioning.
(TA: target anatomy)

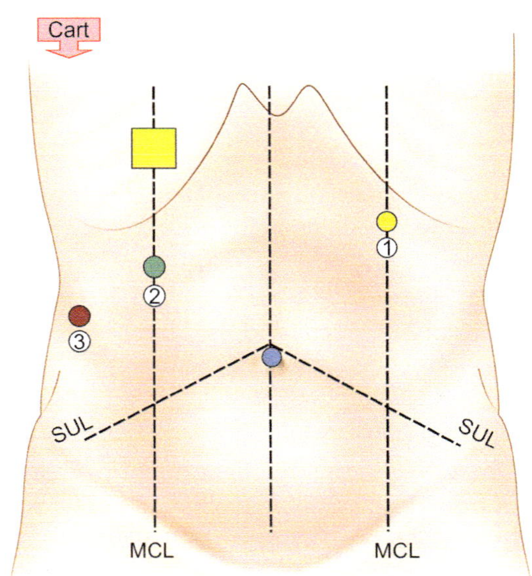

Fig. 54: Position of patient cart and ports.
(MCL: midclavicular line; SUL: spinoumbilical line)

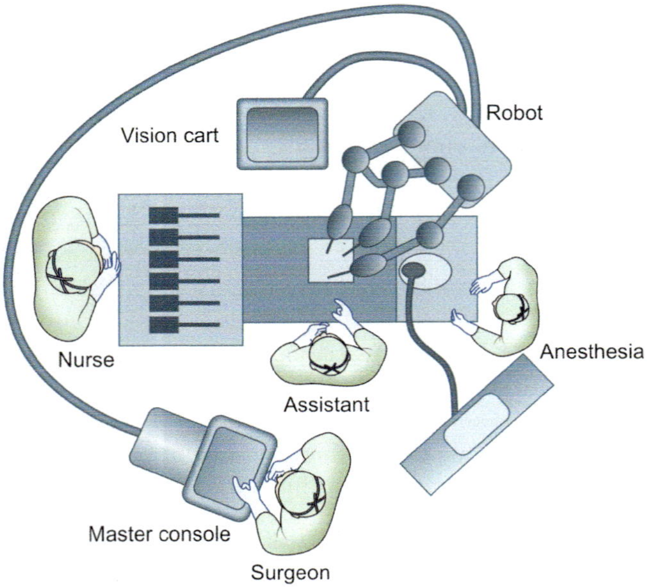

Fig. 55: Operating room setup for cholecystectomy.

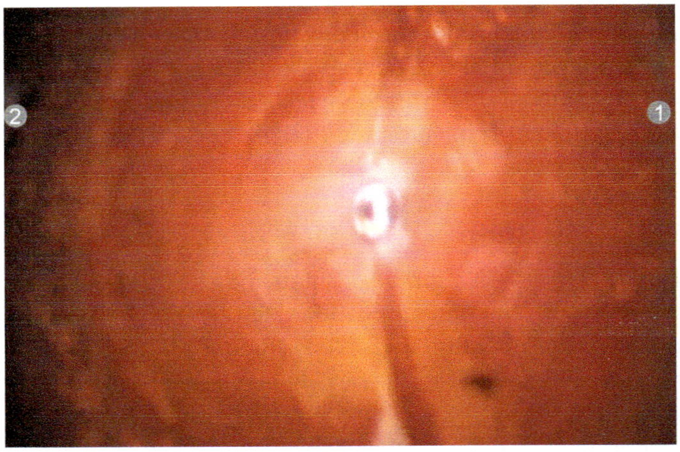

Fig. 56: Camera port insertion under vision with 0° endoscope and Optiview cannula.

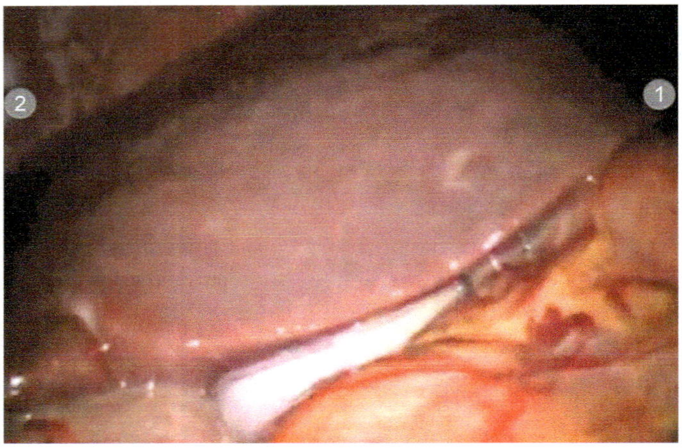

Fig. 57: Diagnostic laparoscopy.

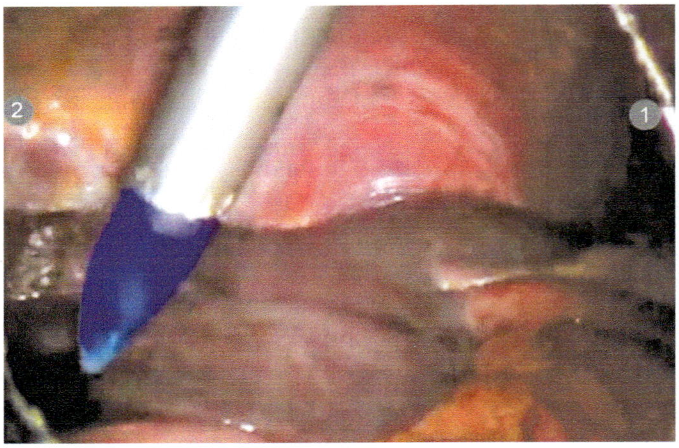

Fig. 58: da Vinci port placement under vision.

A diagnostic laparoscopy is done and gallbladder is visualized **(Fig. 57)**.

Patient is positioned in reverse Trendelenburg position with left tilt. Three da Vinci 8 mm ports are inserted under vision as per the guiding principles described above **(Figs. 58 and 59)**.

Any adhesiolysis, if required, is done at this particular time with standard laparoscopic instruments.

Step 2 (Docking of Robotic Cart)

Patient cart is brought over the right shoulder of the patient. Docking of camera arm is done first followed by instrument arms. The principles of docking are kept in mind and system checkup is done after docking is complete. Instruments are inserted under endoscopic vision such as R1: Maryland dissector and R2 and R3: Prograsp forceps **(Figs. 60 to 62)**.

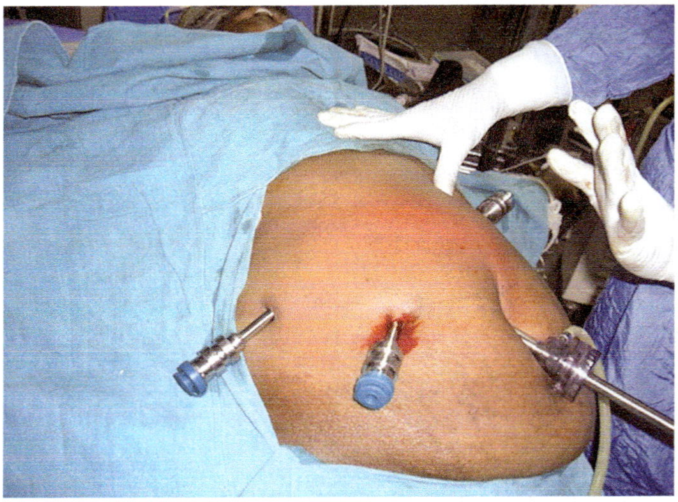

Fig. 59: Final port position for robotic cholecystectomy.

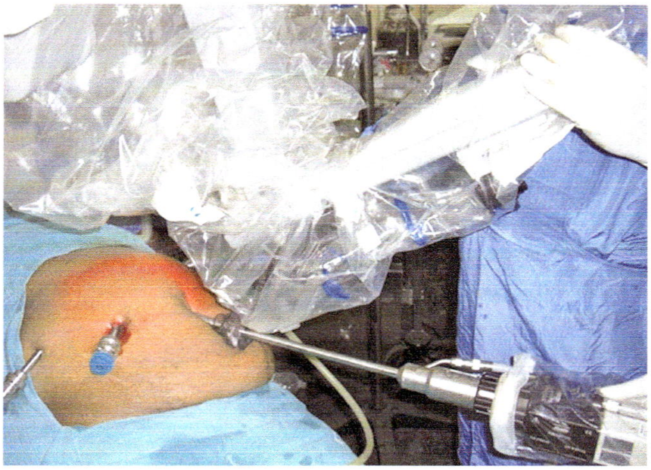

Fig. 60: Docking the camera arm.

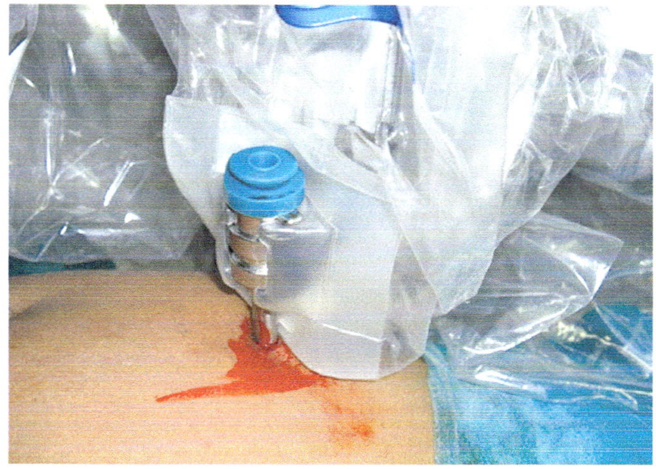

Fig. 61: Docking the instrument cannula to the instrument arm.

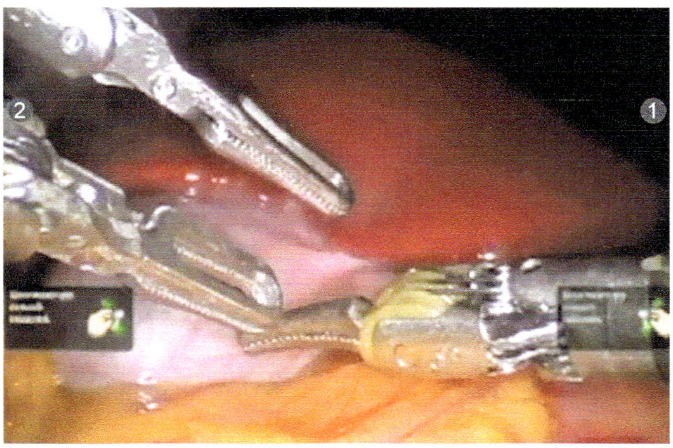

Fig. 62: Insert the instruments under endoscopic vision.

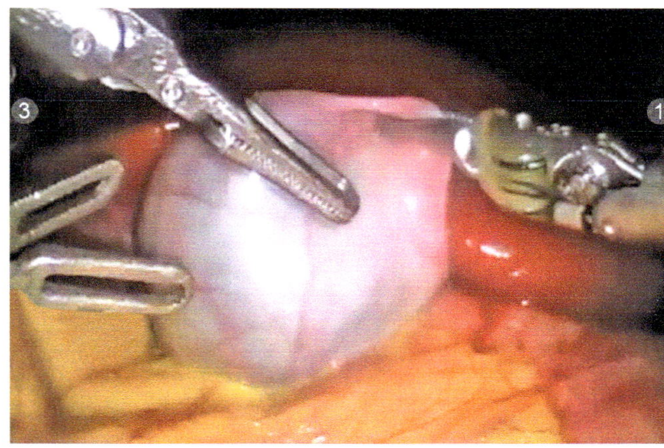

Fig. 63: Holding the fundus with R1 Maryland dissector so as to enable R3 grasping forceps to retract it.

Step 3

Fundus is grasped with prograsp forceps (R3) and pushed toward the right shoulder of the patient **(Figs. 63 and 64)**. This traction is constant once the arm is locked unlike in laparoscopy where it depends on the expertise of the holding assistant. Care should be taken to avoid injury to diaphragm because of inadvertent slippage of fundus from the grasper. Due to lack of haptic feedback to the main surgeon, it can go unnoticed and cause trauma to diaphragm.

Step 4

Hartmann's is grasped with prograsp forceps (R2) and Calot's triangle is dissected with Maryland EndoWrist instruments (R1). Seven degrees of freedom in the EndoWrist instruments give a distinct advantage in this dissection **(Figs. 65 to 69)**.

Step 5

Cystic duct and artery are dissected completely. Clips are applied with EndoWrist hemolock clip applicator (R1) **(Figs. 70 to 73)**.

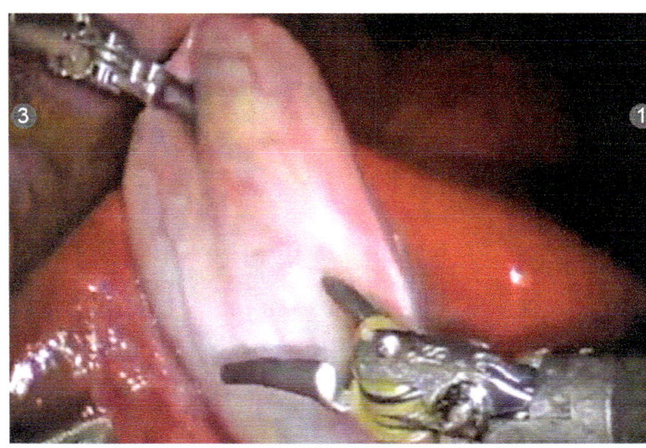

Fig. 64: Pushing the fundus toward the right shoulder.

Step 6

The cystic duct and artery are divided with the EndoWrist scissors (R1) in between the clips **(Figs. 74 to 78)**. The EndoWrist movements enable the surgeon to cut precisely in the direction required.

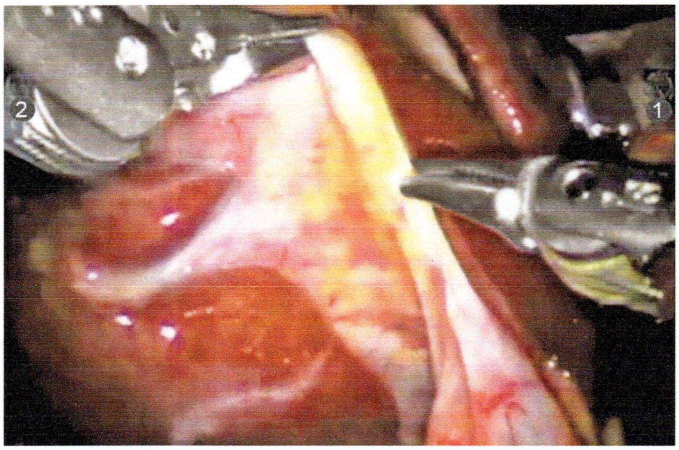

Fig. 65: Hartmann's is grasped by R2 and Calot's triangle being dissected by Maryland in R1.

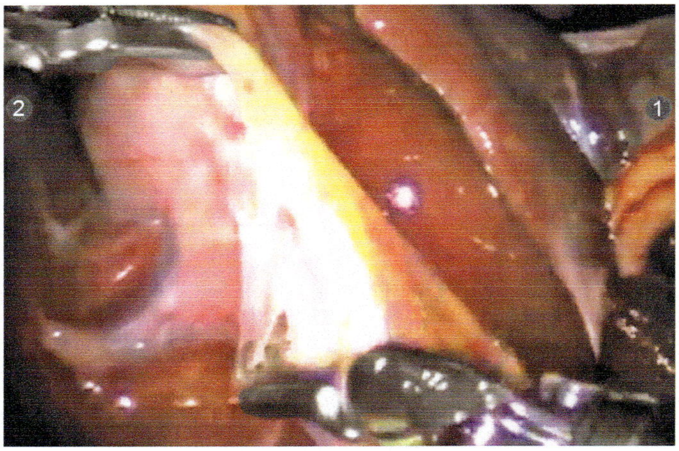

Fig. 66: Posterior peritoneum being dissected off the Calot's triangle.

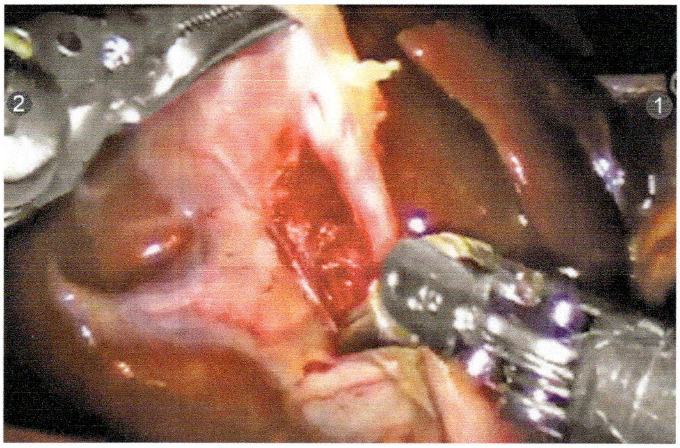

Fig. 67: Posterior window creation.

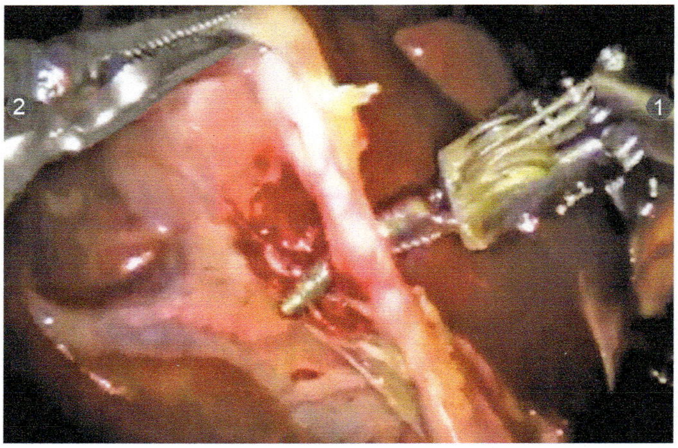

Fig. 68: Cystic duct being dissected using the degrees of freedom of the Maryland dissector.

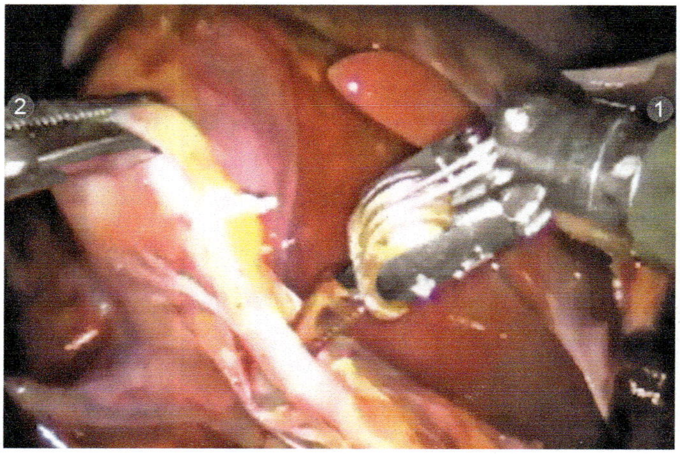

Fig. 69: Window made posterior to cystic duct.

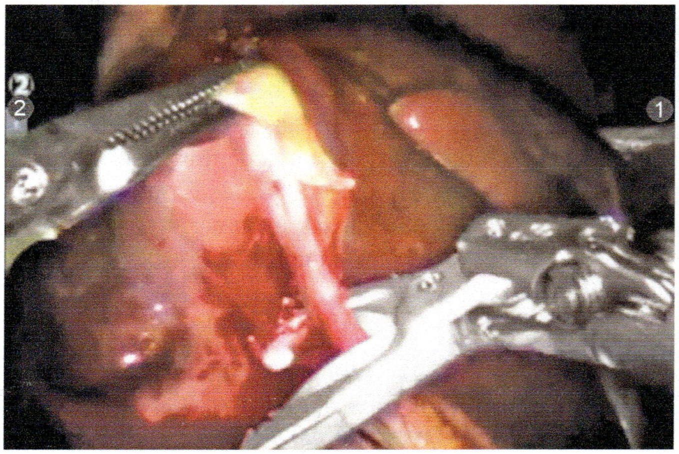

Fig. 70: Clip being applied by robotic clip applicator. The degrees of freedom can be used for optimum clip application.

Step 7

The gallbladder is dissected off the gallbladder fossa **(Figs. 79 and 80)** with the help of hook electrode with monopolar cautery (R1). The EndoWrist function of the hook provides a great deal of versatile movements, which aid in this step of surgery.

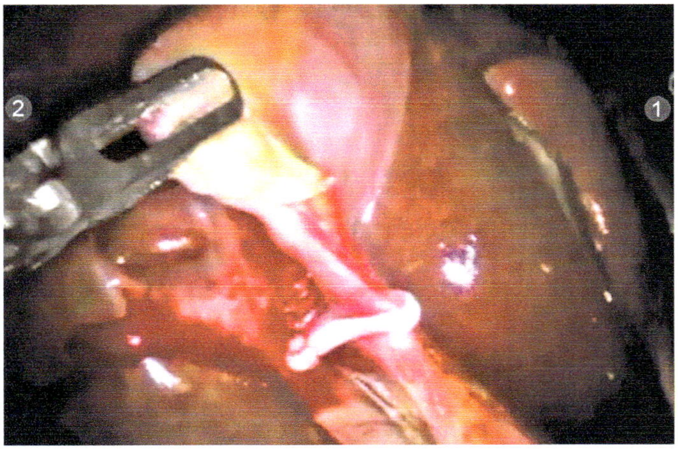

Fig. 71: Clip applied to cystic duct.

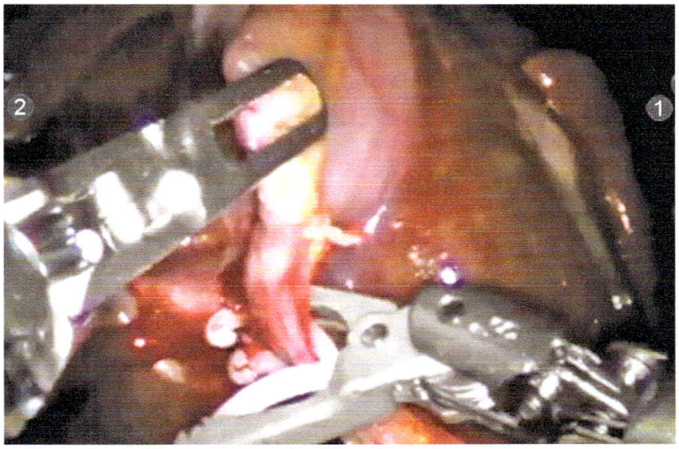

Fig. 72: Second clip being applied.

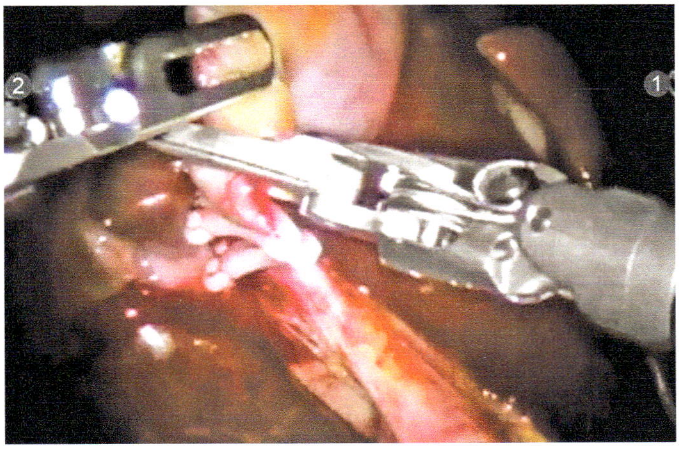

Fig. 73: Third clip being applied.

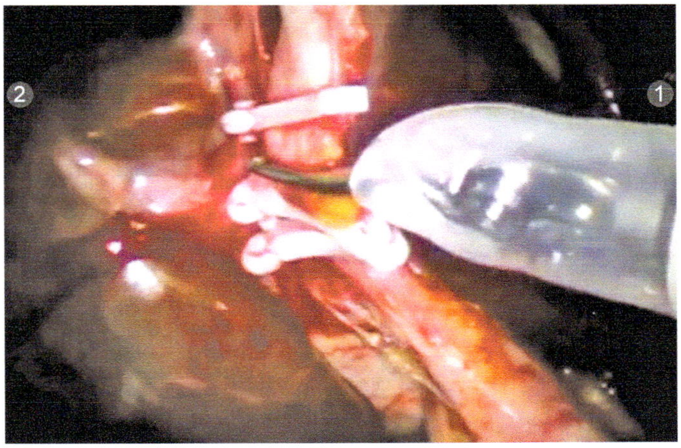

Fig. 74: Cystic duct being divided with scissors.

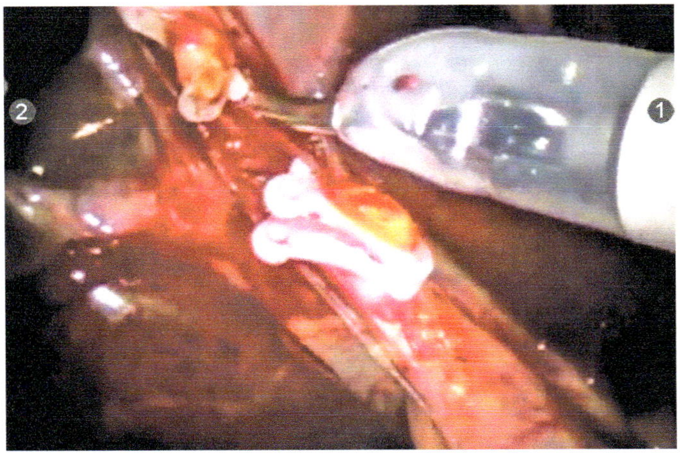

Fig. 75: Cystic duct divided.

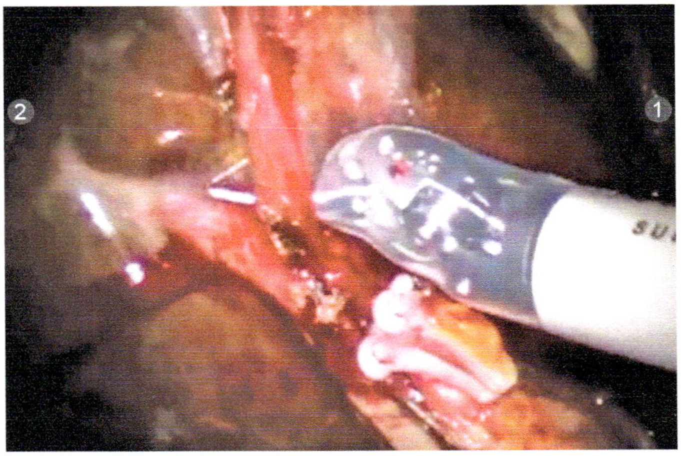

Fig. 76: Cystic artery dissected.

Step 8

Just before taking off the gallbladder from the fossa, it is retracted cephalad and the gallbladder fossa is inspected for any bleed or bile leak **(Fig. 81)**.

Step 9

The R3 arm is undocked and Endobag is inserted by the patient-side assistant surgeon using standard laparoscopic grasper. Any suction/irrigation can also be done by the

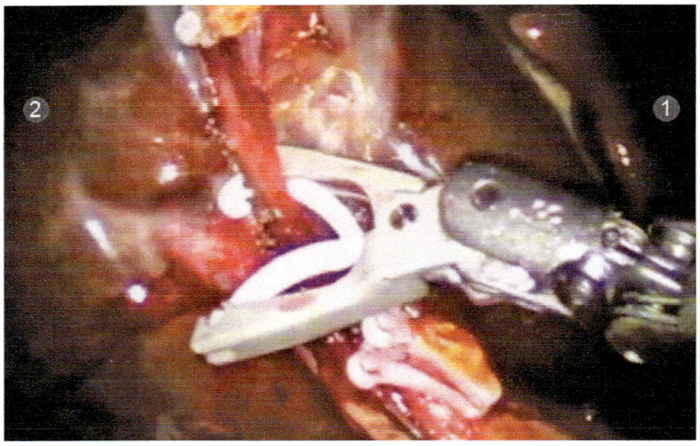

Fig. 77: Clip applied on cystic artery.

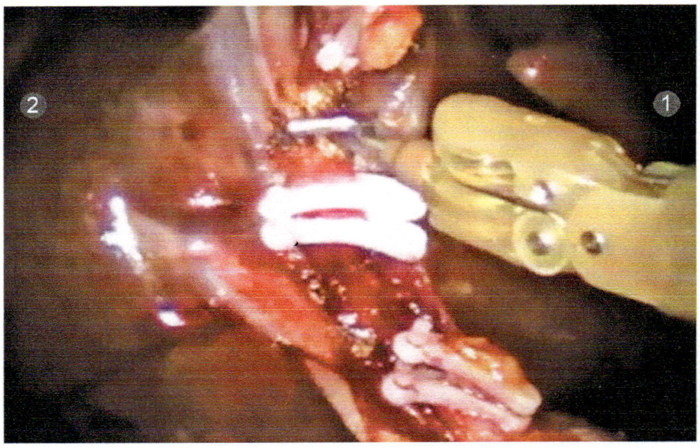

Fig. 78: Cystic artery being divided with EndoWrist hook.

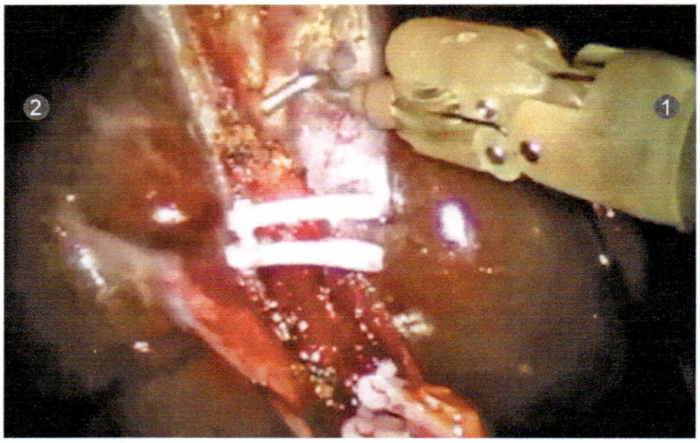

Fig. 79: Dissection of gallbladder (GB) of GB fossa commenced.

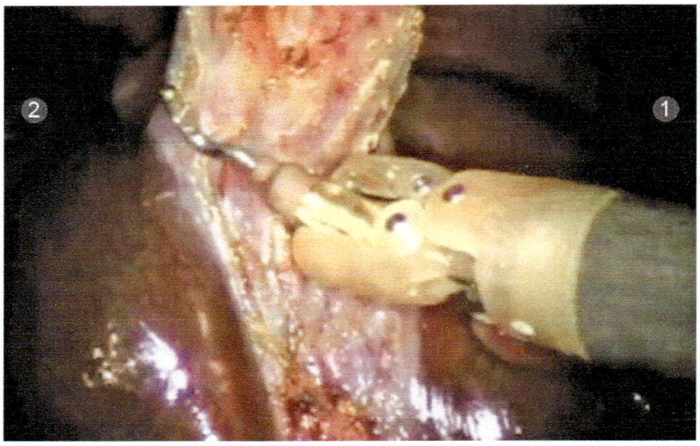

Fig. 80: Dissection done in a vascular plane.

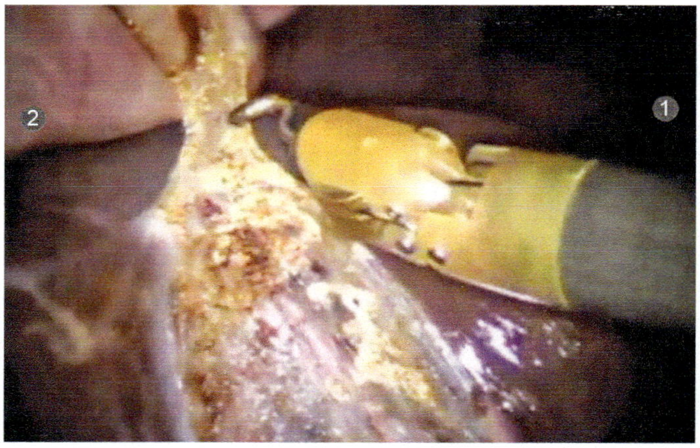

Fig. 81: Inspection of gallbladder (GB) fossa.

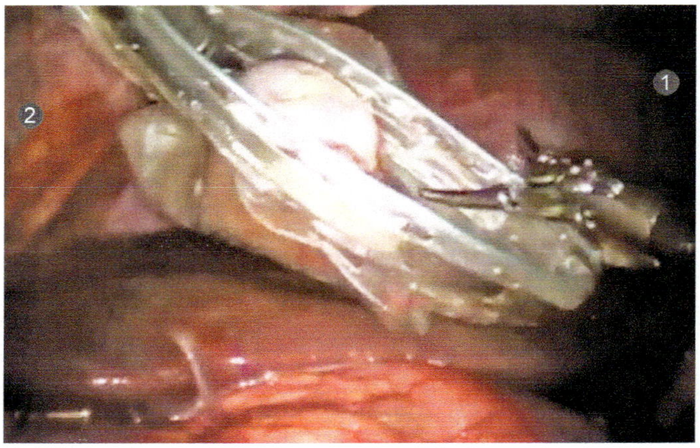

Fig. 82: Gallbladder placed in Endobag.

assistant surgeon by undocking R3. Gallbladder is placed in the Endobag and extracted out **(Figs. 82 and 83)**.

Step 10

Check for hemostasis and clip position. Remove instruments and ports under vision. Incisions are closed in layers.

Discussion

Laparoscopic cholecystectomy for treatment of biliary colic is a relatively straightforward, routine procedure. It will be difficult to defend the use of a highly developed and expensive surgical tool that requires additional time for preparation and larger incisions for the trocars, especially

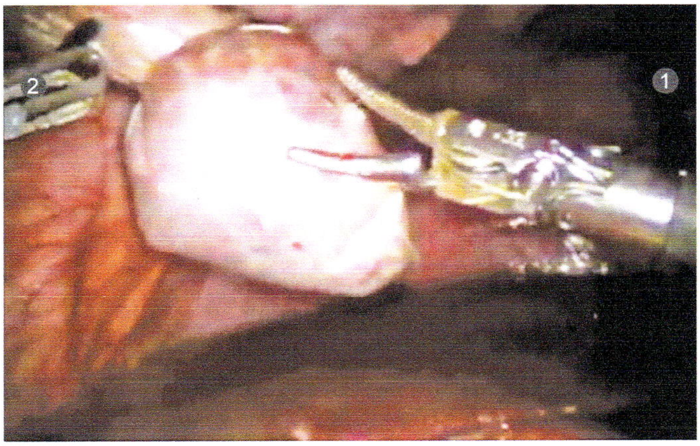

Fig. 83: Gallbladder (GB) being extracted out.

while advantages of such tools are hard to prove for this specific procedure.

There are two situations in which robotics can be applied to this particular procedure:

1. Complicated gallstone disease such as acute cholecystitis, common bile duct (CBD) exploration, or choledochoenterostomy
2. Ideal learning and teaching environment for gastrointestinal robot-assisted surgery.

Advantages

Robotic instruments clearly provide superiority in some aspects of the surgery. The increased degrees of freedom (wrist action) allow the surgeon to easily reach behind structures and negotiate difficult surgical angles. The ergonomics of the operating surgeon can be significantly improved by operating in the sitting position and facing directly forward toward the 3D operative image. These can be of value in cases of acute and chronic cholecystitis, where vision is impaired by inflammation, where there is an increased tendency for diffuse bleeding in the dissection field, and edema and fibrosis make the dissection difficult.

By adjusting movement scaling, surgeon tremor can be significantly reduced; thereby, increasing operative precision. The translation of the surgeon's hand and wrist movements is reliable and can be scaled down to improve precision and increase steadiness.

Limitations

There is a need for more variety in type and size of robotic trocars. The robotic arms are bulky, taking up significant space and limiting the capability of the surgical assistant. Furthermore, the da Vinci system is not attached to the operating table, so the position of the table cannot be changed without undocking the instrument and camera. The robotic arms lack haptic feedback, so the surgeon must rely on visual cues to avoid stretching and damaging tissue or suture. Financially, surgical robotic systems remain quite expensive and are associated with significant operating cost. Current robotic systems and instrumentation are still considered to be first generation and should improve as the technology evolves.

Conclusion

Robotic cholecystectomy is feasible and safe. There is a significant learning curve (around 20–30 cases) to gain experience for setting up the robotic instrumentation, which appears to be much less steep for the actual use of the machine.

It is unlikely that robotic cholecystectomy will be routinely performed in the near future. Further studies are needed to identify the benefits to the patient and compare it to the additional cost of robotic cholecystectomy before routine application of this technique can be justified. However, robotic cholecystectomy may prove its value in cases of complex gallstone disease and is an excellent procedure for teaching the basics of robotic surgery.

ROBOTIC CORONARY BYPASS SURGERY

Four ports are used and robotic arm is introduced. One of the arms contains telescope, which sends 12–15 times magnified clear image on the monitor. Another arm is for a stabilizer, which is used to hold the diseased coronary artery in place while bypass is performed. The other two remaining right and left instrument is used to perform microvascular anastomosis. Currently, robotic coronary bypass surgery should be considered only for the patient who have single vessel disease but in near future, we have hope to perform double or even triple bypass surgery **(Fig. 84)**.

The attached instruments are controlled by the surgeon, who sits at an adjacent console. Several passive mechanical devices, primarily used to hold the telescope, have been developed as assistants for general laparoscopic surgery. They successfully reduce the stress on the surgeon by eliminating the inadvertent movements of a human assistant, which can be distracting and disorienting.

More and more surgeries from prostate to heart are being performed by doctors remotely guiding robotic arms. In such procedures, the surgeon's hands never enter the patient. After the initial incisions are made, robotic arms wielding a tiny camera and surgical tools make the snips, stanch the blood flow, and sew up inside when all is done. The surgeon sits at a console usually in the operating room, although the technology would allow a doctor to operate on a patient on the other side of the world peering into binocular-like lenses at views provided by the camera inside the patient. The doctor guides the robot's work by twisting his wrists in stirrup-like handles, moving his thumb and forefinger in scissor-like loops, or tapping foot pedals to focus the camera or move a robotic arm.

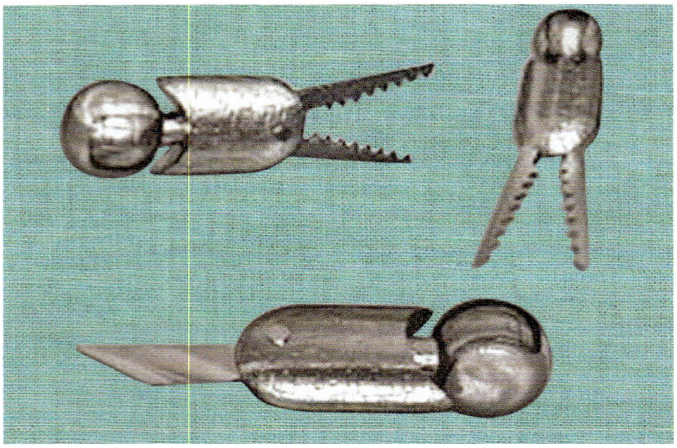

Fig. 84: Instruments used by the da Vinci surgical system.

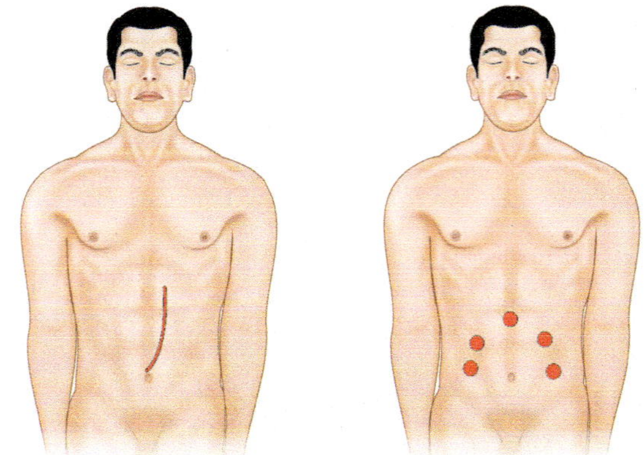

Fig. 85: Comparison between open and da Vinci prostatectomy.

ROBOTIC PROSTATECTOMY

The most common robotic surgery is radical prostatectomy. Its use has grown from just 1,500 procedures in 2000 to an estimated 20,000 last year. More than 8,000 prostate glands were removed robotically last year, up from 36 in 2000. The procedure accounted for >10% of the 75,000 prostatectomies done in 2004. Busy professionals like the fact that they can be out of the hospital in a day, versus two or three for open surgery, and resume normal activities in 1 week rather than 6 weeks. Cutting nerves around the prostate can lead to incontinence or impotence, so precision is important. Between 25 and 60% of conventional prostatectomy, patients suffer from postoperative impotence. Small studies of robotic surgery have shown at least a short-term benefit in terms of impotence and incontinence.

Not every patient is a candidate. Complicated cases when the patient is very sick, needs multiple procedures, or has had previous chest surgery are not suited to robotics. Nor can a heart transplant or artificial heart implant bed one this way. If the complication arises, the patient may windup being opened. So, patients who want robotics smaller scars and quicker recovery times will need to ask hard questions. Find out how many times, the procedure you need has been done robotically and what the advantages and disadvantages are. Just as important, ask how many robotic surgeries, the doctor who will do yours has performed. In real life, you want the force of experience to be with you.

For qualified candidates, the robotic prostatectomy offers numerous potential benefits over the traditional open prostatectomy, including **(Fig. 85)**:

- Shorter hospital stay
- Less pain
- Less risk of infection
- Less blood loss and transfusions
- Less scarring
- Faster recovery
- Quicker return to normal activities.

While still a technology that is in its infancy, the use of robots to assist in surgery is becoming more and more widespread. There are now large case series reported in the literature that show possible benefits to the patient in terms of recovery from such surgeries as prostate and cardiac procedures. Additionally, as these systems continue to develop, improved technology and software provide the surgeon with "assistance" that improves precision and accuracy **(Figs. 86A to D)**.

Robotic technology requires a tremendous financial investment, so you might not see it at every community hospital in the near future. However, as with all technology, the price will likely fall quickly as the applications are expanded, as more widespread adoption occurs and as the field of robotics experiences additional breakthroughs. For now, many major academic institutions are beginning to purchase and deploy these systems.

Technology allows amazing things to be accomplished. Robotic surgery is a new and expensive tool that is beginning to see adoption. MIS with a robot and without bypass is the next logical step in the development of cardiac surgery. It is beginning to show clear benefits for patients and this means that it will likely become more and more popular with time and as the price falls.

ROBOTIC VERSUS LAPAROSCOPIC PROSTATECTOMY

In laparoscopy, the surgeon uses long instruments through small openings and maneuvers them with direct hand contact. Robotic systems use even more delicate instruments that possess two additional degrees of movement excursion (for a total of six, as with a human hand). Comfortably seated at the robot console, the surgeon can maneuver the instruments via a computer interface.

Laparoscopic radical prostatectomy is associated with a steep learning curve. Even in the hands of expert surgeons, laparoscopic radical prostatectomy requires extensive

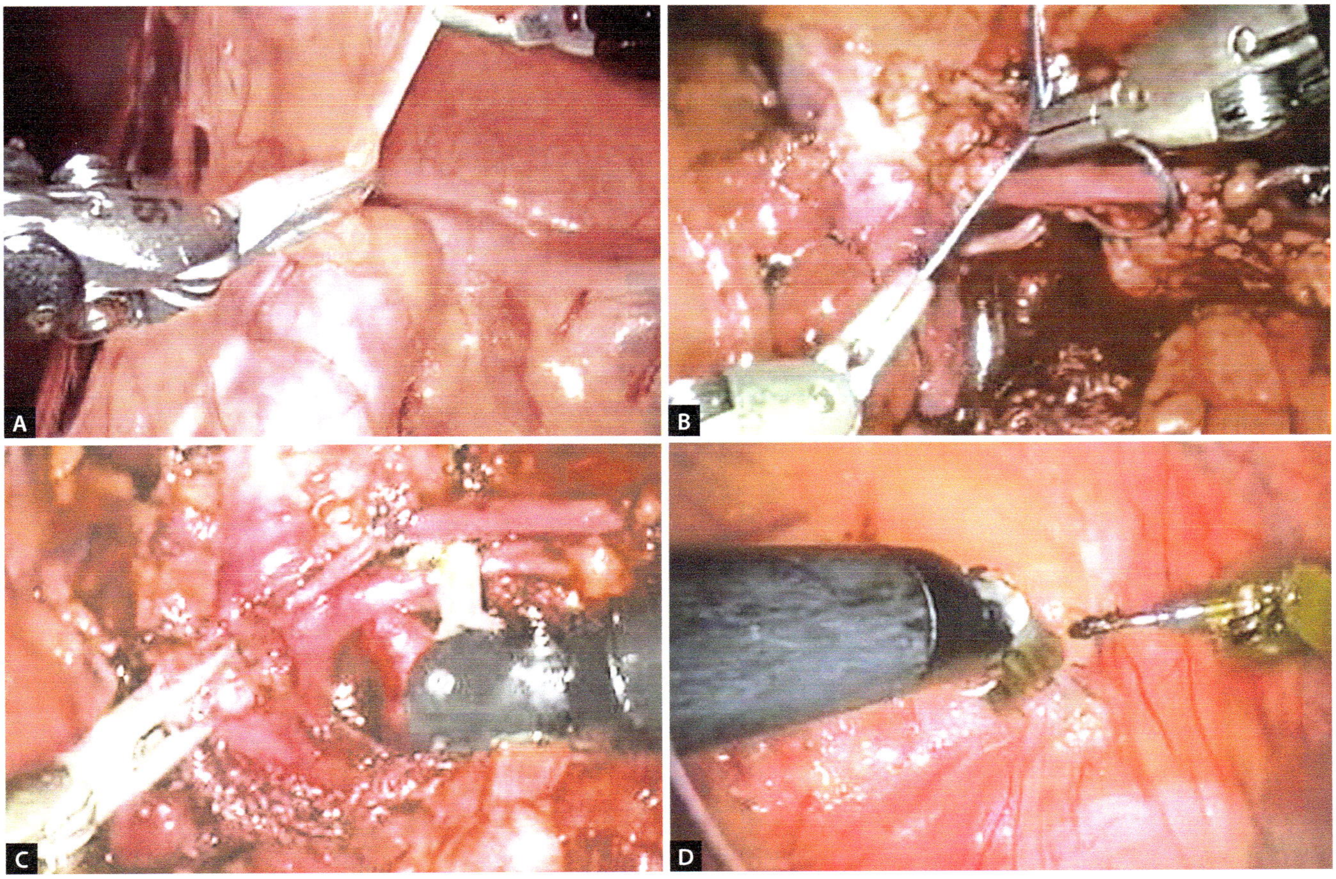

Figs. 86A to D: Robotic-assisted nephrectomy.

learning; approximately 40 cases are needed to master this technique. In contrast, the learning of robotic prostatectomy seems to be more intuitive and less demanding.

Robotic prostatectomy is a safe, effective, and reproducible technique for removing the prostate. In most patients, it can be performed within 1.5–2 hours with minimal blood loss and few complications. The procedure incorporates principles of both laparoscopic and open radical prostatectomy. The patients enjoy benefits of surgical treatment in the setting of less invasion, minimal pain, limited blood loss, and early functional and overall recovery.

NEW SURGICAL ROBOTS

Senhance Surgical System

Robotic-assisted digital laparoscopy (Senhance Surgical System) provides a digitized interface between the surgeon and the patient designed to increase surgeon control and reduce surgical variability. The physical open architecture of the system is composed of independent robotic-assisted manipulator arms that are compatible with conventional trocars and familiar laparoscopic instruments and, thus, taking advantage of the existing operating room and surgical suite ecosystem **(Fig. 87)**.

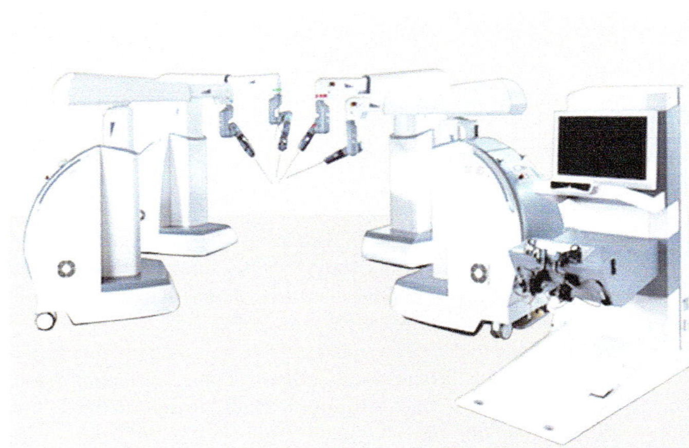

Fig. 87: Senhance surgical robot system.

Avatera Surgical System

The Avatera robotic surgical system gained CE mark last month for use in keyhole surgery, with its initial focus on gynecology and urology. It consists of the main surgical robot and its control unit and various endoscopes and instruments **(Fig. 88)**.

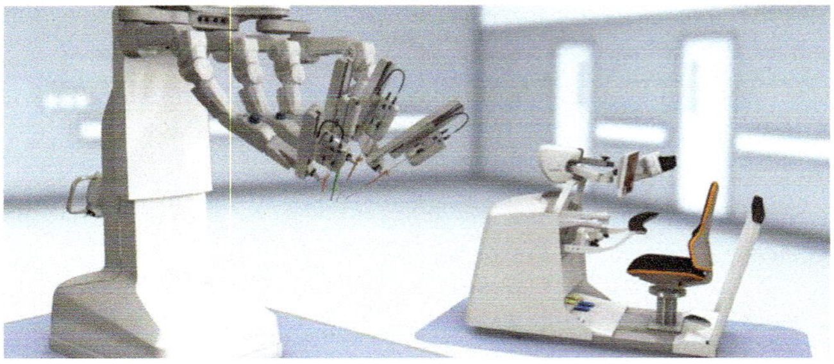

Fig. 88: The Avatera robotic surgical system.

Indian Robotic Surgical System

The SSI MANTRA is made in India. Surgical robot is the brainchild of cardiac surgeon Dr Sudhir Srivastava and was developed in an Atal Incubation Centre. It has conducted 18 successful surgeries and the cost is likely to be one-fourth of leading global competitor, da Vinci robot **(Fig. 89)**.

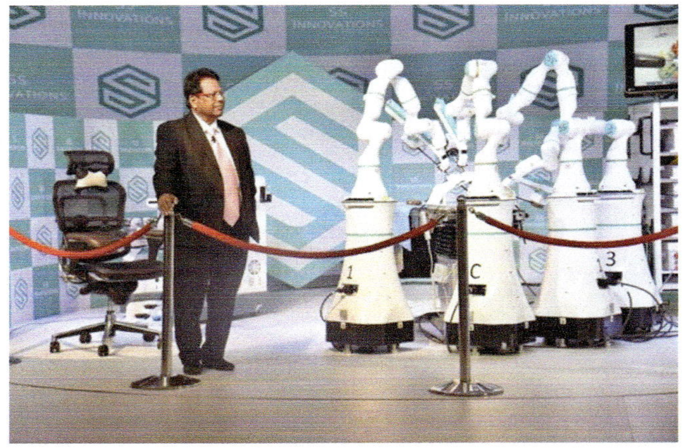

Fig. 89: SSI MANTRA is made in India surgical robot.

Artificial intelligence is a buzzword on everyone's lips today. Johnson & Johnson has partnered with Google to form Verb Surgical, which is developing a "digital surgery program". While it is still quite early in development, it is expected to include advancements in data analytics, machine learning, and connectivity. A recent study from this device reported on completely autonomous suturing using the robot in an animal model. Artificial intelligence could also potentially play a significant role in presurgical planning, intraoperative 3D imaging, and navigation allowing for even more precise and subtle operations. People expect that ultimately robots will replace surgeons and actually perform the surgery. Nevertheless, it is believed that this still remains well in the future. However, given the speed at which artificial intelligence research is progressing, you never know when surgeons' jobs could be under complete hand of surgical robot.

BIBLIOGRAPHY

1. Berguer R. Surgery and ergonomics. Arch Surg. 1999;134:1011-6.
2. Berguer R, Rab GT, Abu-Ghaida H, Alarcon A, Chung J. A comparison of surgeons' posture during laparoscopic and open surgical procedures. Surg Endosc. 1997;11:21-39.
3. Beurger R, Rember M, Beckley D. Laparoscopic instruments cause increased forearm fatigue: a subjective and objective comparison of open and laparoscopic techniques. Minim Invasive Ther Allied Tech. 1997;6:36-40.
4. Buess GF, Schurr MO, Fischer SC. Robotics and allied technologies in endoscopic surgery. Arch Surg. 2000;132:229-35.
5. Cadière GB, Himpens J, Germany O, Izizaw R, Degueldre M, Vandromme J, et al. Feasibility of robotic laparoscopic surgery: 146 cases. World J Surg. 2001;25:1467-77.
6. Cadière GB, Himpens J, Bruyns J. How to avoid esophageal perforation while performing laparoscopic dissection of the hiatus. Surg Endosc. 1995;9:450-2.
7. Cadière GB, Himpens J, Vertruyen M, Favretti F. The world's first obesity surgery performed by a surgeon at a distance. Obes Surg. 1999;9:206-9.
8. Cadière GB, Houben JJ, Bruyns J, Himpens J, Panzer JM, Gelin M. Laparoscopic Nissen fundoplication technique and preliminary results. Br J Surg. 1994;81:400-3.
9. Chan A, Chung S, Yim A, Lau J, Ng E, Li A. Comparison of two-dimensional vs three-dimensional camera systems in laparoscopic surgery. Surg Endosc. 1997;11:438-40.
10. Cheah WK, Lenzi JE, So J, Dong F, Kum CK, Goh P. Evaluation of a head-mounted display (HMD) in the performance of a simulated laparoscopic task. Surg Endosc. 2001;15:990-1.
11. Davies B. A review of robotics in surgery. Proc Inst Mech Eng. 2000;214:129-40.
12. Dion YM, Gaillard F. Visual integration of data and basic motor skills under laparoscopy. Influence of 2-D and 3-D video-camera systems. Surg Endosc. 1997;11:995-1000.
13. Dosis A, Bello F, Rockall T, Munz Y, Moorthy K, Martin S, et al. ROVIMAS: a Software Package for Assessing Surgical Skills Using the da Vinci Telemanipulator System. Birmingham: IEEE Publisher; 2003.
14. Felger JE, Nifong LW, Chitwood WR. The evolution of and early experience with robot-assisted mitral valve surgery. Surg Laparosc Endosc Percutan Tech. 2002;12:58-63.
15. Gallagher AG, Satava RM. Virtual reality as a metric for the assessment of laparoscopic psychomotor skills. Learning curves and reliability measures. Surg Endosc. 2002;16:1746-52.
16. Garcia-Ruiz A, Gagner M, Miller JH, Steiner CP, Hahn JF. Manual vs robotically assisted laparoscopic surgery in the performance of basic manipulation and suturing tasks. Arch Surg. 1998;133:957-61.
17. Garcia-Ruiz A, Smedira NG, Loop FD, Hahn JF, Miller JH, Steiner CP, et al. Robotic surgical instruments for dexterity enhancement in thoracoscopic coronary artery bypass graft. J Laparoendosc Adv Surg Tech A. 1997;7:277-83.
18. Hanna GB, Cuschieri A. Influence of two-dimensional and three-dimensional imaging on endoscopic bowel suturing. World J Surg. 2000;24:444-9.
19. Hernandez JD, Bann SD, Munz Y, Moorthy K, Datta V, Martin S, et al. The learning curve of a simulated surgical task using the da Vinci telemanipulator system. Br J Surg. 2002;89:17-8.
20. Himpens J, Leman G, Cadière GB. Telesurgical laparoscopic cholecystectomy. Surg Endosc. 1998;12:1091.
21. Johns DB, Brewer JD, Soper NJ. The influence of three-dimensional video systems on laparoscopic task performance. Surg Laparosc Endosc. 1996;6:191-7.
22. Kim VB, Chapman WHH, Albrecht RJ, Bailey BM, Young JA, Nifong LW, et al. Early experience with telemanipulative robot-assisted laparoscopic cholecystectomy using da Vinci. Surg Laparosc Endosc Percutan Tech. 2002;12:33-40.
23. McDougall EM, Soble JJ, Wolf JS, Nakada SY, Elashry OM, Clayman RV. Comparison of three-dimensional and two-dimensional laparoscopic video systems. J Endoural. 1996;10: 371-4.

24. Mentges B, Buess G, Schäfer D, Manncke K, Becker HD. Local therapy of rectal tumors. Dis Colon Rectum. 1996;39:886-92.
25. Mueller MD, Camartin C, Dreher E, Hanggi W. Three-dimensional laparoscopy: gadget or progress? A randomized trial on the efficacy of three-dimensional laparoscopy. Surg Endosc. 1999;13:469-72.
26. Munz Y, Hernandez H, Bann S, Bello F, Dosis A, Martin S, et al. The advantages of 3D visualization in surgical performance with the da Vinci telemanipulation system. J Soc Laparosc Surg. 2002;6:264-94.
27. Satava RM. Emerging technologies for surgery in the 21st century. Arch Surg. 1999;134:1197-202.
28. Shea JA, Healey MJ, Berlin JA, Clarke JR, Malet PF, Staroscik RN, et al. Mortality and complications associated with laparoscopic cholecystectomy: a meta-analysis. Ann Surg. 1996;224:609-20.
29. Taffinder N, Smith S, Mair J, Russell R, Darzi A. Can a computer measure surgical precision? Reliability, validity and feasibility of the ICSAD. Surg Endosc. 1999;13:81.
30. Voorhorst FA, Overbeeke CJ, Smets GJ. Spatial perception during laparoscopy: implementing action-perception coupling. Stud Health Technol Inform. 1997;39:379-86.
31. Wappler M. Medical manipulators: a realistic concept? Minim Invasive Ther. 1995;4:261-6.
32. Williams LF, Chapman WC, Bonau RA, McGee EC, Boyd RW, Jacobs JK. Comparison of laparoscopic cholecystectomy with open cholecystectomy in a single center. Am J Surg. 1993;165:459-65.
33. Yohannes P, Rotariu P, Pinto P, Smith AD, Lee BR. Comparison of robotic versus laparoscopic skills: is there a difference in the learning curve? Urology. 2002;60:39-45.

CHAPTER 48

Transanal Endoscopic Microsurgery

INTRODUCTION

Transanal endoscopic microsurgery (TEM) was developed by Professor Gerhard Buess from Tübingen, Germany and it became available for widespread use in 1983 **(Fig. 1)**. A surgeon's ability to remove rectal lesions transanally is limited by access and exposure with conventional instruments usually restricting the surgeon to the distal 6–7 cm of rectum. When transanal excision is not possible, the traditional transabdominal approach, a major surgical procedure, is necessary. TEM, with its longer reach and enhanced visibility of the entire rectum, extends the boundaries of transanal surgery, giving appropriately selected patients a minimally invasive surgical option with a faster and virtually pain-free recovery.

Transanal endoscopic microsurgery allows for local excision of rectal neoplasm with greater exposure than transanal excision and less morbidity than transabdominal approaches. Supporters of the TEM technique praise the excellent exposure of the rectum and the minimal invasiveness as opposed to conventional surgical techniques. The arrival of TEM was associated with an increase in the number of operations for rectal cancer; however, the use of TEM remained constant relative to radical resections. Use of TEM resection alone is appropriate for all adenomas and cancers staged Tis and T1. Use of TEM alone is not an appropriate treatment for T2 cancers.

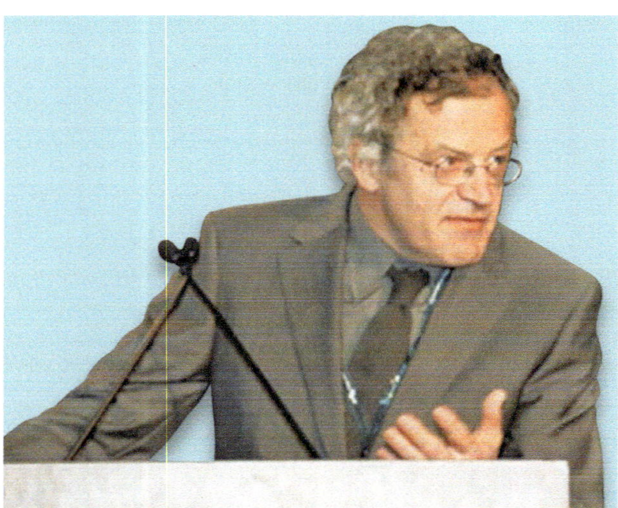

Fig. 1: Inventor of transanal endoscopic microsurgery (TEM) technology.

Local excision of rectal neoplasms is an accepted method of treating selected lesions and can be accomplished through either a transanal approach or a posterior proctotomy. The former is hindered by poor exposure and visibility of lesions in the middle and upper rectum. While the latter approach does give somewhat improved exposure of these more cephalad tumors, it may be complicated by fecal fistulae or sphincter impairment. TEM has emerged as a better technique for removing lesions in the middle and upper rectum and it obviates the need for a posterior proctotomy. Furthermore, the transanal rectoscope extends the boundaries of transanal surgery by providing access to lesions previously inaccessible with conventional means. The net result is an operative approach to rectal lesions that are not hindered by the poor exposure and limited reach associated with conventional retractors.

Virtually any adenoma of any size or degree of circumferential involvement can be removed with TEM. Adenomas are removed with a 5-mm margin of normal mucosa and dissection is undertaken in the submucosal plane. For large adenomas or those that have firm areas within them or previous histological evidence of atypia or dysplasia, the risk of harboring an occult cancer is increased; for such lesions, it is generally recommended that a full-thickness excision can be performed. Other benign indications for TEM include transrectal rectopexy for prolapse, for which there has been limited experience to date, and correction of anastomotic strictures by stricturoplasty.

INDICATIONS OF TRANSANAL ENDOSCOPIC MICROSURGERY

Benign

- Rectal polyps
- Carcinoid tumors
- Retrorectal masses
- Anastomotic strictures
- Extrasphincteric fistulae
- Pelvic abscesses.

Malignant

- Malignant rectal polyps
- T1-T2 rectal cancer
- Palliative excision of T3 cancer.

INSTRUMENTS

The basic TEM instrumentation includes the combined endosurgical unit, which regulates carbon dioxide insufflation, saline irrigation, and suction. The rectoscope is 40 mm in diameter and is available in lengths of 12 and 20 cm **(Fig. 2)**. Once the rectoscope is inserted to the desired location within the rectum, it is secured to the operating room table with a double ball-and-socket supporting arm **(Figs. 3A and B)**. During the dissection, the supporting arm is moved frequently to maintain direct visibility of the lesion. The end of the rectoscope is sealed with an airtight facepiece that has five entry ports. These ports, in turn, are sealed by rubber caps and sleeves, so that the various instruments necessary for the dissection can be inserted. One of the big advantages of TEM is binocular vision **(Figs. 4 and 5)**. The binocular stereoscopic eyepiece is inserted through one of the ports and it has an accessory scope for video hookup. The various instruments needed are suction catheter, a needle-tipped high-frequency electrical knife, tissue graspers that are oriented to the right or left, scissors, and a needle holder. The suction catheter, tissue graspers, and needle-tipped knife can all be connected to the cautery unit, which greatly facilitate control of hemorrhage and coagulation of bleeding vessels **(Figs. 6 to 8)**.

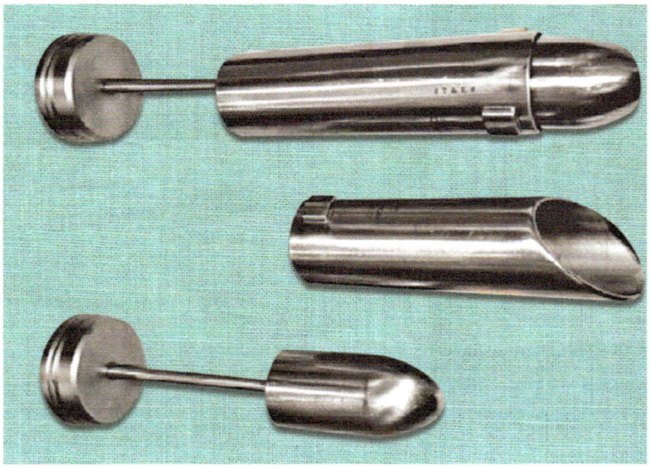

Fig. 2: 40 mm proctoscope.

PATIENT POSITIONING IN TRANSANAL ENDOSCOPIC MICROSURGERY

Position of lesion determines positioning of patient on the operating room table **(Figs. 9A to D)**. The patient should be positioned in such a way that the lesion should be made to be in the 6 o'clock position for the operator **(Fig. 10)**.

Therefore, the position of the patient in the operating room is dependent on tumor location. Since the bevel of the rectoscope must face downward, patients with anterior lesions are placed in the prone position, whereas patients with posterior lesions are placed in the lithotomy position. Patients with lateral lesions are placed accordingly into the appropriate decubitus position.

TRANSANAL ENDOSCOPIC MICROSURGERY PROCEDURES (FIGS. 11 TO 15)

Properly selected rectal cancers can also be removed with TEM; for such lesions, a 1 cm margin of normal tissue surrounding the lesion should be obtained. A full-thickness excision is mandatory to accurately stage the depth of penetration and unpredictable in its location. TEM is a safe technique and having low number of complications; however, this procedure is not a license to disregard established criteria for local excision of cancers. The exceptions to this may be tumor size and location.

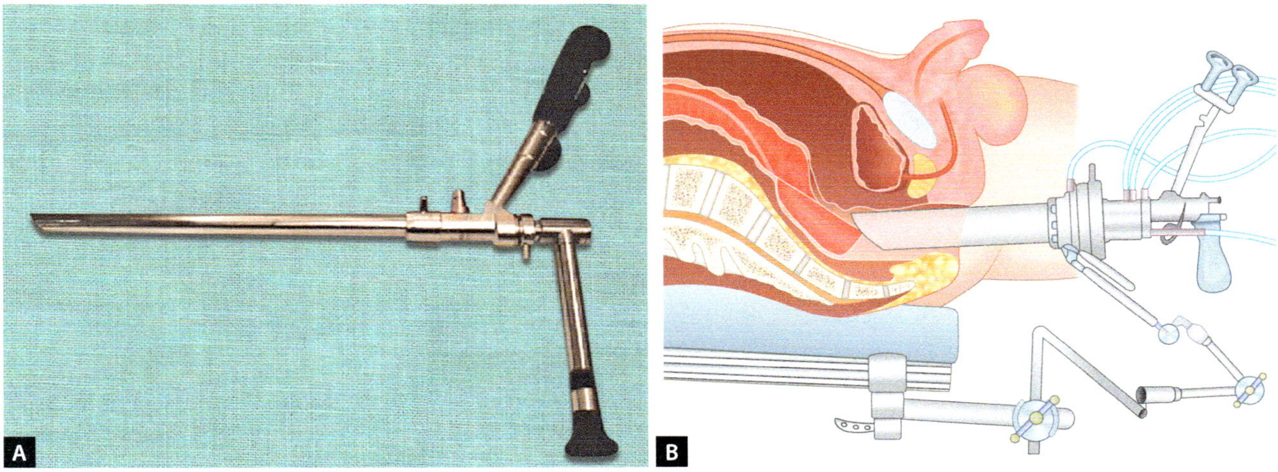

Figs. 3A and B: Stereoscope used in transanal endoscopic microsurgery (TEM).

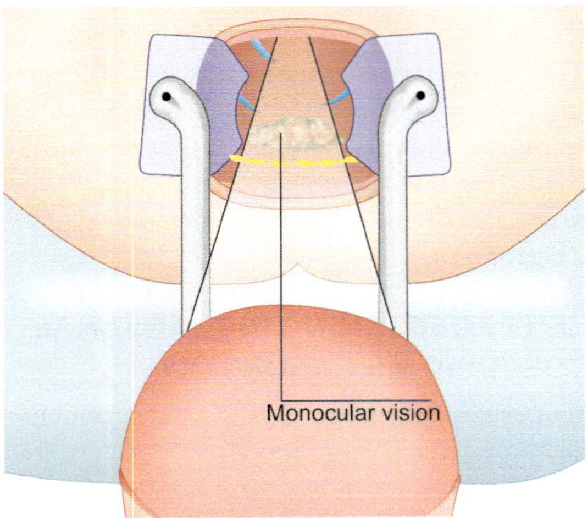

Fig. 4: Monocular vision in laparoscopy.

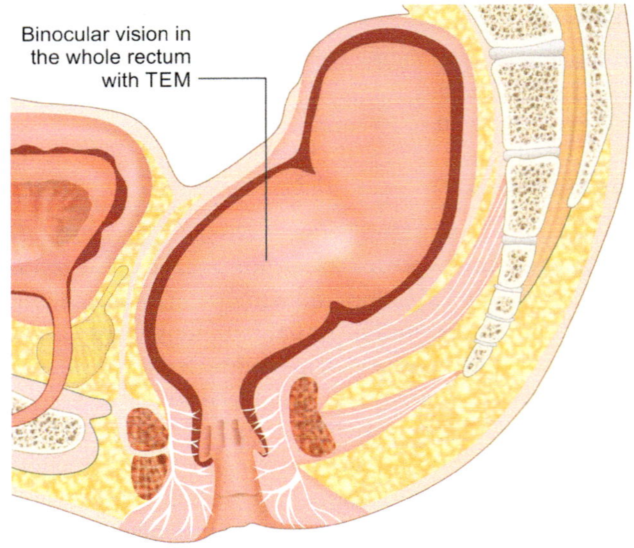

Fig. 5: Stereoscopic vision in transanal endoscopic microsurgery (TEM).

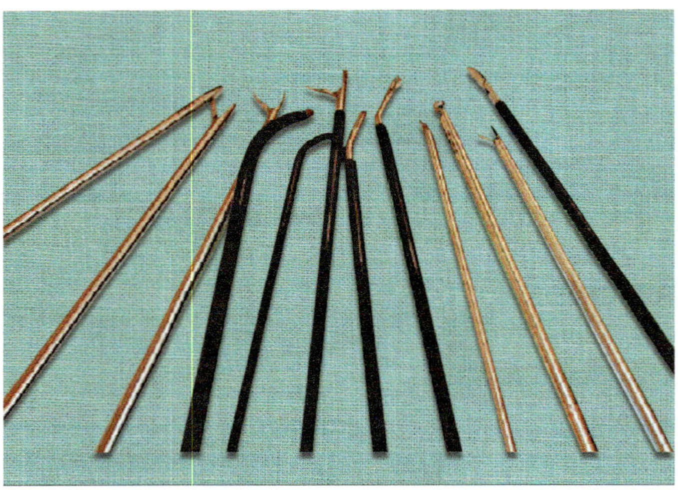

Fig. 6: Fine curve tipped instruments for transanal endoscopic microsurgery (TEM).

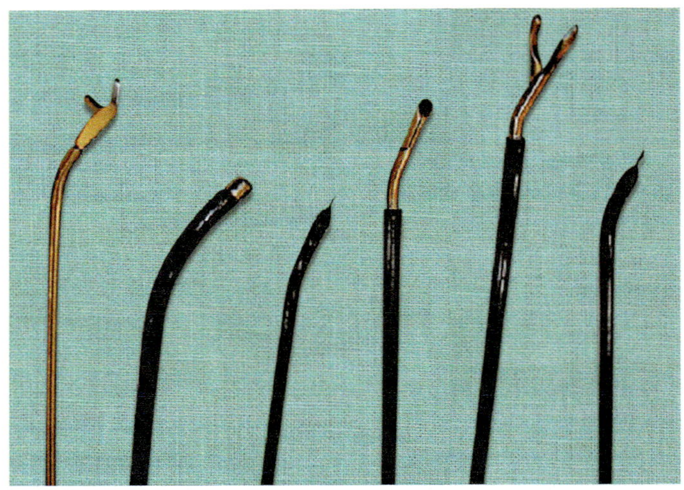

Fig. 7: Needle holders and electrosurgical instruments used in transanal endoscopic microsurgery (TEM).

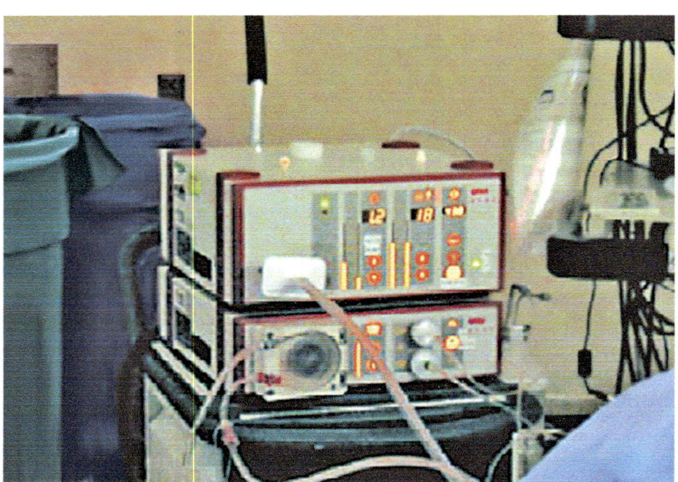

Fig. 8: Insufflator used in transanal endoscopic microsurgery (TEM).

With its superior optics, constant rectal distention, and longer instrument casing, TEM is not limited to small, distally located lesions. Because of the magnification capabilities of the TEM equipment—about 30 times greater than normal—we are able to better visualize the lesion and get very good margins. This minimizes the chances of the patient needing a colostomy, which can sometimes result with open surgery, even with benign lesions. One may argue that cancers within the middle and upper rectum should all be treated with low anterior resection (LAR); however, if we accept the criteria for local excision as being appropriate for lesions in the distal rectum, we must embrace them as well for lesions in the middle and upper rectum. Currently, TEM has not had a significant impact on the treatment of rectal cancer. If, however, preoperative chemotherapy and radiation become the standard of care and have the effect of

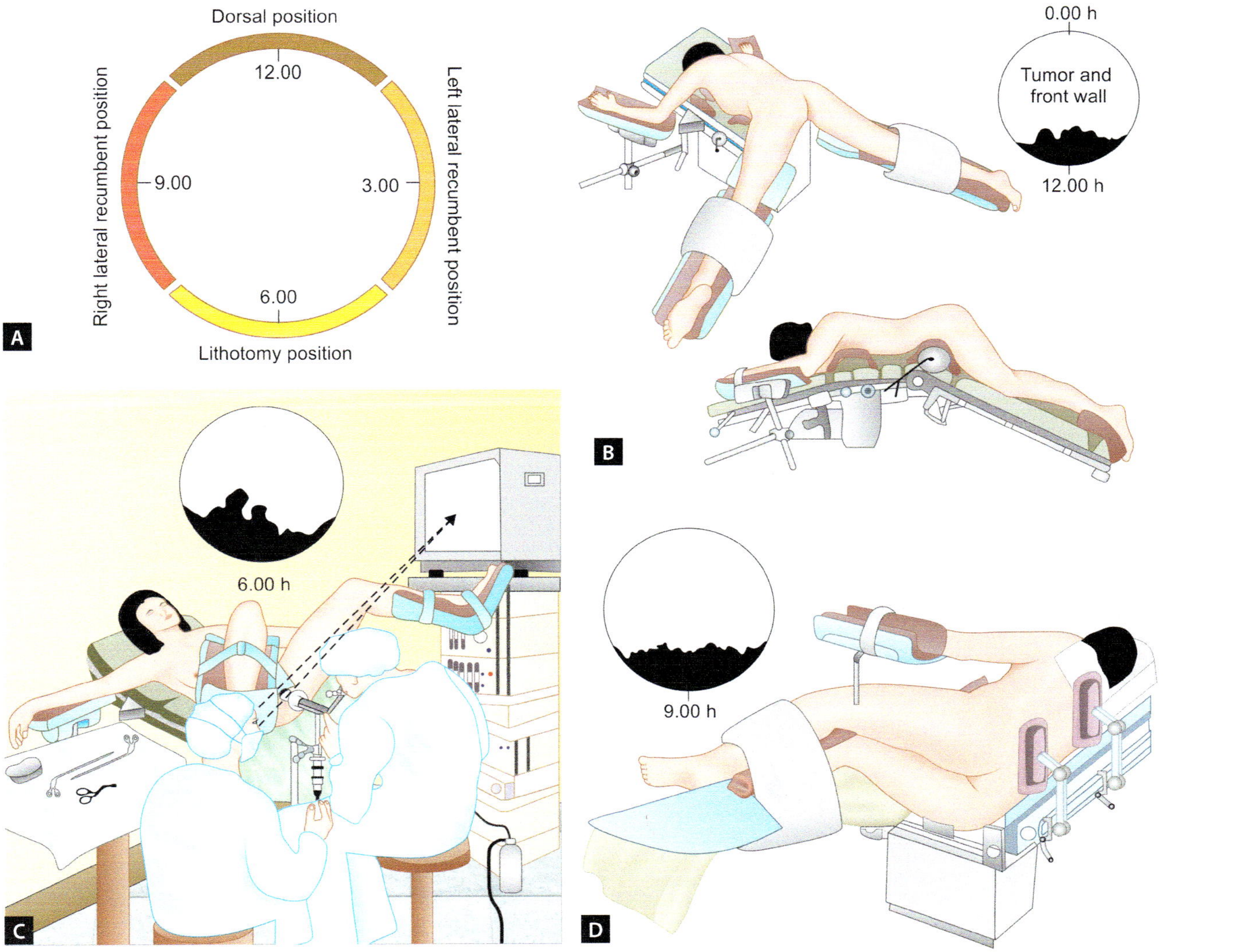

Figs. 9A to D: Positioning of patient for transanal endoscopic microsurgery (TEM).

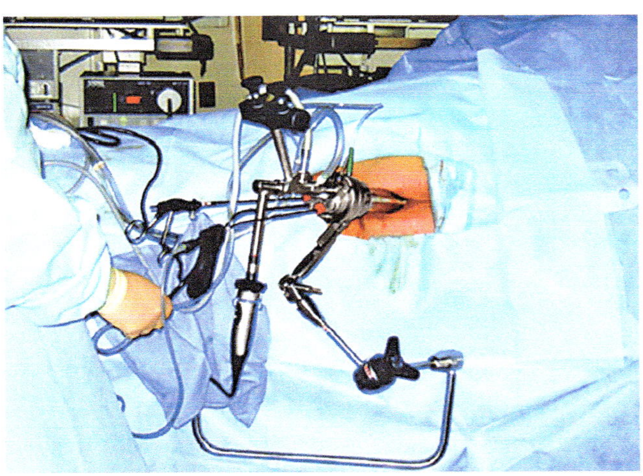

Fig. 10: Patient position for lesion at right lateral position.

causing a downgrade of tumor stage, low shrinking tumors, and even inducing a complete remission, TEM may have an increased role. However, this remains to be seen and can only be answered with further studies.

Data presented at the annual meeting of the American Society of Colon and Rectal Surgeons last July also suggests that TEM offers certain advantages over the more standard procedure. In a retrospective study that compared transanal excision with TEM for both benign and malignant rectal masses, the TEM procedure was much more likely to result in a complete resection and yields negative margins compared with transanal excision (88% vs. 71%). This was true whether the lesion was benign or malignant. It was also more likely to produce an intact, nonfragmented specimen compared with transanal excision (94% vs. 63%) making it easier for pathological evaluation.

The rate of recurrence, both local and distant, was also lower in patients who had undergone TEM compared with transanal excision (5% vs. 25%). This was particularly true for rates of local recurrence, which were significantly lower for both benign and malignant lesions following TEM (4% vs. 20%). The rate of complications was similar between both groups.

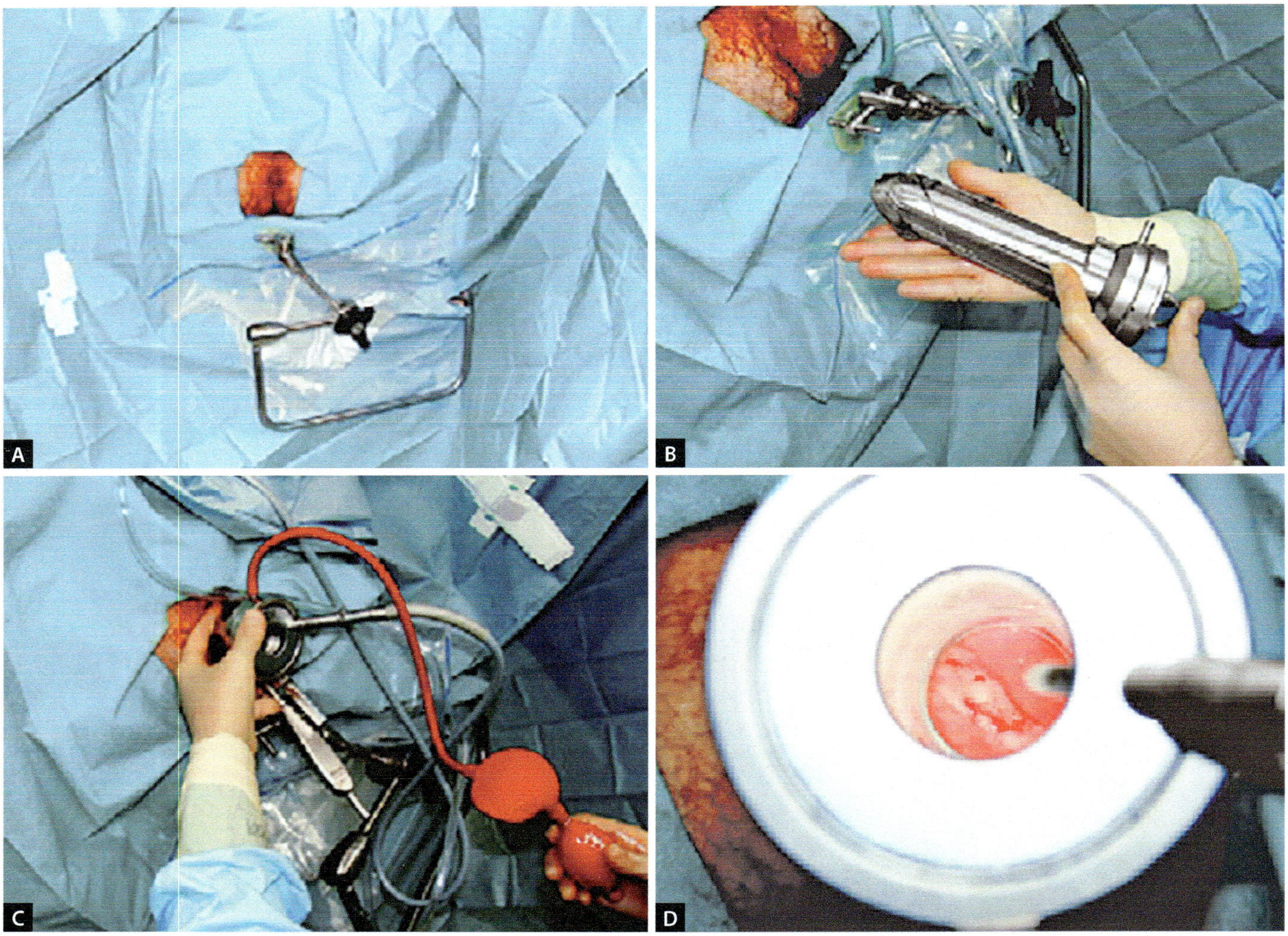

Figs. 11A to D: Setting up instruments in transanal endoscopic microsurgery (TEM) to start procedure.

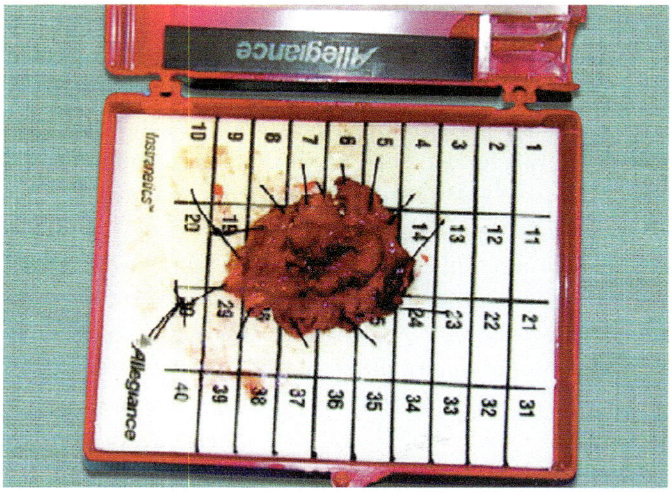

Fig. 12: Resected tissue through transanal endoscopic microsurgery (TEM).

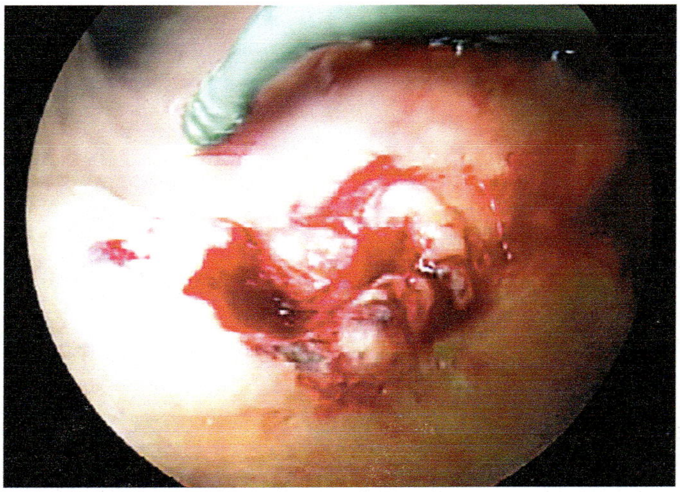

Fig. 13: Marking of margin of tissue in transanal endoscopic microsurgery (TEM).

COMMON COMPLICATIONS

- Perforation of intraperitoneal rectal wall—unable to close using TEM in 3.9%
- Required LAR or diversion (one patient)
- Early mild incontinence/soiling in 2.6% resolved by 10 weeks.

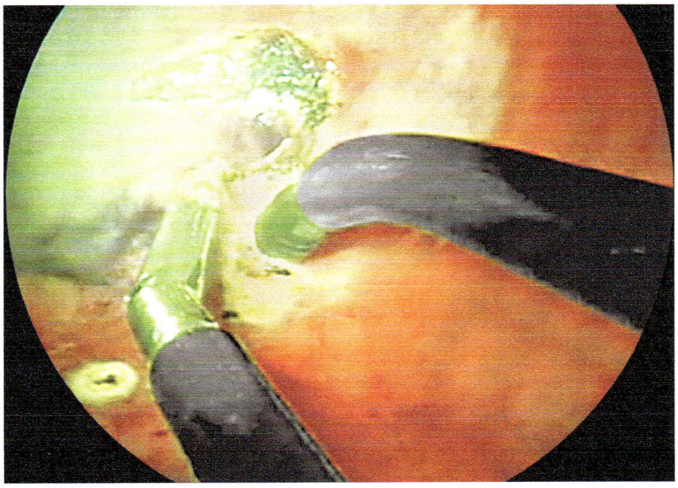

Fig. 14: Excision of malignant tissue in transanal endoscopic microsurgery (TEM).

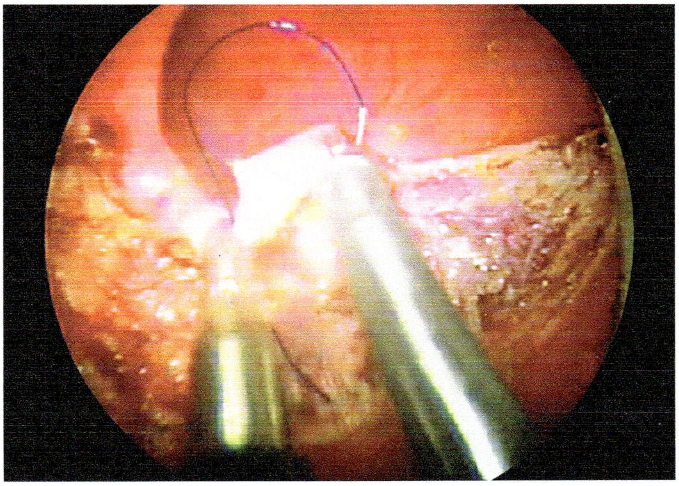

Fig. 15: Suturing in transanal endoscopic microsurgery (TEM).

CONCLUSION

The cost of the TEM equipment must be mentioned. The capital outlay of >$50,000 is considerable. That is why, you have to have the volume to justify this much expense. However, this is offset by several factors. There is no doubt that some surgeons will argue about how many patients have rectal lesions that are definitely reachable only with the TEM system. These patients are clearly saved a transabdominal rectal excision and realize a very significant cost saving. In addition, there are no disposable costs per case and the equipment is robust, requiring minimal maintenance (our own system is now 10-year-old). The imaging stack is compatible with the laparoscopic surgical system available in most operating suites. However, in view of the limited number of patients undergoing a TEM in a tertiary referral center, we believe that this is not a suitable approach for every colorectal unit and suggests that only larger centers would have enough patients to justify the costs. TEM is appropriate for a very specific patient population that includes patients with rectal benign or early cancer with no lymph node involvement. However, in this setting, the benefits are such that this technique has a rightful place as part of the colorectal surgeon's operative armamentarium.

BIBLIOGRAPHY

1. Beuss G, Mentges B, Manncke K, Starlinger M, Becker HD. Technique and results of transanal microsurgery in early rectal cancer. Am J Surg. 1992;163:63-9.
2. Beuss G. Review. Transanal endoscopic microsurgery (TEM). JR Coll Surg Edinb. 1993;38:239-45.
3. Bleday R. Local excision of rectal cancer. World J Surg. 1997; 21:706-14.
4. Bouvet M, Milas M, Giaceo GG, Cleary KR, Jnajan NA, Skibber JM. Predictors of recurrence after local excision and postoperative chemoradiotherapy of adenocarcinoma of the rectum. Ann Surg Oncol. 1999;6:26-32.
5. Chakravarti A, Compton CC, Shellito PC, Wood WC, Landry J, Machuta SR, et al. Long-term follow-up of patients with rectal cancer managed by local excision with and without adjuvant irradiation. Ann Surg. 1999;230:49-54.
6. Enker WE, Merchant N, Cohen AM, Lanouette NM, Swallow C, Guillem J, et al. Safety and efficacy of low anterior resection for rectal cancer. Ann Surg. 1999;230:544-54.
7. Fielding LP, Philips RKS, Fry JS, Hittinger R. Prediction of outcome after curative surgery for large bowel cancer. Lancet. 1986;2:904-6.
8. Fielding LP, Philips RKS, Hittinger R. Factors influencing mortality after curative resection for large bowel cancer in elderly patients. Lancet. 1989;1:595-7.
9. Geraghty JM, Williams CB, Talbot IC. Malignant colorectal polyps, venous invasion and successful treatment by endoscopic polypectomy. Gut. 1991;32:774-8.
10. Guillem JG, Paty PB, Cohen AM. Surgical treatment of colorectal cancer. CA Cancer J Clin. 1997;47:113-28.
11. Hermanek P. A pathologist's point of view on endoscopically removed polyps of the colon and rectum. Acta Hepatogastroenterol. 1978;25:169-70.
12. Hurst PA, Proust WG, Kelly JM, Bannister JJ, Walker RT. Local recurrence after low anterior resection using the staple gun. Br J Surg. 1982;69:275-6.
13. Isbister WH. Colorectal cancer surgery in the elderly: an audit of surgery in octogenarians. Aust N Z J Surg. 1997;67:557-61.
14. Jehle EC, Haehnael T, Starlinger MJ, Becker HD. Alterations of anal sphincter functions following transanal endoscopic microsurgery (TEM) for rectal tumours. Gastroenterology. 1992;102:365.
15. Karanjia ND, Schache DJ, North WRS, Heald RJ. 'Close shave' in anterior resection. Br J Surg. 1990;77:510-2.
16. Killingback M. Local excision of carcinoma of the rectum: indications. World J Surg. 1992;16:437-46.
17. Matheson NA, McIntosh CA, Krukowski ZH. Continuing experience with single layer appositional anastomosis in the large bowel. Br J Surg. 1985;70:S104-6.
18. McArdle CS, Hole D, Hansell D, Blumgart LH, Wood CB. Prospective study of colorectal cancer in the west of Scotland: ten year follow-up. Br J Surg. 1990;77:280-2.
19. Mella J, Biffin A, Radcliffe AG, Stamatakis JD, Steele RJC. Population based audit of colorectal cancer management in two UK health regions. Br J Surg. 1997;84:1731-6.
20. Mellow M. Neoplasms. In: Raskin J, Nord HJ (Eds). Colonoscopy: Principles and Techniques. New York: Igaku-Shoin Ltd; 1995. pp. 345-56.

21. Mentges B, Buess G, Effinger G, Manncke K, Becker HD. Indications and results of local treatment of rectal cancer. Br J Surg. 1997;84:348-51.
22. Mentges B, Buess G, Schafer D, Manncke K, Becker HD. Local therapy for rectal tumours. Dis Colon Rectum. 1996;39:886-92.
23. Minsky BD, Enker WE, Cohen AM, Lauwers G. Clinicopathological features in rectal cancer treated by local excision and postoperative radiation therapy. Radiat Med. 1995;13:235-41.
24. Muldoon JP. Treatment of benign tumours of the rectum. Clin Gastroenterol. 1975;4:563-70.
25. Ota DM, Skibber J, Rich TA. MD Anderson Cancer Center experience with local excision and multimodality therapy for rectal cancer. Surg Oncol Clin North Am. 1992;1:147-52.
26. Saclarides TJ. Transanal endoscopic microsurgery. Surg Clin North Am. 1997;77:229-39.
27. Saclarides TJ. Transanal endoscopic microsurgery: a single surgeon's experience. Arch Surg. 1998;133:595-8.
28. Taylor RH, Hay JH, Larsson SN. Transanal local excision of selected low rectal cancers. Am J Surg. 1998;175:360-3.
29. Willett CG, Compton CC, Shelito PC, Efird JT. Selection factors for local excision or abdominoperineal resection of early stage rectal cancer. Cancer. 1994;73:2716-20.
30. Winde G, Nottberg H, Keller R, Schmid KW, Bunte H. Surgical cure for early rectal carcinomas (T1): transanal endoscopic microsurgery vs. anterior resection. Dis Colon Rectum. 1996; 39:969-76.

CHAPTER 49 Future of Minimal Access Surgery

INTRODUCTION

The future laparoscopic technology includes three-dimensional virtual reality and expands the scanning rate from 525 lines of resolution to 1,000 or 1,200 lines per frame and the quality of picture would be twice better than existing system.

With virtual reality, a three-dimensional computer image is presented through liquid crystal glasses.

The future of three-dimensional images is not far away and many instrument companies have prototype in the field **(Fig. 1)**.

Laparoscopic surgery is growing in such a speed that three-dimensional image projection system is going to replace the conventional monitor in near future and surgeon will get a virtual image in air just above the body of patient. This new projection system will abolish all the limitation of current two-dimensional images without depth perception.

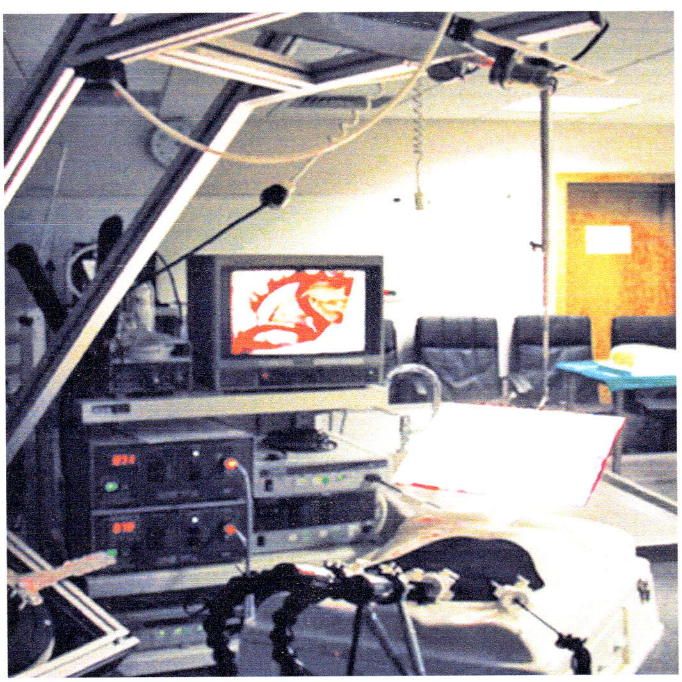

Fig. 1: Hologram projection system.

NATURAL ORIFICE TRANSLUMINAL ENDOSCOPIC SURGERY

Over the past 10 years, the major drive in surgery has been the development and application of minimal access approaches to traditional operations. This philosophy has crossed all surgical specialties and has had a major impact on training, technological developments, and patient care.

In general surgery, the emphasis has been on laparoscopic techniques, which can now be applied to the majority of intra-abdominal procedures. Evidence suggests that the reduction in trauma to the abdominal wall and the physiology of the pneumoperitoneum have a positive impact on patients undergoing abdominal operations.

Although still not widely applied, these techniques have put surgeons on notice that flexible endoscopy may become an important component of their practice.

Surgeons have gone beyond the luminal confines of the gastrointestinal tract to perform intra-abdominal procedures. With existing flexible endoscopic instrumentation, the wall of the stomach is punctured and an endoscope is advanced into the peritoneal cavity to perform various procedures; thus far, the use of this technique for diagnostic exploration, liver biopsy, cholecystectomy, splenectomy, and tubal ligation has been reported in animal models. Recently, transvaginal endoscopic cholecystectomy is performed in France **(Figs. 2A to F)**.

After the intervention is finished, the scope is pulled back into the stomach and the puncture is closed. Several videos have been shown at scientific meetings that suggest that at least transgastric appendectomy has been performed in humans. Other natural orifices, such as the anus or vagina, also allow access to the peritoneal cavity **(Figs. 3A to C)**. Although in its infancy, the performance of natural orifice transluminal endoscopic surgery (NOTES) may, thus, further revolutionize the field of abdominal surgery.

Obvious questions are raised by the possibilities of NOTES:

- Is there any clinical advantage to avoiding incisions in the abdominal wall? Can the visceral wall be closed safely and reliably?

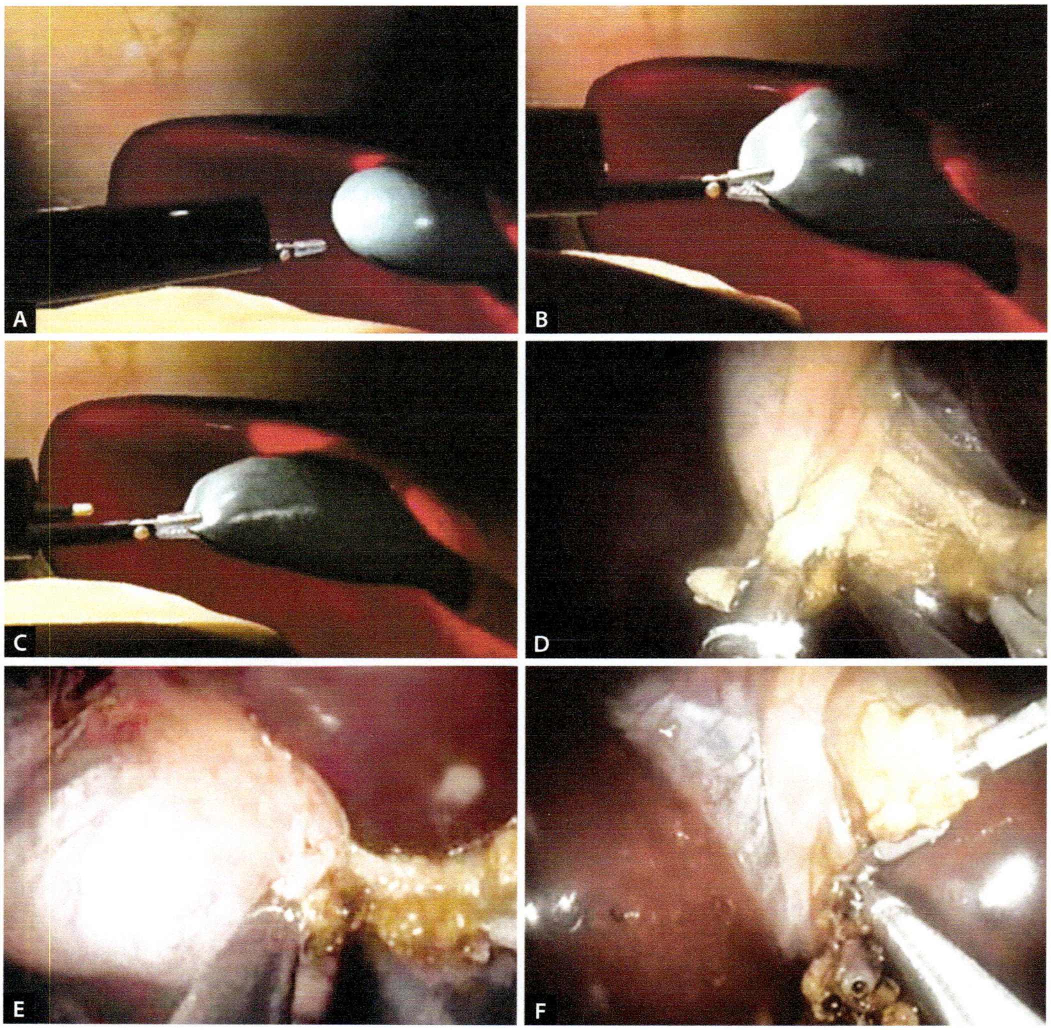

Figs. 2A to F: Transvaginal cholecystectomy.

- Does the flora of the natural orifice lead more to peritoneal infection?
- Who should perform these procedures and how should the individuals be trained in NOTES?

The Society of American Gastrointestinal and Endoscopic Surgeons (SAGES) and gastroenterologists from the American Society for Gastrointestinal Endoscopy (ASGE) held a summit meeting to build a conceptual framework for the initial safe application of NOTES procedures. It was acknowledged that the development of NOTES further blurred the lines between the traditional boundaries of gastrointestinal surgeons and endoscopists. Several broad concepts and principles were agreed upon and will soon be published in detail in a whitepaper.

Safe Application of Natural Orifice Transluminal Endoscopic Surgery

The concepts included the following: initially, NOTES should be performed by a team of experienced laparoscopic surgeons and interventional endoscopists in an operating room. Clinical procedures should be done under Institutional Review Board Supervision and entered into a prospective outcomes database. Basic research is needed to assess the physiologic alterations caused by the visceral puncture and the bacteriology of the peritoneal cavity following transluminal interventions. Collaboration with industry is critical to the development of effective instruments allowing traction/countertraction and stable optical platforms as well as the means to control hemostasis, securely close the visceral wall, and perform suturing functions and gastrointestinal anastomoses.

The roots of NOTES have been established, but work is still needed to refine techniques, verify safety, and document efficacy. With continued research, NOTES may prove to be a sound method with clinical benefit to patients. Appropriate scientific scrutiny, collaboration among gastrointestinal interventionalists, and effective means of training for these techniques will be critical on emerging technologies.

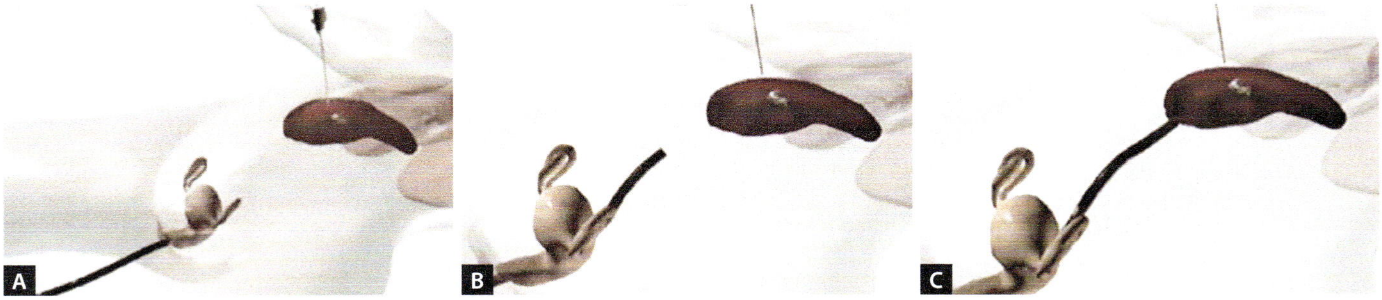

Figs. 3A to C: Introduction of operative endoscope through the vaginal orifice.

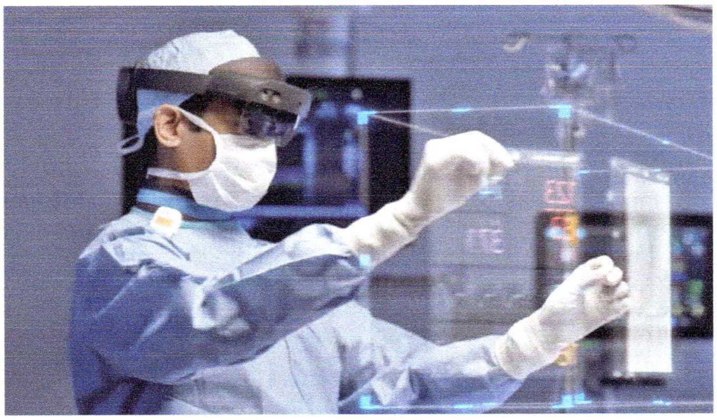

Fig. 4: Augmented reality in minimal access surgery.

AUGMENTED REALITY IN MINIMAL ACCESS SURGERY

Augmented reality is slowly emerging in minimal access surgery around the world to help the laparoscopic and robotic surgeons and the operating team **(Fig. 4)**. We have seen surgeons wearing the Google glass and as technology evolves, both in terms of devices and software, we are seeing an extension in applications. Reaching a truly augmented surgeon through augmented reality will require few more years. For the time being, augmented reality and virtual reality are becoming more and more common in minimal access surgical training and in the preparation of laparoscopic surgery, letting the surgeon to practice on a virtual patient that mirrors, accurately, the real patient. The development of augmented reality devices allows minimal access surgeon to incorporate data visualization into diagnostic and treatment procedures to improve work efficiency, safety, and cost and to enhance surgical outcome.

BIBLIOGRAPHY

1. Badiali G, Ferrari V, Cutolo F, Freschi C, Caramella D, Bianchi A, et al. Augmented reality as an aid in maxillofacial surgery: validation of a wearable system allowing maxillary repositioning. J Craniomaxillofac Surg. 2014;42:1970-6.
2. Callovini G, Sherkat S, Callovini G, Gazzeri R. Frameless nonstereotactic image-guided surgery of supratentorial lesions: introduction to a safe and inexpensive technique. J Neurol Surg A Cent Eur Neurosurg. 2014;75:365-70.
3. Davis MC, Can DD, Pindrik J, Rocque BG, Johnston JM. Virtual interactive presence in global surgical education: international collaboration through augmented reality. World Neurosurg. 2016;86:103-11.
4. Gavaghan K, Oliveira-Santos T, Peterhans M, Reyes M, Kim H, Anderegg S, et al. Evaluation of a portable image overlay projector for the visualisation of surgical navigation data: phantom studies. Int J Comput Assist Radiol Surg. 2012;7:547-56.
5. Gavaghan KA, Peterhans M, Oliveira-Santos T, Weber S. A portable image overlay projection device for computer-aided open liver surgery. IEEE Trans Biomed Eng. 2011;58:1855-64.
6. Gonzalez SJ, Guo YH, Lee MC. Feasibility of augmented reality glasses for real-time, 3-dimensional (3D) intraoperative guidance. J Am Coll Surg. 2014;219:S64.
7. Ieiri S, Uemura M, Konishi K, Souzaki R, Nagao Y, Tsutsumi N, et al. Augmented reality navigation system for laparoscopic splenectomy in children based on preoperative CT image using optical tracking device. Pediatr Surg Int. 2012;28:341-6.
8. Inoue D, Cho B, Mori M, Kikkawa Y, Amano T, Nakamizo A, et al. Preliminary study on the clinical application of augmented reality neuronavigation. J Neurol Surg A Cent Eur Neurosurg. 2013;74:71-6.
9. Kang X, Azizian M, Wilson E, Wu K, Martin AD, Kane TD, et al. Stereoscopic augmented reality for laparoscopic surgery. Surg Endosc. 2014;28:2227-35.
10. Kenngott HG, Wagner M, Gondan M, Nickel F, Nolden M, Fetzer A, et al. Real-time image guidance in laparoscopic liver surgery: first clinical experience with a guidance system based on intraoperative CT imaging. Surg Endosc. 2014;28:933-40.
11. Kersten-Oertel M, Gerard I, Drouin S, Mok K, Sirhan D, Sinclair DS, et al. Augmented reality in neurovascular surgery: feasibility and first uses in the operating room. Int J Comput Assist Radiol Surg. 2015;10:1823-36.
12. Kocev B, Ritter F, Linsen L. Projector-based surgeon-computer interaction on deformable surfaces. Int J Comput Assist Radiol Surg. 2014;9:301-12.
13. Kranzfelder M, Bauer M, Magg M. Image-guided surgery. Endosk Heute. 2014;27:154-8.
14. Lahanas V, Loukas C, Smailis N, Georgiou E. A novel augmented reality simulator for skills assessment in minimal invasive surgery. Surg Endosc. 2015;29:2224-34.
15. LeBlanc F, Champagne BJ, Augestad KM, Neary PC, Senagore AJ, Ellis CN, et al. A comparison of human cadaver and augmented reality simulator models for straight laparoscopic colorectal skills acquisition training. J Am Coll Surg. 2010;211:250-5.
16. Lelos N, Campos P, Sugand K, Bailey C, Mirza K. Augmented reality dynamic holography for neurology. J Neurol Neurosurg Psychiatr. 2014;85:1.
17. Marescaux J, Diana M. Inventing the future of surgery. World J Surg. 2015;39:615-22.

18. Nam WH, Kang DG, Lee D, Lee JY, Ra JB. Automatic registration between 3D intraoperative ultrasound and preoperative CT images of the liver based on robust edge matching. Phys Med Biol. 2012;57:69-91.
19. Okamoto T, Onda S, Matsumoto M, Gocho T, Futagawa Y, Fujioka S, et al. Utility of augmented reality system in hepatobiliary surgery. J Hepatobiliary Pancreat Sci. 2013;20:249-53.
20. Okamoto T, Onda S, Yanaga K, Suzuki N, Hattori A. Clinical application of navigation surgery using augmented reality in the abdominal field. Surg Today. 2015;45:397-406.
21. Pessaux P, Diana M, Soler L, Piardi T, Mutter D, Marescaux J. Robotic duodenopancreatectomy assisted with augmented reality and real-time fluorescence guidance. Surg Endosc. 2014;28:2493-8.
22. Pessaux P, Diana M, Soler L, Piardi T, Mutter D, Marescaux J. Towards cybernetic surgery: robotic and augmented reality-assisted liver segmentectomy. Langenbecks Arch Surg. 2015; 400:381-5.
23. Profeta AC, Schilling C, McGurk M. Augmented reality visualization in head and neck surgery: an overview of recent findings in sentinel node biopsy and future perspectives. Br J Oral Maxillofac Surg. 2016;54:694-6.
24. Shakur SF, Luciano CJ, Kania P, Roitberg BZ, Banerjee PP, Slavin KV, et al. Usefulness of a virtual reality percutaneous trigeminal rhizotomy simulator in neurosurgical training. Neurosurgery. 2015;11:420-5.
25. Shekhar R, Dandekar O, Bhat V, Philip M, Lei P, Godinez C, et al. Live augmented reality: a new visualization method for laparoscopic surgery using continuous volumetric computed tomography. Surg Endosc. 2010;24:1976-85.
26. Shenai MB, Dillavou M, Shum C, Ross D, Tubbs RS, Shih A, et al. Virtual interactive presence and augmented reality (VIPAR) for remote surgical assistance. Neurosurgery. 2011;68:200-7.
27. Sugimoto M, Yasuda H, Koda K, Suzuki M, Yamazaki M, Tezuka T, et al. Image overlay navigation by markerless surface registration in gastrointestinal, hepatobiliary and pancreatic surgery. J Hepatobiliary Pancreat Sci. 2010;17:629-36.
28. Tabrizi LB, Mahvash M. Augmented reality-guided neurosurgery: accuracy and intraoperative application of an image projection technique. J Neurosurg. 2015;123:206-11.
29. Tsutsumi N, Tomikawa M, Uemura M, Akahoshi T, Nagao Y, Konishi K, et al. Image-guided laparoscopic surgery in an open MRI operating theater. Surg Endosc. 2013;27:2178-84.
30. Vemuri AS, Wu JCH, Liu KC, Wu HS. Deformable three-dimensional model architecture for interactive augmented reality in minimally invasive surgery. Surg Endosc. 2012;26:3655-62.
31. Vera AM, Russo M, Mohsin A, Tsuda S. Augmented reality telementoring (ART) platform: a randomized controlled trial to assess the efficacy of a new surgical education technology. Surg Endosc. 2014;28:3467-72.
32. Watanabe E, Satoh M, Konno T, Hirai M, Yamaguchi T. The transvisible navigator: a see-through neuronavigation system using augmented reality. World Neurosurg. 2016;87:399-405.
33. Wen R, Chui CK, Ong SH, Lim KB, Chang SKY. Projection-based visual guidance for robot-aided RF needle insertion. Int J Comput Assist Radiol Surg. 2013;8:1015-25.
34. Yoshino M, Saito T, Kin T, Nakagawa D, Nakatomi H, Oyama H, et al. A microscopic optically tracking navigation system that uses high-resolution 3D computer graphics. Neurol Med Chir (Tokyo). 2015;55:674-9.

CHAPTER 50

Troubleshooting and Checklist

SAFETY CHECKLIST OF MINIMAL ACCESS SURGERY

In minimal access surgery, surgeon uses a variety of instrument and techniques to operate with less damage to the body than with open surgery. In general, minimally invasive surgery is associated with less pain, a shorter hospital stays, and fewer complications, but many safety considerations should be kept in mind. Following checklist should be kept in operation theater and theater staff should be carefully access this checklist **(Fig. 1)**.

What would you do if the following situations occurred during a laparoscopic surgery?

The field turns pink or yellow:

- White balancing may not be initially before inserting the telescope into the abdomen. White balance the camera should be done after withdrawing it
- There may be wrongly connected RGB cable. The RGB cable should be checked for proper connection
- Low voltage can sometimes alter the color

MIS safety checklist

1. Prepatient entry

A. Circulating nurse duties

Parameter	Actions
Surgeon preference card	☐ Reviewed
OR table position	☐ Correct orientation and weight capacity
	☐ Bean bag mattress (if indicated)
	☐ Table accessories (e.g., spreader bars/leg supports/foot board as indicated)
	☐ Positioned for fluoroscopy if indicated
Power sources	☐ Connected and linked to all devices
CO_2 insufflator	☐ Check CO_2 volume, pressure and flow
	☐ Backup cylinder and accessories (wrench and key) in place Filter for CO_2 unit or tubing
Video monitors	☐ Position per procedure
	☐ Test pattern present
Suction/irrigation	☐ Cannister set
	☐ Irrigation and pressure bag available
Alarms	☐ Turned on and audible
Video documentation	☐ Recording media available and operational (DVD, print, etc.)

B. Scrub person duties

Parameter	Actions
Reusable instruments	☐ Check movement handles and jaws, all screws present
	☐ Check sealing caps
	☐ Instrument vents closed
	☐ Check cautery insulation
Veress needle	☐ Check plunger/spring action
	☐ Flush needle and stopcock saline solution available
Hasson cannula	☐ Check valves, plunger, and seals
Trocars/ports	☐ Check appropriate size/type
	☐ Close stopcocks
Laparoscope	☐ Size and type per preference
	☐ Check lens clarity
	☐ Antifog solution or warmed saline for lens cleaning

2. After patient entry

Parameter	Actions
Patient position	☐ Secured to OR table, safety straps on
	☐ Pressure sites padded
	☐ Arms out or tucked per procedure
Sequential compression device	☐ On and connected to device
Electrosurgical unit	☐ Ground pad applied
Foot controls	☐ Positioned for surgeon access
Power sources (camera, insufflator, light source, monitors, cautery, ultrasonics, bipolar)	☐ Turned on (on standby)
Miscellaneous	☐ Foley catheter (if indicated)
	☐ Naso-or orogastric tube (bougies if indicated)
Antibiotics	☐ Given as indicated

3. After prep and drape

Parameter	Actions
Electrosurgical unit	☐ Cautery cords connected to unit
Monopolar cautery	☐ Tip protected
Ultrasonic or bipolar device	☐ Connected to unit ☐ Activation test performed
Line connections	☐ Camera cord
	☐ Light source (on standby)
	☐ CO_2 tubing (Connected and flushed)
	☐ Suction/irrigation(suction turned on)
	☐ Smoke evacuation filter connected
Local anesthetic	☐ Syringe labeled and filled with anesthetic of choice needle connected
Fluoroscopy case	☐ Mix and dilute contrast appropriately and label
	☐ Clear tubing, syringe, catheter of air bubbles, label syringes

Fig. 1: Minimally invasive safety checklist.
(CO_2: carbon dioxide; MIS: minimally invasive surgery)

- Bile or blood spillage may turn the field pink or yellow due to staining of field. The inadvertent injury to bowel and spillage of bowel content may cause the field to turn yellow.

Sudden blackout:

- The cause of sudden blackout may be due to fused bulb of light source. Switch of light source should be turn to use backup bulb
- There may be disconnected camera or monitor cable or the fuse of camera blown due to fluctuation in voltage. The fuse and connection of camera and monitor should be checked
- The tip of the telescope may be touching any object completely, so there is no way for light to come out. The telescope should be repositioned.

Poor definition of picture:

- The poor picture may be due to soiled lens with blood or other body fluids. It should be cleaned with warm water
- The camera may not be white balanced or focused properly. The fine tuning of camera should be tried. The proper white balance of camera is necessary to get a good quality picture. White balancing of camera should be done by placing the telescope 6 cm away from a complete white gauge piece or tissue paper
- Excessive blood in the operative field resulting in absorption of light and poor field is one of the causes of poor vision of operating field. Proper irrigation and suction should be tried to get a clear view.

What action would you take to control marked intra-abdominal bleeding from a trocar site?

For immediate control:

- With inserted trocar, pressure should be applied on the bleeding site either from outside or using a pledget from within under vision
- A Foley catheter can be inserted and the balloon can be inflated and pulled up creating a tamponade effect
- A purse string suture can be taken around the incision of trocar and tightened to check the bleeding
- A clamp can be applied to the port site till the bleeding is controlled.

For more permanent control:

- The bleeding vessel can be sutured from within under vision or controlled with diathermy or a full-thickness bite can be taken externally at the region of the bleeding vessel
- The incision can be extended and the vessel can be found by proper debridement and then bleeding vessel should be ligated.

What action would you take if trocar injury to a large vessel occurs?

- The trocar should be left in place. The adequate resuscitative measures should be taken (such as blood should be at hand for the transfusion)
- Urgent laparotomy should be performed and repair of the vessel with adequate exposure should be done
- The help of a vascular surgeon should be asked.

What would you do following a sudden collapse of the patient during an endoscopic procedure?

Possible causes for the collapse could be:

- Vasovagal shock due to peritoneal irritation
- Carbon dioxide (CO_2) embolism either by direct entry of gas into vessel or through absorption
- Hypercarbia due to systemic CO_2 absorption results in respiratory acidosis and pulmonary hypertension leading to cardiac dysrhythmia
- *Arrhythmias*: Atrioventricular (AV) dissociation, junctional rhythm, sinus bradycardia, and asystole due to vagal response to peritoneal stretching.

Insufflation should be stopped and abdomen should be deflated. The patient should be kept in a head-down and right-up position (steep left lateral Trendelenburg position) and 100% oxygen (O_2) should be administered. The blood gas levels should be analyzed and corrected accordingly. The gas in the right ventricle should be removed with a central venous catheter, if possible. If there is any arrhythmia and atropine, antiarrhythmic should be given. In case of ventricular fibrillation, there may be need of DC defibrillator.

What would you select the pressure insufflator at the start of diagnostic laparoscopy in an adult healthy patient?

If general anesthesia is employed, the starting flow rate is set at 1 L/min, pressure 12 mm Hg, and volume 2–3 L.

During diagnostic laparoscopy under local anesthesia, insufflation is begun at a flow rate of 1 L/min, initial low pressure 2–3 mm Hg, and volume not exceeding 2 L.

What would you do when?

High pressure is registered when CO_2 is insufflated in the VN before the needle has been placed in the body:

- Veress needle may be blocked
- The gas tap may not be opened
- Gas tube may be kinked

The tap should be checked for right direction and the needle should be flushed with saline to ensure that it is not blocked. The faulty Veress needle should be changed.

High pressures (10 or 15 mm Hg) are obtained during insufflation at 1 L/min:

- The needle may be in the wrong plane and not in the peritoneal cavity
- Gas tap or needle may be partially blocked.

Right plane of insertion of needle should be checked by the saline drop test and negative aspiration test. If the problem continues, than needle should be withdrawn and reinserted.

What would you do if after insufflation and on insertion of the telescope?

You saw gas in the greater omentum: If there is gas in the greater omentum, the probability is that either the Veress needle or the trocar has entered and insufflated gas into it. There is an increased risk of systemic absorption of CO_2 resulting in embolism. The necessary precautions to prevent this should be taken. Antithrombotics (heparin) should be given, the patient should be tilted head down and left lateral, and 100% O_2 should be given for inspiration.

Only fat is seen and there is no crepitant in the abdominal wall: The telescope is probably in the omentum and should be withdrawn and any possible injury to the omental vessel should be checked.

What action would you take when?

You are unable to advance trocar into abdomen: If the trocar is a disposable one, confirm whether the blade tip is charged and reintroduced. Alternatively, the tip may get discharged halfway. The trocar should be removed, recharged, and inserted again. If it is a reusable trocar, the tip may be blunt in which case it would be better to use a different sharp trocar.

The tip of the obturator is seen entering the abdominal cavity during insertion of a secondary trocar: The skin incision may be small, so the trocar has to be removed, the incision should be extended, and the trocar should be reinserted.

List the safety mechanisms of different types of trocars.

Blunt (Hasson) trocar—blunt with insertion under direct vision. This type of trocar works on the safety of direct vision: Some disposable trocars have a sharp blade with a spring loaded safety shield, which cover the blade tip once the peritoneal cavity is entered. This spring loaded spring mechanism reduces the risk of injury to the underlying viscera by the blade tip.

Other disposable trocars require charging before insertion and when the tip enters the peritoneal cavity, the blade tip retracts inside.

Reusable trocars have triangular and conical tips. The triangular tips are sharper and tend to cause more vascular injury.

Some disposable trocars have a screw-shaped cannula, which has to be inserted like a screw, which enables the surgeon to have more control over the force with which he inserts the trocar. These have an additional advantage of not slipping out during the procedure.

Nonbladed obturator is used in some trocars for careful insertion where the problem of charging the blade tip and its potency does not arise.

Visiport is a mechanism in which the telescope is inserted into the cannula and the gun is fired through the abdominal wall visualizing each layer until the peritoneal cavity is reached. The trocars are, thus, inserted under vision layer-by-layer.

Radially dilating trocars are also available. It has the advantage of entry through a very small incision and then incision can be dilated with the serial dilator.

Ultrasonically activated trocar system is used in some high-risk patients. It consists of an ultrasonic generator and a transducer attached to the trocar spike.

The sharp pyramidal tip is activated with a frequency of 23.5 kHz and amplitude of 150 µm. The trocar fits a 5-mm plastic sheath that is introduced inside a 10-mm dilator whose tip is conical.

List the factors that contribute to increase the risk of complications with using Veress needle.

- Faulty needle—dysfunctional spring tip
- Wrong method of insertion
- Not guarding the needle and not inserting like a dart
- Uncontrolled forceful insertion of needle
- Wrong angle of insertion, i.e., directing straight down instead of toward the pelvic cavity
- Excessive force from shoulder rather than wrist while inserting
- Previous abdominal surgery and scarred abdomen
- *Thin scaphoid individual*: Risk of deep entry
- *Spinal deformities*: Kyphoscoliosis
- Late pregnancy
- Morbid obesity
- Organomegaly
- Portal hypertension.

PROCEDURE CHECKLISTS: VERESS NEEDLE INSERTION

Check and Set the Insufflator

Pressure Level and Flow Rate

Initial flow rates should be set at around 1 L/min. Optimal exposure is obtained with intra-abdominal pressures of 12.0–16.0 mm Hg. Lower pressures (e.g., 10 mm Hg) may give adequate visualization, especially in women with lax abdominal walls. This causes less stretching of the diaphragm, possibly reducing postoperative pain. Low pressure pneumoperitoneum may be used in conjunction with techniques to lift the abdominal wall in patients with impaired respiratory or cardiac states. An initial setting of 10.0–15.0 mm Hg is recommended for routine procedures.

- Connect gas supply to Veress needle
- Check gas flow, needle patency, and spring loaded central blunt stylet
- Palpation test
- Assessment of abdominal wall thickness by palpation with the fingers down to the aorta
- Make a small skin incision
- Tension abdominal wall and insert needle.

The safest technique is to hold the needle at a point along its shaft at a distance from the tip, which equates with that estimated by palpation as the abdominal wall thickness. The other hand holds up the abdominal wall, providing countertension as the needle is "threaded" in. You should be able to feel the needle puncture two distinct layers. Once the sharp tip enters the peritoneal cavity, the spring loaded blunt stylet is released with an audible (palpable) click.

Check that the Needle is in the Correct Position

A number of tests exist to confirm correct positioning of the needle tip.

- *Aspiration*: Uses a saline-filled syringe
- *Saline drop test*: Uses a drop of saline in the Veress needle hub
- *Negative pressure test*: Retraction of the anterior abdominal wall
- Early insufflation pressures
- *Volume test*: Approximate 3 L of gas are required to reach pressures of 10 mm Hg.

If an extraperitoneal position is suspected, the needle can be withdrawn and repositioned. The number of passes required should be recorded. If a small amount of blood is aspirated, reinsertion is justified. If large amounts of blood escape up the needle, laparotomy is indicated. If bowel content is aspirated, the needle is withdrawn and reinserted in another location. Subsequent inspection and adequate treatment for bowel injury are mandatory.

Insufflate

After a minimum of 1 L of gas has been insufflated and needle position has been confirmed, the rate may be increased for more rapid filling. Periodic checks should be made of symmetric distension and abdominal resonance. Once the desired pressure has been reached, close the gas tap on the needle and withdraw it.

Uses of the Diathermy Hook

- Use a metal trocar
- Pass the hook through an introducer tube or manually open the valve of the cannula to protect the hook from damage. Trumpet-type valves necessitate the use of the introducer
- Select the tissue to be divided. You may require inserting the hooks tip parallel to the margin of the structure and then rotating it in a way to hook up tissue. You may need to use sweeping movements to separate the tissues. Do not lift too large an amount of tissue. Several small "bites" are more effective and safer. Work away from important structures
- Inspect the tissue on the hook
- Be aware of possible additional contact points
- The camera operator may need to withdraw slightly to prevent the lens being splattered
- Coagulate and/or cut the tissue on the hook
- Control any possible overshoot
- Continued dissection using this technique may require the hook to be cleaned of charred material withdraw and clean with the supplied implement until clean. Smoke is generated if charring occurs, this can obscure the field. Open at a point of the cannula to allow gas to escape from the abdomen. This will automatically be replaced by fresh gas from the insufflator
- When dissection is finished, watch the hook into the introducer tube as tissue may accidentally catch up and get damaged
- Open the cannula valve, if necessary, to prevent damage to the hook.

Introduction of a Pledget into the Abdominal Cavity

- Atraumatic, ratcheted grasper or a spiked biopsy forceps are passed through the introducer tube externally
- The pledget is placed in the open jaws, making sure that enough pledget is placed between the jaws for a secure grip and enough pledget protrudes, so that, in use, the grasper does not act on the tissues
- The grip is secured by closing the jaws, doing up the racket, and as an added precaution against intra-abdominal loss, an elastic band is used to ensure closure is maintained
- The pledget is then completely withdrawn into the introducer tube
- The introducer tube is passed through a large cannula into the abdominal cavity
- The pledget can now be extruded from the introducer and used.

Retrieval of a Pledget from the Abdominal Cavity

- When the pledget is no longer required, it is withdrawn inside the introducer tube. It is extremely important that the camera follows the instrument and the pledget is seen to enter the tube
- The tube can then be withdrawn from the cannula
- The pledget is extruded from the lower end and released from the grasper.

Application of Metal Clips

Is clip appropriate or would it be better to use a ligature?

- Load the clip applicator
- Insert through an appropriate cannula
- Place the jaws around the structure to be ligated
- Check for correct placement by observing from different angles or rotating the instrument
- Partially close the instrument (this traps the tissue to be ligated and it can again be checked)
- Firmly close the jaws
- Open and withdraw. Single clips should not be trusted for vessels of any size.

How do laparoscopy on the abdomen with previous scar?

The patient with previous abdominal surgery is at high risk for minimal access surgery. In these patients, following techniques should be used:

- *The open insufflation technique*:
  - Hasson technique
  - Fielding technique
- Pneumoperitoneum should be created with a Veress needle by selecting an alternate site of insertion distant from the old abdominal incision
- Insufflations with a Veress needle inserted in posterior vaginal fornix or transuterus route
- Insertion of optical trocar—primary port.

Hasson Technique

This is a very safe technique to enter the abdomen, especially in patients with scarred abdomen from multiple previous surgeries.

This is an open technique where surgeon can see what he is doing. It is performed in an area of the abdomen distant from previous scars and likely to be free of adhesions. After the induction of anesthesia, 1 cm horizontal incision is made. Blunt dissection is carried out until the underlying fascia is identified. The fascia is elevated with a pair of Kocher clamps. Adherent subcutaneous tissue is gently dissected free. It is then incised to permit entry of trocar into the peritoneal cavity. Two heavy, absorbable sutures are placed on either side of the fascial incision just like repair of umbilical hernia. Care must be taken when applying these sutures not to injure the underlying viscera. The Kocher clamps are next removed and 10 mm blunt trocar is advanced into the peritoneal cavity. The obturator is removed and the sleeve is secured in position with the previously placed two sutures. The sleeve of the trocar is wrapped with Vaseline gauze to prevent leakage of insufflated gas around the trocar.

Open Fielding Technique

This technique developed by Fielding in 1992 involves a small incision over the everted umbilicus at a point where the skin and peritoneum are adjacent. Pneumoperitoneum can be created using Fielding technique in patients with abdominal incisions from previous surgery, providing there is no midline incision, portal hypertension, and recanalized umbilical vein, and umbilical abnormalities such as urachal cyst sinus, or umbilical hernia are present. A suture is not usually required to prevent gas leakage because the umbilicus has been everted (so the angle of insertion of the laparoscopic port becomes oblique) and the incision required is relatively small. However, one may be needed to stabilize the port. Thorough skin preparation of the umbilicus is carried out and the everted umbilicus (with toothed grasping forceps) is incised from the apex in a caudal direction. Two small retractors are inserted to expose the cylindrical umbilical tube running from the undersurface of the umbilical skin down to the linea alba. This tube is then cut from its apex downward toward its junction with the linea alba. Further blunt dissection through this plane permits direct entry into the peritoneum. Once the peritoneal cavity is breached, the laparoscopic port (without trocar) can then be inserted directly and insufflations started. A blunt internal trocar facilitates insertion of this port and an external grip that can be attached to the port to secure it in position.

Advantages of Using the Open Technique

- The incidence of injury to adhered organ, although not eliminated, is significantly reduced by entry into the peritoneal cavity under direct vision
- There is a decreased risk of injury to the retroperitoneal vessels. The obturator is blunt and the angle of entry allows the surge onto maneuver the cannulas at an angle, which avoids viscera, while still assuring peritoneal placement
- The risk of extraperitoneal insufflations is eliminated. Placement under direct vision ensures that insufflation of gas is actually into the peritoneal cavity
- The likelihood of hernia formation is decreased because the fascia is closed as part of the technique
- In experienced hands, the open technique is cost-effective. The Hasson technique does not increase the operative time required, creating a pneumoperitoneum and may even lessen it.

Alternative Sites for Introducing Veress Needle

For avoiding the injury to the adhered portion of bowel in the patient with previous abdominal surgeries, the alternative site for the introduction of Veress needle can be chosen other than umbilicus.

For Previous Laparotomy with Midline Incision

For a previously operated abdomen with a midline incision, Veress needle should be placed in the upper left quadrant of the abdomen just lateral to the rectus sheath. The preperitoneal space in hypochondriac region is more easily insufflated than at the umbilicus. The Veress needle at hypochondriac region needs to be passed more deeply into the abdomen in order to enter the peritoneal cavity because all the layers of abdomen are present here and there is a thick layer of muscle as well. The right upper quadrant should be avoided because of the size of the liver and the presence of the falciform ligament. There is some report of injury to liver if the liver is enlarged or the careless insertion of Veress needle to right hypochondrium is performed.

For a Previous Laparotomy with Upper Midline Incision

In patient with scar on the upper midline of abdomen, the Veress needle should be placed in the right lower quadrant; the left lower quadrant should generally be avoided since in older patients, there are usually sigmoid adhesions in the left lower quadrant.

For Previously Operated Abdomen with a Solitary Incision in an Upper or Lower Abdominal Quadrant

In a patient with the scar in the upper or lower abdominal quadrant, the Veress needle should be passed in the opposite abdominal quadrant just lateral to the rectus muscle. The left lower and right upper quadrant should be avoided, if it is possible.

For Patient with Previously Operated Abdomen in Multiple Quadrants

In these patients, a Veress needle or open cannula in an area farthest from the existing abdominal scar should be used. When there is any confusion regarding the presence of adhesion inside the abdomen where Veress needle has to go, the open cannula technique should be used.

Transvaginal or Transuterine Insufflation

Some surgeons prefer to introduce Veress needle through the posterior fornix or through the uterus in female with previous abdominal surgery. Although this method of pneumoperitoneum is now very popular, the placement of a needle via the posterior fornix has been demonstrated to be safe. If this route of pneumoperitoneum has been chosen, then the needle must be placed in the midline about 1.75 cm behind the junction of the vaginal vault and smooth epithelium of external os **(Figs. 2A and B)**.

Insufflation with an Optical Trocar (Visiport)

This is one of the techniques used for performing laparoscopic procedures in patient with previous scarred abdomen. An incision of 1 cm long is made in the area of the abdominal wall distant from the previous scars. The Littlewood forceps are used to elevate the abdomen. The Visiport optical trocar is introduced with telescope. The optical trocar is advanced slowly through the different planes of the abdominal wall. The blade at the tip of the Visiport cuts the tissue, which is visible so there is very less chance of injury to intra-abdominal organ, if the surgeon is experienced.

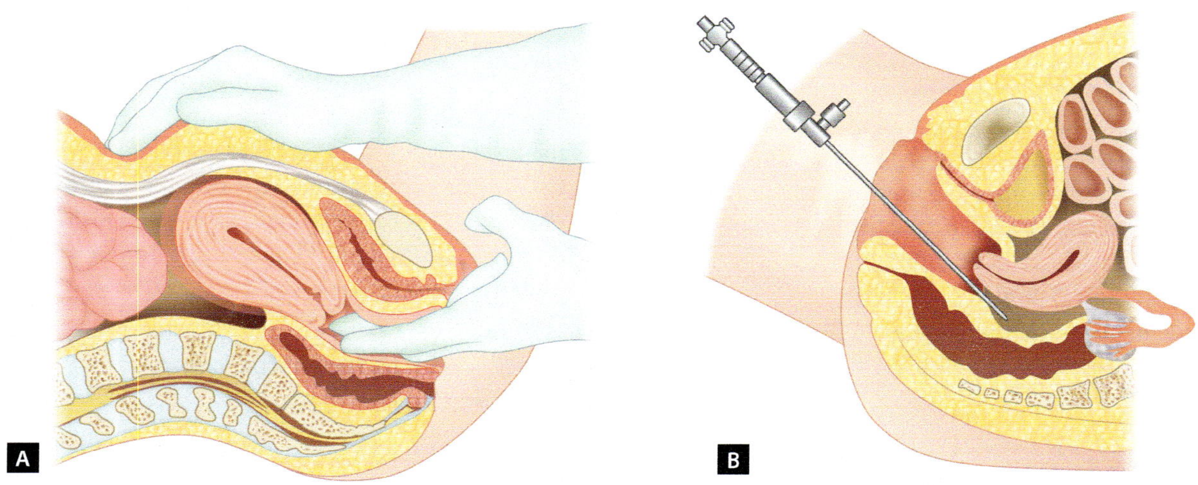

Figs. 2A and B: Transvaginal route of insufflation.

BIBLIOGRAPHY

1. Cataldo PA. Transanal endoscopic microsurgery. Surg Clin North Am. 2006;86:915-25.
2. Fleshman J, Marcello P, Stamos MJ, Wexner SD. Focus Group on Laparoscopic Colectomy Education as endorsed by the American Society of Colon and Rectal Surgeons (ASCRS) and the Society of American Gastrointestinal and Endoscopic Surgeons (SAGES): guidelines for laparoscopic colectomy course. Surg Endosc. 2006;20:1162-7.
3. Gavagan JA, Whiteford MH, Swanstrom LL. Full-thickness intraperitoneal excision by transanal endoscopic microsurgery does not increase short-term complications. Am J Surg. 2004;187:630-4.
4. Heald RJ, Husband EM, Ryall RD. The mesorectum in rectal cancer surgery: the clue to pelvic recurrence? Br J Surg. 1982;69:613-6.
5. Jagannath SB, Kantsevoy SV, Vaughn CA, Chung SS, Cotton PB, Gostout CJ, et al. Peroral transgastric endoscopic ligation of fallopian tubes with long-term survival in a porcine model. Gastrointest Endosc. 2005;61:449-53.
6. Kantsevoy SV, Jagannath SB, Niiyama H, Chung SS, Cotton PB, Gostout CJ, et al. Endoscopic gastrojejunostomy with survival in a porcine model. Gastrointest Endosc. 2005;62:287-92.
7. Lezoche E, Guerrieri M, Paganini AM, D'Ambrosio G, Baldarelli M, Lezoche G, et al. Transanal endoscopic versus total mesorectal laparoscopic resections of T2-N0 low rectal cancers after neoadjuvant treatment: a prospective randomized trial with a 3-year minimum follow-up period. Surg Endosc. 2005;19: 751-6.
8. Pai RD, Fong DG, Bundga ME, Odze RD, Rattner DW, Thompson CC. Transcolonic endoscopic cholecystectomy: a NOTES survival study in a porcine model (with video). Gastrointest Endosc. 2006;64:428-34.
9. Park PO, Bergstrom M, Ikeda K, Fritscher-Ravens A, Swain P. Experimental studies of transgastric gallbladder surgery: cholecystectomy and cholecystogastric anastomosis (videos). Gastrointest Endosc. 2005;61:601-6.
10. Rattner D, Kalloo A, ASGE/SAGES Working Group. ASGE/SAGES Working Group on Natural Orifice Translumenal Endoscopic Surgery. October 2005. Surg Endosc. 2006;20:329-33.
11. Swanstrom LL, Smiley P, Zelko J, Cagle L. Videoendoscopic transanal-rectal tumor excision. Am J Surg. 1997;173:383-5.
12. Wagh MS, Merrifield BF, Thompson CC. Survival studies after endoscopic transgastric oophorectomy and tubectomy in a porcine model. Gastrointest Endosc. 2006;63:473-8.

Index

Page numbers followed by *b* refer to box, *f* refer to figure, and *t* refer to table.

D

E

H

I

J

K

L

M

N

O

T

W

X

Z